COLORECTAL CANCER

COLORECTAL CANCER
A Clinical Guide to Therapy

HARRY BLEIBERG, MD, PhD

Department of Gastroenterology and Medical Oncology,
Institut Jules Bordet, Brussels, Belgium

Gastrointestinal Oncology Service,
Memorial Sloan-Kettering Cancer Center, New York,
USA

PHILIPPE ROUGIER, MD, PhD

Department of Gastroenterology and Digestive Oncology,
Hôpital Ambroise Paré, Boulogne, France

Department of Medical Oncology/Hematology,
Kliniken Essen-Mitte, Essen, Germany

© 2002 Martin Dunitz Ltd, a member of the Taylor & Francis group

First published in the United Kingdom in 2002
by Martin Dunitz Ltd, The Livery House, 7–9 Pratt Street, London NW1 0AE

Tel.:   +44 (0) 20 74822202
Fax.:   +44 (0) 20 72670159
E-mail: info@dunitz.co.uk
Website: http://www.dunitz.co.uk

Although every effort has been made to ensure that all owners of copyright material have been acknowledged in this publication, we would be glad to acknowledge in subsequent reprints or editions any omissions brought to our attention.

Although every effort has been made to ensure that drug doses and other information are presented accurately in this publication, the ultimate responsibility rests with the prescribing physician. Neither the publishers nor the authors can be held responsible for errors or for any consequences arising from the use of information contained herein. For detailed prescribing information or instructions on the use of any product or procedure discussed herein, please consult the prescribing information or instructional material issued by the manufacturer.

A CIP record for this book is available from the British Library.

ISBN 1-85317-808-X

Distributed in the USA by
Fulfilment Center
Taylor & Francis
7625 Empire Drive
Florence, KY 41042, USA
Toll Free Tel.: +1 800 634 7064
E-mail: cserve@routledge_ny.com

Distributed in Canada by
Taylor & Francis
74 Rolark Drive
Scarborough, Ontario M1R 4G2, Canada
Toll Free Tel.: +1 877 226 2237
E-mail: tal_fran@istar.ca

Distributed in the rest of the world by
ITPS Limited
Cheriton House
North Way
Andover, Hampshire SP10 5BE, UK
Tel.: +44 (0)1264 332424
E-mail: reception@itps.co.uk

Composition by Wearset Ltd, Boldon, Tyne and Wear

Printed and bound in Great Britain by Biddles Limited, Guildford and King's Lynn

Contents

PART 8 NEW APPROACHES TO TREATMENT

PART 9 SPECIAL ISSUES IN COLORECTAL CANCER

Preface

The last few years have witnessed dramatic progress in the understanding and the treatment of colorectal cancer. New concepts have emerged, new treatment options have been identified and new standards established.

In this new book, building on the success of the 1998 title, *Management of Colorectal Cancer*, we have tried to cover the many aspects of colorectal cancer: epidemiology, genetics, screening, prognosis, chemoprevention, surgery, radiotherapy, chemotherapy, targeted therapies, and other special issues such as quality of life and cost assessment. Each of these areas has been subdivided into a number of specific topics, discussed in depth by well-known experts in the field. We wanted this book to be representative of research activity and clinical approaches in both the USA and in Europe, and American and European researchers have contributed to its content. In areas where the American and European approaches are significantly different, we have presented separate discussions (Chapters 22, 23, 56, 57, 59 and 60), with some controversis being argued by their original protagonists.

What have been the major developments in this field over the last few years? Surgery offers new technical approaches. In rectal cancer, resection of the rectum including total excision of the mesorectum has become widely accepted, with a local recurrence rate decreased to less than 10%, as compared with more than 30% previously observed. In colon cancer, minimal invasive surgery has arisen as a potential oncologically valuable approach (Chapters 10 and 11). For liver metastases, there are data suggesting that with the use of appropriate perioperative chemotherapy, patients with non-resectable liver metastases could be rendered resectable and have a similar survival to those with resectable lesions at presentation. Moreover, new ablative techniques for destroying surgically non-resectable liver lesions appear to offer new opportunities for the complete eradication of liver metastases (Chapters 33 and 34). Eventually, chemotherapy consisting of hepatic arterial floxuridine after resection or ablation of colorectal liver metastases appears to have the potential to further improve survival (Chapter 36).

Over the last two years, it has been demonstrated that combination chemotherapy including 5-FU/leucovorin bolus or infusion with irinotecan or oxaliplatin has a statistically significant impact on survival-related parameters (Chapters 56 and 57). Second-line treatment after failure of a previous 5-FU/leucovorin-based regimen is now part of our current clinical practice (Chapter 58).

Where are we going from here? In about two years, we should obtain the results of the randomized studies investigating the role of adjuvant 5-FU/leucovorin with irinotecan or oxaliplatin in stage III colon cancer. The adjuvant treatment of stage II colon cancer will remain controversial until the results of new properly designed studies are available (Chapters 13 and 14).

The rapid advances in the understanding of the molecular genetic causes of cancer are revolutionizing our approach to colorectal cancer treatment. Measurement of molecular parameters may have an impact on prognosis and prediction of outcome (Chapter 37). The corresponding technologies for performing these analyses and the design of targeted therapies will open, hopefully, a new era in the treatment of colorectal cancer (Chapters 62–64).

Harry Bleiberg
Nancy Kemeny
Philippe Rougier
Hansjochen Wilke

Contributors

Marc J Abramowicz MD, PhD
Department of Medical Genetics
University Hospital Erasme – ULB
Route de Lennik 808
B–1070 Brussels
Belgium

Wolf Achterrath MD
Aventis GmbH
Konigsteiner Strasse
65812 Bad Soden
Germany

René Adam MD, PhD
Hepatobiliary Center
Hôpital Paul Brousse
94804 Villejuif Cedex
France

Clare Adams MA, FRCS
Department of Surgery
University of Birmingham
Queen Elizabeth Hospital
Birmingham B15 2TH
UK

Norwood Anderson MD
Medical Oncology
The Cancer Center of Boston
125 Parker Hill Avenue
Boston, MA 02120
USA

Thierry André MD
Hôpital Tenon
4 rue de la Chine
75020 Paris
France

Enrique Aranda MD, PhD
Medical Oncology Unit
Hospital Clinico y Provincial Reina Sofia
14004 Córdoba
Spain

Arie Ariche MD
Hashalom 128
BP 1311
85025 Meitar
Israel

Pascal Artru MD
Service of Internal Medicine/Oncology
Hôpital Saint-Antoine
184 du Faubourg Saint-Antoine
75571 Paris
France

Eli Avisar MD
Division of Surgical Oncology
University of Pittsburgh Medical Center
300 Kaufman Building
3471 Fifth Avenue
Pittsburgh, PA 15213–3221
USA

Daniel Azoulay MD
Hepatobiliary Center
Hôpital Paul Brousse
94804 Villejuif Cedex
France

Robert Benamouzig MD, PhD
Hepato-Gastroenterology Department
Hôpital Avicenne
125 Rue de Stalingrad
93009 Bobigny Cedex
France

Anne-Marie Benhamiche MD
Registre Bourguignon des Cancers Digestifs
Faculté de Médecine
21079 Dijon Cedex
France

Giordano D Beretta MD
Unit of Medical Oncology
Ospedale Riuniti
Largo Barozzi, 1
24128 Bergamo
Italy

Anton Bilchik MD, PhD, FACS
Department of Surgery
John Wayne Cancer Institute
Santa Monica, CA 90404
USA

Henri Bismuth MD, FACS
Hepatobiliary Center
Hôpital Paul Brousse
94804 Villejuif Cedex
France

Harry Bleiberg MD, PhD
Department of Gastroenterology and
Medical Oncology
Institut Jules Bordet
Rue Héger-Bordet 1
B-1000 Brussels
Belgium

Michèle Boisdron-Celle PharmD, PhD
Centre Paul Papin
2 rue Moll
49033 Angers Cedex 01
France

Fred T Bosman MD, PhD
Institut Universitaire de Pathologie
Bugnon 25
CH-1011 Lausanne
Switzerland

Jean-François Bosset MD
Radiotherapy Department
Besançon University Hospital
25030 Besançon Cedex
France

Jean Bourhis MD, PhD
Department of Radiotherapy
Institut Gustave-Roussy
39 rue Camille Desmoulins
94805 Villejuif Cedex
France

Peter Boyle FRSE
Division of Epidemiology and Biostatistics
European Institute of Oncology
Via Ripamonti 435
20141 Milan
Italy

Marc Buyse ScD
International Drug Development Institute
B-1050 Brussels
Belgium

Guy-Bernard Cadière MD, PhD
Department of Gastrointestinal Surgery
University Hospital Saint Pierre (ULB)
Rue Haute 322
B-1000 Brussels
Belgium

Denis Castaing MD
Hepatobiliary Center
Hôpital Paul Brousse
94804 Villejuif Cedex
France

Thomas Cecil BM, FRCS
Colorectal Research Unit
North Hampshire Hospital
Basingstoke RG24 9NA
UK

Ming-Jen Chen MD
CRC Institute for Cancer Studies
Clinical Research Block
Univesity of Birmingham
Edgbaston
Birmingham B15 2TT
UK

Andrés Cervantes MD, PhD
Department of Haematology
and Medical Oncology
Hospital Clinic Universitari
46010 Valencia
Spain

Stephen Chaney MD
Department of Biochemistry and Biophysics
Lineberger Comprehensive Cancer Center
Chapel Hill, NC 27514
USA

Guy A Chung-Faye MD
CRC Institute for Cancer Studies
Clinical Research Block
Univesity of Birmingham
Edgbaston
Birmingham B15 2TT
UK

David Cunningham MD, FRCP
GI and Lymphoma Units
The Royal Marsden NHS Trust
Downs Road
Surrey SM2 5PT
UK

Esteban Cvitkovic MD
Service des Maladies Sanguines
Immunitaires et Tumorales
Hôpital Paul Brousse
94807 Villejuif Cedex
France

Frédéric Daenen MD
Division of Nuclear Medicine
University Hospital
Sart Tilman, B35
B-4000 Liege 1
Belgium

Aimery de Gramont MD
Service of Internal Medicine/Oncology
Hôpital Saint-Antoine
184 du Faubourg Saint-Antoine
75571 Paris
France

Marian Delgado MD
Hepatobiliary Center
Hôpital Paul Brousse
94804 Villejuif Cedex
France

Richard Devine MD
Department of Colorectal Surgery
Mayo Clinic and Mayo Medical School
Rochester, MN 55905
USA

Robert B Diasio MD
Department of Medicine and Pharmacology
Comprehensive Cancer Center
University of Alabama at Birmingham
Birmingham, AL 35294
USA

Eduardo Díaz-Rubio MD, PhD
Department of Medical Oncology
Hospital Clinico de San Carlos
28040 Madrid
Spain

Don S Dizon MD
Department of Gastrointestinal Oncology
Memorial Sloan-Kettering Cancer Center
1275 York Avenue
New York, NY 10021
USA

Robert F Dondelinger MD
Division of Medical Imaging
University Hospital
Sart Tilman, B35
B-4000 Liege 1
Belgium

Roger Dozois MD
Department of Colorectal Surgery
Mayo Clinic and Mayo Medical School
Rochester, MN 55905
USA

Peter C Enzinger MD
Dana Farber Cancer Institute
44 Binney Street
Boston, MA 02115-6084
USA

Charles Erlichman MD
Department of Oncology
Mayo Cancer Center
200 First Street SW
Rochester, MN 55905
USA

Francois Eschwège MD
Department of Radiotherapy
Institut Gustave-Roussy
39 rue Camille Desmoulins
94805 Villejuif Cedex
France

Jean Faivre MD
Registre Bourguignon des Cancers Digestifs
Faculté de Médecine
21079 Dijon Cedex
France

John W Fielding MD, FRCS
Department of Surgery
University of Birmingham
Queen Elizabeth Hospital
Birmingham B15 2TH
UK

Yuman Fong MD
Department of Surgery
Memorial Sloan-Kettering Cancer Center
1275 York Avenue
New York, NY 10021
USA

Hugo ER Ford MA, MRCP
CRC Centre for Cancer Therapeutics
The Royal Marsden NHS Trust
Downs Road
Surrey SM2 5PT
UK

Evleyn S Fox, CANP
Division of Hematology/Oncology
Vincent T Lombardi Cancer Research Center
Georgetown University Medical Center
3800 Reservior Road, NW
Washington, DC 20007-2197
USA

Erick Gamelin MD, PhD
Centre Paul Papin
2 rue Moll
49033 Angers Cedex 01
France

Diamon Gangji MD, PhD
RUBIO, Department of Medical Oncology
Erasme Hospital
808 Route de Lennik
B-1070 Brussels
Belgium

Sylvie Giachetti MD
Chronotherapy Unit and INSERM E0118
Institut du Cancer et d'Immunogénétique
Hôpital Paul Brousse
94807 Villejuif Cedex
France

Bengt Glimelius MD, PhD
Department of Oncology, Radiotherapy and Clinical Immunology
University Hospital
SE- 751 85 Uppsala
Sweden

Ali Goharin MD
Department of Digestive Surgery
Institut Gustave-Roussy
39 rue Camille Desmoulins
94805 Villejuif Cedex
France

Richard M Goldberg MD
Division of Medcial Oncology
Department of Oncology
Mayo Clinic
200 First Street SW
Rochester, MN 55905-0001
USA

François Goldwasser MD, PhD
Medical Oncology Unit
Hôpital Cochin, AP-HP
27 rue du Faubourg Saint-Jacques
75014 Paris
France

Jean L Grem MD, FACP
National Cancer Institute
Nationl Naval Medical Center
8901 Wisconsin Avenue
Bethesda, MD 20889-5105
USA

David L Grinblatt MD
Section of Hematology/Oncology
Department of Medicine
University of Chicago
5841 S Maryland Avenue, MC1000
Chicago, IL 60637
USA

François Guinet MD
Hepatobiliary Center
Cancer Service
Hôpital Paul Brousse
94804 Villejuif Cedex
France

Leonard L Gunderson MD, MS
Division of Radiation Oncology
Mayo Clinic and Mayo Medical School
Rochester, MN 55905
USA

Michael J Haddock MD
Division of Radiation Oncology
Mayo Clinic and Mayo Medical School
Rochester, MN 55905
USA

Richard J Heald OBE, MChir, FRCS
Colorectal Research Unit
North Hampshire Hospital
Basingstoke RG24 9NA
UK

Stefan Heinrich MD
Department of General and Vascular Surgery
JW Goethe University
Theodor-Stern-Kai 7
60590 Frankfurt
Germany

Patrice Hérait MD
Cvitkovic and Associates
94270 Kremlin-Bicetre
France

Paul Hermanek MD
Emeritus Professor of Surgical Pathology
Friedrich-Alexander-Universität
Krankenhausstrasse 12
D- 91054 Erlangen
Germany

Jacques M Himpens MD
Department of Gastrointestinal Surgery
University Hospital Saint Pierre (ULB)
Rue Haute 322
B-1000 Brussels
Belgium

Steven N Hochwald MD
Department of Surgery
University of Florida College of Medicine
Gainesville, FL 32610
USA

Paulo M Hoff MD
Center for Clinical Studies in Cancer
Hospital Albert Einstein
Avenue Albert Einstein 627/701
São Paulo 05651-901
Brazil

Roland Hustinx MD
Division of Nuclear Medicine
University Hospital
Sart Tilman, B35
B-4000 Liège 1
Belgium

Paul Jacobs PhD
RUBIO, Department of Medical Oncology
Erasme Hospital
808 Route de Lennik
B-1070 Brussels
Belgium

Nancy Kemeny MD
Gastrointestinal Oncology Service
Memorial Sloan-Kettering Cancer Center
1275 York Avenue
New York, NY 10021
USA

David J Kerr MD, DSc, FRCP
CRC Institute for Cancer Studies
Clinical Research Block
University of Birmingham
Edgbaston
Birmingham B15 2TT
UK

Claus-Henning Köhne MD
Medizinische Klinik und Poliklinik I
Universitätsklinikum Carl Gustav Carus
der TU-Dresden
Fetscherstrasse 74
01309 Dresden
Germany

Marcel Krulik MD
Service of Internal Medicine/Oncology
Hôpital Saint-Antoine
184 du Faubourg Saint-Antoine
75571 Paris
France

Francis Kunstlinger MD
Hepatobiliary Center
Hôpital Paul Brousse
94804 Villejuif Cedex
France

Roberto Labianca MD
Unit of Medical Oncology
Ospedale Riuniti
Largo Barozzi, 1
24128 Bergamo
Italy

Philippe Lasser MD
Department of Digestive Surgery
Institut Gustave-Roussy
39 rue Camille Desmoulins
94805 Villejuif Cedex
France

Cynthia Gail Leichman MD
Albany Medical Center
47 New Scotland Avenue
Albany, NY 12208
USA

Maria Elena Leon MD
Division of Epidemiology and Biostatistics
European Institute of Oncology
Via Ripamonti 435
20141 Milan
Italy

Francis Lévi MD PhD
Chronotherapy Unit and INSERM E0118
Institut du Cancer et d'Immunogénétique
Hôpital Paul Brousse
94807 Villejuif Cedex
France

Jacob J Lokich MD
Medical Oncology
The Cancer Center of Boston
125 Parker Hill Avenue
Boston, MA 02120
USA

Matthias Lorenz MD
Department of General and Vascular Surgery
JW Goethe University
Theodor-Stern-Kai 7
60590 Frankfurt
Germany

Christophe Louvet MD
Service of Internal Medicine/Oncology
Hôpital Saint-Antoine
184 du Faubourg Saint-Antoine
75571 Paris
France

Antoine Lusinchi MD
Department of Radiotherapy
Institut Gustave-Roussy
39 rue Camille Desmoulins
94805 Villejuif Cedex
France

John S Macdonald MD
Division of Medical Oncology
Saint Vincents Comprehensive Cancer Center
325 West 15th Street
New York, NY 10011
USA

Frédérique Maindrault-Goebel MD
Service of Internal Medicine/Oncology
Hôpital Saint-Antoine
184 du Faubourg Saint-Antoine
75571 Paris
France

Philippe Maingon MD
Radiotherapy Department
Centre Georges-François Leclerc
21034 Dijon Cedex
France

Robert Malafosse MD
Centre for Digestive Sugery
Hôpital Ambroise Paré
92104 Boulogne Cedex
France

Harvey Mamon MD
Department of Radiation Oncology
Massachusetts General Hospital
100 Blossom Street
Boston, MA 0244-2617
USA

Eleftherios Mamounas MD
Aultman Hospital Cancer Center
2600 6th Street, SW
Canton, OH 44710
USA

Georges Mantion MD
Department of Surgery
Besançon University Hospital
25030 Besançon Cedex
France

John L Marshall MD
Divison of Hematology/Oncology
Vincent T Lombardi Cancer Research Center
Georgetown University Medical Center
3800 Reservior Road, NW
Washington, DC 20007-2197
USA

Robert J Mayer MD
Dana Farber Cancer Institute
44 Binney Street
Boston, MA 02115-6084
USA

Hans-Joachim Meyer MD
Clinic for Visceral & Transplant Surgery
Hannover Medical School
Carl-Neuberg-Strasse 1
30625 Hannover
Germany

Rachel SJ Midgley MRCP
CRC Institute for Cancer Studies
Univesity of Birmingham
Edgbaston
Birmingham B15 2TT
UK

Brendan J Moran MCh, FRCS
Colorectal Research Unit
North Hampshire Hospital
Basingstoke RG24 9NA
UK

Dion G Morton MD, FRCS
Department of Surgery
University of Birmingham
Queen Elizabeth Hospital
Birmingham B15 2TH
UK

Heidi Nelson MD
Division of Colon and Rectal Surgery
Mayo Clinic and Mayo Medical School
200 First Street SW
Rochester, MN 55905
USA

Niels Neymark MD
Health Economics Unit
EORTC Data Center
Avenue E Mounier 83
B-1200 Brussels
Belgium

Bernard Nordlinger MD
Centre for Digestive Surgery
Hôpital Ambroise Paré
92104 Boulogne Cedex
France

John MA Northover MS, FRCS
Imperial Cancer Research Fund
Colorectal Cancer Unit
St Mark's Hospital
Northwick Park
Harrow
Middlesex HA1 3UJ
UK

Michael J O'Connell MD
Division of Medical Oncology
Mayo Clinic
Rochester, MN 55905
USA

Lars Påhlman MD, PhD
Colorectal Unit
Department of Surgery
University Hospital
SE- 751 85 Uppsala
Sweden

Didier Peiffert MD, PhD
Radiation Oncology Department
Centre Alexis Vautrin
54500 Vandoeuvre-les-Nancy
France

John Pemberton MD
Division of Colorectal Surgery
Mayo Clinic and Mayo Medical School
Rochester, MN 55905
USA

Christophe Penna MD
Centre for Digestive Sugery
Hôpital Ambroise Paré
92104 Boulogne Cedex
France

M Adelaide Pessi MD
Unit of Medical Oncology
Ospedale Riuniti
Largo Barozzi, 1
24128 Bergamo
Italy

Pascal Pledbols MD, PhD
Department of Medical Oncology
Hôpital Henri Mondor
Assistance Publique – Hôpitaux de Paris
9400 Créteil
France

Jean-Pierre Pignon MD PhD
Department of Biostatistics and Epidemiology
Institut Gustave-Roussy
94805 Villejuif Cedex
France

Rudolf Raab MD
Department of Abdominal and
Transplantation Surgery
Hannover Medical School
Konstanty-Gutschow-Strasse 8
30625 Hannover
Germany

Eric Raymond MD
Department of Medicine
Insitut Gustave-Roussy
94805 Villejuif Cedex
France

Jose I Restrepo MD
Clinica Soma
Calle 51 no. 45–93 of 215
Medellin, Columbia
South America

Vincent Richard MD
RUBIO, Department of Medical Oncology
Erasme Hospital
808 Route de Lennik
B-1070 Brussels
Belgium

Pierre Rigo MD
Division of Nuclear Medicine
University Hospital
Sart Tilman, B35
B-4000 Liège 1
Belgium

Philippe Rougier MD, PhD
Department of Gastroenterology
and Digestive Oncology
Hôpital Ambroise Paré
CHU Paris-Ouest
9 avenue Charles de Gaulle
92100 Boulogne Cedex
France

Youcef M Rustum PhD
Scientific Affairs and Graduate Education
Roswell Park Cancer Institute
Buffalo, NY 14263
USA

Sukamal Saha MD, FACS, FRCS(C)
Department of Surgery and Anatomy
McLaren Regional Medical Center
Michigan State University
Flint, MI 48532-3685
USA

Daniel J Sargent PhD
Department of Oncology
Mayo Cancer Center
200 First Street SW
Rochester, MN 55905
USA

Steven Schild MD
Division of Radiation Oncology
Mayo Clinic and Mayo Medical School
Rochester, MN 55905
USA

Richard L Schilsky MD
Division of Biological Sciences
University of Chicago
5841 S Maryland Avenue, MC1000
Chicago, IL 60637
USA

Alberto F Sobrero MD
Medical Oncology
University of Udine
Piazza S Maria 1
33100 Udine
Italy

Paul H Sugarbaker MD, FACS, FRCS
Surgical Oncology
The Washington Cancer Institute
110 Irving Street NW
Washington, DC 20010
USA

Melanie Thomas MD
Division of Cancer Medicine
MD Anderson Cancer Center
1515 Holcombe Boulevard
Houston, TX 77030-4095
USA

Christophe Tournigand MD
Service of Internal Medicine/Oncology
Hôpital Saint-Antoine
184 du Faubourg Saint-Antoine
75571 Paris
France

Eric Van Cutsem MD, PhD
Department of Internal Medicine
University Hospital Gasthuisberg
Herestraat 49
B-3000 Leuven
Belgium

Udo Vanhoefer MD, PhD
Department of Internal Medicine (Cancer Research)
West German Cancer Center
University of Essen Medical School
45122 Essen
Germany

Thierry Velu MD, PhD
RUBIO, Department of Medical Oncology
Erasme Hospital
808 Route de Lennik
B-1070 Brussels
Belgium

Chris Verslype MD
Department of Internal Medicine
University Hospital Gasthuisberg
Herestraat 49
B-3000 Leuven
Belgium

Uwe Werner MD
Department of Abdominal and
Transplantation Surgery
Hannover Medical School
Konstanty-Gutschow-Strasse 8
30625 Hannover
Germany

Samuel Wieand PhD
Department of UPCI-Biostatistics Facility
Suite 325
Sterling Plaza
201 North Craig Street
Pittsburgh, PA 15213
USA

David Wiese MD, PhD
Department of Pathology
McLaren Regional Medical Center
Michigan State University
Flint, MI 48532-3685
USA

Hansjochen Wilke MD
Innere Klinik/Onkologie
Kliniken Essen-Mitte
Ev. Huyssens-Stiftung
45136 Essen
Germany

Christopher G Willett MD
Department of Radiation Oncology
Massachusetts General Hospital
100 Blossom Street
Boston, MA 0244-2617
USA

Jacques A Wils MD
Department of Oncology
Laurentius Hospital
6043 CV Roermond
The Netherlands

Sidney J Winawer MD
Gastroenterology and Nutrition Service
Department of Medicine
Memorial Sloan-Kettering Cancer Center
1275 York Avenue
New York, NY 10021
USA

Bruce Wolff, MD
Division of Colorectal Surgery
Mayo Clinic and Mayo Medical School
Rochester, MN 55905
USA

Norman Wolmark MD
Department of Human Oncology
Allegheny General Hospital
320 North Avenue
Pittsburgh, PA 15212-4772
USA

Tonia Young-Fadok MD
Division of Colorectal Surgery
Mayo Clinic and Mayo Medical School
Rochester, MN 55905
USA

Ann G Zauber PhD
Department of Epidemiology and Biostatistics
Memorial Sloan-Kettering Cancer Center
1275 York Avenue
New York, NY 10021
USA

Part 1

Background and Epidemiology

1

Biology of colorectal cancer: An overview of genetic factors

Marc J Abramowicz

CANCER IS A GENETIC DISEASE IN A SOMATIC CELL

From a genetic vantage point, there are two types of cells in diploid organisms such as humans: germinal cells and somatic cells. Germinal cells consist of sperm, ova, and their precursors produced in the germline. All other cells are somatic. All somatic cells contain essentially the same two copies of the 40 000 genes or so that make up the human genome – one copy from the mother and one copy from the father of the individual. Ova and sperm cells contain only one copy. After fertilization, the zygote owns two copies, and divides to develop into a new individual, with a germline and somatic cell lines.

Mutations may occur anytime at any location in the genome, but only those mutations present in germ cells can be passed on to the offspring of a patient. Such mutations underlie familial predisposition to cancer. Somatic mutations, while not transmitted to offspring, will be transmitted to daughter cells when the mutated cell divides. Such mutations underlie tumour progression. Cancer is best viewed as a genetic disease in a somatic cell and all daughter cells arising from its clonal expansion.

It is important to realize that most somatic mutations will not result in cancer. As more than 90% of mammalian genomic DNA apparently has no function, many mutations produce no effect. Mutations in functional DNA may be neutral – or they may be harmful and kill the cell, which will be replaced by division of a neighbouring cell. Only those mutations that affect genes involved directly or indirectly in the control of cell proliferation and promote it will be tumorigenic. Such mutations are relatively rare, but once present, are selected in a Darwinian way, because they allow clonal expansion of the mutated cell over non-mutated cells. Additional tumorigenic

mutations will occur that will be selected in the same way for increasing malignancy, since only those that allow an even more rapid growth will lead to the emergence of a subclone that will eventually come to medical attention. Neoplasms thus progress step by step by accumulation of perhaps 5–10 mutations in the clonal and subclonal descendants of a somatic cell.

Mutations that activate cell proliferation are relatively rare, so the spontaneous occurrence of 5–10 mutations in one cell is unlikely and not expected to explain the observed incidence of cancer, even though the clonal expansion of the initially mutated somatic cell increases the target for additional mutations. Therefore it has been postulated that cancer must also involve some mechanism that increases the rate of mutation – the so-called mutator phenotype. This is an instability of the genome which neoplastic cells acquire early in their progression. It is believed that the mutator-phenotype-associated increased mutation rate is random, and produces mutations that promote cell proliferation as well as neutral and harmful mutations that may result in cell death. As Vogelstein commented, cancer needs the 'just right instability' for progression.

MANY MOLECULAR STEPS OF COLORECTAL CANCER PROGRESSION HAVE BEEN ELUCIDATED

Colorectal cancer happens to be the model in which multistep tumour progression has been best understood and validated in molecular terms. In a now classic study of the late 1980s, Vogelstein and co-workers[1] correlated the histology of adenoma-to-carcinoma progression with four chromosomal changes found in tumours, as compared with non-tumoral chromosomes from the same patients. In the following decade, the genes involved at these four chromosomal loci have been identified and extensively characterized. One of them, called APC for 'adenomatous polyposis coli', turned out to be pivotal. One important function of APC is that of a negative regulator of β-catenin,[2] via stimulation of β-catenin phosphorylation by GSK3 and subsequent ubiquitination and degradation by the proteasome. β-Catenin itself is a multifunction protein. It is able to bind E-cadherin, a transmembrane cell adhesion molecule, and also contains a transcription transactivation domain. When bound to TCF7L2, a transcription factor that binds DNA at sequence-specific sites but lacks a transcription activator domain, β-catenin recruits RNA polymerase II molecules and drives transcription of specific genes, including oncogenes and PPARδ (see below). The lack of functional APC protein, or the deletion of its β-catenin-binding domain, or the mutation of an amino acid of β-catenin that is phosphorylated by GSK3 in the presence of APC, all lead to overactivity of the β-catenin/TCF7L2 transcriptional activation pathway and promote proliferation of the intestinal cell.[2,3]

Interestingly, much of our knowledge of APC in common colorectal cancer comes from studies in a very rare, hereditary form of cancer, familial adenomatous polyposis. Indeed, in their 1988 paper, Vogelstein et al[1] had already reported that chromosomal changes were the same, regardless of whether adenomas or carcinomas had occurred sporadically in a patient or in the context of familial polyposis. This will be discussed in some detail later in this chapter.

The current model of genetic changes associated with tumorigenesis in about 85% of colorectal cancers involves the sequential alteration of the genes APC, K-RAS, DCC/CMAD4/JVB18 (whose loci are close to one another on chromosome 18) and p53.[3] This represents the genotype of tumour cells, i.e. the genetic changes associated with colorectal tumorigenesis, and correlates with their phenotype, i.e. their pathologic stage and clinical expression.

ENVIRONMENTAL AND GENETIC FACTORS MODULATE THE COURSE OF TUMOUR PROGRESSION

Polymorphisms or mutations in other genes, such as MOM1,[4] may modulate phenotypic (histologic and clinical) expression of the tumorigenic mutations that make up the tumour genotype. Environmental factors, such as aspirin or perhaps the fat content of the diet, can also modulate the phenotypic expression of the tumour genotype. These environmental factors exert their effects via proteins that are expressed in the intestinal cells and are of course encoded by genes. For example, eicosanoids and some lipid molecules are ligands for PPARδ, a nuclear protein that binds to specific sites in DNA and activates the expression of some genes that in turn stimulate intestinal cell proliferation.[5] In this model (whose in vivo significance is not yet established), the PPARδ gene is a mediator of the modulatory effect of environmental substances, but is not a part of the genotypic changes acquired by the tumour. It is presently unknown whether naturally occurring variants, i.e. polymorphisms, of the PPARδ gene provide protection or susceptibility to colorectal tumour progression in individuals who carry them, but one is entitled to speculate that polymorphisms in some genes do bestow normal subjects throughout life with various degrees of susceptibility to cancer, and modulate their responses to diet and chemopreventive agents such as aspirin. Such susceptibility is inborn, but its inheritance is complex, as opposed to simple Mendelian inheritance, because it is due to the combination of several genetic variants that are inherited independently.

MIN AND CIN: TWO MUTATOR PHENOTYPES

The type of genomic instability associated with 85% of adenomas that progress to carcinomas is called chromosomal instability (CIN).[1,6] It is characterized by large genomic rearrangements such as chromosomal translocation, amplification or deletion of chromosomal segments, or other types of allelic losses, accompanied by loss of heterozygosity (LOH) for nearby polymorphic markers of DNA. The molecular mechanisms underlying CIN are largely unknown. Tumours that display CIN may be referred to as CIN+ or LOH+. In the remaining 15% of adenomas, another type of mutator phenotype is found, called microsatellite instability (MIN).[7] This consists of an increased rate of point mutations affecting one or a few base pairs of DNA apparently at random throughout the genome, which can be easily demonstrated at the level of microsatellites, i.e. short DNA sequences that are repeated in tandem at well-defined loci throughout the genome. Although MIN can occur at occasional loci in any tumour, high-frequency MIN, i.e. at 40% or more of microsatellite loci, indicates MIN as the mutator phenotype. The molecular mechanism underlying MIN is a tumour-cell-acquired deficiency of a biochemical enzymatic system called mismatch repair (MMR), which normally corrects point mutations introduced by DNA polymerase in daughter DNA strands during DNA replication (replication errors, RER). The mismatch repair enzymatic system is made up of at least five subunits, MLH1, MSH2, MSH6 (GTBP), PMS1, and PMS2, each of which is encoded by a different gene.[8] MSI[+] tumours are more frequent in the right colon.[7]

The presence of MIN indicates a distinct mutational pathway in colorectal adenomas, which, however, shares features with the classical, chromosomal-instability-associated pathway. For example, the loss of APC-mediated β-catenin decay seems essential in both pathways – however, it results from loss of function of the *APC* gene in almost all tumours with CIN but from point mutations of the β-catenin gene, causing resistance to APC-dependent phosphorylation and subsequent decay,[2] in many tumours with MIN.[9] On the other hand, late MIN[+] tumours often show inactivating mutations of the type II transferring growth factor β (TGF-β) receptor, which are rare in late CIN[+] tumours, which conversely have a high rate of *p53* gene mutation and allelic loss.[10] Interestingly, most of the type II TGF-β receptor gene mutations in MIN[+] tumours affect a sequence of 10 repeating adenines, i.e. a very small microsatellite within the coding sequence of the gene. TGF-β inhibits the growth of epithelial cells, and cells from colon neoplasms often stop responding to TGF-β as they become more malignant. The gene for its type II receptor thus behaves as an anti-oncogene, whose mutation is tumorigenic.

Apart from tumorigenic mutations, random mutations in other genes might lead to aberrantly expressed proteins eliciting immune responses, which might explain the lymphocytic infiltrates that are often found in MIN[+] tumours.[11]

The distinct genetic changes, histologic findings, and distribution in the colon of the 15% subset of MIN[+] colorectal tumours are associated with lower pathologic stage at diagnosis, less propensity to metastasize independently of pathologic stage, and better prognosis, so these tumours might require a different and possibly less aggressive scheme of therapy.[12]

In addition to 15% of sporadic colorectal tumours, MIN is found in over 95% of tumours arising in hereditary non-polyposis colorectal cancer, the most frequent form of inherited colorectal cancer, as will be discussed below. The MIN-associated better prognosis seems to apply to inherited as well as to sporadic colorectal cancer.[11]

HEREDITARY CANCER SYNDROMES ARE DUE TO GERMLINE MUTATIONS IN GENES THAT ARE MUTATED SOMATICALLY IN SPORADIC CANCERS

Some cancers run in families as a result of autosomal dominant inheritance, i.e. each affected individual has a 50% chance of transmitting the cancer predisposition to each offspring, regardless of sex. Mendelian theory predicts that such predisposition is due to a mutation in one of the two copies (the two alleles) of a particular gene. In 1971, on the basis of comparisons between inherited and sporadic forms of a very rare cancer, retinoblastoma, Knudson proposed the 'two-hit' hypothesis (reviewed in reference 13). This was later validated by molecular studies, and is also applicable to other tumours, in particular to colorectal cancer. According to the two-hit hypothesis, both alleles of a given gene must be mutated in order for a cell to undergo malignant transformation. In sporadic retinoblastoma, both alleles must mutate in the same somatic cell – that is, *two* mutations of the same locus must occur independently in the same cell; this is a rare event that will take a long time to occur. In hereditary retinoblastoma, a mutated allele is passed through the germline, and hence is present in all somatic cells since birth (actually since fertilization). Therefore, in order for any somatic cell of the retina to undergo malignant transformation, only *one* mutation, of the second allele, is necessary. Such a 'second hit' is not a very rare event – which explains why both eyes are almost always affected in familial retinoblastoma.

Knudson's two-hit hypothesis explains why hereditary cancers display three particular features: familial inheritance, early onset, and multiplicity of primary tumours. It assumes that the molecular steps of tumour progression are identical in familial and sporadic cancers. The model is now understood on the basis of germline mutations in tumour supressor genes, also called anti-oncogenes.

HEREDITARY COLORECTAL CANCER SYNDROMES

Familial adenomatous polyposis (FAP) and hereditary non-polyposis colorectal cancer (HNPCC) are the main inherited colorectal cancer syndromes. Both are due to mutations in tumour suppressor genes and are transmitted as autosomal dominant traits in affected families. Both are characterized by multiple adenomas and early-onset cancer, and both exhibit the sequence of adenoma-to-carcinoma progression.

They do, however, display distinct mutator pheno-types, with CIN and MIN being found in FAP-derived tumours and HNPCC-derived tumours respectively. Other rare syndromes, such as juvenile polyposis, Peutz–Jeghers syndrome, Cowden's disease, and neurofibromatosis, are associated with non-adenomatous tumours and will not be discussed in this chapter.

Familial adenomatous polyposis (FAP)

FAP is found in about 1/7000 individuals and in perhaps up to 1% of all patients with colorectal cancer. Around adolescence, FAP patients develop hundreds to thousands of adenomatous polyps, mainly in the left colon, each of which progresses to carcinoma. The median age at cancer diagnosis in FAP, if untreated, is 42 years.[3] The only curative treatment is colectomy – either proctocolectomy or colectomy with ileorectal anastomosis. Polyposis is inherited as an autosomal dominant trait linked to chromosome 5q21 and is due to germline, heterozygous mutation of the *APC* gene located there,[14,15] with most disease-causing mutations resulting in a truncated protein product.[16] At the somatic level, cell growth leading to adenoma progression is initiated by loss of the second, wild-type *APC* allele, followed by other genetic changes in a context of CIN.[1] Some extracolonic manifestations, such as benign subcutaneous tumours and mandibular osteomas (Gardner syndrome), may be found in some patients while being absent in affected relatives bearing the same *APC* gene mutation. Conversely, foci of congenital hyperplasia of the retinal pigmentary epithelium (CHRPEs), when present, breed true, i.e. co-segregate in affected members of the family, which indicates that CHRPEs are caused by the *APC* gene mutation itself rather than by other factors in FAP patients.[17]

Analyses of germline *APC* mutations in other FAP families allowed delineation of other types of relationships between genotype and phenotype. Mutations clustering near the 5′ end (left end) of the *APC* gene, and a few other mutations, cause an attenuated form of polyposis, which is associated with a smaller number of polyps and a later onset of cancer.[18] Conversely, mutations located between codons 1250 and 1464 cause profuse, earlier-onset polyposis, with frequent upper gastrointestinal polyps, and a high risk of peritoneal desmoid formation after laparotomy, leading some experts to recommend total proctocolectomy rather than ileorectal anastomosis and surveillance of the remaining rectum in affected patients.[19]

In classic polyposis (as opposed to attenuated polyposis), the penetrance of the mutation, i.e. the fraction of mutation carriers who become ill, is virtually complete unless the patient dies of another cause early in life. In about 25% of new cases, the family history is negative for polyposis, consistent with a new mutation of the *APC* gene in the patient, which may often be demonstrated if both biological parents are available for a retrospective mutation analysis. Penetrance may be less than 100% in attenuated polyposis. Interestingly, a mutation of the *APC* gene has been described whose penetrance is very incomplete, causing perhaps a twofold increased risk for colorectal cancer.[20] It consists of a thymine-to-adenine substitution that creates a poly-adenine tract within the gene. This alteration, transmitted through the germline, can be viewed as a premutation at the somatic level, because the poly-adenine tract is mitotically hypermutable.

Hereditary non-polyposis colorectal cancer (HNPCC)

HNPCC, or the Lynch syndrome, is thought to underlie 5–10% of all colorectal cancers. It differs from FAP in three aspects. Firstly, cancer in HNPCC is not heralded by a benign phenotypic finding that would allow a specific diagnosis. Secondly, penetrance is incomplete, around 80%. Thirdly, a mutation in any of several genes may cause the syndrome, and in a given family it is impossible to tell which is the relevant gene. Current diagnostic methods consist of a systematic analysis of all genes involved in patients suspected to have HNPCC. Five genes are known, *MLH1*, *MSH2*, *PMS1*, *PMS2*, and *MSH6* (*GTBP*), which encode subunits of the multienzyme complex responsible for mismatch repair (MMR) of DNA. *MLH1* and *MSH2* are the most clinically significant – each of which is found mutated in about 35% of HNPCC families.[8] The first hit is an inactivating mutation transmitted through the germline, and the second hit consists of somatic inactivation of the second allele, resulting in a deficiency of the MMR machinery. This correlates with MIN being found in 95% of HNPCC tumours. Tumours from *MSH6*-linked HNPCC may, however, be associated with low levels of MSI.[21] HNPCC tumours occur preferentially in the proximal colon. Once initiated, the adenoma-to-carcinoma progression is fast (see later in this chapter).[3]

Because of incomplete penetrance of the mutation and because of the small size of many families, especially in industrialized countries, HNPCC may not appear to be familial. Conversely, because of the high frequency of sporadic colorectal cancer in the general population, familial cases are often merely coincidental. Therefore several attempts have been made to devise selective criteria that would discriminate HNPCC from sporadic cases. In outbred populations with no significant founder effects, as opposed to more inbred populations such as the Finnish population,[22] the best clinical criteria are probably those known as the Amsterdam criteria: at least three family members in at least two successive generations must have colorectal cancer; at least one must be diagnosed before the age of 50 years; and polyposis must be excluded.[8] The benefit of systematic mutation analyses of MMR genes in familial or early-onset cases that do not fulfil the Amsterdam criteria is a matter of debate, because these analyses are labour-intensive. Conversely, the assessment of MIN in tumours is relatively easy, and this phenotypic sign, although not specific, may help sort further HNPCC cases.[22]

Adenomas in HNPCC are relatively frequent in the right colon. HNPCC patients have a 30% risk of additional synchronous or metachronous cancers, and extracolonic cancers are frequent in HNPCC; for example, endometrial cancer occurs in 20–40% of female mutation carriers.[8,22,23]

GENETIC COUNSELLING IN HEREDITARY COLORECTAL CANCER

Once a diagnosis of polyposis has been made, relatives must be informed of their risk of inheriting the syndrome, which is transmitted as an autosomal dominant trait. Specifically, each child of an affected patient has a 50% chance of bearing the mutation and hence of developing the disease sometime in life. Siblings have the same 50% risk, except for cases due to new mutations, which can usually be suspected on the basis of a negative family history. DNA analysis of a blood sample from a patient with demonstrated polyposis should be considered the first step in evaluating the risk in relatives. Current techniques detect germline mutations of *APC* in over 80% of families. Finding the mutation in the proband allows for presymptomatic diagnosis in at-risk relatives, with a caveat in a minority of families where the pathogenic nature of the mutation is questionable, i.e. when a mutation is found that does not result in truncation of the protein product. In such cases, and in families where no mutation can be found, an indirect genetic approach can be used provided that other relatives are available for blood sampling and are informative in a strategy of genetic linkage analysis. The latter consists of studying the familial transmission of

polymorphic DNA markers of the genomic region of chromosome 5 that encompasses the *APC* gene, in order to find a marker whose transmission parallels that of polyposis in the given family. In a minority of families, neither a direct search for *APC* mutation nor an indirect study of linkage to the *APC* locus will be informative, and all at-risk relatives must be offered the same endoscopy screening measures as relatives who are found to carry the mutation in informative families. Most authors consider that prophylactic colectomy must not be performed before the occurrence of polyps. Guidelines for surveillance hinge on flexible sigmoidoscopy once or twice per year, starting at age 10 years, and every 3–5 years after age 40 years in the rare mutation carriers who do not develop multiple polyps by that age. Upper endoscopy, with examination of the Vater ampulla, is recommended every 3 years after age 20 years.

Genetic counselling of patients and at-risk relatives is essential, as well as psychological support. It is hoped that the prognosis of mutation carriers will change in the next decade with the availability of efficient chemoprophylaxis, perhaps based on cyclooxygenase-2 inhibitors.[24]

In HNPCC families, the risk of inheriting the mutation from an affected parent is also 50%, but the subsequent risk of developing a cancer is about 80% for colon cancer and is less for extracolonic tumours, for example 20–40% for endometrial cancer in women. The causal mutation can be found with current techniques in about 70% of families.[8,22,23] In the remaining families, genetic linkage is usually impossible because of genetic heterogeneity, i.e. because any one of the several MMR genes could be involved and it is not possible to tell which one should be studied by linkage analysis, although some attempts are promising.[25] Mutation carriers and at-risk relatives whose carrier status is unknown should have colonic surveillance based on colonoscopy once a year starting at age 20–25 years, as well as pelvic echography in women starting at age 25–30 years. Genetic counselling is required in patients as well as in at-risk relatives.

HEREDITARY CANCER SYNDROMES HIGHLIGHT ASPECTS OF COLORECTAL CANCER TUMORIGENESIS

The mean age at diagnosis of cancer in FAP and in HNPCC is similar, at around 42 years – and thus about 25 years earlier than in sporadic adenocarcinomas. This is consistent with clinical and animal data showing that in FAP, adenomas appear early in life and progress at the same rate as sporadic adenomas

– in contrast to HNPCC, where adenomas appear on average at the same age as sporadic adenomas but progress rapidly to carcinomas. These observations can be confronted with molecular data, yielding a model of gatekeeper and caretaker genes.[3] Loss of the normal APC protein occurs very early in sporadic adenomas (at least in those with CIN) – in fact as early as at the stage of aberrant crypt foci, consistent with a role in tumour initiation. APC can be viewed as the gene responsible for maintaining a constant cell number in renewing intestinal cells, i.e. a gatekeeper gene, and loss of APC is the major single event that results in a permanent imbalance of cell division over cell death. This correlates with the clonal expansion and adenoma formation in FAP patients each time an intestinal cell suffers a second hit (Knudson's model), and hence in the early appearance of multiple adenomas. Furthermore, virtually every FAP family known to date is linked to a mutation of APC on chromosome 5, indicating that APC is the only gene whose product acts as a gatekeeper in intestinal cells. Conversely, the initiation of adenomas is not accelerated in HNPCC patients, since they do not harbour germline APC mutations, but, once initiated, any adenoma cell having suffered a second hit in the corresponding MMR gene will acquire the MIN mutator phenotype, i.e. much earlier than in sporadic adenomas. The loss of MMR may occur before tumour initiation, and remain silent until then. This model of gatekeeper (APC) and caretakers (MMR subunits) is probably valid for other types of sporadic and inherited cancers, such as breast/ovarian cancer,[26] but may be more complex: for instance, APC might display a caretaker function in addition to its gatekeeper role (R Fodde, personal communication).

MANY COLORECTAL CANCERS ARE MULTIFACTORIAL IN ORIGIN RATHER THAN SPORADIC OR HEREDITARY

Sporadic and hereditary cancers probably represent the extremes of a continuum. Hereditary cancers, perhaps 5–10% of all colorectal cancers, result from a strong predisposition that is inherited through the germline as an autosomal dominant trait, and this corresponds to a single mutation in a gatekeeper or a caretaker gene as discussed above. It is clear, however, that many more colon and rectum cancers, like breast cancers and prostate cancers, display significant albeit not Mendelian heritability.[27] This may result from partial mutations in hereditary cancer genes, such as the poly-adenine tract mutation of the

APC gene discussed above,[20] resulting in an increased relative risk for colorectal cancer, transmitted in families as an autosomal dominant trait. Many more cases probably arise on a multigenic basis, i.e. an inborn genetic pattern due to a particular combination of genetic variants that are frequent in the population and are otherwise harmless (genetic polymorphisms). As each polymorphism is transmitted independently to offspring in families, multigenic traits show some familial clustering but do not follow the dominant or recessive laws of Mendel as single-gene traits do. It is currently unclear whether genetic polymorphisms implicated in multigenic cancer heredity affect the same genes implicated in hereditary cancers and/or other genes, but it is likely (as mentioned above) that the unique biochemical identity of each individual, due to his or her unique genome make-up, plays a role in the response to diet and other environmental factors acting on the intestine.

FUTURE TRENDS

Genetic analysis of neoplasms may help optimize therapy

The MIN phenotype is an independent prognostic factor associated with better outcome in colorectal cancer, and may be associated with different sensitivities to chemotherapeutic agents,[12] so it is likely that a MIN search will be part of the clinical work-up of colorectal tumours in the future. Other genetic changes in tumours are likely to become included in routine staging and grading as well.

MIN[+] tumours are more frequent in the right colon, and the presence of MIN significantly increases the risk of a further, metachronous tumour in colorectal cancer patients.[28] Further studies should address whether MIN in an adenoma screened from the general population in the left colon indicates the need for right colonoscopy, especially in Europe, where right-sided tumours are less frequent than in America or Japan.

Regarding the rare hereditary syndromes, some APC mutations in FAP seem to warrant more aggressive initial surgical treatment,[19] making molecular analysis a useful contribution in medical decision making, in addition of course to its role in genetic counselling and surveillance of at-risk relatives. In suspected HNPCC cases, the identification of a germline MMR gene mutation is paramount for surveillance in relatives. In the future, it is likely that biochemical profiling of the patient, using a combination of genetic tests, will help adjust adjuvant chemotherapy.

Chemoprevention

Several classes of drugs have been found to decrease the incidence of adenomas or colorectal cancers in various target groups; these include non-steroidal anti-inflammatory drugs, calcium salts, folic acid, and oestrogens (reviewed by Jänne and Mayer[29]). For example, a cyclooxygenase-2 inhibitor showed promise during a 6-month trial in FAP patients in terms of reducing the number of polyps.[24] It remains unclear, however, whether this approach is effective in reducing morbidity and mortality in FAP, and how it applies to lower-risk patients. From a general viewpoint, the perspective of chemoprevention in FAP or other high-risk patients in the future warrants caution when contemplating radical options of surgical prophylaxis in young mutation carriers with no polyps.

DNA chips

High-density microarrays of DNA probes coupled to automated laser reading and direct input to computer (DNA chips) is a developing technology for testing up to 100 000 mutations or polymorphisms in a given subject in a reasonable time, which would allow complex genetic profiling either of tumours, or of individuals. Possible applications include adjustment of treatment according to tumour genotype, adjustment of adjuvant chemotherapy according to patient's phenotype (genetic pharmacology), and stratification of the general population with regard to risk of multigenic cancer in order to better target prevention.

REFERENCES

1. Vogelstein B, Fearon ER, Hamilton SR et al, Genetic alterations during colorectal-tumor development. *N Engl J Med* 1988; **319**: 525–32.
2. Morin PJ, Sparks AB, Korinek V et al, Activation of beta-catenin-Tcf signaling in colon cancer by mutations in beta-catenin or APC. *Science* 1997; **275**: 1787–90.
3. Kinzler KW, Vogelstein B, Lessons from hereditary colorectal cancer. *Cell* 1996; **87**: 159–70.
4. Cormier RT, Hong KH, Halberg RB et al, Secretory phospholipase Plag2g2a confers resistance to intestinal tumorigenesis. *Nature Genet* 1997; **17**: 88–91.
5. Wu GD, A nuclear receptor to prevent colon cancer. *N Engl J Med* 2000; **342**: 651–3.
6. Lengauer C, Kinzler KW, Vogelstein B, Genetic instability in colorectal cancer. *Nature* 1997; **386**: 623–7.
7. Thibodeau SN, Bren G, Schaid D, Microsatellite instability in cancer of the proximal colon. *Science* 1993; **260**: 816–19.
8. Wijnen JT, Vasen HFA, Meera Khan P et al, Clinical findings with implications for genetic testing in families with clustering of colorectal cancer. *N Engl J Med* 1998; **339**: 511–18.
9. Mirabelli-Primdahl L, Gryfe R, Kim H et al, Beta-catenin mutations are specific for colorectal carcinomas with microsatellite instability but occur in endometrial carcinomas irrespective of mutator pathway. *Cancer Res* 1999; **59**: 3346–51.
10. Markowitz S, Wang J, Myeroff L et al, Inactivation of the type II TGF-b receptor in colon cancer cells with microsatellite instability. *Science* 1995; **268**: 1336–8.
11. Offit K, Genetic prognostic markers for colorectal cancer. *N Engl J Med* 2000; **342**: 124–5.
12. Gryfe R, Kim H, Hsieh ETK et al, Tumor microsatellite instability and clinical outcome in young patients with colorectal cancer. *N Engl J Med* 2000; **342**: 69–77.
13. Knudson AG, Antioncogenes and human cancer. *Proc Natl Acad Sci USA* 1993; **90**: 10914–21.
14. Groden J, Thliveris A, Samowitz W et al, Identification and characterization of the familial adenomatous polyposis coli gene. *Cell* 1991; **66**: 589–600.
15. Nishisho I, Nakamura Y, Miyoshi Y et al, Mutations of chromosome 5q21 genes in FAP and colorectal cancer patients. *Science* 1991; **253**: 665–9.
16. Powell SM, Petersen GM, Krush AJ et al, Molecular diagnosis of familial adenomatous polyposis. *N Engl J Med* 1993; **329**: 1982–7.
17. Olschwang S, Tiret A, Laurent-Puig P et al, Restriction of ocular fundus lesion to a specific subgroup of APC mutations in adenomatous polyposis coli patients. *Cell* 1993; **75**: 959–68.
18. Spirio L, Olschwang S, Groden J et al, Alleles of the APC gene: an attenuated form of familial polyposis. *Cell* 1993; **75**: 951–7.
19. Vasen HF, van der Luijt RB, Slors JF et al, Molecular genetic tests as a guide to surgical management of familial adenomatous polyposis. *Lancet* 1996; **348**: 433–5.
20. Laken SJ, Petersen GM, Gruber SB et al, Familial colorectal cancer in Ashkenazim due to a hypermutable tract in APC. *Nature Genet* 1997; **17**: 79–83.
21. Kolodner RD, Tytell JD, Schmeits JL et al, Germ-line MSH6 mutations in colorectal cancer families. *Cancer Res* 1999; **59**: 5068–74.
22. Salovaara R, Loukola A, Kristo P et al, Population-based molecular detection of hereditary nonpolyposis colorectal cancer. *J Clin Oncol* 2000; **18**: 2193–200.
23. Loukola A, de la Chapele A, Aaltonen LA. Strategies to screen for hereditary non polyposis colorectal cancer. *J Med Genet* 1999; **36**: 819–22.
24. Steinbach G, Lynch PM, Phillips RKS et al, The effect of Celecoxib, an cyclooxygenase-2 inhibitor, in familial adenomatous polyposis. *N Engl J Med* 2000; **342**: 1946–52.
25. Yan H, Papadopoulos N, Marra G et al, Conversion of diploidy to haploidy. *Nature* 2000; **403**: 723–4.
26. Kinzler KW, Vogelstein B, Gatekeepers and caretakers. *Nature* 1997; **386**: 761–3.
27. Lichtenstein P, Niels V, Holm NV et al, Environmental and heritable factors in the causation of cancer – analyses of cohorts of twins from Sweden, Denmark, and Finland. *N Engl J Med* 2000; **343**: 78–85.
28. Masubuchi S, Konishi F, Togashi K et al, The significance of microsatellite instability in predicting the development of metachronous multiple colorectal carcinomas in patients with nonfamilial colorectal carcinoma. *Cancer* 1999; **85**: 1917–24.
29. Jänne PA, Mayer RJ, Primary care: chemoprevention of colorectal cancer. *N Engl J Med* 2000; **342**: 1960–8.

2

Recent developments in the epidemiology of colorectal cancer

Peter Boyle, Maria Elena Leon

INTRODUCTION

Colorectal cancer is the fourth commonest form of cancer which occurs worldwide, with an estimated 782 900 new cases diagnosed in 1990.[1] Global, age-standardized rates of colorectal cancer (ICD9 153 and 154) incidence are slightly higher in men than in women (19.4 and 15.3 per 100 000 respectively).[1] The disease is most frequent in occidental countries, and particularly so in North America, Australia, New Zealand, and parts of Europe. The incidence of this malignancy shows considerable variation among racially or ethnically defined populations in multiracial/ethnic countries. The diseases of colon and rectal cancer appear to be distinct, but, unfortunately, there are recognized difficulties in distinguishing colon and rectal cancer in mortality statistics for a variety of reasons.[2] Wherever possible in this chapter, the distinction between colon and rectum will be preserved.

Colon cancer is a disease of economically 'developed' countries. Before 60 years of age, the disease is slightly more common in women, whereas it is more frequent in men thereafter.[3] In men, eight of the ten highest age-standardized incidence rates of colon cancer are recorded in population groups in the USA, with Canada, Japan, and New Zealand completing the group (Table 2.1). It is of potentially considerable significance that these high rates are to be found in a variety of population groups, including Blacks in Detroit (34.9 per 100 000), Los Angeles (34.8), San Francisco (33.8), Atlanta (32.4), and New Orleans (31.4), Japanese and Whites in Hawaii (34.4 and 32.7, respectively), and non-Maori in New Zealand (31.2). More recent data from the USA on colorectal incidence and mortality rates from 1992 to 1998, age-adjusted to the 1970 US standard population, confirm the racial/ethnic gradient of this dis-

ease. In detail, incidence rates (per 100 000) reported for Blacks, Whites, Asian/Pacific Islanders, American Indian/Alaskan, and Hispanics are 50.1, 42.9, 38.2, 28.6, and 28.4, respectively.[4] Worldwide, in men, the lowest incidence rates are found in a variety of population groups in the developing countries, with the lowest rate being reported in Setif, Algeria (0.4 per 100 000). In women, the group of highest incidence rates includes population groups in New Zealand and North America, with the lowest rates being recorded in Algeria and India (Table 2.1). In each sex, a number of low-rate regions are found in India.[5]

Ethnic and racial differences in colon cancer as well as studies on migrants suggest that environmental factors play a major role in the aetiology of the disease. In Israel, male Jews born in Europe or America are at higher risk for colon cancer than those born in Africa or Asia, and a change in risk in the offspring of Japanese who had migrated to the USA heralded by Haenszel and Kurihara[6] has taken place, the incidence rates approaching or surpassing those in Whites in the same population and being three or four times higher than among Japanese in Japan.

Incidence rates of colon cancer have increased worldwide since 1985, particularly in men,[1] with the exception of North America. In areas formerly at low risk, the number of left-sided tumours has shown a greater increase.[7] In Australia, between 1973 and 1993, colorectal cancer occurred most frequently in the sigmoid colon and the rectum. In the right colon, cancer occurred most commonly in the caecum. From 1973 to 1993, incidence rates increased in the right colon (by 2.8% per annum in men and 2.0% per annum in women) and in the left colon (1.6% in men and 0.7% in women). The incidence rates also increased for cancer of the rectum, by 2.0% per

Table 2.1 Ten highest and ten lowest average, annual, all ages, age-standardized, incidence rates per 100 000 population for colon cancer in men and women worldwide around the early 1990s. Data are abstracted from Parkin et al.[5]

Colon, male ICD9 153 Registry	Cases	Rate	Colon, female ICD9 153 Registry	Cases	Rate
USA, Detroit: Black	806	34.9	New Zealand: non-Maori	3650	29.6
USA, Los Angeles: Black	771	34.8	Canada, Newfoundland	503	28.1
USA, Hawaii: Japanese	462	34.4	USA, San Francisco: Black	408	27.9
USA, San Francisco: Black	353	33.8	USA, Detroit: Black	899	27.9
USA, Hawaii: White	293	32.7	USA, San Francisco: Japanese	57	27.0
USA, Atlanta: Black	300	32.4	USA, Los Angeles: Black	860	26.5
Japan, Hiroshima	939	31.6	USA, Atlanta: Black	400	26.1
Canada, Newfoundland	504	31.4	USA, New Orleans: Black	314	25.8
USA, New Orleans: Black	247	31.4	Canada, Nova Scotia	1028	25.2
New Zealand: non-Maori	3045	31.2	USA, Connecticut: Black	188	25.2
Thailand, Chiang Mai	139	4.1	Vietnam, Hanoi	81	2.9
Ecuador, Quito	64	3.9	Kuwait: non-Kuwaiti	13	2.2
Kuwait: Kuwaiti	22	3.5	India, Bangalore	128	2.0
Uganda, Kyadondo	16	3.1	China, Qidong	79	2.0
Mali, Bamako	22	3.1	Mali, Bamako	13	1.4
China, Qidong	64	2.1	India, Madras	84	1.3
India, Madras	122	1.8	India, Karunagappally	5	1.3
India, Karunagappally	5	1.4	India, Trivandrum	8	1.0
India, Barshi, Paranda	6	0.7	Algeria, Setif	7	0.6
Algeria, Setif	4	0.4	India, Barshi, Paranda	4	0.4

annum in men and by 0.7% per annum in women.[8] More complex patterns are seen in high-risk countries. Rates for cancer of the ascending (right) colon have increased from 1992 to 1998 in the USA.[4] This finding is believed to be due to improvements in diagnosis, increased 'screening' with sigmoidoscopy, and removal of pre-cancerous lesions from the descending (left) colon.

The colorectal mortality rate is decreasing in the USA. Disease detection at earlier stages due to screening practices and the availability of more efficient treatment regimes have driven a reduction in cancer death. Still, average annual colorectal cancer death rates in the USA have shown higher rates in Blacks for both sexes (27.2 and 19.5 in Black males and females and 20.1 and 13.7 in White males and

females).[4] In other parts of the world, increasing rates are observed in the Nordic countries, while, in England and Wales, mortality rates are declining in all age groups in both sexes.

DESCRIPTIVE EPIDEMIOLOGY OF CANCER OF THE RECTUM (ICD9 154)

Although somewhat less frequent than colon cancer, rectal cancer shows many features of colon cancer in its geographic distribution. In contrast to colon cancer, rectal cancer is more common in men, with a sex ratio of 1.5 to 2.0. Little difference exists in the incidence rates between Western countries of North America, Europe, and Australia, with rates in the range of 8 to 20 for men and 5 to 11 for women. In contrast, the mortality rates in the USA are among the lowest in developed countries, with large declines in mortality rates in Blacks and Whites for both sexes and very little change in incidence. This is believed to be artefactual, since half the patients diagnosed with rectal cancer have their deaths certified to colon cancer.[9,10] Elsewhere, time trends are not consistent with rising rates in Japan and declining rates in Denmark and in England and Wales.

The highest incidence rates of rectal cancer in men are found in the Yukon in Canada (33.7 per 100 000) and in Bohemia and Moravia in the Czech Republic (24.2 per 100 000). There is little geographic pattern to the highest-rate regions, which contain a diversity of populations in the USA, Hungary, Italy, France, Australia, Canada, and Israel (Table 2.2). An unexpected feature of these data is the high incidence rates found in Japanese men in San Francisco (19.3) and Hawaii (19.0). In women, the highest rates are lower than those in men, and there is a variety of population groups among the highest incidence rates. In each sex, there is a variety of population groups from the developing world among the regions with the lowest rates (Table 2.2).

Unlike colon cancer, mortality from rectal cancer has not risen much in Japanese migrants to the USA.[6] Polish migrants have shown an increased risk for both sites.[11]

Table 2.2 Ten highest and ten lowest average, annual, all ages, age-standardized, incidence rates per 100 000 population for rectal cancer in men and women worldwide around the early 1990s. Data are abstracted from Parkin et al.[5]

Rectum, male ICD9 154 Registry	Cases	Rate	Rectum, female ICD9 154 Registry	Cases	Rate
Canada, Yukon	25	33.7	Canada, Yukon	12	14.4
Czech Republic	7970	24.2	Israel: Jews born in Europe	1053	12.8
Zimbabwe, Harare: European	23	22.4	Czech Republic	5602	11.6
France, Haut-Rhin	446	21.5	South Australia	673	11.4
Slovakia	2984	20.6	Israel: all Jews	1533	11.4
New Zealand: non-Maori	1955	20.1	France, Haut-Rhin	343	11.2
Japan, Hiroshima	576	19.4	New Zealand: non-Maori	1362	11.2
USA, San Francisco: Japanese	28	19.3	Australia, Victoria	1876	11.0
Australia, Victoria	2610	19.2	Australian Capital Territory	74	11.0
USA, Hawaii: Japanese	235	19.0	Germany, Saarland	691	10.9
India, Bangalore	212	3.1	Vietnam, Hanoi	70	2.4
Israel: non-Jews	31	3.1	Algeria, Setif	27	2.3
Thailand, Chiang Mai	101	3.1	India, Trivandrum	18	2.3
India, Trivandrum	21	3.0	Kuwait: non-Kuwaiti	13	2.3
Thailand, Khon Kaen	63	3.0	Thailand, Khon Kaen	48	1.9
Mali, Bamako	26	2.9	Kuwait: Kuwaitis	11	1.9
Brazil, Belem	30	2.8	Uganda, Kyadondo	11	1.8
Algeria, Setif	24	2.6	India, Barshi, Paranda, Bhum	10	1.1
India, Barshi, Paranda, Bhum	23	2.6	Mali, Bamako	8	0.7
India, Karunagappally	6	1.6	India, Karunagappally	1	0.3

TEMPORAL TRENDS IN COLORECTAL CANCER MORTALITY (ICD9 153 AND ICD9 154)

In 1990, there were 437 000 colorectal cancer deaths reported worldwide.[12] The major problem in comparison of death rates from colon and rectal cancer separately between populations is the problem of attribution of 'vaguely' defined cancers on the death certificate. The root of the problem was the habit of any death ascribed by the certifying physician as 'cancer of the large intestine' being classified to the three-digit code for colon: this of course could have been a rectal cancer. For this and several other reasons, it is preferable to investigate mortality from colon and rectal cancer together as a single entity. However, there is a recognized loss of information that could be available if mortality data were of a higher quality.

In Canada, the truncated and overall age-adjusted mortality rates remained relatively stable in men until the earlier 1970s, and have been decreasing ever since. In women, both the truncated and overall age-adjusted mortality rates have been decreasing since 1955. Birth cohort examination shows that the rates have been stable or decreasing in successive birth cohorts in men and women for the age groups examined, although the decrease in rates was more pronounced in women. Canada is one of the few countries outside the Nordic countries where national incidence and mortality data are available.[13] Colorectal cancer incidence, and mortality, rates are higher by about 50% in men compared with women. In each gender group, the incidence and mortality rates increased to a peak in the mid-1980s, and the all-ages rates have subsequently declined (Figure 2.1).

In Japan, both the truncated and overall age-adjusted mortality rates have been increasing in both men and women since 1955. Examination of rate by birth cohorts suggests a consistent increase in rates in successive birth cohorts born before 1940 in both sexes. For cohorts born after 1940, the rates seem to have levelled off, and may have even declined in both sexes.[14]

In the former Czechoslovakia, both the truncated and overall age-adjusted mortality rates have been increasing in both men and women since 1955. Birth cohort examination indicates an increase in rates in successive birth cohorts in both sexes, although the rates in younger age groups seem to be levelling off.

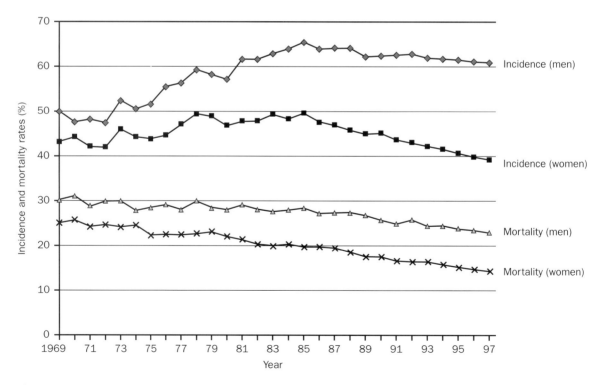

Figure 2.1 Colorectal cancer incidence and mortality in men and women in Canada.

In Poland, both the truncated and overall age-adjusted mortality rates have been increasing since 1959 in both men and women. Examination by birth cohorts suggests an increase in rates in successive birth cohorts for almost all age groups examined, and in both sexes.

In Germany, both the truncated and overall age-adjusted mortality rates increased between 1955 and 1979. Thereafter, the rates in women have been decreasing – more so in the truncated rates. In men, after a brief and slight decrease between 1980 and 1983, the rates seem to have increased again in the last few years. Birth cohort examination shows an increase in rates for earlier birth cohorts and a decrease in recent birth cohorts at all age groups examined, and in both men and women.

In the UK, the overall age-adjusted mortality rates experienced a slight decrease in men since 1955, although the truncated rates remain relatively unchanged. In women, both the truncated and overall age-adjusted mortality rates have been decreasing during the entire study period. Birth cohort examination by birth cohorts shows similar rates in successive birth cohorts born before 1930 and a slight decrease in those born after. In women, the rates have been decreasing in successive birth cohorts for all the age groups examined.

In Denmark, there is no clear overall time trend for either truncated or overall age-adjusted mortality rates in men since 1955. In women, however, a slight decrease was observed for both truncated and overall age-adjusted mortality rates during the entire study period. Birth cohort examination suggests that the rates are similar in men and decreasing in women in successive birth cohorts.

In Australia, both the truncated and overall age-adjusted mortality rates have been increasing in men since 1955, although the increase in the overall age-adjusted mortality rates seems to have slowed down over the last few years. In women, a slight decrease was observed for both truncated and overall age-adjusted mortality rates since the early 1970s. Birth cohort examination shows an increase in rates in successive birth cohorts born before 1935 in men and a decrease in rates in those born after. In women, the rates are similar or have been decreasing in successive birth cohorts for most of the age groups examined, except for the age groups between 40 and 49, where a slight increase in rates in successive birth cohorts was observed. Interesting data have been published regarding a comprehensive analysis of the descriptive epidemiology of colorectal cancer in New South Wales.[8]

Colorectal cancer was the second most common cancer reported in men and women in New South Wales in 1993.[8] The age-standardized incidence rates in men and women in 1993 were 46.1 and 31.0 respectively: this is considerably lower than the incidence rates in Canada (Figure 2.1). From 1973 to 1993, the incidence rates rose by an average of 1.9% per annum in men and 0.9% in women while mortality was steady in men and fell by 0.9% in women. These increases in incidence in men occurred over the age of 45 and in women between the ages of 45 and 74. The overall mortality rate in men remained stable despite a fall in rates in younger men. In women, the fall in mortality of 0.9% per annum could be attributed to falls in the very youngest and oldest age groups.[8]

In Italy, the mortality rate for colorectal cancer in both men and women has been increasing steadily since 1955. Since 1980, there has been a levelling-off in rates in women, particularly in the truncated age range.

For comparison purposes, incidence data from colon and rectal cancer have been combined (Table 2.3): this allows one to realize more clearly the impact of colorectal cancer on communities worldwide. For colorectal cancer, the highest incidence rates in men are reported from Japanese communities in Hawaii (53.5), non-Maoris in New Zealand (51.3) and Japanese in Hiroshima (51.0). The lowest rates are found in various developing countries, with the range between the lowest rate (3.1 in Karunagappally, India) and the highest (53.5 in Hawaiian Japanese) being considerable. Similar patterns and differences exist in women (Table 2.3).

ANALYTICAL EPIDEMIOLOGY

Most colorectal cancers, between two-thirds and 90%, arise from benign, adenomatous polyps lining the wall of the bowel, with those that grow to a large size and have a villous appearance or contain dysplastic cells being the most likely to progress to cancer.[15] The development of colorectal cancer is a multistep process involving genetic mutations in mucosal cells, the activation of tumour-promoting genes, and the loss of genes that suppress tumour formation.[16] The natural history and the role of several risk factors in the aetiology of colorectal cancer are becoming more clearly understood,[17,18] and the genetic events involved in colorectal cancer susceptibility are being uncovered with increasing frequency:[19,20] the recent rate of progress in our understanding of the genetics of colorectal cancer is impressive.[21,22] Few specific risk factors of a non-

Table 2.3 Ten highest and ten lowest average, annual, all ages, age-standardized, incidence rates per 100 000 population for colon and rectal cancer combined in men and women worldwide around the early 1990s. Data are abstracted from Parkin et al.[5]

Colorectum, male ICD9 153/154 Registry	Cases	Rate	Colorectum, female ICD9 153/154 Registry	Cases	Rate
USA, Hawaii: Japanese	697	53.5	New Zealand: non-Maori	5012	40.8
New Zealand: non-Maori	5000	51.3	Canada, Newfoundland	678	38.3
Japan, Hiroshima	1515	51.0	USA, Detroit: Black	1172	36.6
France, Haut-Rhin	1041	49.9	USA, Los Angeles: Black	1182	36.5
Italy, Trieste	547	49.4	USA, San Francisco: Black	527	36.4
France, Bas-Rhin	1445	49.2	Israel, Jews born in America or Europe	3034	35.8
Canada, Yukon	39	49.0	USA, San Francisco: Japanese	76	35.4
USA, Detroit: Black	1100	48.3	USA, Atlanta: Black	529	35.0
Czech Republic	15906	48.2	Canada, Nova Scotia	1400	35.0
USA, Los Angeles: Black	1061	47.9	South Australia	2047	34.2
Brazil, Belem	73	7.3	Thailand, Khon Kaen	129	5.2
Ecuador, Quito	123	7.2	Uganda, Kyadondo	26	5.1
Thailand, Chiang Mai	240	7.2	India, Bangalore	300	4.8
Mali, Bamako	48	6.0	Kuwait: non-Kuwaiti	26	4.5
India, Madras	367	5.6	India, Madras	258	4.1
India, Bangalore	374	5.5	India, Trivandrum	26	3.3
India, Trivandrum	38	5.4	Algeria, Setif	34	2.9
India, Barshi, Paranda, Bhum	29	3.3	Mali, Bamako	21	2.1
Algeria, Setif	28	3.1	India, Karunagappally	6	1.6
India, Karunagappally	11	3.1	India, Barshi, Paranda, Bhum	14	1.5

dietary origin have been established for colorectal cancer; inflammatory bowel diseases and familial polyposis syndromes produce a high risk of colorectal cancer in affected individuals, but account for only a small proportion of the overall incidence of colorectal cancer.[23,24]

PHYSICAL ACTIVITY, BODY MASS INDEX, AND ENERGY INTAKE

There appears to be strong evidence from epidemiological studies that men with high occupational or recreational physical activity appear to be at a lower risk of colon cancer.[25] Such evidence comes from follow-up studies of cohorts who are physically active

or who have physically demanding jobs, as well as from case–control studies that have assessed physical activity, by, for example, measurement of resting heart rate, or by questionnaire. The association remains even after control for potential confounding factors such as diet and body mass index (BMI).

The relationship between risk of colorectal cancer and self-reported occupational and recreational physical activity has been investigated in a population-based cohort in Norway.[26] Physical activity at a level equivalent to walking four hours per week was associated with a decreased risk of colon cancer among women when compared with the (referent) sedentary group (relative risk, RR, 0.62; 95% confidence interval, CI 0.40–0.97): this was particularly marked in the proximal colon (RR 0.51; 95% CI

0.28–0.93). The trend in reducing risk with increased physical activity was similar in women and in men aged over 45 years.[26]

The Nurses' Health Study quantified time spent on physical activity during leisure time as well as the energy equivalent spent during such activity (metabolic equivalents, MET).[27] Women who spent more than 21 MET-hours per week on leisure-time physical activity had a relative risk of colon cancer that was almost half that of women who spent less than 2 MET-hours per week (RR 0.54; 95% CI 0.33–0.90).[27] Women who had a BMI >29 kg/m^2 had a relative risk of colon cancer that was increased by about one-half (RR 1.45; 95% CI 1.02–2.07) compared with women who had a BMI <21 kg/m^2. The trend in risk showed an increasing trend with increasing waist-to-hip ratio (RR 1.48; 95% CI 0.88–2.49) for comparison of the highest quintile ratio (>0.833) with the lowest (<0.728). The significant inverse association between leisure-time physical activity and the risk of colon cancer in women resembles the association previously described in men. Increasing physical activity and maintaining lean body weight should be regarded as preventive practices to reduce the risk of developing colon cancer.

Furthermore, physical activity appears to modify the association between dietary factors and colon cancer. The risk of colon cancer with increased fat intake has been reported to be higher in sedentary as opposed to active men.[28]

It has been a fairly consistent finding in studies that have examined the issue that energy intake is higher in cases of colorectal cancer than in the comparison group: the mechanism is, however, complex.[29] Physically active individuals are likely to consume more energy, but recent studies suggest that physical activity reduces colorectal cancer risk.[28,30,31] Some attention has been given to the study of such factors in the development of adenomas, the benign lesions from which the majority of colorectal cancers develop. A case–control study was conducted among patients seen at three colonoscopy practices in New York City: all patients had a history of adenomas.[32] Men in the upper quarter of BMI were found to have an increased risk of recurrent adenomas: the odds ratios were found to be 2.2, 1.9, and 1.9, respectively, in the second, third, and fourth quarter of BMI compared with the lowest quarter. However, no effect was found in women. This either detracts from the findings given the lack of internal consistency or indicates that there is a true biological interaction: in any event, this issue deserves further study.

A case–control study of new adenoma cases and adenoma-free controls demonstrated that physical activity in leisure protected women against colorectal adenomas. There was no evidence of a protective effect of work activity among either women or men, although men who participated in no sport were at an increased risk for adenomas (odds ratio, OR, 1.68; 95% CI 0.93–3.20).[33]

Giovannucci et al[34] took the opportunity to examine the effects of physical activity, BMI, and the pattern of adipose distribution on the risk of colorectal adenomas. Within the Nurses' Health study, 13 057 female nurses, aged 40–65 years in 1986, had an endoscopy between 1986 and 1992. During this period, 439 were newly diagnosed with adenomas of the distal colorectum. After controlling for age, prior endoscopy, parental history of colorectal cancer, smoking, aspirin use, and dietary intake, physical activity was associated inversely with the risk of large adenomas ($\geq$1 cm) in the distal colon (RR 0.57; 95% CI 0.30–1.08), comparing high and low quintiles of average weekly energy expenditure from leisure activities. Much of this benefit came from activities of moderate intensity, such as brisk walking.

Additionally, BMI was associated directly with risk of large adenomas in the distal colon (RR 2.21; 95% CI 1.18–4.16) for BMI $\geq$29 kg/m^2 compared with BMI values <21 kg/m^2. The relationships between BMI or physical activity were considerably weaker for rectal adenomas.[34] This study indicates a similar association between physical activity and occurrence of adenomas in many respects similar to that for colorectal cancer. Exercise appears to protect against adenomas and colorectal cancer, and increasing BMI serves to increase the risk of both.

The reason for such an inverse association has not been identified, but has been postulated as being the effect of exercise on bowel transit time,[35] the immune system,[36] or serum cholesterol and bile acid metabolism.[37] The same consistent results have not been reported until recently on studies in women, but one possible explanation is that the weaker variation in, for example, occupational activity among women may make such an association more difficult to detect. Also, infrequent bowel movements, directly related to bowel transit time, have not been associated with an increased risk of colorectal cancer in women,[38] whether or not physical activity affects transit time.

The available data, however, show no consistent association between obesity and colorectal cancer risk (although analysis and interpretation of this factor is difficult in retrospective studies, where weight loss may be a sign of the disease), although there is now evidence that there may be an association with adenomas. This positive effect of energy does not appear to be merely the result of overeating, therefore, and may reflect differences in metabolic efficiency. (If the possibility that the association with energy intake is a methodological artefact is excluded – since it seems unlikely that such a consistent finding would emerge from such a variety of study designs in a diversity of population groups – then it would imply that individuals who utilize energy more efficiently may be at a lower risk of colorectal cancer.)

DIETARY AND NUTRITIONAL PRACTICES

A diet rich in fruit and vegetables has been associated with a reduced risk of colorectal cancer in many, but not all, observational studies.[39] The association between fruit and vegetable consumption and the incidence of colon and rectal cancers has been studied in two cohorts: the Nurses' Health Study (88 764 women) and the Health Professionals' Follow-up Study (47 325 men).[40] Assessment of the diet was completed during different calendar years in women and men, during which a total of 1 743 645 person-years of follow-up were accrued and 937 cases of colon cancer were identified. No association was found between colon cancer incidence and fruit and vegetable consumption. For women and men combined, a difference in fruit and vegetable consumption of one additional serving per day was associated with a covariate-adjusted relative risk of greater magnitude but lacking statistical significance (RR 1.02; 95% CI 0.98–1.05).[40]

This apparent lack of association between consumption of fruits and vegetables and colorectal cancer risk contradicts a widely accepted relationship between nutritional practices and chronic disease risk. Another association under scrutiny is that between fat intake and colorectal cancer risk. There appears to be consistent evidence from epidemiological studies that intake of dietary fat and meat is positively related to colorectal cancer risk: this evidence is obtained from ecological studies, animal experiments, and case–control and cohort studies. *Many of these studies have failed to demonstrate that the association observed with fat intake is independent of energy intake*. Willett et al[41] published the results obtained from the US Nurses' Health Study involving follow-up of 88 751 women aged 34–59 who were without cancer or inflammatory bowel diseases at recruitment. After adjustment for total energy intake, consumption of animal fat was found to be associated with increased colon cancer risk. The trend in risk was highly significant ($p = 0.01$), with the relative

risk in the highest compared with the lowest quintile being 1.89 (95% CI 1.13–3.15). No association was found with vegetable fat. The relative risk of colon cancer in women who ate beef, pork, or lamb as a main dish every day was 2.49 (95% CI 1.24–5.03), compared with those women reporting consumption less than once per month. The authors interpreted their data as providing evidence for the hypothesis that a high intake of animal fat increases the risk of colon cancer, and they supported existing recommendations to substitute fish and chicken for meats high in fat.[41] However, with an increasing amount of information becoming available from prospective studies, there is only weak evidence of an association between fat intake and colorectal cancer risk.[42] Nevertheless, there is still evidence of a positive association coming out from retrospective studies, such as that from Italy.[43] Clearly, some further work is required on this particular topic.

The study by Willett et al[41] provides the best epidemiological evidence to date identifying increased meat consumption as a risk factor for colon cancer, independently of its contribution to fat intake and total caloric intake. Laboratory evidence is available that strongly suggests that cooked meats may be carcinogenic, particularly with regard to aminoimidazoazarenes (AIAs), which are produced when meats are cooked.[44,45] As well as being highly mutagenic in bacterial assays, there is now evidence that AIAs are mammalian carcinogens, since feeding experiments in mice have produced tumours in various anatomical sites.[46] However, the situation is not entirely straightforward: for example, it has been shown that anticarcinogenic compounds are produced in fried ground beef.[47] Thus, in the same food, the potential exists to have mixtures of potentially carcinogenic and anti-carcinogenic substances.

A recently published meta-analysis of 13 prospective studies looking at meat consumption and colorectal cancer risk has reported an increased risk (12–17%) with a daily increase of 100 g of all meat or red meat. The risk was higher (49%) with a daily increase of 25 g of processed meat.[48] Again, in a second study published in parallel, high intake of carcinogenic compounds produced when meat is well cooked at high temperatures has been associated with an increased risk of colorectal adenomas.[49]

Whittemore et al[28] performed a case–control study of Chinese in North America and China, thus ingeniously utilizing the large difference in risk of colorectal cancer that exists between the two continents. Colorectal cancer risk in both continents was increased with increasing intake of total intake of energy, and specifically by saturated fat: however, no relationship was found with other sources of energy in the diet. Colon cancer risk was elevated among men employed in sedentary occupations, and, in both continents and in each sex, the risks for cancer of the colon and rectum increased with increased time spent sitting: the association between colorectal cancer risk and saturated fat was stronger among the sedentary than the active. Risk among sedentary Chinese Americans of either sex increased more than fourfold from the lowest to the highest category of saturated fat intake. Among migrants to North America, risk increased with increasing time spent in North America. Attributable risk calculations suggest that, if these associations are causal, then saturated fat intakes exceeding 10 g/day, particularly in combination with physical inactivity, could account for 60% of colorectal cancer incidence among Chinese-American men and 40% among Chinese-American women.[28]

The specific fatty acids in the diet may also be important: animal experiments have suggested that linoleic acid (an n − 6 polyunsaturated fatty acid) promotes colorectal carcinogenesis[50,51] and that a low-fat diet rich in eicosapentaenoic acid (an n − 3 polyunsaturated fatty acid) has an inhibitory effect on colon cancer.[52] However, there have been no consistent findings from epidemiological studies regarding n − 3 and n − 6 fatty acids and colorectal cancer risk.

Among protective dietary factors, the original hypothesis of the effect of dietary fibre was based on a clinical/pathological observation and a hypothesized mechanism whereby increasing intake of dietary fibre increases faecal bulk and reduces transit time. More recent thinking suggests that this mechanism may not be as relevant to colorectal carcinogenesis as previously thought.[53] The term 'fibre' encompasses many components, each of which has specific physiological functions. The commonest classification is into the insoluble, non-degradable constituents (mainly present in cereal fibre) and the soluble, degradable constituents such as pectin and plant gums (mainly present in fruits and vegetables). Epidemiological studies have reported differences in the effect of these components. For example, Tuyns et al[54] and Kune et al[55] found a protective effect for total dietary fibre intake in case–control studies, and the same was found in one prospective study.[56] However, a large number of studies could find no such protective effect (see Willett[29] for a review). The large majority of studies in humans have found no protective effect of fibre from cereals, but have consistently found a protective effect of fibre from vegetable and, perhaps, fruit sources,[29,39] and dietary diversity has been shown to be an important element in this protection.[57] This could conceivably reflect an association with other components of fruits and vegetables, with 'fibre' intake acting merely as an indicator of consumption.

Two randomized studies, conducted in the USA, looking at dietary interventions and the risk of recurrent adenomatous polyps have recently revealed no protective effect from fibre. The dietary interventions in question were, for the Polyp Prevention Trial,[58] to have either intensive counselling to follow a low-fat, high-fibre, fruit and vegetable diet or to be given a brochure on healthy eating, and, for the Wheat Bran Fiber Study,[59] to have a high wheat bran fibre cereal supplement (13.5 g of fibre in 2/3 cup of cereal per day) or low wheat bran fibre cereal supplement (2 g of fibre in 2/3 cup cereal per day). The latter study reports that increasing dietary fibre will not reduce the risk of developing colorectal cancer, although praising the benefits of high-fibre diets for the prevention of other chronic conditions. A possible explanation for the observed null results in both studies may be a short follow-up period, precluding the detection of cancerous lesions that require a longer time before emerging.

A potential pathway for this protective association has been investigated in a novel epidemiological study design.[60] Cruciferous vegetable intake exhibited a significant inverse association with colorectal cancer risk (OR 0.59; 95% CI 0.34–1.02). When tumours were characterized by p53 overexpression (p53-positive) aetiological heterogeneity was suggested for family history of colorectal cancer (OR 0.39; 95% CI 0.16–0.93), intake of cruciferous vegetables (test for trend, $p = 0.12$) and beef consumption (test for trend, $p = 0.08$). Cruciferous vegetable consumption exhibited a significant association when p53-positive cases were compared with controls (OR 0.37; 95% CI 0.17–0.82). When p53-negative cases were compared with controls, a significant increase in risk was observed for family history of cancer (OR 4.46; 95% CI 2.36–8.43) and beef consumption (OR 3.17; 95% CI 1.83–11.28). The authors concluded that the p53-dependent (positive) pathway was characterized by an inverse association with cruciferous vegetable intake and that p53-independent tumours were characterized by family history and beef consumption.[60]

Recent studies have found that insulin-like growth factor 1 (IGF-1) levels correlate with risk of cancer in several sites (prostate and colorectal cancer in men, breast in premenopausal women, and lung in men and women). Prediagnostic plasma levels of IGF-1 and IGFBP-3 (which possesses an opposing effect) have been assessed in association with the risk of colorectal cancer and adenoma in women in the Nurses' Health Study.[61] The study indicates that high levels of circulating IGF-1 and particularly low levels of IGFBP-3 are associated independently with an elevated risk of large or tubulovillous/villous colorectal adenoma and cancer.[61]

Insulin and insulin-like growth factors can stimulate proliferation of colorectal cells, and high intakes of refined carbohydrates and markers of insulin resistance are associated with colorectal cancer. A case–control study on colorectal cancer conducted in Italy was employed to test the insulin/colon cancer hypothesis by determining whether the dietary glycaemic index and the glycaemic load are associated with colorectal cancer risk. Average daily dietary glycaemic index and glycaemic load were calculated, and fibre intake was estimated from a validated food frequency questionnaire. Direct associations with colorectal cancer risk emerged for glycaemic index (OR in highest versus lowest quintile 1.7; 95% CI 1.4–2.0) and glycaemic load (OR 1.8; 95% CI 1.5–2.2), after allowance for socio-demographic factors, physical activity, number of daily meals, and intakes of fibre, alcohol, and energy. Odds ratios were more elevated for cancer of the colon than rectum. Being overweight and having a low intake of fibre from vegetables and fruit appeared to amplify the adverse consequences of high glycaemic load.[62]

The role of a variety of various micronutrients in colorectal cancer risk has been examined as well. Calcium has been proposed on theoretical grounds as potentially having a modifying role in colorectal carcinogenesis,[63] but little supporting evidence was immediately forthcoming from epidemiological studies,[64] although these early studies in humans are of limited value because of questionable study design or inadequacy of the estimation of diet.

To investigate this hypothesis, an intervention trial of colorectal adenoma recurrence was established in North America.[65,66] This trial[66] involved 930 subjects (mean age 61 years; 72% men) with a recent history of colorectal adenomas, randomly assigned to receive either calcium carbonate (3 g (1.2 g of elemental calcium) daily) or placebo, with follow-up colonoscopies 1 and 4 years after the qualifying examination. Subjects in the calcium group had a lower risk of recurrent adenomas detected at 1-year or 4-year colonoscopy. Among the 913 subjects who underwent at least one study colonoscopy, the adjusted risk ratio for any recurrence of adenoma on the calcium supplementation group as compared with placebo was 0.85 (95% CI 0.74–0.98). The main analysis was based on the 832 subjects (409 in the cal-

cium group and 423 in the placebo group) who completed both follow-up examinations. At least one adenoma was diagnosed between the first and second follow up endoscopies in 127 subjects in the calcium group (31%) and 159 subjects in the placebo group (38%); there was a reduction in risk of recurrent adenoma of about one-fifth associated with calcium supplementation (OR 0.81; 95% CI 0.67–0.99). The adjusted ratio of the average number of adenomas in the calcium group to that in the placebo group was 0.76 (95% CI 0.60–0.96). The effect of calcium was independent of initial dietary fat and calcium intake.

In another study, conducted in Europe, 665 patients with a history of colorectal adenomas were randomly assigned to three treatment groups, one of which used calcium but in a different form to that employed in North America (calcium gluconolactate and carbonate (2 g elemental calcium daily)).[67] Participants had a colonoscopy after 3 years of follow-up. Among the 552 participants who completed the follow-up examination, 94 had stopped treatment early. At least one adenoma developed in 28 (15.9%) of 176 patients in the calcium group, 58 (29.3%) of 198 in the fibre group, and 36 (20.2%) of 178 in the placebo group. The adjusted odds ratio for recurrence was reduced by one-third for calcium treatment (OR 0.66; 95% CI 0.38–1.17), and was increased (OR 1.67; 95% CI 1.01–2.76) for patients in the group allocated to fibre. The odds ratio associated with the fibre treatment was significantly higher in participants with baseline dietary calcium intake above the median than in those with intake below the median. The findings suggested to the authors that supplementation with fibre (in the form of ispaghula husk) may have adverse effects on colorectal adenoma recurrence, especially in patients with high dietary calcium intake. However, once again, calcium supplementation was associated with a modest (although in this case non-significant) reduction in the risk of adenoma recurrence. This hypothesis is worth further study on a larger scale, despite the clear problems in investigating such dietary hypotheses.[68]

Both body iron stores and dietary iron intake have been reported to increase the risk of colorectal neoplasms. The potential association between serum ferritin concentration and recurrence of colorectal adenomas was assessed among 733 individuals with baseline determinations of ferritin as part of a multi-centre clinical trial of antioxidant supplements for adenoma prevention.[69] This study demonstrated no statistically significant linear association between log ferritin concentration and adenoma recurrence

($p = 0.33$). Dietary intake of iron and red meat was inversely associated with adenoma recurrence among participants with replete iron stores but not consistently associated among those with non-replete stores.[69] These findings suggest that any role of iron stores and dietary iron in influencing the risk of colorectal adenoma recurrence is likely to be complex and difficult to disentangle.

One of the major reasons why such trials and studies can be difficult to interpret relates to off-study use of vitamins and minerals, which are probably becoming more common and certainly vary from country to country. During the course of a colorectal neoplasia chemoprevention trial using aspirin in a group of colorectal carcinoma survivors, Sandler et al[70] obtained information on the use of vitamins, minerals, and supplements at baseline and every 6 months. One or more supplements were used at some time by 55% of subjects. Among those who took supplements, 66% took more than one and 13% took five or more. The mean number of supplements taken was 2.6 (1.7 standard deviation). Vitamins were the most commonly used (49%), followed by minerals (22%), botanicals (13%), and others (5%). Calcium (16%) was the most frequent mineral. Among users, there were no differences in supplement use by age or gender. However, it is clear that this is a major factor that needs to be taken into account in the design (e.g. assessing sample size correctly) and interpretation phase of such intervention studies.

A number of studies have reported positive associations with alcohol consumption and colorectal cancer risk,[71] but it remains to be proven whether the putative association is with alcohol per se and not with the caloric contribution of alcohol or due to influences in the components of diet in alcohol drinkers. There is some experimental evidence that vitamin E and selenium may be protective against colon tumours,[50] and there is support for the hypothesis that β-carotene protects also.[29] Lactobacilli, found in some dairy products, may have a favourable effect on the intestine.[72] In 1988, the IARC considered that 12 case–control studies of sufficient quality have addressed the issue of coffee consumption and the risk of colorectal cancer, and 11 of these have indicated inverse (protective) associations.[73] No association has been found with tea drinking or caffeine intake from all sources considered. A recent meta-analysis looked at the comparison between 'high' and 'low' consumption in 12 retrospective and 5 prospective studies. A protective effect was suggested from retrospective studies but not confirmed by published prospective studies.[74]

TOBACCO SMOKING AND COLORECTAL CANCER RISK

The large bowel has not historically been considered as a site where the risk of cancer is linked to cigarette smoking,[75] although it has been suggested that it may be an independent risk factor that may be specifically associated with the early stages of colorectal epidemiology.[76] A more recent review of all epidemiological evidence has indicated the strength and consistency of this finding.[77] Giovannucci[77] concluded that 21 out of 22 studies found that long-term, heavy cigarette smokers have a two- to threefold elevated risk of colorectal adenoma. The risk of large adenomas, those that present a high risk of colorectal cancer within a relatively short time frame, was elevated in smokers in all 12 studies that examined this association.

The studies of smoking and colorectal cancer risk conducted earlier in the 1950s through to the 1970s did not show consistently any association, and led review groups to consider that, based on the available evidence, there was no association demonstrated (see e.g. reference 75). However, 27 studies in various countries, including the large majority of those that have been conducted in the past two decades, show a consistent association between tobacco use (essentially cigarette smoking) and colorectal cancer. In the USA, 15 of 16 studies conducted after 1970 in middle-aged and elderly men and, in the 1990s, in women demonstrate such an association. Giovannucci[77] considered that this temporal pattern is consistent with an induction period of three to four decades between exposure and the development of clinical colorectal cancer. Overall, accumulating evidence, much within the past decade, strongly supports the addition of colorectal cancer to the list of tobacco-associated malignancies. Such an association has biological plausibility, since carcinogens from tobacco could reach the colorectal mucosa through either the alimentary tract or the circulatory system, and could then damage or alter expression of cancer-related genes. It appears likely that up to one in five colorectal cancers in the USA may be associated with such exposure.

HORMONE REPLACEMENT THERAPY

There is increasing evidence supporting (an originally unexpected) association between use of hormone replacement therapy (HRT) and a reduced risk of colorectal cancer. A Medline search was used to identify observational studies published between

January 1974 and December 1993 for a meta-analysis.[78] The overall risk for colorectal cancer and oestrogen replacement therapy was 0.92 (95% CI 0.74–1.5). There was no separate effect when colon and rectal cancer were considered as separate entities.[78] Subsequent to this report, there have been further studies published.

A case–control study from Seattle, USA among 193 women aged 30–62 years with colon cancer and an equal number of controls was conducted to examine the relationship between colon cancer and female hormone use.[79] Use of non-contraceptive hormones after the age of 40 years was associated with a reduced risk of colon cancer (OR 0.60; 95% CI 0.35–1.01). The risk among women with five or more years of use was 0.47 (95% CI 0.24–0.91).[79]

Colorectal cancer mortality was examined in some detail in the American Cancer Society Prospective Study. With the risk set to 1.0 among women who reported to be never-users of HRT (the referent group), the risk associated with ever-use was 0.69 (95% CI 0.60–0.79).[80] Relative to the risk in never-users, the risk associated with less than 1 year of use of HRT was 0.81 (95% CI 0.63–1.03), with between 2 and 5 years of use it was 0.76 (95% CI 0.61–0.95), with between 6 and 10 years of use it was 0.55 (95% CI 0.39–0.77), and for 11 or more years of use it was 0.54 (95% CI 0.39–0.76).

Of 19 published studies of HRT and colorectal cancer risk, 10 support an inverse association and the remaining 5 show a significant reduction in risk. The risk seems lowest among long-term users. Although there are still some contradictions in the available literature, it appears likely that use of HRT reduces the risk of colorectal cancer in women. The risk appears to halve with 5–10 years of such use. The role of unopposed as compared with combination HRT is an open issue for colorectal cancer.

More recently published studies add evidence of a protective effect of HRT use and risk of colon cancer or mortality from colon cancer. Use of HRT, present or past, has been associated with an increased short-term survival after diagnosis with colon cancer in postmenopausal women,[81] a 50% reduction in the risk of colon cancer,[82] and protection against microsatellite-instability-positive tumours.[83] A meta-analysis of HRT use and colon cancer has found that there is a protective effect and that this effect is stronger in current or recent users and among users of more than 5 years' duration.[84] Despite these encouraging findings, it is important to emphasize that women using HRT tend to adopt lifestyle choices that confer protection from colon cancer or other chronic conditions, such that confounding

cannot be excluded with certainty from studies assessing HRT as a protective factor in colon cancer. For example, the practice of exercise involving increased physical activity, increased consumption of fruits and vegetables, and reduced fat intake and/or past screening (colonoscopy, sigmoidoscopy, or occult blood test) tend to be followed more often by women who are HRT ever-users than by never-users.[82] Beral and colleagues,[85] in their review of the use of HRT and the subsequent risk of cancer, advocate caution in over-interpreting the suggested protective effect in colon cancer.

PROSPECTS FOR CHEMOPREVENTION

It is well known that individuals with adenomata, particularly large adenomata, are at increased risk of second or subsequent polyps. Selective recruitment from such a population would have intrinsic attractions. Firstly, subsequent disease risk is raised and therefore the numbers requiring recruitment would be reduced. Secondly, the chances of patients adhering to treatment schedules would be likely to be raised because of their primary disease profiles. Data obtained in such a study would in essence be concentrated upon rates of adenoma development, with little emphasis upon cancer occurrence, and not upon cancer behaviour, since few invasive cancers would be likely to be detected. Nevertheless, such a study has obvious attractions: colorectal polyps present one of the most useful intermediate endpoints (biomarkers) at the present time.

Any agents chosen for study should be capable of long-term administration, and should be largely if not completely free of adverse effects. In addition, there should be plausible epidemiological and/or biological evidence in favour of their ability to inhibit polyp development and/or retard tumour growth. Finally, it should be possible to combine their use with that of antimitotic drugs, so that a single trial could consider adjuvant therapy as well as adjuvant chemoprevention. The requirement of adverse-effect-free treatment that can be given continuously for very prolonged periods makes novel chemical entities unpromising candidates.

Candidates include at least vitamin A or β-carotene, vitamin C, vitamin D, vitamin E, calcium supplements, folate, anti-inflammatory drugs, and H_2 antagonists.[86] Relatively novel chemical entities such as protease inhibitors are at an earlier stage of development, making prolonged treatment too speculative a possibility. Taken overall, there are suggestions of benefit for all of the above compounds (some stronger than others) in reducing the risk of developing colorectal cancer and/or in preventing polyp occurrence. Effects on secondary spread are little understood, except that anti-inflammatory agents have been used clinically in the past in trying to inhibit osteolysis. (See also discussion of this topic in Chapter 5.)

NON-STEROIDAL ANTI-INFLAMMATORY DRUGS

There is abundant evidence that the use of non-steroidal anti-inflammatory drugs (NSAIDs) is associated with reduced risks of colorectal cancer and adenomatous polyps.[87–91] Effects have been demonstrated consistently, though not completely uniformly, are evident in case–control and cohort studies, and appear to be related to dose and duration of treatment.[86] These effects are biologically plausible: (i) NSAID use appears to prevent or reduce the frequency of carcinogen-induced animal colon tumours;[92–94] (ii) NSAIDs appear to reduce growth rates in colon cancer cell lines; and (iii) polyp formation in familial adenomatous polyposis coli (FAP) appears to be retarded.[95,96] For example, in a randomized trial of the use of sulindac in FAP, among nine patients taking the drug, six had complete regression of rectal polyps and three partial regression; in the placebo group, polyps increased in five, remained unchanged in two, and decreased in the remaining two.[95]

The use of these drugs is attractive because they are licensed for use in humans and their effects, outside the issue of cancer prevention, are well understood. There is little evidence on the basis of trials that NSAIDs can prevent cancer recurrence. The use of indomethacin or other cyclooxygenase antagonists has been suggested to improve natural killer cell activity, and to enhance non-specific immunotherapy of experimental lung tumour metastases.[97–99] In a randomized study in cervical cancer in 160 patients, the use of indomethacin enhanced survival of those given radiation treatment by 27% at 5 years and 41% at 10 years.[100]

There is a very good case for a controlled trial of NSAIDs in the prevention of colorectal cancer.[101] If such a treatment trial were to be undertaken, then the benefits and risks would need to be understood, and an appropriate dose chosen for an appropriate agent. The available evidence indicates that both aspirin and non-aspirin NSAIDs may be of value, although aspirin may be the more effective – at least as judged by calculated odds ratios. Note, however, that published data give little clinically useful data on doses required: although the US Physicians' Health Study suggests that 325 mg of aspirin on alternate days may be relatively ineffective.[102] Aspirin is known to have additional potential cardiovascular benefits through inhibiting platelet cyclooxygenase irreversibly, though similar benefits are likely to be obtained with (for example) regular indomethacin use.

NSAIDs have classic adverse effects on the kidney (interstitial nephritis), skin (rash and photosensitivity), lung (predispose to asthma), and liver (hepatitis – particularly with diclofenac). However, none of these, individually or collectively, is as frequent as gastrointestinal bleeding from peptic ulcers and, to a lesser extent, from the colon. Risks vary by up to 20-fold between agents and by up to 10-fold by dose.[103] Risks can almost certainly be reduced by using enteric-coated drugs, but available evidence has generally been obtained with standard preparations. Whether it would be wise to alter deliberately the delivery pattern in treating large-bowel disease is unclear. Enteric-coated preparations are probably completely absorbed in the small bowel, and non-enteric-coated in the stomach and small bowel, so differences may be immaterial. Since in the US Physicians' Health Study, low-dose aspirin (325 mg on alternate days) appeared relatively ineffective in preventing colon cancer, doses of at least 325 mg daily may be required. It is unclear, however, whether in that study the follow-up was sufficiently prolonged. Risk reduction in US nurses only became apparent after 20 years of continuous use.[104] Consequently, the US Physicians' Study may have also had a less than optimal intervention period.

COX-2 INHIBITORS

Considerations of chemopreventive strategies need to remain focused on the condition being dealt with. As Sporn[105] pointed out, the disease is *carcinogenesis* and not *cancer*, and nowhere is this process better understood than in the case of colorectal cancer. Although the mode of action of NSAIDs in reducing the incidence of colon cancer is not entirely understood, there are some strong clues, including a body of clinical evidence and recent experimental evidence demonstrating the effect of NSAIDs on colorectal carcinogenesis. NSAIDs have demonstrated effects on the modulation of several putative biomarkers of colorectal cancer in rats treated with azoxymethane, including the formation of aberrant crypt foci (ACF) and oncogene (*myc*, *ras*, *p53*) expression. NSAIDs also inhibit the production of prostaglandins, and other eicosanoids, from arachidonic acid by the cyclooxygenase (COX) component of prostaglandin synthase. There is considerable evidence that prostaglandin E_2 (PGE_2) induces cellular proliferation and may also suppress immune surveillance and killing of malignant cells. High levels of PGE_2 can also cause downregulation of the signal transduction mechanisms responsible for maintaining the differentiated state of the cell.

It has been established that two isoforms of COX exist. The COX-1 isoform is expressed constitutively throughout normal human tissues, including the kidney and gastric mucosa, where the prostaglandins produced are thought to play a protective role. The COX-2 isoform is an inducible form of cyclooxygenase found in very low levels in normal tissues and in greatly increased levels in inflamed tissues.

NSAIDs reduce the incidence of colorectal cancer in humans and in animal models, and COX-2 expression is increased in animal models of colorectal cancer and FAP (the AOM rat and the MIN mouse). COX-2 inhibitors are chemopreventive in animal models of colorectal cancer in AOM-induced ACF and tumour models and in knockout mice.[86]

In addition, NSAIDs reduce mucosal prostaglandins and cause ulcers, which can result in bleeding, perforation, or outlet obstruction; exogenous prostaglandins reduce both endoscopic ulcers and ulcer complications by about 50% over 6 months. Celecoxib, a new COX-2 inhibitor, could be expected to reduce the frequency of ulcers as a complication of therapy. It has been examined in the context of colorectal cancer control in a variety of different study designs: (i) a preclinical efficacy study on rats; (ii) a control diet versus an experimental diet (containing celecoxib) for 2 weeks; and (iii) rats injected with carcinogen at 2 weeks and evaluated at 50 weeks. Celecoxib inhibited the incidence of colorectal tumours by 93% and multiplicity by 97%, and the results exceeded those seen with NSAIDs in studies of similar design and with a decreased number of side-effects.

SUMMARY AND CONCLUSIONS

Colorectal cancer is the fourth commonest form of cancer worldwide, with an estimated 782 900 new cases diagnosed in 1990.[1] High incidence rates are found in Western Europe, North America, and Australasia, and intermediate rates in Eastern Europe, with the lowest rates being found in sub-Saharal Africa.[3] The disease is not uniformly fatal although there are large differences in survival

according to the stage of disease. In advanced colorectal cancer in which curative resection is possible, the 5-year survival rate in Dukes B is 45%, dropping to 30% in Dukes C.[106] The 5-year survival rate in resected Dukes A is around 80%, and survival following simple resection of an adenomatous pedunculated polyp containing carcinoma in situ (or severe dysplasia) or intramucosal carcinoma is generally close to 100%. It is estimated that there are, however, still 394 000 deaths from colorectal cancer worldwide annually.[12]

The large differences in survival between early- and late-stage disease clearly indicate the advantage in detecting colorectal cancer at an early stage. The simplest advice is to ensure that any change in bowel habits or unexpected presence of blood in the stool should be investigated. Faecal Occult Blood Testing (FOBT) is aimed at the detection of early asymptomatic cancer, and is based on the assumption that such cancers will bleed and that small quantities of blood lost in the stool may be detected chemically or immunologically. A significant reduction in colorectal cancer mortality with annual testing using Hemoccult has been reported.[107] The cumulative annual mortality rate in the group screened annually was 5.88 per 1000, compared with 8.83 in the control group and 8.33 in the group screened biennially. The results are of considerable importance, but it is difficult to ignore the observation that 38% of those screened annually and 28% of those screened biennially underwent at least one colonoscopy during the study period, although it is somewhat reassuring that the incidence of colorectal cancer was so similar in the three groups (23, 23, and 26 per 1000 for those screened annually, those screened biennially, and those in the control group, respectively). The authors considered that the likely effect of colonoscopy, in removing polyps, had not yet affected the incidence and mortality from colorectal cancer.

FOBT has been reported from case–control studies to reduce colorectal cancer mortality rates by 31%[108] and 57% (in women).[109] In a non-randomized study, it was shown that annual rigid sigmoidoscopy and FOBT, rather than sigmoidoscopy alone, was associated with a reduction in colorectal cancer mortality.[110] There have now been three randomized trials of FOBT, each demonstrating a reduction in colorectal cancer mortality. Mandel et al[107] reported a reduction of 33% in colorectal cancer mortality after 13 years in subjects who were offered annual screening with FOBT, but a non-significant reduction (of 6%) in those who were offered biennial screening. In two more recent studies, from Nottingham, UK[111] and Denmark,[112] the colorectal cancer mortality rates in the group offered biennial FOBT were respectively 0.85 and 0.82 times the rates in the control population. An (approximate) combined analysis of these latter studies produces a relative risk of colorectal cancer death of 0.84 (95% CI 0.75– 0.94).[113]

These findings are important confirmation that FOBT screening may be effective in the prevention of death from colorectal cancer. There are both advantages and disadvantages to FOBT. On the one hand, it is low-cost, although the investigation of false positives (around 1–3% per test) certainly increases the cost, and it 'examines' the entire colon and rectum. However, FOBT is currently characterized by a low sensitivity (with around 40% of cancers and 80% of adenomas being missed by the test[114,115]) and by detecting colorectal cancers at the later stages in the natural history during which lesions bleed, which leads to a short lead-time and the requirement for frequent testing. Rehydration of slides results in increased positivity but also an increased number of colonoscopies and a decreased specificity of the test. The costs must be weighed against the benefits before public health policy on this topic is formulated.[107]

An important development recently has been the demonstration that after 18 years there is a significant reduction in the incidence of colorectal cancer in subjects randomized to the Hemoccult arm of the Minnesota study.[116] Mandel and colleagues[116] followed the participants in the Minnesota Colon Cancer Control Study for 18 years. A total of 46 551 people, most of whom were 50–80 years old, were enrolled between 1975 and 1978, and were randomly assigned to annual screening, biennial screening, or usual care (the control group). During the 18-year follow-up period, 1359 new cases of colorectal cancer were identified: 417 in the annual-screening group, 435 in the biennial-screening group, and 507 in the control group. The cumulative incidence ratios for colorectal cancer in the screening groups as compared with the control group were 0.80 (95% CI 0.70–0.90) and 0.83 (95% CI 0.73–0.94) for the annual-screening and biennial-screening groups, respectively. For both screening groups, the number of positive slides was associated with the positive predictive value both for colorectal cancer and for adenomatous polyps at least 1 cm in diameter. The authors concluded that the use of either annual or biennial FOBT significantly reduces the incidence of colorectal cancer.[116]

Until a randomized controlled trial has been undertaken and reported, the efficacy of flexible sigmoidoscopy as a screening test for preventing death from colorectal cancer will remain unproved. However, there is now a good deal of evidence supporting infrequent sigmoidoscopy as a potentially effective screening modality for colorectal cancer. Impressive reductions in rectal cancer and cancer of the proximal colon have been reported from demonstration studies: an 85% reduction in 21 000 subjects undergoing 'clearing' proctosigmoidoscopy followed by annual proctosigmoidoscopy, with removal of all lesions detected;[117] a 70% reduction in the risk of colorectal cancer for 10 years following sigmoidoscopy;[118] an 80% reduction in incidence following examination mostly performed by flexible sigmoidoscopy;[119] and an 85% reduction of rectal cancers achieved by the removal of adenomas.[120] Although the initial examination may be expensive, there is the advantage that polyps may be removed at the time of the initial procedure and no follow-up visits will be required. Use of a 65 cm flexible sigmoidoscope appears to be the most effective proposition at the present time, since this avoids the more complicated colonoscopy and yet still covers over two-thirds of the large intestine.

There are some extremely important issues to address in the area of colorectal cancer screening:

- *Should FOBT now be recommended as a population screening method?* This decision depends on many factors, including the value placed on the magnitude of the mortality reduction, the false-positive rate associated with Hemoccult testing, the acceptance of the test to the general population and the economic costs involved.
- *Should consideration be given to other screening modalities for colorectal cancer?* Screening with sigmoidoscopy has been demonstrated in case–control and non-randomized studies to reduce the incidence and mortality from colorectal cancer by over 50%.[118,121,122] FOBT does not appear to reduce the incidence of colorectal cancer.
- *Since a large proportion of individuals tested for faecal occult blood have positive tests and are referred for colonoscopy, could it prove effective to bypass FOBT and go directly to a screening colonoscopy? Or flexible sigmoidoscopy?* This latter strategy is currently being assessed in a large randomized trial, and it is a clear reflection of the tremendous potential for colorectal cancer early detection by screening, which is clearly outlined in detail elsewhere.[123] This should continue to be a priority research activity at present.

The classical concept of risk of colorectal cancer being increased by increased consumption of fat, protein, and meat and to be reduced by increased consumption of fruits and vegetables[124] is currently being challenged as more epidemiological data become available. It has been hypothesized that alterations to serum triglycerides and/or plasma glucose could be one possible vehicle for the effects of various aetiological factors.[125] Thus there are prospects for primary prevention, although it is difficult to know how to successfully bring about such large-scale alterations to the diets of large proportions of populations. The large bowel has not been traditionally considered as a site where the risk of cancer is linked to cigarette smoking,[75] although more recent evidence strongly points to the existence of such an association between cigarette smoking and an increased risk of both adenomatous polyps and colorectal cancer.[77] There is also interesting evidence suggesting that specific chemopreventive strategies could prove useful in the prevention of colorectal cancer.[86]

While there are many questions to be resolved, it is apparent that colorectal cancer is becoming increasingly understood and prospects for prevention are becoming apparent. Making colorectal cancer a form of cancer for which a large proportion of deaths may be preventable[122] is a success for epidemiology. Achieving colorectal cancer control is the immediate challenge.

ACKNOWLEDGEMENT

It is a pleasure to acknowledge that this work was conducted within the framework of support by the Italian Association for Cancer Research (*Associazone Italiana per la Ricerca sul Cancro*).

REFERENCES

1. Parkin DM, Pisani P, Ferlay J, Estimates of the worldwide incidence of 25 major cancers in 1990. *Int J Cancer* 1999; **80:** 827–41.
2. Boyle P, Relative value of incidence and mortality data in cancer research. *Rec Res Cancer Res* 1989; **114:** 41–63.
3. Boyle P, Zaridze DG, Smans M, Descriptive epidemiology of colorectal cancer. *Int J Cancer* 1985; **36:** 9–18.
4. Howe HL, Wingo PA, Thun MJ et al, Annual report to the nation on the status of cancer (1973 through 1998), featuring cancers with recent increasing trends. *J Natl Cancer Inst* 2001; **93:** 824–42.
5. Parkin DM, Whelan S, Ferlay L et al (Eds), *Cancer Incidence in Five Continents*, Vol VII. Lyon: IARC Scientific Publication 143, 1997.
6. Haenszel W, Kurihara M, Studies of Japanese migrants I. Mortality from cancer and other diseases among Japanese in the United States. *J Natl Cancer Inst* 1968; **40:** 43–68.
7. Haenszel N, Correa P, Cancer of the colon and rectum and adenomatous polyps. A review of epidemiologic findings. *Cancer* 1971; **28:** 14–24.
8. Bell J, Coates M, Day P, Armstrong BK, *Colorectal Cancer in New South Wales in 1972 to 1993*. Sydney: Cancer Council, New South Wales Health Department, 1996.
9. *National Cancer Institute: 1985 Annual Cancer Statistics Review*. Bethesda, MD: NIH Publication 86-2789, 1986.
10. *National Cancer Institute: 1987 Annual Cancer Statistics Review, Including Cancer Trends 1950–1985*. Bethesda, MD: NIH Publication 88-2789, 1988.
11. Staszewski J, Migrant studies in alimentary tract cancer. *Rec Results Cancer Res* 1972; **39:** 85–97.
12. Pisani P, Parkin DM, Bray F, Ferlay J, Estimates of the worldwide mortality from 25 major cancers in 1990. *Int J Cancer* 1999; **83:** 18–29.
13. *Canadian National Cancer Statistics 1997*. Toronto: National Cancer Institute of Canada, 1997.
14. Boyle P, La Vecchia C, Negri E et al, Trends in diet-related cancers in Japan: a conundrum? Lancet 1993; **342:** 752.
15. Peipens LA, Sandler RS, Epidemiology of colorectal adenomas. *Epidemiol Rev* 1994; **16:** 273–97.
16. Vogelstein B, Fearon ER, Hamilton SR et al, Genetic alterations during colorectal-tumour development. *N Engl J Med* 1988; **319:** 525–32.
17. Fearon ER, Vogelstein B, A genetic model for colorectal tumorigenesis. *Cell* 1990; **61:** 759–67.
18. Morotomi M, Guillem J, LoGerfo P, Weinstein IB, Production of diacylglycerol, an activator of protein kinase C, by human intestinal microflora. *Cancer Res* 1990; **50:** 3595–9.
19. Bodmer WF, Balley CJ, Bodmer J et al, Localization of the gene for familial adenomatous polyposis on chromosome 5. *Nature* 1987; **328:** 614–18.
20. Hall NR, Murday VA, Chapman P et al, Genetic linkage in Muir–Torre syndrome to the same chromosomal region as cancer family syndrome. *Eur J Cancer* 1994; **30:** 180–2.
21. Bishop DT, Thomas HJW, The genetics of colorectal cancer. *Cancer Surv* 1990; **9:** 585–604.
22. Bishop DT, Hall NR, The genetics of colorectal cancer. *Eur J Cancer* 1990; **30:** 1946–56.
23. Cohen AM, Minsky BD, Schilsky RL, Colon cancer. In: *Cancer: Principles and Practice of Oncology*, 4th edn. (deVita VT, Hellman S, Rosenberg SA, eds). Philadelphia: JB Lippincott, 1993.
24. McMichael AJ, Giles GG, Colorectal cancer. In: *Cancer Surveys: Trends in Incidence and Mortality* (Doll R, Fraumeni JF, Muir CS, eds). Cold Spring Harbor, NY: Cold Spring Harbor Press, 1994: 77–98.
25. Shephard RJ, Exercise in the prevention and treatment of cancer – an update. *Sports Med* 1993; **15:** 258–80.
26. Thune I, Lund E, Physical activity and risk of colorectal cancer in men and women. *Br J Cancer* 1996; **73:** 1134–40.
27. Martinez ME, Giovannucci E, Spiegelman D et al, Leisure-time physical activity, body size, and colon cancer in women. Nurses' Health Study Research Group. *J Natl Cancer Inst* 1997; **89:** 948–55.
28. Whittemore AS, Wu-Williams AH, Lee M et al, Diet, physical activity and colorectal cancer among Chinese in North America and China. *J Natl Cancer Inst* 1990; **82:** 915–26.
29. Willett WC, The search for the causes of breast and colon cancer. *Nature* 1989; **338:** 389–94.
30. Vena JE, Graham S, Zielezny M et al, Occupational exercise and risk of cancer. *Am J Clin Nutr* 1987; **45:** 318–27.
31. Slattery ML, Schumacher ML, Smith KR et al, Physical activity, diet and role of colon cancer in Utah. *Am J Epidemiol* 1988; **128:** 989–99.
32. Davidow Al, Neugut AL, Jacobsen JS et al, Recurrent adenomatous polyps and body mass index. *Cancer Epidemiol Biomark Prev* 1996; **5:** 313–15
33. Sandler RS, Pritchard ML, Bangiwala SI, Physical activity and

the risk of colorectal adenomas. *Epidemiology* 1995; **6:** 602–6.

34. Giovannucci E, Colditz GA, Stampfer MJ, Willett WC, Physical activity, obesity and risk of colorectal cancer in women (United States). *Cancer Causes Contr* 1996; **7:** 253–63.

35. Holdstock DJ, Misiewicz JJ, Smith T et al, Propulsion (mass movements) in the human colon and its relationship to meals and somatic activity. *Gut* 1970; **11:** 91–9.

36. Simon HB, The immunology of exercise. *JAMA* 1984; **252:** 2735–8.

37. Bartram HP, Wynder EL, Physical activity and colon cancer risk? Physiological consideration. *Am J Gastroenterol* 1989; **84:** 109–12.

38. Dukas L, Willett WC, Colditz GA et al, Prospective study of bowel movement, laxative use, and risk of colorectal cancer among women. *Am J Epidemiol* 2000; **151:** 958–64.

39. Steinmetz KA, Potter JD, Vegetable, fruit, and cancer I. Epidemiology. *Cancer Causes Contr* 1991; **2:** 325–58.

40. Michels KB, Giovannucci E, Joshipura KJ et al, Prospective study of fruit and vegetable consumption and incidence of colon and rectal cancers. *J Natl Cancer Inst* 2000; **92:** 1740–52.

41. Willett WC, Stampfer MJ, Colditz GA et al, Relation of meat, fat, and fiber intake to the risk of colon cancer in a prospective study among women. *N Engl J Med* 1990; **323:** 1664–72.

42. Willett WC, Diet and cancer: one view at the start of the millennium. *Cancer Epidemiol Biomark Prev* 2001; **10:** 3–8.

43. Franceschi S, Favero A, The role of energy and fat in cancers of the breast and colon-rectum in a southern European population. *Ann Oncol* 1999; **10** (Suppl 6): 61–3.

44. Sugimura T, Past, present and future of mutagens in cooked foods. *Environ Health Perspect* 1986; **67:** 5–10.

45. Felton JS, Knize MG, Shen NH et al, Identification of the mutagens in cooked beef. *Environ Health Perspect* 1986; **67:** 17–24.

46. Schiffman MH, Felton JS, Fried foods and the risk of colon cancer. *Am J Epidemiol* 1990; **131:** 376–8.

47. Ha WI, Grim NK, Periza MW, Anticarcinogenics from fried ground beef: heat-altered derivatives of linoleic acid. *Carcinogenesis* 1987; **8:** 1881–7.

48. Sandhu MS, White I, McPherson K, Systematic review of the prospective cohort studies on meat consumption and colorectal cancer risk: a meta-analytical approach. *Cancer Epidemiol Biomark Prev* 2001; **10:** 439–46.

49. Sinha R, Kulldorff M, Chow WH et al, Dietary intake of heterocyclic amines, meat-derived mutagenic activity, and risk of colorectal adenomas. *Cancer Epidemiol Biomark Prev* 2001; **10:** 559–62.

50. Zaridze DG, Environmental etiology of large-bowel cancer. *J Natl Cancer Inst* 1983; **70:** 389–400.

51. Sakaguchi M, Hiramatsu Y, Takada H et al, Effect of dietary unsaturated and saturated fats on azoxymethane-induced colon carcinogenesis in rats. *Cancer Res* 1984; **44:** 1472–7.

52. Minoura YT, Takata T, Sakaguchi M et al, Effect of dietary eicosapentaenoic acid on azoxymethane induced colon carcinogenesis in rats. *Cancer Res* 1988; **46:** 4790–4.

53. Kritchevsky D, Diet, nutrition and cancer: the role of fibre. *Cancer* 1986; **58:** 1830-6.

54. Tuyns AJ, Haeltermann M, Kaaks R, Colorectal cancer and the intake of nutrients: oliogosaccharides are a risk factor, fats are not. A case–control study in Belgium. *Nutr Cancer* 1987; **10:** 181–96.

55. Kune S, Kune GA, Watson LF, Case–control study of dietary aetiological factors: the Melbourne colorectal cancer study. *Nutr Cancer* 1987; **9:** 21–42.

56. Heilbrun LK, Hankin JH, Nomura AMY et al, Colon cancer and dietary fat, phosphorous and calcium in Hawaiian-Japanese men. *Am J Clin Nutr* 1986; **43:** 306–9.

57. Fernandez E, d'Avanzo B, Negri E, Franceschi S, La Vecchia C,

Diet diversity and the risk of colorectal cancer in northern Italy. *Cancer Epidemiol Biomark Prev* 1996; **5:** 433–6.

58. Schatzkin A, Lanza E, Corle D et al, Lack of effect of low-fat, high-fiber diet on the recurrence of colorectal adenomas. *N Engl J Med* 2000; **342:** 1149–55.

59. Alberts DS, Martinez ME, Roe D et al, Lack of effect of a high-fiber cereal supplement on the recurrence of colorectal adenomas. *N Engl J Med* 2000; **342:** 1156–62.

60. Freedman AN, Michalek AM, Marshall JR et al, Familial and nutritional risk factors for p53 overexpression in colorectal cancer. *Cancer Epidemiol Biomark Prev* 1996; **5:** 285–91.

61. Giovannucci E, Pollak MN, Platz EA et al, A prospective study of plasma insulin-like growth factor-1 and binding protein-3 and risk of colorectal neoplasia in women. *Cancer Epidemiol Biomarkers Prev* 2000; **9:** 345–9.

62. Franceschi S, Dal Maso L, Augustin L et al, Dietary glycemic load and colorectal cancer risk. *Ann Oncol* 2001; **12:** 173–8.

63. Newmark HL, Wargovich MJ, Bruce WR, Colon cancer and dietary fat, phosphate and calcium: a hypothesis. *J Natl Cancer Inst* 1984; **72:** 1323–5.

64. Sorenson AW, Slattery ML, Ford MH, Calcium and colon cancer: a review. *Nutr Cancer* 1988; **11:** 135–45.

65. Baron JA, Beach M, Mandel JS et al, Calcium supplements and colorectal adenomas. Polyp Prevention Study Group. *Ann NY Acad Sci* 1999; **889:** 138–45.

66. Baron JA, Beach M, Mandel JS et al, Calcium supplements for the prevention of colorectal adenomas. Calcium Polyp Prevention Study Group. *N Engl J Med* 1999; **340:** 101–7

67. Bonithon-Kopp C, Kronborg O, Giacosa A et al, Calcium and fibre supplementation in prevention of colorectal adenoma recurrence: a randomised intervention trial. European Cancer Prevention Organisation Study Group. *Lancet* 2000; **356:** 1300–6.

68. Byers T, Diet, colorectal adenomas, and colorectal cancer. *N Engl J Med* 2000; **342:** 1206–7.

69. Tseng M, Greenberg ER, Sandler RS et al, Serum ferritin concentration and recurrence of colorectal adenoma. *Cancer Epidemiol Biomark Prev* 2000; **9:** 625–30.

70. Sandler RS, Halabi S, Kaplan EB et al, Use of vitamins, minerals, and nutritional supplements by participants in a chemoprevention trial. *Cancer* 2001; **91:** 1040–5.

71. Longnecker MP, Orza MJ, Adams ME et al, A meta-analysis of alcoholic beverage consumption in relation to risk of colorectal cancer. *Cancer Causes Contr* 1990; **1:** 59–68.

72. Goldin BR, Gorbach SL, The effect of milk and lactobacillus feeding on human intestinal bacterial enzyme activity. *Am J Clin Nutr* 1984; **39:** 756–61.

73. *IARC Monographs on the Evaluation of the Carcinogenic Risk of Chemicals to Man.* Vol 44. *Coffee, Tea, Mate, Methylxanthines (Caffeine, Theophylline, Theobromine) and Methylglyoxal.* Lyon: International Agency for Research on Cancers, 1988.

74. Giovannucci E, Meta-analysis of coffee consumption and risk of colorectal cancer. *Am J Epidemiol* 1998; **147:** 1043–52.

75. *IARC Monographs on the Evaluation of the Carcinogenic Risk of Chemicals to Man.* Vol 38. *Tobacco Smoking,* Lyon: International Agency for Research on Cancers, 1986.

76. Giovannucci E, Colditz GA, Strampfer MJ et al, A prospective study of cigarette smoking and risk of colorectal adenoma and colorectal cancer in U.S. women. *J Natl Cancer Inst* 1994; **86:** 192–9.

77. Giovannucci E, An updated review of the epidemiological evidence that cigarette smoking increases risk of colorectal cancer. *Cancer Epidemiol Biomark Prev* 2001; **10:** 725–31.

78. MacLennan SC, MacLennan AH, Ryan P, Colorectal cancer and oestrogen replacement therapy: a meta-analysis of epidemiological studies. *Med J Austr* 1991; **162:** 491–3.

79. Jacobs EJ, White E, Weiss NS, Exogenous hormones, reproductive history and colon cancer. *Cancer Causes Contr* 1994; **5:** 359–66.

80. Calle EE, Miracle-McMahill HL, Thun MJ, Heath CW, Estrogen replacement therapy and risk of fatal colon cancer in a prospective cohort of postmenopausal women. *J Natl Cancer Inst* 1995; **87:** 517–23.

81. Slattery ML, Anderson K, Samowitz W et al, Hormone replacement therapy and improved survival among postmenopausal women diagnosed with colon cancer (USA). *Cancer Causes Contr* 1999; **10:** 467–73.

82. Prihartono N, Palmer JR, Louik C et al, A case–control study of use of postmenopausal female hormone supplements in relation to the risk of large bowel cancer. *Cancer Epidemiol Biomark Prev* 2000; **9:** 443–7.

83. Slattery ML, Potter JD, Curtin K et al, Estrogens reduce and withdrawal of estrogens increase risk of microsatellite instability-positive colon cancer. *Cancer Res* 2001; **61:** 126–30.

84. Hebert-Croteau N, A meta-analysis of hormone replacement therapy and colon cancer in women. *Cancer Epidemiol Biomark Prev* 1998; **7:** 653–9.

85. Beral V, Banks E, Reeves G, Appleby P, Use of HRT and the subsequent risk of cancer. *J Epidemiol Biostat* 1999; **4:** 191–215.

86. Langman MJS, Boyle P, Chemoprevention of colorectal cancer. *Gut* 1998; **43:** 578–85.

87. Pelag I, Maibach HT, Brown SH, Wilcox CM, Aspirin and non-steroidal anti-inflammatory drug use and the risk of subsequent colorectal cancer. *Arch Intern Med* 1994; **154:** 394–9.

88. Rosenberg L, Palmer JR, Zauber AG et al, A hypothesis: non-steroidal anti-inflammatory drugs reduce the incidence of large bowel cancer. *J Natl Cancer Inst* 1991; **83:** 355–8.

89. Kune GA, Kune S, Watson JF, Colorectal cancer risk, chronic illnesses, operations and medications: case control results from the Melbourne Colorectal Cancer Study. *Cancer Res* 1988; **48:** 4399–404.

90. Giovannucci E, Rimm EB, Stampfer MJ et al, Aspirin use and the risk of colorectal cancer and adenoma in male health professionals. *Ann Intern Med* 1994; **121:** 241–6.

91. Logan RF, Little J, Hawtin PG, Hardcastle JD, Effect of aspirin and non-steroidal anti-inflammatory drugs on colorectal adenomas: case control study of subjects participating in the Nottingham faecal occult blood screening programme. *BMJ* 1993; **307:** 285–9.

92. Narisawa T, Sato M, Tani M, Takahashi I, Inhibition of development of methylnitrosourea induced colonic tumours by peroral administration of indomethacin. *Jpn J Cancer Res* 1982; **73:** 377–81.

93. Reddy BS, Rao CV, Rivenson A, Kelloff G, Inhibitory effect of aspirin on azoxymethane-induced colorectal carcinogenesis in F344 rats. *Carcinogenesis* 1993; **14:** 1493–7.

94. Skinner SA, Penny AG, O'Brien PE, Sulindac inhibits the rate of growth and appearance of colon tumours in rats. *Arch Surg* 1991; **126:** 1094–6.

95. Labayle D, Fischer D, Vielh P et al, Sulindac causes regression of rectal polyps in familial adenomatous polyposis. *Gastroenterology* 1991; **101:** 307–11.

96. Giardiello FM, Hamilton SR, Krush AJ et al, Treatment of colonic and rectal adenomas with sulindac in familial adenomatous polyposis. *N Engl J Med* 1993; **328:** 1313–16.

97. Lala PK, Parhar RS, Singh P, Indomethacin therapy abrogates the prostaglandin mediated suppression of natural killer activity in tumorbearing mice and prevents tumor metastasis. *Cell Immunol* 1986; **99:** 108–18.

98. Narisawa T, Takahashi M, Masuda T et al, Prevention of peritoneal carcinomatosis recurrence with a prostaglandin synthesis inhibitor, indomethacin. *Gan To Kagaku Ryoho* 1987; **14:** 2496–501.

99. Schultz RM, Altorn MG, Potentiation of non-specific immunotherapy of experimental lung metastases by indomethacin. *J Immunopharmacol* 1983; **5:** 277–80.

100. Weppelmann B, Monkemeier D, The influence of prostaglandin antagonists on radiation therapy of carcinoma of the cervix. *Gynecol Oncol* 1984; **17:** 196–9.

101. Farmer KC, Goulston K, Macrae F, Aspirin and non-steroidal anti-inflammatory drugs in the chemoprevention of colorectal cancer. *Med J Austr* 1993; **159:** 649–50.

102. Gann PH, Manson J, Glynn RJ et al, Low-dose aspirin and incidence of colorectal tumours in a randomised trial. *J Natl Cancer Inst* 1993; **85:** 1220–4.

103. Langman MJS, Weil J, Wainwright P et al, Risks of bleeding peptic ulcer associated with individual non-steroidal anti-inflammatory drugs. *Lancet* 1994; **343:** 1075–8.

104. Giovannucci E, Egan KM, Hunter DJ et al, Aspirin and the risk of colorectal cancer in women. *N Engl J Med* 1995; **333:** 609–14.

105. Sporn M, Chemoprevention of cancer. *Lancet* 1993; **342:** 1211–13.

106. Morson BC, *Gastrointestinal Pathology.* Oxford: Blackwell Scientific, 1979.

107. Mandel JS, Bond JH, Church TR et al, Reducing mortality from colorectal cancer by screening for fecal occult blood. *N Engl J Med* 1993; **328:** 1365–71.

108. Selby JV, Friedman GD, Quesenberry CP, Weiss NS, Effect of fecal occult blood testing on mortality from colorectal cancer: a case–control study. *Ann Intern Med* 1993; **118:** 1294–7.

109. Wahrendorf J, Robra BP, Wiebelt H et al, Effectiveness of colorectal cancer screening: a population-based case–control study in Saarland, Germany. *Eur J Cancer Prev* 1993; **1:** 221–7.

110. Winawer SJ, Flehinger BJ, Schottenfeld D, Miller DG, Screening for colorectal cancer by screening with fecal occult blood testing and sigmoidoscopy. *J Natl Cancer Inst* 1993; **85:** 1311–18.

111. Hardcastle JD, Chamberlain JO, Robinson MHE et al, Randomised controlled trial of faecal-occult-blood screening for colorectal cancer. *Lancet* 1996; **348:** 1472–7.

112. Kronberg O, Fenger C, Olsen J, Jorgensen OD, Sondergaard O, Randomised study of screening for colorectal cancer with faecal-occult-blood test. *Lancet* 1996; **348:** 1467–71.

113. Hardcastle JD, Screening for colorectal cancer. *Lancet* 1997; **349:** 358.

114. Rozen P, Ron E, Fireman Z et al, The relative value of fecal occult blood tests and flexible sigmoidoscopy in screening for large bowel neoplasia. *Cancer* 1987; **60:** 2553–8.

115. Allison J, Feldman R, Tekawa I, Hemocult screening in detecting colorectal neoplasm. *Ann Intern Med* 1990; **112:** 328–33.

116. Mandel JS, Church TR, Bond JH et al, The effect of fecal occult-blood screening on the incidence of colorectal cancer. *N Engl J Med* 2000; **343:** 1603–7.

117. Gilbertson VA, Nelms JM, The prevention of invasive cancer of the rectum. *Cancer* 1978; **41:** 1137–9.

118. Selby JV, Friedman GD, Quesenberry CP et al, A case–control study of screening sigmoidoscopy and mortality from colorectal cancer. *N Engl J Med* 1992; **26:** 653–7.

119. Newcomb PA, Norfleet RG, Storer BE, Surawicz TS, Marcus PM, Screening sigmoidoscopy and colorectal cancer mortality. *J Natl Cancer Inst* 1992; **84:** 1572–5.

120. Atkin WS, Morson BC, Cuzick J, Long-term risk of colorectal cancer after excision of rectosigmoid adenomas. *N Engl J Med* 1992; **326:** 658–62.

121. Greenberg R, Baron J, Prospects for preventing colorectal cancer death. *J Natl Cancer Inst* 1993; **85:** 1182–4.

122. Boyle P, Progress in preventing death from colorectal cancer (Editorial). *Br J Cancer* 1995; **72:** 528–30.

123. Mandel J, Colon and rectal cancer. In: *Cancer Screening.*

(Reintgen DS, Clark RA, eds). St Louis, MO: Mosby, 1996: 55–96.

124. Potter JD, Slattery ML, Bostwick RM, Gapstur SM, Colon cancer: a review of the epidemiology. *Epidemiol Rev* 1993; **15:** 499–545.

125. McKeown-Eyssen G, Epidemiology of colorectal cancer revisited: Are serum triglycerides and/or plasma glucose associated with risk. *Cancer Epidemiol Biomark Prev* 1994; **3:** 687–95.

Part 2

Prevention and Screening

3

Hemoccult as an approach to colorectal cancer screening

Jean Faivre, Anne-Marie Benhamiche

INTRODUCTION

The World Health Organization (WHO)[1] and the Council of Europe[2] have both published principles regarding screening as a tool for cancer prevention and early detection. Screening is the testing of healthy people for diseases that have so far not given rise to symptoms. Colorectal cancer fulfils the conditions that have been defined for mass screening: it is a major cause of morbidity and mortality in industrialized countries, with an estimated number of 198 000 new cases reported in the 15 member states of the European Union in 1995.[3] Despite advances in diagnostic techniques and treatment, the 5-year survival rates remain poor.[4] However, colorectal cancer can be cured if detected at an early age, and in certain cases can be prevented by the removal of adenomas. Considerable research efforts have been launched over the last 15 years to evaluate the ability of screening tests to decrease colorectal cancer mortality and incidence. Currently, the simplest screening method for colorectal cancer is periodic stool testing for occult blood. The most extensively evaluated test is the Hemoccult II (Smith Kline Diagnostic, California). The purpose of this chapter is to consider the evidence for screening for colorectal cancer based on published studies.

FAECAL OCCULT BLOOD TESTS

Most available faecal occult blood tests are guaiac-based tests that detect the peroxidase-like activity of haemoglobin. Among these, the only test that has been extensively evaluated is the Hemoccult II test. This test is easy to perform: two slides are prepared from three consecutive stool samples. It is also inexpensive and without great inconvenience to the individual. In patients who screen positive, a total colonoscopy must follow. The positivity rate of the Hemoccult test in the initial screen when it is performed without diet restriction and is non-rehydrated is 2%.[5–7] On subsequent screenings, it varies between 1% and 1.5%. The positivity rate is slightly lower with diet restrictions (around 1%), but these may decrease compliance. Positivity is much higher with rehydrated tests (between 6% and 10%).[8,9] Rehydration is not recommended by the manufacturer, and is not used in most screening programmes. It increases sensitivity but decreases specificity, making the predictive accuracy of a positive test very low. The positive predictive value for a positive non-rehydrated test is about 10% for colorectal cancer, and ranges between 30% and 40% for adenomas. The sensitivity of the test is estimated to be around 50% and its specificity to be 98%.[10] More complex faecal occult blood tests, particularly immunochemical tests specific for human haemoglobin, have been developed. Although they are more sensitive, their specificity at a population level is not well established. If the detection of occult blood in the faeces is low enough to induce a positivity rate of the test of over 3%, it will not be suitable for mass screening. Such an elevated rate would induce unnecessary and therefore undesirable colonoscopies, which could cause severe complications for otherwise-healthy participants.

RESULTS OF CASE–CONTROL STUDIES

One possible method for evaluating the efficacy of screening is a case–control approach in areas where screening is already widely carried out. The screening history in subjects who died of a colorectal cancer is compared with those of controls. Six case–control studies have been conducted in order to estimate the efficacy of screening with faecal occult blood tests with regard to colorectal cancer.[11–16] The screening test was the Hemoccult test in five studies and an immunological test in one study. Although some discrepancies can be observed, the studies suggest a 30–40% theoretical reduction in colorectal cancer mortality among those who participate in the screening test (Table 3.1). It must not be forgotten that case–control studies compare participants with non-participants and that they provide an indication of reduction in risk independently of compliance rate. This means that the results are valid for a 100% compliance rate. However, the difficulty of controlling for all relevant confounding factors could still limit the accuracy of these studies.

RESULTS OF CONTROLLED STUDIES

Five trials were undertaken to evaluate the effect of screening on colorectal cancer mortality with the Hemoccult test (Table 3.2). One study was performed on volunteers (the Minnesota study), while the four others were population-based. Four trials were randomized studies (Minnesota, Funen, Nottingham,

and Göteborg). In the fifth study, in Burgundy, small, neighbourhood-sized geographical areas were allocated to either the screening or the control group.

Together with the efficacy of the screening test, compliance is a major determinant in the effectiveness of a screening programme. Compliance was highest in the Minnesota study, which was performed on volunteers. In the annually screened group: 90% completed at least one screening and 75% all the screening rounds.[9] Such results cannot be expected in a general population. Trials in volunteers overestimate the mortality reduction that can be achieved in a general population. In the European population-based studies, compliance with the first screening was 67% in Funen, 66% in Göteborg, and 53% in Nottingham and in Burgundy. The proportion of the population screened at least once was 67%, 68%, 60%, and 69% respectively. In total, 46% completed five screenings in Funen, while 31% did so in Burgundy. In Nottingham, 37% completed all screenings, i.e. three to six according to the period of recruitment. Screening was limited to two rounds in Göteborg. The method of delivery of the screening test affected compliance. The participation rate in the UK and in Nordic countries was achieved by mailing the test with one or two reminders. When mailing the test, compliance rates were much lower in France: between 26% and 34%, according to the screening campaign.[7] Our data indicate that in

		Percentage of subjects screened		
	Ref	Cases	Controls	Odds ratio[a]
California	12	31.5	42.8	0.7 (0.5–0.9)
Saarland	11			
Males		17.8	15.0	1.2 (0.7–0.9)
Females		16.2	29.4	0.5 (0.3–0.8)
Seattle	13	8.3	15.6	0.5 (0.3–0.9)
Japan	14	5.9	12.1	0.4 (0.2–0.9)
Florence	16	22.3	28.5	0.6 (0.4–0.9)
Burgundy	15	49.4	61.1	0.7 (0.5–0.9)

Table 3.1 Results of case–control studies

[a]Range in parentheses.

Table 3.2 Population-based trials of Hemoccult screening for colorectal cancer

	Funen, Denmark	Nottingham, UK	Göteborg, Sweden	Burgundy, France
Study population	61 933	152 850	68 308	91 553
Age (years)	45–74	50–74	60–64	45–74
Screening test	Hemoccult, unhydrated, biennially	Hemoccult, unhydrated, biennially	Hemoccult, unhydrated, 2 rounds	Hemoccult, unhydrated, biennially
Complete screening	67% did at least 1 screen, 46% completed 5 screens	60% did at least 1 screen, 38% completed all (3–6) screens	68% did at least 1 screen, 60% completed the 2 screening rounds	69% did at least 1 screen, 37% completed 5 screens
Positivity rate (1st screen)	1.0%	2.1%	6.3%	2.1%
Positive predictive value for colorectal cancer	12.2%	11.5%	4.7%	11.4%
Proportion of colorectal cancer, TNM stage I	Screen 22% Control 11%	Screen 20% Control 11%	?	Screen 29% Control 21%
Years of trial follow-up	10	Median 7.8	Median 8.3	9
Relative risk (and 95% confidence interval) of colorectal cancer death with screening	0.82 (0.68–0.99)	0.85 (0.74–0.99)	0.88 (0.69–1.12)	0.86 (0.71–1.03)

France, mailing cannot be used alone. Active participation of primary-care physicians is crucial in obtaining a high participation rate. Offering the test during a routine consultation resulted in a participation rate of over 85%. These data suggest that in France and probably in all Latin countries, it is mandatory to have general practitioners participate actively in the screening programmes.

In all trials, it can be seen that screen-detected cancers are picked up at a less advanced stage than in controls. In the European trials, the proportion of TNM stage I cancers was about 40%. The drift toward detecting less advanced stages of the disease is maintained when the test group as a whole is compared with the control group. These data do not represent a sufficient argument in favour of the effectiveness of screening. There are a number of biases. Slowly growing tumours are more likely to be picked up by screening (length bias). Screening may hasten the diagnosis of incurable cancers, giving a longer lifespan to the disease without actually prolonging it (lead-time bias), and subjects who participate in screenings can be at lower risk (selection bias). To exclude these confusion factors, the effectiveness of a screening programme should be evaluated in terms of the number of cancer deaths prevented. Available data provide clear evidence that biennial screening with a Hemoccult test can reduce mortality from colorectal cancer. The Minnesota study reported a 21% reduction (relative risk (RR) 0.79, 95% confidence interval (CI) 0.62–0.97) with an 18-year follow-up.[17] The Funen study reported an 18% reduction (RR 0.82, 95% CI 0.68–0.98)[5] with a 10-year follow-up, the Nottingham study a 15% reduction (RR 0.85, 95% CI 0.74–0.99)[6] with a mean 7.8-year follow-up, and the Burgundy study a 14% reduction (RR 0.86, 95% CI 0.71–1.03) with a 9-year follow-up.[18] A recent meta-analysis of randomized Hemoccult test trials showed a 16% reduction in colorectal cancer mortality.[19]

IMPLEMENTATION OF COLORECTAL CANCER SCREENING

When colorectal cancer screening is undertaken, it should be offered only in organized programmes, with quality insurance at all levels and good information available to participants about benefits and risks. Opportunistic screening activities are not acceptable, since they may not achieve the potential benefits and may cause unnecessary negative side-effects. The reduction of colorectal cancer mortality achieved in trials depends on the screening frequency, the number of screens that each person has, the completeness of the follow-up after a positive test, and the benefit of early treatment. Colorectal cancer screening will be effective only if the results obtained in trials are reproduced in routine health care. This means that performance indicators should be monitored regularly: compliance must be over 50%, the positivity rate of the screening test must be between 1% and 3%, the colonoscopy rate in these subjects must be over 90%, and among explored subjects about 10% must have a cancer and 30–40% an adenoma. This analysis can be more precise if the screening database is linked to cancer registry data. In particular, interval cancers are easily monitored. The running of an organized screening programme requires a computer-generated list of all persons to be targeted by screening, and computerized data on all screening tests and on the assessment of results, final diagnosis, and treatments performed.

CONCLUSIONS

There is unequivocal evidence from case–control studies and controlled studies that repeated faecal occult blood testing with unrehydrated Hemoccult II reduces colorectal cancer mortality. To achieve a significant mortality reduction of at least 15%, initial compliance with the screening test must be over 50%, and participation in the successive screening campaigns (at least every 2 years) must be high, as must compliance with colonoscopy in positive screens. This is why a rigid organization with a call–recall system and a quality assurance evaluation is necessary in order to achieve effectiveness. According to the Consensus Position Statement of the cancer experts of the 15 countries of the European Union, adopted after the Vienna Conference (November 1999), there is now sufficient evidence to recommend the implementation of well-organized population-based faecal occult blood screening with the Hemoccult II repeated at least every 2 years in asymptomatic adults over 50 years of age, with colonoscopy in positive screens as a first step in reducing colorectal cancer mortality.[20] These conclusions may be modified in the future by the evaluation of new faecal occult blood tests or by the use of endoscopy as a screening tool. Whether society can afford screening with Hemoccult II is a political question, but the relatively few flaws in the test should not be a factor in the decision to fund screening campaigns using the Hemoccult II. It is well established that a substantial number of deaths from colorectal cancer can be avoided by screening with this method, and it is the only strategy for which effectiveness has been demonstrated up to now.

REFERENCES

1. Wilson JMG, Jungner G, *Principles and Practice of Screening for Disease*. Geneva: World Health Organization, Public Health Paper 34, 1968.
2. Council of Europe: Committee of Ministers, *On Screening as a Tool of Preventive Medicine*. Strasbourg: Council of Europe, Recommendation R (94) 11, 1994.
3. Ferlay J, Bray F, Sankila R, Parkin DM (eds), *EUCAN – Cancer Incidence, Mortality and Prevalence in the European Union*. Lyon: IARC Cancer Base No. 4, 1999.
4. Berrino F, Sant M, Verdecchia A et al, *Survival of Cancer Patients*

in Europe. The EUROCARE Study. Lyon: IARC Scientific Publication No. 132, 1995.

5. Kronborg O, Fenger C, Olsen J et al, Randomized study of screening for colorectal cancer with faecal-occult-blood test. *Lancet* 1996; **348:** 1467–71.

6. Hardcastle JD, Chamberlain JO, Robinson MHE et al, Randomized controlled trial of faecal-occult-blood screening for colorectal cancer. *Lancet* 1996; **348:** 1472–7.

7. Tazi MA, Faivre J, Dassonville F et al, Participation in faecal occult blood screening for colorectal cancer in a well defined French population: results of five screening rounds from 1988 to 1996. *J Med Screening* 1997; **4:** 147–51.

8. Kewenter J, Brevenge H, Engaras B et al, Results of screening, rescreening, and follow-up in a prospective randomized study for detection of colorectal cancer by faecal occult blood testing. Results of 68,308 subjects. *Scand J Gastroenterol* 1994; **29:** 468–73.

9. Mandel JS, Bond JH, Church TR et al, Reducing mortality from colorectal cancer by screening for faecal occult blood. *N Engl J Med* 1993; **328:** 1365–71.

10. Launoy F, Smith TC, Duffy SW, Bouvier V, Colorectal cancer mass screening: estimation of faecal occult blood test sensitivity taking into account cancer mean sojourn time. *Int J Cancer* 1997; **73:** 220–4.

11. Warhendorf J, Robra BP, Wiebelt H et al, Effectiveness of colorectal cancer screening: results from a population-based case-control study in Saarland, Germany. *Eur J Cancer Prev* 1993; **2:** 221–7.

12. Selby JV, Friedman GD, Quesenberry CP, Weiss NS, Effect of fecal occult blood testing on mortality from colorectal cancer. *Ann Intern Med* 1993; **104:** 1661–8.

13. Lazovich D, Weiss NS, Stevens NG et al, A case–control study to evaluate efficacy of screening for faecal occult blood. *J Med Screening* 1995; **2:** 84–9.

14. Saito H, Soma Y, Koeda J et al, Reduction in risk of mortality from colorectal cancer by fecal occult blood screening with immunochemical hemagglutination test. A case–control study. *Int J Cancer* 1995; **61:** 465–9.

15. Faivre J, Tazi MA, El Mrini T et al, Faecal occult blood screening and reduction of colorectal cancer mortality: a case–control study. *Br J Cancer* 1999; **79:** 680–3.

16. Zappa M, Castiglione G, Grazzini G et al, Effect of faecal occult blood testing on colorectal mortality: result of a population-based case–control study in district of Florence, Italy. *Int J Cancer* 1997; **73:** 208–10

17. Mandel JS, Church TR, Ederer F, Bond JF, Colorectal cancer mortality effectiveness of biennial screening for faecal occult blood. *J Natl Cancer Inst* 1999; **91:** 434–7.

18. Faivre J, Tazi MA, Milan C et al, Controlled trial of faecal occult blood screening for colorectal cancer in Burgundy (France). Results of the first 9 years. *Gastroenterology* 1999; **116:** A400.

19. Towler B, Irwig L, Glasziou P et al, A systematic review of the effects of screening for colorectal cancer using the faecal occult blood test, Hemoccult. *BMJ* 1998; **317:** 559–65.

20. Advisory Committee on Cancer Prevention, Recommendations on cancer screening in the European Union. *Eur J Cancer* 2000; **36:** 1673–8.

4

Screening colonoscopy

Ann G Zauber, Sidney J Winawer

INTRODUCTION

Colorectal cancer is the second leading cause of cancer mortality and the fourth most commonly diagnosed cancer in the USA, where in 2001, we expect that 135 400 men and women will be diagnosed with colorectal cancer and that 56 700 people will die of this disease.[1] We expect approximately 945 000 new cases of colorectal cancer and 492 000 deaths due to colorectal cancer worldwide.[2] Colorectal cancer affects both men and women in approximately equal numbers. It may be possible to dramatically reduce the incidence and mortality of this cancer with the technology now available that can identify and remove precursor adenomatous polyps. Colonoscopy screening has the potential for a larger reduction in colorectal cancer mortality than that achieved by fecal occult blood testing or sigmoidoscopy screening.[3] Recently, colonoscopy complication rates have become substantially reduced,[4] fees for colonoscopy have been lowered, and the procedure has become more widely available in many countries. Cost analyses based on estimated effects suggest that screening colonoscopy every 10 years is as cost-effective as standard screening.[5] Currently, we have evidence from observational studies that colonoscopic polypectomy can reduce colorectal cancer incidence. Stronger evidence for this preventative strategy will require a randomized controlled trial to assess whether a colonoscopy screening is efficacious and what is the magnitude and duration of the reduction in colorectal cancer incidence and mortality with the intervention of colonoscopy screening. The evidence for the prevention of colorectal cancer by colonoscopy is presented in this chapter.

RATIONALE FOR COLORECTAL CANCER SCREENING

Population screening for disease is recommended only if the disease is a public health burden, the natural history of the disease is known, the preclinical phase of the disease can be detected, intervention in the preclinical phase is effective, and the screening modalities are acceptable to those at risk.[6] Colonoscopy screening to prevent colorectal cancer satisfies all these conditions. The rationale and issues related to this approach are given below for colorectal cancer.

ADENOMA–ADENOCARCINOMA SEQUENCE

It is now generally accepted that colorectal cancer largely arises from a precursor lesion, the adenomatous polyp. The concept of progression from adenoma to adenocarcinoma, the adenoma–carcinoma sequence, is based on evidence from autopsy, clinical, epidemiological, and molecular genetic studies.[7,8] The prevalence of adenomas in persons aged 55 years or over in Western countries is 30–40%, based on autopsy studies.[9] Because of their malignant potential, polyps are currently removed when detected, and progression to cancer cannot be observed. In a retrospective cohort of 226 patients from the Mayo Clinic who were diagnosed with a polyp greater than or equal to 1 cm on barium enema in the precolonoscopy era, 3% of polyps enlarged and the accumulated risk of colorectal cancer in 5, 10, and 20 years was 4%, 14%, and 35%, respectively. The incidence of colorectal cancer in these patients was four times that of the general population.[10,11]

CURRENT CHOICES FOR COLORECTAL CANCER SCREENING TESTS

The long progression from adenoma to adenocarcinoma of 10–20 years on average provides a long window of opportunity for intervention.[4] The different screening tests for prevention of colorectal cancer address different aspects of this long process. For example, a fecal occult blood test is unlikely to detect a small polyp with a low propensity to bleed. However, a fecal occult blood test is more likely to detect larger polyps, early cancers, and late-stage cancers with a high propensity to bleed. Flexible sigmoidoscopy can detect polyps of all sizes, as well as colorectal cancer provided the neoplasm is within the reach of the flexible sigmoidoscope. Colonoscopy can detect polyps and neoplasia of all sizes in all regions, but requires a more extensive preparation than that for flexible sigmoidoscopy.

Fecal occult blood test (FOBT)

Recent evidence from randomized controlled trials has demonstrated that colorectal cancer mortality can be reduced by 15–33% by screening for stool blood.[12–15] The reduction is primarily due to the detection of early-stage cancer.[4] Although these results are promising, there are concerns about the sensitivity for the detection of cancer by the commonly used stool blood tests.[16,17] Several major organizations have recommended that the stool blood test be offered annually to men and women over age 50 years, by itself or in conjunction with flexible sigmoidoscopy every 5 years.[4,18,19]

Flexible sigmoidoscopy

Retrospective studies have suggested that screening sigmoidoscopy can reduce rectosigmoid colorectal cancer mortality by 60% and overall colorectal cancer mortality by at least 30%.[20,21] The basis for this benefit is not completely clear, but is probably related to the detection of early-stage cancer and the finding and removal of precancerous adenomatous polyps. The American Cancer Society (ACS) guidelines include flexible sigmoidoscopy alone as an acceptable option for colorectal cancer screening in average-risk populations but state their preference is to combine flexible sigmoidoscopy every 5 years with an annual fecal occult blood test. The ACS position is that either an annual fecal occult blood test or flexible sigmoidoscopy every 5 years is preferable to no screening at all, but the combination of the two tests is preferred compared with either test alone.[19]

Double-contrast barium enema

A double-contrast barium enema every 5 years is included as one of five options for colorectal cancer screening in average-risk populations by the most recent screening guidelines of the ACS and others.[4,19] However double-contrast barium enema failed to detect 52% of adenomas over 1 cm in size detected by colonoscopy in a blinded comparison.[22]

Screening colonoscopy

The goal of colorectal cancer screening is to detect early-stage curable cancers and premalignant adenomatous polyps. Stool blood testing is a poor test for polyp detection, and sigmoidoscopy will detect polyps only in the distal portion of the bowel. Flexible sigmoidoscopy fails to identify up to 50% of people with proximal adenomas.[23–28] Recently, there has been a proximal shift of colorectal neoplasia.[29] African-Americans and older women are more likely to have proximal neoplasia, which would not be detected by flexible sigmoidoscopy.[30] There is also much interest in the possibility of non-polypoid or flat lesions giving rise to colorectal cancer.[31,32] Endoscopy is required to detect and remove such lesions.

The National Polyp Study demonstrated prospectively a dramatic reduction (76–90%) in expected colorectal incidence following colonoscopic polypectomy in patients with newly diagnosed adenomas.[3] These results suggest that colonoscopy screening could provide a large reduction in colorectal cancer incidence and mortality, by finding and removing adenomas in the entire colon. These findings suggest that for colorectal cancer screening we can and should emphasize detection and removal of the precursor lesion before a cancer has developed.[33] The ACS and the Agency for Health Care Policy Research/American Gastroenterological Association Guidelines include screening colonoscopy as an option for the average-risk population. However, screening colonoscopy is the preferred screening option of the American College of Gastroenterology and others.[34–36]

EVIDENCE FOR SCREENING COLONOSCOPY

If the adenoma–carcinoma sequence is valid, removal of adenomas should interrupt this sequence, and this should in turn result in a decreased incidence of colorectal cancer and ultimately a decreased mortality. The effectiveness of colonoscopic polypectomy was demonstrated by several observational studies. The National Polyp Study prospectively followed 1418 patients who had a complete colonoscopy during which one or more newly diagnosed colorectal adenomas were removed.[3] The observed incidence rate of colorectal cancer in the National Polyp Study cohort following polypectomy was compared with the expected rates, which were based on three reference groups, including one general population registry and two cohorts in which colonic polyps were not removed. Five colorectal cancers were detected at surveillance, in comparison with an expected number of 21 based on general population (SEER) rates and 43–48 expected in a polyp-bearing population with no further intervention. These comparisons of observed to expected corresponded to a reduction in colorectal cancer incidence of 76–90% with colonoscopic polypectomy (Figure 4.1). A retrospective cohort study in Italy also demonstrated a 66% reduction in colorectal cancer incidence relative to the general population following colonoscopic polypectomy.[37,38] This study demonstrated the effectiveness of colonoscopic polypectomy in standard clinical practice to reduce colorectal cancer incidence. In a case–control study from Kaiser Permanente, screening with rigid sigmoidoscopy was associated with a 60% reduction in

mortality of colorectal cancer within the reach of the scope.[20] The reduction in risk was observed even for screening intervals up to 10 years. Similar results were reported in another sigmoidoscopy case–control study.[21] A large US Veterans Affairs case–control study of endoscopy also showed a reduction in colorectal cancer incidence.[39] A prospective study of US male health professionals has also shown that screening endoscopy (primarily flexible sigmoidoscopy) is associated with a lower risk for all colorectal cancer (42% reduction) and for distal colon or rectal cancer (60% reduction).[40] Atkin et al[41] reported a 60% reduction in rectal cancer in men following adenoma removal in the St Mark's cohort. Women in this cohort had an excess risk of rectal cancer because of incomplete removal of rectal adenomas.

The feasibility of screening colonoscopy has been demonstrated by Lieberman et al[27] and by Imperiale et al[28] in two special populations. Lieberman et al[27] reported on the clinical findings of screening colonoscopy in 3196 patients from 13 Veterans Affairs Medical Centers in the USA. At the initial screening colonoscopy, one or more neoplastic lesions were detected in 38% of the patients, and an adenoma with a diameter of 10 mm or more or with villous features was detected in 8% of patients. Lieberman et al[27] also reported that 52% of those

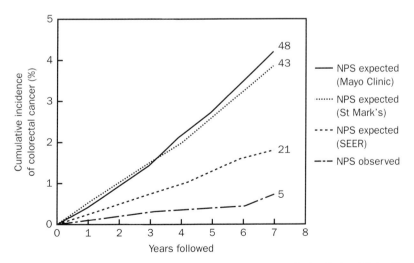

Figure 4.1 The observed and expected cumulative incidence of colorectal cancer in the National Polyp Study (NPS) is presented, with the scale given on the left vertical axis. The number of colorectal cancers expected and observed are given on the curves. The expected rates are based on a comparison with the general population (SEER) and with two historical cohorts in which patients with polyps were ascertained but not removed and followed over time for the occurrence of colorectal cancer. (Adapted from Winawer et al, *N Engl J Med* 1993; 329: 177–81[3], with permission. © 1993 Massachusetts Medical Society. All rights reserved.)

patients with advanced neoplasia in the right colon had no distal lesions. Imperiale et al[28] reported the clinical findings for screening colonoscopy on 1994 volunteers drawn from employees, retirees, and family members of employees of Eli Lilly. They also concluded that about half the cases of advanced proximal neoplasia would be missed if colonoscopy were confined to those with distal polyps. Rex et al[42] reported the findings from screening colonoscopy on 210 asymptomatic average-risk people aged 50–75 years with a negative fecal occult blood test. Fifty-three (25%) of the subjects had adenomas and two had cancers. Rogge et al[24] have shown that screening colonoscopy can be accomplished at a low cost and in large numbers in a corporate program, but have not evaluated the acceptability and compliance of this procedure in the general population. They found adenomas in 34% of 639 patients, and 6 carcinomas.[24]

SCREENING INTERVALS FOR COLONOSCOPY

Current screening guidelines state that colonoscopy screening should begin at age 50 years in the average-risk population and should be repeated every 10 years for those with negative findings.[4,19,34] The choice of a 10-year repeat screening is based (1) on the long natural history of the adenoma–adenocarcinoma sequence[4] and (2) on the Kaiser Permanente study by Selby et al[20] that showed screening with rigid proctoscopy provided protection from colorectal cancer death at a site within reach of the rigid scope for up to 10 years. There is great interest in the possibility of a once-in-a-lifetime screening colonoscopy, but this option should be tested in a randomized controlled trial. Atkin et al[43,44] are currently conducting a randomized controlled trial of once-in-a-lifetime screening flexible sigmoidoscopy in the UK for reduction of colorectal cancer mortality. We know that endoscopy examination can miss detecting adenomas, particularly small adenomas. Hixson et al[45] and Rex et al[46] showed in tandem colonoscopy studies that few large adenomas are missed by colonoscopy but that 20–25% of smaller adenomas (those less than 1 cm) are missed.

SURVEILLANCE FOLLOWING COLONOSCOPY SCREENING

The National Polyp Study was designed to assess the timing of surveillance intervals following initial polypectomy of an adenomatous polyp. Patients were randomized to surveillance colonoscopy at 1 and 3 years after initial colonoscopy or to surveillance colonoscopy after 3 years. The percentage of patients with advanced adenomas (an adenoma of size larger than 1 cm or with high-grade dysplasia or a malignant polyp) was 3.3% whether the patient had surveillance colonoscopy at 1 and 3 years or only at 3 years.[47] These findings form the basis for the suggested surveillance interval of 3 years after the initial colonoscopy for those with an initial colonoscopy. Further analysis of the National Polyp Study data suggests that the adenoma patient at baseline can be classified on the basis of the initial examination findings as low- or high-risk for subsequent advanced adenomas. The low-risk adenoma patients could be encouraged to extend the surveillance interval to 6 or more years.[47,48] The most recent ACS guidelines have adopted recommendations for different surveillance intervals depending on baseline risk factors.[19] Rex et al[49] performed surveillance colonoscopy 5 years after a normal colonoscopy in a cohort of 154 patients. Only one patient had a polyp greater than 1 cm on follow-up. These findings suggest that the surveillance interval following a normal colonoscopy could be extended beyond 5 years, and provide evidence for the current guidelines suggesting 10-year surveillance for those with a normal colonoscopy.

ACCEPTABILITY OF SCREENING COLONOSCOPY IN THE GENERAL POPULATION

Patient compliance with screening colonoscopy is an important consideration, particularly for an invasive test such as colonoscopy. Compliance should be enhanced when the general population understands that screening colonoscopy can prevent colorectal cancer by removing polyps before the development of cancer. Elwood et al[50] found that colonoscopy was as acceptable to subjects, more comfortable, less embarrassing and only slightly more costly compared to sigmoidoscopy. Atkin et al[43] reported the results of their pilot study for a once-offered flexible sigmoidoscopy trial in the UK in asymptomatic people. They used a two-step recruitment design, and found that 75% of those who agreed to participate in the study and were assigned to screening flexible sigmoidoscopy actually had the flexible sigmoidoscopy examination. They also found that 60% of those asked did join the randomized trial. These levels of participation are higher than that obtained by Schroy et al,[51] who offered free sigmoidoscopy screening to employees of the city of Boston. Of those who returned a postcard expressing interest, 35%

were screened with flexible sigmoidoscopy. Vernon[52] reviewed participation in colorectal cancer screening and concluded that at present it is not known whether or not a high percentage of persons would undergo screening colonoscopy if offered the opportunity. Currently, only 21% of the US population over age 50 years reported having had a fecal occult blood test in the past year and 34% had had a flexible sigmoidoscopy within the previous 5 years as reported by the Behaviorial Risk Factor Surveillance System (BRFSS) for 1999. Consequently, considerably less than 50% of average-risk Americans aged 50 years or more have had an appropriate colorectal cancer screening test.[53]

COST–EFFECTIVENESS OF SCREENING COLONOSCOPY

Screening colonoscopy is attractive on a cost–effectiveness basis. Analyses suggest that screening colonoscopy is as cost-effective as that of annual screening mammography if colonoscopy is only performed every 10 years.[5,54–56] These analyses are based on a number of assumptions, including the long natural history of the adenoma–adenocarcinoma sequence, with an average time of progression of approximately 10 years. Marshall et al[57] suggested that the cost of colonoscopic surveillance has a marked effect on the costs for any screening strategy that evaluates the positive screening test with a subsequent colonoscopy examination. Consequently, extending the colonoscopy surveillance intervals for those at lower risk could have dramatic savings in health dollars.

ALTERNATIVES TO COLONOSCOPY SCREENING

Other alternatives to screening colonoscopy are annual stool blood testing and screening sigmoidoscopy with or without stool blood testing. The reduction in colorectal cancer mortality with stool blood testing is a result primarily of cancer detection. Colonoscopy screening would result in cancer prevention primarily by adenoma detection and removal. Flexible sigmoidoscopy is being evaluated in the USA in the multicenter NCI-supported PLCO (prostate, lung, colorectal, ovary) trial[58] and in the UK in a large multicenter trial.[43,44] The UK investigators have estimated a possible colorectal mortality reduction as high as 45% by sigmoidoscopy, which is not as high as that anticipated for colonoscopy

screening.[44] The results from these trials will not be available until at least the year 2008. Reported observations in the USA indicate that sigmoidoscopy will fail to identify a significant proportion of people with proximal neoplasia.[27,28]

New colorectal cancer screening tests are under development, but will need to be evaluated thoroughly before being used in clinical practice for the average-risk population. Alternatives to screening colonoscopy include targeting genetically susceptible individuals for colonoscopy. However, identification of inherited genetic syndromes is possible in only 5–6% of individuals at risk for colorectal cancer (familial adenomatous polyposis (FAP) and known hereditary non-polyposis colorectal cancer (HNPCC)).[59] Inherited *APC* mutations reported in Ashkenazi Jews in the general population require further study.[60] Virtual colonoscopy[61,62] has been recently proposed as another alternative screening option, but must be evaluated for its efficacy and effectiveness before being used as a screening tool.[63] The possibility of using a multitarget assay system to detect altered human DNA in stool has been proposed by Ahlquist et al,[64] and further testing of this procedure is currently under study. Dong et al[65] have suggested that a small panel of genetic markers in stool might potentially detect as many as 70% of colorectal cancers. However they note that additional work is required to determine the sensitivity and specificity of these markers for colorectal neoplasia in asymptomatic patients.[65,66] A chemopreventative agent, the cyclooxygenase-2 inhibitor drug celecoxib, can reduce the number and size of adenomas in familial adenomatous polyposis.[67] Randomized controlled trials are currently underway to assess how this agent affects colorectal cancer risk in a more general population setting.

CONCLUSIONS

Our present understanding of the adenoma–carcinoma sequence and the currently available clinical tools provide a basis for a powerful approach to the prevention of a major cancer. It is likely that colorectal cancer incidence and mortality can be reduced by detecting and removing the premalignant lesions, adenomatous polyps. There is considerable evidence that the natural history of colorectal cancer as it evolves from the adenomatous polyp is very long. There is also considerable evidence that once the colon is cleared of all neoplastic lesions, most patients do not need intensive follow-up surveillance. In addition, the vast majority of the general population have not accepted current colorectal cancer screening with fecal occult blood tests and flexible sigmoidoscopy, which needs to be performed on a regular basis and has limited effectiveness. Although screening colonoscopy offers the promise of dramatically reducing colorectal cancer incidence, there are major challenges to the wide implementation of this approach, including public acceptance and available medical resources.

ACKNOWLEDGEMENT

This work was supported by the Tavel-Reznick Fund.

REFERENCES

1. Greenlee RT, Hill-Harmon MB, Thun M, *Cancer statistics, 2001. CA Cancer J Clin* 2001; **51:** 15–36.
2. Ferlay J, Bray F, Pisani P, Parkin DM, *Globocan 2000: Cancer Incidence, Mortality and Prevalence Worldwide. Version 1.0. IARC Cancer Base No. 5.* Lyon: IARC Press, 2001/WHO Globocan.
3. Winawer SJ, Zauber AG, Ho MN et al, Prevention of colorectal cancer by colonoscopic polypectomy. *N Engl J Med* 1993; **329:** 1977–81.
4. Winawer SJ, Fletcher R, Miller L et al, Colorectal cancer screening: clinical guidelines and rationale. *Gastroenterology* 1997; **112:** 594–642.
5. Wagner JL, Tunis S, Brown M et al, The cost–effectiveness of colorectal cancer screening in average risk adults. In: *Prevention and Early Detection of Colorectal Cancer* (G Young, P Rozen, B Levin, eds). Philadelphia: WB Saunders, 1996: 321–56.
6. Shapiro S, Goals of screening. *Cancer* 1992; **70:** 1252–8.
7. Morson B, Genesis of colorectal cancer. In: *Clinics in Gastroenterology* (Sherlock P, Zamcheck N, eds). Philadelphia: WB Saunders, 1976: 505–25.
8. Vogelstein B, Fearon E, Hamilton S et al, Genetic alterations during colorectal tumor development. *N Engl J Med* 1988; **319:** 525–32.
9. Eide TJ, Stalsberg H, Polyps of the large intestine in Northern Norway. *Cancer* 1978; **42:** 2839–48.
10. Stryker SJ, Wolff BG, Culp CE et al, Natural history of untreated colonic polyps. *Gastroenterology* 1987; **93:** 1009–13.
11. Otchy D, Ransohoff D, Wolff B et al, Metachronous colon cancer in persons who have had a large adenomatous polyp. *Am J Gastroenterol* 1996; **91:** 448–54.
12. Mandel JS, Bond JH, Church TR, Reducing mortality from colorectal cancer by screening for fecal occult blood. *N Engl J Med* 1993; **328:** 1365–71.
13. Mandel JS, Church TR, Ederer F et al, Colorectal cancer mortality: the effectiveness of biennial screening for fecal occult blood. *J Natl Cancer Inst* 1999; **91:** 434–7.
14. Hardcastle JD, Chamberlain J, Robinson M et al, Randomized controlled trial of faecal-occult blood screening for colorectal cancer. *Lancet* 1996; **348:** 1472–7.
15. Kronborg O, Fenger C, Olsen J et al, Randomised study of screening for colorectal cancer with faecal-occult blood test. *Lancet* 1996; **348:** 1467–71.
16. Allison JE, Teckawa IS, Ranson LJ, Adrain AL, A comparison of fecal occult-blood tests for colorectal-cancer screening. *N Engl J Med* 1996; **334:** 155–9.
17. Ransohoff D, Lang C, Suggested technique for fecal occult blood testing and interpretation in colorectal cancer screening. Clinical guideline: Part 1. *Ann Intern Med* 1997; **126:** 808–22.
18. US Preventive Services Task Force, *Guide to Clinical Preventive Services.* Alexandria, VA: International Medical Publishing, 1996.
19. Smith RA, von Eschenbach AC, Wender R et al, American Cancer Society Guidelines for the Early Detection of Cancer: update of early detection guidelines for prostate, colorectal, and endometrial cancers. *CA Cancer J Clin* 2001; **51:** 38–75.
20. Selby JV, Friedman GD, Quesenberry PJ, Weiss NS, A case–control study of screening sigmoidoscopy and mortality from colorectal cancer. *N Engl J Med* 1992; **326:** 653–7.
21. Newcomb PA, Norfleet RG, Storer BE et al, Screening sigmoidoscopy and colorectal cancer mortality. *J Natl Cancer Inst* 1992; **84:** 1572–5.
22. Winawer SJ, Stewart ET, Zauber AG et al, A comparison of colonoscopy and double-contrast barium enema for surveillance after polypectomy. National Polyp Study Work Group. *N Engl J Med* 2000; **342:** 1766–72.
23. Lieberman D, Smith F, Screening for colon malignancy with colonoscopy. *Am J Gastroenterol* 1991; **86:** 946–51.
24. Rogge JD, Elmore MF, Mahoney SJ et al, Low-cost, office-based, screening colonoscopy. *Am J Gastroenterol* 1994; **89:** 1775–80.
25. Foutch PG, Mai H, Parky K et al, Flexible sigmoidoscopy may be ineffective for secondary prevention of colorectal cancer in asymptomatic average-risk men. *Dig Dis Sci* 1991; **36:** 924–8.
26. Zarchy TM, Ershoff D, Do characteristics of adenomas on flexible sigmoidoscopy predict advanced lesions on baseline colonoscopy? *Gastroenterology* 1994; **106:** 1501–4.
27. Lieberman DA, Weiss DG, Bond JH et al, Use of colonoscopy to screen asymptomatic adults for colorectal cancer. *N Engl J Med* 2000; **343:** 162–8.
28. Imperiale TF, Wagner DR, Lin CY et al, Risk of advanced proximal neoplasms in asymptomatic adults according to the distal colorectal findings. *N Engl J Med* 2000; **343:** 169–74.
29. Devesa SS, Chow WH, Variation in colorectal cancer incidence in the United States by subsite of origin. *Cancer* 1993; **71:** 3819–26.
30. Rex DK, Khan AM, Shah P et al, Screening colonoscopy in asymptomatic average-risk African Americans. *Gastrointest Endosc* 2000; **51:** 524–7.
31. Kudo S, Endoscopic mucosal resection of flat and depressed types of early colorectal cancer. *Endoscopy* 1993; **25:** 455–61.
32. Rembacken BJ, Fujii T, Cairns A et al, Flat and depressed colonic neoplasms: a prospective study of 1000 colonoscopies in the UK. *Lancet* 2000; **355:** 1211–14.
33. Atkin WS, Whynes DK, Improving the cost–effectiveness of colorectal cancer screening. *J Natl Cancer Inst* 2000; **92:** 513–14.
34. Rex DK, Johnson DA, Lieberman DA et al, Colorectal Cancer Prevention 2000: Screening Recommendations of the American College of Gastroenterology. *Am J Gastroenterol* 2000; **95:** 868–77.
35. Rex DK, Sigmoidoscopy or colonoscopy: which way are we headed? *Am J Gastroenterol* 2000; **95:** 1116–18.
36. Lieberman D, Colonoscopy as a mass screening tool. *Eur J Gastroenterol Hepatol* 1998; **10:** 225–9.
37. Citarda F, Tomaselli G, Capocaccia R et al, The Italian Multicentre Study Group. Efficacy in standard clinical practice of colonoscopic polypectomy in reducing colorectal cancer incidence. *Gut* 2001; **48:** 812–15.
38. Winawer SJ, Zauber AG, Colonoscopic polypectomy and the incidence of colorectal cancer. *Gut* 2001; **48:** 753–6.
39. Muller AD, Sonnenberg A, Prevention of colorectal cancer by flexible endoscopy and polypectomy. *Ann Intern Med* 1995; **123:** 904–10.

40. Kavanagh AM, Giovannucci E, Fuchs CS, Colditz GA, Screening endoscopy and risk of colorectal cancer in United States men. *Cancer Causes Control* 1998; **9:** 455–61.

41. Atkin WS, Morson BC, Cuzick J, Long-term risk of colorectal cancer after excision of rectosigmoid adenomas. *N Engl J Med* 1992: **326:** 658–62.

42. Rex DK, Lehman GA, Hawes RH et al, Screening colonoscopy in asymptomatic average-risk persons with negative fecal occult blood tests. *Gastroenterology* 1991; **100:** 64–7.

43. Atkin WS, Hart A, Edwards R et al, Uptake, yield of neoplasia and adverse effects of flexible sigmoidoscopy screening. *Gut* 1998; **42:** 229–31.

44. Atkin SW, Cuzick J, Northover JMA, Whynes DK. Prevention of colorectal cancer by once-only sigmoidoscopy. *Lancet* 1993; **341:** 736–40.

45. Hixson LJ, Fennerty MB, Sampliner RE et al, Prospective study of the frequency and size distribution of polyps missed by colonoscopy. *J Natl Cancer Inst* 1990; **82:** 1769–72.

46. Rex DK, Cutler CS, Lemmel GT et al, Colonoscopic miss rate of adenomas determined by back-to-back colonoscopies. *Gastroenterology* 1997; **112:** 24–8.

47. Winawer SJ, Zauber AG, O'Brien MJ et al, Randomized comparison of surveillance intervals after colonoscopic removal of newly diagnosed adenomatous polyps. *N Engl J Med* 1993; **328:** 901–6.

48. Zauber AG, Winawer SJ, Bond J et al, Can surveillance intervals be lengthened following colonoscopic polypectomy? *Gastroenterology* 1997; **112:** A50.

49. Rex DK, Cummings OW, Helper DJ et al, 5-year incidence of adenomas after negative colonoscopy in asymptomatic average-risk persons. *Gastroenterology* 1996; **111:** 1178–81.

50. Elwood J, Ali G, Schlup M et al, Flexible sigmoidoscopy or colonoscopy for colorectal screening: a randomized trial of performance and acceptability. *Cancer Detect Prev* 1995; **19:** 337–47.

51. Schroy P 3, Wilson S, Afshal N, Feasibility of high-volume screening sigmoidoscopy using a flexible fiberoptic endoscope and a disposable sheath system. *Am J Gastroenterol* 1996; **91:** 1331–7.

52. Vernon S, Participation in colorectal cancer screening: a review. *J Natl Inst Cancer* 1997; **89:** 1406–22.

53. MMWR, *Trends in screening for colorectal cancer – United States, 1997 and 1999. Morb Mort Weekly Rep* 2001; **50:** 162–6.

54. Lieberman D, Cost–effectiveness of colon cancer screening. *J Gastroenterol* 1991; **86:** 1789–94.

55. Sonnenberg A, Delco F, Inadomi JM, Cost–effectiveness of colonoscopy in screening for colorectal cancer. *Ann Intern Med* 2000; **133:** 573–84.

56. Frazier A, Colditz GA, Fuchs CS, Kuntz KM, Cost–effectiveness of screening colorectal cancer in the general population. *JAMA* 2000; **284:** 1954–61.

57. Marshall JR, Fay D, Lance P, Potential costs of flexible sigmoidoscopy based colorectal cancer screening. *Gastroenterology* 1996; **111:** 1411–17.

58. Gohagan K, Prorok PC, Kramer BS et al, The prostate, lung, colorectal, and ovarian cancer screening trial of the National Cancer Institute. *Cancer* 1995; **75:** 1869–73.

59. Burt RW, Colon cancer screening. *Gastroenterology* 2000; **119:** 837–53.

60. Laken S, Petersen G, Gruber S et al, Familial colorectal cancer in Ashkenazim due to a hypermutable tract in *APC. Nature Genet* 1998; **17:** 79–83.

61. Hara AK, Johnson CD, Reed JE et al, Detection of colorectal polyps by computed tomographic colography: feasibility of a novel technique. *Gastroenterology* 1996; **110:** 284–90.

62. Fenlon HM, Nunes DP, Schroy PC III et al, A comparison of virtual and conventional colonoscopy for the detection of colorectal polyps. *N Engl J Med* 1999; **341:** 1496–503.

63. Bond JH, Virtual colonoscopy – promising, but not ready for widespread use. *N Engl J Med* 1999; **341:** 1540–2.

64. Ahlquist DA, Skoletsky JE, Boynton KA et al, Colorectal cancer screening by detection of altered human DNA in stool: feasibility of a multi-target assay system. *Gastroenterology* 2000; **119:** 1219–27.

65. Dong SM, Traverso G, Johnson C et al, Detecting colorectal cancer in stool with the use of multiple genetic targets. *J Natl Cancer Inst* 2001; **93:** 858–65.

66. Atkin W, Martin JP, Stool DNA-based colorectal cancer detection: finding the needle in the haystack. *J Natl Cancer Inst* 2001; **93:** 798–9.

67. Steinbach G, Lynch PM, Phillips RKS et al, The effect of celecoxib, a cyclooxygenase-2 inhibitor, in familial adenomatous polyposis. *N Engl J Med* 2000; **342:** 1946–52.

5
Chemoprevention of colorectal cancer

Robert Benamouzig

INTRODUCTION

Cancer chemoprevention consists in the use of chemical agents to prevent or inhibit the development of carcinogenesis. This intervention can take place at any level throughout the spectrum of carcinogenesis, from the first molecular abnormalities occurring in morphologically normal colonic epithelial cells to the invasive-carcinoma stage. However, in contrast to chemotherapy, the aim is not to cure an already developed tumour. Chemoprevention can also be used, secondarily, to reduce tumour recurrence or the formation of new tumours in patients already treated for a colorectal cancer. Dietary prevention of cancer is not strictly considered to be chemoprevention – except when it concerns particular, isolated, compounds (vitamins, calcium, specific components of food). The use of this restricted definition allows us to consider chemoprevention agents as pharmaceuticals.

CHEMOPREVENTION: CONCEPT AND METHODS

In primary or secondary prevention, the efficacy and low toxicity of an agent must be demonstrated before it is administered to a large population. At present, there is not enough definite evidence for any agent used for chemoprevention to envisage its systematic use in medical practice. The ongoing assessment of several candidate drugs by double-blind, placebo-controlled, randomized studies will contribute to confirmation of their efficacy.[1] As for any pharmaceutical compound, the toxico-pharmaco-clinical development of chemopreventive agents involves phase I, phase II, and phase III trials. Phase I trials assess safety and pharmacodynamic and pharmacokinetic properties with single-dose and multiple-dose studies for periods of a few days to one year. Phase II trials assess efficacy by double-blinded, randomized studies using intermediate (surrogate) biomarkers correlated with tumour incidence, such as, for example, colonic cell-proliferation assessment. Phase III trials are double-blinded randomized studies assessing clinical efficacy on occurrence or recurrence of tumours.[2]

The usual approach consists in assessing the efficacy of the tested compound in patients with a history of adenomatous polyps who have a high risk of recurrence. The selection of this subgroup of patients at high risk of developing new adenomas permits an evaluation on smaller cohorts than if the population was not selected. Randomization of at least 600 patients is necessary to demonstrate with a good rate of success (80%) a 35% decrease in the development of colorectal adenomas, after a 3-year period. To be able to assess such a population, one must be able to recruit an initial population of about 1500 eligible subjects, considering that about 50% will volunteer. Trials can include patients with familial adenomatous polyposis (FAP), but this could then make it difficult to extrapolate results to the general population.[3] Among the numerous agents tested, we shall only consider compounds used in humans. Data on menopausal hormone replacement therapy will not be presented here, and nor will those on dietary fibre, but see the discussion on these topics in Chapter 2.

ASPIRIN AND OTHER NON-STEROIDAL ANTI-INFLAMMATORY DRUGS

Numerous experimental and epidemiological evidence shows the chemopreventive efficacy of a regular consumption of aspirin and/or non-steroidal anti-inflammatory drugs (NSAIDs) on the occurrence of colorectal cancer (see also Chapter 2).

Preclinical data on animal models

Aspirin, sulindac, piroxicam, indomethacin, ibuprofen,

and ketoprofen inhibit colon tumours induced by azoxymethane (AOM) or other agents in rodents[4] as well as carcinogenesis related to *APC* gene mutations in the Min mouse model.[5] This effect is dose-related and can be observed from the aberrant crypt foci step.[6]

Sulindac, familial adenomatous polyposis, and sporadic polyps

Sulindac, at a dose of 100–400 mg/day, reduces the number and the size of colonic polyps in patients with FAP, who previously had or had not undergone colectomy.[4] The efficacy of sulindac administered rectally has been assessed more recently. An initial treatment of two suppositories of 150 mg delivered per day has a similar efficacy to oral treatment. It is then possible to decrease doses progressively, the minimal effective dose being in the range of 50–100 mg/day.[7] There are few data on sulindac efficacy for longer periods.[8] The effect of sulindac is only temporary, and polyp recurrence is observed a few months after the interruption of treatment[9] but these polyps regress if the treatment is resumed. However, three cases of rectal carcinoma were reported during sulindac treatment.[10,11] These observations were in patients who presented a regression of their polyps – which suggests that this drug could be ineffective when tumour proliferation is too advanced. These cases prompt caution about the relevance of using this drug.

Sulindac efficacy on sporadic polyps seems likely, but should be confirmed because of the contradictory results of the two available studies.[12,13] The occurrence of potentially severe haemorrhagic accidents precludes prophylactic strategies with this compound.[14]

Sulindac sulfone, a metabolite of sulindac that can increase the rate of apoptosis, is under investigation.[15–17]

Epidemiological data

Several case–control and cohort studies have investigated the relation between aspirin or NSAID consumption and colorectal carcinoma or polyps. Several studies have also been conducted in patients with rheumatoid polyarthritis who regularly take NSAIDs and aspirin.

Rheumatoid polyarthritis and colorectal carcinoma

In two Swedish and Finnish trials, conducted on respectively 11 863 and 9469 patients with rheumatoid polyarthritis, 40% and 30% reductions in the risk of colon and rectal carcinoma were noted respectively.[18,19] These data confirm the results of two previous studies conducted in Finland in 46 101 and 1000 patients with rheumatoid polyarthritis.[20,21] A causal relationship between aspirin or NSAID consumption and a reduction in the risk of colorectal carcinoma or polyps remains speculative, and the possibility of bias cannot be excluded.

Case–control studies

Thirteen case–control studies have evaluated the effect of aspirin or NSAIDs on the risk of colorectal carcinoma.[4,22–24] Twelve case–control studies have assessed the effect on the occurrence of colorectal polyps.[4,25,26] Despite methodological limitations, these trials have shown that regular consumption of aspirin and/or NSAIDs is related to a significant reduction in colorectal carcinoma and adenomas. The magnitude of this reduction ranges from 21% to 68% depending on the study, but the median is usually about 40%. Even when aspirin and/or NSAIDs consumption is regular and over a long period, if it is interrupted for more than one year, the risk reduction seems to disappear. This suggests that the effect of aspirin and NSAIDs is only temporary. A preventative effect is not observed with paracetamol. The effect of aspirin and NSAIDs is seen for both colon and rectum, in both men and women, and whether or not there is a familial history of colorectal cancer. It seems to be positively related to the dose, frequency, and duration of consumption. An aspirin consumption above 325 mg/day and/or for more than 5 years could represent the efficacy threshold below which this effect is not observed.

Cohort studies

Six of the seven cohort studies available suggest that regular consumption of aspirin and/or NSAIDs reduces the risk of colorectal cancer.[4,27] Three cohort studies also suggest that regular consumption of aspirin and/or NSAIDs is protective against polyps.[4] There is a 14–18% risk reduction according to the cohort studies. This reduction is positively related to the frequency of aspirin consumption, particularly above 8–16 doses per month. It is also more pronounced when the duration of exposure is greater than 10 years, and is only significant after 20 years in the Nurse's Health Study. Only one study, conducted on 13 897 retired Californians followed from

1981 to 1989, among whom 111 men and 129 women developed colorectal cancer, shows a small increase in the relative risk of colorectal cancer related to daily aspirin consumption. After adjustment for gender, the association was no longer observed in women, but persisted slightly in men. The characteristics of this study – the elevated mean age of the subjects at inclusion (73 years) and a lack of precision concerning adjustments during analysis – make the results difficult to interpret.

Randomized study

Only one randomized trial is available.[28] This study assessed the effect of aspirin at a dose of 325 mg every other day in 22 071 male physicians in the USA. The Physicians' Health Study was primarily designed to assess the effect of aspirin on the risk of coronary artery disease. The incidence of colorectal cancer and polyps did not differ between the treatment and placebo cohorts after 5 years of treatment. In the treatment cohort, the relative risk of cancer was 1.15 and that of colonic polyps or in situ cancer was 0.86. The 12-year follow-up confirmed these results.[29] The absence of a significant effect of aspirin could be explained by a number of factors: the low incidence of cancer observed ($n = 118$), the population not being representative of the general population (indicated by a high degree of physical activity and an abnormally low rate of cardiovascular disease in the placebo cohort), an insufficient period of aspirin use (5 years), and exclusion of regular aspirin users at the beginning of the study.

Finally, most of the case–control and cohort studies, including more than 20 000 cases of colorectal cancer and more than 2000 cases of colorectal polyps, show that aspirin and/or NSAID consumption is associated with a reduction in the incidence of colorectal polyps and cancer. However, the causal nature of this association cannot be positively asserted. Thus aspirin appears to have a preventive effect, but this remains to be proved by randomized prospective studies. With this aim, a study was initiated in France in January 1997, including 300 patients given 160 or 300 mg lysine acetylsalicylate daily over 4 years. Results are expected in 2002–2003.

Other salicylate metabolites

Treatments with salicylate metabolites are associated with a reduction in the incidence of colorectal cancer in patients with widespread inflammatory colitis.[30,31] This protective effect was confirmed for balsalazide in Min mice.[32]

Cyclooxygenase-2 inhibitors

Cyclooxygenase-2 (COX-2) inhibitors reduce cell proliferation, and may induce an increase in apoptosis in a number of cancerous or adenomatous cell lines.[33] Celecoxib induces a 40% reduction in chemoinduced aberrant cryptic foci in rats.[34] It also induces a 90% reduction in chemoinduced tumours in rats[35] and Min mice,[36] as well as in the growth of colon cancer cells implanted in nude mouse.[37] Celecoxib leads to a reduction in the number and total area of polyps in patients with familial polyposis.[38] These promising results led to the setting up of large multicentre intercontinental clinical trials in subjects with a history of colonic polyadenomas. Results are expected in 2004–2005.[39,40]

Mechanisms

The preventive effect of NSAIDs could be partly related to COX-2 inhibition. COX-2 is induced by different signals, including proinflammatory cytokines such as interleukin-1 (IL-1) or growth factors such as epidermal growth factor (EGF) and transforming growth factor β (TGF-β).[41] Indeed, there is an increase in COX-2 mRNA and protein expression in colon tumour tissue in humans[42–46] and rodents.[47,48] This increase in expression can be observed from the adenomous step.[49,50] It is less pronounced in familial cancers.[51] The cell type(s) involved are still under discussion: epithelial cells for Min mouse adenomas, AOM-induced rat tumours, and human adenomas and cancers, or stromal cells for Min mouse adenomas and AOM-induced tumours in mice.[52–55]

Colon tumour cells with increased COX-2 expression have impaired adherence to the extracellular matrix and a resistance to apoptosis.[56] The increased COX-2 expression is associated with a tumoral neoangiogenesis[57] that is inhibited by NSAIDs, in particular by COX-2 inhibitors.[58]

Knockout experiments with the *COX-2* gene conducted in the polyposis model in Min mice suggest that the *APC* gene could play a major role. Indeed, an 86% reduction in the number of polyps was observed in animals when both alleles of the *COX-2* gene were inactivated.[59] The *APC* gene codes for a protein that regulates the phosphorylation of another cytoplasmic protein, β-catenin. *APC* mutations are thus responsible for an elevation in the cytoplasmic β-catenin level. The excess β-catenin then migrates to the nucleus, where it forms a complex with another protein, TCF-4. This complex induces the expression of a nuclear hormonal receptor, PPARδ, which, in association with the retinoid X receptor RXR, leads to the expression of different growth and proliferation promoter genes. NSAIDs and COX-2 inhibitors act partly by inhibiting the action of PPARδ, correcting abnormalities induced by *APC* gene mutations.[60]

In vitro experiments conducted in cell lines with no cyclooxygenase activity but sensitive to NSAIDs suggest the existence of other pathways independent of the cyclooxygenase one. Among these, the inhibitory action of the NF-κB signal could be significant, as could the action on other nuclear receptors from the PPAR family: PPARα and PPARγ.[61,62]

CALCIUM

Diets rich in calcium and/or vitamins are associated with a lower risk of colorectal cancer and adenomas. Several trials are in progress to assess the protective role of different calcium salts in humans, already well characterized in vitro and in different experimental models in vivo.[63] A randomized study conducted in the USA on 832 patients with a history of colorectal polyadenomas has shown a moderate but significant protective effect of daily supplementation with 3 g of calcium carbonate (equivalent to 1200 mg of elemental calcium) over 4 years on the formation of new adenomas (adjusted relative risk of 0.81, with a 95% confidence interval of 0.67–0.99).[64] The low level of this effect and the negative results observed in a European trial, however, do not support the widespread use of calcium supplementation in the general population.

FOLATE

The protective role of diets rich in fruits and vegetables is accepted. A diet rich in folate is associated with a lower risk of colorectal adenomas and cancer. Supplementation with folic acid reduces the number of chemoinduced tumours in rats.[65] It is also associated with a lower prevalence of precancerous lesions and cancer in patients with ulcerative colitis.[66] This effect is dependent on the polymorphism of one of the enzymes involved in folate metabolism, methyltetrahydrofolate reductase (MTHFR).[67] Assessment of the role of folate in colon carcinogenesis is still in process in a North American phase III study, but systematic supplementation with folate of cereals, flour, pasta, and rice is already done in the USA.[68]

VITAMINS

Several studies have assessed or are in the process of assessing the role of β-carotene and vitamin C or E.[69] A study has shown that supplementation with 25 mg β-carotene, 1 g vitamin C, and 400 mg vitamin E is ineffective with respect to recurrence of colonic polyadenomas.[70] Another trial has assessed the effect of supplementation with 15 mg β-carotene, 150 mg vitamin C, 75 mg vitamin E, 100 µg selenium, and 1.6 g calcium carbonate on the growth of small polyps after 3 years – also with negative results. A third trial has shown no significant effect of supplementation with 50 mg α-tocopherol and 20 mg β-carotene administered over 5–8 years.[72]

DFMO

2-Difluoromethylornithine (DFMO) is a drug that specifically inhibits the activity of ornithine decarboxylase (ODC), the key enzyme in polyamine synthesis, implicated in cell proliferation. Two studies assessing DFMO are in process in the USA.[73]

OTHER COMPOUNDS

Numerous other compounds showing effects in in vitro or in vivo animal studies are being evaluated in preliminary trials. Among these, we shall only mention 3-hydroxy-3-methylglutaryl-coenzyme A, *N*-acetylcysteine, ursodesoxycholic acid, lycopene (found in tomatoes), some flavonoids, and oltipraz (an analogue of dithiolthiones found in cruciferous vegetables such as cabbage and broccoli).

REFERENCES

1. Janne PA, Mayer RJ, Chemoprevention of colorectal cancer. *N Engl J Med* 2000; **342:** 1960–8.
2. Kelloff GJ, Johnson JR, Crowell JA et al, Approaches to the development and marketing approval of drugs that prevent cancer. *Cancer Epidemiol Biomarkers Prev* 1995; **4:** 1–10.
3. Hawk E, Lubet R, Limburg P, Chemoprevention in hereditary colorectal cancer syndromes. *Cancer* 1999; **86:** 2551–63.
4. Benamouzig R, La consommation d'aspirine ou d'anti-inflammatoires non stéroïdiens diminue-t-elle le risque de cancer colique. *Gastroenterol Clin Biol* 1998; **22:** S22–7.
5. Barnes CJ, Lee M, Chemoprevention of spontaneous intestinal adenomas in the adenomatous polyposis coli Min mouse model with aspirin. *Gastroenterology* 1998; **114:** 873–7.
6. Mereto E, Frencia L, Ghia M, Effect of aspirin on incidence and growth of aberrant crypt foci induced in the rat colon by 1,2-dimethylhydrazine. *Cancer Lett* 1994; **76:** 5–9.
7. Winde G, Schmid KW, Brandt B et al, Clinical and genomic

influence of sulindac on rectal mucosa in familial adenomatous polyposis. *Dis Colon Rectum* 1997; **40:** 1156–68.

8. Waddell WR, Ganser GF, Cerise EJ, Loughry RW, Sulindac for polyposis of the colon. *Am J Surg* 1989; **157:** 175–9.

9. Rigau J, Pique JM, Rubio E et al, Effects of long-term sulindac therapy on colonic polyposis. *Ann Intern Med* 1991; **115:** 952–4.

10. Niv Y, Fraser GM, Adenocarcinoma in the rectal segment in familial polyposis coli is not prevented by sulindac therapy. *Gastroenterology* 1994; **107:** 854–7.

11. Lynch HT, Thorson AG, Smyrk T, Rectal cancer after prolonged sulindac chemoprevention. A case report. *Cancer* 1995; **75:** 936–8.

12. Matsuhashi N, Nakajima A, Fukushima Y et al, Effects of sulindac on sporadic colorectal adenomatous polyps. *Gut* 1997; **40:** 344–9.

13. Ladenheim J, Garcia G, Titzer D et al, Effect of sulindac on sporadic colonic polyps. *Gastroenterology* 1995; **108:** 1083–7.

14. Ishikawa H, Akedo I, Suzuki T et al, Adverse effects of sulindac used for prevention of colorectal cancer. *J Natl Cancer Inst* 1997; **89:** 1381.

15. Reddy BS, Kawamori T, Lubet R et al, Chemopreventive effect of *S*-methylmethane thiosulfonate and sulindac administered together during the promotion/progression stages of colon carcinogenesis. *Carcinogenesis* 1999; **20:** 1645–8.

16. Stoner GD, Budd GT, Ganapathi R et al, Sulindac sulfone induced regression of rectal polyps in patients with familial adenomatous polyposis. *Adv Exp Med Biol* 1999; **470:** 45–53.

17. Van Stolk SR, Stoner G, Hayton WL et al, Phase I trial of exisulind (sulindac sulfone, FGN-1) as a chemopreventive agent in patients with familial adenomatous polyposis. *Clin Cancer Res* 2000; **6:** 78–89.

18. Gridley G, McLaughlin JK, Ekbom A et al, Incidence of cancer among patients with rheumatoid arthritis. *J Natl Cancer Inst* 1993; **85:** 307–11.

19. Kauppi M, Pukkala E, Isomaki H, Low incidence of colorectal cancer in patients with rheumatoid arthritis. *Clin Exp Rheumatol* 1996; **14:** 551–3.

20. Isomaki HA, Hakulinen T, Joutsenlahti U, Excess risk of lymphomas, leukemia and myeloma in patients with rheumatoid arthritis. *J Chronic Dis* 1978; **31:** 691–6.

21. Laakso M, Mutro O, Isomaki H, Koota K, Cancer mortality in patients with rheumatoid arthritis. *J Rheumatol* 1986; **13:** 522–6.

22. Collet JP, Sharpe C, Belzile E et al, Colorectal cancer prevention by non-steroidal anti-inflammatory drugs: effects of dosage and timing. *Br J Cancer* 1999; **81:** 62–8.

23. Coogan PF, Rosenberg L, Louik C et al, NSAIDs and risk of colorectal cancer according to presence or absence of family history of the disease. *Cancer Causes Control* 2000; **11:** 249–55.

24. Langman MJ, Cheng KK, Gilman EA, Lancashire RJ, Effect of anti-inflammatory drugs on overall risk of common cancer: case–control study in general practice research database. *BMJ* 2000; **320:** 1642–6.

25. Garcia Rodriguez LA, Huerta-Alvarez C, Reduced incidence of colorectal adenoma among long-term users of nonsteroidal anti-inflammatory drugs: a pooled analysis of published studies and a new population-based study. *Epidemiology* 2000; **11:** 376–81.

26. Breuer-Katchinski B, Nemes K, Rump B et al, Long-term use of nonsteroidal antiinflammatory drugs and the risk of colorectal adenomas. The Colorectal Adenoma Study Group. *Digestion* 2000; **61:** 129–34.

27. Smalley W, Ray WA, Daugherty J, Griffin MR, Use of non-steroidal anti-inflammatory drugs and incidence of colorectal cancer: a population-based study. *Arch Intern Med* 1999; **159:** 161–6.

28. Gann PH, Manson JE, Glynn RJ et al, Low-dose aspirin and incidence of colorectal tumors in a randomized trial. *J Natl Cancer Inst* 1993; **85:** 1220–4.

29. Sturmer T, Glynn RJ, Lee IM et al, Aspirin use and colorectal cancer: post-trial follow-up data from the Physicians' Health Study. *Ann Intern Med* 1998; **128:** 713–20.

30. Pinczowski D, Ekbom A, Baron J et al, Risk factors for colorectal cancer in patients with ulcerative colitis: a case–control study. *Gastroenterology* 1994; **107:** 117–20.

31. Bus PJ, Nagtegaal ID, Verspaget HW et al, Mesalazine-induced apoptosis of colorectal cancer: on the verge of a new chemopreventive era? *Aliment Pharmacol Ther* 1999; **13:** 1397–402.

32. MacGregor DJ, Kim YS, Sleisenger MH, Johnson LK, Chemoprevention of colon cancer carcinogenesis by balsalazide: inhibition of azoxymethane-induced aberrant crypt formation in the rat colon and intestinal tumor formation in the B6-Min/+ mouse. *Int J Oncol* 2000; **17:** 173–9.

33. Elder DJ, Halton DE, Crew TE, Paraskeva C, Apoptosis induction and cyclooxygenase-2 regulation in human colorectal adenoma and carcinoma cell lines by the cyclooxygenase-2-selective non-steroidal anti-inflammatory drug NS-398. *Int J Cancer* 2000; **86:** 553–60.

34. Reddy BS, Rao CV, Seibert K, Evaluation of cyclooxygenase-2 inhibitor for potential chemopreventive properties in colon carcinogenesis. *Cancer Res* 1996; **56:** 4566–9.

35. Kawamori T, Rao CV, Seibert K, Reddy BS, Chemopreventive activity of celecoxib, a specific cyclooxygenase-2 inhibitor, against colon carcinogenesis. *Cancer Res* 1998; **58:** 409–12.

36. Sasai H, Masaki M, Wakitani K, Suppression of polypogenesis in a new mouse strain with a truncated Apc(Delta474) by a novel COX-2 inhibitor, JTE-522. *Carcinogenesis* 2000; **21:** 953–8.

37. Sheng H, Shao J, Kirkland SC et al, Inhibition of human colon cancer cell growth by selective inhibition of cyclooxygenase-2. *J Clin Invest* 1997; **99:** 2254–9.

38. Steinbach G, Lynch PM, Phillips RK et al, The effect of celecoxib, a cyclooxygenase-2 inhibitor, in familial adenomatous polyposis. *N Engl J Med* 2000; **342:** 1946–52.

39. Dannenberg AJ, Zakim D, Chemoprevention of colorectal cancer through inhibition of cyclooxygenase-2. *Semin Oncol* 1999; **26:** 499–504.

40. Reddy BS, Hirose Y, Lubet R et al, Chemoprevention of colon cancer by specific cyclooxygenase-2 inhibitor, celecoxib, administered during different stages of carcinogenesis. *Cancer Res* 2000; **60:** 293–7.

41. Fosslien E, Molecular pathology of cyclooxygenase-2 in neoplasia. *Ann Clin Lab Sci* 2000; **30:** 3–21.

42. Eberhart CE, Coffey RJ, Radhika A et al, Upregulation of cyclooxygenase 2 gene expression in human colorectal adenomas and adenocarcinomas. *Gastroenterology* 1994; **107:** 1183–8.

43. Kargman SL, O'Neill GP, Vickers PJ et al, Expression of prostaglandin G/H synthase-1 and -2 protein in human colon cancer. *Cancer Res* 1995; **55:** 2556–9.

44. Sano H, Kawahito Y, Wilder RL et al, Expression of cyclooxygenase-1 and -2 in human colorectal cancer. *Cancer Res* 1995; **55:** 3785–9.

45. Kutchera W, Jones DA, Matsunami N et al, Prostaglandin H synthase 2 is expressed abnormally in human colon cancer: evidence for a transcriptional effect. *Proc Natl Acad Sci USA* 1996; **93:** 4816–20.

46. Sakuma K, Fujimori T, Hirabayashi K, Ternao A, Cyclooxygenase (COX)-2 immunoreactivity and relationship to p53 and Ki-67 expression in colorectal cancer. *J Gastroenterol* 1999; **34:** 189–94.

47. DuBois RN, Radhika A, Reddy BS, Entingh AJ, Increased cyclooxygenase-2 levels in carcinogen-induced rat colonic tumors. *Gastroenterology* 1996; **110:** 1259–62.

48. Singh J, Hamid R, Reddy BS, Dietary fat and colon cancer: modulation of cyclooxygenase-2 by types and amount of dietary fat during the postinitiation stage of colon carcinogenesis. *Cancer Res* 1997; **57:** 3465–70.

49. Maekawa M, Sugano K, Sano H et al, Increased expression of cyclooxygenase-2 to -1 in human colorectal cancers and adenomas, but not in hyperplastic polyps. *Jpn J Clin Oncol* 1998; **28:** 421–6.

50. Hao X, Bishop AE, Wallace M et al, Early expression of cyclooxygenase-2 during sporadic colorectal carcinogenesis. *J Pathol* 1999; **187:** 295–301.

51. Sinicrope FA, Lemoine M, Xi L et al, Reduced expression of cyclooxygenase 2 proteins in hereditary nonpolyposis colorectal cancers relative to sporadic cancers. *Gastroenterology* 1999; **117:** 350–8.

52. Chapple KS, Cartwright EJ, Hawcroft G et al, Localization of cyclooxygenase-2 in human sporadic colorectal adenomas. *Am J Pathol* 2000; **156:** 545–53.

53. Hull MA, Booth JK, Tisbury A et al, Cyclooxygenase 2 is upregulated and localized to macrophages in the intestine of Min mice. *Br J Cancer* 1999; **79:** 1399–405.

54. Shattuck BR, Lamps LW, Heppner GK et al, Differential expression of matrilysin and cyclooxygenase-2 in intestinal and colorectal neoplasms. *Mol Carcinogen* 1999; **24:** 177–87.

55. Bamba H, Ota S, Kato A et al, High expression of cyclooxygenase-2 in macrophages of human colonic adenoma. *Int J Cancer* 1999; **83:** 470–5.

56. Tsuji M, DuBois RN, Alterations in cellular adhesion and apoptosis in epithelial cells overexpressing prostaglandin endoperoxide synthase 2. *Cell* 1995; **83:** 493–501.

57. Prescott SM, Fitzpatrick FA, Cyclooxygenase-2 and carcinogenesis. *Biochim Biophys Acta* 2000; **1470:** M69–78.

58. Jones MK, Wang H, Peskar BM et al, Inhibition of angiogenesis by nonsteroidal anti-inflammatory drugs: insight into mechanisms and implications for cancer growth and ulcer healing. *Nature Med* 1999; **5:** 1418–23.

59. Oshima M, Dinchuk JE, Kargman SL et al, Suppression of intestinal polyposis in Apc delta716 knockout mice by inhibition of cyclooxygenase 2 (COX-2). *Cell* 1996; **87:** 803–9.

60. Wu GD, A nuclear receptor to prevent colon cancer. *N Engl J Med* 2000; **342:** 651–3.

61. Grilli M, Pizzi M, Memo M, Spano P, Neuroprotection by aspirin and sodium salicylate through blockade of NF-kappaB activation. *Science* 1996; **274:** 1383–5.

62. Yamamoto Y, Yin MJ, Lin KM, Gaynor RB, Sulindac inhibits activation of the NF-kappaB pathway. *J Biol Chem* 1999; **274:** 27307–14.

63. Faivre J, Bonithon KC, Chemoprevention of colorectal cancer: recent results. *Cancer Res* 1999; **151:** 122–33.

64. Baron JA, Beach M, Mandel JS et al, Calcium supplements for the prevention of colorectal adenomas. Calcium Polyp Prevention Study Group. *N Engl J Med* 1999; **340:** 101–7.

65. Cravo ML, Mason JB, Dayal Y et al, Folate deficiency enhances the development of colonic neoplasia in dimethylhydrazine-treated rats. *Cancer Res* 1992; **52:** 5002–6.

66. Lashner BA, Heidenreich PA, Su GL et al, Effect of folate supplementation on the incidence of dysplasia and cancer in chronic ulcerative colitis. A case–control study. *Gastroenterology* 1989; **97:** 255–9.

67. Ma J, Stampfer MJ, Giovannucci E et al, Methylenetetrahydrofolate reductase polymorphism, dietary interactions, and risk of colorectal cancer. *Cancer Res* 1997; **57:** 1098–102.

68. Mills JL, Fortification of foods with folic acid – How much is enough? *N Engl J Med* 2000; **342:** 1442–5.

69. Hennekens CH, Buring JE, Manson JE et al, Lack of effect of long-term supplementation with beta carotene on the incidence of malignant neoplasms and cardiovascular disease. *N Engl J Med* 1996; **334:** 1145–9.

70. Greenberg ER, Baron JA, Tosteson TD et al, A clinical trial of antioxidant vitamins to prevent colorectal adenoma. Polyp Prevention Study Group. *N Engl J Med* 1994; **331:** 141–7.

71. Hofstad B, Almendingen K, Vatn M et al, Growth and recurrence of colorectal polyps: a double-blind 3-year intervention with calcium and antioxidants. *Digestion* 1998; **59:** 148–56.

72. Albanes D, Malila N, Taylor PR et al, Effects of supplemental alpha-tocopherol and beta-carotene on colorectal cancer: results from a controlled trial (Finland). *Cancer Causes Control* 2000; **11:** 197–205.

73. Meyskens FJ, Gerner EW, Development of difluoromethylornithine (DFMO) as a chemoprevention agent. *Clin Cancer Res* 1999; **5:** 945–51.

Part 3

Pathology and Prognostic Factors

6

Pathology of colorectal cancer

Paul Hermanek

INTRODUCTION

In this chapter, we shall deal only with those areas of pathology that are relevant for treatment decisions, analysis of treatment results and quality management. Thus we do not include diagnosis and differential diagnosis, epidemiology, genetics, precancerous conditions and lesions, causal and formal pathogenesis, and the dysplasia–carcinoma sequence. Because 95% of all malignant tumours of the colon and rectum are carcinomas, predominantly the pathology of carcinomas will be discussed, and only in the last section will a short overview be given of the other, very uncommon, malignant tumours (endocrine, mesenchymal and lymphoid).

DEFINITION OF CARCINOMA IN THE COLON AND RECTUM

In contrast to the stomach or the small intestine, a neoplasm in the colon and rectum has metastatic potential only after invasion of at least the submucosa. Thus, for the colorectum in the biological and clinical sense, carcinoma is present only after the submucosa has been invaded. Such lesions are termed invasive carcinomas.

Between dysplasia in the general definition of an intraepithelial lesion and an invasive carcinoma as defined above, we find an intermediate step of malignant progression, namely a neoplastic lesion that shows invasive growth into the lamina propria or between the fibres of the muscularis mucosae, but does not reach the submucosa. According to clinical experience, lymph-node metastasis is not to be expected in these 'mucosal' or 'intramucosal' lesions.[1] Thus

Morson[2] recommended that the use of the word 'carcinoma' should be restricted to that stage of the dysplasia–carcinoma sequence that has crossed the line of the muscularis mucosae with invasion of the submucosa. We use this nomenclature in the following.

Unfortunately, outside the UK and the German-speaking countries, the term 'carcinoma' is not used uniformly. Thus, in any cancer statistics and in any report of treatment results, one has to make sure whether the data relate to invasive carcinoma only or include high-grade dysplasia (non-invasive carcinoma) too.

SITE DISTRIBUTION

The pathologies of carcinoma of the colon and rectum are essentially the same, although there are differences in epidemiology and etiology. In the literature, the definitions of colon and rectum vary. This renders comparisons difficult and explains some differences among data. According to the updated International Documentation System for Colorectal Cancer (IDS for CRC),[3,4] carcinomas that have a lower border of the tumour 16 cm or less from the anal verge (measured by a rigid rectosigmoidoscope) are classified as rectal carcinomas. Using this definition, in high-incidence areas, about 50% of all colorectal carcinomas are located in the rectum, 25% in the sigmoid colon and 25% in the remaining parts of the colon. However, during the past two decades, a slow change in the distribution, with a shift to the right, has been reported in some, but not all, high-incidence countries. In this context, it is interesting that in low-incidence countries the proportion of carcinomas of the right colon is relatively high.

GROSS MORPHOLOGY

Early carcinomas of the colon and rectum, i.e. tumours limited to the submucosa, present in most cases as polypoid (exophytic) lesions, pedunculated, semipedunculated or sessile. Sometimes flat lesions are observed with no or only slight elevation (not more than twice the height of mucosa). In such flat lesions, a slight central depression may also be present.

Advanced carcinomas (invading beyond the submucosa) present in four types, similar to the Borrmann categories of gastric carcinoma:

- polypoid (protuberant);
- ulcerated, with sharply demarcated margins;
- ulcerated, without definite borders;
- diffusely infiltrating.

In contrast to gastric carcinoma, the latter two types are uncommon; the ulcerated tumour with sharply demarcated margins is by far the most common type, followed by the polypoid type as second.

HISTOMORPHOLOGY

Histological typing

The present World Health Organization (WHO) classification is shown in Table 6.1. Adenocarcinoma and mucinous adenocarcinoma (sometimes still termed mucoid or colloid adeno- carcinoma) account for 90–95% of carcinomas; all other types are uncommon. Mucinous adenocarcinomas are more frequently observed in the colon (about 15%) than in the rectum (about 10%).

Some adenocarcinomas show areas with abundant mucus production. However, unless mucus contributes to more than 50% of the tumour bulk, the tumour should still be classified as adenocarcinoma. Also, the presence of scattered Paneth cells and endocrine cells or of small foci of squamous differentiation does not influence the classification. Signet-ring cells may also be present in mucinous adenocarcinomas. However, more than 50% of the tumour should comprise signet-ring cells before it is classified as signet-ring cell carcinoma. The uncommon undifferentiated carcinoma (former designations: carcinoma simplex, anaplastic, trabecular carcinoma) should be distinguished from poorly differentiated adenocarcinoma, high-grade endocrine carcinoma (small-cell carcinoma), lymphoma and leukaemic deposits by use of mucin stains and immunohistochemistry.

Extremely uncommon carcinomas not listed in the WHO classification, and reported in only a few cases, include clear cell (hypernephroid) carcinoma, spindle cell carcinoma, choriocarcinoma, melanotic adenocarcinoma, carcinomas arising in endometriosis, calcified adenocarcinoma, giant cell carcinoma and Paneth-cell-rich papillary adenocarcinoma.

Histological grading

Histopathological grading of tumours is performed to provide some indication of their aggressiveness, which may in turn relate to prognosis and/or treatment choice.

The traditional system of grading distinguishes four grades:

G1 well-differentiated: a carcinoma with histological and cellular features that closely resemble normal epithelium;
G2 moderately differentiated: a carcinoma intermediate between G1 and G3;
G3 poorly differentiated: a carcinoma with histological or cellular features that only barely resemble normal epithelium (there must be at least some gland formation or mucus production);
G4 undifferentiated: no glandular or squamous differentiation at all (thus G4 applies in the colon and rectum to undifferentiated carcinoma only, see Table 6.1).

The WHO classification[5] also provides a grading system, with two classes:

- low-grade, encompassing G1 and G2;
- high-grade, including G3 and G4.

This grading system fulfils all clinical requirements, and can be performed with higher reproducibility. Thus we prefer grading with only two categories. When a carcinoma shows different grades of differentiation, the higher grade should determine the final categorization. Thus a carcinoma that shows both low- and high-grade areas should be classified as high-grade. However, the disorganized glands seen commonly at the advancing edge of the carcinoma should not be considered as high-grade malignancy. High-grade carcinomas account for 20–25% of resected carcinomas.

Table 6.1 Histological typing and grading: WHO classification[5,6]

Type	ICD-O code	Definition	Grading system (G1–4)	Low/high (L/H)
Adenocarcinoma	8140/3	Glandular epithelium, tubular and/or villous	1–3	L/H
Mucinous adenocarcinoma	8480/3	More than 50% extracellular mucin	1–3	L/H
Signet-ring cell carcinoma	8490/3	More than 50% signet-ring cells (intracytoplasmatic mucin)	3	H
Squamous cell carcinoma	8070/3	Exclusively squamous differentiation	1–3	L/H
Adenosquamous carcinoma	8560/3	Adenocarcinoma plus squamous cell carcinoma	1–3	L/H
Medullary carcinoma	8510/3	Sheets of malignant cells X (not graded), abundant cytoplasm and prominent infiltration by intraepithelial lymphocytes		
Undifferentiated carcinoma	8020/3	No glandular structure or other features to indicate definite differentiation	4	H

Note: The small cell carcinoma mentioned in the WHO classification[5] is now classified as poorly differentiated endocrine carcinoma[7] (see Figure 6.4).

Additional histological parameters

For describing the histomorphology of an individual colorectal carcinoma, there are some further parameters to be considered:[8–10]

- the character of the invasive margin (pushing or expanding, or well-circumscribed versus irregular diffusely infiltrating);
- peritumoral inflammation;
- the presence of peritumorous lymphoid aggregates;
- fibroblastic stromal resection (desmoplasia);
- invasion of lymphatics (L classification):[11] L0, no lymphatic invasion; L1, lymphatic invasion; LX, lymphatic invasion cannot be assessed;
- venous invasion (V classification):[11] V0, no venous invasion; V1, microscopic venous invasion; V2, macroscopic venous invasion; VX, venous invasion cannot be assessed; in the case of microscopic venous invasion, it is important to distinguish between involvement of intramural veins (submucosa, muscularis propria) and that of extramural veins (beyond muscularis propria);
- invasion of perineural spaces.

In addition, the type of lymph-node reactions may be recorded, because it reflects the host reactions. There may be follicular hyperplasia (in more than 50% or in 50% or less of regional nodes) or paracortical hyperplasia or both.[12]

SPECIAL CLINICAL TYPES OF COLORECTAL CARCINOMA

Hereditary non-polyposis colon cancer (HNPCC)[13,14]

Carcinomas in this hereditary syndrome have a tendency to occur primarily in the right colon and at a much younger age (most cases between 35 and 45 years) than the usual sporadic carcinoma (preferred age 55–65 years). The otherwise uncommon histological feature of medullary carcinoma with numerous tumour-infiltrating lymphocytes (TILs) and marked peritumoral lymphoid reaction is frequently seen. Mucinous adenocarcinomas and high-grade tumours are observed relatively often. There is an increased incidence of metachronous multiple primary tumours. HNPCC accounts for at least 4–6% of all colorectal carcinomas.

Carcinoma arising in familial adenomatous polyposis (FAP)

Less than 1% of colorectal carcinomas arise in FAP and in the 'hereditary flat adenoma syndrome' (HFAS), a variant of FAP, usually with fewer than 100 adenomas, mostly of flat type. The histological features are similar to those of sporadic cancers; however, there is a high proportion of multiple synchronous primary tumours in symptomatic cases (up to a third of cases).

Carcinoma developing in inflammatory bowel disease

Carcinomas in inflammatory bowel disease arise predominantly in extensive ulcerous colitis with a history of 10 years or longer. There are often synchronous multiple carcinomas. The incidence of flat and diffusely infiltrating carcinomas, high-grade tumours, mucinous adenocarcinomas and signet-ring cell carcinomas is higher than in ordinary colorectal carcinomas. Less than 1% of all colorectal carcinomas arise in inflammatory bowel disease.

TUMOUR SPREAD

Knowledge of tumour spread is of paramount importance for surgical procedure in treating colorectal carcinoma. The possible routes of tumour spread are shown in Figure 6.1.

Local spread

The different types of local spread determine the extent of surgical resection, and lead to the demand for avoidance of local tumour spillage.

(a) Extent of resection

In colon carcinoma, the extent of resection is determined by the extent of lymph-node dissection and the vascular supply. However, in rectal carcinoma, the distal margin of clearance may be critical, especially in tumours located in the lower rectum. In this context, it is important that histological examination of rectal carcinomas in curable stages demonstrates that the continuous distal local spread usually extends no more than some millimetres beyond the grossly recognizable margin of the tumour. However, in the perimuscular tissue, discontinuous spread in the form of so-called satellites must be considered. Such microscopic tumour nodules, without residua of lymph-node tissue and not more than 3 mm in diameter, are found in the mesorectum, predominantly in the radial direction, but also distal, some centimetres from the lower tumour margin.

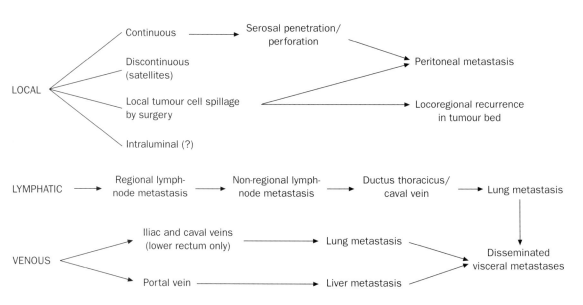

Figure 6.1 Tumour spread.

Thus, low anterior resection for tumours of the middle and lower rectal third has to include total mesorectal excision down to the pelvic floor,[15] while the margin of clearance within the proper wall of the rectum (muscularis propria, submucosa, mucosa) may be limited to 1 cm in situ except in cases of high-grade tumours, which require 2 cm distal margin.[16]

(b) Avoidance of local spillage of tumour cells

A local spillage of tumour cells results in a significantly increased incidence of locoregional recurrence.[17] This is observed in rectal carcinoma after iatrogenic tumour perforation during mobilization or in cases of two-step low anterior resection (first resection with tumour in the distal resection line, further resection with tumour-free resection line) with transsection of tumour tissue. Adherence of a tumour to adjacent organs may be caused by peritumorous inflammation or by tumorous invasion. A respective discrimination by gross inspection or palpation is not possible. In such cases, a primary multivisceral resection is indicated if a curative operation is intended. Any biopsy from the adherence should be avoided, because in cases of tumour invasion, biopsy results in local tumour spillage.[18]

The basis of local therapy

The classical concept for curative oncological surgery is the so-called radical resection, which includes wide resection of the primary together with formal (systematic) regional lymphadenectomy. For selected carcinomas without lymph-node metastases, local procedures such as endoscopic polypectomy or surgical local excision can also be used with curative intention.[19,20] The indication for such procedures is determined by the risk of lymph-node metastasis already present compared with the increased risk of surgical mortality from radical procedures.

The probability of regional lymph-node metastasis depends primarily on histological features of the primary tumour, such as depth of invasion, histological grade and absence or presence of lymphatic invasion. This is shown in Table 6.2, which is based on the careful histological examination of 2720

Table 6.2 Frequency of regional lymph-node metastasis in colorectal carcinoma: pathological findings in radical resection specimens – only cases with resection for cure (R0) (Department of Surgery, University of Erlangen, 1969–1993)

Depth of invasion		Frequency of regional lymph-node metastasis			
		Low-risk histology[a]		High-risk histology[b]	
pT1	Submucosa	5/172	(2.9%)	12/71	(17%)
pT2	Muscularis propria:				
	inner (circular) layer	19/212	(9.0%)	34/93	(37%)
	outer (longitudinal) layer	58/299	(19.4%)	39/97	(40%)
pT3	Subserosa/pericolic/ perirectal tissue; extension beyond muscularis propria:				
	≤5 mm	82/432	(19.0%)	337/522	(64.6%)
	>5 mm	38/142	(26.8%)	290/346	(83.8%)
pT4	Serosa/adjacent	36/126	(28.6%)	149/208	(71.6%)

[a]Low-risk: low grade (G1, 2) *and* no histologically detectable invasion of lymphatics (L0).
[b]High-risk: high grade (G3, 4) *or* histologically detected invasion of lymphatics (L1).

radical tumour resections for cure (R0). It shows that the risk of lymph-node metastasis already present is minimal in pT1 tumours with so-called low-risk histology, i.e. low grade of malignancy (G1, G2) *and* no demonstrable lymphatic invasion (L0). Thus local therapy with curative intent can be considered predominantly for carcinomas of low-risk histology invading the submucosa only. In patients with considerably increased surgical risk, it may also be used for carcinomas invading the inner muscularis propria if low-risk histology is present.

Lymph-node dissection for colon carcinoma

The extent of lymph-node dissection in radical surgery is determined by the lymph drainage. While most parts of the colon drain into one direction, for both flexures and the right and left third of the transverse colon, a bidirectional lymph drainage exists.[21,22] Tumours of the hepatic flexure and the right third of the transverse colon drain into nodes along the right as well as the middle colic artery. Therefore radical resection should be performed as extended right hemicolectomy (right and transverse colectomy), with removal of the nodes along the ileocolic, right and middle colic arteries. The bidirectional lymph drainage of tumours of the splenic flexure and the adjacent left third of the transverse colon and upper third of the descending colon requires an extended left hemicolectomy (left and transverse colectomy) for radical resection.

Lymphatic spread of rectal carcinoma

The main lymph drainage of rectal carcinoma occurs upwards to the nodes along the superior rectal and inferior mesenteric vessels. Skipping of nodes is uncommon, and occurs in about 3% of cases with nodal metastasis (9/234 = 2.8%).[21] In curable cases, retrograde lymph-node metastasis (along the inferior rectal arteries to inguinal nodes) is exceptional. The reports on the incidence of lateral lymphatic spread are controversial. If lateral metastasis is defined as metastasis along the iliac vessels outside the mesorectum, involvement of these nodes in curable cases is obviously rare. Thus an indication for additional lateral dissection of the iliac nodes is at least questionable, in particular when considering the significant morbidity of this procedure.[23]

The extent of dissection upwards is still under discussion (low or high ligature of the inferior mesenteric artery). The analysis of 821 curative radical resections with high ligature revealed involvement of high nodes in about 3% (Department of Surgery, University of Erlangen: 18/590 = 3.1%; multicentre study of the German Study Group on Colo-Rectal Carcinoma (SGCRC): 8/231 = 3.4%). Between 10% and 20% of these patients survive for 5 years;[24] thus high ligature presents a benefit to only about 0.5% of all patients operated on. This explains why in clinical studies an advantage cannot yet be proved.

TUMOUR COMPLICATIONS

Colorectal carcinoma may cause severe acute complications with the need for urgent or emergency surgery, for example acute ileus and/or free perforation or massive bleeding. Ileus and perforation are predominantly observed in colon carcinoma. Patients with such complications have a high surgical risk; in addition, their long-term prognosis is poor. In treatment statistics, these patients should be separated from those with elective surgery.

Other complications, such as fistulas or peritumorous abscesses, are of minor influence on prognosis, but may lead to extended surgery.

CLASSIFICATION OF ANATOMICAL EXTENT BEFORE TREATMENT

In the history of staging, the introduction of a pathological stage classification for rectal carcinoma by Cuthbert Dukes[25] in 1930 was an important step. However, in the following years, the Dukes system was repeatedly modified, indicating that the original system no longer fulfilled modern requirements, and led to considerable confusion.[26] In particular, the Dukes classification does not take into consideration distant metastasis, does not allow the recognition of early carcinomas (limited to the submucosa) and does not consider the number of regional lymph nodes involved. Thus today the anatomical extent of colorectal carcinoma should be classified according to the TNM system. The TNM system was recommended for daily use and clinical trials by the NIH Consensus Conference on Adjuvant Treatment,[27] and was introduced in Germany and the USA for general use in cancer hospitals. The present 5th edition system is shown in Table 6.3. To

Table 6.3 The TNM/pTNM classification[11,31]

The definitions of the clinical classification (TNM) correspond to those of the pathological classification (pTNM).

T/pT – Primary tumour

TX/pTX	Primary tumour cannot be assessed
T0/pT0	No evidence of primary tumour
Tis/pTis	Carcinoma in situ: intraepithelial or invasion of lamina propria[a]
T1/pT1	Tumour invades submucosa
T2/pT2	Tumour invades muscularis propria
T3/pT3	Tumour invades through muscularis propria into subserosa or into non-peritonealized pericolic or perirectal tissues
T4/pT4	Tumour directly invades other organs or structures[b] and/or perforates visceral peritoneum

Notes: [a]This includes cancer cells confined within the glandular basement membrane (intraepithelial) or lamina propria (intramucosal), with no extension through the muscularis mucosae into the submucosa
[b]Direct invasion in T4/pT4 includes invasion of other segments of the colorectum by way of the serosa, e.g. invasion of the sigmoid colon by a carcinoma of the caecum

N/pN – Regional lymph nodes

NX/pNX	Regional lymph nodes cannot be assessed
N0/pN0	No regional lymph-node metastasis
N1/pN1	Metastasis in 1–3 pericolic or perirectal lymph nodes
N2/pN2	Metastasis in 4 or more pericolic or perirectal lymph nodes

Note: A tumour nodule greater than 3 mm in diameter in perirectal or pericolic adipose tissue without histological evidence of a residual lymph node in the nodule is classified as regional perirectal/pericolic lymph-node metastasis. However, a tumour nodule up to 3 mm in diameter is classified in the T category as discontinuous extension, i.e. T3/pT3.

M/pM – Distant metastasis

MX/pMX	Presence of distant metastasis cannot be assessed
M0/pM0	No distant metastasis
M1/pM1	Distant metastasis

Regional lymph nodes

Regional lymph nodes are the pericolic and perirectal and the nodes along the named vascular trunks supporting the various anatomical subsites:

Appendix	ileocolic
Caecum	ileocolic and right colic
Ascending colon	ileocolic, right colic and middle colic
Hepatic flexure	middle colic and right colic
Transverse colon	right colic, middle colic, left colic and inferior mesenteric
Splenic flexure	middle colic, left colic and inferior mesenteric

Table 6.3 continued

Descending colon	left colic and inferior mesenteric
Sigmoid colon and rectosigmoid	left colic, superior rectal (haemorrhoidal) and inferior mesenteric
Rectum	superior rectal (haemorrhoidal), inferior mesenteric and internal iliac

The nodes along the sigmoid arteries are considered pericolic.

Perirectal nodes include the mesorectal (paraproctal), lateral sacral, presacral, sacral promotory (Gerota), middle rectal (haemorrhoidal) and inferior rectal (haemorrhoidal) nodes. Metastasis in the external iliac or common iliac nodes is classified as distant metastasis.

Ramifications (i.e. optional subdivisions of existing TNM/pTNM categories)

pTis[9]	pTic	Intraepithelial carcinoma
	pTim	Intramucosal carcinoma
pT1[9]	pT1a	No evidence of lymphatic or venous invasion
	pT1b	Lymphatic or venous invasion present
pT3[29]	pT3a	Minimal: tumour invades through the muscularis propria into the subserosa or into non-peritonealized pericolic or perirectal tissues, not more than 1 mm beyond the outer border of the muscularis propria
	pT3b	Slight: tumour invades through the muscularis propria into the subserosa or into non-peritonealized pericolic or perirectal tissues, more than 1 mm but not more than 5 mm beyond the outer border of the muscularis propria
	pT3c	Moderate: tumour invades through the muscularis propria into the subserosa or into non-peritonealized pericolic or perirectal tissues, more than 5 mm but not more than 15 mm beyond the outer border of the muscularis propria
	pT3d	Extensive: tumour invades through the muscularis propria into the subserosa or into non-peritonealized pericolic or perirectal tissues, more than 15 mm beyond outer border of the muscularis propria
pT4[29]	pT4a	Invasion of adjacent organs or structures, without perforation of visceral peritoneum
	pT4b	Perforation of visceral peritoneum

classify a tumour according to pTNM (pathological classification), some requirements must be met (Table 6.4). The stage grouping of the TNM system is shown in Figure 6.2.

Micrometastasis and isolated tumour cells[28,30]

Micrometastasis is defined as metastasis 0.2 cm or less in greatest dimension. Cases with only micrometastasis may be identified by the addition of '(mi)' to the pN and/or pM category, e.g. pN1(mi) or pM1(mi). In micrometastasis, tumour cells have penetrated the wall of lymph sinus or blood vessels and there is extrasinusoidal or extravascular proliferation. Micrometastasis has to be distinguished from isolated (disseminated or circulating) tumour cells in lymph nodes, blood or bone marrow or at other distant sites. Isolated tumour cells (single cells or small clusters) may be detected by morphological methods, in particular cytochemistry, or by non-morphological methods such as flow cytometry or polymerase chain reaction (PCR). Because their independent prognostic significance remains to be proven, isolated tumour cells are not considered in the TNM classification. However, positive morphological findings of isolated tumour cells may be indicated by the addition of '(i+)', and positive non-morphological findings by the addition of '(mol+)', e.g. pN0(i+) or M0(mol+).

Table 6.4 Requirements for pT, pN and pM classification[11,29-31]

pT3 or less

Pathological examination of the primary carcinoma removed by short segment (limited) or radical resection *with no gross tumour* at the circumferential (deep, radial, lateral), proximal and distal margins of resection (with or without microscopic involvement), *or* pathological examination of the primary carcinoma removed by endoscopic polypectomy or local excision with histologically tumour-free margins of resection

pT4

Pathological confirmation of perforation of the visceral peritoneum,[a] or microscopic confirmation of invasion of adjacent organs or structures

pN0

Histological examination of a regional lymphadenectomy specimen will ordinarily include 12 or more regional lymph nodes

pN1/2

If the pathology report does not indicate the number of involved nodes, classify as pN1

[a] Pathological confirmation may be achieved from biopsies or resection or by cytology of specimens obtained from the serosa overlying the primary tumour

	(p)M0		(p)M1
	pN0	pN1, 2	
pT1			
	I		
pT2			
		III	IV
pT3			
	II		
pT4			

Figure 6.2 UICC/AJCC stage grouping.[11,31]

CLASSIFICATION OF ANATOMICAL EXTENT AFTER TREATMENT

While TNM and pTNM describe the anatomical extent of cancer before treatment, the residual tumour (R) classification deals with tumour status after treatment. It reflects the effects of therapy, influences further therapeutic procedures and is the strongest predictor of outcome.[11,29] Thus, following tumour resection, first of all, the pathologist has to examine the resection lines to obtain the R classification, which is based on clinical as well as histopathological findings (Figure 6.3). In this regard, the main problem is the examination of the circumferential (lateral, radial), i.e. mesorectal and mesocolon, resection margins. In general, at least two conventional blocks or a large-area (giant) block have to be submitted for histology (for detailed methodic recommendations, see reference 32).

HISTOLOGICAL GRADING OF TUMOUR REGRESSION

In cases of neoadjuvant (preoperative) radio- and/or

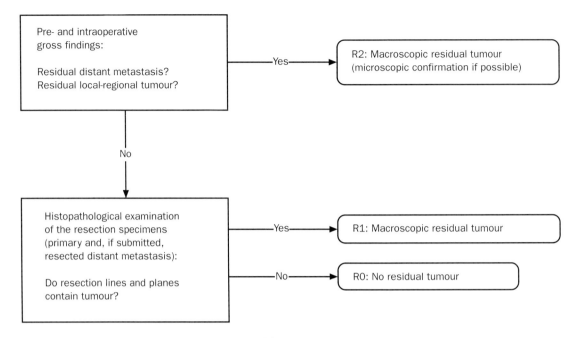

Figure 6.3 UICC/AJCC residual tumour (R) classification.[11,31] From Hermanek et al (eds), *UICC, TNM Supplement 1993. A Commentary on Uniform Use.* Berlin: Springer-Verlag, 1993.

chemotherapy, the pathologist has to assess the tumour response. Unfortunately, there are not yet any internationally agreed systems for describing the regressive changes and staging methods in such cases. A proposal of Dworak et al[33] is used in Germany.[34] Complete regression is possible, but, from our experience, it is very uncommon, provided that the tumour region is carefully worked-up. Thus, for regression grading, detailed statements on work-up should be given to enable estimation of the reliability of findings.

PROGNOSTIC FACTORS

Prognostic factors are variables (covariates) with independent influence on outcome. They may differ according to the various ways of measuring outcome (various endpoints) (e.g. overall survival, disease-free survival, relapse rate and response to treatment) and also for different patient subgroups. The identification of prognostic factors, in particular the acceptance of new prognostic factors, should follow certain rules.[35] Table 6.5 shows the prognostic factors for patients with residual tumour and those with complete resec-

tion of the tumour. They are divided into proven and probable. Only recently have sufficient data become available to demonstrate that surgical treatment and the individual surgeon are independent prognostic factors in colorectal cancer.[36–39]

It should be emphasized that the independent prognostic significance of all biological and molecular factors (factors of the so-called new pathology) remains to be proven.[4,8–10]

Proven as well as probable prognostic factors have to be included in analyses of clinical trials and also in retrospective studies; otherwise the results cannot be accepted without doubt.

THE HISTOPATHOLOGICAL REPORT

The histopathological report has to include all possible information that may be important in relation to tumour classification, description of surgical procedure and prognostic factors. This enables diagnosis, treatment decisions, estimation of prognosis, and analysis of treatment results and of the quality of diagnosis and treatment.

Table 6.5 Prognostic factors in colorectal carcinoma (unfavourable level of covariates is shown in parentheses)

A.   **Patients with residual tumour (R1, R2)**

Proven prognostic factors

Distant metastasis (present)
Localization of residual tumour (distant)
For patients with multiple distant metastases: performance status (increasing ECOG grade, decreasing Karnofsky score)

B.   **Patients with complete resection of tumour (no residual tumour, R0)**

	Proven prognostic factors	Probable prognostic factors
Tumour-related	Anatomical extent: pTNM and stage grouping (higher category) Histological grade (high-grade) Venous invasion (present, predominantly extramural) Histological pattern of tumour margin (infiltrative)	Anatomical site or primary (lower rectum) Tumour perforation/obstruction (present) Lymphatic and perineural invasion (present) Peritumoral lymphoid cells/ lymphoid aggregates (non-conspicuous/absent)
Patient-related	CEA serum level (>5 ng/ml) Comorbid disease (present, higher ASA grade)	Gender (male)
Treatment-related	Surgeon	For subgroups: multimodal therapy (not performed)

Specific recommendations for the content of surgical pathology reports have been published in various countries since the 1980s (an overview is given in reference 40). The minimal data to be included in a present-day surgical pathology report are listed in Table 6.6. It is based on recent publications.[4,41–43] It may be extended (extended programme) in specialized institutions and in clinical studies. This extended programme includes all features with proven or probable prognostic significance (see Table 6.5) and data describing the oncological quality of surgery (see below).

QUALITY MANAGEMENT AND PATHOLOGY

Quality management is a requirement for diagnostic activities in pathology departments as well as for the treatment of cancer and for clinical studies.

Quality management within pathology departments

The methods of quality management within pathology departments have recently been described and summarized by Rosai.[44]

There are indicators of the quality of histopatho-

Table 6.6 Minimal data to be included in surgical pathology reports on colorectal specimens

A. Incision biopsies

Gross description	Number of pieces
Histology	Extension (intraeplthelial/intramucosal/invasion of submucosa)
	Histological type
	Histological grade

B. Polypectomies

Gross description	Number of pieces
	Macroscopic type (flat/sessile/semipedunculated/pedunculated)
	Greatest dimension (without stalk)
Histology: tumour	Histological type
	Histological grade
	Extension (intraepithelial/intramucosal/invasion of submucosa)
	In semipedunculated and pedunculated polyps: extension of invasion of submucosa (none/head/stalk)
	Lymphatic invasion (L classification)
	Venous invasion
Histology: margins	Involvement, minimal distance of tumour from margin (mucosal margins, deep margin)

C. Local excision (submucosal, full-thickness)

Gross description	Number of pieces
	Tumour configuration (exophytic–fungating/endophytic–ulcerative/diffusely infiltrating)
	Greatest dimension of tumour
	Margins: minimal distance of tumour from mucosal and deep margins
Histology: tumour	Histological type
	Histological grade
	Extension (pT classification)
	Lymphatic invasion (L classification)
	Venous invasion (intramural, extramural)
Histology: margins	Involvement, minimal distance of tumour from mucosal and deep margins
Histology: additional pathological findings (e.g. adenoma, dysplasia)	

D. Resection specimens

Gross description: resection specimen	Parts of colorectum removed
	Adjacent organs removed

Table 6.6 continued	
	Number of pieces received (resection en bloc/not en bloc)
	Number of malignant tumours
Gross description: tumour[a]	Localization
	In rectal carcinomas:
	• Site in relation to peritoneal reflection (above/at/below)
	• Site of distal border of tumour (upper/middle/lower third)
	• In case of abdominoperineal excision: distance between distal border of tumour and anal verge/method of measurement[b]
	Greatest dimension
	Tumour perforation (spontaneous/iatrogenic)
Gross descriptions: margins	Minimal distance from proximal and distal margin/method of measurement[b]
	Minimal distance from circumferential (radial, lateral) margin/method of measurement[b]
Histology: tumour[a]	Anatomical extent: pTNM classification
	Number of regional lymph nodes examined
	Number of regional lymph nodes involved
	Apical lymph node status
	Histological type
	Histological grade
	Venous invasion (intramural/extramural)
	Histological pattern of infiltrating margins (pushing–expanding/diffusely infiltrating)
Histology: margins	Involvement, minimal distance[c] for
	• proximal margin[d]
	• distal margin[d]
	• doughnut
	• circumferential (radial, lateral)[c]
	• resected adjacent organs[d]
Histology: additional lesions	Adenoma/dysplasia/familial adenomatous polyposis/ulcerative colitis/other chronic inflammatory bowel diseases/other

[a]In the case of multiple primary tumours, data for the most advanced tumour should be reported.
[b]Measurement on fresh specimen without tension/on fixed specimen, pinned/on fixed specimen, unpinned.
[c]Histological examination may be omitted if a rectal carcinoma does not invade perirectal tissues and if in colonic carcinoma the distance from the circumferential (mesocolic) margin is 15 mm or more.
[d]Histological examination only:
• if distance between border of the tumour and margin is <5 cm on fresh not-stretched specimen or <3 cm on fixed specimen;
• if histological grade is G3 or G4;
• if extensive lymphatic or venous invasion is present.

logical assessment and work-up (Table 6.7). In all pathology departments, the respective data should currently be collected and analysed. Any deviation from the usual values (ranges) and changes in frequencies should lead to careful analysis and response.

Special attention should be paid to careful examination of the circumferential resection margin[32,43] and lymph nodes because of the crucial prognostic significance of the respective findings. With regard to lymph-node examination, Lewin et al[47] stated: 'Evidence of a good nodal dissection is the finding of lymphoid tissue in the 1- to 3-mm range, with a sprinkling of pieces of fibrofatty tissue and small vessels ... Conversely, inadequate sampling is characterized by the finding of only few nodes measuring 1 cm or more.'

Pathology findings in resection specimens indicative of oncological quality of surgery

The most important goal of surgical treatment is to achieve complete tumour resection (R0 resection). Thus the rate of R0 resections related to all patients is an important intermediate indicator of quality. However, there are also some pathological findings on resection specimens that give further information on the oncological quality of surgery:

1. Evidence of local spillage of tumour cells: iatrogenic tumour perforation or tumour resection not en bloc with transection of tumour tissue? (See page 59)
2. Length of resected bowel: limited (segmental) resection or radical resection with ligature of the trunk of the supplying vessels?
3. In cases of colon carcinomas with multidirectional lymph drainage: dissection of one or two lymph drainage areas?
4. Number of removed lymph nodes (provided that there is an adequate node-examination technique)?
5. In rectal carcinoma of the upper third: distal margin of clearance in muscular wall as well as in mesorectum (no coning) not less than 5 cm in situ corresponding to 3 cm measured on the fresh resection specimen without tension?
6. In rectal carcinoma of the middle and lower third:
   - Careful gross inspection of the surface of the specimen: bilobed appearance of the

correctly mobilized mesorectum with intact smooth surface?
- Distal margin of clearance in muscular wall not less than 1 cm measured on the fresh resection specimen without tension?

Data on all these parameters are needed for a reasonable assessment of the oncological quality of surgical treatment.[43,45,46]

Quality assurance of clinical trials on adjuvant and neoadjuvant therapy: the surgical pathologist's point of view

From the point of view of a surgical pathologist who has spent many years directing a tumour registry and has intensively investigated prognostic factors in colorectal carcinoma, it is remarkable how many of the protocols on adjuvant or neoadjuvant therapy have failed to adequately consider quality assurance with regard to pathology and surgical treatment.[4,48]

In adjuvant treatment, the quality of pathological examination of resection specimens influences the selection of patients and thus the results. Therefore data indicating the quality of pathology (Table 6.7) must always be included in reports on respective clinical trials. The frequency of all tumour resections, of resections without and with microscopic residual tumour (R0, R1), and the pN classification for *all* patients seen at the institution(s) during the study period must be stated. This information indicates the general surgical attitude as well as the quality of pathological examination.

Tumour classification according to international recommendations is an important indicator of the quality of oncological studies. Any comparison of results will be made impossible by authors who do not classify their tumours according to the generally accepted international systems.

In presentation of results, a pooling of substages with different prognosis should be avoided. For stage III, a subdivision into the prognostically different subgroups pN1 versus pN2 is necessary: the 5-year survival rates are significantly different: for rectal carcinoma, observed 47% versus 34%, relative 59% versus 41% ($p < 0.05$); for colon carcinoma, observed 50% versus 34%, relative 68% versus 44% ($p < 0.01$).[49] Therefore, in studies with a limited number of patients, different treatment results for stage

Table 6.7 Quality indicators for pathological diagnosis (modified from references 45 and 46)

Parameter	Range		Indicative of
	Colon	Rectum	
Tumour type:			
Mucinous adenocarcinoma/frequency	~15%	~10%	Adherence to WHO classification
Tumour grade:			
High-grade/frequency	————20–25%————		
R classification:			
Frequency of R1 related to resections considered as complete by the surgeon	0–5%	5–10 (~20)%	Carefulness of histological examination of resection lines[a]
Regional lymph nodes:			
• Frequency of node-positive cases related to radical resections for cure (RO resections)	————40–50%————		Carefulness of histological examination of regional lymph-node drainage area[a]
• Number of examined nodes in radical standard resections for cure (RO)[b,c]/mean	————20–30————		
• Frequency of cases with fewer than 12 nodes[c]	————<5%————		

[a]Also influenced by the surgeon.
[b]Radical standard resection is defined as bowel resection with formal dissection of a single lymph-drainage area.
[c]Except cases with neoadjuvant therapy.

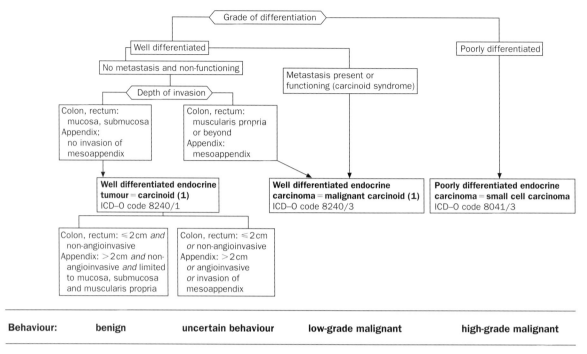

Behaviour: **benign**   **uncertain behaviour**   **low-grade malignant**   **high-grade malignant**

Note: (1) Well-differentiated endocrine tumours and carcinomas may be subdivided according to hormone production into serotonin-producing (ICD–O code 8241/1 or 3), enteroglucagon-producing (ICD–O 8157/1 or 3) and others.

Figure 6.4 WHO classification of endocrine tumours of appendix, colon and rectum.[7]

III may be explicable by different proportions of the substages.

In each report of results, the distribution of proven and probable *independent prognostic factors* (Table 6.6) is mandatory. In particular, the prognostic significance of the surgical treatment and the individual surgeon (see page 68) is extremely important in multicentre studies on adjuvant and neoadjuvant treatment. In such studies, quality assessment of surgery is crucial. However, in the most recent studies, surgery is still inadequately described, and thus the results of such studies are doubtful.[4,39] Therefore, for trials of adjuvant and neoadjuvant treatment, the surgical treatment has to be described in detail; the individual surgeon should of course be documented, by local code,[3] and stratification according to institution and individual surgeon should be considered.[48]

MALIGNANT TUMOURS OTHER THAN CARCINOMAS

Traditionally, *carcinoid tumours* have been separated from epithelial tumours and considered as endocrine or neuroendocrine neoplasms. Figure 6.4 shows the recently published WHO classification.[7] The criteria for assignment to the various tumour types are different for tumours of the appendix and for those of the colon and rectum.

Most endocrine tumours of the appendix are localized at the distal tip, and cause local symptoms leading to appendectomy. Most tumours produce serotonin and show benign behaviour. The uncommon malignant carcinoids require radical right hemicolectomy.

In the colon and rectum, the latter is the preferred site of endocrine tumours. They are mostly small asymptomatic well-differentiated tumours (carcinoids). They produce mainly enteroglucagon; definite hyperfunctional syndromes are mostly absent. Tumours less than 1–2 cm and limited to mucosa and submucosa are usually treated and cured by local excision, while in larger tumours and those invading beyond the submucosa, radical resection as in carcinomas is indicated. Colonic carcinoid tumours are usually larger and therefore more frequently malignant than those of the rectum. In about 5% of cases, multiple primary tumours are present. The course in the case of distant metastasis is often surprisingly prolonged; thus surgical treatment should be considered for patients with distant metastasis too.

Exocrine tumours frequently show a minority of dispersed endocrine cells. *Mixed exocrine–endocrine carcinomas* should be diagnosed only in the case of quantitatively balanced amounts of endocrine and exocrine components.

About 1% of all malignant colorectal tumours are *leiomyosarcomas* or so-called *gastrointestinal stromal tumours* (GIST). The latter term is a collective name for tumours in which an assignment as myogenic or neurogenic is not reliably possible.

Kaposi sarcoma in the colon and rectum is usually observed in patients with AIDS and Kaposi sarcoma of the skin or lymph nodes. In most cases, the involvement of the large intestine is clinically silent. Other malignant mesenchymal tumours are extremely rare.

Some *malignant melanomas* in the rectum (without involvement of the anal region) have been reported.

Primary colorectal lymphomas (no evidence of liver, spleen, non-mesenteric lymph node or bone marrow involvement at the time of presentation) are very rare, most cases involving the ileocaecal region and the rectum. Sometimes an association with ulcerous colitis or Crohn's disease has been observed. Grossly, a nodular or polypoid mass or a diffuse infiltrate may be present. The classification is not yet standardized.

For further details on non-carcinomatous malignant tumours see references 47 and 50.

REFERENCES

1. Fenoglio-Preiser CM, The distribution of large intestine lymphatics: relationship to risk of metastasis from carcinomas of the large intestine. In: *Adenomas Containing Carcinoma of the Large Bowel: Advances in Diagnosis and Therapy* (Fenoglio-Preiser CM, Rossini FP, eds). New York/Verona: Raven Cortina International, 1985.

2. Morson BC, *The Pathogenesis of Colorectal Cancer.* Philadelphia: WB Saunders, 1978.

3. Fielding LP, Arsenault PA, Chapuis PH et al, Clinicopathological staging for colorectal cancer: an International Documentation System (IDS) and an International Comprehensive Anatomical Terminology (ICAT). *J Gastroenterol Hepatol* 1991; **6:** 325–44.

4. Soreide O, Norstein J, Fielding LP, Silen W, International standardization and documentation of the treatment of rectal cancer. In: *Rectal Cancer Surgery. Optimisation – Standardisation – Documentation* (Soreide O, Norstein J, eds). Berlin: Springer-Verlag, 1997.

5. Jass JR, Sobin LH, *Histological Typing of Intestinal Tumours*, 2nd edn. WHO International Histological Classification of Tumours. Berlin: Springer-Verlag, 1989.

6. Hamilton SR, Aaltonen LA (eds), *Pathology and Genetics of Tumours of the Digestive System: World Health Organization Classification of Tumours.* Lyon: IARC, 2000.

7. Solcia E, Klöppel G, Sobin LH, *Histological Typing of Endocrine Tumours*, 2nd edn. WHO International Histological Classification of Tumours. Berlin: Springer-Verlag, 1999.

8. Hermanek P, Sobin LH, Colorectal carcinoma. In: *Prognostic Factors in Cancer* (Hermanek P, Gospodarowicz MK, Henson DE, Hutter RVP, Sobin LH, eds). Berlin: Springer-Verlag, 1995.

9. Compton C, Fenoglio-Preiser CM, Pettigrew N, Fielding LP, American Joint Committee on Cancer Prognostic Factors Consensus Conference: Colorectal Working Group. *Cancer* 2000; **88:** 1739–57.

10. Hobday TJ, Erlichman C, Colorectal cancer. In: *UICC: Prognostic Factors in Cancer*, 2nd edn (Gospodarowicz MK, Henson DE, Hutter RVP et al, eds). New York: Wiley, 2001.

11. Sobin LH, Wittekind C (eds), *UICC TNM Classification of Malignant Tumours*, 5th edn. New York: Wiley, 1999.

12. Dworak O, Morphology of lymph nodes in the resected rectum of patients with rectal carcinoma. *Pathol Res Pract* 1991; **187:** 1020–4.

13. Green SE, Bradburn DM, Varma JS, Burn J, Hereditary non-polyposis colorectal cancer. *Int J Colorect Dis* 1998; **13:** 3–12.

14. Lynch HT, Lynch JF, Genetics of colorectal cancer. *Digestion* 1998; **59:** 481–92.

15. Heald RJ, Ryall RD, Husband E, The mesorectum in rectal cancer surgery: clue to pelvic recurrence. *Br J Surg* 1982; **69:** 613–16.

16. Hohenberger W, Hermanek P Jr, Hermanek P, Gall FP, Decision-making in curative rectum carcinoma surgery. *Onkologie* 1992; **15:** 209–20.

17. Zirngibl H, Husemann B, Hermanek P, Intraoperative spillage of tumor cells in surgery for rectal cancer. *Dis Colon Rectum* 1990; **33:** 610–14.

18. Hermanek P Jr, Multiviscerale Resektion beim kolorektalen Karzinom-Erfahrungen der SGKRK-Studie. *Langenbecks Arch Chir* 1992; Suppl II (Kongreßber): 95–100.

19. Gall FP, Hermanek P, Update of the German experience with local excision of rectal cancer. *Surg Oncol Clin North Am* 1992; **1:** 99–109.

20. Hermanek P, Marzoli GP (eds), *Lokale Therapie des Rektumkarzinoms. Verfahren in kurativer Intention.* Berlin: Springer-Verlag, 1994.

21. Hermanek P, Giedl J, Neues aus der chirurgischen Pathologie des kolorektalen Karzinoms. *Wien med Wschr* 1988; **138:** 292–6.

22. Jatzko G, Lisberg P, Wette V, Improving survival rates for patients with colorectal cancer. *Br J Surg* 1992; **79:** 588–91.

23. Scholefield JH, Northover JMA, Surgical management of rectal

cancer. *Br J Surg* 1995; **82:** 745–8.

24. Pezim ME, Nicholls RJ, Survival after high or low ligation of the inferior mesenteric artery during curative surgery for rectal cancer. *Ann Surg* 1984; **200:** 729–33.

25. Dukes CE, The spread of cancer of the rectum. *Br J Surg* 1930; **12:** 643–8.

26. Kyriakos M, The President's cancer, the Dukes classification, and confusion. *Arch Path Labor Med* 1985; **109:** 1063–6.

27. NIH Consensus Conference, Adjuvant therapy for patients with colon and rectal cancer. *JAMA* 1990; **264:** 1444–50.

28. Hermanek P, Hutter RVP, Sobin LH, Wittekind Ch, Classification of isolated tumor cells and micrometastasis. Communication International Union Against Cancer. *Cancer* 1999; **86:** 2668–73.

29. Hermanek P, Henson DE, Hutter RVP, Sobin LH (eds), *UICC, TNM Supplement 1993. A Commentary on Uniform Use.* Berlin: Springer-Verlag, 1993.

30. Wittekind C, Henson DE, Hutter RVP, Sobin LH (eds), *UICC: TNM Supplement, 2nd edn.* New York: Wiley, 2001.

31. Fleming ID, Cooper JS, Henson DE et al (eds), *American Joint Committee on Cancer (AJCC) Cancer Staging Manual*, 5th edn. Philadelphia/New York: Lippincott-Raven, 1997.

32. Hermanek P, Wittekind Ch, The pathologist and the residual tumor (R) classification. *Pathol Res Pract* 1994; **190:** 115–23.

33. Dworak O, Keilholz L, Hoffmann A, Pathological features of rectal cancer after preoperative radiochemotherapy. *Int J Colorect Dis* 1997; **12:** 19–23.

34. Wagner G, Hermanek P, *Organspezifische Tumordokumentation.* Berlin: Springer-Verlag, 1995.

35. Hermanek P, Prognostic factor research in oncology. *J Clin Epidemiol* 1999; **52:** 371–4.

36. McArdle CS, Hole D, Impact of variability among surgeons on postoperative morbidity and mortality and ultimate survival. *BMJ* 1991; **302:** 1501–5.

37. Kessler H, Mansmann U, Hermanek P Jr et al, for the Study Group Colo-Rectal Carcinoma (SGCRC), Does the surgeon affect outcome in colon carcinoma? *Semin Colon Rectal Surg* 1998; **9:** 233–40.

38. Kessler H, Hermanek P, for the Study Group Colo-Rectal Carcinoma (SGCRC), Outcomes in rectal cancer surgery are directly related to technical factors. *Semin Colon Rectal Surg* 1998; **9:** 247–53.

39. Hermanek P, Impact of surgeon's technique on outcome after treatment of rectal carcinoma. *Dis Colon Rectum* 1999; **42:** 559–62.

40. Hermanek P (ed), *Diagnostische Standards. Lungen-, Magen-, Pankreas- und kolorektales Karzinom.* München: W Zuckschwerdt, 1995.

41. Association of Directors of Anatomical and Surgical Pathology, Recommendations for the reporting of resected large intestinal carcinomas. *Hum Pathol* 1996; **27:** 5–8.

42. Compton CC, Henson DE, Hutter RVP et al, for Members of the Cancer Committee, College of American Pathologists, Updated protocol for the examination of specimens removed from patients with colorectal carcinoma. *Arch Pathol Lab Med* 1997; **121:** 1247–54.

43. Quirke Ph, The pathologist, the surgeon and colorectal cancer – Get it right because it matters. *Progr Pathol* 1998; **4:** 201–13.

44. Rosai J, *Ackerman's Surgical Pathology*, 8th edn. St Louis, MO: Mosby, 1996.

45. Hermanek P, Qualitätsmanagment bei Diagnose und Therapie kolorektaler Karzinome. *Leber Magen Darm* 1996; **26:** 20–4.

46. Hermanek P, Qualität der Chirurgie aus der Sicht des Pathologen. In: *Rektumkarzinom: Das Konzept der Totalen Mesorektalen Exzision* (Büchler MW, Heald RJ, Maurer CA, Ulrich B, eds). Basel: Karger, 1998.

47. Lewin KJ, Riddell RH, Weinstein WM, *Gastrointestinal Pathology and its Clinical Implications.* Tokyo: Igaku-Shoin, 1992.

48. Hermanek P, Data collection aspects for the design of adjuvant treatment protocols in colorectal carcinoma. *Onkologie* 1991; **14:** 491–7.

49. Hermanek P, Long-term results of a German prospective multicenter study on colo-rectal cancer. In: *Recent Advances in Management of Digestive Cancer* (Takahashi T, ed). Tokyo: Springer-Verlag, 1993.

50. Fenoglio-Preiser CM, Noffsinger AE, Stemmermann GN et al, *Gastrointestinal Pathology*, 2nd edn. Philadelphia/New York: Lippincott-Raven, 1999.

7

Sentinel lymph-node mapping in colorectal cancer

Sukamal Saha, Anton Bilchik, David Wiese

INTRODUCTION

Colorectal cancer remains the fourth leading cause of cancer-related death worldwide, with the most recent published account of 783 000 new cases in 1990 causing about 437 000 deaths globally.[1] In the USA, it is the third most common cause of cancer-related mortality, with an estimated 129 400 new cases diagnosed in 1999 and 56 600 deaths.[2]

Lymph-node metastasis remains one of the most powerful and predictive prognostic factors for survival in most solid tumors, including colorectal cancer. Success of treatment is greatly influenced by appropriate staging of the disease. The basis of colorectal cancer staging depends upon evaluation of the primary tumor in the bowel as well as assessment of the regional lymph nodes in the adjacent mesentery for the presence of metastasis. Although the extent of resection for a particular tumor in the large bowel is fairly standardized, nodal staging is highly dependent on harvesting the lymph nodes from the adjacent mesentery and their pathologic assessment for metastatic disease. This undoubtedly varies greatly between pathologists and laboratories. Small (<5 mm) lymph nodes often may be missed, and lymph nodes draining directly from the primary tumor may not be harvested at all.[3] Although a technician can take over 1000 6 μm-thick sections from a 10 mm lymph node, usually only one or two such sections per lymph node are examined by the pathologist – and this is often considered the standard of care. Thus, there is a great probability that small metastatic lymph nodes, as well as those containing micrometastases, are being missed by routine pathologic examination.

About 55% of patients with colorectal cancers initially present with disease confined to the bowel wall (American Joint Committee on Cancer (AJCC) stage I or II disease). These patients are usually not treated with adjuvant chemotherapy outside a protocol, because of the paucity of data showing a survival advantage.[4] Nonetheless, about 20–30% of patients with so-called localized disease (AJCC stage I or II) develop systemic metastases within 5 years of diagnosis.[4] It is possible that failure to identify micrometastatic disease by routine pathologic examination of the lymph nodes may play a role in understaging the disease. Thus, patients with missed nodal disease may not receive chemotherapy, and this may have a negative impact on their survival. Various methods have been described in order to increase the yield of occult micrometastases in the lymph nodes (i.e. serial sectioning,[5] the fat clearing technique,[6] the pinning and stretching method,[7] immunohistochemistry,[8] etc.). Although such techniques are useful, they remain extremely labor-intensive and costly, and thus have not been adapted as standard pathologic practice.

The 'sentinel lymph node' (SLN) concept was originally proposed by Cabanas in 1977 for patients with carcinoma of the penis,[9] and was popularized by Morton and his colleagues for patients with melanoma.[10] The SLN is the first node on the direct lymphatic pathway from the primary tumor. Thus, the SLN is the first one (or few) lymph nodes most likely to harbor metastatic cells when a regional nodal metastasis takes place. Numerous publications in the last seven or eight years have described the usefulness of the SLN mapping technique for the diagnosis of nodal micrometastases in melanoma and breast cancers.[11–13] Morton and colleagues have shown that in patients with malignant melanoma, the status of SLNs reflects the histologic features of the remainder of the lymphatic basin with more than 98% accuracy.[10] Many authors have confirmed since then the validity of accurate staging by the SLN mapping technique in melanoma and breast cancer.[11-13] The identification of one to four such SLNs in the direct lymphatic pathway from the primary tumor allows the pathologist to perform meticulous histologic and immunohistochemical studies by multi-level microsections. Such a detailed analysis of all the lymph nodes resected would be extremely cost-prohibitive. Yet analysis of these few 'high-risk' SLNs would greatly enhance the diagnosis of nodal micrometastases that could have been missed by routine pathologic examinations. Patients who are upstaged by the diagnosis of occult micrometastases in the SLNs may then receive adjuvant chemotherapy, and this may lead to an increase in survival.

PERSONAL SERIES

For the first time in the world, our group has performed a prospective study for SLN mapping in patients with colorectal cancer.[14] The purpose of the study was fourfold: (1) to determine the feasibility of SLN mapping using isosulfan blue dye (Lymphazurin 1%; Ben Venue Labs, Inc., Bedford, OH); (2) to assess the accuracy of the SLNs in determining the status of regional nodes; (3) to identify any aberrant mesenteric lymphatic drainage patterns; (4) to assess the limitations of the technique in patients with colorectal cancer.

PATIENTS AND METHODS

From October 1996 to March 1999, 101 consecutive patients with the diagnosis of colorectal cancer were prospectively entered into the study. There were 48 males and 53 females, with ages ranging from 36 to 97 years (mean 71 years). Preoperative evaluation included a complete history and physical examination, complete blood counts, liver function study, carcinoembryonic antigen (CEA), colonoscopy, and computed tomography of the abdomen and pelvis. At operation, the abdomen was explored to confirm the site of the primary tumor and any distant metastases. Some mobilization of the bowel away from the tumor was needed to deliver the bowel adjoining the

tumor near the surface. Mesenteric dissection was kept at a minimum to prevent disruption of the lymphatic pathway. With a tuberculin syringe, 1–2 ml of isosulfan blue dye was injected subserosally around the tumor in a circumferential manner without injecting into the lumen. For low- and mid-rectal lesions, the tumor was visualized through a proctoscope, and approximately 2 ml of the dye was injected transanally in the submucous layer using a spinal needle. Within 5–10 minutes of injection, the dye then travels via the lymphatics to the nearby lymph nodes and turns them pale to dark blue. The first one to four such blue nodes near the tumor with the most direct drainage from the primary tumor are considered as SLN(s). The SLNs, as they turn blue, can be better visualized on the posterior or retroperitoneal surface of the mesentery (Figure 7.1), usually lying along the main feeding vessels. They are marked with sutures as 1st, 2nd, 3rd, or 4th SLN(s), and are not removed immediately. Once these nodes have been marked with suture, a standard oncologic resection with segmental colectomy and regional lymphadenectomy is performed. The identification of the SLNs may be difficult in patients with thick mesentery, where some cautery dissection may be needed to expose the SLNs. For mid- to low-rectal lesions, immediate bedside dissection of the specimen to identify the most directly draining blue lymph node(s) adjacent to the tumor is done to mark the SLN(s).

PATHOLOGIC EVALUATION

Pathologic examination of the SLNs is critical for accurate staging of the disease. Once the SLNs have been tagged with suture in the operative suite, the entire specimen is sent to the pathology laboratory. The SLNs are dissected free from the specimen. These lymph nodes are sectioned grossly at about 2–3 mm intervals, and are blocked separately in individual cassettes. The remainder of the specimen is dissected and sampled for routine evaluation by standard pathologic methods. It is recommended that pericolic mesenteric tissue be post-fixed in Carnoy's fluid for 2–14 hours to assist in the identification of additional non-SLNs. On average, a total of 15–20 lymph nodes should be recovered from a standard colorectal resection specimen.

For each SLN, usually a total of 10 sections are cut through the blocks, at a thickness of 4 μm each about

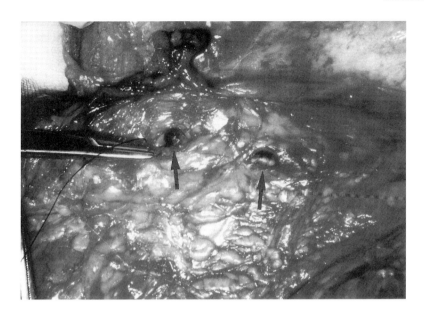

Figure 7.1 Two blue SLNs (arrows) on the retroperitoneal surface of the mesentery, in a patient with ascending colon cancer, being marked with suture.

20–40 μm apart. One of the sections, usually at the 5th level, is immunostained for the demonstration of low-molecular-weight cytokeratin (AE-1; Ventana, Tucson, AZ). The other sections are stained routinely with hematoxylin and eosin (H&E).

RESULTS

Of the 101 consecutive patients in this study, 90 had colon and 11 had rectal cancer. The numbers and actual locations of the primary tumors were as follows: cecum 17; right colon 28; transverse colon 11; splenic flexure 2; left colon 2; sigmoid colon 20; rectosigmoid colon 10; rectum 11. The SLN mapping technique successfully identified one to four SLN(s) in 100 (99%) of the 101 patients. One patient with a low rectal cancer was treated with preoperative chemo-radiotherapy. No SLN was identified in this patient, although 1 of 43 lymph nodes was positive for metastasis. The analysis that follows is based on results for the remaining 100 consecutive patients, in all of whom at least one SLN was identified. A total of 1642 lymph nodes (mean 16.4 per patient) were examined, of which 165 (mean 1.6 per patient) lymph nodes were identified as SLN(s). The distribution and pattern of nodal metastases are shown in Table 7.1. As in melanoma and breast cancer, more than

one SLN was found in 54% of patients. In 58 (95%) of the 61 patients, the SLNs, as well as all non-SLNs, were without any metastasis. In the other 3 patients, the SLNs were negative, but 5 non-SLNs were positive for metastases (skip metastases). In 39 patients, the SLNs had metastases; of these, in 19 patients, the SLNs were the only site of metastasis, with all other non-SLNs being negative. In 10 of these 39 patients, micrometastases were found only in one or two microsections of a single SLN (Figure 7.2) (four were confirmed only by immunohistochemistry). These 10% of patients therefore had occult micrometastases.

In 2 patients, the SLN mapping technique detected an aberrant lymphatic pathway, thus altering the extent of surgery. Overall, the specificity of SLN mapping for colorectal cancer in our series of 100 patients was 100%, with a sensitivity of 93% and a negative predictive value of 95%. Solitary metastasis in one SLN, as was found in 19% of patients, may have upstaged these patients from AJCC stage I/II to stage III, and they may then benefit from adjuvant chemotherapy.

To evaluate whether the higher incidence of micrometastases in the SLNs, as opposed to the non-SLNs, might be due to an increased number of microsectionings of the SLNs, all non-SLNs, as well as SLNs from the first 25 consecutive patients, were

Table 7.1 Distribution of numbers and incidence of metastases in the SLNs

Total number of patients with SLN(s)	100/101 (99%)
Total number of lymph nodes	1642 (16.4 per patient)
Total number of SLNs	165 (1.6 per patient)

One SLN	46%
Two SLNs	44%
Three SLNs	9%
Four SLNs	1%

Patients with negative SLN	61%
Patients with positive SLN	39%
Patients with negative SLN and positive non-SLNs	3% (skip metastases)
Patients with solitary metastasis in SLN	19%
Patients with isolated micrometastases in SLN	10%
Patients with positive immunohistochemistry and negative H&E	4%

sectioned at 10 levels. Of the 390 lymph nodes examined (average 15.6 per patient), 13 (36%) of the 36 SLNs were positive for metastases, while only 24 (7%) of the 354 non-SLNs had metastases. When all the initially negative non-SLNs were sectioned at 10 levels and reexamined, only 0.6% (2 of 330 lymph nodes) revealed previously undetected micrometastases.[15] These results not only confirm the well-known fact that the distribution of metastases is reflective of the lymphatic drainage, but also confirm that there may be no further benefit in performing multilevel sections of the non-SLNs in standard practice.

ROLE OF LAPAROSCOPY IN SLN MAPPING FOR COLORECTAL CANCER

Laparoscopic colon surgery is increasingly being used for benign conditions. The reported benefits for this technique include reduction in cost and improvement in quality of life. Its role in malignancy is unclear. Inadequate resection, leaving behind metastatic lymph nodes, and port-site recurrences are among the arguments given against laparoscopic colon resection for colorectal cancer. We therefore evaluated the potential role of lymphatic mapping in laparoscopic colon resection for cancer. Seven patients with early colon cancer (malignant polyps, T1–T2 lesions) underwent lymphatic mapping. After the abdomen was insufflated to a pressure of 15 mmHg, a laparoscope was inserted into the abdominal cavity. A colonoscope was then introduced transrectally and the lumen of the colon was transilluminated. An endobabcock was placed around the colon distal to the tip of the colonoscope to facilitate visualization of the tumor or primary site. Isosulfan blue dye 0.5–1 ml was then injected submucosally at the periphery of the tumor or the polypectomy site at four quadrants via the colonoscope. The primary site was then identified and the blue lymphatic channel followed to the SLN(s) by the laparoscope. The SLN(s) were identified and marked with a suture or a clip. Following this, a standard laparoscopic colectomy was performed, including the tagged SLN(s) within the resected specimen.

Colonoscopic injection and the lymphatic mapping added approximately 20 minutes to the operating time. In all seven cases, the primary site and an average of two SLNs per patient were identified. The SLN correctly identified the nodal status of the entire

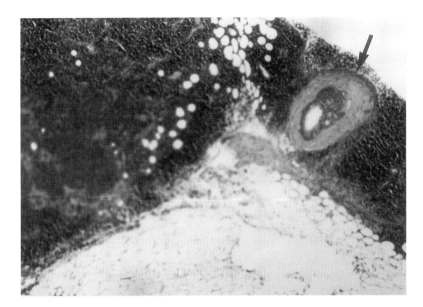

Figure 7.2 Micrometastasis (arrow) seen in a solitary 7 mm SLN after multilevel microsection (×40).

resected specimen in all cases. In one case, the mapping demonstrated aberrant drainage that altered the margins of resection. In another case, the SLN was negative by H&E but positive by cytokeratin, thereby upstaging this patient from AJCC stage I to stage III disease. Thus, this laparoscopic technique may be used to identify the primary site, demonstrate aberrant lymphatic pathways, and identify the most important lymph node (SLN) draining the primary site.

ULTRASTAGING BY IMMUNOHISTOCHEMISTRY AND RT-PCR

Although H&E staining is the gold standard for the diagnosis of metastasis in the lymph nodes, 15–20% of the cases of occult micrometastasis may be missed by routine H&E examination.

Multiple studies have been published[7,16–18] regarding the method of immunostaining with cytokeratin for the diagnosis of occult nodal micrometastasis. Immunohistochemical studies can be performed on paraffin-embedded tissue samples. The interpretation of a positive reaction requires that the positive staining be present in cells that exhibit a malignant cytologic feature, preferably in cellular clusters in a subcapsular sinus location (Figure 7.3). The possibility of benign epithelial inclusions must be eliminated

before accepting a positive staining result.

An even more sensitive molecular technique using the reverse-transcriptase polymerase chain reaction (RT-PCR) has been developed to further upstage node-negative patients.[19] It is extremely important to avoid contamination of the SLNs by tumor cells at the time of pathologic dissection in order to avoid a false-positive result.

Since it is not practical to perform RT-PCR on all resected lymph nodes, we applied this technology to the SLNs. Specific primers targeting mRNA expression of tumor markers expressed in colon cancer were used. The advantage of this multiple-marker RT-PCR assay is that even though these tumors can be heterogeneous, the possibility of detection of micrometastases is increased. We have demonstrated concordance between the primary tumor and the SLNs, and 30% of patients were upstaged in this study.[20]

CONCLUSIONS

Multiple studies have confirmed the high accuracy of the SLN mapping technique in correctly predicting the presence of micrometastases in regional lymph nodes of patients with malignant melanoma and breast cancer.[10–13]

The first report of the SLN mapping technique in

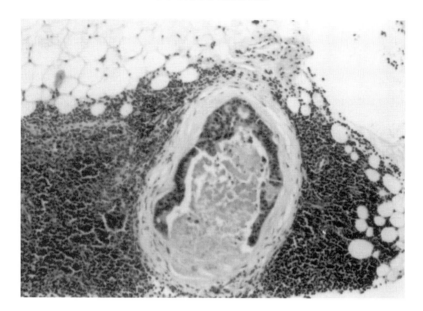

Figure 7.3 Positive immunohistochemistry stain for cytokeratin in a solitary SLN (×100).

colorectal cancer was given by our group in 1997 at the annual meeting of the Society of Surgical Oncology.[21] Since then, our studies have further confirmed that, as in melanoma and breast cancer, SLNs can be localized in a high (99%) number of cases with a high degree of accuracy (97%) in colorectal cancer patients. The only failure of identification of an SLN in a patient with low-rectal cancer may be due to submucosal fibrosis of the lymphatics resulting from neoadjuvant radiotherapy. Despite the technical difficulty associated with peritumoral injection of the dye in rectal tumors, SLN mapping was successful in 10 (91%) of 11 patients with rectal cancer as compared with all patients with colon cancer. Three patients with skip metastases in this series included one patient with two closely situated primary tumors, one patient with perforated carcinoma, and one patient with previous colon surgery. Thus, potential limitations of this technique in colorectal cancer may include previous surgery, radiation therapy, perforation, and possibly multiple primaries.

In both melanoma and breast cancer, a combination of radionuclide dye and isosulfan blue dye is used for optimal SLN mapping in most reported series. Radionuclide dye was unnecessary for SLN mapping in colorectal cancer, which reduces the cost of the procedure ($31 per vial of the dye). Furthermore, the majority of the SLNs were found within 7 cm of the primary tumor site within the mesentery. The proximity to the primary site could lead to a 'shine-through' effect, reducing the sensitivity of the radioactivity of the SLNs. Owing to this and other logistic problems involved with the use of radiolabeled material in the operating room, no attempt was made to use this for SLN mapping in colorectal cancer. Unlike melanoma and breast cancer, a much shorter learning curve is anticipated in performing this technique because of the ease in identifying the blue nodes and most general surgeons' relative familiarity with performing routine colorectal surgery.

One of the main advantages of SLN mapping in patients with melanoma and breast cancer is that it allows the surgeon to avoid routine radical lymphadenectomy in patients with negative SLNs. In our study, no attempt was made to perform less than a standard oncologic colon resection. Instead, our focus was to identify the few 'high-risk' SLNs that have the highest probability of harboring micrometastases. Pathologists can then perform more meticulous examinations on these few nodes by means of multilevel microsections. Indeed, 19% of patients may have been upstaged to AJCC stage III disease. In particular, micrometastases seen in one or two microsections of a single SLN, in 10% of patients, most probably would have been missed by conventional pathologic examination. Thus, these patients truly were upstaged from AJCC stage I/II to stage III. Patients whose disease is upstaged on discovery of such micrometastases can be offered adjuvant chemotherapy, with the potential for improved survival.

The prognostic significance of occult micrometastases has been confirmed in many studies for breast cancer[22] and melanoma.[11] As this technique identifies a significant number (19%) of cases of colorectal cancer with occult micrometastases, we believe that effective systemic chemotherapy may play an important role in changing the prognosis of these patients. The implication of RT-PCR analysis for micrometastasis in colorectal cancer is evolving. Liefers et al[23] have shown a significant survival advantage for RT-PCR-negative patients with stage II colorectal cancer as opposed to RT-PCR-positive patients (5-year survival rates of 75% versus 36%). Owing to its potential in predicting this survival advantage, an ongoing RT-PCR study is being done for patients undergoing SLN mapping, the results of which will be published soon.

As the application of SLN mapping is being expanded for other solid neoplasms,[24] we hope that its use in colorectal cancer will become part of the standard practice of the general surgeon, given its simplicity, high accuracy, and low cost, and its aid to pathologists in focusing their attention on one to four nodes for detailed analysis, thereby upstaging a significant number of patients. A larger multi-institution study is warranted to evaluate the potential implications of the SLN mapping technique in colorectal cancer patients for appropriate therapeutic planning and to determine its impact on survival.

REFERENCES

1. Parkin DN, Pisani P, Ferlay J, Global cancer statistics. *CA Cancer J Clin* 1999; **49:** 33–64.
2. Landis SH, Murray T, Bolden S et al, Cancer statistics 1999. *CA Cancer J Clin* 1999; **49:** 8–31.
3. Rodriguez-Bigas MA, Maamoun S, Weber TK et al, Clinical significance of colorectal cancer: metastases in lymph nodes <5 mm in size. *Ann Surg Oncol* 1996; **3:** 124–30.
4. Cohen AM, Kelsen D, Saltz L et al, Adjuvant therapy for colorectal cancer. *Curr Prob Cancer* 1998; **22:** 5–77.
5. Pickreen JW, Significance of occult metastases, a study of breast cancer. *Cancer* 1961; **14:** 1261–71.
6. Cawthorn SJ, Gibbs NM, Marks CG, Clearance technique for the detection of lymph nodes in colorectal cancer. *Br J Surg* 1986; **73:** 58–60.
7. Crucitti F, Doglietto GB, Bellantone R et al, Accurate specimen preparation and examination is mandatory to detect lymph nodes and avoid understaging in colorectal cancer. *J Surg Oncol* 1992; **51:** 153–8.
8. Greenson JK, Isenhart CE, Rice R et al, Identification of occult micrometastases in pericolic lymph nodes of Dukes' B colorectal cancer patients using monoclonal antibodies against cytokeratin and CC49. *Cancer* 1994; **73:** 563–9.
9. Cabanas RM, An approach for treatment of penile carcinoma. *Cancer* 1977; **39:** 456–66.
10. Morton DL, Wen DR, Wong JH et al, Technical details of intraoperative lymphatic mapping for early stage melanoma. *Arch Surg* 1992; **127:** 392–9.
11. Reintgen D, Haddad F, Pendas S et al, Lymphatic mapping and sentinel lymph node biopsy. *Sci Am* 1998; **17:** 1–17.
12. Guiliano AE, Kirgan DM, Guenther JM et al, Lymphatic mapping and sentinel lymphadenectomy for breast cancer. *Ann Surg* 1994; **220:** 391–401.
13. Cox CE, Haddad F, Bass S et al, Lymphatic mapping in the treatment of breast cancer. *Oncology* 1998; **12:** 1283–98.
14. Saha S, Accurate staging of colorectal cancer by SLN mapping – a prospective study. In: Post Graduate Course 22, *Annual Meeting American College of Surgeons, 1999*: 34–7.
15. Wiese D, Saha S, Badin J, Sentinel lymph node mapping in staging of colorectal cancer. *Am J Clin Pathol* 1999; **112:** 542 (abstract).
16. Bertoglio S, Percivale P, Gambini C et al, Cytokeratin immunostaining reveals micrometastasis in negative hematoxylin–eosin lymph nodes of resected stage I–II (PT2–pT3) colorectal cancer. *J Chemother* 1997; **9:** 119–20.
17. Oberg A, Stenling R, Tavelin B, Lindmark G, Are lymph node micrometastases of any clinical significance in Dukes' stages A and B colorectal cancer? *Dis Colon Rectum* 1998; **41:** 1244–9.
18. Broll R, Schauer V, Schimmelpenning H et al, Prognostic relevance of occult tumor cells in lymph nodes of colorectal carcinomas. *Dis Colon Rectum* 1997; **40:** 1465–71.
19. Mori M, Mimori K, Inoue H et al, Detection of cancer micrometastases in lymph nodes by reverse transcriptase polymerase chain reaction. *Cancer Res* 1995; **55:** 3417–20.
20. Bilchik AJ, Saha S, Wiese D et al, Molecular staging of early colon cancer on the basis of sentinel node analysis: a multicenter phase II trial. *J Clin Oncol* 2001; **19:** 1128–36.
21. Saha S, Ganatra BK, Gauthier J et al, Localizations of sentinel lymph node (SLN) in colon cancer – a feasibility study. In: *Cancer Symposium (Abstract Book – Society of Surgical Oncology)*, 1997: 54.
22. International Ludwig Breast Cancer Study Group, Prognostic importance of occult axillary lymph node micrometastases from breast cancers. *Lancet* 1990; **335:** 1565–8.
23. Liefers G, Cleton-Jansen C, Van de Velde C et al, Micrometastases and survival in stage II colorectal cancer. *N Engl J Med* 1998; **339:** 223–8.
24. Bilchik A, Giuliano A, Essner R et al, Universal application of intraoperative lymphatic mapping and sentinel lymphadenectomy in solid neoplasms. *Cancer J Sci Am* 1998; **4:** 351–8.

8

Postoperative histopathological evaluation: Implications for prognosis?

Fred T Bosman

INTRODUCTION

Histopathological examination of biopsy and surgical specimens plays an important role in the clinical management of patients with colorectal cancer. In order to establish a final diagnosis in endoscopically suspected cancer, histological examination of small biopsy specimens is indispensable. To verify the nature of a polyp, histological examination of the endoscopic resection specimen is important. When a carcinoma is found in a polyp, the depth of invasion and the status of the resection margins will also indicate whether or not additional treatment might be necessary. Examination of surgical resection specimens of colorectal carcinoma is performed in order to verify the diagnosis, determine the stage and grade of the tumour, and establish the lymph node status and the completeness of the resection. It is the purpose of this chapter to briefly review the pathological procedures concerning the work-up of a resection specimen and to discuss in depth which pathological parameters play a role in clinical decision making and to what extent this may change in the (near) future.

PATHOLOGICAL EXAMINATION OF A SURGICAL RESECTION SPECIMEN

Careful macroscopy is an essential first step in the work-up of a resection specimen. The work-up will differ significantly between colectomy and rectal resection specimens. Whatever the origin of the specimen, inspection of the lateral margins of resection is important. When the macroscopic tumour margin is less than 5 cm from the lateral resection margin, histological examination of this margin is essential. Serial sectioning of the tumour mass is important to judge the depth of infiltration into the bowel wall. Tissue samples will be taken of the area of deepest infiltration. For colectomy specimens, the orientation of serial sectioning is less important. For rectal resection specimens, this has to be perpendicular to the axis of the lumen after marking of the circumferential surface. Detailed examination of the minimal distance between the circumferential (inked) margin and the point of deepest infiltration is important.[1] Pericolic/rectal fat will be carefully dissected in order to obtain a maximum number of lymph nodes for histological examination. To facilitate the detection of lymph nodes, clearance of the fat can be very helpful.[2] Much has been said and written about the minimum number of lymph nodes to be sampled for reliable lymph-node staging. A minimum of six nodes is important.[3] The sites of lymph nodes will be carefully recorded:[4] adjacent to the tumour, proximal to the tumour, distal to the tumour, and in the resection margin – along the larger vessels.

Microscopy will reveal the nature of the tumour (usually an adenocarcinoma), the subtype (mucinous or colloid carcinoma can be distinguished as subtypes), and the degree of differentiation, which is conventionally graded as well, moderately, and poorly differentiated. Modern histochemical and molecular techniques allow a more detailed description of the characteristics of the tumour, as will be discussed later. The depth of invasion will be recorded for colon carcinomas and the minimal distance between the invasion front and the circumferential margin for rectal tumours.[5] Additional relevant parameters are the pattern of extension (pushing or invasive), angio-invasion, perineural invasion, and lymphoid inflammatory response.[6–8] The resection margins will be histologically examined, as well as the lymph nodes. For standard procedures, one section of all lymph nodes found will be studied without special techniques, such as immuno-histochemistry. The number of positive lymph nodes relative to the total number per level will be recorded. All of these parameters will be included in the final conclusion, which will end with a classification of the tumour according to stage. It is our standard procedure to stage the tumours according to the Astler–Collier modification of the original Dukes classification, to the TNM classification, and to the Jass classification, although the latter is not universally applied. A comparison of the first two staging systems is provided in Figure 8.1.

PROGNOSTIC SIGNIFICANCE OF CLASSICAL PARAMETERS

It is generally recognized that tumour stage, conventionally expressed in the Dukes classification, is the most powerful predictor of final outcome.[12] There is a clear tendency towards use of the TNM system, in particular with stage grouping according to the American Joint Committee on Cancer (AJCC).[13] The latter staging system is almost congruent with the Dukes classification. The 5-year survival rate according to Dukes stage is presented in Table 8.1. The

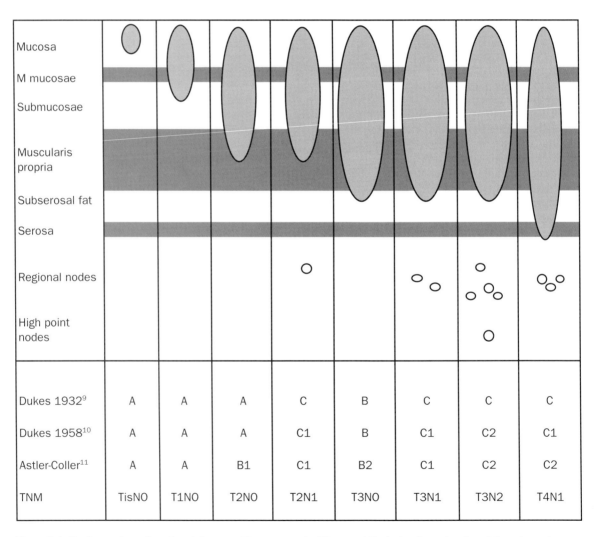

Dukes 1932[9]	A	A	A	C	B	C	C	C
Dukes 1958[10]	A	A	A	C1	B	C1	C2	C1
Astler-Coller[11]	A	A	B1	C1	B2	C1	C2	C2
TNM	TisN0	T1N0	T2N0	T2N1	T3N0	T3N1	T3N2	T4N1

Figure 8.1 Staging systems for colorectal cancer. The upper part of the panel illustrates the extension of the primary tumour through the layers of the bowel wall.[9–11]

Table 8.1 Survival rates for colorectal cancer according to the Dukes and TNM classifications			
Dukes stage	5-year survival rate (%)	TNM stage	5-year survival rate (%)
A	80	0	75
		I (A + B)	
B	65	II	60
C	25	III	30
D	10	IV	5

Dukes and the TNM classifications do not take angio-invasion, perineural invasion and lymphoid inflammatory response into account. The TNM classification supplies a subdivision of the N status. Although there is a generally shared feeling that the prognosis decreases with more positive nodes and more widespread nodal involvement, this has not been adequately validated.[4] Venous invasion is a prognostically useful characteristic of proven value, and ought to be included in prognostic algorithms.[5,14] This might also be true for perineural invasion, although this has not been adequately proven. Lymphocytic infiltration, as proposed by Shepherd et al,[8] has also been used by others,[7,15] but has not been proven to be consistently valid as a prognostic parameter, partly because its grading lacks reproducibility. In rectal cancer, the minimal distance to the circumferential margin of resection is an important predictor for recurrent disease. This has led to the use of this parameter as a decisive element in determining whether or not postoperative adjuvant radiotherapy might be necessary.[16]

PROGNOSTIC SIGNIFICANCE OF NEWER TUMOUR PARAMETERS

The introduction into diagnostic histopathology of methods developed in cell and molecular biology has enabled a much more detailed analysis of tumour cell characteristics. These developments include histochemical staining – which allows detailed characterization of differentiation at the level of proteins and mRNA, of proliferation and apoptotic activity, and of invasive behaviour and metastatic spread – and also molecular genetic analysis – which allows detailed characterization of genetic aberrations in the tumour cells. Many of these new parameters have already been proven of prognostic relevance in retro-

spective studies. Very few have been used as discriminating parameters in clinical management, however.

Parameters related to invasion and metastasis

The impact of lymph-node metastases on prognosis has been an important reason why several groups have studied the yield of lymph-node metastases by immunohistochemical staining for micrometastases, mostly using antibodies against cytokeratins. Several studies have indeed shown that this approach yields micrometastases in 25% of cases that could have otherwise been classified as node-negative.[17,18] The impact of this result on prognosis, however, is not yet resolved. Jeffers et al[17] did not find any relationship between lymph-node micrometastases and prognosis, whereas Greenson et al[18] found better prognosis in Dukes B patients without metastases than in those with micrometastases. There is a strong tendency towards the introduction of polymerase chain reaction (PCR)-based methods for the analysis of tumour spread, not only in lymph nodes but also systemically via the circulation.[19] In most of these studies, PCR is used to detect mRNA coding either for cytokeratins[20] or for carcinoembryonic antigen (CEA).[21,22] Using such an approach, Liefers et al[23] found 50% of histologically node-negative cases to harbour tumour cells. Whether or not the detected cells were passing through the lymph node or had already established a growing metastasis cannot be determined, since this approach does not allow histological verification of the assayed sample. Some authors claim that such 'micrometastases' have prognostic impact.[23,24] Others have been unable to confirm this.[25] The same holds true for the PCR detection of circulating tumour cells.[26] Only careful prospective studies using such parameters will tell whether or not these sensitive assays might contribute to the clinical management of the disease.

In line with the importance of metastases, invasive behaviour of the tumour or cellular characteristics indicative of invasive behaviour have been studied in detail. An interesting approach was proposed by Hase et al,[27] who distinguished between two patterns of invasion: irregular tumour cell budding at the invasive front versus a straight 'pushing' tumour margin. Irregular budding invasion was associated with a poorer survival, even after stratification for Dukes stage. The problem with these parameters is that they can only be assessed more or less subjectively, which lacks reproducibility. For this reason, such parameters will not solve problems of staging.

With the rapidly advancing insights into the mechanisms of tumour cell invasion, numerous attempts have already been made to develop new prognostic parameters based upon the molecular actors involved in this highly complex process. Invasion implies *proteolytic degradation of the extracellular matrix* surrounding the tumour cells, a *stromal response* to this aggressive tumour cell behaviour, *dissolution of intercellular adhesion*, which is mediated by cell adhesion molecules, and *migration through the extracellular matrix*, which involves cell–matrix interaction and activation of the tumour cell cytoskeleton. All of these processes have been studied in connection with prognosis.

Matrix proteases belonging to the plasminogen activator (PA)–plasmin system have been studied repeatedly as prognostic factors in colorectal cancer.[28–30] Urokinase (uPA) staining appeared to be predictive for the development of liver metastases.[28,29] Ganesh et al[30] determined the components of the system, including uPA, tissue plasminogen activator (tPA), and the inhibitors PAI-1 and PAI-2 by immunoassay. A high ratio of uPA in cancer tissue to tPA in normal tissue and a high level of PAI-2 were predictive of poor outcome. Murray et al[31] found expression of matrix metalloproteinase 1 (MMP-1), an interstitial collagenase, to be associated with poor prognosis. Sunami et al,[32] however, found better prognosis for high MMP-1 expressing cancers.

Stromal response, in terms of basement membrane deposition in the tumour centre, was studied by Havenith et al[32] and subsequently by Offerhaus et al.[34] Consistently, an extensive deposition of basement membrane material around tumour cell nests was indicative of a favourable prognosis. This phenomenon has been explained in terms of a protective effect of the host response against the tumour. A somewhat contrasting observation is the association of a pronounced desmoplastic response at the tumour edge with unfavourable prognosis.[35] Microvessel formation, indicating active angiogenesis, is an integral element of the stromal response. Abdalla et al[36] found high microvessel counts to be correlated with good prognosis. In multivariate analysis, however, this parameter was not an independent predictor.[37]

Extensive attention has been paid to expression of cell adhesion molecules and prognosis, following the observation that loss of E-cadherin expression in carcinoma cells in model systems induced invasive behaviour. The E-cadherin–catenin complex plays an important structural role in linking desmosomes with the cytoskeleton. The *APC* gene, whose mutations are responsible for familial adenomatous polyposis coli (FAP), is also implicated in the interaction of the E-cadherin–catenin complex with the cytoskeleton.[38] E-cadherin normally uses β-catenin as a link with the cytoskeleton. Apart from their role in this complex and thus in cell–cell adhesion, β-catenin and *APC* also function in the Wnt signalling pathway, which is almost invariably disturbed in colorectal cancer.[39] Mutations in *APC* or the β-catenin gene inhibit their complex-forming capacity, which results in accumulation of β-catenin in the cytoplasm and the nucleus. In the nucleus, β-catenin activates the transcription factors Lef/Tcf, and cell proliferation ensues.

The prognostic value of expression of members of the E-cadherin–catenin complex has recently been studied. It has become clear that cadherin mutations are rare, its apparent loss of expression during invasion being due to downregulated expression.[40] Mutations of the β-catenin gene occur regularly. Expression levels essentially parallel the differentiation level of the tumours. A prognostic value was reported for E-cadherin expression in colorectal cancer, but this was largely accounted for by tumour grade.[41,42] Interestingly, patterns of expression were almost identical in primary lesions and in the corresponding metastases.[43,44] A practical limitation of E-cadherin expression is that loss of immunohistochemical staining is rather difficult to score. As yet, the E-cadherin–catenin complex and the Wnt signalling pathway are more of tumour biological than of clinical interest.

The CD44 family of hyaluronan receptors has attracted much attention, following reports that expression of splice variants of CD44 (most notably the v6 variant) is correlated with unfavourable prognosis.[45] Several papers have confirmed the value of CD44v6 expression as an independent prognostic variable,[46] but this has been contested, leaving the value of CD44v6 expression somewhat disputed.[47] Another group of genes with a disputed role in colorectal cancer prognosis are the *nm23* genes. Loss of expression of *nm23* has been reported to correlate with the occurrence of distant metastases in colorectal cancer,[48] but others have been unable to confirm this finding.[49] A newly discovered gene that seems to be implicated in colorectal cancer metastasis is *Drg-1*. Its potential clinical use, however, remains to be established.[50]

Parameters related to proliferation and apoptosis

Tumour behaviour is determined to a significant extent by the capacity of the cancer cells to multiply and hence increase tumour volume. In recent years, it has become clear that not only cell proliferation but also cell loss determines the rate of volume increase of a tumour. Cell loss is largely determined by apoptosis, i.e. programmed cell death.

Several possibilities are available for the determination of proliferative activity. The most conventional is a mitotic count, but this is not a very reliable parameter. Through cytometric analysis of cellular DNA content, the fraction of cancer cells in S phase of the cell cycle can be determined. This technique has some limitations, however. Tumour cell populations tend to have multiple stem lines with variable DNA content, which makes the determination of an S-phase fraction unreliable. Also, when paraffin-embedded material is analysed, which has become the most frequently applied method, determination of the S-phase fraction is unreliable.[51] Nonetheless, prognostic significance of a high S-phase fraction has been reported.[52]

Cell-cycle regulators have been studied to some extent in colorectal cancer in a prognostic context. Palmqvist et al[53] reported a strong correlation between p27/Kip1 expression and prognosis and Handa et al[54] found a similar correlation for cyclin A. Analysis of cell proliferation has become popular with the introduction of the immunohistochemical methods to determine the growth fraction of a tumour cell population. The best available technique is labelling of the Ki-67 antigen, using the MIB-1 antibody in paraffin sections. Using these techniques, multivariate analysis of patient populations has shown that cancer cell proliferative index is an independent predictor of tumour behaviour.[55]

Techniques are now also available for the histochemical staining of apoptotic cells. These techniques rely on detection of internucleosomal DNA fragmen-

tation, which is an early phenomenon in apoptotic cells. This so-called in situ nick-end labelling (ISEL or TUNEL) has been used by several investigators. The findings are not yet conclusive, but tend to favour a positive correlation between higher apoptotic index and better prognosis.[56] Much has become known about the molecular events that precede apoptosis. In the regulating pathways, the tumour suppressor gene *TP53* (also known as *p53*, and encoding the p53 protein) and the oncogene *bcl-2* are involved. *TP53* blocks the cell cycle in a genetically damaged cell in order to allow DNA repair. When the damage is irreparable, *TP53* induces apoptosis. In contrast, upregulation of *bcl-2* expression blocks apoptosis. Against this background, the prognostic value of *TP53* and *bcl-2* expression has been evaluated. High *TP53* expression has been found to be correlated with poor prognosis,[57,58] and such a correlation for *bcl-2* has also been found[59] – although this has been contested by others.[60] As it is likely that response to chemo- and radiotherapy involves the apoptotic pathway, it might be possible to use *TP53* and *bcl-2* expression to predict tumour response to these therapeutic modalities. Mutated *TP53* and high *bcl-2* expression would block the apoptotic pathway and render the tumour cell therapy-resistant. Indications that this approach might be clinically valid have been published.[61] Also, expression of *p21*, which is induced by p53 activation, is independently correlated with survival,[62] and likewise *p21* expression correlates with a response to radiotherapy.[63]

Parameters related to tumour cell differentiation

Conventionally, in grading of carcinomas, cytonuclear features (nuclear pleomorphism and hyperchromasia, and cytoplasmic characteristics) as well as architecture (formation of glands, cell stratification, and polarity) are taken into account. This subjective appraisal is usually translated into three grades: well, moderately and poorly differentiated. Grading has been reported to be prognostically significant. However, conventional purely morphological grading is not very reproducible, and was of only borderline prognostic significance in a study of prognostic variables.[6] A plausible alternative to subjective grading would be analysis of the expression of characteristic products of terminally differentiated cells. For goblet cells, a variety of antibodies allow the detection of mucin production. For columnar resorptive cells, staining for microvillus-associated proteins such as villin, or of membrane-associated disaccharidases such as sucrase isomaltase, can be used. Lysozyme is an adequate marker for Paneth cells, and chromogranin A for endocrine cells. In many studies, the prognostic significance of these markers, either singly or in combination, has been investigated.[64] In general, tumours with highly differentiated cells tend to have a more favourable prognosis than those with predominantly undifferentiated cells. In contrast, several studies have indicated that tumours with endocrine cells tend to behave more aggressively.[65,66] The search for differentiation-related prognostic markers has clearly not yielded any markers whose impact comes close to that of tumour stage. From a conceptual point of view, this may be explained by the fact that differentiation takes only tumour cell characteristics into account, whereas stage- and growth-related parameters reflect the interaction between cancer cells and the host. An exciting new possibility for analysis of tumour differentiation is gene expression profiling by cDNA arrays. With this new technology, the expression of thousand of genes can be mapped in one test.[67]

Parameters related to oncogenes and tumour suppressor genes

Colorectal cancer is probably the most intensely studied tumour type with regard to molecular genetic abnormalities. Pioneering work by Vogelstein's group led to the development of a model for the molecular events responsible for colorectal carcinogenesis.[68,69] This concept has led in turn to intensive searches for diagnostic and prognostic uses of these molecular parameters. The prognostic value of TP53 and bcl-2 and their potential use for the prediction of response to chemo- and radiotherapy have been briefly mentioned above. Surprisingly, for general use in the diagnosis and prognosis of colorectal cancer, molecular genetic parameters have had as yet very limited impact.

Gross genetic abnormalities, as reflected in cellular DNA content, have been studied repeatedly in the last decades. Ploidy analysis has become relatively simple, and this parameter could be useful, especially since it reflects an end stage in the development of the neoplasm and thus combines the effects of various individual genetic abnormalities. Most studies indicate that tumour ploidy is correlated with patient survival.[70,71] Tumour ploidy has, however, been found to be correlated with parameters including tumour stage, grade, and proliferative activity, and therefore its impact as an independent prognostic indicator has been limited.[72]

In several studies, the presence of TP53 mutations and of immunohistochemical expression of the p53 protein has been correlated with an unfavourable prognosis. The results are rather conflicting, because some investigators found a significant correlation,[73] which, however, was not confirmed by others.[60,62] The p53-induced p21 gene has been reported as an independent predictor of favourable outcome.[60] Interestingly, anti-p53 autoantibodies have been identified in the circulation of colorectal cancer patients. Anti-p53 antibody-positive patients had a significantly worse outcome.[74]

Of all genetic abnormalities associated with colorectal cancer, TP53 and Ki-ras mutations have received most attention. Also mutations in the Ki-ras gene have been found to be of prognostic significance: tumours with Ki-ras mutations (about 50%) were prognostically more unfavourable than those without[75,76] – even more so when these were combined with TP53 mutations. Also in this respect, there is much controversy in the literature. A meta-analysis of a large number of cases showed Ki-ras mutations as such to be associated with increased risk of relapse and death, but with a more pronounced effect for a G-to-T mutation of codon 12.[77] Recent data indicate that considerable genetic heterogeneity exists in colorectal neoplasms, which calls for more extensive sampling of tumours for molecular genetic abnormalities.[78] Given the fact that Ki-ras mutations have been identified even in preneoplastic, non-dysplastic lesions, it is unlikely that as a single parameter they will have important prognostic significance.

Of some of the other genes that figure in the Vogelstein model – APC, MCC ('mutated in colorectal cancer') and DCC ('deleted in colorectal cancer')[68,69] – a role in tumour behaviour still needs to be established. These are large genes with a wide scattering of point mutations, which makes their analysis cumbersome and time-consuming. They have, as yet, not been studied in a sufficient number of patients to allow any firm conclusions regarding their prognostic role. Jen et al[6] identified an important role for a gene on 18q, which might be the DCC gene at this locus. SMAD4 is also in this locus, and has been recently identified as a metastasis predictor.[79] The story will certainly not end with the genes discussed above. The discovery of the genes responsible for the Lynch syndrome, a family of genes playing a role in mismatch repair, has led to studies on the roles of microsatellite instability (which reflects defects in these genes) in the diagnosis and prognosis of colorectal cancer. It has become clear that microsatellite instability occurs in most Lynch-syndrome-associated colorectal carcinomas, and also in a limited proportion (about 15%) of sporadic colorectal cancers, but it also occurs in non-neoplastic (e.g. inflammatory) conditions.[80] Some authors[81] have reported improved survival for microsatellite-unstable tumours, whereas others[82,83] have found no such correlation. An important function of microsatellite analysis might be in screening for mismatch-repair gene defects, prior to the more cumbersome sequencing of the *hMLH1* gene.[84] Other genes will follow. Worldwide, the search for new genetic defects in neoplastic diseases, including colorectal cancer, is on, and this will undoubtedly lead to the discovery of new prognostic factors.

CONCLUSIONS

Where does this impressive collection of new tumour cell characteristics leave us with the management of today's colorectal cancer patients? For the Dukes A, C, and D categories the problem is less urgent. For Dukes B patients, however, the possibility of progressive disease is far from remote, which calls for identification of high-risk groups to be included in adjuvant treatment protocols. The general risk profile is clear. A Dukes B tumour that has infiltrating borders, is angio-invasive, induces the expression of collagenase type IV, is mutated in *TP53* and Ki-*ras*, has lost E-cadherin expression but gained expression of CD44v6, is *bcl-2*-positive, has a high proliferative index, is aneuploid, and shows loss of heterozygosity of 18q runs a very high risk for recurrent disease. It is not yet clear which combination of these parameters is the most predictive. Nor do we know whether long-term survival will be improved if adjuvant therapy is administered on the basis of the expression of a set of unfavourable markers. Additional clinical research will be necessary to bring tumour biological research into the realm of everyday clinical application. Given the implications of a large number of genes for the determination of tumour behaviour, expression profiling by the cDNA array approach holds high promise. Prospective studies as to the clinical utility of molecular prognostic markers are urgently needed.

REFERENCES

1. Adam IJ, Mohamdee MO, Martin IG et al, Role of circumferential margin involvement in the local recurrence of rectal cancer. *Lancet* 1994; **344:** 707–11.

2. Cawthorn SJ, Gibbs NM, Marks CG. Clearance technique for the detection of lymph nodes in colorectal cancer. *Br J Surg* 1986; **73:** 58–60.

3. Caplin S, Cerottini JP, Bosman FT et al, For patients with Dukes' B (TNM Stage II) colorectal carcinoma, examination of six or fewer lymph nodes is related to poor prognosis. *Cancer* 1998; **83:** 666–72.

4. Shida H, Ban K, Matsumoto M et al, Prognostic significance of location of lymph node metastases in colorectal cancer. *Dis Colon Rectum* 1992; **35:** 1046–50.

5. Compton CC, Pathology report in colon cancer: What is prognostically important? *Dig Dis* 1999; **17:** 67–79.

6. Jen J, Kim H, Piantadosi S et al, Allelic loss of chromosome 18q and prognosis in colorectal cancer. *N Engl J Med* 1994; **331:** 213–21.

7. Harrison JC, Dean PJ, el-Zeky F, Vander Zwaag R, Impact of the Crohn's-like lymphoid reaction on staging of right-sided colon cancer: results of multivariate analysis. *Hum Pathol* 1995; **26:** 31–8.

8. Shepherd NA, Saraga EP, Love SB, Jass JR, Prognostic factors in colonic cancer. *Histopathology* 1989; **14:** 613–20.

9. Dukes CE, The classification of carcinoma of the rectum. *J Pathol Bacteriol* 1932; **35:** 323–32.

10. Dukes CE, Bussey HJR, The spread of rectal cancer and its effect on prognosis. *Br J Cancer* 1958; **12:** 309–20.

11. Astler VB, Coller FA, The prognostic significance of direct extension of carcinoma of the colon and rectum. *Ann Surg* 1954; **139:** 846–54.

12. Deans GT, Parks TG, Rowlands BJ, Spence RA, Prognostic factors in colorectal cancer. *Br J Surg* 1992; **79:** 608–13.

13. American Joint Committee on Cancer (AJCC), *Manual for Staging of Cancer*, 4th edn (Beahrs OH, Henson DE, Hutter RVP, Kennedy JB, eds). Philadelphia: Lippincott, 1992.

14. De Quay N, Cerottini JP, Albe X et al, Prognosis in Duke's B colorectal carcinoma: the Jass classification revisited. *Eur J Surg* 1999; **165:** 588–92.

15. Di Giorgio A, Botti C, Tocchi A et al, The influence of tumor lymphocytic infiltration on long term survival of surgically treated colorectal cancer patients. *Int Surg* 1992; **77:** 256–60.

16. de Haas-Kock DF, Baeten CG, Jager JJ et al, Prognostic significance of radial margins of clearance in rectal cancer. *Br J Surg* 1996; **83:** 781–5.

17. Jeffers MD, O'Dowd GM, Mulcahy H et al, The prognostic significance of immunohistochemically detected lymph node micrometastases in colorectal carcinoma. *J Pathol* 1994; **172:** 183–7.

18. Greenson JK, Isenhart CE, Rice R et al, Identification of occult micrometastases in pericolic lymph nodes of Dukes' B colorectal cancer patients using monoclonal antibodies against cytokeratin and CC49. Correlation with long-term survival. *Cancer* 1994; **73:** 563–9.

19. Hardingham JE, Hewett PJ, Sage RE et al, Molecular detection of blood-borne epithelial cells in colorectal cancer patients and in patients with benign bowel disease. *Int J Cancer* 2000; **89:** 8–13.

20. Yun K, Merrie AE, Gunn J et al, Keratin 20 is a specific marker of submicroscopic lymph node metastases in colorectal cancer: validation by K-RAS mutations. *J Pathol* 2000; **191:** 21–6.

21. Futamura M, Takagi Y, Koumura H et al, Spread of colorectal cancer micrometastases in regional lymph nodes by reverse transcriptase-polymerase chain reactions for carcinoembryonic antigen and cytokeratin 20. *J Surg Oncol* 1998; **68:** 34–40.

22. Liefers GJ, Tollenaar RA, Cleton-Jansen AM, Molecular detection of minimal residual disease in colorectal and breast cancer. *Histopathology* 1999; **34:** 385–90.

23. Liefers GJ, Cleton-Jansen AM, van de Velde CJ et al, Micrometastases and survival in stage II colorectal cancer. *N Engl J Med* 1998; **339:** 223–8.

24. Sanchez-Cespedes M, Esteller M, Hibi K et al, Molecular detection of neoplastic cells in lymph nodes of metastatic colorectal

cancer patients predicts recurrence. *Clin Cancer Res* 1999; **5:** 2450–4.

25. Nakanishi Y, Ochiai A, Yamauchi Y et al, Clinical implications of lymph node micrometastases in patients with colorectal cancers. A case control study. *Oncology* 1999; **57:** 276–80.

26. Wharton RQ, Jonas SK, Glover C et al, Increased detection of circulating tumor cells in the blood of colorectal carcinoma patients using two reverse transcription–PCR assays and multiple blood samples. *Clin Cancer Res* 1999; **5:** 4158–63.

27. Hase K, Shatney C, Johnson D et al, Prognostic value of tumor 'budding' in patients with colorectal cancer. *Dis Colon Rectum* 1993; **36:** 627–35.

28. Mulcahy HE, Duffy MJ, Gibbons D et al, Urokinase-type plasminogen activator and outcome in Dukes' B colorectal cancer. *Lancet* 1994; **344:** 583–4.

29. Sato T, Nishimura G, Yonemura Y et al, Association of immunohistochemical detection of urokinase-type plasminogen activator with metastasis and prognosis in colorectal cancer. *Oncology* 1995; **52:** 347–52.

30. Ganesh S, Sier CF, Griffioen G et al, Prognostic relevance of plasminogen activators and their inhibitors in colorectal cancer. *Cancer Res* 1994; **54:** 4065–71.

31. Murray GI, Duncan ME, O'Neil P et al, Matrix metalloproteinase-1 is associated with poor prognosis in colorectal cancer. *Nature Med* 1996; **2:** 461–2.

32. Sunami E, Tsuno N, Osada T et al, MMP-1 is a prognostic marker for hematogenous metastasis of colorectal cancer. *Oncologist* 2000; **5:** 108–14.

33. Havenith MG, Arends JW, Simon R et al, Type IV collagen immunoreactivity in colorectal cancer. Prognostic value of basement membrane deposition. *Cancer* 1988; **62:** 2207–11.

34. Offerhaus GJ, Giardiello FM, Bruijn JA et al, The value of immunohistochemistry for collagen IV expression in colorectal carcinomas. *Cancer* 1991; **67:** 99–105.

35. Halvorsen TB, Seim E, Association between invasiveness, inflammatory reaction, desmoplasia and survival in colorectal cancer. *J Clin Pathol* 1989; **42:** 162–6.

36. Abdalla SA, Behzad F, Bsharah S et al, Prognostic relevance of microvessel density in colorectal tumours. *Oncol Rep* 1999; **6:** 839–42.

37. Galindo Gallego M, Fernandez Acerno MJ, Sanz Ortega J, Aljama J, Vascular enumeration as prognosticator for colorectal carcinoma. *Eur J Cancer* 2000; **36:** 55–60.

38. Su LK, Vogelstein B, Kinzler KW, Association of the APC tumor suppressor protein with catenins. *Science* 1993; **262:** 1734–7.

39. Arends JW, Molecular interactions in the Vogelstein model of colorectal carcinoma. *J Pathol* 2000; **190:** 412–16.

40. Streit M, Schmidt R, Hilgenfeld RU et al, Adhesion receptors in malignant transformation and dissemination of gastrointestinal tumors. *J Mol Med* 1996; **74:** 253–68.

41. Dorudi S, Sheffield JP, Poulsom R et al, E-cadherin expression in colorectal cancer. An immunocytochemical and in situ hybridization study. *Am J Pathol* 1993; **142:** 981–6.

42. Dorudi S, Hanby AM, Poulsom R et al, Level of expression of E-cadherin mRNA in colorectal cancer correlates with clinical outcome. *Br J Cancer* 1995; **71:** 614–16.

43. van der Wurff AA, Arends JW, van der Linden EP et al, L-CAM expression in lymph node and liver metastases of colorectal carcinomas. *J Pathol* 1994; **172:** 177–81.

44. van der Wurff AA, ten Kate J, van der Linden EP et al, L-CAM expression in normal, premalignant, and malignant colon mucosa. *J Pathol* 1992; **168:** 287–91.

45. Yamaguchi A, Urano T, Goi T et al, Expression of a CD44 variant containing exons 8 to 10 is a useful independent factor for the prediction of prognosis in colorectal cancer patients. *J Clin Oncol* 1996; **14:** 1122–7.

46. Mulder JW, Kruyt PM, Sewnath M et al, Colorectal cancer prognosis and expression of exon-v6-containing CD44 proteins. *Lancet* 1994; **344:** 1470–2.

47. Gotley D, Fawcett J, Walsh M et al, Expression of alternatively spliced variants of the cell adhesion molecule CD44 is not related to tumor progression in colorectal cancer. *Clin Exp Metastasis* 1996; **145:** 28.

48. Cohn KH, Wang FS, Desoto-LaPaix F et al, Association of nm23-H1 allelic deletions with distant metastases in colorectal carcinoma. *Lancet* 1991; **338:** 722–4.

49. Ichikawa W, Positive relationship between expression of CD44 and hepatic metastases in colorectal cancer. *Pathobiology* 1994; **62:** 172–9.

50. Guan RJ, Ford HL, Fu Y et al, Drg-1 as a differentiation-related, putative metastatic suppressor gene in human colon cancer. *Cancer Res* 2000; **60:** 749–55.

51. Yamazoe Y, Maetani S, Nishikawa T et al, The prognostic role of the DNA ploidy pattern in colorectal cancer analysis using paraffin-embedded tissue by an improved method. *Surg Today* 1994; **24:** 30–6.

52. Schutte B, Reynders MM, Wiggers T et al, Retrospective analysis of the prognostic significance of DNA content and proliferative activity in large bowel carcinoma. *Cancer Res* 1987; **47:** 5494–6.

53. Palmqvist R, Stenling R, Oberg A, Landberg G, Prognostic significance of p27(Kip1) expression in colorectal cancer: a clinico-pathological characterization. *J Pathol* 1999; **188:** 18–23.

54. Handa K, Yamakawa M, Takeda H et al, Expression of cell cycle markers in colorectal carcinoma: superiority of cyclin A as an indicator of poor prognosis. *Int J Cancer* 1999; **84:** 225–33.

55. Chen YT, Henk MJ, Carney KJ et al, Prognostic significance of tumor markers in colorectal cancer patients: DNA index, S-phase fraction, p53 expression and Ki-67 index. *J Gastrointest Surg* 1997; **1:** 266–73.

56. Baretton GB, Diebold J, Christoforis G et al, Apoptosis and immunohistochemical bcl-2 expression in colorectal adenomas and carcinomas. Aspects of carcinogenesis and prognostic significance. *Cancer* 1996; **77:** 255–64.

57. Goh HS, Yao J, Smith DR, p53 point mutation and survival in colorectal cancer patients. *Cancer Res* 1995; **55:** 5217–21.

58. Hamelin R, Laurent-Puig P, Olschwang S et al, Association of p53 mutations with short survival in colorectal cancer. *Gastroenterology* 1994; **106:** 42–8.

59. Ofner D, Riehemann K, Maier H et al, Immunohistochemically detectable bcl-2 expression in colorectal carcinoma: correlation with tumour stage and patient survival. *Br J Cancer* 1995; **72:** 981–5.

60. Pereira H, Silva S, Juliao R et al, Prognostic markers for colorectal cancer: expression of p53 and BCL2. *World J Surg* 1997; **21:** 210–13.

61. Watson AJ, Merritt AJ, Jones LS et al, Evidence of reciprocity of bcl-2 and p53 expression in human colorectal adenomas and carcinomas. *Br J Cancer* 1996; **73:** 889–95.

62. Zirbes TK, Baldus SE, Moenig SP et al, Prognostic impact of p21/waf1/cip1 in colorectal cancer. *Int J Cancer* 2000; **89:** 14–18.

63. Qiu H, Sirivongs P, Rothenberger M et al, Molecular prognostic factors in rectal cancer treated by radiation and surgery. *Dis Colon Rectum* 2000; **43:** 451–9.

64. Ho SB, Itzkowitz SH, Friera AM et al, Cell lineage markers in premalignant and malignant colonic mucosa. *Gastroenterology* 1989; **97:** 392–404.

65. Hamada Y, Oishi A, Shoji T et al, Endocrine cells and prognosis in patients with colorectal carcinoma. *Cancer* 1992; **69:** 2641–6.

66. de Bruine AP, Wiggers T, Beek C et al, Endocrine cells in colorectal adenocarcinomas: incidence, hormone profile and prognostic relevance. *Int J Cancer* 1993; **54:** 765–71.

67. Backert S, Gelos M, Kobalz U et al, Differential gene expression

in colon carcinoma cells and tissues detected with a cDNA array. *Int J Cancer* 1999; **82**: 868–74.

68. Fearon ER, Vogelstein B, A genetic model for colorectal tumorigenesis. *Cell* 1990; **61**: 759–67.

69. Kinzler KW, Vogelstein B, Lessons from hereditary colorectal cancer. *Cell* 1996; **87**: 159–70.

70. Chapman MA, Hardcastle JD, Armitage NC, Five-year prospective study of DNA tumor ploidy and colorectal cancer survival. *Cancer* 1995; **76**: 383–7.

71. Baretton G, Gille J, Oevermann E, Lohrs U, Flow-cytometric analysis of the DNA-content in paraffin-embedded tissue from colorectal carcinomas and its prognostic significance. *Virchows Arch B, Cell Pathol Mol Pathol* 1991, **60**. 123–31

72. Sun XF, Carstensen JM, Stal O et al, Prognostic significance of p53 expression in relation to DNA ploidy in colorectal adenocarcinoma. *Virchows Arch A, Pathol Anat Histopathol* 1993; **423**: 443–8.

73. Kahlenberg MS, Stoler DL, Rodriguez-Bigas MA et al, p53 tumor suppressor gene mutations predict decreased survival of patients with sporadic colorectal carcinoma. *Cancer* 2000; **88**: 1814–19.

74. Shiota G, Ishida M, Noguchi N et al, Circulating p53 antibody in patients with colorectal cancer: relation to clinicopathologic features and survival. *Dig Dis Sci* 2000; **45**: 122–8.

75. Bell SM, Scott N, Cross D et al, Prognostic value of p53 overexpression and c-Ki-ras gene mutations in colorectal cancer. *Gastroenterology* 1993; **104**: 57–64.

76. Thebo JS, Senagore AJ, Reinhold DS, Stapleton SR, Molecular staging of colorectal cancer: K-ras mutation analysis of lymph nodes upstages Dukes B patients. *Dis Colon Rectum* 2000; **43**: 155–9.

77. Andreyev HJ, Norman AR, Cunningham D et al, Kirsten ras mutations in patients with colorectal cancer: the multicenter 'RASCAL' study. *J Natl Cancer Inst* 1998; **90**: 675–84.

78. Shibata D, Schaeffer J, Li ZH et al, Genetic heterogeneity of the c-K-ras locus in colorectal adenomas but not in adenocarcinomas. *J Natl Cancer Inst* 1993; **85**: 1058–63.

79. Tarafa G, Villanueva A, Farre L et al, DCC and SMAD4 alterations in human colorectal and pancreatic tumor dissemination. *Oncogene* 2000; **19**: 546–55.

80. Bubb VJ, Curtis LJ, Cunningham C et al, Microsatellite instability and the role of hMSH2 in sporadic colorectal cancer. *Oncogene* 1996; **12**: 2641–9.

81. Gonzalez-Garcia I, Moreno V, Navarro M et al, Standardized approach for microsatellite instability detection in colorectal carcinomas. *J Natl Cancer Inst* 2000; **92**: 544–9.

82. Curran B, Lenehan K, Mulcahy H et al, Replication error phenotype, clinicopathological variables, and patient outcome in Dukes' B stage II (T3,N0,M0) colorectal cancer. *Gut* 2000; **46**: 200–4.

83. Messerini L, Ciantelli M, Baglioni S et al, Prognostic significance of microsatellite instability in sporadic mucinous colorectal cancers. *Hum Pathol* 1999; **30**: 629–34.

84. Aaltonen LA, Salovaara R, Kristo P et al, Incidence of non-polyposis colorectal cancer and the feasibility of molecular screening for the disease. *N Engl J Med* 1998; **338**: 1481–7.

Part 4

Management of Localized Disease

9

Surgery for colon cancer

Clare Adams, John W Fielding, Dion G Morton

INTRODUCTION

Surgical treatment of colon cancer would appear to have come a long way from the first resection and anastomosis performed by Reybard in 1833. However, despite multidisciplinary treatment advances, there has been little improvement in overall 5-year survival for over 30 years. Radical surgery still remains the only potentially curative treatment for this common cancer.

The general surgical principles for colonic resection in the treatment of colorectal cancer have changed little in recent history. Improvements in resuscitation, antibiotic treatment, and anaesthesia have allowed the surgeon to be more radical, especially in the emergency setting. These improvements in supportive care have at the same time increased the prominence of surgery in treatment-related morbidity. As mortality has fallen, so surgeons have increasingly looked at morbidity, in particular at the necessity for stoma formation. Stomas are most often required for emergency patients who present with peritonitis or obstruction. On-table lavage or subtotal colectomy can now provide 'stoma-free' alternatives for selected patients, even in the emergency setting.

The key outcome measures in the treatment of colon cancer are still 5-year survival and 2-year local recurrence rates. The stage of disease at the time of presentation is the most influential factor affecting 5-year survival. Conversely, the local recurrence rate is greatly influenced by obstruction/perforation at the time of presentation. Surgical technique has also been implicated in influencing the local recurrence rate,[1] particularly for the resection of rectal tumours.[2]

Our ability to assess the likely success of surgical treatment at the time of operation remains limited, but new intraoperative investigations such as radioimmune-guided surgery (RIGS) and intraoperative ultrasound (IOUS) may prove to be suitably sensitive tools with which to assess tumour clearance and help to guide adjuvant therapy.

The frequency of emergency presentation in many series remains over 30%, which is a disappointingly high figure. It is to be hoped that increased public awareness, and perhaps screening, could reduce the frequency of emergency presentation and so reduce the associated morbidity and mortality.

This chapter sets out to address the issues concerning safe radical surgery for curative treatment of colon cancer, in both the elective and emergency settings, and discusses some of the new developments that may influence its management in forthcoming years.

ELECTIVE SURGERY

Elective surgery for colorectal cancer is undertaken in 65–85% of operative cases, with the remainder presenting as emergencies. Surgery may be carried out with either curative or palliative intent. Palliative resection is usually considered for the treatment of advanced colon cancer, even in the presence of metastases, in order to prevent the late complications of obstruction and perforation. Palliative surgery may involve a local resection of the primary tumour, or occasionally bypass of a locally advanced lesion.

Outcome is considerably influenced by the mode of presentation and the nature of the surgery. Radical surgery in the elective setting results in a 5-year survival rate more than twice that for emergency surgery (Table 9.1). Further improvements in outcome for colorectal cancer will depend upon maximizing the number of patients on whom elective radical resection can be performed.

In the absence of distant metastases or diffuse peritoneal spread, which is relatively rare, radical resection should be considered, since it offers the only curative therapeutic option. The overall 5-year

Table 9.1 Presentation and outcome in patients with colorectal cancer (data adapted from references 3–5)

Mode of presentation	Percentages of all patients	Resection performed (%)	In-hospital mortality (%)	5-year survival rate (%)
Elective surgery	60	>95	5	50
Emergency	25	70	20	25
Non-operative	15	—	40	<5

survival rate in patients undergoing curative surgery is over 50% in most series. Even in locally advanced lesions, in which local structures are invaded, a 5-year survival rate approaching 30% can be achieved.[6]

The main focus of this section will be on radical elective surgery.

Preoperative assessment

Effective treatment requires a multidisciplinary care team. The gastroenterologist, medical oncologist, and stomatherapist may all need to be involved in the planning of treatment. The management plan should also be discussed with the general practitioner, the community nurse, and, in selected cases, the social services and the palliative care team, so that adequate support can be provided once the patient is discharged from hospital.

Preoperative evaluation must include evaluation of any comorbid medical factors, as well as determining the extent of disease. Comorbid medical illness rarely precludes surgical treatment, since local resection provides the most effective symptomatic control. Elective surgery can be delayed for treatment for reversible conditions and for stabilizing chronic disease.

Preoperatively, it is advised that patients undergo either a double contrast barium enema or a total colonoscopy in order to exclude synchronous tumours. These have been estimated to occur in 6% of cases, of which 50% lie outside the range of resection.[7] Colonoscopy has the advantage over barium enema of providing access for biopsy and histological confirmation of any tumour. It is also more effective in detecting small adenomas. This is most important in the small group of young patients with familial predisposition in whom the presence of satellite adenomas can be an indication for an extended colectomy to facilitate subsequent control of metachronous disease.

Preoperative staging of the primary tumour for colon tumours is less likely to influence management than in the case of rectal cancer. However, contrast-enhanced computed tomography (CT) scanning of the liver to look for metastases should be performed as an adjunct to intraoperative assessment of the liver. Intraoperative palpation of the liver has been repeatedly shown to underestimate the presence of metastases. This is of particular importance in colorectal cancer, since over 50% of distant metastases first present in the liver.[8] Accurate staging of liver metastases is becoming increasingly important with the development of locoregional intrahepatic arterial chemotherapy and hepatic resection as adjuvant therapeutic options following primary resection. Intraoperative ultrasonography has been reported as being more specific than preoperative CT scanning for the detection of liver metastases,[9] and is being more widely used in an attempt to improve perioperative staging. Preoperative serum carcinoembryonic antigen (CEA) estimation has also been advocated, since a subsequent postoperative rise in this level can be the first sign of early recurrence. Elevated CEA levels have been found in patients with recurrent tumour in whom preoperative serum levels had been normal, suggesting that this follow-up investigation can be useful regardless of the preoperative serum level.[10]

Resection technique

In the elective setting, where preoperative bowel preparation has been performed, primary anastomosis should be feasible, and a protecting temporary stoma is rarely required for colonic lesions.

The principles of radical surgical resection for colon cancer remain the same regardless of the site of the primary tumour, namely ligation of the major vascular pedicle, obtaining tumour-free margins, and resection of any contiguous organs involved by tumour. Ligation of the major vascular pedicle allows for wide excision of the lymph nodes draining the tumour. In a formal hemicolectomy, the proximal resection margin is usually determined by the level of the major vascular ligation (Figure 9.1). In a left hemicolectomy, ligation of the inferior mesenteric artery flush with the aortic origin has been strongly advocated.[11] No resultant increase in survival has been shown, and, notably, no long-term survivors among patients with apical node metastases have been reported.[12] A wide resection, including the vascular pedicle, will, however, provide the maximum number of lymph nodes and so help in accurate tumour staging. More recently, subtotal colectomy has been advocated for young patients (<50 years), and for those patients with synchronous tumours (Figure 9.2), in order to reduce the risk of developing metachronous cancer later in life. Except for those

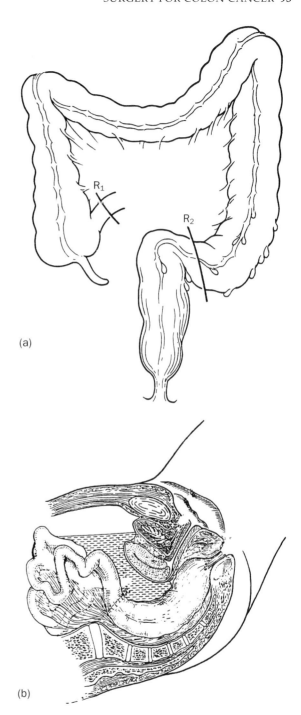

(a)

(b)

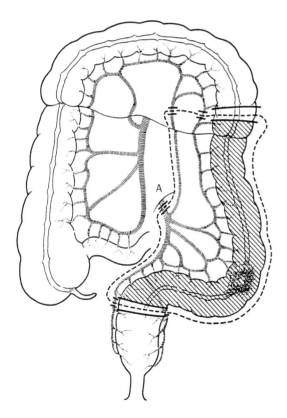

Figure 9.1 Left hemicolectomy. The diagram shows the limits of resection for a sigmoid carcinoma. High ligation of the inferior mesenteric artery (A) is performed in order to remove the lymphatics draining the tumour. The blood supply to the colon is maintained via the marginal artery. Reproduced with permission from Keighley MRB, Williams NS, *Surgery of the Anus, Rectum and Colon*. London: WB Saunders, 1993.

Figure 9.2 A subtotal colectomy and ileorectal anastomosis. The limits of resections are shown in (a): R_1–R_2. An end-to-end ileorectal anastomosis is shown in (b). Retaining the rectum preserves the reservoir and reduces problems with postoperative diarrhoea. Reproduced with permission from Keighley MRB, Williams NS, *Surgery of the Anus, Rectum and Colon*. London: WB Saunders, 1993.

patients with a known inherited syndrome, this approach, as yet, has no proven benefit in terms of reduced cancer recurrence rates and prolonged survival. It may, in fact, be the case that regular colonoscopic follow-up, with polypectomy where required, is as effective in preventing metachronous tumours, and could have a lower resultant morbidity, particularly in terms of subsequent frequency of bowel action.

For over 40 years, surgeons have been concerned that tumour mobilization and manipulation could cause metachronous tumours by local tumour-cell seeding and also cause distant metastatic spread.[13,14] These early reports encouraged the development of the 'no-touch technique', in which the vascular supply to the colon is ligated and the colonic lumen occluded by tapes prior to mobilization of the tumour. Molecular biological techniques have demonstrated that the 'no-touch technique' significantly reduces the frequency of circulating tumour cell spread into the portal blood during surgical manipulation.[15] The viability of these cells and their clinical significance remains controversial. One early report showed an increased disease-free interval compared with historical controls.[16] A more recent prospective randomized trial found a trend towards a reduced number and greater time to the development of liver metastases in a no-touch isolation group, but these differences did not reach statistical significance.[17] The findings from these studies suggest there may be a limited benefit from this approach.

Although many surgeons would advocate intrarectal irrigation with cytotoxic agent during a low anterior resection, in a colonic resection where the distal resection margin is usually further away from the tumour, the potential benefits are unclear. Recurrent tumour at the site of the colonic anastomosis is rarely seen following curative resection for colon tumours. The main focus of attention in colonic resections for cancer is in obtaining node clearance.

It has generally been argued that lymph node invasion occurs in a stepwise fashion, involving first the paracolic nodes before spread to the mesenteric vessel nodes and so to the para-aortic nodes. Skip lesions are now recognized,[18] re-emphasizing the importance of multiple node sampling by the histopathologist, for accurate staging of the tumours. Radical resection is therefore required not only for tumour clearance, but also to provide adequate lymph node samples for histology. This is now influencing patient selection for adjuvant chemotherapy, and so, although high arterial ligation may confer little survival benefit to the patient from primary surgery, its benefit in the future is likely to be seen in more appropriate selection for adjuvant treatment. A similar myth – that distant metastases will only occur after lymph node involvement – has also been dispelled,[19] emphasizing the importance of optimal perioperative assessment for liver metastases.

Prophylactic colectomy

Prophylactic colectomy has been well established in the treatment of longstanding total colitis and of familial adenomatous polyposis. The development of restorative proctocolectomy has provided a continent option for the treatment of these patients (Figure 9.3). Advances in our understanding of the molecular genetics of other inherited cancer syndromes, most notably hereditary non-polyposis colorectal cancer (HNPCC),[20] have considerably increased the number of patients for whom prophylactic colectomy can be considered.[21] In HNPCC families, the tumours are predominantly right-sided, and so rectal resection is not usually required. The therapeutic options are colonoscopic surveillance and polypectomy or subtotal colectomy and ileorectal anastomosis, with subsequent follow-up surveillance of the rectal stump. Because of the high risk of colorectal cancer (>80% lifetime risk) and the significant risk of interval cancer development during colonoscopic surveillance,[22] increasing numbers of known gene carriers are likely to request prophylactic colectomy. Other tumours are also commonly seen in HNPCC families, notably ovarian and endometrial carcinomas. The benefits of synchronous prophylactic hysterectomy and oophorectomy in postmenopausal female family members are uncertain, and further work is required in HNPCC families to clarify these issues.

Minimally invasive surgery

The development of new laparoscopic instruments has encouraged their application in colorectal cancer surgery. Prior to 1993, more than 1500 laparoscopic colectomies had been reported in the literature, about half of which were for colorectal cancer. The enthusiasm for this approach lay in the perceived reduced early morbidity associated with a colectomy. Reports have demonstrated a significantly shorter hospital stay, and suggested more rapid recovery measurable up to 4 months postoperatively in patients operated on laparoscopically in comparison with those receiving open resection for colorectal cancer.[23] There remains considerable concern about

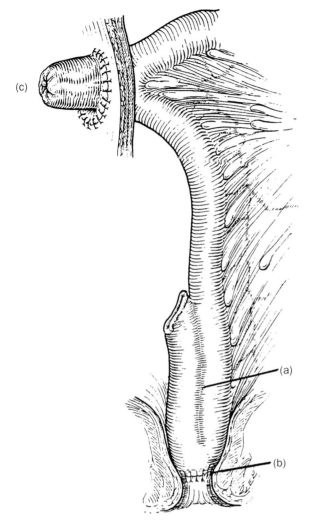

(c)

(a)

(b)

Figure 9.3 Restorative protocolectomy. Following the removal of the whole colon and rectum, a neo-reservoir is fashioned from the terminal ileum (a). Continuity is restored by anastomosis to the anal canal (b). The anastomosis is usually protected by a temporary loop ileostomy (c). Reproduced with permission from Keighley MRB, Williams NS, *Surgery of the Anus, Rectum and Colon*. London: WB Saunders, 1993.

recurrence is independent of the site of removal of the resected specimen. Factors contributing to port-site tumour growth include spillage of malignant cells as a result of advanced-tumour perforation or rough tissue handling; a breach in the mechanical and chemical barriers provided by the peritoneum; wound contamination by direct inoculation or extraction of specimens; and a favourable local milieu for tumour growth at the port site provided by inflammatory mediators and by growth and angiogenic factors. Carbon dioxide may play a role in certain tumour lines in which it may be a stimulating factor.[25]

Strict adherence to oncological principles of surgery, careful dissection techniques, wound protection, and lavage of port sites with cytocidal agent will all improve the outcome of laparoscopic surgery for colon cancer. However, it is generally agreed that laparoscopic colectomy for neoplastic disease should be restricted to clinical trials. The 5-year results of the ongoing American national cooperative trials should address many of the concerns about laparoscopic colorectal cancer resections.

Surgery in the elderly

Major efforts to reduce colorectal-cancer-related mortality are being undertaken by health services worldwide. These currently focus on the implementation of presymptomatic diagnosis in order to downstage disease at the time of presentation and the development of adjuvant chemotherapeutic regimens to increase long-term survival in patients who have undergone attempted curative surgery for locally advanced disease. These two approaches have both been shown to be of proven efficacy in randomized controlled trials. It must be remembered, however, that elderly patients are largely excluded from screening and adjuvant chemotherapy, and, in an increasingly elderly population, the benefits of these advances will be diluted in the total patient population.

The incidence of colorectal cancer approximately doubles with each decade from 40 to 80 years, and two-thirds of colorectal cancer patients are now over 65 years old at the time of diagnosis. In an ageing population, this figure can be expected to rise.[26] Guidelines for the treatment of elderly patients are clearly required. In a multicentre review, Samet et al[27] found that as few as 54% of patients over 75 years of age received definitive surgery for colorectal cancer. A large number of studies in elderly patients have been reported.[28] Comorbid disease and emer-

the ability to achieve wide tumour clearance with this technique. It seems likely that such technical problems will be overcome.

A second area of concern is that of port-site recurrence, which has been reported in up to 4% of cases.[24] This problem appears to be directly related to the laparoscopic approach, and has been reported even in association with early-stage disease. The site of

Table 9.2 Surgery in the elderly: five series from the British Isles reviewing the outcome of surgery for colorectal cancer in elderly patients (all patients were 70 years of age or older)

Ref	Year of publication	Median year of diagnosis	No. of patients	Perioperative mortality rate (%)	5-year survival rate (%)
30	1984	1972	327	29	26
31	1983	1977	288	19	—
32	1989	1978	1147	12	—
33	1988	1982	171	6	48
34	1994	1984	225	5	52

gency presentation have been shown to significantly influence survival,[29] but these studies have failed to show any relationship between age at presentation and perioperative mortality or age-adjusted 5-year survival. These findings support the use of radical surgery in elderly patients. The high incidence of comorbid disease requires that these patients be carefully assessed prior to surgery. Reversible risk factors have been identified in up to 60% of elderly patients presenting with colorectal cancer,[29] highlighting the importance of preoperative assessment. In five series reported from the British Isles between 1982 and 1994, a considerable reduction in perioperative mortality rate (Table 9.2) and a resultant rise in 5-year survival rate are seen over the 13 years.[30–34]

These figures appear to reflect the impact of careful preoperative assessment and improved perioperative patient care over the 20-year period. Inadequate primary surgery in the elderly population is likely to result in increased morbidity and an increase in subsequent emergency treatment, with resulting higher costs to the health services. Adequate primary surgery for elderly patients is required, even if they are excluded from the potential benefits of screening and adjuvant therapy programmes.

EMERGENCY SURGERY

Between 16% and 35% of patients with colorectal cancer present as emergencies. The early mortality in this group of patients is three times that of elective cases, and the overall 5-year survival rate is just over 10%.[35,36] As a consequence, the main emphasis in the treatment of these patients is on minimizing early mortality. Achieving long-term cure is necessarily of secondary importance. The poor outcome for these patients has stimulated a wide range of therapeutic options. There remains a lack of consensus as to the optimal surgical management. It is clear, however, that minimizing the number of patients presenting as emergencies could produce a profound improvement in survival for patients with colorectal cancer, and should be a focus of attention for health care services in the future.

The commonest reasons for emergency presentation are obstruction or perforation of the colon. Massive rectal bleeding is an unusual event in colorectal cancer, being more commonly associated with bleeding from diverticular disease or angiodysplasia.

In the presence of free peritonitis, primary resection with colonic anastomosis is associated with a high risk of anastomotic dehiscence and potentially lethal consequences.[37] In such a situation, formation of an end stoma, usually with resection of the tumour and perforated bowel, is the accepted therapeutic option.

Aggressive preoperative resuscitation with intravenous fluids and antibiotics is of paramount importance in the emergency setting. Because this is often an elderly population, a postoperative intensive care bed should be sought. In the frailer patient, preoperative resuscitation with central pressure monitoring in a high-dependency unit may be required.

The optimal treatment for patients with a localized perforation, or a left-colonic obstruction, is more controversial. Some form of large-bowel decompression should be considered for all obstructed patients, since, even in extremis, it provides the only effective palliative option.

Confirmation of obstruction should be obtained preoperatively by a single-contrast enema in order to exclude pseudo-obstruction.

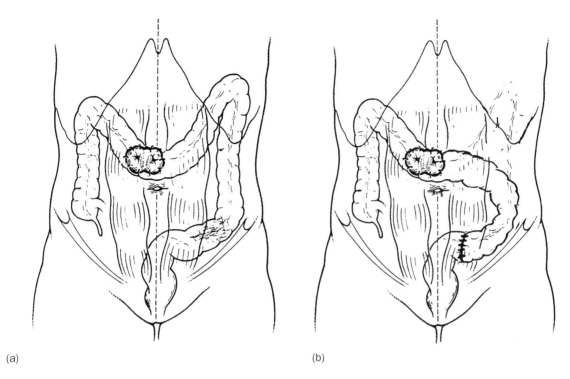

(a)　　　　　　　　　　　　　　　　　　　(b)

Figure 9.4 Three-stage procedure. An obstructing carcinoma in the sigmoid colon is shown. The colon is decompressed by fashioning a transverse loop colostomy (a). In the second procedure, the tumour is resected and a primary anastomosis fashioned (b). In the third stage, the loop colostomy is closed (not shown). Reproduced with permission from Keighley MRB, Williams NS, *Surgery of the Anus, Rectum and Colon*. London: WB Saunders, 1993.

Originally, a three-stage surgical approach (Figure 9.4) was used, despite a reported cumulative post-operative mortality as high as 30%,[38] and a correspondingly high surgical morbidity. These poor results cast doubt on the advisability of delayed resection. An initial temporary loop colostomy has a reported mortality of over 5%,[39] and an associated morbidity of at least 20%. The major complication rate is in excess of 10% for subsequent closure of these colostomies, and less serious complications, notably prolapse and retraction, are not uncommon events. Poor long-term survival figures associated with the three-stage procedure, coupled with high cumulative morbidity and mortality following subsequent resection and closure of the stoma, has prompted surgeons to attempt primary resection at the time of initial operations.[40]

During the 1970s, primary resection of left-sided obstructing tumours, with formation of an end colostomy, was more frequently performed. This is known as Hartmann's procedure (Figure 9.5).[41] This procedure combines the advantages of resection of the disease at the time of first operation with an over-

all shorter hospital stay than a three-stage procedure.[40,42] Retrospective series have reported comparable perioperative morbidity and mortality for the two- and three-stage procedures[43] (Table 9.3).

The major perceived disadvantage of Hartmann's resection is the relatively low rate of stoma closure (60%) in the secondary procedure.[54] The technical feasibility of laparoscopic reversal of Hartmann's procedure is now established,[55] and it seems possible that this could reduce the perioperative morbidity associated with the secondary stoma closure.

In addition to the high mortality from emergency surgery for colorectal cancer, surgeons have been concerned about the high rates of stoma formation and the associated morbidity, in terms of both complications from the stoma and the psychological and functional impact upon this largely elderly patient population. These factors have pushed surgeons towards performing primary anastomosis and avoidance of a stoma. The description of on-table colonic lavage prior to anastomosis of previously unprepared bowel[56,57] resulted in a resurgence of this

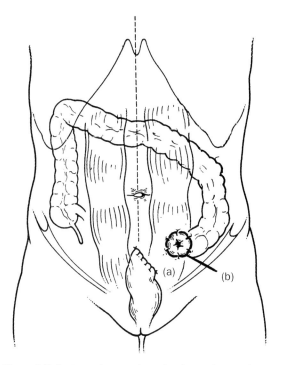

Figure 9.5 Hartmann's procedure. An obstructing carcinoma of the sigmoid colon has been resected. The rectal stump is closed (a) and an end colostomy fashioned (b). Reproduced with permission from Keighley MRB, Williams NS, *Surgery of the Anus, Rectum and Colon.* London: WB Saunders, 1993.

approach (Figure 9.6).[58] It is now recognized that this is a major procedure that cannot be undertaken lightly, particularly in elderly unfit patients.[48] It is of interest that the importance of mechanical bowel preparation is not entirely proven.[59] Its major advantage is a likely reduction in clinical complications in the event of anastomotic leak. The consensus remains that a clean prepared bowel is likely to confer an additional measure of safety and perhaps reduce intraoperative contamination. Reported leak rates following on-table lavage are less than 5%,[60,61] but are generally from retrospective studies in selected patients and are unlikely to reflect the overall leak rate were this procedure more widely performed. The duration of hospital stay is reduced by this technique, and the crude 5-year survival rate is acceptable.[46] In their audit of emergency for colorectal cancer, Runkel et al[62] reported significantly improved postoperative and long-term outcome after performing more aggressive emergency surgery – increasingly performing radical lymphadenectomy and replacing staged procedures with primary resection and on-table colonic lavage. The outcome for emergency patients improved to such an extent that regression analysis no longer found timing of surgery (emergency versus elective) to be a significant prognostic factor for curative resections.

An alternative to on-table lavage is subtotal colectomy and ileo-sigmoid anastomosis.[51,63] This proce-

Table 9.3 Outcome after emergency surgery for obstructed colorectal cancer					
Procedure	No. of patients[a]	Overall mortality rate (%)	Permanent stoma rate (%)	Length of hospital stay (days)	Ref
Three-stage resection	195 (5)	11	25	34[b]	39, 42, 44–46
Hartmann's resection	295 (5)	11	30	30[b]	40, 42, 47–49
Primary anastomosis	42 (6)	5	—	16	47, 48, 50–53

- There is a notable fall in the length of hospital stay between two- and three-stage procedures, and one-stage resection and anastomosis.
- The number of cases in the one-stage series is considerably smaller, indicating a higher degree of case selection for these more major procedures.

[a] Number of series in parentheses.
[b] In those undergoing reversal of their stoma.

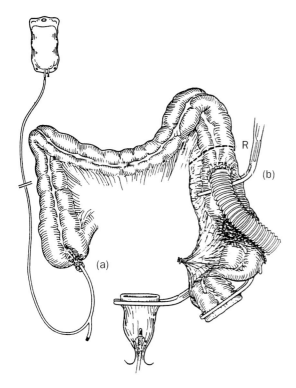

Figure 9.6 On-table lavage. An obstructing carcinoma of the descending colon is being resected. The proximal bowel is washed out by antegrade lavage. A catheter is placed in the caecum via the appendix stump (a). The effluent is collected via plastic tubing as shown (b). Following lavage, the left colon is resected (R), and a primary anastomosis fashioned. Reproduced with permission from Keighley MRB, Williams NS, *Surgery of the Anus, Rectum and Colon*. London: WB Saunders, 1993.

dure has the advantage of removing the distended bowel, and is particularly suitable for cases in which the bowel wall has been compromised by distension. The operative mortality rate is reported as less than 10%, and the reported anastomotic leakage rate is considerably less than 5%.[64,65] One prospective study has compared on-table lavage with subtotal colectomy,[66] and no difference in mortality has been identified between the two groups. The main concern about subtotal colectomy involves the technical demands of the operation, but, with an experienced surgeon, in selected patients, this does not appear to be a clinical problem. One area of concern is that of uncontrollable diarrhoea as a consequence of the extensive resection. Most reports suggest that this is not a major clinical problem with patients having a bowel frequency of no more than three times a day.[66]

The literature would suggest that good results from these more aggressive procedures are likely to result from careful patient selection.

Since all surgical options give much poorer results in the emergency setting, ideal management obviates emergency surgery during the acute stage of obstruction. A 'blow-hole' caecostomy has been advocated for the management of obstruction.[67] It provides a minimally invasive option that can be carried out under local anaesthetic for high-risk patients in order to stabilize them prior to more major surgery. This had previously lost favour because of incomplete decompression and leakage, resulting in peritonitis. The use of a large-gauge Foley catheter with regular irrigation every few hours to prevent blockage, and careful suturing of the caecum to the abdominal wall, make this option safer. It is, however, generally considered an unreliable method of decompression, and has associated heavy demands on nursing attention.

Metallic endoprostheses have been used in recent years to overcome acute neoplastic obstruction of the left and transverse colon.[68] Stent placement does not require anaesthesia or analgesia. As a definitive palliative treatment, the technique provides good results and clear benefits to a selected group of patients.[69] Before surgery, staging of disease, even on an outpatient basis, and scheduling of elective surgery after optimal colonic preparation can be accomplished with a stent in place. Worldwide experience of this technique is still limited, and further evaluation will be required.

SURGERY FOR LOCOREGIONAL RECURRENCE

The commonest site for recurrent colon cancer is the liver (Figure 9.7), and most resectable recurrences occur here.[8] Locoregional recurrence is seen in a little over 10% of cases, but is linked to 30% of deaths.[70] Diffuse peritoneal disease is seen in a further 10% of cases, but is clearly not amenable to salvage surgery. Cohort series suggest that only about 10% of cases with locoregional recurrence are potentially resectable at the time of symptomatic presentation. Early diagnosis of asymptomatic recurrence has therefore been explored in order to increase the potential for attempted curative surgery.

Early studies in this field were based on a second-look laparotomy.[71] In an early series from Minnesota of 377 patients undergoing potentially curative surgery, 110 patients underwent re-look laparotomy, of whom 40 were found to have residual/recurrent cancer. Seven patients with recurrent disease

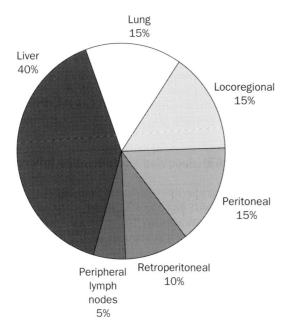

Figure 9.7 The relative frequency at different sites following attempted curative resection for colon cancer.

ultimately were rendered disease-free for more than 5 years. However, six patients died as a result of their surgery, and no benefit could be demonstrated from this approach.

A more selective approach to second-look surgery has subsequently been advocated. Intensive follow-up by colonoscopy, CT scanning, and serum CEA testing is widely employed. For patients who are then found to have evidence of recurrence, a second-look laparotomy has been advocated.

A more recent series[72] of 120 patients having surgery for locally recurrent colorectal cancer reported a 5-year disease-free survival without recurrence rate of 22% for curative resection. Although palliative resection did not improve survival when compared with supportive management only, it can improve the quality of life. The authors conclude that resections are justifiable wherever possible.

Serum CEA levels have been investigated for the early diagnosis of asymptomatic recurrence. An inverse relationship between CEA level and resectability of the recurrent tumour at subsequent operation has been demonstrated,[73] translating into improved survival with lower CEA levels.[74] However, a prospective randomized trial found that although raised CEA was the first indicator of recurrent disease in 80% of patients with liver metastases,

this figure was only 46% for sites other than the liver. CEA was particularly unreliable as a predictor of pelvic and peritoneal recurrence.[75] This suggests that CEA levels are insufficiently sensitive to identify 'early' locoregional recurrence. Preliminary reports using follow-up magnetic resonance imaging (MRI) and positron emission tomography (PET) scanning are inconclusive, but warrant further investigation.[76]

Radioimmuno-guided surgery (RIGS) provides a novel method of intraoperative assessment of tumour spread,[77] and it could complement preoperative staging. The principal of this technique is to use a gamma-detecting probe in order to detect the presence and location of a radioisotope-labelled tumour-associated antibody. A multicentre phase III trial has been reported,[78] supporting the use of this imaging modality for localization of disease for surgical excision and for determination of surgical resectability. One potential use of this system is in identifying, at the time of operation, the limit of involvement of the draining lymphatics and so help to define the small group of patients who may benefit from salvage surgery for recurrent tumour.

Follow-up surveillance of the liver for recurrent disease can be justified outside clinical trials. A meta-analysis of papers that compare intensive follow-up with less frequent follow-up[79] has concluded that intensive follow-up with estimation of CEA levels for early detection of resectable recurrence improves the 5-year survival rate by 9%. However, optimal follow-up protocols have yet to be established, particularly regarding intensive surveillance for extrahepatic recurrence. There is clearly a need for further work in the field of follow-up and surveillance in colorectal cancer management.

CONCLUSIONS

Although there has been little recent change in surgical technique in the treatment of colon cancer, there has been increased clarity in terms of optimal surgical management. Radical surgery has been demonstrated to provide the optimal treatment, even in an elderly population, and, provided that the patient's preoperative condition is stabilized, such surgery can be safely undertaken, even in the presence of significant comorbid disease. The importance of radical surgery is in providing accurate disease staging as well as providing local control of disease. The importance of accurate staging will increase in the foreseeable future as novel adjuvant therapeutic regimens become available.

There will be an increase in the number of prophylactic colectomies performed, particularly in patients carrying mutations in the genes causing hereditary non-polyposis colorectal cancer. Such prophylactic surgery will be suitable for laparoscopic resection, particularly as improved instrumentation becomes available. One area that has been under-investigated is how the health services will cope with an increasingly elderly population, for whom presymptomatic diagnosis and aggressive adjuvant therapy may not be appropriate or feasible.

Preoperative investigation has, as yet, had little impact upon colon cancer management. Novel intra-operative assessment by ultrasound scanning, and radioimmune-guided surgery, may result in some changes in practice. They may facilitate more accurate intraoperative staging of disease and help to select for locoregional therapy, such as the placement of peritoneal catheters, hepatic artery and portal vein cannulae, or intraoperative radiotherapy.

There remains a considerable proportion of patients for whom current therapeutic options are either unsuccessful or inappropriate: 25% of patients present as emergencies, and a further 15% are deemed unfit for any surgical intervention. In order to make any sizeable impact on overall morbidity and mortality, earlier diagnosis is required for these patients. It is hoped that increased public awareness, combined with presymptomatic diagnosis by surveillance of high-risk groups, and screening of defined age groups in the community, will go some way towards addressing this problem.

REFERENCES

1. McArdle CS, Hole D, Impact of variability among surgeons on postoperative morbidity and mortality and ultimate survival. *BMJ* 1991; **302:** 1501–5.
2. Heald RJ, Ryall RD, Recurrence and survival after total mesorectal excision for rectal cancer. *Lancet* 1986; **i:** 1479–82.
3. Allum WH, Slaney G, McConkey CC, Powell J, Cancer of the colon and rectum in the West Midlands, 1957–1981. *Br J Surg* 1994; **81:** 1060–3.
4. McArdle CS, Hole D, Hansell D et al, Prospective study of colorectal cancer in the west of Scotland: 10-year follow-up. *Br J Surg* 1990; **77:** 280–2.
5. Scott NA, Jeacock J, Kingston RD, Risk factors in patients presenting as an emergency with colorectal cancer. *Br J Surg* 1995; **82:** 321–3.
6. Durdey P, Williams NS, The effect of malignant and inflammatory fixation of rectal carcinoma on prognosis after rectal excision. *Br J Surg* 1984; **71:** 787–90.
7. Barillari P, Ramacciato G, De Angelis R et al, Effect of preoperative colonoscopy on the incidence of synchronous and metachronous neoplasms. *Acta Chir Scand* 1990; **156:** 163–6.
8. Martin EW, Minton JP, Carey LC, CEA-directed second-look surgery in the asymptomatic patient after primary resection of colorectal carcinoma. *Ann Surg* 1985; **202:** 310–17.
9. Paul MA, Mulder LS, Cuesta MA et al, Impact of intraoperative ultrasonography on treatment strategy for colorectal cancer. *Br J Surg* 1994; **81:** 1660–3.
10. Zeng Z, Cohen AM, Urmacher C, Usefulness of carcinoembryonic antigen monitoring despite normal preoperative values in node-positive colon cancer patients. *Dis Colon Rectum* 1993; **36:** 1063–8.
11. Bacon HE, Kubchandani I, The rationale of aortico-pelvic lymphadenectomy and high ligation of the inferior mesenteric artery for carcinoma of the left half of the colon and rectum. *Surg Gynecol Obstet* 1964; **118:** 503–9.
12. Grinnell RS, Results of ligation of inferior mesenteric artery at the aorta in resection of carcinoma of the descending and sigmoid colon and rectum. *Surg Gynecol Obstet* 1965; **121:** 1031–5.
13. Cole WH, Packard D, Southwick HW, Cancer of the colon and special reference to prevention of recurrence. *JAMA* 1954; **155:** 1549–55.
14. McGraw EA, Lars JP, Cole WH, Free malignant cells in relation to recurrence of cancer of the colon. *JAMA* 1964; **154:** 1251–4.
15. Hayashi N, Egami H, Kai M et al, No-touch isolation technique reduces intraoperative shedding of tumor cells into the portal vein during resection of colorectal cancer. *Surgery* 1999; **125:** 369–74.
16. Turnbull RB Jr, Kyle K, Watson FR, Spratt J, Cancer of the colon: the influence of the no-touch isolation technic on survival rates. *Ann Surg* 1967; **166:** 420–7.
17. Wiggers T, Jeekel J, Arends JW et al, No-touch isolation technique in colon cancer: a controlled prospective trial. *Br J Surg* 1988; **75:** 409–15.
18. Jinnai D, Quoted in: *Surgery of the Anus, Rectum and Colon*, 4th edn (Goligher JC, ed). London: Baillière Tindall, 1984: 447.
19. Finlay IG, Meek DR, Gray HW et al, Incidence and detection of occult hepatic metastases in colorectal carcinoma. *BMJ* 1982; **284:** 803–5.
20. Mecklin JP, Jarvinen HJ, Hakkiluoto A et al, Frequency of hereditary nonpolyposis colorectal cancer. A prospective multicenter study in Finland. *Dis Colon Rectum* 1995; **38:** 588–93.
21. Lynch HT, Is there a role for prophylactic subtotal colectomy among hereditary nonpolyposis colorectal cancer germline mutation carriers? *Dis Colon Rectum* 1996; **39:** 109–10.
22. Vasen HF, Taal BG, Nagengast FM et al, Hereditary nonpolyposis colorectal cancer: results of long-term surveillance in 50 families. *Eur J Cancer* 1995; **31A:** 1145–8.
23. Psaila J, Bulley SH, Ewings P et al, Outcome following laparoscopic resection for colorectal cancer. *Br J Surg* 1998; **85:** 662–4.
24. Wexner SD, Cohen SM, Port site metastases after laparoscopic colorectal surgery for cure of malignancy. *Br J Surg* 1995; **82:** 295–8.
25. Raymond MA, Schneider C, Kostle S et al, The pathogenesis of portsite recurrence. *J Gastrointest Surg* 1998; **2:** 406–14.
26. DeCosse JJ, Tsioulias GJ, Jacobson JS, Colorectal cancer: detection, treatment, and rehabilitation. *CA Cancer J Clin* 1994; **44:** 27–42.
27. Samet J, Hunt WC, Key C et al, Choice of cancer therapy varies with age of patient. *JAMA* 1986; **255:** 3385–90.
28. McGinnis LS, Surgical treatment options for colorectal cancer. *Cancer* 1994; **74**(7 Suppl): 2147–50.
29. Fitzgerald SD, Longo WE, Daniel GL, Vernava AM, Advanced colorectal neoplasia in the high-risk elderly patient: Is surgical resection justified? *Dis Colon Rectum* 1993; **36:** 161–6.
30. Umpleby HC, Bristol JB, Rainey JB, Williamson RC, Survival of 727 patients with single carcinomas of the large bowel. *Dis Colon Rectum* 1984; **27:** 803–10.
31. Edwards RT, Bransom CJ, Crosby DL, Pathy MS, Colorectal carcinoma in the elderly: a geriatric and surgical practice compared. *Age Ageing* 1983; **12:** 256–62.

32. Fielding LP, Phillips RK, Hittinger R, Factors influencing mortality after curative resection for large bowel cancer in elderly patients. *Lancet* 1989; **i**: 595–7.

33. Irvin TT, Prognosis of colorectal cancer in the elderly. *Br J Surg* 1988; **75**: 419–21.

34. Mulcahy HE, Patchett SE, Daly L, O'Donoghue DP, Prognosis of elderly patients with large bowel cancer. *Br J Surg* 1994; **81**: 736–8.

35. Fielding LP, Wells BW, Survival after primary and after staged resection for large bowel obstruction caused by cancer. *Br J Surg* 1974; **61**: 16–18.

36. Aldridge MC, Phillips RK, Hittinger R et al, Influence of tumour site on presentation, management and subsequent outcome in large bowel cancer. *Br J Surg* 1986; **73**: 663–70.

37. Irvin TT, Greaney MG, The treatment of colonic cancer presenting with intestinal obstruction. *Br J Surg* 1977; **64**: 741–4.

38. Clark J, Hall AW, Moossa AR, Treatment of obstructing cancer of the colon and rectum. *Surg Gynecol Obstet* 1975; **141**: 541–4.

39. Gutman M, Kaplan O, Skornick Y et al, Proximal colostomy: still an effective emergency measure in obstructing carcinoma of the large bowel. *J Surg Oncol* 1989; **41**: 210–12.

40. Dixon AR, Holmes JT, Hartmann's procedure for carcinoma of rectum and distal sigmoid colon: 5-year audit. *J R Coll Surg Edinb* 1990; **35**: 166–8.

41. Adams WJ, Mann LJ, Bokey EL et al, Hartmann's procedure for carcinoma of the rectum and sigmoid colon. *Aust NZ J Surg* 1992; **62**: 200–2.

42. Gandrup P, Lund L, Balslev I, Surgical treatment of acute malignant large bowel obstruction. *Eur J Surg* 1992; **158**: 427–30.

43. Mileski WJ, Rege RV, Joehl RJ, Nahrwold DL, Rates of morbidity and mortality after closure of loop and end colostomy. *Surg Gynecol Obstet* 1990; **171**: 17–21.

44. de Almeida AM, Gracias CW, dos Santos NM, Aldeia FJ, Surgical management of acute, malignant obstruction of the left colon with colostomy. *Acta Med Port* 1991; **4**: 257–62 (in Portuguese).

45. Malafosse M, Goujard F, Gallot D, Sezeur A, Treatment of acute obstruction due to left colonic cancer. *Chirurgie* 1989; **115**(Suppl 2): 123–6 (in French).

46. Sjodahl R, Franzen T, Nystrom PO, Primary versus staged resection for acute obstructing colorectal carcinoma. *Br J Surg* 1992; **79**: 685–8.

47. Ambrosetti P, Borst F, Robert J et al, Single-stage excision anastomosis of left colonic obstruction excision treated as an emergency. *Chirurgie* 1989; **115**(Suppl 2): I–VII (in French).

48. Koruth NM, Krukowski ZH, Youngson GG et al, Intra-operative colonic irrigation in the management of left-sided large bowel emergencies. *Br J Surg* 1985; **72**: 708–11.

49. Pearce NW, Scott SD, Karran SJ, Timing and method of reversal of Hartmann's procedure. *Br J Surg* 1992; **79**: 839–41.

50. Amsterdam E, Krispin M, Primary resection with colocolostomy for obstructive carcinoma of the left side of the colon. *Am J Surg* 1985; **150**: 558–60.

51. Dorudi S, Wilson NM, Heddle RM, Primary restorative colectomy in malignant left-sided large bowel obstruction. *Ann R Coll Surg Engl* 1990; **72**: 393–5.

52. Hong JC, Hwang DM, Wang YH, Intraoperative antegrade colon irrigation – in the management of obstructing left-sided colon cancer. *Kao-Hsiung i Hsueh Ko Hsueh Tsa Chih [Kaohsiung J Med Sci]* 1989; **5**: 309–13 (in Chinese).

53. Murray JJ, Schoetz DJ Jr, Coller JA et al, Intraoperative colonic lavage and primary anastomosis in nonelective colon resection. *Dis Colon Rectum* 1991; **34**: 527–31.

54. Koruth NM, Hunter DC, Krukowski ZH, Matheson NA, Immediate resection in emergency large bowel surgery: a 7 year audit. *Br J Surg* 1985; **72**: 703–7.

55. Gorey TF, O'Connell PR, Waldron D et al, Laparoscopically assisted reversal of Hartmann's procedure. *Br J Surg* 1993; **80**: 109.

56. Radcliffe AG, Dudley HA, Intraoperative antegrade irrigation of the large intestine. *Surg Gynecol Obstet* 1983; **156**: 721–3.

57. Dudley HA, Radcliffe AG, McGeehan D, Intraoperative irrigation of the colon to permit primary anastomosis. *Br J Surg* 1980; **67**: 80–1.

58. White CM, Macfie J, Immediate colectomy and primary anastomosis for acute obstruction due to carcinoma of the left colon and rectum. *Dis Colon Rectum* 1985; **28**: 155–7.

59. Duthie GS, Foster ME, Price-Thomas JM, Leaper DJ, Bowel preparation or not for elective colorectal surgery. *J R Coll Surg Edinb* 1990; **35**: 169–71.

60. Konishi F, Muto T, Kanazawa K, Morioka Y, Intraoperative irrigation and primary resection for obstructing lesions of the left colon. *Int J Colorectal Dis* 1988; **3**: 204–6.

61. Yu BM, Surgical treatment of acute intestinal obstruction caused by large bowel carcinoma. *Chung-Hua Wai Ko Tsa Chih [Chin J Surg]* 1989; **27**: 285–6; 443 (in Chinese).

62. Runkel NS, Hinz U, Lehnert T et al, Improved outcome after emergency surgery for cancer of the large intestine. *Br J Surg* 1998; **85**: 1260–5.

63. Hughes ES, McDermott FT, Polglase AL, Nottle P, Total and subtotal colectomy for colonic obstruction. *Dis Colon Rectum* 1985; **28**: 162–3.

64. Wilson RG, Gollock JM, Obstructing carcinoma of the left colon managed by subtotal colectomy. *J R Coll Surg Edinb* 1989; **34**: 25–6.

65. Stephenson BM, Shandall AA, Farouk R, Griffith G, Malignant left-sided large bowel obstruction managed by subtotal/total colectomy. *Br J Surg* 1990; **77**: 1098–102.

66. Arnaud JP, Bergamaschi R, Emergency subtotal/total colectomy with anastomosis for acutely obstructed carcinoma of the left colon. *Dis Colon Rectum* 1994; **37**: 685–8.

67. Salim AS, Percutaneous decompression and irrigation for large bowel obstruction. New approach. *Dis Colon Rectum* 1991; **34**: 973–80; discussion 978–80.

68. Mainar A, De Gregorio Ariza MA, Tejero E et al, Acute colorectal obstruction: treatment with self-expandable metallic stents before scheduled surgery – results of a multicenter study. *Radiology* 1999; **210**: 65–9.

69. De Gregorio MA, Mainar A, Tiger E et al, Acute colorectal obstruction: stent placement for palliative treatment – results of a multicenter study. *Radiology* 1998; **209**: 117–20.

70. Gilbert JM, Jeffrey I, Evans M, Kark AE, Sites of recurrent tumour after 'curative' colorectal surgery: implications for adjuvant therapy. *Br J Surg* 1984; **71**: 203–5.

71. Wangensteen OH, Sosin H, How can the outlook in alimentary tract cancer be improved? *Am J Surg* 1968; **115**: 7–16.

72. Delpero JR, Pol B, Le Treut P et al, Surgical resection of locally recurrent colorectal adenocarcinoma. *Br J Surg* 1998; **85**: 372–6.

73. Schneebaum S, Arnold MW, Young D et al, Role of carcinoembryonic antigen in predicting resectability of recurrent colorectal cancer. *Dis Colon Rectum* 1993; **36**: 810–15.

74. Bakalakos EA, Burak WE Jr, Young DC, Martin EW Jr, Is carcino-embryonic antigen useful in the follow-up management of patients with colorectal liver metastases? *Am J Surg* 1999; **177**: 2–6.

75. McCall JL, Black RB, Rich CA et al, The value of serum carcinoembryonic antigen in predicting recurrent disease following curative resection of colorectal cancer. *Dis Colon Rectum* 1994; **37**: 875–81.

76. Beets G, Penninckx F, Schiepers C et al, Clinical value of whole-body positron emission tomography with [^{18}F]fluorodeoxyglucose in recurrent colorectal cancer. *Br J Surg* 1994; **81**: 1666–70.

77. Thurston MO, Majzisik CM, History and development of radioimmunoguided surgery. *Semin Colon Rectal Surg* 1995; **6:** 185–91.

78. Wolff BG, Bolton J, Baum R et al, Radioimmunoscintigraphy of recurrent metastatic or occult colorectal cancer with technetium Tc^{99m} 88BV59H21-ZV67-66 (HumaSPECT®-Tc), a totally human monoclonal antibody. *Dis Colon Rectum* 1998; **41:** 953–62.

79. Bruinvels DJ, Stigglebout AM, Kievit J et al, Follow-up of patients with colorectal cancer. A meta-analysis. *Ann Surg* 1994; **219:** 174–82.

10

Laparoscopic left colectomy for cancer

Guy-Bernard Cadière, Jacques M Himpens

INTRODUCTION

Reports of trocar-site recurrences and recurrences on the mini-laparotomy scar after laparoscopic colon resection jeopardize the future of this novel mode of treatment for colon cancer. Considering, however, the significant immediate benefit for the patient, laparoscopic colon resection for cancer is still performed. In order to evaluate the feasibility of this technique as well as its safety, three questions should be asked.

1. Does laparoscopy increase the risk of parietal metastasis?
2. Is a laparoscopic resection oncologically sufficient?
3. Are recurrence rate and survival different with laparoscopy versus conventional resection?

The answers to these questions seem to be in favour of the laparoscopic approach. Several studies have demonstrated that the incidence of parietal metastasis is no higher with laparoscopy than with classic resection. Moreover, the resection margins after laparoscopic resection seem to be equivalent to or even better than with conventional treatment. The Clinical Outcomes of Surgical Therapy (COST) study, analysing the 3-year follow-up and comparing it with the US National Cancer Institute (NCI) statistics of colon resection, could not find any significant difference between the two approaches.

Despite the fact that follow-up is still insufficient, it seems that laparoscopic colectomy is a safe and reliable technique in the treatment of colon cancer. This procedure should, however, be performed in the context of clinical trials until larger series and longer follow-ups are available.

TECHNIQUE

A number of guidelines should be followed when performing laparoscopic colon resection:

1. Stable trocars must be used, thereby reducing local parietal trauma.
2. The tumour itself should not be mobilized, but rather a no-touch technique should be used.
3. Vascular control should be achieved at the beginning of the procedure.
4. Tumour exclusion plus bowel lumen occlusion proximally as well as distally should be performed.
5. The extraction site through which the sample is withdrawn should be protected.
6. The resection should be no smaller than with the conventional approach.
7. Preoperative lavage should be avoided as much as possible, so as not to scatter tumour cells.

Laparoscopic colon resection is a complex endeavour since it involves wide dissection, causing frequent tool and camera changes.

Preparation of the patient

Bowel preparation is essential – not only for obtaining a clean colon but also for avoiding dilated small bowel. The patient should be put on a residue-poor diet for 8 days; 48 hours before the procedure, 3 litres of polyethylene glycol should be ingested. An additional 1 or 2 litres of polyethylene glycol should be drunk the day before the procedure. With this regimen, colon preparation should be satisfactory and the small bowel should not be dilated.

Placement of the patient

The patient is in a so-called lithotomy position, with the arms along the body. A nasogastric tube and an indwelling Foley catheter are in place, the surgeon and the first assistant are located to the right of the patient, and the scrub nurse is placed between the legs of the patient (Figure 10.1). The video monitor is directly in front of the surgeon, at the level of the patient's left thigh, so that surgeon, optical system, operative field, and monitor are approximately on the same axis. Scissors, the aspiration cannula, and the clip applier are placed in a pocket, which is fixed on the patient's right thigh.

Placement of trocars and tools

Four trocars are used for this procedure (Figure 10.2). The first 10 mm trocar is placed 1 cm cephalad of the umbilicus, and will harbour the optical system. A second 5 mm trocar is inserted in the right lower quadrant on the midclavicular line. This trocar opening can be enlarged if needed in order to allow the introduction of linear cutting and stapling devices. A third 5 mm trocar is placed on the right midclavicular line at the level of the umbilicus. A fourth 5 mm trocar is placed in the left upper quadrant approximately at the level of the umbilicus on the left midclavicular line. An additional 5 mm trocar can be placed in a suprapubic position, if it is desired to perform stapling and extraction from this side. The second trocar allows the introduction of scissors or of a coagulating hook, held in the surgeon's right hand. The third trocar harbours the grasping forceps, which will be kept in the surgeon's left hand. The fourth trocar in the left upper quadrant will harbour an atraumatic grasper.

Exploration of the abdominal cavity

If problems in localizing the tumour are expected, a preoperative colonoscopy can be performed. However, it is preferable to have the gastroenterologist mark the tumour preoperatively with methylene blue or with China ink. The problem with perioperative colonoscopy is that air insufflation – necessary for visualization with the colonoscope – will reduce the field of view for the surgeon.

Once the surgeon has spotted the tumour site, the entire abdominal cavity is checked in order to rule out metastatic disease.

Exposure of the left colon

The patient is put in a 10° Trendelenburg position with a 20° roll to the right. The surgeon stays to the right of the patient or shifts to between the legs. The

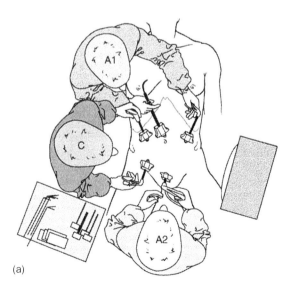

(a)

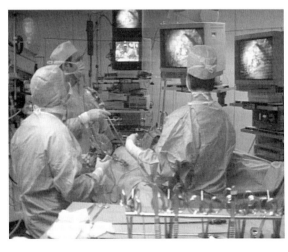

(b)

Figure 10.1 (a,b) Placement of the patient and the team: first assistant (A1); surgeon (C); scrub nurse (A2).

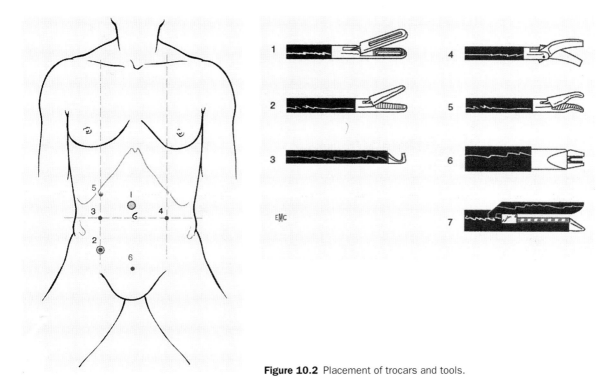

Figure 10.2 Placement of trocars and tools.

larger omentum is reflected on the anterior side of the stomach and tucked in front of the left liver lobe, thereby exposing the transverse colon. The Trendelenburg tilt is then increased to 30°. The small-bowel loops are pulled cephalad and tucked in a supramesocolic position, so that the entire meso-colon, the third duodenum, and the angle of Treitz are clearly visible. It is sometimes necessary to maintain the small bowel in the supramesocolic position by using a grasper from the fourth (left upper quadrant) trocar. This grasper snaps the small bowel about 20 cm distal to the angle of Treitz, and creates a hinge that maintains the small bowel in its desired position.

Exposure of the pelvis necessitates clearance of terminal ileum and caecum. If necessary, an additional grasper can be placed through a fifth trocar placed on the right midclavicular line about 8–10 cm proximal to the third trocar. This grasper picks up the distal ileum about 30 cm proximal to the ileocaecal valve, and will keep the last small bowel loops as well as the caecum in the right lower quadrant in an orthostatic fashion (Figure 10.3).

In female patients, exposure of the pelvis can be favourably influenced by retracting the uterus with a percutaneously inserted transuterine stitch.

It is impossible to expose the entire left colon from midtransversum down to the upper part of the rectum at the same time. The procedure has to be subdivided into two steps: first dissection of the splenic angle and then dissection of left colon and rectosigmoid.

Strategy of left colectomy

The strategy of left colectomy is identical in the case of cancer or benign colitis. First, Toldt's fascia must be dissected, together with the perirectal fascia. Second, the left paracolic gutter must be severed. Third, Douglas' pouch must be incised. Fourth, the mesorectum and distal rectum must be transsected, and fifth, the proximal colon must be transsected as well. In order to separate the colon and mesocolon from the retroperitoneum, it is necessary to incise the parietal peritoneum along the aorta, dissect the lower mesenteric artery and lower mesenteric vein, and finally sever the neural branches coming from the periaortic plexus that innervate the mesocolon.

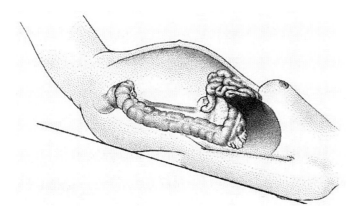

Figure 10.3 Exposure of the left colon: the patient is in full Trendelenburg position and the small bowel loops are pulled cephalad.

Incision of the mesocolic peritoneal sheet

The peritoneal sheet at the root of the left mesocolon is grasped by the forceps, and is incised with scissors from distal to proximal, starting at the sacral promontory, and continuing along the aorta up to the third part of the duodenum. The incision is then taken to the patient's left, aiming towards the splenic angle, thereby crossing the path of the inferior mesenteric vein, on its way to the lower border of the pancreas.

Ligation of inferomesenteric artery and vein

The grasper in the fourth (left upper quadrant) trocar grasps the mesosigmoid, which is pulled cephalad towards the patient's left (Figure 10.4). This manoeuvre puts the inferior mesenteric artery under traction. The root of this artery is then clearly visible at approximately 1–3 cm distal to the third part of the duodenum. The grasper is then repositioned so as to pick up the peritoneum exactly at the level of this artery. If it is decided not to mobilize the splenic angle, the artery is severed just distal to the origin of the left colic artery.

When the patient is obese, a significant dissection is needed to reveal the artery. The dissection is performed with the coagulating hook. The periarterial neural plexus should be left posteriorly, away from the specimen. The periarterial lymph nodes, however, should be included in the specimen. A needle holder is introduced in the second trocar, and looped around the artery, and the artery is then tied using an intracorporeal knotting technique. Additional clips can be placed for safety.

The inferior mesenteric vein is clipped at the lower border of the pancreas.

Separation of Toldt's fascia

Unlike the case of open surgery, the incision of the left colic gutter is delayed until later in the procedure. The purpose of this delay is to avoid the left colon dropping medially and obscuring the operative field. Moreover, with the surgeon being positioned to the patient's right, it is logical to keep the dissection of the most remote part of the operative field towards the end of the dissection.

The correct technique to separate Toldt's fascia (the adherent left mesocolon) is to grasp the distal part of the inferior mesenteric artery, which is lifted anteriorly. This is done by the surgeon's left hand, with the right hand dissecting very carefully with the tip of the scissors in the direction pointing towards the patient's left shoulder. The correct plane of dissection is the one that leaves anteriorly only the ante-

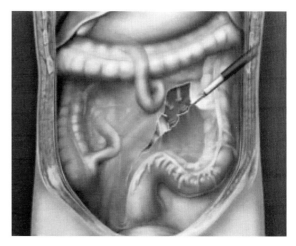

Figure 10.4 Incision of the mesocolic peritoneal sheet and ligation of the inferomesenteric artery and vein.

rior peritoneal sheet, the veins, the arteries, and the nerves. Automatically, the left ureter and Gerota's fascia will be left posteriorly. The general shape of the dissection is a pyramid with the forceps from the fourth trocar at the apex (Figure 10.5).

The superior limit of dissection is the inferior border of the pancreas. The left limit is the left paracolic gutter. The next step of the dissection is oriented distally. Small branches from the neural plexus going towards the left colon and the sigmoid must be severed at this stage.

Dissection of the pararectal fascia

Dissection of the pararectal fascia is initiated at the level of the sacral promontory (Figure 10.6). The correct plane of dissection is continuous with the plane of Toldt's fascia. The most obvious danger is to start dissecting too posteriorly into the presacral space, which would expose the presacral veins, which are easily torn. If the correct space is entered, however, dissection is bloodless. The space located between the visceral sheet of the peritoneum and the parietal sheet is located anterior to the left and right hypogastric nerves, which must be seen and parietalized during the dissection.

Incision of the left colic gutter

The forceps in the fourth trocar pulls the sigmoid loop towards the right upper quadrant. The peritoneal

reflection is held with the forceps in the third trocar. This provides counter-traction, which facilitates dissection with scissors coming from the second trocar. Incision is continued from distal to proximal, i.e. from the iliac vessels at the level of the sacral promontory all the way up to the splenic angle. This incision joins the previously dissected posterior mesocolon. Subsequently incision is oriented distally towards the left side of the rectum (Figure 10.7). The ureter is again visualized and

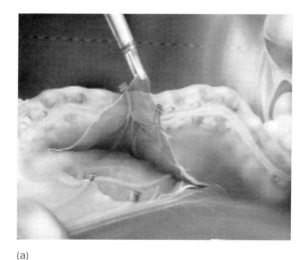

(a)

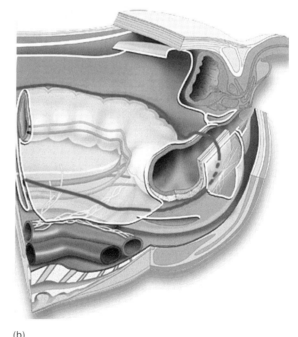

(b)

Figure 10.6 (a,b) Further stages in the separation of the Toldt's fascia.

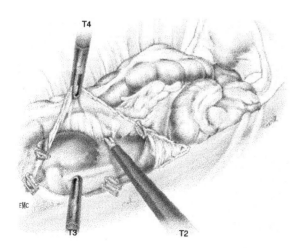

Figure 10.5 The beginning of the separation of the Toldt's fascia.

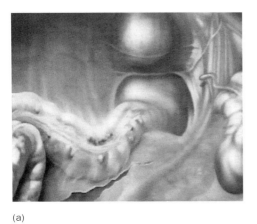

(a)

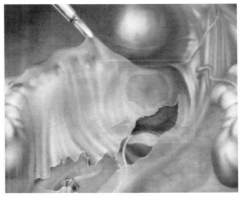

(b)

Figure 10.7 (a,b) Dissection of the parietal fascia.

left posteriorly. Dissection finally joins the perirectal fascia located at the left side of the rectum.

Incision of Douglas pouch

The grasper in the fourth trocar pulls the upper rectum to the left of the patient. The grasper in the third trocar grasps the peritoneal sheet overlying the bladder, and pulls it anteriorly. The peritoneal reflection is severed from right to left. The prerectal space located between the colon and Denonvilliers' fascia is opened and the anterior side of the rectum is exposed (Figure 10.8).

Dissection of the mesorectum

At the chosen level for transection, the muscular layer of the rectum is exposed on its entire circumference (Figure 10.9). The dissection can be performed with scissors, with a coagulating hook, or with an ultrasonic scalpel. The superior haemorroidal vessels are coagulated or clipped.

Transsection of the rectum

The second trocar located at the superior and anterior

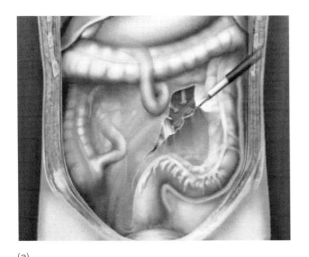

(a)

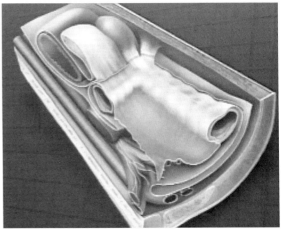

(b)

Figure 10.8 (a) Incision of the left colic gutter; (b) incision of the parietocolic and splenocolic ligament.

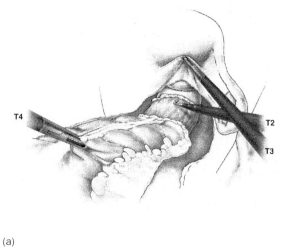

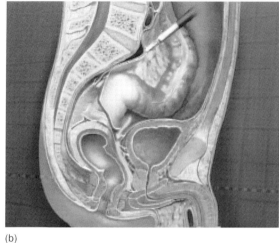

(a)

(b)

Figure 10.9 (a,b) Incision of Douglas pouch.

iliac spine is replaced by a 12 mm trocar, which allows the introduction of a linear cutting and stapling device (Figure 10.10). Alternatively, this device can also be introduced in a suprapubic position if the stapler is flexible. It is essential that the stapling device be perpendicular to the rectum. If this is not the case then transsection of the rectum is very difficult.

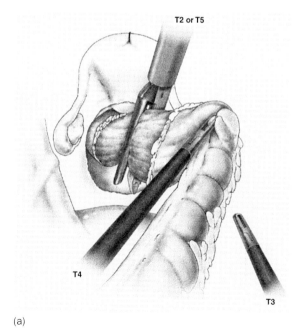

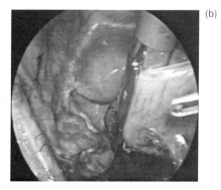

(b)

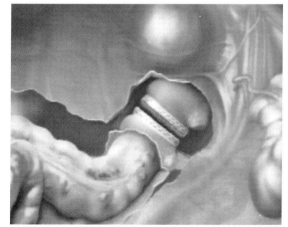

(c)

(a)

Figure 10.10 (a–c) Transsection of the rectum.

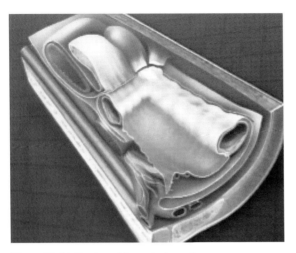

Figure 10.11 Freeing of the splenic angle.

Freeing of the splenic angle, laparoscopic anatomy of the splenic angle

Freeing of the splenic angle allows one to obtain more slack with the proximal colon, which guarantees a tension-free anastomosis. Freeing of this angle can be performed either by simple severence of the peritoneal attachments of the colon at that level or by additionally cutting the root of the left mesocolon, care being taken to spare the midcolic artery. The direction of dissection can be either from medial to lateral or the opposite.

Freeing of the splenic angle from medial to lateral (Figure 10.11)

The posterior attachments of the colon at the splenic level are severed after opening Toldt's fascia as previously described. Posterior dissection is performed from medial to lateral while the surgeon is holding the root of the left mesocolon in a ventral direction, with Gerota's fascia and the anterior side of the pancreas being left posteriorly. It is essential not to dissect in too posterior a direction, to avoid injury to the pancreas or indeed opening of the retropancreatic space.

Dissection of Toldt's fascia is continued along the lower border of the pancreas up to the splenic angle and the left paracolic gutter. The bursa can be opened at this level by severance of the anterior layer of the transverse mesocolon. In order to continue the dissection, surgeon and patient must be put in a different position: the patient is put in a reversed

Trendelenburg position. The lateral roll is maintained. The surgeon is now placed between the patient's legs. Dissection of the greater omentum is initiated at the left side of the transverse colon, a little lateral of the midline, and is continued towards the splenic angle. The bursa must be opened at this stage in order to allow good visualization of the blood vessels in the transverse mesocolon, which must be preserved. This step of the dissection is straightforward, good traction and countertraction being obtained by ventral traction of the omentum and posterior traction of the transverse colon.

Mobilization of the splenic angle from lateral to medial

The patient is placed in a slightly reversed Trendelenburg position with 20° lateral roll. The surgeon is positioned between the patient's legs. The surgeon's right hand is holding the scissors introduced in the fourth trocar, while the left-hand atraumatic grasper, introduced in the second trocar, is pulling the colon distally and to the right.

If it is simply desired to mobilize the splenic angle with the aim of a limited resection, as for a benign polyp, the colo-omental attachments are first best severed from right to left (from midtransversum towards the splenic angle). Subsequently, the left gutter, the phrenocolic ligament (from proximal to distal), and finally the left mesocolonic posterior attachments are severed, while the surgeon pulls the colon towards the right lower quadrant with the atraumatic grasper, in the second trocar.

Transsection of the left mesocolon

The left mesocolon is incised at the chosen level. Drummond's arcade is spared. Even though some surgeons only transsect the mesocolon while exteriorizing the specimen, the present technique avoids troublesome haematomas created by forceful pulling while exteriorizing. The transsected mesocolon also provides additional slack. The proximal colon section is prepared for anastomosis outside the peritoneal cavity.

Extraction and resection of the tumour

The specimen is extracted through a mini-laparotomy obtained by enlarging a trocar opening in the right lower quadrant or suprapubically. It is

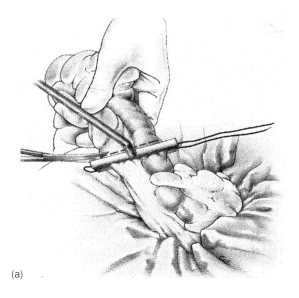

(a)

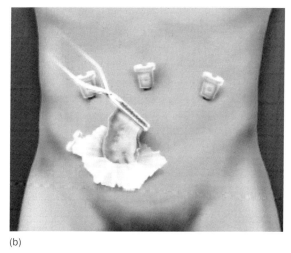

(b)

Figure 10.12 (a,b) Proximal transsection of the colon.

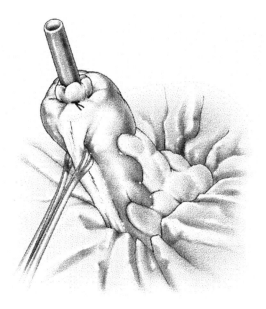

(a)

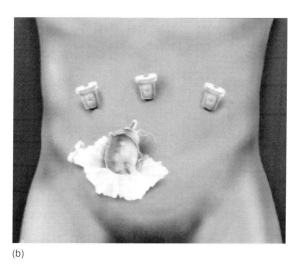

(b)

Figure 10.13 (a,b) Purse string on the anvil of a circular stapler.

extremely important to protect the wound with a plastic sleeve in order to avoid soiling by tumour cells or faecal material. The proximal transsection level of the colon is dissected free of all fat and small vessels. The bowel is then transsected and removed (Figure 10.12).

The anvil of a circular stapler is introduced in the bowel lumen and a purse string performed. The bowel is replaced intraperitoneally and the mini-laparotomy is closed in layers (Figure 10.13).

Anastomosis

The circular stapler is introduced transanally and a conventional circular stapled anastomosis is performed through the distal staple line. The resected doughnuts are checked for completeness (Figure 10.14). The anastomosis must be free of traction and well vascularized. It can be tested for air leaks after its immersion under saline.

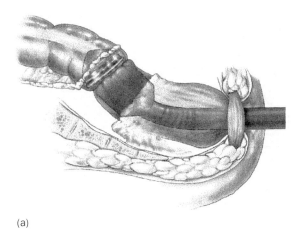

(a)

Figure 10.14 (a,b) Circular stapled anastomosis.

(b)

Postoperative evolution

The nasogastric tube is removed in the recovery room. Oral feedings are resumed on postoperative day 2, and the patient is discharged on the fifth post-operative day.

BIBLIOGRAPHY

1. Cady J, Godefroy J, Sibaud O, La résection anastomose coeliochirurgicale dans la sigmoidite diverticulaire et ses complications à propos de soixante-cinq cas. *Chirurgie* 1996; **121:** 350–4.

2. Cooperman A, Zucker KA, Laparoscopic guided intestinal surgery. In: *Surgical Laparoscopy* (Zucker KA, Bailey RW, Reddick EJ, eds). St Louis, MO: Quality Medical Publications: 259–310.

3. Falk PM, Beart RW, Wexner SD et al, Laparoscopic colectomy: a critical appraisal. *Dis Colon Rectum* 1993; **36:** 91–7.

4. Franklin ME, Ramos R, Rosenthal D, Schuessler W, Laparoscopic colonic procedures. *World J Surg* 1993; **17:** 51–6.

5. Franklin ME, Laparoscopic management of colorectal disease. The United States experience. *Dig Surg* 1995; **12:** 284–7.

6. Gallot D, Les colectomies pour maladies diverticulaires. In: *Encylopédie de Médecine et Chirurgie. Techniques Chirurgicales: Chirurgie Digestive.* Paris, 1988.

7. Goligher JC (ed), *Surgery of the Anus, Rectum and Colon,* 4th edn. London: Baillière Tindall, 1984.

8. Jacobs M, Verdeja GD, Golstein DS, Minimally invasive colon resection. *Surg Laparosc Endosc;* **2:** 144–50.

9. Knight ChD, Griffen D, An improved technique for low anterior resection of the rectum using the EEA stapler. *Surgery* 1982; **88:** 710–14.

10. Lamy J, Louis R, Michotey G et al, *Nouveau Traité de Technique Chirurgicale,* Tome XI. Paris: Masson, 1976: 454–60.

11. Leroy J, Laparoscopic colorectal resection. Technical aspects after 150 operations. *Osp Maggiore;* **88(3):** 262–6.

12. Lumley JW, Fielding GA, Rhodes M et al, Laparoscopic assisted colorectal surgery. Lessons learned from 240 consecutive patients. *Dis Colon Rectum* 1996; **39:** 155–9.

13. Mariette D, Sbai-Idrissi S, Bobocescu E et al, La colectomie coelio-préparée: technique et résultats. *J Chir* 1996; **133:** 3–5.

14. Parneix M, Zaranis C, Apport et place de la viscéro-synthèse dans la chirurgie conservatrice sphinctérienne du cancer rectal. A propos de 80 anastomoses coloanales ou colo-rectales sous-péritonéale. *Lyon Chir* 1990; **86:** 198–200.

15. Redwine DB, Sharpe DR, Laparoscopic segmental resection of the sigmoid colon for endometriosis. *J Laparoendosc Surg* 1991; **1:** 217–20.

16. Trebuchet G, Le Calvet JL, Launois B, Traitement coelio-chirurgical des sigmoïdites diverticulaires. *Chirurgie* 1996; **121:** 89–90.

17. Wexner SD, Cohen SM, Johansen OB et al, Laparoscopic colorectal surgery: a prospective assessment and current perspective. *Br J Surg* 1993; **80:** 87–90.

18. Wexner SD, Reissman P, Pfeifer J et al, Laparoscopic colorectal surgery: analysis of 140 cases. *Surg Endosc* 1996; **10:** 133–6.

19. Cadière G-B, Himpens J, Left colectomy for cancer. In: *Management of Colorectal Cancer* (Bleiberg H, Rougier Ph, Wilke H-J, eds). London: Martin Dunitz, 1998: 93–102.

20. Cadière G-B, Leroy J, Drouard F et al, Colectomie gauche pour cancer par voie laparoscopique. *J Coelio-Chir* 1994; **12:** 17–22.

21. Vertruyen M, Cadière G-B, Himpens J, Bruyns J, Colectomie pour cancer par coelioscopie. *J Pathol Digest* 1996; **6:** 47.

11

Minimal invasive surgery for colon cancer: Where do we stand?

José I Restrepo, Heidi Nelson

INTRODUCTION

Limited retrospective and prospective data suggest that early recurrence is similar in open and laparoscopic colectomy for cancer. This has softened the skepticism triggered by the increased rates of wound and trocar-site tumor implantation reported initially. Enthusiasm for the treatment of colon cancer with minimally invasive surgery and the stated oncologic concerns have prompted the initiation of trials around the world. Currently, there are eight prospective, national, and international trials defining whether laparoscopic colectomy has advantages over the open counterpart, and whether it compromises oncologic outcomes. These trials share the same aims: evaluation of the safety of the procedure, the quality of life, the cancer outcome, and cost analysis. The US National Institutes of Health (NIH) Laparoscopic versus Open Colectomy for Cancer Trial opened accrual in 1994, and has served as a model for others. Preliminary reports are encouraging, although final results are still not available. Only after these studies have been completed will the role of laparoscopic colectomy for cancer (LCC) be determined. Currently, the American Society of Colon and Rectal Surgery, as well as other national professional societies, recommend that laparoscopic colorectal surgery for cancer with curative intent should only be done in the setting of a randomized, prospective trial.

BENEFITS OF LAPAROSCOPIC TECHNIQUES

Large-bowel laparoscopic surgery is unique in the sense that the colon is a large and mobile organ that requires resection and anastomosis. For this reason, most centers perform laparoscopic-assisted colectomy (LAC) rather than a total laparoscopic procedure. Because of the diversity of procedures, high conversion rates, and early experiences, the benefits of LAC were initially obscured. Significant reductions in postoperative pain, narcotic use, and recovery time, without any apparent compromise of safety or costs, make this procedure attractive to both patients and surgeons. Physiologic and immunologic advantages make it even more appealing, especially for cancer.

Recovery time

Recovery has been consistently shorter with LAC. This encompasses the hospital length of stay (LoS) and the time required to resume normal activity and work. LAC reduces postoperative ileus, as shown by early passage of flatus, first bowel movement, and tolerance of regular diet. Overall LoS reductions range from 2 to 5 days.[1–5] In colon cancer trials, similar results are found, with a reduction ranging from 2 to 7 days.[4] Most prospective randomized trials support these results,[2,6] although others do not.[7] Diminished ileus is a major determinant for an earlier discharge. This earlier resumption of bowel function could result from reduced pain[8] and narcotic requirements,[7] or from less intestinal manipulation during surgery. Animal models have not supported the role of psychological conditioning[9] as the only explanation. Furthermore, earlier feeding in open colorectal surgery has been associated with decreased LoS.[10] Although selection bias cannot be avoided in laparoscopy, reported data from prospective randomized trials suggest that the benefits are real.

Besides reducing the LoS, the time required to return to an active and independent life is also reduced.[10] This has an economic impact, which is an issue that needs to be considered. Of particular interest are reports of recovery advantages for LAC compared with an open procedure in the elderly.[11] Stocchi and colleagues[12] found that there was a significant preservation of independence at discharge (94% for laparoscopic versus 76% for open) besides a 3-day decrease in the LoS in patients over 75 years old. The most frequent indication for surgery in this series was colon cancer. The fact that elderly patients were more likely to return to independent living has not only social and psychological impact, but economic implications as well.

Long-term benefits

As a consequence of diminished adhesions from laparoscopic colon procedures,[13] a lower incidence of small-bowel obstruction is to be expected, which may have an impact on the long-term patient benefits. Experimental trials with longer follow-up need to examine this critically. In laparoscopic colectomy, an early reduction of small-bowel obstruction, as a complication, has been observed.[4]

Financial benefits

LAC has been proven feasible, meaning that it can be performed safely and cost-effectively. Results regarding its financial benefits have been conflicting, because many variables are involved. Higher costs are mainly derived from increased operative times, high conversion rates, and the improper use of disposable instruments. Reduced LoS and late complications with limited use of analgesics may influence costs. Earlier return to an active life should also be considered. For a complete analysis, both direct and indirect costs must be accounted for.

Costs and conversion

Costs for both laparoscopic and open procedures are similar, although there is a greater financial burden if the laparoscopic approach has to be converted.[14] Reasons for opening a patient can be gathered in three groups: technical factors, intraoperative complications, and disease-related reasons. The overall conversion rate ranges from 3%[15] to 41%,[5] with 20% being acceptable at the present time. This variability is a reflection of the learning curve. Dean et al,[16] in the Mayo Clinic, reported a weight above 90 kg as a factor for conversion. Adhesions from previous surgery are a frequent cause too. In cancer, conversion rates are similar to benign ones,[7,17–19] and in this setting, reasons to open the patient include extensive tumors, neoplasm low in the rectum, and the presence of bowel distention. Most conversion factors should be identified preoperatively, and early conversion should be opted for in order to achieve cost-effectiveness.

Costs and operating time

It is noteworthy that laparoscopic colon surgery is associated with longer operating times. These are dependent on the experience of the operator and on the frequency of conversion; both factors should improve with exposure to the technique. The reported LAC mean operating time is variable and highly dependent on the learning curve,[20,21] with late experiences reporting well below 190 minutes.[22]

The number of cases required for a surgeon to be proficient doing LAC is variable;[23,24] plateaus have been observed at 10–20 cases.[1,5] This significantly influences conversion rates and operative times, which are the main determinants of costs. Command of the surgical technique is reflected in a significant economy due to reduction of operative time and conversion frequency.

Other potential benefits

Cosmesis

Although cosmesis is clearly secondary to safety or oncologic results, it is an important patient-related benefit implicated in quality of life. A superior cosmetic result for laparoscopic colon surgery has been reported.[25] In laparoscopic-assisted ileocolic resection for Crohn's disease, the cosmetic score was significantly higher than for the open counterpart;[26] body image correlated strongly with cosmesis. Since port placement in colon surgery is flexible, there is a possibility of enhanced aesthetics. The cosmetic effect can be improved if skin folds, creases, and the umbilicus are used for the incisions.

Physiologic advantages

Cardiovascular and pulmonary alterations during a CO_2 pneumoperitoneum have been delineated. Reduced cardiac output and blood pressure with increased systemic vascular resistance, pulmonary hypertension, and metabolic acidosis are expected. No significant harmful CO_2 effects are proven, and alternatives such as helium or nitrous oxide are available. With safe use of pneumoperitoneum, no adverse consequences should be observed. However, laparoscopic procedures are contraindicated if significant deterioration of the cardiac or pulmonary reserve is found.

The pulmonary function is less disturbed following minimally invasive procedures.[27] The gastrointestinal physiologic advantages have been discussed. Milsom and colleagues[7] report a faster recovery of the pulmonary and gastrointestinal function following laparoscopic cancer resection.

Immunologic advantages

This aspect is particularly relevant, since patients with malignancies are often nutritionally compromised. The traumatic injury that occurs with large abdominal incisions has been shown to adversely affect the immune function.[28] Studies have demonstrated less impairment of the immune response in patients undergoing LAC compared with conventional procedures, although this has not been proved for colon cancer.[29] Harmon et al[30] showed that there was a reduction in the interleukin-6 response in laparoscopic procedures compared with open ones; this is evidence of decreased physiologic stress. Postoperative cell-mediated immune function has been also shown to be better preserved in laparoscopic cases.[31] An improved delayed-type hypersensitivity reaction[31] has been associated with laparoscopic procedures in a murine model. These studies suggest that laparoscopic techniques might be beneficial in cancer patients in terms of preservation of the immune function.

So far, the theoretic immunologic benefits have not been reflected in improved septic or oncologic clinical outcomes, and more investigation is needed. A Northern European study will determine the immune status of patients undergoing LCC in order to find if there is any association between immunologic response and survival. It has also been suggested that since there might be a reduced laparoscopic postoperative immunosuppression, adjuvant chemotherapy may be introduced earlier.[32]

MORBIDITY AND MORTALITY

Mortality rates in colon cancer trials comparing laparoscopic and open procedures are similar, and usually below 1.5% (Table 11.1).[2–4,7,19,33–36] Morbidity rates are in the range 8–24% for laparoscopic surgery versus 14–22% for conventional surgery (Table 11.1).[2–4,7,19,33–36] This similarity points toward the relative safety of the laparoscopic technique for colon cancer, and is comparable to the situation for benign cases.[3,4,36] Strict recording of minor complications explains the higher complication rate in the Bokey et al[37] series in right colectomy for cancer. There are fewer wound infections for laparoscopic procedures,[4,37] and reduced pulmonary complications are also reported.[4,27,38] Interestingly, there are few descriptions of complications specific to the laparoscopic procedure, such as trocar-related injuries. A small-bowel perforation not detected at the time of operation[17] and small-intestine necrosis secondary to a trocar hernia have been reported.[35] Unique to minimally invasive surgery is the resection of inadequate or erroneous

Table 11.1 Mortality and morbidity rates for laparoscopic versus open surgery for colon cancer

Authors	Year	No. of patients (lap/open)	Morbidity rate (%) (lap/open)	Mortality rate (%) (lap/open)
Hoffman et al[3]	1994	80/53	13/—	0/0
Lacy et al[2]	1995	25/26	8/30	4.0/0
Franklin et al[4]	1996	191/264	17/23	NS
Leung et al[17]	1997	50/50	26/32	2.0/6.0
Bouvet et al[33]	1998	53/57	24/21	1.0/0
Khalili et al[34]	1998	76/90	19/22	1.2/0
Milsom et al[7]	1998	42/38	15/15	0.9/0.9
Melloti et al[35]	1999	163/—	15/—	0/—
Santoro et al[36]	1999	50/50	20/14	0/0

NS, not stated.

segments of the intestine, which can be avoided with accurate preoperative localization or with simultaneous colonoscopy.

RISKS (ONCOLOGIC CONCERNS)

Although there is enough evidence to support the role of laparoscopy in benign colon disease, its position in curing cancer has not been determined. Laparoscopic palliation for advanced tumors is without controversy. This approach also has an accepted role in the diagnosis and staging of colon tumors – specifically to detect peritoneal dissemination and response to chemo-radiation.

The safety of the laparoscopic approach for malignant disease is the point of greatest concern. While they are attractive because of the multiple patient-related benefits, laparoscopic techniques could not be justified were they to result in increased tumor recurrence. Issues regarding the adequacy of resection, lymph node retrieval, and staging have been raised. The question of port-site recurrence due to altered tumor spread by pneumoperitoneum has prompted research and the initiation of controlled trials. Strict oncologic principles are to be adhered to, such as minimal tumor manipulation, en bloc resection, and clear surgical margins. The specimen should be delivered using wound protection, and the pneumoperitoneum should be released through the cannulas to protect the incisions. Finally, wounds must be meticulously irrigated.

Staging the liver

The main limitation of laparoscopic surgery is the loss of the surgeon's tactile ability, which partially precludes the evaluation of the liver during colon cancer cases. Preoperative studies such as computed tomography (CT) scan or ultrasound are therefore imperative. The question whether laparoscopic visualization and preoperative imaging are as accurate as an exploratory laparotomy in determining extension of the tumor needs to be answered. The recent introduction of laparoscopic ultrasound can improve diagnostic efficacy and compensate for this limitation.

Extent of resection

Laparoscopic resection must include adequate tumor-free margins and lymph node retrieval in order to be as effective as open colectomy. The extent of laparoscopic resection has been investigated in terms of tumor margins, lymph node yield, extent of mesenteric removal, and level of vascular pedicle ligation. Analysis of data demonstrates that equivalent margins have been achieved.[4,37] Radial clearance for T3 and T4 tumors is still considered a challenge for laparoscopic surgeons, and most studies do not include this point. Lymph node harvests from collected series are similar within institutions for laparoscopic and conventional surgery (Table 11.2).[3,4,6,7,14,37,39–43]

Pattern of recurrence

As already indicated, wound and trocar-site tumor implantation rates of between 2.5%[44] and 21%[45] after laparoscopic colectomy were much higher than those accepted for open surgery (0.8–2.5%[46,47]). The presence of trocar-site metastases in patients with curable disease[48] has been the most serious hindrance regarding LCC.[49] Not all recurrences have developed at the port through which the specimen was retrieved, and many were in patients with Dukes B and C lesions. These data have severely questioned the adequacy of LCC, and have demanded clinical trials, as well as research in animals and in vitro.

Current series have consistently reported rates of this type of recurrence under 1.3% (Table 11.3);[4,7,17,33,34,36,38,50–52] most recent ones are lower than 1%. This highlights the importance of an adequate laparoscopic technique (effect of the learning curve) together with a better understanding of how pneumoperitoneum influences trocar-site tumor implantation. Prospective, randomized trials do not report trocar- or wound-site recurrence,[6,7,52] probably as a reflection of an improved surgical technique.

Careful manipulation of the tumor and avoidance of specimen rupture may decrease tumor-cell dissemination. Recommendations, such as avoiding pneumoperitoneum leaks and protecting[53] and irrigating wounds, have proven effective. Gasless laparoscopy is an alternative that warrants further investigation.[54]

In summary, wound and incisional metastases seem to be multifactorial. Some animal studies have shown that pneumoperitoneum tends to increase the spread of carcinoma cells from the peritoneal cavity to the port sites.[55] Direct contact and hematogenous and lymphatic dissemination are other possible routes. Wound implantation can also reflect the behavior of the tumor. There is conflicting clinical and experimental evidence in relation to an

Table 11.2 Lymph node retrieval for open versus laparoscopic surgery for colon cancer

Authors	Year	No. of patients (lap/open)	Lymph nodes[a]	
			Laparoscopy	Open
Hoffman et al[3]	1994	32/31	8.0	6.1
Musser et al[41]	1994	17/24	10.6	7.9
Van Ye et al[14]	1994	14/20	10.5 (0–32)	7.6 (2–19)
Fine et al[39]	1995	30/—	8.7–10	10
Saba et al[65]	1995	20/15	6 (0–21)	10 (2–27)
Tucker et al[43]	1995	20/15	8.7	6.4
Bockey et al[37]	1996	28/33	17	16
Franklin et al[4]	1996	191/214	37	32
Gellman et al[40]	1996	58/38	9.3	9.5
Moore et al[66]	1996	30/34	16.9 (4–56)	15.9 (4–30)
Stage et al[6]	1997	15/14	7 (3–14)	8 (4–15)
Khalili et al[34]	1998	74/90	12	16
Milsom et al[7]	1998	42/38	19 (5–59)	25 (4–74)
Psaila et al[42]	1998	25/29	7	7.7
Leung et al[17b]	1999	50/50	9 (2–28)	8 (3–25)

[a] Range in parentheses.
[b] Rectosigmoid tumors only.

Table 11.3 Port-site and wound implants after laparoscopic surgery for colon cancer

Authors	Year	Study design[a]	Wound implants (implants/No. patients)	%
Guillou et al[67]	1993	NS	1/57	1.8
Berends et al[45]	1994	P	3/14	21.0
Boulez[44]	1996	NS	3/117	2.5
Fleshman et al[50] (COST)	1996	Registry	4/372	1.1
Franklin et al[4]	1996	P	0/191	0
Vukasin et al[68]	1996	Registry	5/451	1.1
Fielding et al[38]	1997	P	2/149	1.3
Stage et al[6]	1997	PR	0/15	0
Bouvet et al[33]	1998	P	0/91	0
Khalili et al[34]	1998	R	0/80	0
Lacy et al[52]	1998	PR	0/31	0
Milsom et al[7]	1998	PR	0/42	0
Bohm et al[51]	1999	P	0/68	0
Leung et al[17]	1999	R	1/147	0.68
Melotti et al[35]	1999	P	2/163	1.2
Santoro et al[36]	1999	P	1/57	0.7

[a] NS, not stated; R, retrospective; P, prospective; PR, prospective randomized.

increased incidence of metastasis following the laparoscopic approach. Only results from multicenter, controlled trials evaluating the pattern of tumor spread with long-term follow-up will help clarify this issue.

TRIALS FOR CANCER

Retrospective and prospective non-randomized trials

Initially, data from retrospective and prospective non-randomized trials were analyzed in order to determine the role of LCC.[4,50,56,57] Because of limitations on sample size and design, evidence from them was not conclusive. Results from these trials suggest that length of bowel and amount of lymph nodes removed were similar. Also, tumor rate recurrence and overall and stage-specific survival were comparable, although follow-up was limited. Results from these studies indicate that it is right to engage patients in large, multicenter studies in order to disclose the safety and benefits of LCC. Since 1998, retrospective[17,34] and prospective non-randomized trials[33,35,36,58] have reported favorable oncologic results and benefits; they support previous studies having a longer follow-up.

Up to 1994, the Clinical Outcomes of Surgical Therapy (COST)[50] study group reviewed their early experience on 372 patients who underwent laparoscopic resection for cancer. They concluded that early outcome was comparable and that long-term follow-up was needed. As a result, the COST group initiated a phase III randomized trial[59] comparing laparoscopic-assisted with open colectomy for cancer.

Prospective randomized trials

To date, results from three prospective, randomized trials on laparoscopic versus open colectomy for cancer have been published (Table 11.4),[6,7,22,52] with partial data available on the NIH Trial.[22] These studies vary in their inclusion criteria, sample size, endpoints, and follow-up.[6] Lacy et al[52] describe similar overall recurrence rates for both approaches. Milsom et al[7] reported two abdominal wall recurrences in the open colectomy group; these patients had disseminated disease. Stage et al[6] focused their research on immunologic outcome. As previously mentioned, none of these studies described laparoscopic trocar or wound metastasis. These experimental trials confirmed previous results, and lead to the conclusion that additional follow-up is needed before it can be determined whether or not the laparoscopic approach influences survival.

National Cancer Institute trial and other international trials (http:\\ncctg.mayo.edu/lapcolon)

To date there are seven international prospective randomized trials evaluating laparoscopic resection of colon cancer: the US NIH-supported trial, the UK Medical Research Council (MRC) CLASSIC trial, the Dutch–North European study (COLOR trial), and trials in Spain, Germany, Brazil, and New Zealand.

Table 11.4 Prospective randomized trials for laparoscopic surgery for colon cancer

Authors	Year started	No. of patients (lap/open)	Follow-up (months)[a]	Overall recurrences (lap/open)
Stage et al[6]	—	15/14	14 (7–19)[b]	—
Lacy et al[52]	1993	31/40	21.4 (13–41)[b]	5 of 31/6 of 40 (16%/15%)
Milsom et al[7]	1993	42/38	18 (1–46)/20 (3–48)[c]	4 of 42/6 of 38 (9.5%/15.8%)
Stocchi and Nelson[22] (NIH trial)	1994	205/203	—[d]	—[d]

[a] Range in parentheses.
[b] Both groups.
[c] Laparoscopic/open.
[d] Data not available for analysis.

(Table 11.5). Because of their expected patient accrual, they will be able to determine quality of life, cost–effectiveness, and cost–utility.

The NIH trial, sponsored by the US National Cancer Institute (NCI), has influenced other interna-tional investigations (Table 11.6). Initiated in 1994 by the COST group, it is designed to answer two unre-solved issues: first, if comparable information on tumor staging is being obtained with laparoscopic or open approaches; and, second, whether the pattern

---

Table 11.5 International trials investigating laparoscopic surgery for colon cancer[a]

Country	Principal investigator	Start date	Sites of resection	No. of patients
New Zealand	PJ Bagshaw	1998	Colon	1260
The Netherlands	HJ Bonjer	1997	Colon	1500
UK	PJ Guillou	1996	Colon and rectum	1000
Germany	F Kockerling	1995	Colon and rectum	1200
Brazil	JS Souza	1993	Colon and rectum	800
Spain	AM Lacy	1993	Colon	250
USA	H Nelson	1994	Colon	1200

[a] Reprinted from Stocchi L, Nelson H, *J Surg Oncol* 1998; **68:** 225–67,[22] with permission of the Mayo Foundation.

Table 11.6 Current accrual from the NIH prospective, randomized trial[a,b]

	No. of patients analyzed	Open	Laparoscopic
Total No. of patients accrued	408	203	205
Mean age (years)		69	67
Gender (% females)		52	48
ASA I/II (%)		87	87
ASA III (%)		13	13
Procedures performed	356	151	154
Right colectomy		77	83
Left colectomy		8	10
Sigmoid colectomy		60	57
Other		6	4
Stage distribution	305	151	154
Stage 0		10	5
Stage I		40	58
Stage II		57	45
Stage III		39	42
Stage IV		5	4
Patients with known previous abdominal surgery		53/151	60/154

[a] Reprinted from Stocchi L, Nelson H, *J Surg Oncol* 1998; **68:** 225–67,[22] with permission of the Mayo Foundation.
[b] More details available at http:\\ncctg.mayo.edu/lapcolon

of recurrence is different. It will also determine if the safety, survival, cost–effectiveness, and quality of life are equivalent. Only patients with right, left, and sigmoid tumors are included. The surgeons involved have done at least 20 laparoscopic colon cancer cases with adherence to proper oncologic practices. Patients are being recruited in 47 institutions in the USA and Canada, and 8 major cooperative oncology groups are participating.

To date, 850 patients have been accrued and preliminary data are available on 408 (Table 11.6). The Quality of Life accrual is complete and a formal analysis will be forthcoming in the very near future. Although survival rates are still too premature to be compared, parameters of adequate resection have been reviewed. Mesenteric length, lymph nodes retrieved, bowel length, and tumor margins were similar with the two techniques. As is standard for large cooperative group trials, a confidential review by the NCI Data Monitoring Committee is underway.

FUTURE DIRECTIONS

Laparoscopic ultrasound

As mentioned earlier, laparoscopic ultrasound (LUS) can compensate for the minimally invasive tactile limitation and improve diagnostic accuracy, allowing evaluation of the liver parenchyma. Since it has only been recently introduced, it was not included in the developing phases of the experimental trials.

There are few reports on the experience with LUS in staging patients undergoing colon cancer resection.[60] Goletti et al[61] used LUS to stage colorectal cancer in 33 patients. They reported a 100% overall liver staging accuracy and 94% sensitivity for nodal metastases, which resulted in changing their therapeutic program in 33% of cases.

Still, the morbidity, accuracy, and time required to perform LUS-guided biopsies need to be tested. Issues such as an increase in operative time, ability to diminish exploratory laparotomy rates, and cost-effectiveness need to be evaluated. Increasing resident exposure in LUS (imaging the biliary tree, liver, and pancreas) will reduce the learning curve associated with it. Recent improvements, such as multifrequency capability and flexible probes, make this technology more appealing. LUS will likely become a standard tool during laparoscopic cancer procedures in the near future.

Laparoscopic rectal cancer surgery

The reported benefits for laparoscopic low anterior and abdominal–perineal resections (APR) for rectal cancer are the same as for LAC, i.e. cosmetic advantages with reduced narcotic use and recovery time. Comparable conversion and complication rates are also reported.

Concerns about adequate removal of the mesorectum and radial margins for rectal tumors with the laparoscopic approach have been raised. It has been stated that complete removal of the mesorectum, clearance of pelvic sidewalls, and proximal ligation of the inferior mesenteric artery are possible.[62] Additionally, laparoscopy may also improve the visualization of the pelvis and help better preserve the autonomic nervous system. Case–control studies have shown no differences in survival, recurrence, and cancer-related mortality in laparoscopic versus open rectal cancer surgeries.[63] Fleshman et al,[64] in a multicenter control trial involving 42 laparoscopic APRs, found comparable tumor recurrence and survival rates with a 2-year follow-up.

Laparoscopic rectal tumor resection involving the abdomen and perineum awaits further evaluation. High complication rates have been described.[17] To date, it has been shown that this approach is technically feasible and that oncologic short-term outcome does not differ from that achieved by open techniques. Sample sizes are still small, and follow-up is short.

CONCLUSIONS

Laparoscopic colorectal procedures can be performed safely and efficiently. That is, morbidity and mortality rates are comparable to those achieved with conventional colectomy; conversion frequency and operating times can be reasonable. Because of improved technology and surgeons' expertise, more laparoscopic clinical applications are anticipated.

In colon cancer, minimally invasive surgery has established itself as a useful alternative for staging and palliation. When considering cure, the procedure is still controversial and under study, even though retrospective and prospective trials show encouraging short-term results. Since questions remain – mainly related to port-site recurrence and long-term survival – it is recommended that patients be enrolled in controlled trials. The role of laparoscopic surgery in the cure of colon cancer remains to be confidently defined by the ongoing studies. Preliminary data from the NIH trial suggest that laparoscopic colectomy for cancer adheres to oncologic principles. Additional issues, such as its immunologic advantage, need further testing. We expect that future data will support the use of laparoscopy over open colectomy for cancer, and we anticipate that minimally invasive colon cancer resection will become the standard procedure in the near future.

REFERENCES

1. Peters WR, Bartels TL, Minimally invasive colectomy: Are the potential benefits realized? *Dis Colon Rectum* 1993; **36:** 751–6.
2. Lacy AM, Garcia-Valdecasas JC, Pique JM et al, Short-term outcome analysis of a randomized study comparing laparoscopic vs open colectomy for colon cancer. *Surg Endosc* 1995; **9:** 1101–5.
3. Hoffman GC, Baker JW, Fitchett CW, Vansant JH, Laparoscopic-assisted colectomy. Initial experience. *Ann Surg* 1994; **219:** 732–40.
4. Franklin ME Jr, Rosenthal D, Abrego-Medina D et al, Prospective comparison of open vs. laparoscopic colon surgery for carcinoma. Five-year results. *Dis Colon Rectum* 1996; **39:** S35–46.
5. Falk PM, Beart RW Jr, Wexner SD et al, Laparoscopic colectomy: a critical appraisal. *Dis Colon Rectum* 1993; **36:** 28–34.
6. Stage JG, Schulze S, Moller P et al, Prospective randomized study of laparoscopic versus open colonic resection for adenocarcinoma. *Br J Surg* 1997; **84:** 391–6.
7. Milsom JW, Bohm B, Hammerhofer KA et al, A prospective, randomized trial comparing laparoscopic versus conventional techniques in colorectal cancer surgery: a preliminary report. *J Am Coll Surg* 1998; **187:** 46–54.
8. Schwenk W, Bohm B, Muller JM, Postoperative pain and fatigue after laparoscopic or conventional colorectal resections. A prospective randomized trial. *Surg Endosc* 1998; **12:** 1131–6.
9. Davies W, Kollmorgen CF, Tu QM et al, Laparoscopic colectomy shortens postoperative ileus in a canine model. *Surgery* 1997; **121:** 550–5.
10. Fleshman JW, Fry RD, Birnbaum EH, Kodner IJ, Laparoscopic-assisted and minilaparotomy approaches to colorectal diseases are similar in early outcome. *Dis Colon Rectum* 1996; **39:** 15–22.
11. Stewart BT, Stitz RW, Lumley JW, Laparoscopically assisted colorectal surgery in the elderly. *Br J Surg* 1999; **86:** 938–41.
12. Stocchi L, Nelson H, Young-Fadok T et al, Laparoscopic versus open colectomy in the elderly; a matched-control study. *Dis Colon Rectum* 1999; **42:** A21.
13. Bessler M, Whelan RL, Halverson A et al, Controlled trial of laparoscopic-assisted vs open colon resection in a porcine model. *Surg Endosc* 1996; **10:** 732–5.
14. Van Ye TM, Cattey RP, Henry LG, Laparoscopically assisted colon resections compare favorably with open technique. *Surg Laparosc Endosc* 1994; **4:** 25–31.
15. Zucker KA, Pitcher DE, Martin DT, Ford RS, Laparoscopic-assisted colon resection. *Surg Endosc* 1994; **8:** 12–17.
16. Dean PA, Beart RW Jr, Nelson H et al, Laparoscopic-assisted segmental colectomy: early Mayo Clinic experience. *Mayo Clin Proc* 1994; **69:** 834–40.
17. Leung KL, Yiu RY, Lai PB et al, Laparoscopic-assisted resection of colorectal carcinoma: five-year audit. *Dis Colon Rectum* 1999; **42:** 327–32.
18. Santoro E, Carlini M, Carboni F, Feroce A, Laparoscopic total proctocolectomy with ileal J pouch–anal anastomosis. *Hepatogastroenterology* 1999; **46:** 894–9.
19. Leung KL, Kwok SP, Lau WY et al, Laparoscopic-assisted resection of rectosigmoid carcinoma. Immediate and medium-term results. *Arch Surg* 1997; **132:** 761–4.
20. Jansen A, Laparoscopic-assisted colon resection. Evolution from an experimental technique to a standardized surgical procedure. *Ann Chir Gynaecol* 1994; **83:** 86–91.
21. Wishner JD, Baker JW Jr, Hoffman GC et al, Laparoscopic-assisted colectomy. The learning curve. *Surg Endosc* 1995; **9:** 1179–83.
22. Stocchi L, Nelson H, Laparoscopic colectomy for colon cancer: trial update. *J Surg Oncol* 1998; **68:** 255–67.
23. Bennett CL, Stryker SJ, Ferreira MR et al, The learning curve for laparoscopic colorectal surgery. Preliminary results from a prospective analysis of 1194 laparoscopic-assisted colectomies. *Arch Surg* 1997; **132:** 41–4 [Erratum 781].
24. Simons AJ, Anthone GJ, Ortega AE et al, Laparoscopic-assisted colectomy learning curve. *Dis Colon Rectum* 1995; **38:** 600–3.
25. Ramos JM, Beart RW Jr, Goes R et al, Role of laparoscopy in colorectal surgery. A prospective evaluation of 200 cases. *Dis Colon Rectum* 1995; **38:** 494–501.
26. Dunker MS, Stiggelbout AM, van Hogezand RA et al, Cosmesis and body image after laparoscopic-assisted and open ileocolic resection for Crohn's disease. *Surg Endosc* 1998; **12:** 1334–40.
27. Schwenk W, Bohm B, Witt C et al, Pulmonary function following laparoscopic or conventional colorectal resection: a randomized controlled evaluation. *Arch Surg* 1999; **134:** 6–12.
28. Slade MS, Simmons RL, Yunis E, Greenberg LJ, Immuno-depression after major surgery in normal patients. *Surgery* 1975; **78:** 363–72.
29. Hewitt PM, Ip SM, Kwok SP et al, Laparoscopic-assisted vs. open surgery for colorectal cancer: comparative study of immune effects. *Dis Colon Rectum* 1998; **41:** 901–9.
30. Harmon GD, Senagore AJ, Kilbride MJ, Warzynski MJ, Interleukin-6 response to laparoscopic and open colectomy. *Dis Colon Rectum* 1994; **37:** 754–9.
31. Allendorf JD, Bessler M, Whelan RL et al, Postoperative immune function varies inversely with the degree of surgical trauma in a murine model. *Surg Endosc* 1997; **11:** 427–30.
32. Young-Fadok TM, Talac R, Nelson H, Laparoscopic colectomy for cancer: the need for trials. *Semin Colon Rectal Surg* 1999; **10:** 94–101.
33. Bouvet M, Mansfield PF, Skibber JM et al, Clinical, pathologic, and economic parameters of laparoscopic colon resection for cancer. *Am J Surg* 1998; **176:** 554–8.
34. Khalili TM, Fleshner PR, Hiatt JR et al, Colorectal cancer: comparison of laparoscopic with open approaches. *Dis Colon Rectum* 1998; **41:** 832–8.
35. Melotti G, Tamborrino E, Lazzaretti MG et al, Laparoscopic surgery for colorectal cancer. *Semin Surg Oncol* 1999; **16:** 332–6.
36. Santoro E, Carlini M, Carboni F, Feroce A, Colorectal carcinoma: laparoscopic versus traditional open surgery. A clinical trial. *Hepatogastroenterology* 1999; **46:** 900–4.
37. Bokey EL, Moore JW, Chapuis PH, Newland RC, Morbidity and mortality following laparoscopic-assisted right hemicolectomy for cancer. *Dis Colon Rectum* 1996; **39:** S24–8.
38. Fielding GA, Lumley J, Nathanson L et al, Laparoscopic colectomy. *Surg Endosc* 1997; **11:** 745–9.
39. Fine AP, Lanasa S, Gannon MP et al, Laparoscopic colon surgery: report of a series. *Am Surg* 1995; **61:** 412–16.
40. Gellman L, Salky B, Edye M, Laparoscopic assisted colectomy. *Surg Endosc* 1996; **10:** 1041–4.
41. Musser DJ, Boorse RC, Madera F, Reed JF III, Laparoscopic colectomy: At what cost? *Surg Laparosc Endosc* 1994; **4:** 1–5.
42. Psaila J, Bulley SH, Ewings P et al, Outcome following laparoscopic resection for colorectal cancer. *Br J Surg* 1998; **85:** 662–4.
43. Tucker JG, Ambroze WL, Orangio GR et al, Laparoscopically

assisted bowel surgery. Analysis of 114 cases. *Surg Endosc* 1995; **9:** 297–300.

44. Boulez J, Surgery of colorectal cancer by laparoscopic approach. *Ann Chir* 1996; **50:** 219–30 (in French).

45. Berends FJ, Kazemier G, Bonjer HJ, Lange JF, Subcutaneous metastases after laparoscopic colectomy. *Lancet* 1994; **344:** 58.

46. Reilly WT, Nelson H, Schroeder G et al, Wound recurrence following conventional treatment of colorectal cancer. A rare but perhaps underestimated problem. *Dis Colon Rectum* 1996; **39:** 200–7.

47. Cass AW, Million RR, Pfaff WW, Patterns of recurrence following surgery alone for adenocarcinoma of the colon and rectum. *Cancer* 1976; **37:** 2861–5.

48. Prasad A, Avery C, Foley RJ, Abdominal wall metastases following laparoscopy. *Br J Surg* 1994; **81:** 1697.

49. Ortega AE, Beart RW Jr, Steele GD Jr et al, Laparoscopic Bowel Surgery Registry. Preliminary results. *Dis Colon Rectum* 1995; **38:** 681–5.

50. Fleshman JW, Nelson H, Peters WR et al, Early results of laparoscopic surgery for colorectal cancer. Retrospective analysis of 372 patients treated by the Clinical Outcomes of Surgical Therapy (COST) study group. *Dis Colon Rectum* 1996; **39:** S53–8.

51. Bohm B, Schwenk W, Muller JM, Long-term results after laparoscopic resection of colorectal carcinoma. *Chirurg* 1999; **70:** 453–5 (in German).

52. Lacy AM, Delgado S, Garcia-Valdecasas JC et al, Port site metastases and recurrence after laparoscopic colectomy. A randomized trial. *Surg Endosc* 1998; **12:** 1039–42.

53. Allardyce R, Morreau P, Bagshaw P, Tumor cell distribution following laparoscopic colectomy in a porcine model. *Dis Colon Rectum* 1996; **39:** S47–52.

54. Watson DI, Mathew G, Ellis T et al, Gasless laparoscopy may reduce the risk of port-site metastases following laparascopic tumor surgery. *Arch Surg* 1997; **132:** 166–8.

55. Jones DB, Guo LW, Reinhard MK et al, Impact of pneumoperitoneum on trocar site implantation of colon cancer in hamster model. *Dis Colon Rectum* 1995; **38:** 1182–8.

56. Hoffman GC, Baker JW, Doxey JB et al, Minimally invasive surgery for colorectal cancer. Initial follow-up. *Ann Surg* 1996; **223:** 790–6.

57. Lord SA, Larach SW, Ferrara A et al, Laparoscopic resections for colorectal carcinoma. A three-year experience. *Dis Colon Rectum* 1996; **39:** 148–54.

58. Kockerling F, Reymond MA, Schneider C et al, Prospective multicenter study of the quality of oncologic resections in patients undergoing laparoscopic colorectal surgery for cancer. The Laparoscopic Colorectal Surgery Study Group. *Dis Colon Rectum* 1998; **41:** 963–70.

59. Nelson H, Weeks JC, Wieand HS, Proposed phase III trial comparing laparoscopic-assisted colectomy versus open colectomy for colon cancer. *J Natl Cancer Inst Monogr* 1995; **19:** 51–6.

60. Foley EF, Kolecki RV, Schirmer BD, The accuracy of laparoscopic ultrasound in the detection of colorectal cancer liver metastases. *Am J Surg* 1998; **176:** 262–4.

61. Goletti O, Celona G, Galatioto C et al, Is laparoscopic sonography a reliable and sensitive procedure for staging colorectal cancer? A comparative study. *Surg Endosc* 1998; **12:** 1236–41.

62. Decanini C, Milsom JW, Bohm B, Fazio VW, Laparoscopic oncologic abdominoperineal resection. *Dis Colon Rectum* 1994; **37:** 552–8.

63. Schwandner O, Schiedeck TH, Killaitis C, Bruch HP, A case–control study comparing laparoscopic versus open surgery for rectosigmoidal and rectal cancer. *Int J Colorectal Dis* 1999; **14:** 158–63.

64. Fleshman JW, Wexner SD, Anvari M et al, Laparoscopic vs. open abdominoperineal resection for cancer. *Dis Colon Rectum* 1999; **42:** 930–9.

65. Saba AK, Kerlakian GM, Kasper GC, Hearn AT, Laparoscopic assisted colectomies versus open colectomy. *J Laparoendosc Surg* 1995; **5:** 1–6.

66. Moore JW, Bokey EL, Newland RC, Chapuis PH, Lymphovascular clearance in laparoscopically assisted right hemicolectomy is similar to open surgery. *Aust NZ J Surg* 1996; **66:** 605–7.

67. Guillou PJ, Darzi A, Monson JR, Experience with laparoscopic colorectal surgery for malignant disease. *Surg Oncol* 1993; **2**(Suppl 1): 43–9.

68. Vukasin P, Ortega AE, Greene FL et al, Wound recurrence following laparoscopic colon cancer resection. Results of the American Society of Colon and Rectal Surgeons Laparoscopic Registry. *Dis Colon Rectum* 1996; **39:** S20–3.

12

Systemic adjuvant therapy of colon cancer

Rachel Midgley

INTRODUCTION

Despite the improvements in surgical technique and postoperative care that are outlined in other chapters of this book, colorectal cancer (CRC) continues to kill 95 000 people in Europe alone each year. Approximately one-fifth of the 150 000 annual newly diagnosed cases have metastatic spread at diagnosis, and chemotherapy at this stage can, at best, improve quality of life and prolong life by 6–12 months.[1] The remaining 80% of patients have no macroscopic evidence of residual tumour post resection. However, more than half of these subsequently develop recurrence and die of their disease.[2] This is a result of viable tumour cells that have metastasized prior to the operation but that are undetectable by our current scanning techniques. Adjuvant chemotherapy administered after a presumed curative operation aims to target these micrometastases and to eradicate them before they can grow into functional tumour masses. Colorectal cancer is just one of a number of solid tumours where this adjuvant stratagem has proven to be effective.

A number of animal experiments have indicated that the presence of a primary tumour can inhibit the growth of synchronous metastases.[3] Theoretically, removal of the primary could stimulate proliferation of any residual cells, boosting the growth fraction and rendering the cells more susceptible to the S-phase-specific effects of chemotherapy in the immediate postoperative period. Therefore it is reasonable to predict that early adjuvant therapy might confer a greater benefit, although this has not been rigorously tested in clinical trials to date.

Choice of route and scheduling of chemotherapy have also been topics of hot debate. These decisions may be based on scientific principles and knowledge of the natural history of the disease. The process of metastasis in colorectal cancer has been explained in two models. First, tumour may spread in a stepped or sequential manner via the portal vein to the liver, and thereafter to distant sites. In this case, one might predict that local administration of chemotherapy via the portal vein might be most efficacious in the adjuvant setting. This is more fully explored in Chapter 15. Alternatively, tumour may disseminate simultaneously via blood and lymph to various organs, with destination determined by specific patterns of cell surface recognition molecules. If so, then systemically intravenous administered chemotherapy may be most appropriate.

This chapter illustrates how the above principles have been applied in the development of adjuvant therapy, specifically concentrating on *systemic* cytotoxic administration in *colon* cancer.

HISTORY OF ADJUVANT THERAPY FOR COLORECTAL CANCER

Adjuvant chemotherapy for colorectal cancer has been a focus of interest for more than three decades, with 5-fluorouracil (5-FU) remaining the prime cytotoxic agent. Many of the early trials were underpowered and retrospective, and no improvement in disease-free survival (DFS) or overall survival (OS) was demonstrated.

The last 10 years has brought more promising results. In 1988, the National Surgical Adjuvant Breast and Bowel Project (NSABP) published data from their first colon cancer study, Protocol C-01.[4] In this study, 773 patients were randomized to receive surgery alone (394 patients) or surgery plus chemotherapy in the form of intravenous 5-FU, semustine (methyl-CCNU) and vincristine (379 patients). At 5-year follow-up, patients treated with surgery alone had 1.29 times the risk of developing recurrence ($p = 0.02$) and 1.31 times the likelihood of dying ($p = 0.05$) compared with patients treated with surgery plus adjuvant chemotherapy.[4] Similar positive results were reported by the North Central Cancer Treatment Group (NCCTG) and Mayo Clinic when comparing surgery versus surgery plus 5-FU/levamisole (LEV).[5]

NATIONAL INSTITUTES OF HEALTH (NIH) AND THE CONSENSUS STATEMENT

Despite the positive results outlined above, there was still nihilism surrounding the use of adjuvant therapy for CRC. However, this changed when Moertel et al[6] reported significant benefit for patients receiving adjuvant chemotherapy in the Intergroup trial. In this trial, 318 patients with stage B colorectal malignancy were randomized to surgical treatment alone or surgery followed by 5-FU/LEV. Also, 929 patients with stage C disease received surgery alone, surgery plus levamisole, or surgery plus 5-FU/LEV.[6] Of the patients treated with levamisole alone, 92% continued treatment for at least 90% of the intended 12-month period (or until death or disease progression intervened), compared with 70% of patients receiving the 5-FU/LEV regimen. In the latter group, the median length of chemotherapy in those who stopped treatment prematurely was 5 months. This disparity may be a consequence of augmented toxicity of the combination. For stage C patients, a 33% reduction in the odds of death and a 41% reduction in recurrence risk were demonstrated in the cohort treated with 5-FU/LEV compared with surgery alone. At 3.5-year follow-up, the overall survival percentages were 77% and 55% in treated and control groups respectively.[6] Levamisole as a single agent produced no extra benefit over surgery alone. Toxicity of levamisole alone comprised arthralgia, myalgia, and a metallic taste in the mouth. Side-effects of the combination appeared similar to those previously experienced with 5-FU alone, and included gastrointestinal toxicity (nausea, vomiting, diarrhoea, and stomatitis), dermatitis, and leukopenia. Only the bone marrow effects necessitated dose limitation.

Investigators then began to question the contribution of levamisole to the overall cytotoxic effects. First, levamisole as a single agent produced no benefit over purely surgical intervention. Second, in advanced CRC, 5-FU/LEV did not improve response rates compared with 5-FU alone. Last, there is no substantive evidence for a mechanism of biological synergy between 5-FU and levamisole.

However, despite these reservations, the Intergroup results provoked the NIH statement:[7]

- All stage III patients who are unable to enter a clinical trial should be offered therapy with 5-FU

and LEV as administered in the Intergroup trial, unless medical or psychosocial contraindications exist.

A similar statement was released from the Seventh Kings Fund Forum in London in the same year, advising that any patient who could not be randomized into the ongoing national AXIS trial of adjuvant treatment should be considered for 5-FU/LEV.[8]

MODULATION OF 5-FU BY FOLINIC ACID (LEUCOVORIN)

In 1991, Gray et al[9] published a meta-analysis of the early 5-FU-inclusive adjuvant CRC trials, and concluded that adjuvant chemotherapy may reduce the odds of death in CRC by 10–15%. In an attempt to improve these results, scientists and oncologists turned again to the biochemistry of 5-FU. 5-FU is a long established cytotoxic with activity against a range of solid tumours. It is metabolized to fluorodeoxyuridine monophosphate (FdUMP) in the cell, and it is this active metabolite that binds to and inhibits the target enzyme thymidylate synthase, thus preventing the formation of thymidine, an important building block in DNA synthesis. This mode of action renders it S-phase-specific. Binding to thymidylate synthase and stabilization of the covalent ternary compound thus formed is maximal in the presence of the reduced folate 5,10-methylenetetrahydrofolate ($5,10$-CH_2FH_4).

It is postulated that in some tumour cells, the amount of folate may be insufficient to permit optimal cytotoxicity of 5-FU. It is this supposition that underlies the theory of effectiveness of folinic acid (FA, leucovorin), which has become established as a biological modulator in trials of 5-FU adjuvant treatment. Folinic acid is a mixture of the stereoisomers 6-L,D-5-formyltetrahydrofolate that replenishes the depleted cellular stores, enhancing and prolonging the activity of 5-FU (Figure 12.1).

This theoretical optimization of cytotoxicity has been borne out in practice. First, in 1992, Buyse et al[10] published a meta-analysis of trials comparing intravenous 5-FU alone with intravenous 5-FU/FA in the treatment of advanced CRC. Response rates in the combination regimen group were almost twice that observed in the single-agent arm (23% versus 11%, odds ratio 0.45, $p < 10^{-7}$). Subsequently, three large randomized phase III trials have produced confirmatory evidence of improved survival in the adjuvant setting for 5-FU/FA patients compared with controls. These results are summarized in Table 12.1.

Table 12.1 Summary of three recent trials comparing 5-FU/FA against control in the adjuvant treatment of colon cancer

Trial (number in study); randomized comparison; follow-up period	Disease-free survival rate (%)		Overall survival rate (%)	
	5 FU/FA	Control	5 FU/FA	Control
Overview of French, Italian, and Canadian Trials (1493 patients); 5-FU/HDFA versus observation; 3-year follow-up	71	62 ($p < 0.0001$)	83	78 ($p = 0.03$)
Intergroup study (309 patients); 5-FU/LDFA versus observation; 5-year follow-up	74	58 ($p = 0.004$)	74	63 ($p = 0.02$)
NSABP Protocol C-03 (1080 patients); 5-FU/HDFA versus MOF; 3-year follow-up	73	64 ($p = 0.0004$)	84	77 ($p = 0.003$)

Abbreviations: 5-FU, 5-fluorouracil; FA, folinic acid; LD, low-dose; HD, high-dose; MOF, semustine/vincristine/5-FU.

The pooled IMPACT study (Italy, France, and Canada) compared 5-FU/high-dose FA (HDFA: 200 mg/m^2) with observation alone.[11] Chemotherapy significantly reduced mortality by 22% (95% confidence intervals (CI) 3–38; $p = 0.029$) and events and recurrences by 35% (95% CI 22–46; $p < 0.0001$), increasing the 3-year DFS rate from 62% to 71% and the OS rate from 78% to 83%.

The National Cancer Institute (NCI)/NCCTG randomized 317 patients with high-risk Dukes B or Dukes C CRC between chemotherapy (6 cycles of 5-FU (425 mg/m^2) plus FA (20 mg/m^2) by rapid intravenous injection daily for 5 consecutive days every 4 weeks) and observation.[12] At 5-year follow-up, the chemotherapy group experienced statistically significant improvements in DFS rate (74% versus 58%, $p = 0.004$) and OS rate (74% versus 63%, $p = 0.02$) compared with the surgery-alone group.

Finally, the NSABP Protocol C-03 compared 5-FU/HDFA (500 mg/m^2) with MOF (semustine, vincristine, 5-FU) – an established regimen used in previous trials.[13] The 3-year DFS and OS rates in the 5-FU/FA group were significantly greater than in the MOF group (73% versus 64%, $p = 0.0004$, and 84% versus 77%, $p = 0.003$). This reflected a 32% reduction in mortality in the 5-FU/FA arm compared with controls.

More recently, results from the NSABP Protocol C-04 have been published, and indicate a DFS advantage for 5-FU/FA (weekly or Roswell/ Gastrointestinal Tumour Study Group (GITSG) schedule) over 5-FU/LEV.[14] Table 12.2 outlines these results. Odds ratios of less than 1.0 suggest shorter DFS or OS intervals than those observed in the control group (5-FU/FA). The 5-FU/FA combination is more effective than the 5-FU/LEV regimen. In addition, 5-FU/FA does not appear to significantly increase toxicity compared with 5-FU alone or 5-FU/LEV. Therefore the extra benefit is at little extra cost to the patient. However, it is worth considering at this point what is the most appropriate dose of folinic acid. The latter is relatively much more expensive than 5-FU, and hence the lowest dose that is proven to be efficacious should be utilized. This question has been addressed in the certain arm of the QUASAR trial. This has randomized more than 5000 stage C patients to 5-FU with or without levamisole plus high- or low-dose folinic acid (HDFA versus LDFA). The early results suggest that LDFA is as efficacious as HDFA, but with a reduction in toxicity – particularly severe mucositis and diarrhoea.[15]

Overall, the available evidence suggests that

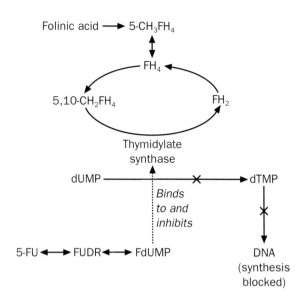

Figure 12.1 Intracellular metabolism and mechanism of action of 5-FU and its modulation by folinic acid. 5-FU is metabolized to FdUMP, which binds to and inhibits the enzyme thymidylate synthase. The ability of 5-FU to inhibit the enzyme is enhanced by the presence of $5,10\text{-}CH_2FH_4$, which can be synthesized from folinic acid, and which stabilizes the formation of a covalent ternary complex between FdUMP and thymidylate synthase.

Key: FUDR, fluorodeoxyuridine; FdUMP, fluorodeoxyuridine monophosphate; dUMP, deoxyuridine monophosphate; dTMP, thymidylate; $5,10\text{-}CH_2FH_4$, 5,10-methylenetetrahydrofolate; FH_2, dihydrofolate; $5\text{-}CH_3FH_4$, 5-methyltetrahydrofolate; FH_4, tetrahydrofolate.

adjuvant therapy for Dukes C colon cancer is definitely worthwhile, with an overall absolute survival improvement of at least 5% (and possibly as much as 20%).

ADJUVANT THERAPY FOR DUKES B COLON CANCER

In contrast to Dukes C colon cancer, there is not yet convincing evidence of benefit from adjuvant chemotherapy for Dukes B colon cancer. The ratio of Dukes B to Dukes C patients seen by oncologists is about 1 : 3. Furthermore the prognosis for Dukes B patients is substantially better than for Dukes C patients. For these two reasons, many of the early trials that analysed Dukes B patients as a subset were underpowered and statistically incapable of detecting a true survival difference. Moertel et al[6] did randomize 318 Dukes B patients to 5-FU/LEV or observation alone, and showed no difference in sur-

vival. The IMPACT trials included 841 patients with Dukes B disease, randomizing between 5-FU/HDFA and control, and, again, no survival difference was observed. However, the NSABP group have recently published pooled results from four randomized trials (Protocols C-01, C-02, C-03, and C-04), including data from 1567 Dukes B patients. This retrospective and statistically complex analysis indicates DFS and OS benefits in the Dukes B patients similar to those observed in Dukes C by the same trials group.[16] In the absence of convincing data from prospectively randomized trials, it is reasonable to assume that there is a continuous spectrum of biological risk of relapse rather than the categorical approach taken with the Dukes staging system. It may be postulated that certain high-risk subsets of Dukes B colon patients are more likely to benefit from adjuvant cytotoxics. Positive predictors of poor prognosis include perforation, obstruction, contiguous organ involvement, DNA ploidy, and a high proliferation

Table 12.2 Summary of results from NSABP Protocol C-04				
	5-year DFS rate (%)	**Cumulative odds**	**5-year survival rate (%)**	**Cumulative odds**
5-FU/FA	64	—	74	—
5-FU/FA/LEV	64	0.98	72	0.93
5-FU/LEV	60	0.83 ($p < 0.05$)	69	0.79 ($p < 0.05$)

Abbreviations: DFS, disease-free survival; 5-FU, 5-fluorouracil; FA, folinic acid; LEV, levamisole.

index. In an attempt to answer the questions surrounding the use of adjuvant therapy in Dukes B patients, randomization continues into the uncertain arm of QUASAR, termed QUASAR1. This trial randomizes Dukes B colon cancer patients and rectal cancer patients, after curative surgery, to 5-FU/LDFA or observation alone. More than 2000 of the target 2500 patients have been recruited.

IMPROVING ADJUVANT THERAPY OF COLORECTAL CANCER

Improvements in adjuvant therapy of CRC aim to improve survival outcomes for patients, whilst keeping costs, in terms of patient quality of life and financial implications, to a minimum. How might this be achieved?

Infusional 5-FU

5-FU has a short plasma half-life of 8–14 minutes, and is differentially cytotoxic to cells in S phase. Therefore a logical prediction might be that continuous infusion of 5-FU could increase the proportion of susceptible cells and augment cytotoxicity. A meta-analysis of six randomized trials comparing continuous-infusion with bolus 5-FU in advanced CRC demonstrated a higher response rate (22% versus 14%) and a small improvement in overall survival (12.1 months versus 11.3 months, $p = 0.04$). The pattern of toxicity was also significantly different, with decreased rates of mucositis, neutropenia, and diarrhoea, but a significantly increased risk of hand–foot syndrome.[17] As a consequence of these promising results, systemic infusional chemotherapy is now being assessed in the adjuvant setting. It is important to note that infusional therapy may incur extra costs in terms of PICC/Hickman-line insertions, training for staff, and possible complications from the central venous catheters such as thrombosis and infection.

Adjuvant infusional chemotherapy via the portal vein (PVI) has also been assessed. In theory, high first-pass metabolism should extract most of the drug locally in the liver, producing high regional dose intensity at a common metastatic site but with little systemic escape and therefore reduced toxicity. Results have been conflicting, but early data from the largest trial to date, the AXIS trial, which randomized 4000 patients between PVI and surgery alone, failed to demonstrate any significant difference between the two arms.[18] This form of treatment is covered in detail in Chapter 15.

Oral fluoropyrimidines

To improve the quality of life and to drive down the human resource costs of administering chemotherapy, there has been a trend towards developing oral fluoropyrimidines to replace the conventional intravenous 5-FU. Although work in this area was initially hampered by the reportedly extremely erratic oral bioavailability of 5-FU (ranging from 0% to 80%), interest has been rekindled with the results of randomized trials of oral UFT (uracil/tegafur) plus folinic acid and the 5-FU prodrug capecitabine against the standard Mayo 5-FU regimen.[19,20] In these trials, 2400 advanced CRC patients were randomized, and equivalence between the Mayo regimen and the oral agents in terms of response rates and overall survival was demonstrated. Differential toxicity was noted, with decreased mucositis and decreased hospitalization rates, but increased hand–foot syndrome, in the oral-agent arms. Hence the pattern of toxicity is similar to that observed with infusional regimens. It is clear that oral agents will be particularly suitable for the adjuvant field, where patients are extremely keen to achieve normality and return to work. They will be tested in this setting in the near future.

Cytotoxics with alternative mechanisms of action

It is increasingly apparent that biological and pharmacodynamic modulation of 5-FU, and the use of other thymidylate synthase inhibitors, are likely to produce only marginal improvements in survival for CRC. Therefore novel chemotherapy agents, exploiting different cellular mechanisms, are being developed. Two of these drugs will be addressed briefly here.

Irinotecan

Irinotecan (CPT-11) is a semisynthetic camptothecin, which works by inhibiting topoisomerase I, and which, in early trials, showed modest activity as a single agent in previously untreated advanced CRC *and* non-cross-resistance with 5-FU. Indeed, in phase II trials with irinotecan in 5-FU-pretreated patients, the results appeared as good as those obtained in chemotherapy-naive patients, with response rates of 13–18% and 19% respectively. Subsequently, two phase III studies compared irinotecan with best supportive care, or with second-line infusional 5-FU for patients with 5-FU-resistant disease.[21,22] Both trials showed statistically significant benefits, with median improvements in survival of 2.9 and 2.3 months respectively. The major toxicity of irinotecan is diarrhoea, which is biphasic – an immediate acute cholinergic diarrhoea during treatment administration, which can be effectively counteracted and prevented by subcutaneous atropine, and a delayed mucositic diarrhoea, with an onset 7–10 days after treatment. It was recognition of this specific toxicity that initially warned oncologists against the use of irinotecan in combination with 5-FU. However, two large randomized trials have demonstrated that this hesitancy was largely unjustified.

In an American trial, 683 patients were randomized to bolus 5-FU/FA alone, irinotecan alone or the combination 5-FU/FA/irinotecan (IRN). The toxicity of the irinotecan plus 5-FU was less than additive, perhaps even antagonistic, since it was no worse than the same dose and schedule of irinotecan given as a single agent. However, whilst 5-FU/FA alone and irinotecan alone gave almost identical progression-free survivals (PFS) (median 4.4 months versus 4.2 months) and response rates (RR) (22% versus 18%), the results for the 5-FU/FA/IRN combination were significantly improved (PFS = 6.9 months and RR = 40%). This did not translate into improved survival, but conclusions are hampered by significant salvage crossover from single-agent to dual therapy.[23]

In a European trial, 387 patients were randomized to receive infusional 5-FU/FA with or without irinotecan. In this trial, toxicity was significantly increased with the addition of irinotecan, but efficacy was also significantly augmented, with increased time to progression (TTP) (median 6.7 months versus 4.4 months, $p = 0.01$), improved RR (41% versus 23%, $p < 0.001$), and improved overall survival (16.8 months versus 14.0 months, $p = 0.03$).[24]

Oxaliplatin
Oxaliplatin is a third-generation platinum compound, which induces DNA crosslinking and apoptotic cell death, and also showed promising early activity. From inception, this drug has been used in combination with 5-FU for two reasons. First, in vitro experiments suggested 5-FU/oxaliplatin (OX) synergy, and, second, the toxicity profiles of the two agents did not appear to overlap. In early phase II experiments, the RR for single-agent oxaliplatin in 106 5-FU-resistant patients was 10%, whilst a RR of 46% was seen among 46 5-FU-pretreated patients when they received an intensive 5-FU/FA/OX schedule.[25] However, there have been no randomized trials powered to assess the effect of second-line oxaliplatin on survival.

With these promising results in advanced disease,

and with our increasing knowledge and experience of the toxicities of these novel agents, their translation into the adjuvant setting is imminent.

INNOVATIVE THERAPEUTIC INNOVATIONS IN THE ADJUVANT TREATMENT OF CRC

Our evolving understanding of the biology of CRC, and in particular, recognition of genes that are switched on or off during carcinogenesis and of proteins that are preferentially expressed in CRC cells, is being translated into innovative immunotherapy and gene therapy techniques.

Immunotherapy

Traditionally, CRC has not been an obvious target for immunotherapy – especially bulky metastatic disease that is unlikely to respond to any immunological manipulation. In the adjuvant setting, where micrometastatic clusters of cells reside in mesenchymal tissues, surrounded by granulocytes, macrophages, and killer cells, all effecting ready initiation of antibody-induced mechanisms of cytotoxicity and all potent inducers of apoptosis, the situation looks more promising. In the early 1980s, an anti-idiotypic anticolorectal cancer IgG2A antibody was developed. It induced cellular cytotoxicity with human effector cells and prevented outgrowth of xenotransplanted human tumour cells in athymic mice. Toxicity studies in advanced CRC in 1991 suggested that it was well tolerated. Riethmuller and colleagues[26] performed a randomized study of the antibody, compared with surgery alone as adjuvant therapy in 189 patients with stage C CRC. The 5-year survival rate was significantly improved in the antibody-treated group (51% versus 36%, $p = 0.025$). The antibody is now being tested in combination with 5-FU/FA for Dukes C colon cancer patients and, as a single agent, compared with observation alone, in Dukes B colon cancer patients.

Gene therapy

There are a myriad of gene therapy techniques that are presently being explored in the context of CRC. Most of these are explained in detail in Chapter 63. One example of these, VDEPT (virus-directed enzyme prodrug therapy), is briefly illustrated here. The concept of VDEPT is to virally transduce the tumour cell with an enzyme (such as cytosine deami-

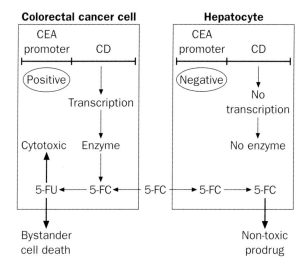

Figure 12.2 VDEPT and colorectal cancer.

Key: CEA, carcinoembryonic antigen; CD, cytosine deaminase; 5-FU, 5-fluorouracil; 5-FC, 5-fluorocytosine.

nase, CD) capable of converting an inactive prodrug (5-fluorocytosine, 5-FC) into an active cytotoxic species (5-FU). Tumour cell specificity is created by splicing in the 5′ transcriptional regulatory sequences of the human carcinoembryonic antigen (CEA) gene (Figure 12.2). This promoter sequence effectively functions as an on–off switch, so that the downstream structural gene is transcribed only by cells that synthesize CEA, i.e. CRC cells. Hence tumour cells expressing CD convert 5-FC to 5-FU, and the high concentrations produced diffuse into and kill immediately neighbouring cells – the so-called bystander effect – leaving less proximate healthy cells intact. Clinical trials using this approach are planned, with regional delivery of the viral vector, with the CEA–CD construct, to patients with hepatic metastases, followed by oral administration of 5-FC.

CONCLUSIONS

Systemic adjuvant therapy of colorectal cancer is a rapidly expanding field. Having explored the use of 5-FU to the full, attention is now focusing upon improving outcomes, using cytotoxics with different mechanisms of action, and by utilizing innovative techniques that are being translated from basic bench research to the bedside.

ACKNOWLEDGEMENTS

This work was supported by the UK Cancer Research Campaign and the UK Medical Research Council.

REFERENCES

1. Gray R, *Guidance on Commissioning Cancer Services. Improving Outcomes in Colorectal Cancer. The Research Evidence.* London: NHS Executive, Department of Health, 1997.
2. Abulafi AM, Williams NS, Local recurrence of colorectal cancer: the problems, the mechanisms, management and adjuvant treatment. *Br J Surg* 1994; **81:** 7–17.
3. De Wys WD, Studies correlating the growth rate of a tumor and its metastases and providing evidence for tumor-related systemic growth-retarding factors. *Cancer Res* 1972; **32:** 374–9.
4. Wolmark N, Fisher B, Rockette H et al, Post operative adjuvant chemotherapy or BCG for colon cancer: results from NSABP Protocol C-01. *J Natl Cancer Inst* 1988; **80:** 30–6.
5. Laurie JA, Moertel CG, Fleming TR et al, Surgical adjuvant treatment of large bowel cancer; an evaluation of levamisole and the combination of levamisole and 5-FU. A study of the North Central Cancer Treatment Group (NCCTG) and the Mayo Clinic. *J Clin Oncol* 1989; **7:** 1447–56.
6. Moertel CG, Fleming TH, MacDonald JS et al, Levamisole and fluouracil for adjuvant treatment of resected colon cancer. *N Engl J Med* 1990; **322:** 352–8.
7. NIH Consensus Conference, Adjuvant therapy for patients with colon and rectal cancer. *JAMA* 1990; **264:** 1444–50.
8. King's Fund Forum, Cancer of the colon and rectum. *Br J Surg* 1990; **77:** 1063–5.
9. Gray R, James R, Mossman J, Stenning S, AXIS: a suitable case for treatment. *Br J Cancer* 1991; **63:** 841–5.
10. Buyse M, Piedbois P, Rustum Y (Advanced Colorectal Analysis Project), Modulation of 5-fluouracil by leucovorin in patients with advanced colorectal cancer: evidence in terms of response rate. *J Clin Oncol* 1992; **10:** 896–903.
11. IMPACT trial, Efficacy of adjuvant fluouracil and folinic acid in colon cancer. *Lancet* 1995; **345:** 939–44.
12. O'Connell M, Maillard J, Kahn MJ et al, Controlled trial of fluouracil and low-dose leucovorin given for 6 months as post-operative adjuvant therapy for colon cancer. *J Clin Oncol* 1997; **15:** 246–50.
13. Wolmark N, Rockette H, Fisher B et al, The benefit of leucovorin modulated 5-fluouracil as post-operative adjuvant treatment for primary colon cancer: results from the National Surgical Adjuvant Breast and Bowel Project Protocol C-03. *J Clin Oncol* 1993; **11:** 1879–88.
14. Wolmark N, Rockette H, Mamounas EP et al, The relative efficacy of 5-fluorouracil/leucovorin, 5-fluorouracil/levamisole and 5-fluorouracil/leucovorin/levamisole in patients with Dukes B and C carcinoma of the colon: first report of the NSABP Protocol C-04. *Proc Am Soc Clin Oncol* 1996; **15:** 205.
15. QUASAR Collaborative Group, Comparison of fluorouracil with additional levamisole, higher-dose folinic acid, or both, as adjuvant chemotherapy for colorectal cancer: a randomised trial. *Lancet* 2000: **355:** 1588–96.
16. Mamounas EP, Rockette H, Jones J et al, Comparative efficacy of adjuvant chemotherapy in patients with Dukes B vs Dukes C colon cancer: results from NSABP adjuvant studies (C-01, C-02, C-03, C-04). *Proc Am Soc Clin Oncol* 1996; **15:** 461.
17. Anonymous, Efficacy of intravenous continuous infusion of

5-fluorouracil with bolus administration in advanced colorectal cancer. *J Clin Oncol* 1998; **16:** 301–18.

18. James RD, on behalf of the AXIS collaborators, Intraportal 5FU (PVI) and peri-operative radiotherapy (RT) in the adjuvant treatment of colorectal cancer (CRC) – 3681 patients randomised in the UK Coordinating Committee on Cancer Research (UKC-CCR) AXIS trial. *Proc Am Soc Clin Oncol* 1999; **18:** 264.

19. Pazdur R, Douillard J-Y, Skillings JR et al, Multicentre phase III study of 5-fluorouracil (5F) or UFT in combination with leucovorin (LV) in patients with metastatic colorectal cancer. *Proc Am Soc Clin Oncol* 1999; **18:** 1009.

20. Twelves C, Harper P, Van Cutsem E, A phase III trial (SO14796) of Xeloda (capecitabine) in previously untreated advanced/metastatic colorectal cancer. *Proc Am Soc Clin Oncol* 1999; **18:** 1010.

21. Cunningham D, Pyrhonen S, James RD et al, Randomised trial of irinotecan plus supportive care versus supportive care alone after fluorouracil failure for patients with metastatic colorectal cancer. *Lancet* 1998; **352:** 1413–18.

22. Rougier P, van Cutsem E, Bajetta E et al, Randomised trial of irinotecan versus fluorouracil by continuous infusion after fluorouracil failure in patients with metastatic colorectal cancer. *Lancet* 1998; **352:** 1407–12.

23. Saltz L, Locker P, Pirotta N et al, Weekly irinotecan, leucovorin and fluorouracil is superior to daily × 5 LV/FU in patients with previously untreated metastatic colorectal cancer. *Proc Am Soc Clin Oncol* 1999; **18:** 898.

24. Douillar J, Cunningham D, Roth A et al, A randomised phase III trial comparing irinotecan + 5FU/FA to the same schedule of 5FU/FA in patients with metastatic colorectal cancer as frontline chemotherapy. *Proc Am Soc Clin Oncol* 1999; **18:** 899.

25. DeGramont A, Vignoud J, Tournigant C et al, Oxaliplatin with high dose leucovorin and 5-fluorouracil 48-hour continuous infusion in pre-treated metastatic colorectal cancer. *Eur J Cancer* 1997; **33:** 214–19.

26. Riethmuller G, Schneider-Gadicke E, Schmilok G, Randomised trial of monoclonal antibody for adjuvant treatment of resected Dukes C colorectal cancer. *Lancet* 1999; **343:** 1177–83.

13

Adjuvant treatment in Dukes B2 colon cancer: No

Charles Erlichman, Daniel J Sargent

INTRODUCTION

The value of adjuvant chemotherapy in patients with Dukes C carcinoma has been well documented.[1] Based on the results of a variety of randomized clinical trials, adjuvant therapy can both reduce the risk of recurrence and extend survival.[2–5] It is estimated that for every 100 patients treated with adjuvant 5-fluorouracil (5-FU) and leucovorin (folinic acid), 10–12 lives are saved. This benefit, coupled with the definite but typically tolerable toxicity profile, make this approach clinically acceptable. In the case of Dukes B2 carcinoma of the colon, considerable controversy exists regarding the relative benefit of treatment. Some analyses have suggested that adjuvant chemotherapy may be of benefit; others have not.[6–8] The conflicting results are in part related to differences in clinical trial design and differences in methods of statistical analysis. However, the primary reason for the controversy relates to the relatively low occurrence of outcome events, i.e. deaths, and the corresponding need for extremely large sample sizes to delineate an effect when the impact of treatment is small. Nevertheless, in practice, we are faced with the challenge of how to best manage patients who present with Dukes B2 carcinoma of the colon. It is our premise that three questions must be addressed before a rational conclusion can be drawn about the utility of adjuvant chemotherapy in the subset of patients who present with Dukes B2 carcinoma of the colon. The questions are:

- Is there statistically significant evidence that chemotherapy is more effective than no treatment in patients with B2 colon cancer?
- What is the clinical impact of the statistical evidence, whether significant or not?
- What is the clinical cost, i.e. type and severity of toxicity, for the clinical benefit achieved?

We shall address these three questions in order to attempt to formulate a rational conclusion.

IS THERE STATISTICAL EVIDENCE THAT CHEMOTHERAPY IS BETTER THAN NO TREATMENT IN DUKES B2 COLON CANCER?

Individual studies have not clearly demonstrated that statistically significant benefit arises from adjuvant chemotherapy in patients with Dukes B2 colon cancer. A recent analysis of INT-0035, a randomized clinical trial including approximately 1350 patients to determine the role of 5-FU and levamisole in both Dukes B2 and C colon cancer, did not demonstrate any benefit of this therapy in the subgroup of 318 B2 patients.[8] INT-0089, a trial of adjuvant chemotherapy in patients with Dukes high-risk B2 and C carcinoma of the colon, accrued 3759 patients and demonstrated a survival advantage for the combination with 5-FU/leucovorin compared to 5-FU/leucovorin/levamisole in the whole population.[9] In a subset analysis performed post facto, this overall survival benefit was not present in patients with high-risk Dukes B2 disease. However, Dukes B2 patients comprised only 20% of the study population.

Owing to the relatively low rate of relapse in Dukes B2 patients, individual adjuvant therapy trials typically have inadequate statistical power to detect a small to moderate treatment benefit in this population. Therefore, two groups have published analyses that pool data from several clinical trials in order to gain power. The National Surgical Adjuvant Breast and Bowel Project (NSABP) retrospectively investigated the relative reduction in recurrence and mortality comparing Dukes B2 with Dukes C patients in four of its trials (C-01, C-02, C-03, and C-04).[6] Specifically, the NSABP investigators tested whether, in each trial, the magnitude of benefit conveyed by the superior arm was consistent between patients with Dukes B2 and C disease. The conclusion drawn was that the relative reduction of recurrence and mortality in patients with Dukes B2 disease was consistent with that observed in patients with Dukes C disease. These trials, however, were not designed to prospectively evaluate the treatment effect in the B2 subset. In a distinct pooled analysis, the IMPACT group combined data from five trials that compared 5-FU/leucovorin with a no-treatment control group.[7] The trials included in the pooled analysis allowed both Dukes B2 and C patients. The IMPACT analysis, which included the 1016 Dukes B2 patients included on these trials, showed no statistically significant treatment benefit. The observed 5-year survival rate in treated patients was 82%, compared with 80% in untreated patients.

A direct comparison between the results of the NSABP analysis and the IMPACT analysis is difficult. In two of the NSABP studies (C-03 and C-04), the experimental arm was compared with an arm containing treatment; that is, a no-treatment control group was absent. Furthermore, in the other two NSABP trials (C-01 and C-02), the comparison was not of 5-FU/leucovorin versus no treatment but rather of MOF (semustine, vincristine, 5-FU) or portal vein infusion, respectively, versus no treatment. The absolute differences in 5-year survival rates between the two treatment arms from the four NSABP studies are 3%, 12%, 8%, and 4% in C-01, C-02, C-03, and C-04 respectively. The trial with the largest difference (C-02) compared 5-FU delivered by portal vein infusion with a no-treatment control. The difference in treatment efficacy in C-03, which had a 5-FU/leucovorin arm, may be explained by the increased incidence of second primary tumors in the MOF-treated patients (25 second primary tumors in the MOF arm versus 11 in the 5-FU/leucovorin arm). The observed differences of 3% and 4% in C-01 and C-04 respectively are similar to that observed by the IMPACT group. Other differences, which cannot easily be identified, may exist between the patients entered on the NSABP trials and those studies involved in the IMPACT analysis. These include differences in the proportion of patients with poorly differentiated tumors, differences in the proportion of the patients who are elderly, and differences in other prognostic factors, such as bowel obstruction.

More recently, Wolmark et al[10] published the results of C-04, a trial that compared 5-FU/leucovorin with 5-FU/levamisole in both Dukes B2 and C patients. In this article, it was claimed that 5-FU/leucovorin has demonstrable efficacy in both the Dukes B2 and C patient subsets. This is presumably based on a survival difference of 3% at 5 years, i.e. 81% for 5-FU/levamisole versus 84% for 5-FU/leucovorin, resulting in a relative risk of 0.71 comparing 5-FU/leucovorin with 5-FU/levamisole. The disease-free survival rate at 5 years is 75% for 5-FU/leucovorin versus 71% for 5-FU/levamisole, with a relative risk of 0.78 in favor of 5-FU/leucovorin. Although these results are intriguing, only 41% of the patients in this trial had Dukes B2 colon cancer. This raises the question of whether the confidence interval around the relative risks excludes one. A more complete analysis of these data would allow the reader to make an informed decision about the utility of 5-FU/leucovorin in Dukes B2 colon cancer.

Based on our review of the data, in addressing the question of whether there is statistically significant evidence that chemotherapy is better than no treatment in Dukes B2 colon cancer, the answer is that the data are conflicting.

WHAT IS THE CLINICAL IMPACT OF THE STATISTICAL EVIDENCE?

As a measure of clinical relevance, statistical significance is a poor tool. With a sufficiently large sample size, the smallest absolute difference will with certainty become statistically significant. Whereas small absolute differences in 5-year survival rates of 1–3% may be scientifically important and critical to furthering the research field, the clinical implications of such a finding need to be carefully assessed. Based on the final data from Intergroup 0035,[11] adjuvant treatment increased the 5-year survival rate in Dukes C patients by approximately 10%. In other words, it is possible to estimate that 10 lives can be saved for 100 patients treated. Based on the IMPACT analysis, when we examine the data for patients with Dukes B2 carcinoma, only two patients are cured for every 100 treated. A critical evaluation of therapy along these lines necessitates that clinicians discuss with their patients the perceived value to the receiver of the therapy prior to proceeding with treatments, which are potentially toxic.

WHAT IS THE CLINICAL COST OF TREATMENT?

The final question that needs to be addressed in contemplating the value of treatment in Dukes B2 patients is what is the clinical cost of treatment? The answer to this question is multifaceted, since several levels of cost must be considered before administering a potentially toxic therapy. First, what are the expected adverse events that a patient may encounter during and after the therapy? Second, what is the cost of therapy for the number of lives saved? Third, what is the societal cost in terms of time lost from work/family responsibilities? Whereas the answer to the third question is difficult to quantitate, existing data can be used to address the first two questions.

To examine the question of the tolerability of treatment, we examined data on adverse events from several large adjuvant colon trials, as summarized in Table 13.1. Data from these trials were not presented separately for Dukes B2 and C patients, but there is no reason to expect a different toxicity profile in the two patient groups. Based on data from the IMPACT study, in patients treated with 5-FU/leucovorin on a daily × 5 basis, grades 3 and 4 nausea and vomiting occurred in only 4% of patients. Stomatitis was more common in 11% of patients, and diarrhea occurred in 8% of patients. The experience with weekly 5-FU/leucovorin, as reported for studies C-04 and INT-0089, suggests that diarrhea, grade 3 or 4, occurs in 27–30% of patients, stomatitis in 2–4% of patients, and vomiting in 1–5% of patients. Hematologic toxicity was minimal, at less than 3% grades 3 and 4. In both C-04 and INT-0089, treatment-related deaths occurred in approximately 0.5% of cases. Consideration of these data focuses the question of what is the clinical cost of treatment. These rates of adverse events are certainly noteworthy, and must be factored into the clinical decision for each patient. In particular, while toxic deaths were rare on all of these trials, they were present. The trade-off between a gain in 5-year survival rates of 2–4%, at the cost of a toxic death rate of 0.5%, requires careful consideration.

CONCLUSIONS

Based on the available data, we can draw several conclusions. At the present time, we feel that in clinical trials of patients with Dukes B2 cancer, a no-treatment control arm continues to be important and appropriate. Regardless of the presence or absence of a no-treatment control group, future clinical trials in this population will be difficult to complete because of the large sample sizes required to provide adequate power. Timely completion of trials may require studies to be international in scope. In addition, the benefit of treatment, if present at all, is clearly small in absolute magnitude. This fact highlights the need for prognostic and predictive factor marker studies, which may identify subsets most likely to benefit from treatment. The currently accruing CALGB coordinated randomized trial of monoclonal antibody 17-1A versus no treatment illustrates several of these points. The study is open to the entire US Colorectal Intergroup, the National Cancer Institute of Canada Clinical Trials Group, and the European Organization for Research and Treatment of Cancer (EORTC). The study includes extensive substudies investigating possible molecular and pathologic prognostic and/or predictive factors.

For treatment decisions for the individual patient, we believe that there are insufficient data to recommend that adjuvant therapy for Dukes B2 colon cancer become the standard of care. The data based on a number of clinical trials are fairly consistent, and indicate that there may be some merit in treating all patients with Dukes B2 colon cancer in order to save a very small number of lives. However, the strength of the statistical evidence, the limited clinical impact associated with treatment, and the real potential for significant toxicity should be taken into account by

Table 13.1 Percentage of patients with grade ≥3 toxicity by study and arm[a]

	NSABP C-04[10]		INT-0089[9]		IMPACT B2[8]
	5-FU + LV (NSABP)	5-FU + Lev (NSABP)	5-FU + LV (Mayo)	5-FU + LV (NSABP)	5-FU + LV (Mayo)
Overall toxicity	35	28	57	41	Not reported
Diarrhea	27	9	21	30	8
Stomatitis	2	4	3	4	11
Vomiting	5	2	20	1	4

[a]5-FU, 5-fluorouracil; LV, leucovorin (folinic acid); Lev, levamisole; the type of regimen is shown in parentheses.

the informed clinician and patient before embarking on this course.

REFERENCES

1. National Cancer Institute, The efficacy of the group C status of levamisole and 5-FU for patients with Dukes' C colon cancer. National Cancer Institute Update, October 1989.
2. Laurie JA, Moertel CG, Fleming TR et al, Surgical adjuvant therapy of large-bowel cancer: an evaluation of levamisole and the combination of levamisole and 5-FU. *J Clin Oncol* 1989; **7:** 1447–56.
3. Moertel CG, Fleming TR, Macdonald JS et al, Levamisole and 5-FU for adjuvant therapy of resected colon cancer. *N Engl J Med* 1990; **322:** 352–8.
4. International Multicenter Pooled Analysis of Colon Cancer Trials (IMPACT) Investigators, Efficacy of adjuvant fluorouracil and folinic acid in colon cancer. *Lancet* 1995; **345:** 939–44.
5. O'Connell MJ, Mailliard JA, Kahn MJ et al, Controlled trial of fluorouracil and low-dose leucovorin given for 6 months as postoperative adjuvant therapy for colon cancer. *J Clin Oncol* 1997; **15:** 246–50.
6. International Multicentre Pooled Analysis of B2 Colon Cancer Trials (IMPACT B2) Investigators, Efficacy of adjuvant fluorouracil and folinic acid in B2 colon cancer. *J Clin Oncol* 1999; **17:** 1356–63.
7. Mamounas E, Wieand S, Wolmark N et al, Comparative efficacy of adjuvant chemotherapy in patients with Dukes' B versus Dukes' C colon cancer: results from four National Surgical Adjuvant Breast and Bowel Project adjuvant studies (C-01, C-02, C-03, and C-04). *J Clin Oncol* 1999; **17:** 1349–55.
8. Moertel CG, Fleming TR, Macdonald JS et al, Intergroup study of fluorouracil plus levamisole as adjuvant therapy for stage II/Dukes' B2 colon cancer. *J Clin Oncol* 1995; **13:** 2936–43.
9. Haller DG, Catalano DJ, MacDonald JS et al, Fluorouracil (FU), leucovorin (LV) and levamisole (lev) adjuvant therapy for colon cancer: preliminary results of INT-0089. *Proc Am Soc Clin Oncol* 1996; **15:** 211.
10. Wolmark N, Wieand HS, Hyams DM et al, Randomized trial of postoperative adjuvant chemotherapy with or without radiotherapy for carcinoma of the rectum: National Surgical Adjuvant Breast and Bowel Project Protocol R-02. *J Natl Cancer Inst* 2000; **92:** 388–96.
11. Moertel CG, Fleming TR, Macdonald JS et al, 5-FU plus levamisole as effective adjuvant therapy after resection of stage III colon carcinoma: a final report. *Ann Intern Med* 1995; **122:** 321–6.

14

Adjuvant treatment in Dukes B2 colon cancer: Yes

Eleftherios Mamounas, Samuel Wieand, Norman Wolmark

INTRODUCTION

Benefit from administration of adjuvant chemotherapy has been firmly demonstrated in Dukes C colon cancer patients based on convincing results from several large prospective randomized trials.[1–5] However, the value of such therapy is still argued for patients with Dukes B disease. In 1990, the last US National Institutes of Health (NIH) Consensus Development Conference on colorectal adjuvant therapy recommended that patients with Dukes C colon cancer receive adjuvant chemotherapy with 5-fluorouracil (5-FU) and levamisole (5-FU + LEV),[6] but did not recommend any specific adjuvant therapy for patients with Dukes B colon cancer outside of clinical trials. The recommendation was mainly based on results from Intergroup study 0035 demonstrating a significant survival improvement with adjuvant 5-FU + LEV in patients with Dukes C colon cancer but no such improvement in patients with Dukes B disease.[1] The lack of survival benefit in Dukes B patients was confirmed in a subsequent update of this trial,[7,8] although a reduction in recurrence similar to that documented for Dukes C patients was observed.

Since the time of the last NIH Consensus Development Conference, there has been accumulating evidence suggesting that leucovorin-modulated 5-FU (5-FU + LV) is also effective in improving disease-free and overall survival both in patients with Dukes C and in those with Dukes B colon cancer.[4] Randomized trials directly comparing the 5-FU + LV regimen with the 5-FU + LEV regimen have demonstrated superiority for the former.[5,9] Although the majority of patients in these trials had Dukes C tumors, in some trials[4,5] a sizeable proportion of patients (about 40%) had Dukes B disease. In those trials, there was no evidence of a differential treatment effect between Dukes B and Dukes C patients, indicating that adjuvant chemotherapy was effective in both groups.

Two possible explanations can be entertained if one accepts a lack of benefit from adjuvant chemotherapy in Dukes B patients. The first is that a true differential chemotherapy effect exists between patients with Dukes B and those with Dukes C tumors because of inherent biologic differences. The second – and more likely – is that no true differential chemotherapy effect exists, but because of the lower event rate in Dukes B patients, adjuvant clinical trials are underpowered to demonstrate significant survival differences in this subset of patients. Thus, despite a similar relative reduction in the rates of recurrence and cancer-related mortality (a measure of true biologic efficacy of adjuvant chemotherapy), the absolute reduction in recurrence and mortality (a measure of significant clinical benefit from adjuvant chemotherapy) is smaller in Dukes B patients than in Dukes C patients.

This chapter reviews the available evidence from randomized trials on the relative efficacy of adjuvant chemotherapy in Dukes B patients compared with Dukes C patients. The preponderance of the evidence supports the presence of true biologic efficacy of adjuvant chemotherapy in Dukes B patients. The evidence is also supportive of a significant clinical benefit from adjuvant chemotherapy in this group of patients.

SUPPORTING EVIDENCE FOR ADJUVANT CHEMOTHERAPY IN DUKES B PATIENTS

The NSABP experience

Most of the available supporting evidence comes from National Surgical Adjuvant Breast and Bowel

Project (NSABP) trials of adjuvant therapy. The NSABP has historically included Dukes B and C colon cancer patients in all its adjuvant chemotherapy trials. In four such trials (C-01, C-02, C-03, and C-04), a disease-free survival (DFS) and/or survival benefit from chemotherapy (reaching or approaching statistical significance) was demonstrated at 5 years of follow-up between at least two treatment arms. These four trials compared different adjuvant chemotherapy regimens with each other or with no-adjuvant-treatment controls. The relatively large proportion of patients with Dukes B tumors in these studies provides an opportunity to address whether Dukes B colon cancer patients benefit from adjuvant chemotherapy and to what extent when compared with Dukes C patients. Results from the comparison in benefit have been reported in both abstract[10] and article form,[11] and will be summarized here.

The four trials were carried out between 1977 and 1990, and had similar eligibility criteria.[2–5] In C-01, C-03, and C-04, eligible patients had adenocarcinoma of the colon resected with curative intent, with no evidence of gross residual or metastatic disease at the time of laparotomy. Patients with pathologically confirmed tumor extension into adjacent organs were eligible provided that all tumor was removed en bloc with negative resection margins. In C-02, randomization occurred prior to operative exploration. Eligible patients were required to have a potentially curable adenocarcinoma as documented by barium enema or endoscopic biopsy. Those patients having intraoperative extent of disease consistent with Dukes D stage did not receive the randomized treatment, and were treated at the discretion of the participating investigator. In all four trials, patients were classified as having Dukes B tumors if, on pathologic examination, the tumor demonstrated full-thickness penetration of the bowel wall (through the serosa or into the pericolic fat), with no regional lymph-node involvement.[12] Patients were classified as having Dukes C tumors if, on pathologic examination, there was evidence of regional lymph-node involvement. In all four trials, patients presenting with obstruction or contained perforation were eligible, but patients presenting with free perforation were not. Protocol C-01[2] compared adjuvant MOF (methyl-CCNU (semustine), vincristine, and 5-FU) with surgery alone. Protocol C-02[3] compared perioperative administration of portal venous infusion (PVI) of 5-FU with surgery alone. Protocol C-03[4] compared adjuvant 5-FU + LV (high-dose LV weekly regimen) with adjuvant MOF. The MOF regimen was identical to that used in C-01, but was given only for five cycles every 10 weeks. The 5-FU + LV regimen was given for eight cycles

(each given for 6 out of 8 weeks). Protocol C-04[5] compared the same adjuvant 5-FU + LV regimen with 5-FU + LEV (as used in the Intergroup adjuvant trials) and with the combination of 5-FU + LV + LEV. The 5-FU + LEV regimen was given for one year.

The four studies included 3820 patients available for analysis, out of which 1565 (41%) presented with Dukes B and 2255 (59%) with Dukes C tumors. The distribution of patient and tumor characteristics such as age, sex, tumor location, and presence of obstruction, contained perforation or extension into adjacent organs was well balanced between Dukes B and Dukes C patients (Table 14.1). Five-year follow-up results in each of the four trials demonstrated a difference in overall survival for all patients for at least two of the arms (Table 14.2). In C-01, administration of the MOF regimen resulted in a 7% absolute improvement in survival over operation alone ($p = 0.07$). In C-02, perioperative PVI of 5-FU resulted in a 7% absolute improvement in survival over operation alone ($p = 0.08$). In C-03, administration of 5-FU + LV resulted in a 10% improvement in survival over MOF ($p = 0.0008$). And in C-04, administration of 5-FU + LV resulted in a 5% absolute improvement in survival over 5-FU + LEV ($p = 0.06$). The 5-year survival results according to stage of disease indicated that in all four studies the observed difference in overall survival was in the same direction for Dukes B and for Dukes C patients (Table 14.2). In C-01, administration of MOF resulted in a 3% absolute improvement in survival in Dukes B patients ($p = 0.73$) and a 9% absolute improvement in survival in Dukes C patients ($p = 0.05$) compared with surgery alone. In C-02, there was a 12% improvement in survival for Dukes B patients ($p = 0.005$) and a 2% improvement for Dukes C patients ($p = 0.81$) with perioperative PVI of 5-FU compared with surgery alone. In C-03, there was an 8% improvement in survival in Dukes B patients ($p = 0.03$) and an 11% improvement in Dukes C patients ($p = 0.003$) with 5-FU + LV compared with MOF. In C-04, there was a 4% improvement in survival in Dukes B patients ($p = 0.25$) and a 4% improvement in Dukes C patients with 5-FU + LV compared with 5-FU + LEV ($p = 0.21$).

Regardless of Dukes stage, there was always an observed reduction in mortality, recurrence, or DFS event rate from chemotherapy, and, in most cases, the reduction was as great or greater for Dukes B patients as for Dukes C patients (Figure 14.1). Specific results were as follows. In C-01, administration of MOF reduced mortality by 7% in Dukes B patients, compared with 26% in Dukes C patients. In C-02, 7 days of perioperative PVI of 5-FU reduced

Table 14.1 Patient and tumor characteristics according to Dukes stage and combined treatment groups in the combined analysis of NSABP Dukes B and Dukes C patients[a]

	Dukes B			Dukes C		
	All (1565 pts) (%)	Combined group 1 (793 pts) (%)	Combined group 2 (772 pts) (%)	All (2255 pts) (%)	Combined group 1 (1131 pts) (%)	Combined group 2 (1124 pts) (%)
Sex:						
Male	58	57	59	52	54	51
Female	42	43	41	48	46	49
Age:						
<60 years	44	45	44	48	47	49
≥60 years	56	55	56	52	53	51
Location:						
Right colon	40	38	41	41	42	39
Left colon	24	24	24	20	18	22
Sigmoid/rectosigmoid	34	36	33	37	37	37
Multiple/unknown	2	2	2	3	3	2
High-risk characteristics (any of obstruction, perforation or extension to adjacent organs):						
No	74	72	75	71	72	70
Yes	26	28	25	28	27	29
Unknown	<1	<1	—	1	2	1

[a]Adapted with permission from Mamounas EP, Rockette H, Jones J et al, Comparative efficacy of adjuvant chemotherapy in patients with Dukes' B vs. Dukes' C colon cancer: results from four NSABP adjuvant studies (C-01, C-02, C-03, C-04). *J Clin Oncol* 1999; **17**: 1349–55.

mortality by 51% in Dukes B patients, compared with 4% in Dukes C patients. In C-03, 5-FU + LV compared with MOF reduced mortality by 53% in Dukes B patients, compared with 31% in Dukes C patients. In C-04, 5-FU + LV compared with 5-FU + LEV reduced mortality by 21% in Dukes B patients, compared with 14% in Dukes C patients. Results for recurrence or DFS event were similar (Figure 14.1). Thus, in all four studies, the treatment effect was similar between Dukes B and Dukes C patients.

However, because of the limited number of Dukes B and Dukes C patients in each of these trials, in any one trial individually one cannot rule out with confidence a substantial difference in treatment effect according to Dukes stage. To address this particular question, data from these four trials were combined into two treatment groups. *Combined Group 1* included the treatment groups from each trial with the inferior outcome for all patients (the surgery-alone groups in C-01 and C-02, the MOF group in C-03, and the 5-FU + LEV group in C-04). *Combined*

Table 14.2 Five-year overall survival (OS) results in NSABP C-01, C-02, C-03, and C-04 according to stage of disease[a]

Study[b]	All			Dukes B			Dukes C		
	No. of pts	OS rate (%)	p-value	No. of pts	OS rate (%)	p-value	No. of pts	OS rate (%)	p-value
C-01									
Operation	375	60	0.07	166	72	0.73	209	50	0.05
MOF	351	67		150	75		201	59	
C-02									
Operation	343	67	0.08	201	76	0.005	142	56	0.81
PVI 5-FU	340	74		188	88		152	58	
C-03									
MOF	516	66	0.0008	141	84	0.03	375	59	0.003
5-FU + LV	513	76		149	92		364	70	
C-04									
5-FU + LEV	690	70	0.06	285	81	0.25	405	63	0.21
5-FU + LV	692	75		285	85		407	67	

[a]Adapted with permission from Mamounas EP, Rockette H, Jones J et al, Comparative efficacy of adjuvant chemotherapy in patients with Dukes' B vs. Dukes' C colon cancer: results from four NSABP adjuvant studies (C-01, C-02, C-03, C-04). *J Clin Oncol* 1999; **17:** 1349–55.
[b]See text for regimens.

Group 2 included the treatment groups from each trial with the superior outcome for all patients (the MOF group in C-01, the perioperative 5-FU PVI group in C-02, and the 5-FU + LV groups in C-03 and C-04) (Figure 14.2). There were no significant differences in patient and tumor characteristics between Combined Group 1 and Combined Group 2 patients within Dukes stage (Table 14.1). To estimate the differential effect of treatment according to Dukes stage, the cumulative odds of death were calculated in the better-outcome group (Combined Group 2) relative to the worse-outcome group (Combined Group 1) for both Dukes B and Dukes C patients (Figure 14.3). The cumulative odds of death in Dukes B patients were 0.70 (indicating a 30% reduction in death rate for Dukes B patients in Combined Group 2 compared with Dukes B patients in Combined Group 1). In comparison, at 5 years, the cumulative odds of death in Dukes C patients were 0.82 (indicating an 18% reduction in death rate for

Dukes C patients in Combined Group 2 compared with Dukes C patients in Combined Group 1).

Finally, the mortality reduction in Dukes B patients was examined according to the presence or absence of clinical adverse prognostic factors. Twenty-six percent of the Dukes B cohort presented with one of the high-risk characteristics such as obstruction, contained perforation, or direct extension to adjacent organs. The efficacy of adjuvant chemotherapy was evident whether patients presented with or without any of the adverse prognostic factors (Figure 14.4). Patients with none of the high-risk characteristics had a 32% reduction in mortality rate (cumulative odds 0.68); those with one or more high-risk characteristics had a 20% reduction in mortality rate (cumulative odds 0.80). This reduction in mortality rate was translated into an absolute improvement in survival of 5% in each risk category (Combined Group 2 87% versus Combined Group 1 82% in the low-risk category, and Combined Group 2

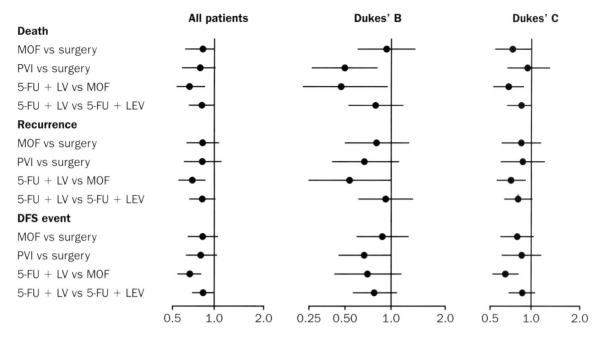

Figure 14.1 Reduction in cumulative odds of death, recurrence, and disease-free survival (DFS) event according to Dukes stage for four NSABP adjuvant colon trials (with 95% confidence intervals). See text for regimens. Adapted with permission from Mamounas EP, Rockette H, Jones J et al, Comparative efficacy of adjuvant chemotherapy in patients with Dukes B vs. Dukes C colon cancer: results from four NSABP adjuvant studies (C-01, C-02, C-03, C-04). *J Clin Oncol* 1999; **17:** 1349–55.

Surgery	(C-01)
Surgery	(C-02)
MOF	(C-03)
5-FU + LEV	(C-04)

Combined Group 1
(1924 patients)

MOF	(C-01)
5-FU PVI	(C-02)
5-FU + LV	(C-03)
5-FU + LV	(C-04)

Combined Group 2
(1896 patients)

Figure 14.2 Combined treatment groups in the combined analysis of NSABP Dukes B and Dukes C patients. See text for regimens. Adapted with permission from Mamounas EP, Rockette H, Jones J et al, Comparative efficacy of adjuvant chemotherapy in patients with Dukes B vs. Dukes C colon cancer: results from four NSABP adjuvant studies (C-01, C-02, C-03, C-04). *J Clin Oncol* 1999; **17:** 1349–55.

75% versus Combined Group 1 70% in the high-risk category).

Other studies

In 1995, Moertel et al[8] reported the results of an Intergroup trial in which 318 Dukes B2 (stage II) patients were randomized to 5-FU + LEV or surgery alone (INT-0035). After 7 years of follow-up, patients receiving 5-FU + LEV had a 31% reduction in recurrence rate. Although this reduction was not statistically significant ($p = 0.10$), this study, by design, was underpowered to detect reductions in recurrence of less than 50%. Thus, these results and those from the NSABP trials are not discordant in terms of colon cancer recurrence. In the Intergroup study, although there was no difference in overall survival, there was a non-significant 20% reduction in the rate of colon-cancer-related deaths in the group receiving 5-FU + LEV. The lack of an overall survival benefit can be partially attributed to the relatively high non-cancer-related death rate in Dukes B patients.

Two other studies have recently examined the relative efficacy of chemotherapy in Dukes B patients. The first,[13] a meta-analysis of 4000 patients participating in 10 studies evaluating the efficacy of short continuous infusion of portal vein chemotherapy, demonstrated that the observed treatment benefit was present both in Dukes A/B patients and in Dukes C patients. The second,[14,15] a pooled analysis of five randomized trials evaluating the efficacy of adjuvant 5-FU + LV in patients with Dukes B colon

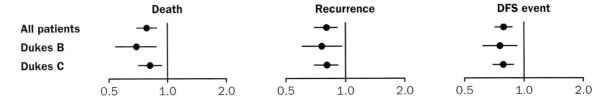

Figure 14.3 Reduction in cumulative odds (Combined Group 2 versus Combined Group 1) of death, recurrence, and disease-free survival (DFS) event according to Dukes stage in the combined analysis of NSABP Dukes B and Dukes C patients (with 95% confidence intervals). Adapted with permission from Mamounas EP, Rockette H, Jones J et al, Comparative efficacy of adjuvant chemotherapy in patients with Dukes B vs. Dukes C colon cancer: results from four NSABP adjuvant studies (C-01, C-02, C-03, C-04). *J Clin Oncol* 1999; **17**: 1349–55.

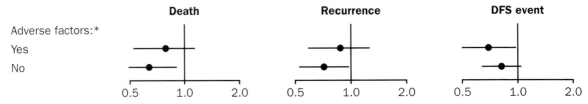

* Obstruction, contained perforation, or extension to adjacent organs

Figure 14.4 Reduction in cumulative odds of death, recurrence, and disease-free survival (DFS) event (Combined Group 2 versus Combined Group 1) according to the presence of adverse clinical prognostic factors in the combined analysis of NSABP Dukes B patients (with 95% confidence intervals). Adapted with permission from Mamounas EP, Rockette H, Jones J et al, Comparative efficacy of adjuvant chemotherapy in patients with Dukes B vs. Dukes C colon cancer: results from four NSABP adjuvant studies (C-01, C-02, C-03, C-04). *J Clin Oncol* 1999; **17**: 1349–55.

cancer, demonstrated a modest improvement in event-free survival and overall survival. In this analysis, 1016 patients with Dukes B colon cancer from five separate trials were randomized to 5-FU + LV or surgery alone. All trials used a regimen of 5-FU at 370–425 mg/m² plus LV 20–200 mg/m² daily for 5 days every 28–35 days, in comparison with the weekly, high-dose LV regimen used in the NSABP studies. A pooled analysis for event-free and overall survival was performed. The median follow-up duration was 5.75 years. There was no significant increase in event-free or overall survival in those patients who received 5-FU + LV. The hazards ratio at 5 years was 0.83 (17% reduction) for event-free survival and 0.86 (14% reduction) for overall survival. The 5-year event-free survival rate was 73% for the surgery-alone group, versus 76% for the group that received adjuvant 5-FU + LV. The 5-year overall survival rate was 80% for the surgery-alone group, versus 82% for the chemotherapy group. The authors of the study concluded that this data set does not support the routine use of 5-

FU + LV in all patients with Dukes B colon cancer. They did state, however, that their study did not have sufficient power at that time to detect the 12% and 14% decreases in point estimates of hazard ratios for event-free and overall survival. They noted that longer follow-up may be needed in order to identify a small benefit from the administration of 5-FU + LV.

COMMENTARY

Those who do not routinely recommend adjuvant chemotherapy for patients with Dukes B colon cancer use two arguments to justify their position. The first relates to the relatively good prognosis of these patients after curative resection alone that could minimize any potential survival gains, particularly in light of the toxicity and cost of adjuvant chemotherapy. The second relates to the possibility of differential effectiveness of adjuvant chemotherapy between Dukes B and Dukes C colon cancer patients, since one cannot assume that the biologic behavior of tumors confined to the bowel wall is the same as that of tumors that involve the regional lymph nodes.

Results from the NSABP trials noted above effectively contradict both these arguments. These findings demonstrate that the 5-year survival of patients with Dukes B colon cancer treated with surgery alone is such that effective adjuvant chemotherapy would be desirable. For other malignancies, such as node-negative breast cancer, adjuvant chemotherapy is recommended in patients with recurrence rates similar to or even lower than those observed in Dukes B colon cancer patients. This is so primarily because a significant body of existing evidence has convinced the oncology community of the efficacy of adjuvant chemotherapy in node-negative breast cancer. Thus, evidence of the effectiveness of adjuvant chemotherapy in Dukes B patients is most important when considering the treatment of these patients. To that extent, the results from the individual NSABP trials and from their combined analysis indicate that adjuvant chemotherapy is biologically as efficacious in patients with Dukes B tumors as in those with Dukes C tumors. Despite the possible limitations inherent in combining several randomized studies that were conducted in different time periods and with changing standards of care, several factors – such as the similarity in eligibility criteria across the studies, the uniformity in follow-up procedures, and the balance in patient and tumor characteristics in the combined treatment groups – lend credibility to the NSABP results.

Some of those who oppose the routine administration of adjuvant chemotherapy in all Dukes B patients agree that such therapy may be indicated only in a subset of patients – those presenting with adverse clinical prognostic factors such as obstruction, contained perforation, or extension into adjacent organs. However, results from the NSABP combined analysis indicate that the benefit from adjuvant chemotherapy in Dukes B patients is independent of the presence or absence of such adverse prognostic factors. Furthermore, the 5-year survival rate for patients in the Combined Group 1 who received less effective therapy and who did not have any of the adverse prognostic factors was only 82%, emphasizing the point that, even in this group of patients, withholding adjuvant chemotherapy is unwarranted.

In summary, a substantial body of evidence supports the view that adjuvant chemotherapy is effective in patients with Dukes B colon cancer to a similar extent as in patients with Dukes C disease. Information from clinical trials further indicates that the benefit from adjuvant chemotherapy seen in Dukes B patients is not confined to those patients at high risk for recurrence but also extends to patients with none of the clinical adverse prognostic factors. The prognosis in the latter group with surgery alone is such that use of systemic adjuvant chemotherapy should be considered.

With the emergence of new molecular and genetic prognostic markers, such as 18q chromosomal deletion,[16] DNA mismatch-repair gene mutations,[17,18] thymidylate synthase levels,[19] and p53 mutations,[20,21] it may be possible in the future to identify subgroups of Dukes B patients with such a good prognosis that adjuvant chemotherapy can be avoided. However, until such biomarkers become validated in prospective studies, all Dukes B patients should be considered for adjuvant chemotherapy after discussion of the risks and benefits from such treatment.

ACKNOWLEDGEMENT

We thank Barbara Good for her editorial assistance with the manuscript.

REFERENCES

1. Moertel CG, Fleming TR, MacDonald JS et al, Levamisole and fluorouracil for adjuvant therapy of resected colon carcinoma. *N Engl J Med* 1990; **322**: 352–8.
2. Wolmark N, Fisher B, Rockette H et al, Postoperative adjuvant chemotherapy or BCG for colon cancer: results from NSABP Protocol C-01. *J Natl Cancer Inst* 1988; **80**: 30–6.
3. Wolmark N, Rockette H, Wickerham DL et al, Adjuvant therapy of Dukes' A, B, and C adenocarcinoma of the colon with portal-vein fluorouracil hepatic infusion: preliminary results from NSABP Protocol C-02. *J Clin Oncol* 1990; **8**: 1466–75.
4. Wolmark N, Rockette H, Fisher B et al, The benefits of leucovorin modulated fluorouracil as postoperative adjuvant therapy for primary colon cancer: results from NSABP Protocol C-03. *J Clin Oncol* 1993; **11**: 1879–87.
5. Wolmark N, Rockette H, Mamounas EP et al, Clinical trial to assess the relative efficacy of fluorouracil and leucovorin, fluorouracil and levamisole, and fluorouracil leucovorin and levamisole in patients with Dukes B and C carcinoma of the colon: results from NSABP C-04. *J Clin Oncol* 1999; **17**: 3553–9.
6. NIH Consensus Conference: Adjuvant therapy for patients with colon and rectal cancer. *JAMA* 1990; **264**: 1444–50.
7. Moertel CG, Fleming TR, MacDonald JS et al, Fluorouracil plus levamisole after resection of stage III colon carcinoma: a final report. *Ann Intern Med* 1995; **122**: 321–6.
8. Moertel CG, Fleming TR, MacDonald JS et al, Intergroup study of fluorouracil plus levamisole as adjuvant therapy for stage II/Dukes' B2 colon cancer. *J Clin Oncol* 1995; **13**: 2936–43.
9. Haller DG, Catalano PJ, MacDonald JS et al, Fluorouracil (FU), leucovorin (LV) and levamisole (LEV) adjuvant therapy for colon cancer: five-year final report of INT-0089. *Proc Am Soc Clin Oncol* 1998; **17**: 256a (Abst 982).
10. Mamounas EP, Rockette H, Jones J et al, Comparative efficacy of adjuvant chemotherapy in patients with Dukes' B vs. Dukes' C

colon cancer: results from four NSABP adjuvant studies (C-01, C-02, C-03, C-04). *Proc Am Soc Clin Oncol* 1996; **15:** 205 (Abst 461).

11. Mamounas E, Wieand S, Wolmark N et al, Comparative efficacy of adjuvant chemotherapy in patients with Dukes' B vs. Dukes' C colon cancer: results from four NSABP adjuvant studies (C-01, C-02, C-03, C-04). *J Clin Oncol* 1999; **17:** 1349–55.

12. Dukes CE, The classification of cancer of the rectum. *J Pathol* 1932; **35:** 323–32.

13. Liver Infusion Meta-analysis Group, Portal vein chemotherapy for colorectal cancer: a meta-analysis of 4000 patients in 10 studies. *J Natl Cancer Inst* 1997; **89:** 497–505.

14. Erlichman C, Marsoni S, Seitz JF et al, Event free and overall survival is increased by FUFA in resected B colon cancer: a pooled analysis of five randomized trials (RCTS). *Proc Am Soc Clin Oncol* 1997; **16:** 280a (Abst 991).

15. International Multicentre Pooled Analysis of B2 Colon Cancer Trials (IMPACT B2) Investigators, Efficacy of adjuvant fluorouracil and folinic acid in B2 colon cancer. *J Clin Oncol* 1999; **17:** 1356–63.

16. Jen J, Kim H, Piantadosi S et al, Allelic loss of chromosome 18q and prognosis in colorectal cancer. *N Engl J Med* 1994; **331:** 213–21.

17. Bronner CE, Baker SM, Morrison PT et al, Mutation in the DNA mismatch repair gene homologue hMLH1 is associated with hereditary non-polyposis colon cancer. *Nature* 1994; **368:** 258–61.

18. Nicolaides NC, Papadopoulos N, Liu B et al, Mutations in two PMS homologues in hereditary nonpolyposis colon cancer. *Nature* 1994; **371:** 75–80.

19. Johnston PG, Fisher ER, Rockette HE et al, The role of thymidylate synthase expression in prognosis and outcome of adjuvant chemotherapy in patients with rectal cancer. *J Clin Oncol* 1994; **12:** 2640–7.

20. Bosari S, Viale G, Possi P et al, Cytoplasmic accumulation of p53 protein: an independent prognostic indicator in colorectal adenocarcinomas. *J Natl Cancer Inst* 1994; **86:** 681–7.

21. Zheng Z-S, Sarkis AS, Zhang Z-F et al, p53 nuclear overexpression: an independent predictor of survival in lymph node positive colorectal cancer patients. *J Clin Oncol* 1994; **12:** 2043–50.

15

Adjuvant intraportal treatment

Roberto F Labianca, Giordano D Beretta, M Adelaide Pessi

INTRODUCTION

Colorectal cancer is one of the most frequent tumours worldwide, ranking third in males and second in females: every year 700 000 new cases are diagnosed and 500 000 patients die from this disease. It is a common opinion that the overall survival related to colorectal cancer has improved only marginally in the last few decades, despite advances in surgery and in early detection: potentially curative resection at disease presentation can be performed in only 70–80% of patients, but, even in these cases, the overall survival rate at 5 years does not exceed 60%, indicating the need for an effective adjuvant treatment.

The use of systemic chemotherapy in this setting is well established, at least in stage III (Dukes C) patients, and is extensively discussed in other chapters of this book. Adjuvant portal vein infusion is another potentially interesting strategy: as the liver is the most common site for spread of colorectal cancer (this organ involvement is macroscopically present on initial cancer diagnosis in 25–30% of patients, with the expected median survival time of these patients being only 6–9 months), it is conceivable that regional chemotherapy, if administered early enough, could inhibit the proliferation of tumour cells. Moreover, the combination of systemic and intraportal therapy appears rational, and could be aimed at increasing the activity of single-modality treatment.

In this chapter the following issues will be discussed: (1) the biological basis for intraportal chemotherapy; (2) the historical Taylor experience; (3) the subsequent confirmatory trials; (4) their inclusion in a comprehensive meta-analysis; (5) the large-scale randomized clinical trial conducted by the European Organization for Research and Treatment of Cancer (EORTC); (6) the most recent contributions, concerning both intraportal treatment alone (the AXIS trial in the UK) and its combination with intravenous therapy (the SMAC trial in Italy and a successive EORTC study).

BIOLOGICAL BASIS

It has been recognized that tumour cells embolize into the portal vein system through the mesenteric vessels, and then invade the liver. Of course, not all circulating cells generate overt metastases, and, in fact, it has been reported that the prognosis of patients with malignant cells in the portal blood is no worse than that of patients without this finding. However, it is possible that metachronous metastases originate from microscopic deposits undetectable at surgery for the primary cancer and therefore that the development of regional chemotherapy capable of eliminating these deposits is warranted.

An important issue with regard to the delivery of antitumour drugs to the liver is vascularity: both the arterial and the portal system play a role in tumour perfusion, and the possible presence of arterioportal and arteriovenous shunting may complicate this pattern. Generally, metastases with diameter less than 1 mm do not display any new vessel formation, while greater deposits are encircled by 'de novo'-shaped vessels that derive from either the arteriolar or the portal tree in a random fashion. As tumour localization grows, reaching a diameter of 5–7 mm, the encircling plexus become more extensive and developed, with a predominance of the arterial circulation and a gradual disappearance of the portal supply. Therefore the arterial route dominates the portal one for established and macroscopically detectable metastatic disease (this observation provides the rationale for the use of locoregional intra-arterial chemotherapy), whereas the portal route is more prominent in the vascularization of micrometastases, and is therefore preferable in the adjuvant setting.

THE PIONEERING EXPERIENCE OF TAYLOR

As early as 1957, Morales et al[1] advocated the use of portal vein infusion of antitumour drugs at the time of resection of colorectal cancer in order to prevent the development of hepatic metastases. In the following years, it became clear that adjuvant therapy should be initiated as soon as possible after surgery, when the tumour burden is minimal and several conditions (such as surgery itself, anaesthetic stress, hypercoagulability, blood transfusions and immunodepression due to surgical manipulation) might facilitate the diffusion of cancer cells.

In 1979, a group of Liverpool surgeons led by Irving Taylor published very interesting results on the use of intraportal chemotherapy in resected colorectal cancer.[2] In a relatively small randomized trial (234 patients), they reported that postoperative infusion of 5-fluorouracil (5-FU) at the dose of 1 g/day, together with heparin (5000 IU/day), for 7 days was able to improve the prognosis of treated patients: at that time (with a mean follow-up of 26 months), 23 patients had died in the control group and 7 in the infusion arm. There was also a significant decrease in the occurrence of liver metastases in the patients treated with portal vein infusion (2, versus 13 in the control group). In a more recent analysis,[3] the same group reported, at a median follow-up of 4 years, significant increases in disease-free survival (DFS) and overall survival (OS) in treated patients (53 patients had died with recurrent disease in the control group and 25 in the infusion group). The relative risk for OS was 0.65, with the most important advantage being obtained in Dukes B colon cancer patients. Once again, the incidence of liver metastases was significantly reduced (5 versus 22 cases) in the treatment group, and this was the main reason for the mortality reduction in patients receiving chemotherapy.

This experience had the merit of demonstrating that the experimental hypotheses about the role of intraportal chemotherapy, performed early after surgical resection of the primary tumour, could be translated into positive clinical results. However, the small number of patients entered in the study made this finding questionable, and required the implementation of confirmatory trials.

CONFIRMATORY TRIALS

After the encouraging results obtained by Taylor, several trials tried to reproduce the efficacy reported by the Liverpool group and to optimize the treatment.

In Switzerland, Metzger et al (on behalf of the Swiss Group of Clinical Cancer Research, SAKK) reported two subsequent updates[4,5] of a multicentre randomized trial, in which a continuous portal infusion of 5-FU (500 mg/m²/24 h for 7 days) plus mitomycin C (MMC) (10 mg/m² h on day 1) was compared with radical surgery alone. A total of 533 patients with histologically proven adenocarcinoma of the colon and rectum who were candidates for a curative en bloc resection and were less than 75 years old were randomized. No significant decrease in liver recurrence rate was observed in these first two reports, even though a significant survival advantage was obtained in patients with Dukes C colon cancer receiving a full dose of chemotherapy. In 1995, the same group published the final results of this trial:[6] at a median follow-up of 8 years, 235 patients had died (108 in the infusion arm and 127 in the control arm), with an increase in 5-year DFS and OS (risk reductions 22% and 26% respectively). Treatment benefits were similar in all subgroups, but the authors confirmed even larger differences for patients with colon cancer and a positive nodal status. Another finding was that, in this population, patients receiving blood transfusions had a significantly shorter DFS (hazard ratio (HR) 1.60), chiefly when more than 4 units of blood products were transfused (HR 2.52). In contrast, patients who had no transfusion and who had been assigned to have portal vein infusion chemotherapy had a significantly longer DFS than patients who had transfusion but no chemotherapy (HR: 0.38).[7]

The same group performed another randomized phase III adjuvant trial with the aim of comparing intraportal versus intravenous short-course perioperative chemotherapy (5-FU, MMC, and heparin were administered in both arms) versus no adjuvant treatment.[8] In this three-arm study, haematological toxicity was evaluated by haemoglobin determination and leukocyte and thrombocyte counts before and during the 10 days after surgery. The authors observed that haemoglobin showed a median decrease of 22% in the control group and that this decrease was worsened significantly by 3% during chemotherapy; leukocytes showed a median decrease of 7% in the control arm, whereas perioperative chemotherapy caused a significantly higher median drop (23% when given through the portal vein and 34% when administered systemically). In contrast, thrombocytes showed a median decrease of 25% in the control group, but chemotherapy was not associated with a significant additional drop. The conclusion was that if drug increases are planned in future trials, the addition of haematopoietic growth factors should be considered. Although the overall results of this trial in a definitive paper are awaited with interest, at the 1998 Meeting of the American Society of Clinical Oncology (ASCO),[9] an analysis after more than 5 years of follow-up was not able to confirm a significant advantage for adjuvant chemotherapy, either intraportal or systemic. With 769 patients randomized, both 5-year DFS and OS rates were comparable in the three groups (60%, 64%, 63% and 68%, 64%, 72%).

In 1990, a Dutch group coordinated by Wereldsma[10] reported the results of a three-arm study in which patients were randomized among 5-FU (1000 mg/24 h for 7 days) plus heparin (5000 U/24 h for 7 days), urokinase (10 000 U/h for 24 h only) or surgery alone. A total of 304 patients were eligible: 102 in the control arm, 99 in the 5-FU plus heparin arm, and 103 in the urokinase arm. With a median follow-up of 44 months, the chemotherapy group showed a significantly lower rate of liver metastases than the other arms (7% versus 23% in the control and 18% in the urokinase group), but DFS and OS were not significantly increased. It is noteworthy that urokinase had no influence on the development of hepatic metastases. As far as toxicity is concerned, the development of septic complications was not related to treatment groups.

A trial by the North Central Cancer Treatment Group (NCCTG) and the Mayo Clinic randomized 220 patients between intraportal infusion of 5-FU plus heparin and control only.[11] After a median follow-up exceeding 5 years, no difference was detected between the two arms in terms of frequency of liver metastases and overall survival. Of course, the quite limited sample size and also the fact that the protocol allowed delay in chemotherapy until the fifth postoperative day represent major drawbacks in the interpretation of these data.

A large randomized trial of intraportal infusion of 5-FU and heparin was published by the National Surgical Adjuvant Breast and Bowel Project (NSABP).[12] Of the 1158 enrolled patients, only 901 were fully evaluable (randomization was performed before surgery and 23% of patients were found ineligible at the resection time). The 5-FU daily dose was 600 mg/m^2, and treatment began 6 hours after surgery. When the trial was published in 1990, survival data after 4 years were mature for only 33% of patients: at that time, a significant difference in DFS rate (74% versus 64%, $p = 0.02$) and a slight but not significant advantage in OS rate (81% versus 73%, $p = 0.07$) were observed in favour of the treated group. As no difference in the frequency of liver metastases was reported between the two arms, the authors stated that the effect of treatment was probably due to a systemic action of the drug and commented upon their results in quite a pessimistic way, which led to some criticism by our group.[13] It should be noted that the follow-up and the analysis of DFS were not complete when the trial was published: further information was included in the meta-analysis (see below), and appeared to show no advantage for intraportal chemotherapy.

In the same period, Fielding et al[14] published the data from a three-arm trial, performed at St Mary's and surrounding hospitals in the UK, comparing controls (145 patients) versus intraportal 5-FU (1000 mg/24 h for 7 days) plus heparin at a dose of 10 000 U/day (130 patients) versus heparin alone (123 patients). They reported that 10.6% of patients in the heparin-alone arm and 18.5% in the 5-FU plus heparin arm failed to complete therapy (chiefly because of premature removal or blockage of the catheter), but they observed no statistically significant difference in the incidence of postoperative complications, even though the control group had a favourable trend in this respect. At a minimal follow-up of 5 years, an increased survival in patients receiving chemotherapy was achieved, but with a significant difference ($p < 0.03$) only in Dukes C; also the frequency of hepatic metastases was lowered. As these differences were greater at 5 years, the authors postulated that most liver metastases appearing in the first 2–3 years after surgery were already present, even if occult, at the moment of primary tumour resection and therefore were vascularized by the hepatic artery. No positive effect for heparin was detected.

The possible systemic effect of perioperative 5-FU was evaluated by Gray et al:[15] the group treated with intraportal chemotherapy, but not the group receiving systemic 5-FU at the same dose, had a lower number of deaths than the control arm.

The Gastrointestinal Tract Cancer Cooperative Group (GITCCG) of the EORTC conducted a three-group randomized trial comparing intraportal 5-FU (500 mg/m^2/day for 7 days) plus heparin versus heparin alone versus surgery alone.[16] A total of 235 patients were enrolled in this trial, which did not show any significant impact on OS rate (5-year figure: 71% in the chemotherapy arm and 69% in the control arm). As the toxic effects were very limited and the accrual was slow, this study was closed and a successor two-arm large-scale trial was started by the same cooperative group (see below).

Other studies have provided ancillary information about the effects of intraportal chemotherapy and have contributed to a better understanding of its mechanism of action. A study in Japan investigated 35 colorectal patients who underwent curative resection, 19 of whom also received adjuvant treatment with intraportal 5-FU and MMC.[17] Natural killer (NK)-cell activity and other immunological parameters were evaluated before and after operation and were compared between the two groups. Marked reductions in NK-cell activity and in the percentages of CD16$^+$ and CD56$^+$ cells were detected postoperatively in the treated group.

The economical implications of intraportal chemotherapy were analysed in a study from Italy.[18] To assess the pharmacoeconomic profile of this adjuvant treatment, the authors carried out an incremental cost–effectiveness analysis on a trial including more than 500 patients, and found that the administration of intraportal chemotherapy implied an incremental cost of $1210 per discontinued life-year saved, giving the best cost–effectiveness profile in comparison with many other pharmacological interventions.

The following general comments can be made about all these and other minor trials[19–21] of intraportal adjuvant chemotherapy: (a) most of the studies were multicentric and, with some exceptions, included rectal cancers as well as colon cancers; (b)

there is a fair degree of consistency regarding the schedule of treatment (5-FU at similar dosages and days of treatment, starting immediately after surgery, and with the addition of MMC in a minority of trials); (c) the effects of anticoagulants were tested in only four protocols, using heparin or urokinase alone; (d) the vast majority of the studies documented improvements in DFS and OS, particularly in Dukes C and colon patients; (e) generally, a significant reduction in the incidence of liver metastases (as reported in the pilot study by Taylor) was not confirmed; suggesting that the positive effect of intraportal chemotherapy could be related to a systemic efficacy of 5-FU; (f) the overall operative mortality in all these trials was about 3–4% and is certainly acceptable, even though some categories of patients should be excluded from this treatment (including insulin-dependent diabetics, individuals with obesity or cardiovascular and pulmonary disease, and patients with evidence of intra-abdominal sepsis at laparotomy or during the early postoperative period).

THE META-ANALYSIS

A first meta-analysis, based on published data only,[22] had postulated a reduction of about one-third in the risk of death for patients receiving intraportal 5-FU infusion, but today this type of analysis is subject to methodological criticism.[23] In 1997, the Liver Infusion Meta-analysis Group coordinated by Piedbois and Buyse published the results of a large systematic revision conducted on about 4000 patients enrolled in 10 studies,[24] most of which have been reviewed above. Data were retrieved for cases included in phase III trials started before 1987 in which 5–7 days of continuous postoperative portal vein infusion were compared with no further treatment after primary tumour resection. The authors confirmed that the most frequent antiproliferative drug was 5-FU, usually administered with heparin, whereas MMC was associated in two trials. In four studies, there was an additional control arm receiving intraportal heparin or urokinase alone, and one trial included a second control group of patients treated with continuous systemic infusion of 5-FU. Survival with and without intraportal chemotherapy was the same for the first 24 months, but it then diverged, with an absolute survival improvement at 5 years of 4.7% ($p = 0.006$). If the original study by Taylor was excluded, this difference decreased to 3.6% but was still significant ($p = 0.04$). If the analysis was restricted to patients with Dukes stage A, B, or C (about 90% of the total), the absolute effect on 5-year survival increased to 6.0% (all trials) or 4.8% (excluding the initial promising study). The meta-analysis confirmed that, in contrast to the very significant reduction in liver metastases reported by Taylor ($p = 0.00000007$), the decreased incidence observed in the nine hypothesis-testing trials was not significant ($p = 0.2$). In the studies with further control groups, there was an advantage in survival for patients treated with cytotoxic portal vein infusion chemotherapy in comparison with non-antiproliferative intraportal drug administration or with systemic chemotherapy. Therefore the authors concluded that 'intraportal infusion of 5-FU, with or without other cytotoxic drugs, for about 1 week after surgery in patients with colorectal cancer may produce an absolute improvement in 5-year survival of a few percent' (it should be emphasized that if a widely practicable adjuvant treatment is able to achieve a 5% increase in long-term OS, this means that its widespread use would avoid many thousands of deaths worldwide each year) and that 'although encouraging, this finding is not statistically secure (in the single studies also a number of inoperable cases were included) and additional evidence from randomized trials involving several thousand more patients (for example, the AXIS trial [see below] and a still ongoing Chinese study in which 8000 patients are foreseen) is needed'.

THE EORTC LARGE-SCALE CLINICAL TRIAL

In this trial,[25] patients were eligible if they presented with a histologically confirmed resectable cancer of the colon or rectum without distant metastases. The exclusion criteria were the usual ones for patients to be included in a study of adjuvant chemotherapy, and radiotherapy (pre- or postoperative) was permitted in rectal cancer if it was deemed necessary by the investigator on the basis of local extension. Randomization was performed before or, preferably, during surgery, and patients were assigned to surgery alone (control group) or the same plus adjuvant treatment. A catheter was inserted in the portal vein during laparotomy: the access to the vein was achieved either by dilatation and cannulation of the umbilical vein or by catheter insertion into portal

vein tributaries. The correct position of the tip was checked by perioperative radiography or by fluorescein infusion, in order to permit a satisfactory perfusion of the two hepatic lobes. In the chemotherapy group, the infusion consisted of 1000 ml 5% dextrose, 5000 IU heparin and 500 mg/m² 5-FU for 24 hours, and was started when the catheter was properly placed, using a continuous-infusion pump rather than a gravity drip. The infusion was given for 7 days, with a careful continuous check-up of the patient.

The main endpoint of the study was overall survival, and, to detect an improvement from 50% to 60% at 5 years after resection, 344 deaths were required, with a global accrual of more than 1000 patients. Between June 1987 and March 1993, 1322 patients were randomized, 977 in EORTC institutions, 258 by GIVIO (Gruppo Italiano per la Valutazione degli Interventi in Oncologia), and 87 by the Japanese Foundation for Cancer Research. Overall, 47 institutions in eight countries participated in the trial. In the 536 patients who started portal vein infusion, catheter complications were observed in 9%, while major toxic effects were detected in only 7%. The median dose of 5-FU was 3454 mg/m² (98.6% of the planned dose). After the 1990 NIH Consensus Conference, Dukes C patients were allowed to receive also adjuvant systemic chemotherapy, but this happened in only 39 cases. After a median follow-up period exceeding 5 years (63 months), and with the total number of expected deaths virtually achieved, the overall survival was similar for the two groups (relative risk of death 1.06). Considering all the randomized patients (intention-to-treat analysis), the estimates of OS rate at 3 years and 5 years were 83% and 73% respectively in the control group and 81% and 72% in the chemotherapy group. Also the estimated DFS rate data were very similar in the two arms (78% and 72% at 3 and 5 years respectively in the control group; 77% and 70% in the treated group), and even the incidence of liver metastases, at first recurrence or later, was essentially the same (79 patients in the control group; 71 in the intraportal group). According to prognostic factors, survival was poorer for older patients, men, patients with rectal cancer, and those with a more advanced Astler–Coller stage.

This study is the largest randomized trial to assess intraportal adjuvant chemotherapy in colorectal cancer, and was not able to find a survival advantage for treated patients. It is interesting to note that if these data were added to the trials included in the meta-analysis, the decrease in the risk of mortality would be no more significant, with an odds ratio increase from 0.89 to 0.92. The authors conclude that 'the intraportal infusion of 5-FU, at a dose of 500 mg/m^2 for 7 days, cannot be recommended as the sole adjuvant treatment for high-risk colorectal cancer after complete surgical excision'.

THE MOST RECENT CONTRIBUTIONS (THE AXIS TRIAL AND THE COMBINATION OF INTRAPORTAL AND SYSTEMIC CHEMOTHERAPY)

At the 1999 ASCO Meeting, data were presented from the large-scale AXIS trial:[26] 3681 patients with colorectal cancer were randomized to intraportal infusion of 5-FU (1 g/24 h for 7 days) plus heparin (5000 U/day for 7 days) or surgery alone. Additionally, rectal cancer patients could be randomized to radiotherapy (choice of pre- or postoperative treatment) or no radiotherapy. With 1426 patients having died and an adequate median follow-up, an estimated survival benefit at 5 years of 2.5% was observed, with a hazard ratio of 0.91 and a greater advantage of colon cancer. Therefore the possible increase in survival due to the addition of intraportal chemotherapy seems lower in comparison with the findings of the meta-analysis; of course, a formal addition of the data of this very large trial to those in the meta-analysis is warranted.

Other trials have investigated whether the addition of intraportal therapy to a standard systemic chemotherapy was able to achieve better results in comparison with the single modalities. In 1992, the EORTC–GITCCG initiated an adjuvant trial[27] in which a double randomization was foreseen: first, patients were allocated to surgery only or to the addition of perioperative chemotherapy (intraportal or intraperitoneal, according to the choice of the individual investigator), then to receive 6-month postoperative chemotherapy with 5-FU plus *l*-leucovorin or 5-FU plus levamisole. This trial was closed to accrual in 1998, with about 2500 patients enrolled; no data are yet available.

Another trial concerning the combination of intraportal and systemic chemotherapy as adjuvant treatment was performed in Italy by GIVIO and ACOI (Associazione dei Chirurghi Ospedalieri Italiani).[28] Between April 1992 and April 1998, 1199 patients were randomized to receive portal vein infusion of 5-FU (500 mg/m^2/day for 7 days after surgery, in combination with heparin) or systemic chemotherapy (*l*-leucovorin 100 mg/m^2 plus 5-FU 370 mg/m^2, both given daily-times-five every 4 weeks) for 6 months or the combination of both. Patients' characteristics were similar across the three arms, with 60% Dukes B, 50% male, and a mean age of 64 years. Systemic and intraportal therapy were completed in 73% and 80% of patients respectively, and both kinds of treatment were well tolerated, the commonest adverse effects being gastrointestinal, without toxic deaths. Currently, at a median follow-up time of 35 months, across the three arms a total of 165 patients died, whereas 237 relapsed. Up to now, no statistically significant difference in DFS ($p = 0.26$) or OS ($p = 0.18$) has been found among the three arms, suggesting the absence of any synergism between regional and systemic treatment. The final analysis will be available at the end of 2001.

Therefore, at the present time, we do not have data supporting the possibility of increasing the activity of the two single modalities through their combination. As the EORTC and the Italian trials display two common arms (intraportal plus systemic and systemic alone treatment), a combined analysis of them appears warranted and should help to give a definitive answer to the question – of course, once the data have become mature enough.

CONCLUSIONS

The findings of the single studies evaluating the role of intraportal chemotherapy as an adjuvant treatment for radically resected colorectal cancer are certainly of great interest: after the initial positive data of Taylor, most of the following confirmatory trials were able to detect a favourable effect on the long-term prognosis of the treated patients, even though the mechanism of action seemed to consist more in a systemic effect than in the expected reduction of liver recurrence. After the strict confirmation of the single-study results by the meta-analysis, many clinicians considered portal vein infusion of 5-FU (together with heparin and possibly with MMC) as a possible step forward in the postoperative treatment of colorectal cancer. This therapy is indeed very simple and is not expensive: catheterization of a tributary of the portal venous system is a quick procedure (adding only 10–15 minutes to the duration of colorectal cancer surgery), 5-FU is one of the cheapest cytotoxic drugs, major side-effects are rare, and usually no extra days of hospitalization are required. Of course, the results could be further improved if a longer period of treatment and/or a higher dose of 5-FU, possibly in combination with other drugs or biomodulators, were employed.

Unfortunately, the results of the most recent trials (the large-scale EORTC study and the AXIS study) have been disappointing, and, considering the large number of patients included, they should reduce the positive impact of the findings of the previous, less extended, studies. In addition, since the combination of intraportal and systemic treatment does not appear able to improve upon the results obtained with the single modalities, intraportal chemotherapy (at least with the low amounts of drug used up to now and the short duration employed in the reported trials) no longer seems quite as promising an approach as it did until recently. Indeed, it is conceivable that, at present, most medical oncologists would prefer to use a systemic adjuvant treatment.

REFERENCES

1. Morales F, Bell M, McDonald GD, Cole WH, The prophylactic treatment of cancer at time of operation. *Ann Surg* 1957; **146:** 588–93.
2. Taylor I, Rowling JT, West C, Adjuvant cytotoxic liver perfusion for colorectal cancer. *Br J Surg* 1979; **66:** 833–7.
3. Taylor I, Machin D, Mullee ME et al, A randomised controlled trial of adjuvant portal vein cytotoxic perfusion in colorectal cancer. *Br J Surg* 1985; **72:** 359–63.
4. Metzger U, Mermillod B, Aeberhard P et al, Intraportal chemotherapy in colorectal carcinoma as an adjuvant modality. *World J Surg* 1987; **11:** 452–8.
5. Metzger U, Laffer U, Castiglione M et al, Adjuvant intraportal chemotherapy for colorectal cancer: 4 year results of the randomized Swiss study. *Proc Am Soc Clin Oncol* 1989; **8:** Abst 105.
6. Swiss Group for Clinical Cancer Research (SAKK), Long-term results of single course of adjuvant intraportal chemotherapy for colorectal cancer. *Lancet* 1995; **345:** 349–53.
7. Swiss Group for Clinical Cancer Research (SAKK), Association between blood transfusion and survival in a randomised multicentre trial of perioperative adjuvant portal chemotherapy in patients with colorectal cancer. *Eur J Surg* 1997; **163:** 693–701.
8. Weber W, Maibach R, Laffer U et al, Early hematological toxicity of adjuvant perioperative intraportal and intravenous chemotherapy with fluorouracil, mitomycin and heparin in colorectal cancer. *Anticancer Res* 1995; **15:** 2197–200.
9. Laffer U, Maibach R, Metzger U et al, Randomized trial of adjuvant perioperative chemotherapy in radically resected colorectal cancer (SAKK 40/87). *Proc Am Soc Clin Oncol* 1998; **17:** Abst 983.
10. Wereldsma JCJ, Bruggink EDM, Meijer WS et al, Adjuvant portal liver infusion in colorectal cancer with 5-fluorouracil/heparin versus urokinase versus control. *Cancer* 1990; **65:** 425–32.
11. Beart RW, Moertel CG, Wieand HS et al, Adjuvant therapy for resectable colorectal carcinoma with fluorouracil administered by portal vein infusion. *Arch Surg* 1990; **125:** 897–901.
12. Wolmark N, Rockette H, Wickerham DL et al, Adjuvant therapy of Dukes' A, B and C adenocarcinoma of the colon with portal-vein fluorouracil hepatic infusion: preliminary results of National Surgical Adjuvant Breast and Bowel Project Protocol C-02. *J Clin Oncol* 1990; **8:** 1466–75.
13. Marsoni S, Torri V, Taiana A et al, Efficacy of intraportal infusion for colon cancer: A fair assessment? *J Clin Oncol* 1991; **9:** 888–9.
14. Fielding LP, Hittinger R, Grace RH et al, Randomised controlled trial of adjuvant chemotherapy by portal vein perfusion after curative resection for colorectal adenocarcinoma. *Lancet* 1992; **340:** 502–6.
15. Gray BN, de Zwart J, Fisher R et al, The Australian and New Zealand trial of adjuvant chemotherapy in colon cancer. In: *Adjuvant Therapy of Cancer*, 5th edn (Salmon SE, ed.). Philadelphia: Grune and Stratton, 1987: 537–46.
16. Nitti D, Wils J, Sahmoud T et al, Final results of a phase III clinical trial on adjuvant intraportal infusion with heparin and 5-fluorouracil (5-FU) in resectable colon cancer (EORTC-GITCCG 1983–1987). *Eur J Cancer* 1997; **33:** 1209–15.
17. Rafique M, Adachi W, Koike S et al, Adverse effects of intraportal chemotherapy on natural killer cell activity in colorectal cancer patients. *J Surg Oncol* 1997; **64:** 324–30.
18. Messori A, Bonistalli L, Costantini M et al, Cost effectiveness of adjuvant intraportal chemotherapy in patients with colorectal cancer. *J Clin Gastroenterol* 1996; **23:** 269–74.
19. Ryan J, Weiden P, Crowley J, Bloch K, Adjuvant portal vein infusion for colorectal cancer: a 3-arm randomized trial. *Proc Am Soc Clin Oncol* 1988; **7:** Abst 95.
20. Schlag P, Saeger HD, Friedl P et al, Perioperative adjuvant intraportal FUDR-chemotherapy does not influence prognosis of colon cancer patients. In: *Proceedings of 6th International Conference on the Adjuvant Therapy of Cancer, 1990.*
21. Kimura O, Kurayoshi K, Hoshino K et al, Prophylactic portal infusion chemotherapy as adjuvant chemotherapy for the prevention of metachronous liver metastases in colorectal cancer. *Surg Today* 1995; **25:** 211–16.
22. Gray R, James R, Mossman J, Stenning S, AXIS – a suitable case for treatment. *Br J Cancer* 1991; **63:** 841–5.
23. Stewart LA, Parmar MK, Meta-analysis of the literature or of individual patient data: Is there a difference? *Lancet* 1993; **341:** 418–22.
24. Liver Infusion Meta-analysis Group, Portal vein chemotherapy for colorectal cancer: a meta-analysis of 4000 patients in 10 studies. *J Natl Cancer Inst* 1997; **89:** 497–505.
25. Rougier P, Sahmoud T, Nitti D et al, Adjuvant portal-vein infusion of fluorouracil and heparin in colorectal cancer: a randomised trial. *Lancet* 1998; **351:** 1677–81.
26. James RD (on behalf of the AXIS collaborators), Intraportal 5FU and perioperative radiotherapy in the adjuvant treatment of colorectal cancer – 3681 patients randomized in the UK Coordinating Committee on Cancer Research (UKCCCR) AXIS trial. *Proc Am Soc Clin Oncol* 1999; **18:** Abst 1013.
27. Rougier P, Nordlinger B, Large scale trial for adjuvant treatment in high risk resected colorectal cancers. Rationale to test the combination of loco-regional and systemic chemotherapy and to compare *l*-leucovorin + 5FU to levamisole + 5FU. *Ann Oncol* 1993; **4**(Suppl): 21–8.
28. Labianca R, Boffi L, Marsoni S et al, A randomized trial of intraportal (IP) versus systemic (SY) versus IP + SY adjuvant chemotherapy in patients with resected Dukes B–C colon carcinoma. *Proc Am Soc Clin Oncol* 1999; **18:** Abst 1014.

16

Adjuvant intraperitoneal chemotherapy

Christophe Penna, Robert Malafosse, Bernard Nordlinger

INTRODUCTION

Colorectal adenocarcinoma is one of the most common malignant diseases worldwide, affecting more than 700 000 individuals each year. Today, 75% of these patients have tumours that may be resected with curative intent, and those with stage I cancer are largely cured by surgery alone, with survival rates of 80–95%.[1–3] For patients with stage II tumours (full-thickness penetration through the bowel wall), the 5-year survival rate ranges from 65% to 75%, while for those with Dukes C (nodal involvement, stage III) it ranges from 40% to 50%.[1–4] These patients are considered at high risk of tumour recurrence, and therefore constitute the target population for current adjuvant therapy. Several large multi-institutional trials have demonstrated a significant reduction in mortality using surgery plus adjuvant systemic chemotherapy compared with surgery alone, particularly in patients with stage III colon cancer.

A recognition of predominant patterns of spread, especially that 50% of recurrences are hepatic metastases and that 20–50% are peritoneal,[5] has provided the impetus for a series of adjuvant locoregional approaches employing portal vein infusion or intraperitoneal perfusion of cytotoxic agents. Adjuvant treatment of colorectal carcinoma soon after resection of all gross disease appears attractive according to several pieces of experimental evidence. Micrometastases are more sensitive to a given drug because of a shorter cell-cycle time, a better accessibility to drugs, and a smaller chance of harbouring resistance.[6,7] Therefore several studies have tried to assess the effectiveness of immediate postoperative intraperitoneal chemotherapy. The treatment, which may be more effective on minimal residual disease, begins soon after completion of curative surgery, and the drugs can be delivered at a high dose concentration at the most common site of recurrence (i.e. peritoneum and liver) with decreased toxic systemic effects. The aim is to obtain, with short treatments, results in the same range as those observed after prolonged systemic chemotherapy, ensuring better compliance and cost benefits, or to associate early regional chemotherapy with delayed long-term systemic treatment and further improve survival.

RATIONALE FOR IMMEDIATE POSTOPERATIVE INTRAPERITONEAL CHEMOTHERAPY

Peritoneal cavity and resection site are common sites of tumour recurrence after initial radical surgical treatment of colorectal cancer.[5,8,9] Intraperitoneal spread of tumour cells can occur prior to surgery by the dissemination of emboli resulting from serosal penetration by cancer or leakage of malignant cells from lymphatics. It can also occur during perioperative mobilization of the tumour and surgical dissection. Finally, fibrin entrapment of intra-abdominal tumour emboli on traumatized peritoneal surface, and tumour promotion of these entrapped cells through growth factors involved in the wound healing process, may also participate in the intraperitoneal diffusion of tumours.[10]

After intraperitoneal administration, high-molecular-weight substances such as chemotherapeutic agents are confined to the abdominal cavity for long periods of time.[11] Intraperitoneal chemotherapy can therefore increase the amount and concentration of drug at the residual tumour, since the peritoneal–plasma barrier causes an increase in the duration of contact between drug and tumour cells. It also decreases the amount of drug in the plasma and reduces the risk of systemic toxicity. Immediate postoperative intraperitoneal chemotherapy can fill the abdominal cavity with a large volume of fluid, which may decrease fibrin accumulation and eliminate tumour cells from the abdomen before they become fixed within scar tissues. The elimination of platelets and monocytes from the abdominal cavity may also reduce the promotion of tumour growth associated with the wound healing process. Another potential advantage of intraperitoneal administration is the absorption of the cytostatic drug via the lymphatics and the portal system, which may be beneficial in the prevention or treatment of hepatic micrometastases.[12] The liver is the most common site of failure following potentially curative surgical resection of primary adenocarcinoma of the colon and rectum. Liver metastases will develop in 40–60% of patients who recur,[13] and are a prominent cause of death. Colorectal liver metastases reach the liver via the portal vein, and such dissemination may occur during surgery.[14] Once established in the liver, micrometastases are fed by portal blood. Administration of a cytotoxic agent using the same route might be more effective than systemic administration. Operative stress and immediate postoperative decrease in immune defences have been shown, in some experimental models, to improve the survival of malignant cells and to facilitate their growth in the liver.[15] Early postoperative administration of chemotherapy might be particularly beneficial, destroying suspected tumour cells in the liver before established tumour growth has taken place.

PHARMACOLOGY AND PHYSIOLOGY OF INTRAPERITONEAL ADMINISTRATION OF CYTOTOXIC DRUGS

The pharmacology and physiology of intraperitoneal drug delivery in the immediate postoperative period have been established following numerous experimental and clinical studies. The peritoneal clearance of a drug is inversely proportional to the square root of its molecular weight. Large molecules such as many chemotherapeutic agents take longer to clear from the peritoneal cavity than smaller ones.[16] Animal studies[17] and intraperitoneal chemotherapy trials in patients with advanced intra-abdominal malignant diseases[18,19] have demonstrated that large volumes of the drug-containing solution are necessary to ensure exposure of the entire peritoneal surface and to overcome much of the resistance to free fluid flow in the abdominal cavity. After intraperitoneal drug delivery, the depth of penetration seems to be extremely limited – ranging from a few cell layers to a few millimetres.[20–22] The tumours to be treated should therefore have small bulk. The major mechanism of extraction of compounds placed into the peritoneal cavity is by way of the portal circulation.[23] Drugs that are metabolized into non-toxic forms during passage through the liver will exhibit a pronounced pharmacokinetic advantage after intraperitoneal installation, and a major portion of the drug will enter the systemic circulation in a non-toxic form. Experimental data suggest that delivery of 5-fluorouracil (5-FU) to the liver after intraperitoneal administration equals the amount of drug entering the liver during intrahepatic artery infusion.[24]

TOLERANCE

Intraperitoneal chemotherapy has been compared with systemic chemotherapy with regard to the frequency of toxic reactions.[25] No difference in the incidence of toxicity was noted between the group of 36 patients who received intraperitoneal 5-FU and the 30 who received intravenous 5-FU with the same schedule. The toxicity of intraperitoneal therapy was limited to local complications such as abdominal pain (mostly due to the volume of fluid instilled). Chemical peritonitis was rare, and when it did occur this was only after prolonged administration of the drug. Effusion of the drug into the subcutaneous tissue has been reported anecdotally.[26,27] While intraperitoneal chemotherapy appears to be more beneficial in the immediate postoperative period (no adhesions, minimal residual disease, hepatic micrometastases), its safety with regard to healing of colonic anastomosis had to be tested. In animal studies, some have found no difference for anastomotic spontaneous rupture or healing strength between rats receiving intraperitoneal chemotherapy starting at day 1, 3, or 7 and controls,[28] while others have found reduced early-postoperative collagen synthesis.[29] Preliminary results of a prospective randomized trial in humans confirmed that early intraperitoneal chemotherapy after surgical resection of high-risk colon cancers was well tolerated and not detrimental to the healing of anastomosis.[30] Two hundred and sixty-seven patients with stage B2 or C colon cancer were randomized to surgery alone (134 patients) or surgery plus 5-FU 600 mg/m^2/24 h intraperitoneally in 1.5 litres of dialysis fluid during 6 days (133 patients). Tolerance was good in 99 patients of the intraperitoneal chemotherapy group. Tolerance was not considered as good in the remaining 34 patients, including 16 with abdominal discomfort and 5 with fever. Hematological and hepatic tolerance was good for the two groups. Overall morbidity was similar in the two groups.

ONCOLOGIC RESULTS

The results of intraperitoneal adjuvant therapy in animal models were promising. In a colon cancer model in rats induced by subcutaneous administration of azoxymethane, 83 rats had isolated colon cancer. Forty-one of those rats with no extra-intestinal involvement were randomized after total colectomy to receive no further treatment or intraperitoneal 5-FU 5 mg/kg/day during 5 consecutive days, beginning 2 weeks after surgery. At the end of the study, 30 rats were evaluable. In the control group, 5 of 18 animals (28%) had peritoneal carcinomatosis and 4 of 18 (22%) had liver metastases. In the treated group, none of the 12 animals had either peritoneal carcinomatosis or liver metastases. Survival analysis was not possible in this model, since rats died because of the metabolic consequences of the total colectomy.[31]

Phase I studies in humans using intraperitoneal 5-FU demonstrated that high levels of the drug uniformly distributed within the peritoneal cavity were obtained providing that the treatment was administered in a large volume of fluid (over 1500 ml). A major fraction of intraperitoneal 5-FU exited from the peritoneal cavity through the portal venous system, and up to 90% was extracted from the blood as it passed from the portal vein into the hepatic venous system.[24] Technical considerations concerning the use of intraperitoneal catheters and drug delivery were also determined.[32]

In 1985, Sugarbaker et al[25] reported the first results of a prospective randomized trial in humans. Sixty-six eligible patients with primary colon or rectal cancer and positive lymph nodes or other poor prognostic signs were randomized into surgery plus intravenous 5-FU (30 patients) or surgery plus intraperitoneal 5-FU (36 patients). Intravenous 5-FU was given as bolus for 5 consecutive days, starting within 2 months of the large-bowel resection, 1 week out of every month for a year. Intraperitoneal 5-FU was administered in 2 litres of solution via a Tenckhoff catheter, using the same schedule as for intravenous 5-FU. Doses of 5-FU were increased each cycle until toxic side-effects occurred. No differences in disease-free survival or overall survival were observed. The median survival was 46.3 months in the intravenous group and 47.5 months in the intraperitoneal group. The percentages of patients who recurred in both arms were virtually identical (37% for intravenous treatment and 36% for intraperitoneal treatment), but the number of patients who recurred with histologically proven peritoneal carcinomatosis was significantly lower in the intraperitoneal 5-FU arm (2 of 10 versus 10 of 11 for the intravenous arm, $p = 0.003$).

In a multicentre trial conducted in Sweden from 1990–1992,[33] 50 patients were randomized to receive adjuvant intraperitoneal 5-FU (500 mg/m^2/day in a small volume of fluid) and intravenous leucovorin (folinic acid: 60 mg/m^2/day) and 51 to receive placebo after curative resection of colorectal cancer. Treatment started on the day after surgery, and continued for 6 days. Surgical complications were similar in both groups, and one anastomotic dehiscence occurred in each arm. Hospital stay was identical, but the time between surgery and the first bowel motion was significantly lower in the placebo arm (4.7 days versus 5.6 days, $p < 0.05$). Toxicity was not significantly different in the two groups; 13% of patients requested termination of treatment, mostly because of abdominal pain. The trial was terminated without survival study after the publication of Moertel's results of adjuvant therapy with 5-FU/levamisole, and a new trial comparing 5-FU/leucovorin versus 5-FU/levamisole with or without leucovorin was started.

In 1998, Scheithauer et al[34] entered 241 patients with resected stage III or high-risk stage II colon cancer into a trial comparing 6 months' intravenous 5-FU and levamisole with 5-FU plus leucovorin given intravenously (days 1–4) and intraperitoneally (days 1–3) every 4 weeks for a total of six courses. After a median follow-up of 4 years, no significant differences were noted between the two treatment regimens in patients with stage II disease. In patients with stage III, a significant improvement in disease-free survival and overall survival was noted in the group receiving systemic plus intraperitoneal treatment, with an estimated 43% reduction in mortality rate. Locoregional recurrences were also markedly reduced in the group treated with systemic and intraperitoneal chemotherapy.

From 1986 to 1991, a multicentre randomized trial was conducted in France to evaluate the results of adjuvant intraperitoneal 5-FU administered during 6 days shortly after curative resection of stage II and II colon cancer.[35] After resection, 267 patients were randomized into two groups. The 133 patients in group 1 underwent resection followed by intraperitoneal administration of 5-FU (0.6 g/m^2/day) for 6 days (days 4–10) and also received 5-FU 1 g intravenously during surgery. The 134 patients in group 2 underwent resection alone. Both groups were comparable. In group 1, 103 patients received the total dose, 18 received a partial dose, and 12 did not receive the chemotherapy. Postoperative abdominal and extra-abdominal complications were similar in both groups; tolerance to treatment was excellent or fair in

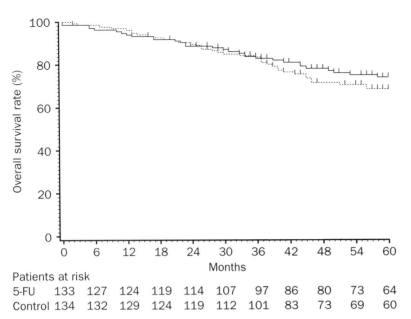

Figure 16.1 Overall survival curves: _____, group 1 intraperitoneal 5-FU; ...., group 2, control. Reprinted from Vaillant J-C, Nordlinger B, Deaffic S et al, Adjuvant intraperitoneal 5-fluorouracil in high-risk colon cancer. A multicenter phase III trial. *Ann Surg* 2000; **231**: 449–56.

Patients at risk	0	6	12	18	24	30	36	42	48	54	60
5-FU	133	127	124	119	114	107	97	86	80	73	64
Control	134	132	129	124	119	112	101	83	73	69	60

97% of patients and poor in 3%. After a median follow-up of 58 months, the 5-year overall survival rates were 74% in group 1 and 69% in group 2 (Figure 16.1); the disease-free survival rates were 68% and 62% respectively. Among patients receiving the full treatment, the 5-year disease-free survival rate was improved in the treatment group in patients with stage II disease (Figure 16.2) but not in those with stage III disease. In this study, chemotherapy with intraperitoneal 5-FU administered during 6 days postoperatively was well tolerated – but was not sufficient to reduce the risk of death significantly. However, the risk of recurrence was reduced for stage II colon cancers.

Overall, the few controlled studies so far available have shown some efficacy of immediate postoperative intraperitoneal chemotherapy alone in node-negative colon cancer and in combination with systemic chemotherapy in stage II colon cancer.

A large-scale trial aiming to test the combination of locoregional and systemic chemotherapy is currently being conducted by the European Organization for Research and Treatment of Cancer. Two thousand patients with stage II or III colon cancer have been randomized postoperatively in order to compare 6 months' intravenous therapy with 5-FU plus either levamisole or leucovorin, with or without immediate postoperative locoregional chemotherapy with 5-FU administered via the portal vein or the peritoneum during 6 days. Preliminary results are due in 2002. Six days' intraperitoneal chemotherapy may prove to be as effective as prolonged intravenous chemotherapy or to add beneficial effects to standard postoperative chemotherapy with 5-FU and levamisole or leucovorin.

SUMMARY AND CONCLUSIONS

The results available concerning intraperitoneal chemotherapy as adjuvant treatment for colorectal cancer in humans represent far too short a period and are too preliminary to allow any definite conclusion to be drawn regarding this mode of treatment. However, these results, added to those of several limited clinical trials using this therapy for other intra-abdominal malignant diseases, suggest some clinical benefit.[36–38] The use of 5-FU in the early postoperative period appears to be well tolerated without detrimental effects on healing of anastomosis. At the present time, there are not enough data to provide a clear-cut consensus on the real benefits of this route of administration. New trials are currently in progress to test new modalities with different drugs or different associations, using both locoregional and systemic treatments, and these may prove to be more effective than systemic chemotherapy alone in the adjuvant treatment of colorectal cancer.

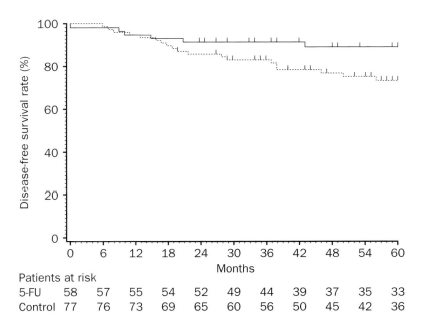

Figure 16.2 Disease-free survival curves of patients with stage II colon cancer: _____, group 1, intraperitoneal 5-FU; ...., group 2 control. Reprinted from Vaillant J-C, Nordlinger B, Deaffic S et al, Adjuvant intraperitoneal 5-fluorouracil in high-risk colon cancer. A multicenter phase III trial. *Ann Surg* 2000; **231**: 449–56.

Patients at risk										
5-FU	58	57	55	54	52	49	44	39	37	35	33
Control	77	76	73	69	65	60	56	50	45	42	36

REFERENCES

1. Gastrointestinal Tumor Study Group, Prolongation of the disease-free interval in surgically treated rectal carcinoma. *N Engl J Med* 1985; **312**: 1465–72.

2. Eisenberg B, DeCosse JJ, Harford F et al, Carcinoma of the colon and rectum: the natural history reviewed in 1,704 patients. *Cancer* 1982; **49**: 1131–4.

3. Floyd CE, Stirling CT, Cohn I Jr, Cancer of the colon, rectum and anus. Review of 1687 cases. *Ann Surg* 1966; **163**: 829–37.

4. Gastrointestinal Tumor Study Group, Adjuvant therapy of colon cancer – results of a prospectively randomized trial. *N Engl J Med* 1984; **310**: 737–43.

5. Sugarbaker PH, Cunliffe WJ, Belliveau J et al, Rationale for integrating early postoperative intraperitoneal chemotherapy into the surgical treatment of gastrointestinal cancer. *Semin Oncol* 1989; **16**(Suppl 6): 83–97.

6. Salmon SE, Kinetics of minimal residual disease. *Rec Results Cancer Res* 1979; **67**: 5–15.

7. Norton L, Simon R, Tumor size, sensitivity to therapy, and design of treatment schedules. *Cancer Treat Rep* 1977; **61**: 1307–17.

8. Minsky BD, Mies C, Rich TA et al, Potentially curative surgery of colon cancer: patterns of failure and survival. *J Clin Oncol* 1988; **6**: 106–18.

9. Gilbert JM, Jeffrey I, Evans M, Kark AE, Sites of recurrent tumour after 'curative' colorectal surgery: implications for adjuvant therapy. *Br J Surg* 1984; **71**: 203–5.

10. Eggermont AM, Steller EP, Marquet RL et al, Local promotion of tumor growth after abdominal surgery is dominant over immunotherapy with interleukin-2 and lymphokine activated killer cells. *Cancer Detect Prev* 1988; **12**: 421–9.

11. Sugarbaker PH, Graves T, DeBruijn EA et al, Rationale for early postoperative intraperitoneal chemotherapy (EPIC) in patients with advanced gastrointestinal cancer. *Cancer Res* 1990; **50**: 5790–4.

12. Taylor I, Brooman P, Rowling JT, Adjuvant liver perfusion in colorectal cancer: initial results of a clinical trial. *BMJ* 1977; **ii**: 1320–2.

13. Cedarmark BJ, Schultz SS, Bakshi S et al, Value of liver scan in the follow-up of patients with adenocarcinoma of the colon and rectum. *Surg Gynecol Obstet* 1977; **144**: 745–8.

14. Fisher ER, Turnbull RB, The cytological demonstration and significance of tumor cells in the mesenteric venous blood in patients with colorectal cancer. *Surg Gynecol Obstet* 1955; **100**: 102–6.

15. Taylor I, Rowling J, West C, Adjuvant cytotoxic liver perfusion for colorectal cancer. *Br J Surg* 1979; **66**: 833–7.

16. Dedrick RL, Meyers CE, Bungay PM et al, Pharmaco-kinetic rationale for peritoneal drug administration in the treatment of ovarian cancer. *Cancer Treat Rep* 1978; **62**: 1–11.

17. Rosenshein N, Blake D, McIntyre PA et al, The effect of volume on the distribution of substances instilled into peritoneal cavity. *Gynecol Oncol* 1978; **6**: 106–10.

18. Howell SB, Pfeifle CE, Wung WE et al, Intraperitoneal cisplatin with systemic thiosulfate protection. *Ann Intern Med* 1982; **97**: 845–51.

19. Dunnick NR, Jones RB, Doppmen JL et al, Intraperitoneal contrast infusion for assessment of intraperitoneal fluid dynamics. *AJR* 1979; **133**: 221–3.

20. Durand RE, Flow cytometry studies of intracellular adriamycin in multicell spheroids in vitro. *Cancer Res* 1981; **41**: 3495–8.

21. Ozols RF, Locker GY, Doroshow JH et al, Pharmacokinetics of Adriamycin and tissue penetration in murine ovarian cancer. *Cancer Res* 1979; **39**: 3209–14.

22. McVie JG, Dikhoff T, Van der Heide J et al, Tissue concentration of platinum after intraperitoneal cisplatin administration in patients. *Proc Am Assoc Cancer Res* 1985; **26**: 162.

23. Lukas G, Brindle S, Greengard P, The route of absorption of intraperitoneally administered compounds. *J Pharmacol Exp Ther* 1971; **178**: 562–6.

24. Speyer JL, Sugarbaker PH, Collins JM et al, Portal levels and

hepatic clearance of 5-fluorouracil after intraperitoneal administration in humans. *Cancer Res* 1981; **41:** 1916–22.

25. Sugarbaker PH, Gianola FJ, Speyer JL et al, Prospective randomized trial of intravenous versus intraperitoneal 5-fluorouracil in patients with advanced primary colon or rectal cancer. *Surgery* 1985; **98:** 414–21.

26. Gianola FJ, Sugarbaker PH, Barofsky I et al, Toxicity studies of adjuvant intravenous versus intraperitoneal 5-FU in patients with advanced primary colon or rectal cancer. *Am J Clin Oncol* 1986; **9:** 1–7.

27. Ozols RF, Young RC, Speyer JL et al, Phase I and pharmacologic studies of adriamycin administered intraperitoneally to patients with ovarian cancer. *Cancer Res* 1982; **42:** 4265–9.

28. Hillan K, Nordlinger B, Ballet F et al, The healing of colonic anastomoses after early intraperitoneal chemotherapy: an experimental study in rats. *J Surg Res* 1988; **44:** 166–71.

29. Martens MF, Hendriks T, Wobbes T, De Pont JJ, Intraperitoneal cytostatics impair early post-operative collagen synthesis in experimental intestinal anastomoses. *Br J Cancer* 1992; **65:** 649–54.

30. Nordlinger B, Bouteloup PY, Favre JP et al, Early postoperative intraperitoneal chemotherapy is feasible and well tolerated in colorectal cancer. A prospective randomized study. *J Cancer Res Clin Oncol* 1990; **116:** 686.

31. Nordlinger B, Puts JP, Hervé JP et al, An experimental model of colon cancer: recurrence after surgery alone or associated with intraperitoneal 5-fluorouracil chemotherapy. *Dis Colon Rectum* 1991; **34:** 658–63.

32. Jenkins J, Sugarbaker PH, Gianola FJ et al, Technical considerations in the use of intraperitoneal chemotherapy administered by Tenckhoff catheter. *Surgery* 1982; **154:** 858–64.

33. Graf W, Westlin J-E, Pahlman L, Glimelius B, Adjuvant intraperitoneal 5-fluorouracil and intravenous leucovorin after colorectal cancer surgery: a randomized phase II placebo-controlled study. *Int J Colorect Dis* 1994; **9:** 35–9.

34. Scheithauer W, Kornek GV, Marczell A et al, Combined intravenous and intraperitoneal chemotherapy with fluorouracil + leucovorin vs fluorouracil + levamisole for adjuvant therapy of resected colon carcinoma. *Br J Cancer* 1998; **77:** 1349–54.

35. Vaillant J-C, Nordlinger B, Deuffic S et al, Adjuvant intraperitoneal 5-fluorouracil in high-risk colon cancer. A multicenter phase III trial. *Ann Surg* 2000; **231:** 449–56.

36. Markman M, Howell SB, Lucas WE et al, Combination intraperitoneal chemotherapy with cisplatin, cytarabine, and doxorubicin for refractory ovarian carcinoma and other malignancies principally confined to the peritoneal cavity. *J Clin Oncol* 1984; **2:** 1321–6.

37. Miller DL, Udelsman R, Sugarbaker PH, Calcification of pseudomyxoma peritonei following intraperitoneal chemotherapy: CT demonstration. *J Comput Assist Tomogr* 1985; **9:** 1123–4.

38. Markman M, Cleary S, Lucas WE et al, Intraperitoneal chemotherapy employing a regimen of cisplatin, cytarabine and bleomycin. *Cancer Treat Rep* 1986; **70:** 755–60.

17

Management of peritoneal surface malignancy from colorectal cancer: The surgeon's role

Paul H Sugarbaker

INTRODUCTION

Oncology as a surgical subspecialty evolved in the midst of a technological revolution in patient care. This discipline expanded from the resection of primary cancer to include the surgical management of metastatic disease. The earliest success with this new concept was with complete resection of locally recurrent colon and rectal cancer.[1,2] Then the resection of liver metastases from the same disease was shown to be of benefit in a selected group of patients.[3] Extension of the concept of complete surgical eradication of metastatic disease to bring about long-term survival to patients with peritoneal surface malignancy has been pioneered by our group.[4,5] Appendix cancer is the paradigm for successful treatment of peritoneal carcinomatosis[6] (see also Chapter 31). The present chapter presents the background, the standardized treatments currently in use, and the selection factors leading to long-term survival with acceptable morbidity and mortality. It is our opinion that prevention and treatment of peritoneal surface dissemination of colon cancer is a surgical responsibility that produces great benefits at acceptable risk and cost.

PRINCIPLES OF MANAGEMENT

The successful treatment of peritoneal surface malignancy requires a combined approach that utilizes peritonectomy procedures and perioperative intraperitoneal chemotherapy. To properly balance the risks and benefits, knowledgeable patient selection is mandatory. Both visceral and parietal peritonectomies are necessary for complete cytoreduction, which is essential for treatment to result in long-term survival. Up to six peritonectomy procedures may be required.[7-9] Their utilization depends on the distribution and extent of invasion of the malignancy disseminated within the peritoneal space. When to pursue cytoreduction and when to accept debulking as the proper treatment may present a difficult surgical judgement.

Rationale for peritonectomy procedures

Peritonectomy procedures are necessary if one is to successfully treat peritoneal surface malignancies with curative intent. Peritonectomy procedures are used in the areas of visible cancer progression in an attempt to leave the patient with only microscopic residual disease. Small tumor nodules are removed using electroevaporation. Involvement of visceral peritoneum frequently requires resection of a portion of the stomach, small intestine, or colorectum.

INTRAPERITONEAL CHEMOTHERAPY

Conceptual changes with intraperitoneal chemotherapy

Modifications of the use of chemotherapy in patients with peritoneal carcinomatosis have occurred and shown favorable results of treatment. A change in *route* of drug administration has occurred. Chemotherapy is given intraperitoneally, or by combined intraperitoneal and intravenous routes. In this new strategy, intravenous chemotherapy alone is rarely indicated. Also, a change in *timing* has occurred in that chemotherapy is used perioperatively. It begins in the operating room and may be continued for the first five postoperative days. Third, a change in *selection* criteria for treatment of abdominal and pelvic malignancy has occurred. With the non-aggressive peritoneal surface mucinous tumors as an exception, the lesion size of peritoneal implants is of great importance. Only patients with small intraperitoneal tumor nodules that have a limited distribution within the abdomen and pelvis are likely to show prolonged benefit. Complete cytoreductive surgery is necessary prior to the intraperitoneal chemotherapy instillation, and this is unlikely for advanced carcinomatosis. Aggressive treatment strategies for an advanced and invasive intraperitoneal malignancy will not produce long-term benefits, and often lead to excessive morbidity or mortality. Treatments to prevent the occurrence or eradicate established seeding must be initiated as early as is possible in the natural history of these diseases in order to achieve the greatest benefits. In most instances, the cytoreduction and intraperitoneal chemotherapy should be considered with the management of the primary cancer.

Peritoneal space to plasma barrier

Intraperitoneal chemotherapy gives high response rates within the abdomen because the 'peritoneal space to plasma barrier' provides dose-intensive therapy.[10] Figure 17.1 shows that high-molecular-weight substances, such as mitomycin C, are confined to the abdominal cavity for long time periods.[11] This means that the exposure of peritoneal surfaces to pharmacologically active molecules can be increased considerably by giving the drugs via the intraperitoneal route rather than the intravenous route.

For the chemotherapy agents used to treat peritoneal carcinomatosis, the area under the curve (AUC) ratios of intraperitoneal to intravenous exposure are favorable. Table 17.1 presents the AUC ratios (intraperitoneal/intravenous) for the drugs in routine clinical use in patients with peritoneal seeding. In our studies, these include 5-fluorouracil (5-FU), mitomycin C, doxorubicin, cisplatin, paclitaxel, and gemcitabine.

One should not assume that the intraperitoneal administration of chemotherapeutic agents eliminates their systemic toxicities. Although the drugs are sequestered within the peritoneal space, they are eventually cleared into the systemic circulation. For this reason, the safe doses of most drugs instilled into the peritoneal cavity are identical to the safe intravenous doses. The exceptions are drugs with hepatic metabolism, such as 5-FU and gemcitabine. An increased dose of approximately 50% is usually possible with 5-FU. The dose for a 5-day course of intravenous 5-FU is approximately 500 mg/m²; for intraperitoneal 5-FU, the dose is 750 mg/m² per day. This considerable (50%) increase in the dose of 5-FU

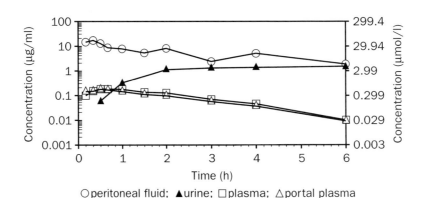

Figure 17.1 High-molecular-weight compounds when instilled into the peritoneal cavity are sequestered at that site for long time periods. The physiologic barrier to the release of intraperitoneal drugs is called the 'peritoneal plasma barrier'. In this experiment, 15 mg of mitomycin C was infused into the cavity as rapidly as possible. Intraperitoneal, intravenous, portal venous, and urine mitomycin C concentrations were determined by HPLC assay. From Sugarbaker PH, Graves T, DeBruijn EA et al, Rationale for early postoperative intraperitoneal chemotherapy (EPIC) in patients with advanced gastrointestinal cancer. *Cancer Res* 1990; **50:** 5790–4 (with permission).

Table 17.1 Area under the curve (AUC) ratios of peritoneal surface exposure to systemic exposure for drugs used to treat intra-abdominal cancer

Drug	Molecular weight (Da)	AUC ratio
5-Fluorouracil	130	250
Mitomycin C	334	75
Doxorubicin	544	500
Cisplatin	300	20
Paclitaxel	808	1000
Gemcitabine	263	50

is of great advantage in treating peritoneal carcinomatosis.

Tumor cell entrapment

The 'tumor cell entrapment' hypothesis explains the rapid progression of peritoneal surface malignancy in patients who undergo treatment using surgery alone. This theory relates the high incidence and rapid progression of peritoneal surface implantation to:

- free intraperitoneal tumor emboli as a result of serosal penetration by cancer;
- leakage of malignant cells from transected lymphatics;
- dissemination of malignant cells directly from the cancer specimen as a result of surgical trauma and backflow of venous blood;
- fibrin entrapment of intra-abdominal tumor emboli on traumatized peritoneal surfaces;
- progression of entrapped tumor cells through growth factors involved in the wound healing process.

These phenomena may cause a high incidence of surgical treatment failure in patients treated for primary gastrointestinal cancer.[11] Also, the reimplantation of malignant cells into peritonectomized surfaces in a reoperative setting must be expected unless intraperitoneal chemotherapy is used.

Chemotherapy employed in the perioperative period not only destroys tumor cells, but also eliminates viable platelets and leukocytes from the peritoneal cavity. This diminishes the promotion of tumor growth associated with the wound healing process. Consequently, the results from use of intraperitoneal chemotherapy show a reduction in local recurrence and peritoneal surface recurrence in

patients with intra-abdominal cancer. Removal of the leukocytes also decreases the ability of the abdomen to resist an infectious process. For this reason, strict aseptic technique is imperative when administering the chemotherapy or handling abdominal tubes and drains.

In order to interrupt this widespread implantation of tumor cells on abdominal and pelvic surfaces, the abdominal cavity is flooded with chemotherapy in a large volume of fluid during the operation (heated intraoperative intraperitoneal chemotherapy with manual distribution) and in the postoperative period (early postoperative intraperitoneal chemotherapy with gravity distribution).

Prior limited benefits with intraperitoneal chemotherapy

The use of intraperitoneal chemotherapy in the past has met with limited success and acceptance by oncologists. There have been three major impediments to greater success:

- limited penetration of drugs into tumor nodules;
- non-uniform drug distribution;
- improper patient selection.

Intracavitary instillation allows very limited penetration of drugs into tumor nodules. Only the outermost layer (approximately 1 mm) of a cancer nodule is penetrated by the chemotherapy. This means that only minute tumor nodules can be definitively treated. In most trials, oncologists have attempted to treat patients with established disease – a group of patients that has caused disappointment in results with intraperitoneal drug use. Microscopic residual disease is the ideal target for intraperitoneal chemotherapy protocols.

A second cause of limited success with intraperitoneal chemotherapy is non-uniform drug distribution. A majority of patients treated by drug instillation into the abdomen or pelvis have had prior surgery, which invariably causes scarring between peritoneal surfaces. The adhesions create multiple barriers to the free access of fluid. Although the instillation of a large volume of fluid will partially overcome the problems created by adhesions, some surface areas will have no access to chemotherapy. Limited access from adhesions is impossible to predict and may increase with repeated installations of chemotherapy.

Non-uniform drug distribution after surgery may result from fibrin entrapment. Surgery causes fibrin deposits on surfaces that have been traumatized by the cancer resection. Free intraperitoneal cancer cells become trapped within the fibrin. The fibrin is infiltrated by platelets, neutrophils, and monocytes as part of the wound healing process. As collagen is laid down, the tumor cells are entrapped within scar tissue. The scar tissue is dense and poorly penetrated by intraperitoneal chemotherapy.

Non-uniform drug distribution may be caused by gravity. Intraperitoneal fluid does not uniformly distribute itself to anterior and posterior peritoneal surfaces. Gravity pulls the fluid to dependent portions of the abdomen; especially the pelvis, paracolic gutters, and the right retrohepatic space. Unless the patient actively pursues frequent changes in position, the surfaces between bowel loops and the anterior abdominal wall will remain relatively untreated.

PATIENT SELECTION FOR TREATMENT

The greatest impediment to lasting benefits from intraperitoneal chemotherapy should be attributed to improper patient selection. A great number of patients with advanced intra-abdominal disease have been treated with minimal benefit. Even with extensive cytoreductive surgery and aggressive intraperitoneal chemotherapy, the patient with extensive disease is not likely to have a lasting benefit. Rapid recurrence of intraperitoneal cancer combined with progression of lymph-node or systemic disease are likely to interfere with long-term survival in these patients. Patients who benefit must have minimal residual disease isolated to peritoneal surfaces that have access to chemotherapy so that complete eradication of disease can occur. In the natural history of this disease, the time of the initiation of treatment has great bearing on the benefits achieved. Asymptomatic patients with small-volume peritoneal surface malignancy must be selected for intraperitoneal chemotherapy protocols.

Clinical assessments of peritoneal surface malignancy

In the past, peritoneal carcinomatosis from colon cancer was considered to be a fatal disease process. The only assessment used was either carcinomatosis present, with a presumed fatal outcome, or carcinomatosis absent, with curative treatment options available. Currently, there are four important clinical assessments of peritoneal surface malignancy that need to be used to select patients who will benefit from treatment protocols. These are (1) histopathology to assess the invasive character of the malignancy; (2) preoperative computed tomography (CT) scan of chest, abdomen, and pelvis; (3) the Peritoneal Cancer Index; (4) the completeness-of-cytoreduction score.

Histopathology to assess invasive character

The biological aggressiveness of a peritoneal surface malignancy will have a profound influence on its treatment options. Non-invasive tumors may have extensive spread on peritoneal surfaces and yet be completely resectable by peritonectomy procedures. Also, these non-invasive malignancies are extremely unlikely to metastasize by lymphatics to lymph nodes or by the blood to the liver and other systemic sites. Therefore, protocols for cytoreductive surgery and intraperitoneal chemotherapy may have a curative intent in patients with a large mass of widely disseminated pseudomyxoma peritonei.[12] Pathology review and an assessment of the invasive or non-aggressive nature of a colonic malignancy is essential to treatment planning.

Preoperative CT scan

The preoperative CT scan of chest, abdomen, and pelvis may be of great value in planning treatments for peritoneal surface malignancy. Systemic metastases can be clinically excluded and pleural surface spread ruled out. Unfortunately, the CT scan should be regarded as an inaccurate test by which to quantitate intestinal type of peritoneal carcinomatosis from adenocarcinoma. The malignant tissue progresses on the peritoneal surfaces, and its shape conforms to the normal contours of the abdominopelvic structures.

This is quite different from the metastatic process in the liver or lung, which progresses as three-dimensional tumor nodules and can be accurately assessed by CT.[13]

However, the CT scan has been of great help in locating and quantitating *mucinous* adenocarcinoma within the peritoneal cavity.[14] These tumors produce copious colloid material that is readily distinguished by shape and by density from normal structures. Using two distinctive radiologic criteria, those patients with resectable mucinous peritoneal carcinomatosis can be selected from those with non-resectable malignancy. This keeps patients who are unlikely to benefit from reoperative surgery from undergoing cytoreductive surgical procedures. The two radiologic criteria found to be most useful are (1) segmental obstruction of small bowel, and (2) the presence of tumor nodules greater than 5 cm in diameter on small bowel surfaces or directly adjacent to small bowel mesentery. These criteria reflect radiologically the biology of the mucinous adenocarcinoma. Obstructed segments of bowel signal an invasive character of malignancy on small-bowel surfaces that would be unlikely to be completely cytoreduced. Mucinous cancer on small bowel or small-bowel mesentery indicates that the mucinous cancer is no longer redistributed. This means that small-bowel surfaces or small-bowel mesentery will

have residual disease after cytoreduction, because these surfaces are impossible to peritonectomize.

Peritoneal Cancer Index

The third assessment of peritoneal surface malignancy is the Peritoneal Cancer Index. This is a quantitative prognostic indicator that integrates both size and distribution of peritoneal implants (Figure 17.2). It should be used in the decision-making process as the abdomen is explored. To arrive at a score, the size of intraperitoneal nodules must be assessed. The lesion size (LS) score should be used. An LS-0 score means that no malignant deposits are visualized. An LS-1 score signifies that tumor nodules less than 0.5 cm are present. The number of nodules is not scored, only the size of the largest nodules. LS-2 signifies that tumor nodules between 0.5 and 5.0 cm are present. LS-3 signifies that tumor nodules greater than 5.0 cm in any dimension are present. If there is a confluence of tumor, the lesion size is scored as 3.

In order to assess the distribution of peritoneal surface disease, the abdominopelvic regions are utilized. For each of these 13 regions, a lesion size score is determined. The summation of the lesion size score in each of the 13 abdominopelvic regions is the

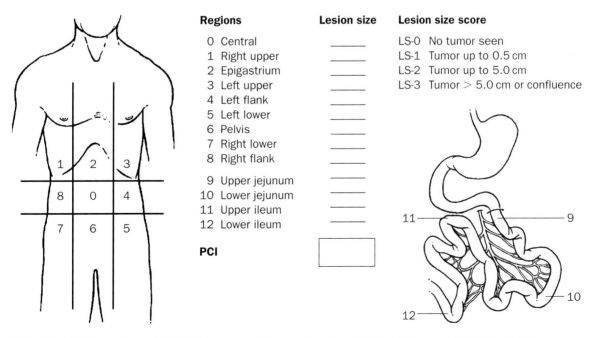

Regions	Lesion size	Lesion size score
0 Central	_____	LS-0 No tumor seen
1 Right upper	_____	LS-1 Tumor up to 0.5 cm
2 Epigastrium	_____	LS-2 Tumor up to 5.0 cm
3 Left upper	_____	LS-3 Tumor > 5.0 cm or confluence
4 Left flank	_____	
5 Left lower	_____	
6 Pelvis	_____	
7 Right lower	_____	
8 Right flank	_____	
9 Upper jejunum	_____	
10 Lower jejunum	_____	
11 Upper ileum	_____	
12 Lower ileum	_____	
PCI		

Figure 17.2 Peritoneal Cancer Index (PCI) is a composite score of lesion size 0–3 in abdominopelvic regions 0–12.

Peritoneal Cancer Index for that patient. The maximum score is 39 (13×3).

The Peritoneal Cancer Index has been validated to date in three separate situations. Gomez and co-workers[15] showed that it could be used to predict long-term survival in patients with peritoneal carcinomatosis from colon cancer having a second cytoreduction. Berthet and co-workers[16] showed that it predicted benefits for treatment of peritoneal sarcomatosis from recurrent visceral or parietal sarcoma. In both clinical studies, the patients with a favorable prognosis had a score of less than 12. Sugarbaker[17] reported a survival of 50% in colon cancer patients with carcinomatosis and a Peritoneal Cancer Index of 10 or less.

There are some caveats regarding the use of the Peritoneal Cancer Index. First, non-invasive malignancy on peritoneal surfaces may be completely cytoreduced. Diseases such as pseudomyxoma peritonei are in this category. With these 'benign tumors', the status of the abdomen and pelvis after cytoreduction may bear no relationship to their status at the time of abdominal exploration. In other words, even though surgeons may find an abdomen with a Peritoneal Cancer Index of 39, it can be converted to an index of 0 by cytoreduction. In these diseases, the prognosis will only be related to the condition of the abdomen after cytoreduction (completeness-of-cytoreduction score, see below).

A second caveat regarding the Peritoneal Cancer Index concerns invasive cancer at crucial anatomic sites. For example, invasive cancer not cleanly resected on the common bile duct will cause a poor prognosis despite a low Peritoneal Cancer Index. Also, unresectable cancer at numerous sites on the small bowel may by itself confer a poor prognosis. Invasive cancer at crucial anatomic sites may function as 'systemic disease equivalent' in assessing prognosis with invasive cancer. Since long-term survival can only occur in patients with complete cytoreduction, residual disease at anatomically crucial sites may negate a favorable score with the Peritoneal Cancer Index.

Completeness-of-cytoreduction score

Another assessment to be used to assess prognosis with peritoneal surface malignancy is the completeness-of-cytoreduction (CC) score. This information is of less value to the surgeon in planning treatments than the Peritoneal Cancer Index. The CC score is not available until after the cytoreduction is complete, rather than as the abdomen is being explored. If it

becomes obvious during exploration that cytoreduction will be incomplete, the surgeon may decide that a palliative debulking that will provide symptomatic relief is appropriate and discontinue plans for an aggressive cytoreduction with intraperitoneal chemotherapy. In both non-invasive and invasive peritoneal surface malignancy, the completeness of cytoreduction score is a major prognostic indicator. It has been shown to function with accuracy in pseudomyxoma peritonei, colon cancer with peritoneal carcinomatosis, and sarcomatosis.[15–18]

The size of peritoneal implants used to determine the CC score may vary with the primary site of the peritoneal carcinomatosis. More chemotherapy-responsive malignancies, such as ovarian cancer, may be eradicated even though larger tumor nodules remain after cytoreduction. For gastrointestinal cancer, the CC score has been defined as follows. A CC-0 score indicates that no peritoneal seeding was exposed during the complete exploration. CC-1 indicates that tumor nodules persisting after cytoreduction are less than 2.5 mm. This is a nodule size thought to be penetrable by intracavity chemotherapy, and would therefore be designated a complete cytoreduction. CC-2 indicates that tumor nodules between 2.5 mm and 2.5 cm are present. CC-3 indicates that tumor nodules larger than 2.5 cm are present or that there is a confluence of unresectable tumor nodules at any site within the abdomen or pelvis. CC-2 and CC-3 cytoreductions are considered incomplete.

PATIENT SELECTION FOR PALLIATIVE SURGERY

Although some patients with peritoneal surface spread of invasive abdominal and pelvic cancer can be treated with a curative approach using cytoreductive surgery and intraperitoneal chemotherapy, others have known incurable recurrent malignancy. These patients will often have life-threatening complications prior to a terminal event. The cause of great suffering and eventual death is often intestinal obstruction and the complications that this condition may initiate: starvation, fistula formation, abscess, and intestinal perforation. The options available to the surgeon to help alleviate adverse symptoms are many. Selection of the treatment that offers the proper risks and benefits can be one of the most difficult of all surgical judgements. For example, some 10–30% of patients with progressive colorectal cancer who develop intestinal obstruction will have adhesions rather than cancer as the cause of obstruction.[19]

If the surgeon elects not to operate, months and even years of good-quality life may be lost. At the other extreme, patients with multiple sites of small-bowel obstruction from cancer may have a major exploratory surgery, develop multiple complications that result in an expensive and long hospitalization, and have little or no benefit. Are there guidelines for proper patient selection? Unfortunately, the clinical information that is available to the surgeon is often inaccurate or even misleading.[13] Precise treatment plans may not be possible in all patients. However, some knowledgeable selection of treatments may be possible.

Work-up in patients with intestinal obstruction and recurrence of colorectal cancer is directed at a determination of the extent of small-bowel involvement, the extent of metastatic disease to liver and systemic sites, and the patient's operative risk. Assessment of the extent of small-bowel involvement may be the most difficult of these three parameters without an exploratory surgical procedure. A major surgical intervention may be appropriate if nutritional independence can be restored. If there is insufficient small bowel available after the relief of obstruction to maintain adequate nutrition, then surgical interventions should be limited to insertion of tubes (gastrostomy or cervical esophagostomy) and ostomy construction. Major exploratory surgery should be avoided if at all possible. Table 17.2 provides the stop signals for surgical palliation of advanced primary or recurrent gastrointestinal cancer.

Attempts to palliate intestinal obstruction from recurrent gastrointestinal cancer by surgery are related to the pattern of dissemination of carcinomatosis.[20] Even with a large volume of cancer recurrence, most of the accumulation of cancer causing obstruction can be found at three specific anatomic sites. These are the gastric outlet, terminal ileum and ileocecal valve region, and the rectosigmoid colon. In patients with a good performance status, aggressive resection of localized disease may offer considerable benefit with acceptable risk. The operations often used are a greater omentectomy, abdominal colectomy, and pelvic peritonectomy with end-ileostomy. In some patients, the greater omentectomy will not restore adequate gastrointestinal drainage, so that a gastrojejunostomy is necessary in order to decompress the stomach. Table 17.3 shows the clinical data used to select patients for abdominal colectomy with end-ileostomy as an approach to intestinal obstruction with recurrent gastrointestinal cancer.

CURRENT METHODOLOGY FOR DELIVERY OF INTRAPERITONEAL CHEMOTHERAPY

Heated intraoperative intraperitoneal chemotherapy

In the operating room, heated intraoperative intraperitoneal chemotherapy is used with continuous manual distribution. Heat is part of the optimizing process, and is used to bring as much dose intensity to the abdominal and pelvic surfaces as is possible. Hyperthermia with intraperitoneal chemotherapy has several advantages. First, heat by itself has more toxicity for cancerous tissue than for normal tissue. This predominant effect on cancer increases as the vascularity of the malignancy decreases. Second, hyperthermia increases the penetration of chemotherapy into tissues. As tissues soften in response to heat, the elevated interstitial pressure of a tumor mass may decrease and allow improved drug penetration. Third, and probably most importantly, heat increases the cytotoxicity of selected chemotherapy agents. This synergism occurs only at the interface of heat and body tissue at the peritoneal surface.

After the cancer resection is complete, the

Table 17.2 Stop signals for surgical palliation (debulking) of advanced primary or recurrent gastrointestinal cancer

1. Poor operative risk so that the patient is unlikely to survive the operation
2. Liver metastasis or clinical evidence of distant disease
3. Inability to clear the primary tumor mass
4. Inability to reestablish gastrointestinal function because of extensive peritoneal seeding

Note: Stop signals 1 and 2 are established preoperatively. Stop signals 3 and 4 are determined after the abdomen has been explored.

Table 17.3 Clinical features that suggest selection of an aggressive versus a conservative surgical approach

	Aggressive resection indicated	Conservative approach favored
Histologic grade	Low	High
History of peritoneal seeding	Absent	Present
CT shows shortening mesentery	Unlikely	Likely
CT shows multiple sites of segmental obstruction	Unlikely	Likely
CT shows tumor nodules >5 cm associated with small bowel	Unlikely	Likely
Large localized cancer recurrence	Likely	Unlikely
Operative risk	Low	High
Short interval between operations	Unlikely	Likely
Mucinous ascites	Likely	Unlikely
Serous or bloody ascites	Unlikely	Likely

Tenckhoff catheter and closed suction drains are placed through the abdominal wall and made watertight with a pursestring suture at the skin. Temperature probes are secured to the skin edge. Using a long-running No. 2 monofilament suture, the skin edges are secured to the self-retaining retractor. A plastic sheet is incorporated into these sutures to create a covering for the abdominal cavity. A slit in the plastic cover is made to allow the surgeon's double-gloved hand access to the abdomen and pelvis (Figure 17.3). During the 90 minutes of perfusion, all the anatomic structures within the peritoneal cavity are uniformly exposed to heat and to chemotherapy. The surgeon gently but continuously manipulates all viscera to keep adherence of peritoneal surfaces to a minimum. Roller pumps force the chemotherapy solution into the abdomen through the Tenckhoff catheter and pull it out through the drains. A heat exchanger keeps the fluid being infused at 42–43°C so that the intraperitoneal fluid is maintained at 41–42°C. A smoke evacuator is used to pull air from beneath the plastic cover through activated charcoal, preventing contamination of air in the operating room by chemotherapy aerosols.

After the intraoperative perfusion is complete, the abdomen is suctioned dry of fluid. The abdomen is then reopened, retractors repositioned, and reconstructive surgery is performed. It should be re-emphasized that no suture lines are constructed until after the chemotherapy perfusion is complete. One exception to this rule is closure of the vaginal cuff to prevent intraperitoneal chemotherapy leakage. The

standardized orders for heated intraoperative intraperitoneal chemotherapy are provided in a practice manual.[21]

REOPERATIVE SURGERY PLUS ADDITIONAL INTRAPERITONEAL CHEMOTHERAPY

As the follow-up of patients with peritoneal surface malignancy progresses, the need for additional operative procedures and additional cycles of intraperitoneal chemotherapy may occur. This seems most evident, at this point in time, with the tumors that do not have a tumor marker by which to monitor for recurrent disease. Peritoneal carcinomatosis from colon cancer is now routinely managed with a second-look operation at 6–9 months.

At the second-look operation, the abdomen is opened widely and all of the peritoneal surfaces are visualized with a complete takedown of all adhesions. Additional cytoreduction is performed, and additional visceral resections may be required. If a CC-1 cytoreduction can again be achieved, then heated intraoperative intraperitoneal chemotherapy is used alone with early postoperative intraperitoneal 5-FU.

If it appears from the re-operation that the initial heated chemotherapy and early postoperative chemotherapy treatments were successful, then the same regimen will be employed again. If there is a 'chemotherapy failure' and recurrent disease is seen in areas that have been previously peritonectomized, then a chemotherapy change would be initiated.[21]

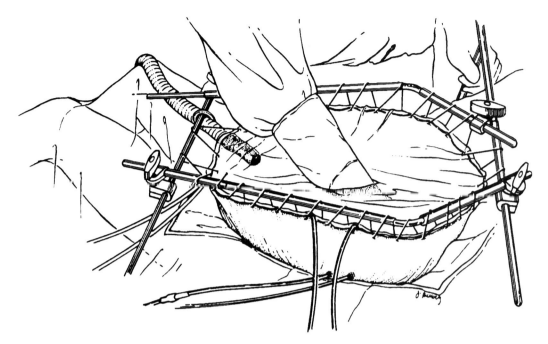

Figure 17.3 Coliseum technique for heated intraoperative intraperitoneal chemotherapy. Surgical manipulation of the abdominal contents after complete resection of cancer assures uniform distribution of heat and chemotherapy.

CLINICAL RESULTS OF TREATMENT

Colon cancer with peritoneal carcinomatosis

To date, approximately 100 patients have been treated who have peritoneal carcinomatosis from colon cancer.[17] The survival of all patients treated is shown in Figure 17.4. The Peritoneal Cancer Index provided a score valuable in selecting patients for treatment (Figure 17.5). In patients who had a complete cytoreduction, there was marked improvement in survival; patients with residual disease show the short survival expected with peritoneal carcinomatosis from colon cancer (Figure 17.6). These data suggest an early aggressive approach to peritoneal surface spread of adenocarcinoma of the colon in selected patients.

Recurrent and obstructing gastrointestinal cancer

Averbach and colleagues looked at their experience with a problematic group of patients. These are patients who developed intestinal obstruction after prior treatment for a gastrointestinal malignancy. With aggressive treatments using second-look surgery, peritonectomy procedures, and intraperitoneal chemotherapy, complete cytoreduction resulted in a 5-year survival in 60% of the patients, while incomplete resection resulted in no 5-year survivals. The patients with appendiceal malignancy had a greatly improved survival as compared with those with colon cancer or other diagnoses. A free interval of greater than 2 years between primary malignancy and the onset of obstruction also correlated favorably with prolonged survival. Only patients with intraperitoneal chemotherapy used in conjunction with cytoreductive surgery were shown to have prolonged survival.[19]

Morbidity and mortality of phase II studies

The morbidity and mortality of 200 consecutive patients who had cytoreductive surgery and heated intraoperative intraperitoneal chemotherapy for peritoneal carcinomatosis have been reported.[22] In these patients, there were three treatment-related deaths (1.5%). Peripancreatitis (6.0%) and fistula (4.5%) were

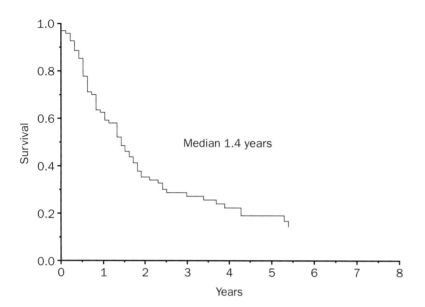

Figure 17.4 Survival of all patients with peritoneal carcinomatosis from colon cancer (95 patients).

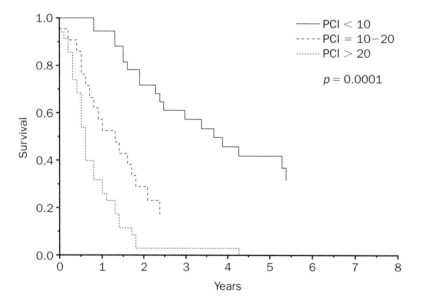

Figure 17.5 Survival of patients with peritoneal carcinomatosis from colon cancer according to the Peritoneal Cancer Index (PCI).

the most common major complications. There were 27.0% of patients with grade 3 or 4 complications (Table 17.4).

Following these treatments, the patient is maintained on parenteral feeding for 2–4 weeks. Approximately 20% of patients, especially those who have had extensive prior surgery or who have a short bowel, will need parenteral feeding after they leave hospital.

ETHICAL CONSIDERATIONS IN CLINICAL STUDIES WITH PERITONEAL SURFACE MALIGNANCY

The sequence of events that should accompany a new program in peritoneal surface malignancy has not yet been defined. The requirements for formal institutional review board approval will vary from one institution to another. The following are guidelines for an evolution of treatment strategies that allows for persistent clinical research.

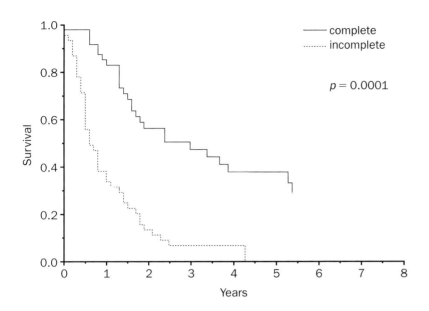

Figure 17.6 Survival of patients with peritoneal carcinomatosis from colon cancer according to completeness of cytoreduction.

$p = 0.0001$

Table 17.4 Morbidity and mortality of 200 treatments of cytoreductive surgery combined with perioperative intraperitoneal chemotherapy

Morbidity	Number	Percentage
Peripancreatitis	12	6.0
Fistula	9	4.5
Postoperative bleeding	9	4.5
Hematologic toxicity	8	4.0
Anastomotic leak	6	3.0
Pulmonary complication	6	3.0
Gastrointestinal toxicity	6	3.0
Pleural effusion tapped	6	3.0
Sterile collection tapped	5	2.5
Pneumothorax	5	2.5
Cardiovascular toxicity	5	2.5
Wound sepsis	5	2.5
Line sepsis	4	2.0
Bile leak	4	2.0
Systemic sepsis	4	2.0
Deep vein thrombosis	2	1.0
Neurologic complication	1	0.5
Pulmonary embolism	1	0.5
Severe pain	0	0.0
Combined grade 3/4 morbidity	54	27.0
Treatment-related mortality	3	1.5

Without exception, adjuvant intraperitoneal chemotherapy studies in patients with primary colorectal cancer must be randomized, and require review by an institutional review board. Also, when a group first attempts to initiate treatment plans with intraperitoneal chemotherapy, the learning curve associated with a new technology is best approached by a start-up protocol approved by an institutional review board. This forces the group to standardize methods and familiarize themselves with the experience of others. Selection criteria to treat patients with a reasonable likelihood of benefit must be evident. A protocol is suggested that allows aggressive cytoreduction and perioperative intraperitoneal chemotherapy in patients with no systemic dissemination and small-volume peritoneal seeding from recurrent colorectal cancer. This omnibus protocol should be utilized over a limited time period to treat 10–20 patients.

Formal protocols should not be required for the treatment of debilitating ascites. Also, the long-term survival of patients with established peritoneal surface malignancy with small volume and limited distribution has been established. After completing the start-up protocols, phase II clinical studies on this group of patients by an oncologic team that has demonstrated experience should proceed without the need for further institutional review board approval. The peritoneal surface spread of most colorectal cancers that have a low Peritoneal Cancer Index and after surgery have a completeness-of-cytoreduction score of 0 or 1 should be routinely treated according to standardized intraperitoneal chemotherapy protocols.

REFERENCES

1. Gunderson LL, Sosin H, Areas of failure found at reoperation (second or symptomatic look) following 'curative surgery' for adenocarcinoma of the rectum: clinicopathologic correlation and implications for adjuvant therapy. *Cancer* 1974; **34:** 1278–92

2. Sugarbaker PH, Surgical management of locally recurrent and metastatic colorectal cancer. In: *Atlas of Surgical Oncology* (Karakousis CP, Copeland EM, Bland QUI, eds). Philadelphia: WB Saunders, 1995: 671–92.

3. Sugarbaker PH, Hughes KA, Surgery for colorectal metastasis to liver. In: *Colorectal Cancer* (Wanebo H, ed). St Louis: Mosby-Year Book, 1993: 405–13.

4. Sugarbaker PH (ed), *Peritoneal Carcinomatosis: Principles of Management*. Boston: Kluwer, 1996.

5. Sugarbaker PH (ed), *Peritoneal Carcinomatosis: Drugs and Diseases*. Boston: Kluwer, 1996.

6. Sugarbaker PH, Chang D, Results of treatment of 385 patients with peritoneal surface spread of appendiceal malignancy. *Ann Surg Oncol* 1999; **6:** 727–31.

7. Sugarbaker PH, Peritonectomy procedures. In: *Peritoneal Carcinomatosis: Principles of Management* (Sugarbaker PH, ed). Boston: Kluwer, 1996: 235–62.

8. Averbach AM, Stephens AD, Sugarbaker PH, Gastric cancer with peritoneal carcinomas; Case report and presentation of a pilot treatment plan. *Surg Rounds* 1996; **19:** 14–21.

9. Sugarbaker PH, Laser-mode electrosurgery. In: *Peritoneal Carcinomatosis: Principles of Management* (Sugarbaker PH, ed). Boston: Kluwer, 1996: 375–85.

10. Jacquet P, Vidal-Jove J, Zhu BW, Sugarbaker PH, Peritoneal carcinomatosis from intraabdominal malignancy: Natural history and new prospects for management. *Acta Belgica Chirurgica* 1994; **94:** 191–7.

11. Sugarbaker PH, Graves T, DeBruijn EA et al, Rationale for early postoperative intraperitoneal chemotherapy (EPIC) in patients with advanced gastrointestinal cancer. *Cancer Res* 1990; **50:** 5790–4.

12. Sugarbaker PH, Ronnett BM, Ancher A et al, Management of pseudomyxoma peritonei of appendiceal origin. *Adv Surg* 1997; **30:** 233–80.

13. Archer A, Sugarbaker PH, Jelinek J, Radiology of peritoneal carcinomatosis. In: *Peritoneal Carcinomatosis: Principles of Management* (Sugarbaker PH, ed). Boston: Kluwer, 1996: 263–88.

14. Jacquet P, Jelinek J, Sugarbaker PH, Abdominal computed tomographic scan in the selection of patients with mucinous peritoneal carcinomatosis for cytoreductive surgery. *J Am College Surg* 1995; **181:** 530–8.

15. Gomez Portilla A, Sugarbaker PH, Chang D, Second-look surgery after cytoreductive and intraperitoneal chemotherapy for peritoneal carcinomatosis from colorectal cancer: analysis of prognostic features. *World J Surg* 1999; **23:** 23–9.

16. Berthet B, Sugarbaker TA, Chang D, Sugarbaker PH, Quantitative methodologies for selection of patients with recurrent abdominopelvic sarcoma for treatment. *Eur J Cancer* 1999; **35:** 413–19.

17. Sugarbaker PH, Successful management of microscopic residual disease in large bowel cancer. *Cancer Chemother Pharmacol* 1999; **43**(Suppl): 15–25.

18. Sugarbaker PH, Schellinx MET, Chang D et al, Peritoneal carcinomatosis from adenocarcinoma of the colon. *World J Surg* 1996; **20:** 585–92.

19. Averbach AM, Sugarbaker PH, Recurrent intraabdominal cancer with intestinal obstruction. *Int Surg* 1995; **80:** 141–6.

20. Sugarbaker PH, Observations concerning cancer spread within the peritoneal cavity and concepts supporting an ordered pathophysiology. In: *Peritoneal Carcinomatosis: Principles of Management* (Sugarbaker PH, ed). Boston: Kluwer, 1996: 79–100.

21. Sugarbaker PH, *Management of Peritoneal Surface Malignancy Using Intraperitoneal Chemotherapy and Cytoreductive Surgery: A Manual for Physicians and Nurses*, 3rd edn. Grand Rapids, MI: Ludann, 1998.

22. Stephens AD, Alderman R, Chang D et al, Morbidity and mortality of 200 treatments with cytoreductive surgery and heated intraoperative intraperitoneal chemotherapy using the coliseum technique. *Ann Surg Oncol* 1999; **6:** 790–6.

18

Surgery for rectal cancer

Rudolf Raab, Hans-Joachim Meyer, Uwe Werner

INTRODUCTION

Rectal carcinoma is still one of the most frequent cancers in so-called developed countries.[1,2] Complete tumour removal is the only measure that gives prospects of cure for the patient. During the last three decades, better survival of all afflicted has been achieved by an increase in the number of curative (i.e. R0) resections and by a decrease in perioperative mortality. Apart from this, in the opinion of many authors,[3–5] no substantial improvement of prognosis has been attained. The most important prognostic factor is the tumour stage according to UICC or Dukes. Next to this the individual surgeon performing the operation is of decisive importance.[6,7] There is a great variability between institutions and surgeons with regard to local recurrence rates and overall results of surgery.[8] Thus, the comments of one of the pioneers in abdominal surgery, the famous German surgeon Johann von Mikulicz, dating from the year 1903 is still valid:[9] *'Wenn wir auch heute schon sagen können, dass das Darmcarcinom eines der dankbarsten Gebiete der Abdominalchirurgie abgiebt, so lassen unsere Resultate doch manches zu wünschen übrig. Sie müssen durch eine Vervollkommnung der Technik besser werden.'* ('Although even today we may say that bowel cancer is one of the most satisfactory fields in abdominal surgery, our results leave much to be desired. They must be improved by a perfection of technique.')

Nowadays, radical resection of the primary lesion is the rule – this is so even in elderly patients and when the entire procedure is only palliative. In general, the resection rate of those operated upon should be near 100% and the operative mortality rate should be below 5%.[10,11] First essentials for operative success are good preparation of the bowel and the use of prophylactic antibiotics. Postoperatively, a close-meshed follow-up is necessary, because early recognized metastases or local recurrences can be reoperated upon in some cases with curative intent, and because in 2–3% of cases a second metachronous carcinoma occurs.[12] Treatment of recurrences and metastases depends on the individual situation. In these cases, interdisciplinary concepts will probably gain more importance in the future.

PREOPERATIVE DIAGNOSTICS

Clinical examination

The preoperative examination of patients forms the basis for surgical therapy. The overall impression of the individual situation is of considerable significance, namely general condition and vitality, as well as the general approach to life on the whole. This can be indicative for basic pre- as well possible intra-operative decisions, for instance with regard to neoadjuvant therapy or to extend or limit radicality. Anamnesis and general physical examination may disclose concomitant diseases that have hitherto been unknown. The family history may provide valuable hints of hereditary diseases or a familial disposition. It is also necessary for a detailed anamnesis to include defaecation habits and differentiated continence capability (e.g. frequency of bowel movement, consistence of bowels, warning period, ability to discriminate, etc.). This is followed by an inspection of the anal region and a digital examination. This is of particular significance, since, compared with apparative sphincter pressure measurement, continence anamnesis and digital examination are very often better aids to the experienced examiner when deciding whether in an individual case continence-maintaining surgery or an intersphincteric resection should be performed.

Obligatory apparative examinations and laboratory tests

Besides the common preparatory measures for the operation, the following examinations should routinely be performed in patients with rectal cancer:

- The tumour marker carcinoembryonic antigen (CEA), and possibly also CA19-9, should be determined. The main purpose of the determination of tumour markers is to get an initial value for postoperative follow-up examinations.[13] Immediate therapeutic consequences may arise if the initial CEA value is very high. Values above 25 µg/l give reasonable suspicion of distant spread; values above 50 µg/l are as good as a proof of bloodborne metastasis.
- Abdominal ultrasonography is the most important measure to exclude liver metastases and ureteral dilatation. With improvements in this method, intravenous pyelography is no longer obligatory, and is only indicated if there is suspicion of ureteral obstruction.
- A chest X-ray should be taken in two planes. Radiographic examination of the chest is generally sufficient to exclude lung metastases. There is no doubt that a computed tomography (CT) scan of the chest has a higher sensitivity. However, considering the small size of lesions that are not seen in the normal X-ray, its specificity is very low. Furthermore, diagnosis of small intrapulmonary lesions will hardly ever be a contraindication to removal of the primary tumour.
- A complete colonoscopy should be performed, with examination of the entire rectum and colon up to the caecum. Endoscopy is the most important measure to localize the tumour and to exclude synchronous adenomas (frequency 25–50%) as well as synchronous carcinomas (frequency about 4%). During endoscopy, a tumour biopsy should be taken to prove the diagnosis. If preoperatively a complete colonoscopy is impossible because of a stenosing tumour, it should be done postoperatively – and in case of any doubt even intraoperatively. To determine the exact distance of the lower edge of the tumour from the anal verge, it is always recommended that the surgeon himself performs an endoscopy with a rigid rectoscope in addition to the colonoscopy. This is because the distance is not infrequently overestimated during examinations with the flexible instrument.
- A double-contrast barium enema is only the second-best method for bowel examination, because no biopsy can be taken. In addition, evacuation of the contrast medium may be delayed or incomplete, especially if there is a stenosis due to the tumour. Remaining barium at the time of the operation might be harmful to the patient if it spills into the abdominal cavity. In the future, CT colonography[14,15] will probably be a good alternative to barium enema if a complete colonoscopy is impossible (see below).

Optional examinations

There are some complementary examinations in rectal cancer. Some of them are not yet (e.g. endorectal ultrasound) or no longer (e.g. intravenous pyelography) part of the routine diagnostic measures:

- It is possible by endorectal ultrasonography to determine the depth of infiltration of the bowel wall (T classification) with an accuracy of about 90%.[16–18] This method serves for preoperative T classification if in early stages (uT1) an operation of limited radicality or in advanced stages (uT4) neoadjuvant therapy is considered.
- A CT scan of the abdomen and the small pelvis may be helpful for planning the operation if there is any suspicion of distant metastases or infiltration of neighbouring organs or structures. However, this is seldom absolutely necessary, because final decisions about extent of the procedure are anyhow only possible intraoperatively. If an abdominal CT scan is indicated, it should be done as spiral (helical) CT, or in the near future possibly as multiplanar spiral CT.[19,20]
- Magnetic resonance imaging (MRI) might give additional information in the case of a T4 tumour, a local recurrence, or metastases. A definitive assessment of its relative importance is not yet possible. There are continuous improvements in both CT and MRI techniques and contrast media. Therefore, an almost optimal imaging of the pelvis with either method can be expected for the future. Possibly, MRI with an endorectal coil and gadolinium enhancement will become an alternative to endorectal ultrasound in the future.[21]
- A CT scan of the chest is indicated if lung metastases are suspected from the chest X-ray, especially if therapeutic consequences would result from the findings (e.g. a lung resection or a limited radical resection of the bowel).
- A cystoscopy is always indicated if there is sus-

picion of an enterovesical fistula or direct tumour infiltration to the urinary bladder. Both occur only rarely.

- Positron emission tomography (PET) using [^{18}F]fluorodeoxyglucose (FDG-PET) allows differentiation between scar and tumour tissue on the basis of their different metabolic activities.[22,23] This may be of clinical importance, especially if local recurrence is supected after extirpation of the rectum.[24,25] In these cases, the sensitivity and specifity of FDG-PET are 96% and 93%, respectively. Therefore, an interdisciplinary German consensus conference 'PET in Oncology' classified this indication as '1a', i.e. in the highest of five categories (1a, appropriate; 1b, mostly acceptable; 2a, helpful; 2b, value as yet unknown; 3, useless).[26]

Methods under clinical evaluation

- CT colonography is a new imaging method for the detection of intraluminal tumours (i.e. polyps or carcinomas). The technique gives three-dimensional endoluminal images. Therefore, a so-called 'virtual colonocopy' has become possible, and may be a substitute if real colonoscopy is not feasible. The first results show that a colon unrevealed by previous colonoscopy could be succesfully examined in more than 90% of patients[14] and that the specificity for adenomas 1 cm in diameter or larger was 89%.[15] These results are as good as or even better than those achieved with barium enema.
- Immunoscintigraphy is used to localize local recurrences or metastases.[18,27] Up to now it has not gained any clinical importance, primarily because of a lack in sensitivity. Moreover, if murine antibodies are used, there is a risk of human anti-mouse antibody (HAMA) formation, which may limit the possible therapeutic use of antibodies in the later course of the disease.

Histological examination

As pointed out above, a histological confirmation of the diagnosis should be aimed at. In the lower third of the rectum, the differentiation between adenocarcinomas and squamous cell carcinomas is of importance because of the different therapeutic approaches towards the two entities. If local excision is considered, a preoperative grading is necesssary, because

operations of limited radicality are contraindicated in high-grade malignancy (G3/G4). In general, the same applies to tumours that show invasion of veins or lymphatic vessels.

SPECIFIC PREOPERATIVE MEASURES

Cleansing of the bowel

The measures for preoperative cleansing of the bowel depend mainly on the degree of stenosis of the bowel lumen. The method of choice is an orthograde lavage,[28,29] which is always possible if there is a flat or ulcerated tumour without significant stenosis. The patient should drink a solution of polyethylene glycol (PEG), which is not absorbable. Thus absorption of great amounts of water can be prevented by an osmotic effect. If the patient is not able to drink the necesssary 3–4 liters of fluid, it may also be given by a feeding tube placed in the duodenum. In this case greater amounts of the solution are needed (6–8 liters or more). The fluid should be at room temperature, and the lavage should be continued until nearly clean liquid is discharged. If cardiac symptoms or crampy pain in the abdomen arise, the lavage should be stopped. Although PEG has no or only negligible side-effects on the cardiovascular system, in cases of severely impaired cardiac or renal function orthograde lavage should be considered contraindicated. If moderate stenosis exists, an attempt with orthograde lavage (possibly fractionated) is justified. Alternatively, the patient is given a fully absorbable diet and daily high enemas for 5–7 days. If there is severe stenosis, the preparation consists of complete parenteral nutrition and repeated high enemas for 1–2 weeks. In addition, intraoperative lavage might be required. The rare cases with a complete ileus necessitate an immediate operation with intraoperative lavage. If this is not possible or not sufficient, a subtotal colectomy must be considered.

Antibiotics

Prophylactic administration of antibiotics is now a routine measure in colorectal surgery.[30] A broad-spectrum antibiotic that is effective also on anaerobes is given as a single shot at the beginning of anaesthesia. Antibiotic treatment should only be continued if there is an ileus, a perforation, or a similar situation with high risk of postoperative infection.

Colostomy

With the patient lying on the operating table, the determination of the best localization for a preternatural anus might be impossible. Therefore, if a temporary or definite colostomy is being considered, the exact possible positions must be marked preoperatively with waterproof ink after examining the patient in the sitting and upright positions.

PRINCIPLES OF SURGICAL MANAGEMENT

The radical operative removal of the primary tumour with its draining lymphatic vessels is the basis of the surgical therapy of colorectal cancer. In our opinion, technical irresectability does not really exist, because there is no neighbouring structure that cannot be resected en bloc with the tumour. Cases in which local R0 resection of primary rectal cancer is not feasible are very infrequent. Furthermore, this can generally only be recognized after crossing the 'point of no return' during the course of the operation. Old age alone is not a contraindication. Radical surgery can be performed safely even in the ninth or tenth decade of life. Because of the secondary complications of the tumour (e.g. perforation, ileus, bleeding, ureteral obstruction, perineal exulceration, and formation of a cloaca), resection is also usually indicated if the intention can only be palliative because of irresectable metastases. Therefore, the only reasons for leaving a tumour in place are the very rare situations of general inoperability, and the judgement that resection is of no value for an individual patient because of a very short expectation of life (<6 months) due to widespread formation of irresectable metastases.

Surgical technique and radicality are of greatest importance.[31–34] No adjuvant therapy can ever make good what one has failed to do surgically. Spacious access is required for a safe and radical operation. We recommend a long median laparotomy. This allows exact exploration of the entire abdomen and the performance of all interventions on colon and rectum, including extension of the resection to other organs. Opening of the abdomen is followed by palpation and inspection of the abdominal organs. Intraoperative ultrasound of the liver is always desirable. Therapeutic decisions must not be based on the presence of liver metastases that are diagnosed by palpation only. When judging the R0 resectability of a tumour, it should be kept in mind that infiltration of surrounding tissues or organs might be mimicked by concomitant inflammation. Only 50–60% of all supposed T4 tumours, in fact, show a crossing of the organ borders histologically. Nevertheless, just the suspicion of infiltration mandates the inclusion of the respective organs or border layers in the resection. As a general rule, a monobloc resection should always be possible. The worst possible incident during operation on colorectal cancer is a tear or cut of the tumour. In these cases, the chance of cure decreases rapidly. In any case of doubt, radicality is more important than preservation of function (e.g. continence, voiding, or sexual function).

Anaesthesiologic management is also an important building block for operative success. Postoperative wound infection rates, for example, can be reduced by higher concentrations of inspired oxygen during the operation.[35]

A negative influence of perioperative blood or plasma substitution on survival is possible.[36] Even if this has not yet been definitively proved, unnecessary transfusions should be avoided by a strict blood-saving operative technique.

Preoperative radiotherapy

Neoadjuvant therapy can be benificial when broad infiltration of neighbouring organs by a tumour in the median or lower third of the rectum is evident or when on examination the tumour is completely fixed (Mason stage IV). Usually this will reduce the size of the tumour, and subsequent surgery can be performed with a reduced risk of the need for an R1 resection or of tearing or cutting into the tumour.

The decision has to be taken with careful consideration of the specific cirumstances in each individual case. The aim is to ascertain improved conditions for the resection, not to transform an 'irresectable' tumour into a resectable one, because, as pointed out above, the actual technical irresectability of a colorectal primary tumour is an extremely rare situation, if it occurs at all. The possibility of management with less operative radicality after preoperative radiotherapy is also very limited. If a rectal tumour actually has infiltrated neighbouring organs (e.g. the bladder or the anterior vaginal wall), then the optimum result would be the presence of fibrous connective tissue at the site treated with radiotherapy, which cannot be distinguished from persisting tumour infiltration intraoperatively. Therefore, the necessity for additional partial or complete resection of the organ concerned remains.

If the decision for neoadjuvant therapy has been taken, the following points should be considered:

- Neoadjuvant combined radio-chemotherapy is probably more efficient than radiotherapy alone because of the radio-sensitizing effect of the chemotherapy, and in addition this will also affect any tumour cells that have already systemically disseminated.
- A significant reduction of tumour size can only be expected after radiation with conventional dose and fractionation for approximately 5 weeks, but not after short-term radiation with 5×5 Gy. As shown by Swedish and Dutch results, short-term radiation can probably reduce the rate of local reccurrence, even with standardized radical surgery including total mesorectal excision. However, this method does not result in notable reduction of a fixed or infiltrating tumour, so that the desired ease of surgery is not achieved.

At present a randomized trial is being conducted in Germany by the university clinics in Hannover (surgery) and Erlangen (radiotherapy). This study is evaluating whether or not principally neoadjuvant radio-chemotherapy for all UICC stage II and III rectal tumours leads to improved results in the sense of prolonged survival, a reduced rate of local recurrence, or an increased rate of sphincter-saving operations. To date, 750 patients have been recruited, and it has already become evident that with this pretreatment the rate of sphincter-saving operations for low rectal tumours can be significantly increased. The first results of the Hannover–Erlangen study regarding survival rate and rate of local recurrence are expected in the year 2002.

Curative surgical interventions for primary rectal cancer

All rectal carcinomas can be removed by one of the two standard procedures, anterior resection or abdominoperineal extirpation, although in some cases limited radicality might be indicated (see below). Spincter-saving resections are increasingly being used. Provided the entire mesorectum is removed, they are as good as or even better than operations sacrificing the anus.[37,38] The definitive decision on sphincter preservation is only possible intraoperatively. It depends on the individual situation and the extension of the tumour. If the tumour is not too big and the sphincter function is normal, there should be a minimum distance of 1 cm between the lower edge of the tumour and the dentate line, the lowest possible level of resection. Thus, the dis-

tance from the anal verge should be at least 3.5–4 cm. If the level of resection is higher than the dentate line, a greater safety margin of approximately 3 cm is necesssary. If the tumour is located in the upper third of the rectum, total mesorectal excision is mostly not necessary. In these cases, the distal margin should be some 5 cm and the mesorectal tissue should be removed to the same length as the bowel wall and with the same circumferential margins as in deeper resections. Usually this requires complete mobilization of the rectum together with the mesorectum from the small pelvis (i.e. excavatio sacralis).

Anterior resection of the rectum

The surgical procedure is now well standardized.[39–41] This is due not least to the efforts of Bill Heald and Warren Enker.[33,42–44] With the patient in a lithotomy position, the operation starts with a midline incision, abdominal exploration, and intraoperative ultrasound examination of the liver. In all operations with curative intent, the inferior mesenteric vessels are divided centrally, the artery at the level of its offspring from the aorta, and the vein at the level of the lower edge of the pancreas. For this purpose, the mobilization of the duodenum with dissection of the ligament of Treitz is required as a first step. After severing the vessels, the sigmoid colon, the descending colon, and the splenic flexure are detached. If this is done keeping strictly within the right plane, there is no need to identify or even snare the left ureter. The colon is divided in the region of the descending or upper sigmoid part. Mobilization of the rectum from the small pelvis requires meticulous care, precision, and attention in order to combine the greatest possible oncological radicality with the greatest possible preservation of sexual and voiding functions. The mesorectum must always be removed completely – at least if the tumour is located in the lower or middle third of the rectum. At the same time, particular care should be taken of the autonomic nerve system, which consists of the superior hypogastric plexus, the right and left hypogastric nerves, the inferior hypogastric plexuses, and subplexuses supplying the different pelvic organs.[45,46] These requirements cannot be fulfilled by mobilizing the rectum in the traditional way dorsally blunt with the surgeon´s hand and laterally by means of clamps and ligatures or even staplers. Instead, only sharp dissection by means of scissors should be used. Electrosurgical dissection with a diathermy knife is also widely used, especially by US surgeons, but this is not really necessary and is associated with a risk of nerve damage. With either method the hypogastric nerves should be identified and preserved, unless they are directly infiltrated by the tumour. Dorsally, the dissection follows a plane right above the fascia of Waldeyer. Lateral to the rectum, the tissue is sharply dissected along the roughly sagittal layer of the internal iliac vessels and the inferior hypogastric plexuses, respectively. Along this way, the only crossing vessels worth mentioning are the middle rectal arteries. Mostly, any bleeding from a middle rectal artery can be stanched by bipolar coagulation – undersewing is seldom necesssary. Only after the dorsal and lateral mobilization has been completed down to the pelvic floor is the bowel detached anteriorly. In doing this, care should be taken not to injure the dorsal wall of the vagina or the seminal vesicles and the prostate, respectively. Nevertheless, if a T4 tumour is suspected, all the respective organs should be included in the monobloc resection.

At the end of the pelvic part of the operation, a definitive decision is made about whether an anterior resection is possible or an abdomino-intersphincteric resection or even an abdominoperineal extirpation of the rectum is necessary. If the resection can be done anteriorly, a right-angled clamp is positioned below the tumour, and the bowel wall is divided below this clamp. After tumour removal we rinse the pelvis and the rectal stump with a cytotoxic solution, and usually with distilled water. This is followed in cases of higher resections by a termino-terminal anastomosis to re-establish bowel continuity. After the more frequent deep resections, we prefer to form a short (5–6 cm) J-pouch of the colon with a pouch–rectal or pouch–anal anastomosis. In both instances, it is unimportant whether the anastomosis is handsewn or done by a circular stapler. The use of staplers presupposes the ability of the standard technique to cope with all possible complications. The double-stapling technique is especially controversial. The increased risk of anastomotic leakage may outweigh the possible advantage of the technique that it is time-saving. The formation of a double-barrelled ileostomy (or transverse colostomy) is always up to the surgeon's discretion. From our point of view, it has proved to be wise to use a protective stoma in all cases of doubt.

Abdomino-intersphincteric resection

For most tumours in the lower third of the rectum, a standard anterior resection is not possible. If the lower edge of the tumour is at least 1 cm above the dentate line and there is no direct infiltration of the levator ani, an intersphincteric resection may be considered.[47–49] The abdominal part of the operation is identical to that described above. However, no right-angled clamp is positioned, and the bowel wall is divided not from above but transanally. After exposing the situs by means of one or two anal retractors (we use two Gelpi retractors positioned crosswise), the mucosa and the internal anal sphincter are divided at the level of the dentate line. The remains of the rectum are released intersphincterically, and the specimen is removed anteriorly. In our opinion, the formation of a colo-anal pouch is of the utmost importance in these cases. The colo-anal pouch gives a functional benefit for the patient for at least the first two postoperative years.[50] Despite such re-creation of a presphincteric reservoir, however, disturbances of continence may occur. Thus only patients with unaltered sphincter function are eligible for this procedure. A transanally handsewn anastomosis is obligatory, because there is no material left that can be used for pursestring suture and stapled anastomosis.

Abdominoperineal extirpation of the rectum

In about 5–10% of tumours of the middle third and about 30–40% of tumours of the lower third of the rectum, the anal sphincter cannot be preserved. Nevertheless, the abdominal part of the operation is again identical to the anterior resection (see above). Following complete anterior mobilization of the rectum, the operation is continued by the same surgeon from a perineal approach. A simultaneous operation with two teams from above and below is incompatible with the demands for oncologically and functionally sufficient surgery as described above. The anus is closed with a pursestring suture. After dividing the skin and the subcutaneous fat, the levator ani is dissected cranio-laterally as far as possible. The preparation begins dorsally with the division of the ano-coccygeal ligament, and is continued laterally. Again the ventral dissection is the last part, because there is the highest risk for damaging the prostatic plexus, the corpora cavernosa plexus or the urethra. The specimen may be removed in either direction, and the perineal wound is closed primarily.

If postoperative radiotherapy is considered or at least possible, care should be taken to keep the small bowel out of the small pelvis. The best way to achieve this goal is by means of anterior resection, because the pelvis is filled with parts of the large bowel, which is not so sensitive to radiation. In the case of an abdominoperineal resection, a pedicled omental graft may be used.[51] Only if this is not possible is an absorbable mesh inserted and fixed between the symphysis and the promontory to prevent the small bowel from descending into the pelvis.[52] However, with this method, a hollow space is left behind in the pelvis, which carries the risk of infection.

RESULTS OF TREATMENT

At Hannover Medical School, we have operated upon 966 patients with primary rectal cancer in the 20-year period from 1971 to 1990. Follow-up was complete until 1995. The median age was 64 years (range 18–87 years). Figure 18.1 shows the frequency in the different age-groups. Overall, most of the tumours were located in the middle third of the rectum, but the proportion of lower tumours was increasing rapidly. In the last 5-year period, we saw about 50% of the tumours in the lower third (Table 18.1). Likewise, an increase in the number of the more advanced stages, especially UICC stage IV, could be observed. Overall, the distribution of the stages was 29.4%, 29.5%, 24.4%, and 16.7% for UICC stages I, II, III, and IV, respectively.

Sphincter-saving resections were performed with increasing frequency. Figure 18.2 shows the development for the different parts of the rectum from the 1970s to the mid-1990s. In the 1990s, only 4% of patients with tumours of the middle rectum and only 38% of those with tumours of the lower rectum underwent an abdominoperineal resection. In 78%,

R0 resections were possible, whereas in 21.2%, only an R2 resection could be performed. This was mostly because of irresectable distant metastases (see Table 18.2). Microscopic residual tumour, i.e. R1 resection, was a rare exception (0.8%). The total complication rate was rather high (41%), but most of the complications were minor ones such as urinary tract or wound infections. Anastomotic leakage occurred in 7.3% and adverse cardio-respiratory events were seen in 8.6%. The operative mortality rate was lowered from 9.9% in the early 1970s to 3.6% in the second half of the 1980s. The remaining deaths were due to cardio-circulatory complications.

The observed overall 5-year survival rate was 47.2% (mortality included). After R0 resection, nearly 60% of all patients survived 5 years, while the rate for non-radical resection was only 3.3% (see Figure 18.3). Besides the R classification, the tumour stage according to UICC was the most important prognostic factor. As shown in Table 18.3, survival rates could be improved significantly over time for stage I and II tumours but not for stage III. Most impressive was the progress in the cases with distant metastases, i.e. UICC stage IV. While three decades ago none of such patients survived, by the end of the 1980s the 5-year survival rate was 8.1% and by the end of the 1990s it was 13.2%. This is an impressive reflection of the success of surgery for liver (and lung) metastases. Thus, estimates that only around 5% of all patients with liver metastases may profit from liver resection appear clearly to be too conservative. Nonetheless, much is left to future efforts in adjuvant, additive, and palliative treatment.

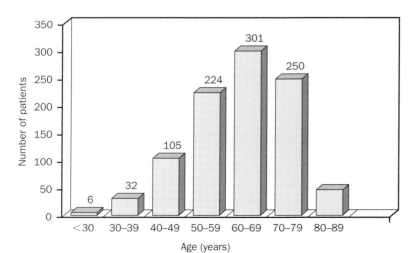

Figure 18.1 Age distribution of patients with primary rectal cancer.

Table 18.1 Relative frequency of cancer in the different parts of the rectum

Period of time	Upper third	Middle third	Lower third
1971–75 (n = 191)	27.7%	53.9%	18.3%
1976–80 (n = 313)	37.1%	39.6%	23.3%
1981–85 (n = 268)	28.7%	38.8%	32.5%
1986–90 (n = 194)	19.6%	32.0%	48.5%
1991–95 (n = 189)	13.8%	36.0%	50.2%
1971–95 (n = 1155)	26.8%	39.9%	33.3%

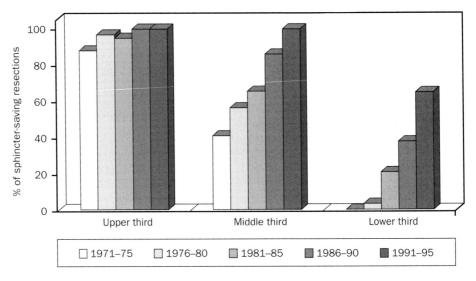

Figure 18.2 Development of the proportion of sphincter-saving resections according to the different parts of the rectum.

Table 18.2 R classification of the operation in relation to UICC stage classification

UICC stage	R0 resection	R1/2 resection
I	98.9%	1.1%
II	96.0%	4.0%
III	92.0%	8.0%
IV	5.8%	94.2%

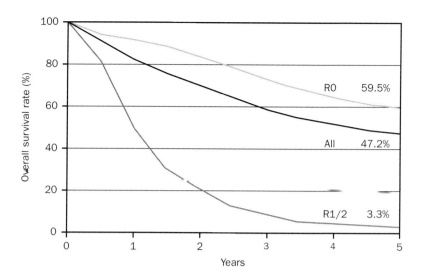

Figure 18.3 Observed overall survival following resection of primary rectal cancer (RO and R1/2 operations; operative mortality included).

Table 18.3 Observed 5-year survival rates following RO resection of primary rectal cancer according to UICC stage classification (operative mortality included)

UICC stage	1971–75	1976–80	1981–85	1986–90	1991–95	1971–1995
I	67.7%	74.3%	83.9%	81.4%	88.6%	76.9%
II	51.0%	57.7%	60.0%	80.0%	76.7%	59.0%
III	40.5%	41.5%	40.3%	39.4%	53.6%	42.6%

PROCEDURES WITH LIMITED RADICALITY

In some cases of rectal cancer, a limited radical approach is sufficient, either with curative intent in early invasive tumours or with palliative intent if there are already irresectable metastases or the patient is inoperable for major abdominal surgery.

Curative intent

Early invasive tumours of the lower and middle third of the rectum may be treated by local excision. A prerequisite is preoperative endoanal ultrasound to determine the T category and histological examination of a tumour biopsy. In uT1 tumours, the risk of lymph-node metastases is around 3%, and therefore within the range of the operative mortality of anterior or abdominoperineal resections. In uT2 tumours, positive nodes are found already in about 20% (see Table 18.4). The situation is analogous for

G3/G4 tumours (high-grade malignancy) and for tumours with a histologically proven invasion of lymph vessels or veins. Postoperative radiation

Table 18.4 pN category in relation to pT category and grading in primary rectal cancer

pT category and grading	Positive lymph nodes (pN1–4)
pT1, G1	3.0%
pT1, G2	3.4%
pT1, G3	(n = 0)
pT2, G1	17.8%
pT2, G2	26.4%
pT2, G3	40.0%

therapy cannot improve the results in patients with T2 or T3 tumours.[53,54] Thus, only patients with well or moderately differentiated uT1 tumours without infiltration into lymph vessels or veins are eligible for a limited excision with curative intent.[55] Exceptions to this rule are possible for patients with uT2 tumours, on the basis of individual considerations. Nevertheless, newer results indicate that the tumour recurrence rates after local excision are higher than expected from previous reports.[56]

Access is transanally, either by a normal anal retractor or by the transanal endoscopic microsurgery (TEM) system according to Buess.[57–59] The tumour is removed by a full-thickness excision of the rectal wall with a portion of perirectal fat and a safety margin of 0.5–1 cm. The defect in the bowel wall is closed by a running or interrupted suture with absorbable material. If definite histological examination of the specimen shows a different result from the initial examination of the biopsy (e.g. a higher T category or a perirectal lymph-node metastasis), then a radical re-operation should be carried out unless there are severe contraindications. An alternative to the transanal approach is the Kraske technique.[60] The tumour is then removed via a parasacral incision and a posterior rectotomy. This approach even allows for segmental resections of the low or middle rectum.

Palliative intent

As has been pointed out, it is very seldom indicated to leave the tumour in place. If a radical operation gives no prospects of cure or at least good palliation, procedures with local destruction or partial ablation of the tumour might be justified. In our institution, the rate of such interventions is below 2% of all rectal cancer patients. Several techniques are described in the literature, including treatment modalities with heat or cryosurgery. We prefer well-aimed local tumour reduction under sight by means of a resectoscope, which is normally used to treat benign prostate hyperplasia. This has several advantages: it is available in all hospitals with a urological department, it is easy to handle, it yields material for a histological examination, the lumen of the rectum can be modelled up to the desired diameter, the method is safe, and it can be repeated under regional anaesthesia as often as necessary.[61]

SURGICAL TREATMENT OF LOCOREGIONAL RECURRENCE

Nearly all cases of anastomotic recurrence and many cases of local recurrence of rectal cancer are caused by the initial procedure, although this cannot be proven for an individual case. Actually, it can be stated that the variability of local recurrence rates between surgeons is in the range of less than 5% to more than 50%. Thus, the surgeon is one of the most important prognostic factors in colorectal cancer, and by far the best method to deal with locoregional recurrence is to avoid it by an adequate technique (i.e. standardized radical resection as described above) during the primary operation.

In most instances, early anastomotic recurrence can be treated sufficiently by a repeated anterior resection. The planes of oncologically correct rectal surgery are very often found untouched during the re-operation of these cases. In many advanced cases with broad extraluminal growth, R0 re-resection is still possible. In our experience, this has given a renewed chance of cure for about 30% of patients. However, such operations are mostly multivisceral resections. Therefore, they should be reserved for specialized centres. Sometimes a complete pelvic exenteration and a sacral resection is needed. These are often desperate interventions that are only justified by the desperate situation of the patient. Thus, it is always the patient's sole decision whether he or she is willing to undergo such extended surgery.

REFERENCES

1. Haenszel W, Correa P, Epidemiology of large bowel cancer. In: *Epidemiology of Cancer of the Digestive Tract* (Correa P, Haenszel W, eds). The Hague: Martinus Nijhoff, 1982: 85–126.

2. Schatzkin A, Schiffman MH, Etiology and prevention: the epidemiologic perspective. In: *Colorectal Cancer* (Wanebo HJ, ed). St Louis, MO: Mosby-Year Book, 1993: 3–19.

3. Enblad P, Adami H-O, Bergström R et al, Improved survival of patients with cancers of the colon and rectum. *J Natl Cancer Inst* 1988; **80**: 568–91.

4. Hawley PR, Rectal carcinoma: surgical progress. *Ann R Coll Surg Engl* 1990; **72**: 168–9.

5. Williams NS, Changing patterns in the treatment of rectal cancer. *Br J Surg* 1989; **76**: 5–6.

6. Fielding LP, Steward-Brown S, Dudley HA, Surgeon-related variables and the clinical trial. *Lancet* 1978; **ii**: 778–9.

7. McArdle CS, Hole D, Impact of variability among surgeons on postoperative morbidity and mortality and ultimate survival. *BMJ* 1991; **302**: 1501–5.

8. Hermanek P Jr, Wiebelt H, Riedl S et al, Studiengruppe Kolorektales Karzinom (SGKRK): Langzeitergebnisse der chirurgischen Therapie des Coloncarcinoms. Ergebnisse der Studiengruppe Kolorektales Karzinom (SGKRK). *Chirurg* 1994; **65**: 287–97.

9. von Mikulicz J, Chirurgische Erfahrungen über das Darmcarcinom. *Arch Klin Chir* 1903; **69:** 28–47.

10. Hermanek P, Wiebelt H, Staimmer D, Riedl S, Prognostic factors of rectum carcinoma – experience of the German Multicenter Study SGCRC. German Study Group Colorectal Carcinoma. *Tumori* 1995; **81**(Suppl 3): 60–4.

11. Northover JMA, Results of curative surgery for colorectal cancer. *Scand J Gastroenterol* 1988; **23**(Suppl 149): 155–8.

12. Raab R, Werner U, Löhlein D, Colorectale Mehrfachcarcinome: Eigenschaften und Langzeitprognose. *Chirurg* 1988; **59:** 96–100.

13. Moore M, Jones DJ, Schofield PF, Harden DG, Current status of tumor markers in large bowel cancer. *World J Surg* 1989; **13:** 52–9.

14. Morrin MM, Kruskal JB, Farrell RJ et al, Endoluminal CT colonography after an incomplete endoscopic colonoscopy. *AJR* 1999; **172:** 913–18.

15. Rex DK, Vining D, Kopecky KK, An initial experience with screening for colon polyps using spiral CT with and without CT colography (virtual colonoscopy). *Gastrointest Endosc* 1999; **50:** 309–13.

16. Beynon J, McC Mortensen NJ, Channer JL, Rigby H, Rectal endosonography accurately predicts depth of penetration in rectal cancer. *Int J Colorect Dis* 1992; **7:** 4–7.

17. Glaser F, Schlag P, Herfarth Ch, Endorectal ultrasonography for the assessment of invasion of rectal tumours and lymph node involvement. *Br J Surg* 1990; **77:** 883–7.

18. Feifel G, Hildebrandt U, New diagnostic imaging in rectal cancer: endosonography and immunoscintigraphy. *World J Surg* 1992; **16:** 841–7.

19. Llaugher J, Palmer J, Perez C et al, The normal and pathologic ischiorectal fossa at CT and MR imaging. *Radiographics* 1998; **18:** 61–82.

20. Schöpf UJ, Becker C, Bruning R et al, Computertomographie des Abdomens mit der Mehrzeilen-Detektor Spiral-CT. *Radiologie* 1999; **39:** 652–61.

21. Drew PJ, Farouk R, Turnbull LW et al, Preoperative magnetic resonance staging of rectal cancer with an endorectal coil and dynamic gadolinium enhancement. *Br J Surg* 1999; **86:** 250–4.

22. Schiepers C, Haustermans K, Geboes K et al, The effect of preoperative radiation therapy on glucose utilization and cell kinetics in patients with primary rectal carcinoma. *Cancer* 1999; **85:** 803–11.

23. Yasuda S, Takahashi W, Takagi S et al, Primary colorectal cancers detected with PET. *Jpn J Clin Oncol* 1998; **28:** 638–40.

24. Takeuchi O, Saito N, Koda K et al, Clinical assessment of positron emission tomography for the diagnosis of local recurrence in colorectal cancer. *Br J Surg* 1999; **86:** 932–7.

25. Franke J, Rosenzweig S, Reinartz P et al, Die Wertigkeit der Positronen-Emissionstomographie (^{18}F-FDG-PET) in der Diagnostik von Rectum-Rezidivcarcinomen. *Chirurg* 2000; **71:** 80–5.

26. Reske SN, Bares R, Büll U et al, Klinische Wertigkeit der Positronen-Emmissions-Tomographie (PET) bei onkologischen Fragestellungen: Ergebnisse einer interdisziplinären Konsensuskonferenz. *Nucl Med* 1996; **35:** 42–52.

27. Hölting T, Schlag P, Steinbächer M et al, The value of immunoscintigraphy for the operative retreatment of colorectal cancer. *Cancer* 1989; **64:** 830–3.

28. DiPalma JA, Brady CE, Colon cleansing for diagnostic and surgical procedures: polyethylene glycol–electrolyte lavage solution. *Am J Gastroenterol* 1989; **84:** 1008–16.

29. Hewitt J, Reeve J, Rigby J, Cox AG, Whole-gut irrigation in preparation for large-bowel surgery. *Lancet* 1973; **ii:** 337–40.

30. Menaker GJ, The use of antibiotics in surgical treatment of the colon. *Surg Gynecol Obstet* 1987; **164:** 581–6.

31. Hermanek P, Sobin LH, Colorectal carcinoma. In: *Prognostic Factors in Cancer* (Hermanek P, Gospodarowicz MK, Henson DE et al, eds). Berlin: Springer-Verlag, 1995: 64–79.

32. Hermanek P, Hohenberger W, The importance of volume in colorectal cancer surgery. *Eur J Surg Oncol* 1996; **22:** 213–15.

33. MacFarlane JK, Ryall RDH, Heald RJ, Mesorectal excision for rectal cancer. *Lancet* 1993; **341:** 457–60.

34. Sugarbaker PH, Corlew S, Influence of surgical techniques on survival in patients with colorectal cancer. *Dis Colon Rectum* 1982; **25:** 545–57.

35. Greif R, Akca O, Horn E-P et al, for the Outcomes Research Group, Supplemental perioperative oxygen to reduce the incidence of surgical wound infection. *N Engl J Med* 2000; **342:** 161–7.

36. Francis DMA, Relationship between blood transfusion and tumour behaviour. *Br J Surg* 1991; **78:** 1420–8.

37. Bozzetti F, Mariani L, Miceli R et al, Cancer of the low and middle rectum: local and distant recurrences, and survival in 350 radically resected patients. *J Surg Oncol* 1996; **62:** 207–13.

38. Jatzko G, Lisborg P, Wette V, Improving survival rates for patients with colorectal cancer. *Br J Surg* 1992; **79:** 588–91.

39. Köckerling F, Gall FP, Chirurgische Standards beim Rektumkarzinom. *Chirurg* 1994; **65:** 593–603.

40. Rosen HR, Schiessel R, Die vordere Rectumresection. *Chirurg* 1996; **67:** 99–109.

41. Stelzner F, Begründung, Technik und Ergebnisse der knappen Kontinenzresektion beim Rektumkarzinom. *Zentralbl Chir* 1992; **117:** 63–6.

42. Heald RJ, Ryall RDH, Husband E, The mesorectum in rectal cancer surgery: clue to pelvic recurrence. *Br J Surg* 1982; **69:** 613–16.

43. Heald RJ, The 'holy plane' of rectal surgery. *J R Soc Med* 1988; **81:** 503–8.

44. Enker WE, Designing the optimal surgery for rectal carcinoma. *Cancer* 1996; **78:** 1847–50.

45. Lepor H, Gregermann M, Crosby R et al, Precise localization of the autonomic nerves from the pelvis plexus to the corpora cavernosa: a detailed anatomical study of the adult male pelvis. *J Urol* 1985; **133:** 207–12.

46. Walsh PC, Schlegel PN, Radical pelvic surgery with preservation of sexual function. *Ann Surg* 1988; **208:** 391–400.

47. Parks AG, Per-anal anastomosis. *World J Surg* 1982; **6:** 531–8.

48. Parks AG, Percy JP, Resection and sutured colo-anal anastomosis for rectal cancer. *Br J Surg* 1982; **69:** 301–4.

49. Schumpelick V, Braun J, Die intersphinctäre Rectumresektion mit radikaler Mesorectumexcision und coloanaler Anastomose. *Chirurg* 1996; **67:** 110–20.

50. Lazorthes F, Chiotasso P, Gamagami RA et al, Late clinical outcome in a randomized prospective comparison of colonic J pouch and straight coloanal anastomosis. *Br J Surg* 1997; **84:** 1449–51.

51. DeLuca FR, Ragins H, Construction of an omental envelope as a method of excluding the small intestine from the field of postoperative irradiation to the pelvis. *Surg Gynecol Obstet* 1985; **160:** 365–6.

52. Kavanah MT, Feldmann MI, Devereux DF, Kondi ES, New surgical approach to minimize radiation-associated small bowel injury in patients with pelvic malignancies requiring surgery and high-dose irradiation. *Cancer* 1985; **56:** 1300–4.

53. Minsky BD, Cohen AM, Enker WE, Mies C, Sphincter preservation in rectal cancer by local excision and local radiation therapy. *Cancer* 1991; **67:** 908–14.

54. Willet CG, Tepper JE, Donnelly S et al, Patterns of failure following local excision and postoperative radiation therapy for invasive rectal adenocarcinoma. *J Clin Oncol* 1989; **7:** 1003–8.

55. Hermanek P, Guggenmoos-Holzmann I, Gall FP, Prognostic factors in rectal carcinoma. A contribution to the further development of tumor classification. *Dis Colon Rectum* 1989; **32:** 593–9.

56. Garcia-Aguilar J, Mellgren A, Sirivongs P et al, Local excision of rectal cancer without adjuvant therapy: a word of caution. *Ann Surg* 2000; **231:** 345–51.

57. Berry AR, Souter RG, Campbell WB et al, Endoscopic transanal resection of rectal tumours – a preliminary report of its use. *Br J Surg* 1990; **77:** 134–7.

58. Buess G, Mentges B, Manncke K et al, Technique and results of transanal endoscopic microsurgery in early rectal cancer. *Am J Surg* 1992; **163:** 63–70.

59. Bueß G, Kayser J, Technik und Indikation zur sphinctererhaltenden transanalen Resektion beim Rectumcarcinom. *Chirurg* 1996; **67:** 121–8.

60. Schildberg FW, Wenk H, Der posteriore Zugang zum Rectum. *Chirurg* 1986; **57:** 779–91.

61. Boeminghaus F, Coburg AJ, Transanale Resektion von obstruierenden Rektumtumoren mittels TUR-Technik (TAR). *Fortschr Gastroenterol Endosk* 1986; **15:** 172–6.

19

Total mesorectal excision: A quality-controlled approach to rectal cancer surgery

Thomas Cecil, Brendan J Moran, Richard J Heald

INTRODUCTION AND HISTORICAL BACKGROUND

Rectal cancer, defined as a tumour with its lower edge less than 15 cm from the anal verge, is a common disease, and accounts for over 30% of all cancers of the large bowel, with approximately 10 000 new cases per year. The rectum is relatively inaccessible, and surgery for rectal cancer is technically demanding, with a high morbidity and mortality for all abdominal procedures. Some early tumours can be treated by either peranal excision or by more recent developments such as transanal endoscopic microsurgery, but over 90% require an abdominal approach by either anterior resection (AR) or abdominoperineal excision (APE). An outstanding feature of rectal cancer surgery is the large variation in the rate of local recurrence: from 3% to 33%.[1] The best results have been consistently reported from units who perform total mesorectal excision (TME) in patients with rectal cancer,[1] a technique popularized by Heald.[2]

The rectum is arbitrarily divided into three portions, the lower rectum (0–6 cm), the middle rectum (7–11 cm), and the upper rectum (12–15 cm). These categories are useful in planning a surgical approach. Most authorities accept that AR with reconstruction is almost always possible in upper-third tumours and in most middle-third tumours. In expert hands, many tumours in the lower rectum can also be safely treated by AR with no oncological disadvantages as compared with APE.[3] Debate continues as to the merits of these operations, especially for tumours of the lower rectum. In the classic surgical textbook, *Rob & Smith's Operative Surgery* (5th edition, 1993), Murray and Veidenheimer[4] claim that abdominoperineal excision is 'the gold standard to which all other operations must be compared ... for all cancers of the lower third and bulky tumours of the middle third'.

Ernest Miles originally described APE in 1907, and outlined his cylindrical concept of cancer spread in all directions particularly in the lymphatics (Figure 19.1).[5] Miles suggested that only the widest possible clearance at the level of the cancer could

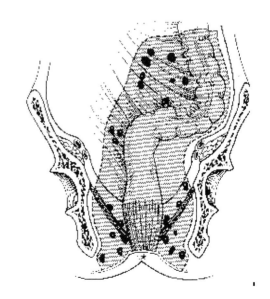

Figure 19.1 Ernest Miles' view of the lymphatic drainage of the rectum, suggesting that the drainage is to nodes below and above the pelvic floor.

have any hope of curing the patient, with a permanent colostomy being the price of cure. The operation was radical in that it removed the cancer with much surrounding tissue, and it was also an operation that could be completed at great speed, often in less than an hour – an important aspect of all surgery in the early part of the twentieth century. However, it paid scant attention to the lymphovascular tissue surrounding the rectum, namely the 'mesorectum', which until recently was ignored by all textbooks of anatomy and operative surgery.[2] The term 'radical' comes from the Latin *radix*, meaning a root. For many plants, if the root is left, the plant will regrow. In cancer terms, this is what the rapid blunt and incomplete dissection of the lymphovascular drainage of the rectum can result in.

Anterior resection was traditionally reserved for the 30–50% of patients in whom the rectal cancer was in the upper part of the rectum. Three important changes in surgical technique have made anterior resection the treatment of choice for 80–90% of all rectal cancer patients:

- the recognition that a margin of clearance of 2 cm of apparently uninvolved intestinal wall beyond the palpable edge of the growth (or possibly less) is adequate, instead of the 5 cm margin previously considered necessary;[6]
- the availability of stapling devices that enable the construction of a safe anastomosis as low as the top of the anal canal;[7]
- the appreciation that a thorough dissection and complete mobilization of the rectum and the cancer is necessary before deciding whether a sphincter-saving operation is possible.

From these changes has arisen the 'TME concept' that adenocarcinoma of the rectum is a supra levator compartment disease (Figure 19.2). The fundamental principle of TME is a precise, careful anatomical dissection in the embryological plane that exists between the mesorectum, derived from the dorsal mesentery, and the parietal presacral fascia. The resultant en bloc dissection of the rectum and its lymphatic drainage provides a radical resection with no roots left behind.

OPERATIVE TECHNIQUE OF TOTAL MESORECTAL EXCISION

The basic principles of TME consist of:

- peri-mesorectal 'holy plane'[8] sharp dissection with diathermy or scissors under direct vision (Figure 19.3);

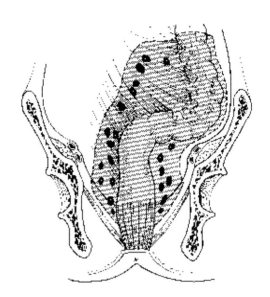

Figure 19.2 Our view of the lymphatic drainage superimposed on Miles' original drawing. It is now generally accepted that infra levator drainage of the rectum does not occur, and we believe that the majority of rectal cancers can be excised in a manner that allows preservation of the sphincter mechanism.

- specimen-orientated surgery, the objective of which is an intact mesorectum with no tearing of the surface and no circumferential margin involvement;
- recognition and preservation of the autonomic nerves on which sexual and bladder function depend;
- a major increase in sphincter preservation and reduction in the number of permanent colostomies.

A careful TME, together with a pouch-to-anus reconstruction, takes 3–5 hours, according to the detail of the patient's build and the particular cancer. In contrast, a traditional APE was often completed in 1 hour.

STEPWISE DESCRIPTION OF THE TECHNIQUE

Surgery should not commence without a bimanual examination under anaesthesia. This is especially important in the female, in order to establish whether the tumour is fully mobile on the posterior vaginal wall. The decision as to whether to excise a part of the posterior vaginal wall is made at this time

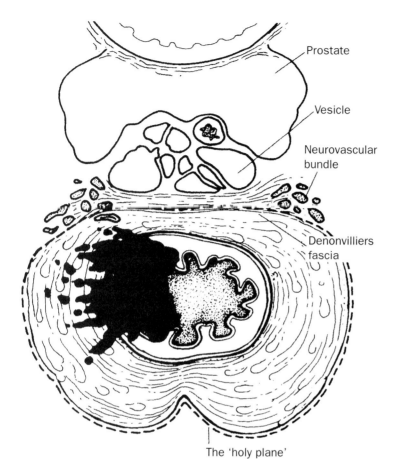

Figure 19.3 A schematic representation of the 'holy plane' in the male.

Prostate

Vesicle

Neurovascular bundle

Denonvilliers fascia

The 'holy plane'

by a combination of rectal and vaginal examination.

A midline incision is made from the pubis to within a few centimetres of the xiphisternum. The small bowel is carefully packed and retracted upwards and to the right. Surgery commences to the left of the sigmoid colon, with the operator standing on the left-hand side of the table. Optimal assistance involves forward three-dimensional traction to identify the plane between the back of the pedicle package and the gonadal vessels, ureter, and preaortic sympathetic nerves. The key to this phase is the recognition of the shiny fascial covered surface of the back of the pedicle with the inferior mesenteric vessels within.

The dissection is extended up to the top of the pedicle package, with separate high ligation of the inferior mesenteric artery and vein. The artery is taken 1–2 cm anterior to the aorta so as to spare the sympathetic nerve plexuses; the vein is divided above its last tributary close to the pancreas. These two high ligations are an integral part of the otherwise-avascular planes, which need to be fol-

lowed for a full mobilization of the splenic flexure.

The sigmoid colon and mesentery are divided well above the cancer (the 'division of convenience'). This is an important step, since complete mobility of the top of the specimen facilitates gentle opening of the peri-mesorectal planes throughout the pelvic dissection.

The areolar tissue of the 'holy plane' is demonstrated by gentle forward traction of the specimen, and dissection is commenced between the shiny posterior surface of the mesorectum and the superior hypogastric plexus as it bifurcates into the hypogastric nerves. Care must be taken to release the hypogastric nerves from the back of the mesorectum, allowing them to drop back onto the sacrum. This plane is extended downwards towards and beyond the tip of the coccyx. The condensation of fascia known as the rectosacral ligament may constitute an apparent barrier to downward progress, requiring positive division with scissors or diathermy. This poses one of the greatest dangers of blunt manual extraction, since the rectosacral ligament may be stronger than the surface fascia over the nodes – thus tearing into the lymphatic field is a real risk.

The plan is extended round to the sides to the so-called 'lateral ligaments'. These remain the subject of much controversy. The following account represents our view of the difficult anatomy in the anterolateral sector. The 'holy plane' is followed downwards and forwards towards the vesicles in the male and the vagina in the female, with the expanding plexiform band of inferior hypogastric plexus outside it but increasingly adherent to it. The key nerves entering this flattened band are the largely sympathetic hypogastric nerves curving distally from the superior plexuses and the 'erigent' parasympathetic nerves coming forwards to it from behind (Figure 19.4). These arise from the front of the roots of the sacral plexus (especially S3 out of sight behind the parietal sidewall fascia). Posteriorly, these 'erigent pillars' from S3 curve forwards outside the parietal fascia but medial to the branches of the internal iliac vessels. A little way behind the vesicles in the male, they pierce the fascia to join the plexus and often contribute nerve branches to the mesorectum and rectum. These 'neural T junctions' are the nearest structures to 'lateral ligaments' that the most careful surgeons will find with precise dissection.

Another structure to be defined by the surgeon during this lateral dissection is the middle rectal artery, which is usually nothing more than a tiny vessel easily obliterated by diathermy. Sato and Sato[9] have shown by careful anatomical studies in cadavers that a true middle rectal artery exists in less than 20% of patients. If one cones in too far medially, one comes across a mesorectal vessel, and if too far laterally, a pelvic sidewall vessel. Neither of these is a true middle rectal vessel, since neither is passing from internal iliac to rectum. It is our belief that most surgeons have in the past thus strayed either outwards into the plexus or inwards into the mesorectum, and created surgical artefacts, which they have called 'lateral ligaments' and 'middle rectal arteries'. If the cancer is actually adherent at this point then 'straying' outwards to the internal iliacs becomes justified, with inevitable damage to the nerve plexus. However, nerve damage can be avoided in the standard TME operation for most cancers.

Anterolaterally and anteriorly following the correct plane forwards will encompass the peritoneal reflection, which remains on the specimen and positively identifies the backs of the seminal vesicles in

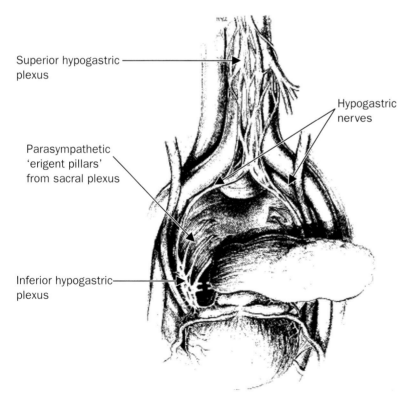

Figure 19.4 Illustration of pelvic nerves.

Superior hypogastric plexus

Hypogastric nerves

Parasympathetic 'erigent pillars' from sacral plexus

Inferior hypogastric plexus

the male and the posterior vaginal wall in the female. Forceful forward retraction on these with a St Mark's retractor will facilitate the development of the areolar space between the vesicles and the smooth front of the mesorectal specimen. We call this smooth surface, which is adherent to and clearly a part of the anterior mesorectum, 'Denonvillier's fascia'. As one works distally, there comes a point where this fascia must be divided transversely as it becomes adherent to the posterior capsule of the prostate. Particular care is necessary during this step to avoid damage to the neurovascular bundles that constitute the distal condensation of the inferior hypogastric plexuses. In a low anterior tumour, this can be exceedingly critical: it is essential to avoid exposing malignant tissue on the front of the specimen whilst the nerves are curving acutely medially.

The anatomy of the insertion of the mesorectal 'package' into the pelvic floor becomes difficult for the surgeon to grasp because of its inaccessibility behind the vesicles and prostate in the male. Careful pursuit of the plane at this level eventually liberates the mesorectal package and takes the operator down to a clean muscle tube, with the 'holy plane' at this level becoming the inter-sphincteric plane.

We use stapling instruments to perform a low anastomosis to the muscle tube and so avoid permanent colostomy. We have developed a preference for the use of a long narrow linear PI 30 stapler (US Surgical, Norwalk, CT) in place of the right-angled clamp (the 'Moran triple-stapling technique').[10] The first PI 30 staple line seals the muscle tube so that the anorectal lumen can be washed out with water as a cytocidal solution. The risk of incorporating viable exfoliated intraluminal cells in the second staple line is thus eliminated, and a second PI 30 is fired through washed bowel, which can then easily be divided between the retracted PI 30 staplers. Only this washed staple line remains within the patient. The first of these two linear staple lines should be safely clear of the palpable distal edge of the cancer. As Morson and others have pointed out, the palpable lower edge of a rectal cancer is usually, though not absolutely invariably, the microscopic edge (B Morson, 1999 personal communication). Downward spread along the muscle tube is not a significant factor in recurrence. A 2 cm clearance is more than adequate, and 1 cm plus the 'doughnut' is acceptable.[11] We routinely construct a stapled colon pouch using a GIA 60 (US Surgical) inserted 5 cm from the end of the fully mobilized colon to create a J pouch. The anvil of the CEEA 31 stapler (US Surgical) is inserted into the same colostomy, which is 'pursestringed' around the shaft. The circular stapler is inserted

transanally and connected to the anvil to form a stapled anastomosis. Care must be taken at this stage to avoid incorporating external sphincter or vagina in the anastomosis.

We perform a thorough abdominal and pelvic lavage using water as a cytocidal agent. We routinely drain the pelvis with two low-pressure suction drains. We protect all low anastomoses with either an anal stent or a defunctioning loop colostomy or ileostomy.

QUALITY CONTROL AND TME

Many quality-control variables can be studied with regard to rectal cancer surgery. Those that have received the most attention, and are probably the most important, are:

- overall survival,
- local recurrence,
- anastomotic leak rates,
- permanent stoma rates.

Morbidity in rectal cancer surgery also arises as a result of damage to the pelvic autonomic nerves, resulting in bladder and sexual dysfunction. Another key feature of quality control specific to TME is 'Quirke-style' histopathology to audit the quality of specimens, which will be discussed later.

Overall survival and local recurrence

Survival and local recurrence rates have been shown in many studies to vary widely between institutions and between surgeons within the same institutions.[12–14] The cure rate from colorectal cancer attributed to the UK by the Eurocare study is only 38%.[15] Similarly, rectal cancer has been reported to have a very high local recurrence rate, the values usually reported being of the order of 20% whether AR or APE is performed.[1] Most local recurrences occur within 2 years, and it seems likely that 'local recurrence' represents residual disease rather than recurrence per se. TME has resulted in the lowest published rates of local recurrence, and this in turn translates into improved long-term survival.[16]

The Basingstoke experience of total mesorectal excision

An update of the Basingstoke results was published in 1998.[16] Of 519 consecutive patients with adenocarcinoma of the rectum undergoing surgical treatment for cure or palliation, 465 (90%) had an AR, with 407

(78%) having a TME. In 58 (11%) patients with a high rectal tumour, circumferential margin resection is performed with trans-mesorectal transection at least 5 cm below the tumour. Of the remaining patients, 37 (7%) had an APE, 10 had a Hartmann's resection, 4 had a local resection and 3 had a laparotomy only. The cancer-specific survival rate of all surgically treated patients was 68% at 5 years and 66% at 10 years. The local recurrence rate was 6% (95% confidence interval, CI, 2–10%) at 5 years and 8% (95% CI 2–14%) at 10 years. In 405 'curative' resections (defined at operation as removal of all macroscopic disease at the time of surgery), the local recurrence rate was 3% (95% CI 0–5%) at 5 years and 4% (95% CI 0–8%) at 10 years. The disease-free survival rate in this group was 80% at 5 years and 78% at 10 years. An analysis of histopathological risk factors for recurrence indicated only the Dukes stage and extramural invasion as variables for systemic recurrence. Only extramural vascular invasion ($p < 0.001$) and Dukes stage ($p < 0.01$) were associated with a higher local recurrence rate. Dukes C cases have been reported to have a particularly high local recurrence rate (Bokey et al:[17] 22.6% hazard ratio 5.5, $p < 0.01$). In a recent analysis of our Dukes C patients, we have found that although lymph node involvement predicts local recurrence, AR with TME in high-risk node-positive cases can achieve local recurrence rates under 10% (Figure 19.5). If surgical priority is given to the difficult task of excision of the whole mesorectum, node status does not predict local recurrence, but remains a predictor of metastases and death. It may be that the local recurrence rate in node-positive disease

provides a useful audit tool for the quality of TME.

This reduction in local recurrence originally proposed by Heald has been achieved by other units adopting TME in the treatment of rectal cancer,[18] and other authors have reported similar low local recurrence rates and improved overall survival with TME.[18–20]

Anastomotic leak rates

Anastomotic leakage is a serious complication following rectal cancer. The lower the anastomoses (particularly below 6 cm), the higher the risk. In 1994, we reported a series of 219 patients with stapled low anastomoses.[21] There were 24 (11%) major leaks with peritonitis or pelvic collections and 14 (6.4%) radiological leaks. All of the major and 13 of the 14 radiological leaks occurred in patients with anastomoses below 6 cm. Other authors have demonstrated the increased risk of leakage for low anastomoses.[22,23] As mentioned above we now routinely use a short colonic J pouch. This has been found in a randomized study of straight versus colon J-pouch anastomosis to significantly reduce leak rates (2% versus 15% for straight; $p = 0.003$).[24] It is proposed that this may be due to a better blood supply in a side-to-end anastomosis, or possibly to the pouch filling the dead space in the pelvis and reducing the chance of pelvic collections. Using a colonic J pouch in conjunction with the Moran triple-stapling technique,[10] the combined clinical and radiological leak rate for our last 100 consecutive rectal

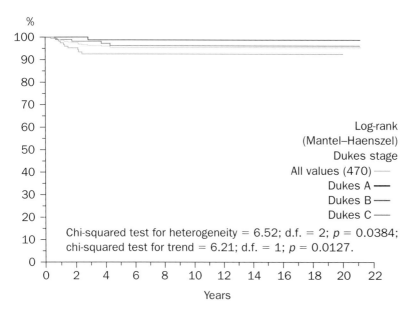

Figure 19.5 Local recurrence rates for Dukes stage in curative AR and TME.

cancers has dropped to 6%, a considerable improvement on our earlier report.

Permanent colostomies

Permanent colostomy rates for rectal cancer vary from 10% to 40% in different series.[25] An important benefit of TME is a marked reduction in the permanent colostomy rate.[3] In our series mentioned above, only 7% of patients with rectal cancer had an APE. Using precise TME combined with the Moran triple-stapling technique,[10] we have found that in over three-quarters of patients with low rectal cancers, sphincter preservation is possible.[3]

Sexual function

Damage to the autonomic nerves during surgery can result in impairment of sexual function. Enker[26] has reviewed several series looking at sexual dysfunction following AR and APE, with impotence occurring in between 25% and 100% of patients. In series with selected patients in whom the autonomic pelvic nerves have been preserved, 80–95% of patients retain sexual function.[26,27] In Basingstoke, we have undertaken a postal survey of all our male rectal cancer patients, regardless of whether we were able to preserve the autonomic nerves at surgery, and found that 70–80% of the functions of erection, ejaculation, penetration, and orgasm are being preserved in those who were active prior to surgery. Age appears to be a predictor of retaining sexual function, with four-fifths of patients under 60 years being active but only three-fifths of patients over 60 remaining active following TME. Clearly, this highlights an important issue that needs to be discussed with patients prior to and following surgery.

THE SURGEON AND THE PATHOLOGIST: 'SPECIMEN-ORIENTATED SURGERY'

The surgical objective in rectal cancer is to produce an intact specimen, with the cancer safely surrounded by the mesorectum, a concept termed 'specimen-orientated surgery'. When 'specimen-orientated surgery' has become the established practice in a unit, the recognition of the features of the TME specimen and the freedom of its margins from cancer involvement become a key factor of audit. In most cases, naked-eye inspection by the surgeon provides the necessary quality control, with further microscopic examination

of the suspected areas of margin involvement being provided by the pathologist.

The surgeon

The optimum TME cancer package consists of an adequate proximal and distal margin of bowel from the tumour (as discussed above). A tapering vascular pedicle at the top of the specimen leads down to the posterior globular, bilobed, lymphovascular mesorectal expansion. The surface of this should be smooth and regular, with no evidence of the surgeon having accidentally breached the mesorectum. Visual inspection of the front of a well-performed TME specimen shows three clear landmarks:

- the cut edge of the peritoneal reflection;
- Denonvillier's fascia, the smooth shiny surface on the anterior mesorectum of the middle third of the rectum;
- the almost-bare anterior aspect of the anorectal muscle in the ultralow anterior resection.

The histopathologist

The pathologist has an important role in the quality control of the TME procedure. Quirke has shown that tumour involvement of the circumferential resection margin (CRM) is highly specific and sensitive in predicting local tumour recurrence.[28] He describes a histological method for examining the rectal cancer specimen, in which transverse slices are taken through the specimen, allowing macroscopic and microscopic assessment of depth of tumour invasion, mesorectal involvement, and circumferential margin involvement. This technique was used to assess 194 patients, of whom 69 (36%) had involvement of the CRM on histopathological examination. These patients were followed prospectively, and 44 developed local recurrence – thus CRM involvement predicted recurrence in 64%. They also compared patients having curative and non-curative operations, and found that, of 141 curative operations, 35 (25%) patients had CRM involvement and 23 of these developed local recurrence (66%). By contrast, only 8% developed local recurrence in the CRM-negative group. Thus, for patients with a curative resection with negative CRM, 90% avoided local recurrence, whereas only 22% of patients with positive CRM were free of local recurrence at 5 years.[29] In examining a wide range of specimens from a wide range of surgeons Quirke[30] notes that 'the most frequent problem is the irregular margin where the surgeon has accidentally left an area of mesorectum behind or lost the plane and cut inwards towards the muscularis propria before finding the correct plane again'. In some of the worse specimens that he has examined, it is possible to see the muscularis propria forming the CRM, which can account for local recurrence after Dukes A tumours.[30] Others have shown similar results,[31–33] with CRM predicting poor outcome. The pathologist can thus help to audit the adequacy of the surgery, which determines the overall outcome for the patient.

SUMMARY

At the start of the new millennium, it is TME that should replace APE as the gold standard to which all other operations must be compared in the treatment of rectal cancer. Whilst clearly the ultimate audit of TME lies in outcome measures such as local recurrence and overall survival, the surgeon is able at the time of surgery to assess the quality of the specimen achieved. This macroscopic assessment is complemented by the pathologist providing feedback as to the adequacy of margins of clearance achieved by the surgeon.

REFERENCES

1. Abulafi AM, Williams N, Local recurrence of colorectal cancer: the problem, mechanisms, management and adjuvant therapy. *Br J Surg* 1994; **81**: 7–19.
2. Heald RJ, Husband EM, Ryall RD, The mesorectum in rectal cancer surgery – the clue to pelvic recurrence? *Br J Surg* 1982; **69**: 613–16.
3. Heald RJ, Smedh RK, Kald A et al, Abdomino-perineal excision of the rectum – an endangered operation. Norman Nigro Lectureship. *Dis Colon Rectum* 1997; **40**: 747–51.
4. Murray JJ, Veidenheimer MC, Abdomino-perineal excision of the rectum. In: *Rob & Smiths's Operative Surgery: Surgery of the Colon and Anus*, 5th edn (Fielding L, Golding S, eds). Oxford: Butterworth–Heinemann, 1993: 472–8.
5. Miles E, *Cancer of the Rectum.* Harrison & Sons. 1923.
6. Williams NS, Dixon MF, Johnston D, Reappraisal of the 5 cm rule of distal excision for carcinoma of the rectum: a study of distal intramural spread and of patients' survival. *Br J Surg* 1983; **70**: 150–4.
7. Moran BJ, Stapling instruments for intestinal anastomosis in colorectal surgery. *Br J Surg* 1996; **83**: 902–9.
8. Heald RJ, The 'Holy Plane' of rectal surgery. *J R Soc Med* 1988; **81**: 503–8.
9. Sato K, Sato T, The vascular and neuronal composition of the lateral ligament of the rectum and the retrosacral fascia. *Surg Radiol Anat* 1991; **13**: 17–22.
10. Moran BJ, Docherty A, Finnis D, Novel stapling technique to facilitate low anterior resection for rectal cancer. *Br J Surg* 1994; **81**: 1230.
11. Karanjia ND, Schache DJ, North WR, Heald RJ, 'Close shave' in anterior resection. *Br J Surg* 1990; **77**: 510–12.
12. Fielding LP, Stewart-Brown S, Blesovsky L, Kearney G, Anastomotic integrity after operations for large bowel cancer; a multicentre study.*BMJ* 1980; **281**: 411–14.
13. McArdle CS, Hole D, Impact of variability amongst surgeons on postoperative morbidity and mortality and ultimate survival. *BMJ* 1991; **302**: 1501–5.
14. Hermanek P, Wiebelt H, Stimmer D, Riedl S, The German Study Group for colorectal cancer. Prognostic factors of rectal cancer – experience of the German multicentre study SGCRC. *Tumori* 1995; **81**: 60–4.
15. Berrıno F, Sant M, Verdecchia A et al (eds), *Survival of Cancer Patients in Europe, the Eurocare Study.* Lyon: International Agency for Research on Cancer, 1995.
16. Heald RJ, Moran BJ, Ryall RDH et al, Rectal cancer: the Basingstoke experience of total mesorectal excision, 1978–1997. *Arch Surg* 1998; **133**: 894–9.
17. Bokey EL, Ojerskog B, Chapuis PH et al, Local recurrence after curative excision of the rectum for cancer without adjuvant therapy: role of total anatomical dissection. *Br J Surg* 1999; **86**: 1164–70.
18. Arbman G, Nilsson E, Hallbook O, Sjodahl R, Local recurrence following total mesorectal excision for rectal cancer. *Br J Surg* 1996; **83**: 375–9.
19. Dixon AR, Maxwell WA, Holmes JT, Carcinoma of the rectum: a 10-year experience. *Br J Surg* 1991; **78**: 308–11.
20. Enker WE, Thaler HT, Cranor ML, Polyak T, Total mesorectal excision in the operative treatment of carcinoma of the rectum. *J Am Coll Surg* 1995; **181**: 335–46.
21. Karanjia ND, Corder AP, Bearn P, Heald RJ, Leakage from stapled low anastomosis after total mesorectal excision for carcinoma of the rectum. *Br J Surg* 1994; **81**: 1224–6.
22. Vignali A, Fazio V, Lavery IC, Factors associated with the occurrence of leaks in stapled rectal anastomoses. *J Am Coll Surg* 1997; **185**: 113–15.
23. Rulier E, Laurent C, Risk factors for anastomotic leakage after resection in rectal cancer. *Br J Surg* 1998; **85**: 335–58.
24. Hallbook O, Pahlman L, Krog M, Randomised comparison of straight and colonic J pouch anastomosis after low anterior resection. *Ann Surg* 1996; **224**: 58–65.
25. Braithwaite BD, Scholefield JH, How does surgical technique affect outcomes in rectal cancer? In: *Challenges in Colorectal Cancer* (Scholefield JH, ed). Oxford: Blackwell Science, 2000: 39–47.
26. Enker WE, Potency, cure, and local control in the operative treatment of rectal cancer. *Arch Surg* 1992; **127**: 1396–401.
27. Masui H, Ike H, Yamaguchi S et al, Male sexual function after autonomic nerve-preserving operation for rectal cancer. *Dis Colon Rectum* 1996; **39**: 1140–5.
28. Quirke P, Durdey P, Dixon MF, Williams NS, Local recurrence of rectal adenocarcinoma due to inadequate surgical resection. Histopathological study of lateral tumour spread and surgical excision. *Lancet* 1986; **ii**: 996–9.
29. Adam IJ, Mohamdee MO, Martin IG, Quirke P, Role of circumferential margin involvement in the local recurrence of rectal cancer. *Lancet* 1994; **344**: 707–11.
30. Quirke P, Limitations of existing systems of staging for rectal cancer, the forgotten margin. In: *Rectal Cancer Research*. Berlin: Springer-Verlag, 1996: 63–81.
31. Cawthorn SJ, Gibbs NM, Marks CG, Clearance technique for detection of lymph nodes in colorectal cancer. *Br J Surg* 1986; **73**: 58–60.
32. de Haas-Kock DF, Baeten CG, Jager JJ, Prognostic significance of radial margins of clearance in rectal cancer. *Br J Surg* 1996; **83**: 781–5.
33. Shepherd NA, Baxter KJ, Love SB, The prognostic importance of peritoneal involvement in colonic cancer: a prospective evaluation. *Gastroenterology* 1997; **112**: 1096–102.

20

Conservative treatment in rectal cancer

Philippe Lasser, Ali Goharin

INTRODUCTION

Local curative treatments for rectal cancer run up against the dogmas of classical cancer surgery, which consider the best treatment to be excision of the affected organ and of the various lymph-node relays dependent on that organ. Effectively, this approach deals only with the tumour, totally disregarding the lymph-node problem. It overlooks possible lymph-node invasion.

Local approaches have a double advantage over classical resection surgery, in that they are less mutilating, especially for lower rectal cancer (avoiding a definitive colostomy), and they are less shocking to the patient. On the other hand, they are subject to local recurrences, which may appear at the tumour site if the resection has been incomplete, or at an undetected and untreated invaded mesorectal lymph node. Indications for these local treatments must be rigorous. Several types of local treatment can be applied.

- *Local excision or resection of the tumour.* This has a great advantage over the other techniques, in that it supplies a specimen for examination by the pathologist, who will be in a position to evaluate the possibility of lymph-node invasion based on a number of histopathological prognostic factors.
- *Destruction of the tumour by radiotherapy (contact therapy), electrocoagulation, laser treatment, or cryosurgery.* These techniques merely destroy the tumour; therefore one cannot accurately assess its in-depth infiltration and make any predictions regarding the risk of lymph-node invasion.

LOCAL RESECTION

Surgical techniques

Several approaches can be used for local resection.

The endoanal (or transanal approach
Two types of local excisions can be performed.[1–4]

- *Submucous excision.* After infiltrating the submucosa with an adrenalized saline solution, the mucosa and submucosa are incised with a scalpel 1 cm from the lower pole of the tumour, until the muscularis is reached. The resection will thus be performed from bottom to top, by gradually lifting the tumour and freeing it from the muscular plane. On the periphery, resection limits must allow for a safety margin of 1 cm. Haemostasis is achieved with an electric scalpel. The surgical wound can be sutured with separate stitches or left open without any risk.
- *Transmural excision (entire rectal wall).* The principle of the resection is the same as above, but it is deeper, affecting the entire thickness of the rectal wall. The perirectal fat is exposed and the rectal muscularis is totally resected. The rectal tumour on its base is referred to the anatomopathologist. Closing the surgical wound is recommended by many surgeons, to avoid infection and secondary haemorrhage, but it is not always feasible. Some surgeons[5–7] electrocoagulate the tumour site extensively to complete haemostasis and to destroy any possible residual tumour.

Excision of the entire rectal wall can only be applied to lower located subdouglasian tumours to avoid peritoneal perforation, and to tumours located on the posterior and lateral surfaces. When the lesion is located on the anterior surface, there is a risk of perforation of the rectovaginal wall in women and a risk of urethral lesions in men. This local resection can be performed with microscopic instruments in a technique called transanal endoscopic microsurgery (TEM), developed by German surgeons.[8]

Other approaches

- *Kraske's retroanal or transsacral route.*[9] The patient is placed in the prone position after section of the anococcygeal body, the coccyx, and finally the last sacral pieces, and the rectum is approached on its posterior face. Incision of the mesorectum and of the rectal wall provides an excellent opening on the anterior and lateral faces.
- The same applies to *York Masson's posterior transsphincteral route*[10] *(posterior anorectomy)*, which involves the total section of the sphincter.

Posterior approach routes are preferable, since they allow exploration of the mesorectum, and the discovery of undetected lymph-node involvement during preoperative examinations. However, they are subject to the formation of rectal fistulas (in 15% of cases),[11] and a temporary colostomy is advisable to avoid this. Kraske's route does not provide an adequate opening for tumours located 6–10 cm up. The endoanal route, therefore, appears preferable to us.

Operating mortality is practically nil according to the various series of publications. Morbidity essentially consists of the falling off of eschars (around postoperative day 5 or 6), which sometimes necessitates repeat surgery. In the Gall and Hermanek series,[1] out of 69 local resections (16 submucous excisions, 31 excisions of the entire wall, and 22 excisions by the transsphincteral route), there were 13 complications necessitating new operations (9%). In the Mentges et al[8] study, the rate of complications requiring surgical reintervention after TEM was 8 out of 113 patients with carcinoma (7%). One might occasionally note the remote development of a variously extensive arc-shaped adhesion, the importance of which depends on the extent of local resection. It rarely hinders transit, and may be sectioned if too extensive.

The tumour, resting on its base, is totally resected, preferably without fragmentation, and is then placed on cork before it is referred to the pathologist, who will evaluate a certain number of prognostic factors, as described by Morson:[12]

- *the degree of parietal infiltration*, using the UICC pTNM classification, which is more precise than Dukes or Aster–Coller: T1 is a tumour invading the mucosa and the submucosa, T2 is a tumour invading the muscularis propria, and T3 is a tumour invading through the muscularis propria into the subserosa;
- *the degree of malignancy* of the tumour, as initially evaluated on preoperative biopsies; local resection is of no benefit in the case of a poorly differentiated tumour;

- *the safety margin*, by making several cuts.

Prognostic factors

What are the macroscopic and anatomopathological features that can be used to determine whether a rectal tumour can benefit from local treatment? They should help in identifying patients without lymph-node invasion.

Macroscopic criteria
Tumour size
Is there a maximum diameter above which local resection is not recommended? What is the relationship between size and risk of lymph-node invasion? Although a smaller tumour will be more amenable to local resection, the diameter of the tumour does not provide information on its in-depth extension. The concept of a 'small tumour' relates to the size of the tumour, and not to its in-depth extension. British and American authors call cancers limited to the submucosa 'early carcinomas'.

In studying the local recurrence rate according to tumour diameter, Killingback[13] notes that among 36 patients, a 12.5% local-recurrence rate was observed in patients with a tumour diameter of less than 3.5 cm, as opposed to a rate of 33% when the diameter was larger than 3.5 cm. This difference, however, was not statistically significant. Most authors estimate that only tumours less than 3 cm in diameter should be resected.

It may be concluded that tumour size is not a major prognostic factor, but a diameter of less than 3 cm seems to be the maximum reasonable size when considering a local resection, since if a 1 cm safety margin is to be preserved around the tumour, the diameter of the surgical wound will be 5 cm. If a larger tumour is involved, the chances are that the minimal safety margin will not be adhered to, which might account for a higher rate of local recurrence.

Macroscopic features of the tumour
Exophytic tumours are only weakly penetrating, as opposed to ulcerated tumours, which show more-rapid in-depth extension. The lymph-node metastasis rate is higher when the tumour is ulcerated than when it is budding.[13,14] However, the ulcerated character of a tumour is not a contraindication to local treatment.[15]

Anatomopathological criteria
Degree of in-depth infiltration of the tumour
This is one of the major factors when considering local treatment. Although the degree of infiltration

can only be determined exactly after resection, a good estimate can be obtained from the preoperative endoscopic sonography and digital examination. Local treatment cannot be evaluated correctly unless the tumour is totally excised. The excision must then remain limited to the wall and not go beyond the muscularis. The risk of lymph-node invasion is closely related to parietal invasion, and is present as soon as the cancer goes beyond the muscularis mucosae.

Three studies[16–18] (Table 20.1) have attempted to evaluate, after 'classical' surgery (low anterior resection or abdominoperineal resection), the risk of lymph-node invasion in relation to parietal invasion for tumours limited to the rectal wall. Thus the local resection of a T1 or T2 tumour may overlook a lymph-node invasion in 12% of T1 tumours (submucosa) and 19% of T2 tumours (muscularis propria). These figures are slightly higher than or comparable to those of Morson et al,[7] which were 11% lymphnode invasion for T1 tumours and 12% for T2 tumours, and those of Hager et al,[2] with 8% for T1 and 17% for T2.

Histopathological differentiation

Tumours are classified into three grades of malignancy according to their degree of differentiation: well-differentiated (grade 1), moderately differentiated (grade 2), and poorly differentiated (grade 3). Some authors add a fourth grade for undifferentiated tumours. The less differentiated the tumour, the higher is the risk of lymph-node invasion. Morson[19] shows a risk of lymph-node invasion of 25% for grade 1 tumours, 50% for grade 2, and 80% for grade 3. This does not take into account the in-depth extension of the tumour. Morson[19] states that the poorly differentiated character of the tumour is a formal contraindication to local treatment, whatever its size and in-depth penetration.

Locke et al,[20] reporting the St Mark's Hospital (London) experience from 1948 to 1984, uphold local resection for well-differentiated (grade 1) tumours, but this technique is inadvisable when the tumour is of intermediate grade (2) or worse (grade 3 or 4). Tanaka et al,[21] in a group of 81 tumours classified as T1, show a risk of lymph-node invasion of 4% for grade 1 tumours and 14% for grade 2.

It may be concluded that one must take into account the histological differentiation of the tumour before considering local resection. All authors agree to eliminate poorly differentiated (grade 3) or undifferentiated (grade 4) tumours. There is no consensus concerning moderately differentiated tumours (grade 2). Serious problems are posed by this type of classification and by the different interpretations by pathologists. Seventy percent of tumours show different differentiation characteristics according to location, and although it is easy to classify tumours in extreme groups (grades 1 and 4), the same does not apply to intermediate groups. Finally, it must be emphasized that the limitations of tumour biopsies do not permit predictions as to the exact histological type. For tumours with a high grade of malignancy, there is only a 40% concordance between biopsy data and thorough examination of the tumour. This shows the importance of a meticulous anatomopathological examination of the entire resection piece for a precise classification.

Other anatomopathological factors

Several authors[1,5,19] have emphasized the negative prognosis of mucinous cancers, which account for 10–20% of rectal cancers, but the published series do not include many of these cases, and it is difficult to draw any definite conclusions regarding the prognosis of these tumours.

More recently, pathologists have emphasized the presence or absence of tumour cells in the lymphatic vessels (lymphatic vessel invasion, LVI) or blood vessels (blood vessel invasion, BVI), although it is often difficult to determine exactly whether it is blood vessels or lymphatic vessels that have been invaded. According to Gall and Hermanek,[1] detection of

Table 20.1 Lymph-node metastasis when the tumour is limited to the rectal wall			
Series	**No. of patients**	**T1 stage**	**T2 stage**
Huddy et al[16]	109	11% (3/27)	23% (19/82)
Lasser et al[17]	123	15% (4/26)	16% (16/97)
Blumberg et al[18]	159	10% (5/48)	17% (19/111)
Total	391	12% (12/101)	19% (54/290)

tumour cells in vessels implies classification of the patient in the high-risk group comparable with poorly differentiated or undifferentiated tumours, and such patients should not receive local treatment. In the Blumberg et al[18] study, tumours were stratified into two groups based on the presence or absence of adverse pathological features (grade, LVI, and BVI): a low-risk group (grade 1 or 2, LVI−BVI−) and a high-risk group (grade 3, LVI+BVI+). High-risk patients had virtually the same lymph-node metastasis rate irrespective of T stage (33% for T1 versus 30% for T2). Low-risk patients with T1 tumours had a 7% rate of lymph-node metastasis, compared with a 14% rate for low-risk patients with T2 tumours (Table 20.2).

The same goes for perinervous tumour sheathing, which is a much more important pathological factor. It is an independent and negative prognostic factor.

Importance of resection margin

Local excision of rectal cancer is acceptable only when tumour resection can be complete and when the risk of lymph-node invasion is minimal.[1] Morson and colleagues[7] have demonstrated the prognostic importance of the resection margin following local resection. They single out three different types of resection: complete resection, incomplete resection (where the resection margin is invaded by tumour), and dubious or uncertain resection (when the pathologist detects tumour cells inside the coagulated peripheral tissues). In a group of 119 patients treated with local resection at St Mark's Hospital, London, they studied the relationship between the local-recurrence and 5-year survival rates and the type of resection (Table 20.3).

Willet et al[22] noted a local-recurrence rate of 33% when the margin was invaded, 15% when the margin was free of tumour, and 9% when resection limits could not be evaluated. Graham et al[23] found a rate of 6% when resection was complete, compared with 52% when resection was incomplete. In our study,[6] the local recurrence rate was zero in 28 patients

---

Table 20.2 Risk of lymph-node metastasis according to pathological factors[18]

Group	All	T1 stage	T2 stage
Low-risk	11% (15/130)	7% (3/42)	14% (12/88)
High-risk	31% (9/29)	33% (2/6)	30% (7/33)

Table 20.3 Risk of recurrence and survival versus resection quality[7]

Quality of local resection	No. of patients	Recurrence rate (%)	Overall 5-year survival rate (%)	Corrected 5-year survival rate[a] (%)
Complete	91	3 (3/91)	82	100
Dubious	14	14 (2/14)	64	96
Incomplete	14	36 (5/14)	57	83
Total	119	8 (10/119)		

[a]Excluding patients who died from causes other than their cancer.

classified as T1, when resection was complete (24 cases) or incomplete (4 cases); while in 11 patients classified as T2, the local recurrence rate with complete resection was zero (7 cases), compared with 50% when resection was incomplete (2/4).

Considering the artefacts secondary to electrocoagulation, one cannot overlook the problems that pathologists face in evaluating the quality of resection. Only highly trained pathologists can adequately classify the quality of resection in the uncertain or dubious group.

Local resection of rectal cancer must be considered only when excision of the tumour can be complete and when the risk of lymph-node invasion is minimal. As previously shown, the risk of lymph-node invasion depends on the degree of tumour wall penetration and the histological differentiation grade. These factors can be evaluated adequately only after complete anatomopathological examination of the resected piece.

Analysis of published data

Local resection alone (Table 20.4)

When the tumour is limited to the submucosa (T1) – grade 1 or 2 – the local-recurrence rate ranges from 0% to 13% and the 5-year survival rate from 90% to 100%. When the tumour invades the muscularis without going beyond (T2) – grade 1 or 2 – the local-recurrence rate ranges from 17% to 44% and the 5-year survival rate from 78% to 82%. Results from

the series of Hager et al[2] are shown in Table 20.5. This clearly shows the importance of in-depth invasion when the tumour is well or moderately differentiated. When the resection is complete, the local recurrence rate is 8% for T1 tumours and 17% for T2 tumours. The metastasis rate is 3% for T1 and 6% for T2. The cancer-related death rate is 0% for T1 and 11% for T2. The 5-year survival rate is 89.6% for T1 and 78% for T2. In this series, 36 patients had a T3 tumour, or a grade 3 or 4 tumour, or an invaded margin, or lymphatic or vascular emboli; Hager et al[2] noted a 24% local-recurrence rate, a 39% cancer-related death rate, and a 15% metastasis rate.

Most authors[27,28] agree in singling out pT1 tumours of grades 1 or 2, LVI−BVI− as the ideal indication for local resection. A randomized study,[29] including 50 patients, compared TEM and anterior resection for T1 tumours, grade 1 or 2. The local-recurrence rate (4%) and the 5-year survival rate (96%) were similar in both groups (24 patients versus 26 patients).

Most authors[27,28] agree in formally contraindicating local resection in T3 tumours or in T1 and T2 tumours with a high-grade malignancy (grade 3). The discussion remains open regarding T2 tumours with a low malignancy grade. In this group, many authors propose postoperative radiotherapy after local resection.

Local resection and postoperative radiotherapy

To reduce and even avoid local recurrence after local resection, a number of authors have proposed

Table 20.4 Literature review: results regarding local resection alone

Series	No. of patients	Invasion level			Local recurrence rate (%)	5-year disease-free survival rate (%)
		T1	**T2**	**T3**		
Morson et al[7]	142	115	20	7	10	93
Whiteway et al[15]	33	12	16	5	12	88
Stearns et al[24]	33	12	16	5	12	84
Killingback et al[13]	34	0	28	6	23	82
Willett et al[22]	29	20	5	4	15	77
Decosse et al[5]	57	25	29	3	—	83
Lasser et al[6]	44	28	15	1	7.5	88
Cuthbertson and Simpson[25]	28	16	12	0	21	100
Biggers et al[26]	234	93	141	0	19	65

Table 20.5 Five-year survival according to T stage in patients with well-differentiated or moderately well-differentiated tumours[2]

Details	Group 1 (T1)	Group 2 (T2)
No. of patients	39	18
Local recurrence rate (%)	8 (3/39)	17 (3/18)
Metastasis rate (%)	3 (1/39)	6 (1/18)
Cancer-related death rate (%)	0	11 (2/18)
5-year survival rate (%)	89.6	78

postoperative radiotherapy for T2 tumours or T1 tumours with adverse pathological factor (grade 2, LVI+BVI+, invaded margin).

The usual doses are around 45 Gy on the entire pelvis, associated with an overdose at the tumour-site level (a total of 60 Gy). Radiotherapy may often be combined with chemotherapy (5-fluorouracil (5-FU) plus leucovorin (folinic acid)). The local recurrence rates reported in the literature for T2 tumours are in the range 0–24%. Results of local resection with postoperative radiotherapy are shown in Table 20.6. Willet et al[22] compared two groups of patients – 40 without radiotherapy and 26 with postoperative radiotherapy – and reported that when the margin was invaded, there was a 33% local-recurrence rate in the first group and a 0% rate in the second group (but the latter included only 6 patients). Chakravarti et al,[37] in a non-randomized study, compared 52 patients with local resection alone and 47 patients with local resection combined with postoperative radiotherapy (26 patients had 5-FU chemotherapy). For T2 tumours, adjuvant radiotherapy reduces the local-recurrence rate at 5 years (33% versus 85%) and improves outcomes in patients with high-risk pathological features, but has no benefit for T1 tumours. Radiotherapy can be proposed for T2 tumours when complementary surgery cannot be performed.

This postoperative radiotherapy is not free from complications. For doses of 53 Gy, McCready et al[38] observed a 29% rate of postoperative complications. These consisted of fistulas in 17% of cases (local excision was performed by the posterior route) and local infection in 12%. Rich et al[39] reported a 50% rate of haemorrhagic rectitis with doses above 60 Gy, but only 6% with doses below 60 Gy.

It may be concluded that the role of postoperative radiotherapy alone or combined with chemotherapy is not yet clearly defined.[40] The series reported in the literature are not homogeneous and the doses delivered are unequal. These adjuvant treatments apply to some T3 tumours that cannot benefit from local resection. Adjuvant radiotherapy can be justified for high-risk T1 tumours (adverse pathological factors) and for low-risk T2 tumours. It might be indicated for certain T2 tumours when their resection is incomplete (invaded margins), or when complementary surgery is risky or an abdominoperineal resection is refused. To define clearly the role of postoperative radiotherapy, it should be possible to perform a randomized therapeutic trial, but this seems hard to achieve, in view of the low number of patients who could benefit from local resection.

Validation of the technique and early screening

This technique applies to few patients. At St Mark's Hospital, London, from 1948 to 1972, 3999 rectal cancers were treated, and only 143 patients (3.6%) had total local resection.[7] The indications for this technique have gradually increased; it was used in only 1.4% of all cases from 1948 to 1952, but this rate went up to 7.5% of all cases from 1968 to 1972.

Local resection of rectal cancer is performed in two steps. First, tumours suitable for local treatment are selected, and then the rationale for this treatment is confirmed after resection and by complete anatomopathological examination of the specimen. Justification for local treatment is based on the quality of resection, the in-depth extension of the tumour, and the degree of histological differentiation. Patients who do not meet the criteria for complete resection should be submitted for further surgery.

Table 20.6 Literature review: results regarding local resection combined with postoperative radiotherapy

Series	No. of patients	Radiotherapy (Gy)	Local-recurrence rate (%)		
			T1	T2	T3
Steele et al[30]	15	45	0 (0/5)	0 (0/10)	—
Jessup et al[31]	12	45	—	0 (0/12)	—
Ota et al[32]	46	45	0 (0/16)	7 (1/15)	20 (3/15)
Minsky et al[33]	??	47	0 (0/4)	17 (2/12)	33 (2/6)
Willett et al[34]	21	45	11 (1/9)	17 (2/12)	—
Wagman et al[35]	39	46	0 (0/6)	24 (6/25)	25 (2/8)
Bouvet et al[36]	65	45	5	20	27

Selection of tumours

- *Digital rectal examination:* local resection must apply to tumors that are easily accessible through digital rectal examination. This is the best way to select tumours. It allows evaluation of the tumour site, the macroscopic character of the tumour, and its mobility in relation to adjacent structures, and makes it possible to look for suspicious lymph nodes in the mesorectum.[41] Digital examination, however, does not permit differentiation between submucous invasion and muscularis invasion. As far as the presence of lymph-node invasion is concerned, digital examination is reliable only half of the time. It may be performed under anaesthesia when examination of the patient proves difficult.
- *Endorectal echography* makes it possible to eliminate any tumours that have extended beyond the muscularis (T3) and any other tumours associated with suspicious lymph nodes in the mesorectum.
- *Preoperative biopsy* makes it possible to accurately evaluate the histological type and degree of differentiation of the tumour, since an accurate classification can only be achieved through examination of the resected piece.

Neither the pelvic scanner nor nuclear magnetic resonance imaging (MRI) are of use for tumour selection. Lymphoscintigraphy has not yet demonstrated its usefulness. Digital rectal examination, endoscopy with biopsy, and endorectal echography allow the selection of tumours for local resection:

- mobile tumours, located at the lower third of the rectum, and with a diameter less than or equal to 3 cm without any palpable or suspicious lymph nodes;
- tumours that do not extend beyond the rectal muscularis, well or moderately differentiated, and ideally located on the posterior or lateral faces.

Local resection is then performed, and the surgeon waits for anatomopathological findings; the patient is advised of the possibility of new surgery should conditions for local resection prove unsatisfactory. Thus the rate of complementary surgery following resection varies according to authors and to initial selection criteria (9–17%).[23] This complementary surgery must be performed if a T3 tumour is involved or in the event of unfavourable prognostic factors (grade 3, LVI+BVI+, perinervous tumoral sheathing), whatever the degree of parietal invasion (T), and finally if resection is incomplete in pT2 tumours. There is no consensus concerning T2 tumours with complete local resection. Some authors will trust surgery alone, while others will perform complementary surgery, and others postoperative radiotherapy. The decision is then conditioned by the age and the general status of the patients, and in the case of non-acceptance of a possible colostomy.

Local resection will be performed alone (absolute indication) if resection is complete in T1 tumours, grade 1 or 2, LVI−BVI− without any complementary treatment.

The decision-making procedure regarding treatment following local resection is summarized in Figure 20.1.

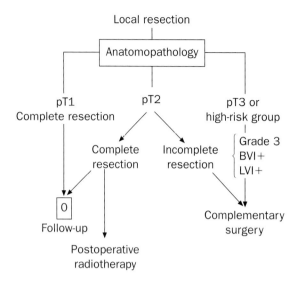

Figure 20.1 Algorithm for deciding on further treatment following local resection.

Follow-up

Local resection of a rectal tumour can only be considered if patients submit to strict follow-up. Salvage surgery following local recurrence will be possible only following an early diagnosis. Graham et al[23] noted a 24% local-recurrence rate following local treatment, with only a 42% rate of complementary salvage surgery (22–100% in the literature). This low rate of complementary surgery can be explained by the lax follow-up and the type of recurrence (lymph-node metastasis in the mesorectum with silent evolution and late diagnosis, and with ineradicable sacral fixation). Gall and Hermanek[1] performed curative complementary surgery in only five cases out of nine (55%).

Patients must be examined every 3 months in the first 2 years, and then every 6 months for the next 5 years. In addition to digital rectal examination and complete clinical examination, an endoscopy, an endorectal echography, and a thoracic radiography should be performed. Should there be the slightest doubt, an examination under anaesthesia should be performed, with deep biopsies. Patients who cannot be adequately followed up will not benefit from local treatment.

CONTACT THERAPY

This treatment, like others (such as electrocoagulation and cryotherapy) that destroy the tumour, does not permit an anatomopathological examination.

Contact therapy has chiefly been developed and used in Lyon by Papillon and colleagues.[42,43]

Technique

The therapy is applied with a Philips RT 50 (50 kV, 12 mA) instrument. The localizer has a diameter of 30 mm at its end, and can slide in a rectoscope. The patient is placed in a genupectoral position, and local anaesthesia of the sphincter is sufficient. The treatment is applied by the radiotherapist alone or assisted by a gastroenterologist, to avoid tube displacement during the treatment. The irradiation time is brief: 1–3 minutes for an output of 20–40 Gy[42,43] or 50 Gy.[44]

Papillon and colleagues give four sessions, spread over 4 weeks with ambulatory patients. The time between sessions makes it possible to assess tumour development during the first 3 weeks, i.e. after two radiotherapy sessions. Some tumours on day 21 are not altered by radiotherapy; they remain indurated and ulcerated, indicating extensive parietal infiltration. In such cases, they cannot be treated by radiotherapy alone, and radical surgery must be performed. It is the third-week test that shows the radiosensitivity of the cancer. Papillon and colleagues make an iridium implantation with a two-tined fork, 1 month after termination of contact therapy, delivering an additional 20–30 Gy at the tumour-site level.

Results

The outstanding series of Papillon and colleagues is reported in Table 20.7.[42] Of the 233 patients cured at year 5, 228 (97%) had normal anal function. There were 14 cases (4.5%) of local recurrence, and 12 cases (3.8%) of lymph-node failure. Of these 26 patients, 7 were saved by salvage therapy.

Among the other series reported in the literature, we may quote Sischy et al[45] (Rochester, NY); after treating 192 patients with contact therapy, with a follow-up of 1–14 years, they find a local-recurrence rate of 6%, and their 5-year survival rate is identical to that of Papillon and colleagues. Horiot et al[46] in Dijon treated 72 patients, with a 5-year survival rate of 78% and a local-recurrence rate of 15%. Finally, Lasser et al[44] find a 5-year survival rate of 72% and a local-recurrence rate of 20%.

Table 20.7 Literature review: results regarding contact therapy

Series	No. of patients	Local-recurrence rate (%)	5-year disease-free survival rate (%)
Papillon and Berard[42]	312	8.3	75
Sischy et al[45]	192	6	75
Roth et al[46]	72	15	70
Lasser et al[44]	42	20	72

Indications

As with local resection, radiotherapists insist on strict selection of patients, and on the importance of close follow-up. According to Lasser et al,[44] tumour size must be less than or equal to 3 cm, which is consistent with the diameter of the rectoscope to which the Philips instrument is connected. Papillon et al state that the tumour must be less than 4–5 cm long (two superimposed irradiation aprons) by 2 cm wide, that is one-quarter of the circumference of the rectal ampulla. In their series, they note that when the diameter is less than 3 cm, the 5-year survival rate is 80%, and goes down to 58% for tumours exceeding 3 cm in diameter. The respective local-recurrence rates are 9% and 17.5%.

Tumours must be well-differentiated or moderately well-differentiated (grade 1 or 2), without any lymph nodes palpable by digital rectal examination or suspected on endorectal echography. In height, they may be located up to 12–14 cm from the anal margin. Anterior-location tumours seem to be an excellent indication for contact therapy as opposed to local resection or to electrocoagulation.

Some juxtasphincteral posterior-seat tumours are not easily accessible for contact therapy. In fact, the rectoscope is hindered by sphincter tonus and canal angulation, and its beam will not entirely reach these tumours.

ELECTROCOAGULATION

Electrocoagulation and fulguration are two features of surgical diathermy, a method that involves destruction of tissues by heat, by means of an electric current running through them. Electrocoagulation has long been used as palliative treatment of inoperable rectal cancers.

Technique

The object of this technique is to destroy the tumour completely if possible, in a single surgical session. The operation is performed with the point of the scalpel[47] or with sharp-edged curettes, to gradually eliminate carbonized and necrotic tissues.[48] First, the healthy mucosa is coagulated for 1 cm at the circumference of the tumour, thus delineating the electrocoagulation area. Once this has been done, digital rectal examination cannot be used to determine the external limits of the tumour, since the coagulated tissues give an impression of rigidity and pseudotumoral infiltration. Destruction of the tumour is done from the surface into depth, and the perirectal fat must be reached. The mean duration of the operation is 1–2 hours. The residual eschar falls off around day 8–10; an endoscopic checkup is then done, and the patient leaves the department. Some authors advocate a new electrocoagulation session around day 10. This is justifiable only if the operator feels that the tumour has not been totally destroyed. Madden and Kandalaft[47] give around four electrocoagulation sessions per patient.

Results

The operative death rate is zero in the series of Crile and Turnbull[48] and Madden and Kandalaft.[47] It is 2% in the Institut Gustave Roussy series.[49] The complication rate is 2–25%. They may consist of haemorrhage when eschars fall out, perforation of the Douglas pouch when the tumour is located too high, abscess of the ischiorectal fossa necessitating drainage by a low route, or transitory sphincteral incontinence when the coagulated tumour was low (juxtasphincteral). Sequelae basically consist of cicatricial stenosis (in 2% of cases), especially with voluminous tumours. The local-recurrence rate is 10–27% and the 5-year survival rate 58–68%.[47–49]

Indications for electrocoagulation[49]

The tumour must not be located too high (because of the risk of perforation of the Douglas pouch) or too low (because of the risk of sphincteral incontinence). It must be on the posterior or lateral faces, since, as with local resection, anterior-seat tumours are prone to rectovaginal fistulas in women and to urethral lesions in men.

CONCLUSIONS

Local excision has the great advantage of providing the pathologist with an item for analysis, as opposed to local destruction techniques (contact therapy and electrocoagulation). Contact therapy has the great advantage of being performed under local anaesthesia on ambulatory patients and without any complications. When patients are strictly selected (budding tumours with a diameter of less than 3 cm, mobile, of grades 1 or 2, without lymph-node invasion: T1 or T2), findings are similar, whether with local resection or contact therapy (local-recurrence rate 8% versus 10%). However, local resection provides the only way to evaluate the exact degree of parietal infiltration. Finally, contact therapy, especially when associated with radiotherapy, can only be administered by highly trained teams.

Local resection would seem advisable, whenever possible. It is intended as curative surgery, with the aim of saving the sphincter and avoiding an abdominoperineal resection. Contact therapy should be restricted to anterior or high-location tumours in elderly patients who do not easily tolerate anaesthesia or hospitalization. The indications for electrocoagulation have gradually diminished, and are now merely the contraindications for other techniques.

Whatever the local treatment used for curative purposes, to quote Papillon, 'the surgeon or radiotherapist must be aware of the responsibility he assumes when agreeing to local treatment of a patient who could be cured by ''traditional radical surgery''. Here, more than anywhere else, the therapist is not entitled to errors.'

REFERENCES

1. Gall FP, Hermanek P, Cancer of the rectum. Local excision. *Surg Clin North Am* 1988; **68**: 1353–65.

2. Hager TH, Gall FP, Hermanek P, Local excision of cancer of the rectum. *Dis Colon Rectum* 1983; **26**: 149–51.

3. Mann CV, Techniques of local surgical excision for rectal carcinoma. *Br J Surg* 1985; **72**(Suppl): 57–8.

4. Nivatvongs S, Wolff B, Technique of per anal excision for carcinoma of the low rectum. *Surg Gynecol Obstet* 1992; **13**: 447–50.

5. Decosse JI, Wong RJ, Quan SHQ et al, Conservative treatment of distal rectal cancer by local excision. *Cancer* 1989; **63**: 219–23.

6. Lasser Ph, Padilla R, Bognel C et al, Traitement conservateur des cancers du bas rectum par tumorectomie et électrocoagulation. A propos de 44 observations. *Cahiers Cancer* 1990; **2**: 8–12.

7. Morson BC, Bussey HJR, Samoorian S, Policy of local excision for early cancer of the colo-rectum. *Gut* 1977; **18**: 1045–50.

8. Mentges B, Buess G, Effinger G et al, Indications and results of local treatment of rectal cancer. *Br J Surg* 1997; **84**: 348–51.

9. O'Brian PH, Kraske's approach to the rectum. *Surg Gynecol Obstet* 1976; **142**: 412–14.

10. Mason Y, Transphincteric approach to rectal lesions. *Ann Surg* 1977; **9**: 171–94.

11. Bleday R, Breen E, Jessup IM et al, Prospective evaluation of local excision for small rectal cancers. *Dis Colon Rectum* 1997; **40**: 388–92.

12. Morson BC, Histological criteria for local excision. *Br J Surg* 1985; **72**(Suppl): 53–4.

13. Killingback MJ, Indications for local excision of rectal cancer. *Br J Surg* 1985; **72**(Suppl): 54–6.

14. Greaney MG, Irvin TT, Criteria for the selection of rectal cancers for local treatment. *Dis Col Rectum* 1977; **20**: 463–6.

15. Whiteway J, Nicholls RJ, Morson BC, The role of surgical local excision in the treatment of rectal cancer. *Br J Surg* 1985; **72**: 694–7.

16. Huddy SPJ, Husband EM, Cook MG et al, Lymph node metastasis in rectal cancer. *Br J Surg* 1993; **80**: 1457–8.

17. Lasser Ph, Bognel C, Elias D et al, Le risque ganglionnaire en cas de cancers du rectum limités à la paroi. Les limites des exérèses locales. *Gastroenterol Clin Biol* 1993; **17**: A180.

18. Blumberg D, Paty PB, Guillem JG et al, All patients with small intra-mural rectal cancer are at risk for lymph node metastasis. *Dis Colon Rectum* 1999; **42**: 881–5.

19. Morson BC, Factors influencing the prognosis of early cancer of the rectum. *Proc R Soc Med* 1996; **59**: 607–8.

20. Lock MR, Ritchie JK, Hawley PR, Reappraisal of radical local excision for carcinoma of the rectum. *Br J Surg* 1993; **80**: 928–9.

21. Tanaka S, Yokota T, Saito D et al, Clinico-pathologic features of early rectal carcinoma and indications for endoscopic treatment. *Dis Colon Rectum* 1995; **39**: 959–63.

22. Willett C, Tepper JE, Donnelly S et al, Patterns of failure following local excision and local excision and post-operative radiation therapy for invasive rectal carcinoma. *J Clin Oncol* 1989; **7**: 1003–8.

23. Graham RA, Garnsey L, Milburn-Jessup J, Local excision of rectal carcinoma. *Am J Surg* 1990; **160**: 306–12.

24. Stearns MW, Sternberg SS, Decosse JJ, Treatment alternatives: localized rectal cancer. *Cancer* 1984; **54**: 2911–14.

25. Cuthbertson AM, Simpson RL, Curative local excision of rectal adenocarcinoma. *Aust NZ J Surg* 1986; **59**: 229–31.

26. Biggers OR, Beart RW, Isltrup DM, Local excision of rectal cancer. *Dis Colon Rectum* 1986; **29**: 374–7.

27. Banerjee AK, Jehle EC, Shorthouse AJ, Buess G, Local excision of rectal tumors. *Br J Surg* 1995; **82**: 1165–73.

28. Andrea KN, Recht A, Busse PM, Sphincter preservation therapy for distal rectal carcinoma. *Cancer* 1997; **70**: 671–83.

29. Winde G, Nottberg H, Keller R et al, Surgical cure for early rectal carcinomas (T1): transanal microsugery vs anterior resection. *Dis Colon Rectum* 1996; **39**: 969–76.

30. Steele G, Busse P, Huberman M et al, A pilot study of sphincter-

sparing management of adenocarcinoma of the rectum. *Arch Surg* 1991; **126:** 696–702.

31. Jessup JM, Bothe A, Stone MD et al, Preservation of sphincter function in rectal carcinoma by a multimodality approach. *Surg Oncol Clin North Am* 1992; **1:** 137–45.

32. Ota DM, Skibber J, Rich TA, M.D. Anderson Cancer Center experience with local excision and multimodality therapy for rectal cancer. *Surg Oncol Clin North Am* 1992; **1:** 147–52.

33. Minsky BD, Enker WE, Cohen AM, Lauwers G, Local excision and post-operative radiation therapy for rectal cancer. *Am J Clin Oncol* 1994; **17:** 411–16.

34. Willet CG, Compton CG, Shellito PC, Efird JT, Selection factors for local excision or abdomino-perineal resection of early stage rectal cancer. *Cancer* 1994; **73:** 2716–20.

35. Wagman R, Minsky B, Cohen AM et al, Conservative management of rectal cancer with local excision and post-operative adjuvant therapy. *Int J Radiat Oncol Biol Phys* 1999; **44:** 841–6.

36. Bouvet M, Milas M, Giacco GG et al, Prediction of recurrence after local excision and post-operative chemoradiation therapy of adenocarcinoma of the rectum. *Ann Surg Oncol* 1996; **6:** 26–32.

37. Chakravarti A, Compton C, Shellito P et al, Long term follow-up of patients with rectal cancer managed by local excision with and without adjuvant radiation. *Ann Surg* 1999; **230:** 49–54.

38. McCready DR, Ota DM, Rich TA et al, Prospective phase I trial of conservative management of low rectal lesions. *Arch Surg* 1989; **124:** 67–70.

39. Rich TA, Weis DR, Mies RS et al, Sphincter preservation in patients with low rectal cancer treated with radiation therapy with or without local excision or fulguration. *Radiology* 1985; **56:** 527–31.

40. Minsky BD, Results of local excision followed by post-operative radiation therapy for rectal cancer. *Radiat Oncol Invest* 1997; **5:** 246–51.

41. Nicholls RJ, York-Mason A, Morson BG et al, The clinical staging of rectal cancer. *Br J Surg* 1982; **69:** 404–9.

42. Papillon J, Berard Ph, Endocavitary irradiation in the conservative treatment of adenocarcinoma of the low rectum. *World J Surg* 1992; **16:** 451–7.

43. Gerard JP, Ayzac L, Coquard R et al, Endocavitary irradiation for early rectal carcinomas (T1–T2). A series of 101 patients treated with the Papillon technique. *Int J Radiat Oncol Biol Phys* 1996; **24:** 775–84.

44. Lasser Ph, Eschwege F, Lacour J et al, Traitement conservateur à but curatif des cancers du rectum. (A propos de 93 observations). In: *Actualités Carcinologiques de l'Institut Gustave-Roussy Paris.* Paris: Masson, 1983; 35–46.

45. Sischy B, Hinsone EJ, Wilkinson DB, Definitive radiation therapy for selected cancers of the rectum. *Br J Surg* 1988; **75:** 901–3.

46. Roth S, Horiot JC, Calais G et al, Prognostic factors in limited rectal cancer treated with intracavitary irradiation. *Int J Radiat Oncol Biol Phys* 1989; **16:** 1445–51.

47. Madden JL, Kandalaft S, Clinical evaluation of electrocoagulation in the treatment of cancer of the rectum. *Am J Surg* 1971; **122:** 347–52.

48. Crile G, Turnbull RB, The role of electrocoagulation in the treatment of carcinoma of the rectum. *Surg Gynecol Obstet* 1972; **135:** 391–6.

49. Lasser Ph, Lacour J, Gadenne C, The place of electrocoagulation in the treatment of cancer of the rectum. *J Exp Clin Cancer Res* 1983; **4:** 427–9.

21

Treatment of locally advanced primary and locally recurrent colorectal cancer

Leonard L Gunderson, Heidi Nelson, Michael G Haddock, Richard Devine, Bruce Wolff, Roger Dozois, Steven Schild, John Pemberton, Tonia Young-Fadok

INTRODUCTION

Combined-modality chemoirradiation is commonly used as a component of treatment in combination with maximum resection for both resectable high-risk and locally advanced or unresectable primary or locally recurrent rectal cancers.[1] With locally unresectable primary or locally recurrent colorectal cancers, standard therapy with surgery, external-beam irradiation (EBRT), and concomitant chemotherapy is often unsuccessful. When intraoperative electron irradiation (IOERT) is added to standard treatment, local control and survival appear to be improved when compared with historical controls in separate analyses from the Mayo Clinic and Massachusetts General Hospital (MGH). Similar results are found in IOERT series from Europe and Japan and in intraoperative high-dose-rate brachytherapy (HDR–IORT) series from the USA and Europe.[1-11] However, maintenance systemic therapy is also needed as a component of treatment, in view of the high rates of systemic failure.

Within the group of patients with locally advanced primary cancers, marked variability in disease extent exists, with no uniform definition of resectability. Depending on the report, a locally advanced cancer can range from a tethered or marginally resectable tumor to a fixed cancer with direct invasion of adjacent organs or structures. The definition may also depend upon whether the assessment of resectability is made clinically (physical examination, radiographs) or at the time of surgery (examination under anesthesia or open exploration with an attempt at resection). The preferred definition of a locally advanced cancer, for the purpose of this chapter, is a cancer that does not appear to be surgically resectable with negative pathologic margins (i.e. there is a high probability on imaging studies or sur-

gical exploration of leaving microscopic or gross residual disease at the resection margin(s) if resection is attempted prior to preoperative chemoirradiation, because of tumor adherence or fixation to that site). Since these patients do poorly with surgery alone, preoperative irradiation plus concomitant chemotherapy (alone or plus maintenance postoperative chemotherapy) has become a component of standard treatment in an attempt to improve treatment outcomes of disease control and survival. This chapter will summarize the evolution of treatment and the role of intraoperative irradiation (IORT) in this group of patients.

Aggressive treatment approaches in patients with local or regional relapse after resection of primary rectal or colon cancers are often not considered. For those institutions that favor an aggressive approach with curative intent in such patients using preoperative EBRT with or without chemotherapy, combined with resection and IORT, justification is found in series that use only the non-IORT components. Data will be presented from US and European non-IORT versus IORT series to allow comparisons of disease control and survival.

PATIENT EVALUATION AND SELECTION

The appropriateness of an aggressive treatment approach with curative intent that may include IORT as a component of treatment should be determined by the surgeon, radiation oncologist, and medical oncologist in the setting of a joint preoperative consultation, whenever feasible. This allows input from all specialties with regard to studies that would be necessary to rule out metastatic disease and useful for both EBRT and IORT planning as well as whether IORT may be an appropriate component of treatment. An informed consent can be obtained with regard to potential benefits and risks, and optimal sequencing of surgery and EBRT can be discussed and determined.

General criteria for the evaluation and selection of patients with locally advanced primary and recurrent colorectal cancers who may be candidates for IORT as a component of treatment have been detailed previously in publications from both the Mayo Clinic and MGH.[2–11] By definition, there must be no contraindications for exploratory surgery. In a majority of patients treated at both institutions, surgery alone would not achieve local control, and EBRT doses needed for local control following subtotal resection or with EBRT alone would exceed normal tissue tolerance. An IORT approach should permit direct irradiation of unresected or marginally resected tumor with single or abutting IORT fields, while allowing surgical displacement or shielding of dose-limiting normal organs or tissue. Patients with documented distant metastases are not usually candidates, since their lifespan is not adequate to evaluate treatment-related effectiveness or tolerance. Exceptions are considered when surgical resection of solitary liver or lung metastasis is feasible and planned, or metastases have been stable for a year or more or have responded excellently to systemic therapy.

The pretreatment patient work-up should include a detailed evaluation of the extent of the locally advanced primary or locally recurrent lesion, combined with studies to rule out hematogenous (liver, lung, or other) or peritoneal spread of disease. In addition to history and physical examination, the routine evaluation includes complete blood count (CBC), liver and renal chemistries, chest film, and carcinoembryonic antigen (CEA). If the rectum is still present, the local evaluation includes digital examination, proctoscopy and/or colonoscopy, and a barium enema study, including cross-table lateral views. When low- or mid-rectal lesions are immobile or fixed, or symptoms suggest pelvic recurrence following abdominoperineal resection, computed tomography (CT) of the pelvis and abdomen can confirm lack of free space between the malignancy and a structure that may be surgically unresectable for cure (i.e. presacrum, pelvic sidewall); such patients should be given preoperative irradiation plus 5-fluorouracil (5-FU)-based chemotherapy prior to an attempt at resection. Extrapelvic spread to para-aortic nodes or liver and the pretreatment status of ureters with regard to the presence or absence of obstruction can also be determined from a CT of the abdomen and pelvis. If hematuria is present or findings on CT or excretory urogram suggest bladder involvement, cystoscopy should be done prior to or on the day of surgical exploration. In patients with cutaneous or perineal fistulae, fistulography may be helpful in determining both size and depth for the purpose of treatment planning of both irradiation and surgical procedures.

TREATMENT FACTORS

Sequencing of treatment modalities

For most patients with locally advanced primary or locally recurrent colorectal cancers, delivery of preoperative concomitant chemoirradiation (45–55 Gy in 1.8–2.0 Gy fractions plus concomitant 5-FU-based chemotherapy) followed by restaging and resection with or without IORT in 3–6 weeks offers the following theoretical advantages over the sequence of resection and IORT followed by postoperative EBRT plus chemotherapy:

1. There is the potential for alteration of implantability of cells that may be disseminated intra-abdominally or systemically at the time of marginal or partial surgical resection.
2. Patients with metastases detected at the restaging work-up or laparotomy can be deleted, thus sparing some patients the potential risks of aggressive surgical resection and IORT.
3. There is the possibility of tumor shrinkage, with an increased probability of achieving a gross total resection.
4. There is a reduction in the treatment interval between the EBRT and IORT components of irradiation (if surgical resection and IORT are done initially and postoperative complications occur, the delay to the EBRT plus chemotherapy component of treatment may be excessive).

If patients present with locally recurrent colorectal cancer after adjuvant treatment that included 45–50 Gy of EBRT, full doses of preoperative EBRT will not be feasible. In such instances, we usually deliver 10–30 Gy in 1.8–2.0 Gy fractions plus concomitant protracted venous infusion 5-FU (PVI 5-FU: 225 mg/m^2/24 h) with surgical exploration and attempted gross total resection plus IORT 1 day to 3 weeks after completion of the preoperative chemoirradiation (advantages 1 and 4 above still hold).

At the present time, at the Mayo Clinic, chemotherapy is instituted simultaneously with EBRT for locally advanced primary and locally recurrent colorectal cancers. The advantage of starting irradiation and chemotherapy simultaneously is that effective local and systemic treatment are instituted simultaneously.[12-15] There is less danger, therefore, that one component of disease will become uncontrollable because of disease progression during single-modality treatment. The disadvantage of starting chemotherapy simultaneously with EBRT is that full-intensity chemotherapy may never be feasible. For tolerance reasons, the intensity of chemotherapy during EBRT is usually less than if chemotherapy precedes EBRT. If further cycles of chemotherapy are given after pelvic EBRT, full-intensity chemotherapy may not be feasible because of alterations in bone marrow reserve.

A potential advantage of altered sequencing of chemotherapy and EBRT (i.e. deliver two or three cycles of multiple-drug chemotherapy before starting combined irradiation/chemotherapy) would be the ability to give full-intensity chemotherapy for at least two or three cycles. This may have an increased impact on occult systemic disease and thereby decrease the ultimate rates of systemic metastases. The danger of starting chemotherapy before EBRT, however, is that the local component of disease may continue to progress and subsequent resection may never be feasible.

Surgical methods, primary unresectable cancers: interaction with irradiation

The objective of surgery is to remove the tumor and primary nodal drainage with as wide a margin around both as is technically feasible and safe. When adjacent organs are involved, they should be removed en bloc with the specimen, assuming that the associated morbidity would be minimal and acceptable to the patient. If a primary rectal cancer is adherent to the prostate or the base of the bladder, it is preferable to use preoperative EBRT plus concomitant chemotherapy followed by gross total resection and supplemental IORT with electrons (IOERT) or high-dose-rate brachytherapy (HDR–IORT). This multimodality approach may allow preservation of the involved organ if favorable downstaging occurs. If a colon cancer is adherent to surrounding organs or structures, en bloc resection of the involved site should usually be performed (an exception may be a sigmoid cancer with adherence to the base of the bladder, for which organ preservation can be achieved as with rectal cancers). Small clips should be placed around areas of adherence and presumed microscopic residual disease for the purpose of

boost-field postoperative EBRT, if IORT options do not exist, and to mark the tumor bed for follow-up evaluation with serial CT studies. With rectal cancers, the pelvic floor should be reconstructed after resection to minimize the amount of small bowel within the true pelvis, and primary or partial closure of the perineum should be performed after abdominoperineal resection to hasten healing and decrease the interval to initiation of postoperative adjuvant treatment.

When deciding whether sphincter-preserving procedures are suitable for rectal lesions, the surgeon and pathologist commonly refer to the distal bowel margin (amount of resected normal bowel below the primary lesion). When lesions extend beyond the entire rectal wall, however, the narrowest transected or dissected surgical margin is often the lateral or anteroposterior margin. Therefore, attention should always be paid to obtaining adequate radial and mesorectal margins.

An anterior resection with reanastomosis can safely be performed following moderate-dose preoperative irradiation (45–50 Gy in 1.8–2 Gy fractions). An unirradiated limb of large bowel should be used for the proximal limb of the anastomosis, with temporary diverting stomas done only on the basis of operative indications (typically for ultralow anterior resection, coloanal anastomoses, or tension on the anastomosis). Published data confirm that this approach results in an acceptably low risk of anastomotic leak.

Surgical methods: locally or regionally recurrent cancers

The intent of surgery for patients with local or regional recurrence is to accomplish a gross total resection, if technically feasible and safe. Although palliation may be a secondary benefit from re-resective surgery in patients with local recurrence, extensive surgical procedures are not advised for purposes of palliation alone, unless disabling complications of sepsis or bleeding are an issue. Patients should, therefore, be evaluated for the possibility of curative intent surgery, with the possibility of metastatic disease excluded and the potential resectability of local disease determined on the basis of preoperative imaging studies.

Pelvic recurrences are typically amenable to re-resection if they are strictly posterior or anterior. Evidence of lateral pelvic sidewall involvement diminishes the chance of complete resection with negative pathologic margins; however, operative assessment and at least an opportunity for resection and IORT is warranted, providing no other contraindications are identified. Although locoregional recurrences that occur above or below S2 of the sacrum are amenable to resection using anterior table sacral resection or distal sacretomy, respectively, the presence of tumor both above and below S2 precludes curative surgery. Similarly, although vascular tumor involvement of either the arterial or venous structures at or distal to the aorta may be resectable, involvement of both structures contraindicates curative surgery in most, if not all, cases.

At the time of surgery, careful assessment for metastatic disease is essential. If possible, it is preferable to determine resectability before critical structures are sacrificed or injured. Adjacent involved organs should be removed en bloc with the specimen if the associated morbidity is acceptable to the patient and physician. When the recurrent tumor is locally adherent to the prostate or base of the bladder, since the side-effects of pelvic exenteration are excessive, it may be preferable to deliver preoperative EBRT and infusional 5-FU (or bolus 5-FU plus leucovorin) followed by gross total resection, with organ preservation, and supplemental IORT to the site of adherence (it may be feasible to spare the organ involved by adherence). However, in view of severe adhesions due to prior surgery and/or adjuvant EBRT, organ preservation is often not technically feasible in the setting of locally recurrent lesions, and exenterative procedures may be necessary in order to accomplish a gross total resection. The option of sparing the bladder should be reserved for those cases where present function is good and there is minimal adherence, such that comparable local regional control could be accomplished with exenteration versus organ-preserving resection plus IORT.

In the setting of pelvic recurrence of rectal cancer, it is rarely possible or reasonable to restore intestinal continuity. Most often, a previous low anterior resection is being converted to an abdominoperineal resection (APR) or a previous APR to a sacretomy or exenteration. In the face of local relapse, it is usually ill-advised to place another anastomosis in this heavily treated field, which is at risk for subsequent local relapse. Rarely, in a highly motivated patient with good sphincter function and a very proximal anastomotic recurrence, it may be reasonable to perform a coloanal anastomosis. Following moderate doses of preoperative EBRT (45–50 Gy) alone or plus concomitant 5-FU-based chemotherapy, anterior resection and primary anastomosis may be safely accomplished if an unirradiated loop of large bowel can be used for the proximal limb of the anastomosis.

Temporary diverting colostomies or ileostomies need be done only if surgical indications exist.

If at the end of resection it is decided that postoperative EBRT is indicated, small titanium or vascular clips should be placed around areas of adherence or residual disease for the purpose of boost-field EBRT. The pelvic floor should be reconstructed after resection to minimize the amount of small bowel within the true pelvis, and primary closure of the perineum should be performed after APR to hasten healing (2–6 weeks versus 2–3 months) and decrease the interval to postoperative EBRT and chemotherapy, if indicated. In patients who have been heavily pretreated or those with large defects, vascularized myocutaneous flap closure should be strongly considered. The muscle closes the dead space of the pelvis, which is typically fibrotic and prone to small-bowel adhesion formation, and the fresh non-irradiated skin ensures perineal healing. For posterior sacretomy wounds, vascularized myocutaneous flap closure has become the standard at the Mayo Clinic.[16]

If patients develop locally recurrent disease following prior adjuvant EBRT, preoperative and postoperative EBRT options are limited at the time of retreatment unless pelvic reconstruction can be accomplished to displace small bowel (omentum, mesh, other). In previously irradiated patients, IORT as salvage is usually feasible only in the setting of gross–total resection of disease, and extended organ resection (anterior exenteration, distal sacretomy, etc.) may be necessary in order to achieve total resection.

Irradiation factors

EBRT alone or plus concomitant chemotherapy

The method of EBRT in previously unirradiated patients has been fairly consistent in most single-institution and group colorectal IORT studies. In the Mayo Clinic and MGH IOERT trials, doses of 45–55 Gy are delivered in 1.8 Gy fractions, 5 days per week over 5–6 weeks in previously unirradiated patients. For pelvic lesions, treatments are given with linear accelerators using ≥ 10 MV photons and four field-shaped EBRT techniques.[3–6,8–11] With extrapelvic lesions, unresected or residual disease plus 3–5 cm margins of normal tissue are included to 45 Gy, usually with parallel-opposed fields. Reduced fields with 2–3 cm margins are treated to 50–55 Gy. When chemotherapy is given during EBRT, 5-FU is given either as a single drug in daily PVI (225 mg/m²/24 h

7 days per week or until intolerance[14]) or in combination with leucovorin in bolus injections (5-FU 400 mg/m^2 plus leucovorin 20 mg/m^2 intravenous push for 4 consecutive days during the first week of EBRT and 3–4 days during the last week[15]).

In previously irradiated patients, only partial-dose EBRT can be given as a component of treatment.[11,17] Since marginal resection is usually the surgical option, it is preferable that low-dose EBRT be given prior to an attempt at resection unless the patient presents with fixed small-bowel loops within a prior high-dose EBRT field. Initially, Mayo Clinic patients in retreatment situations received EBRT alone or EBRT plus bolus 5-FU (with or without leucovorin). Currently, patients receive 20–30 Gy in 1.8–2.00 Gy fractions plus PVI 5-FU (225 mg/m^2/24 h). With concomitant bolus 5-FU plus EBRT, surgery would need to be delayed for 2 weeks or more after delivery of the bolus 5-FU to allow the white blood cell (WBC) and platelet nadirs to have been reached. With PVI 5-FU at 225 mg/m^2, patients can proceed directly to surgical resection after completion of the combined EBRT plus concomitant chemotherapy, if indicated or desired.

IOERT

EBRT is supplemented by IOERT at the joint discretion of the surgeon and radiation oncologist as discussed previously. The radiation oncologist joins the surgeon at the time of surgical exploration or resection to help determine both the feasibility of a subsequent IOERT boost and the size and shape of the IOERT applicator. If surgical exploration precedes EBRT and residual or unresectable disease remains after an attempt at resection, a similar intraoperative assessment for IOERT can be performed.

After APR, optimal IOERT field exposure is determined with regard to an abdominal (Figure 21.1a–d) versus a perineal approach (Figure 21.1e) and prone versus supine or lithotomy patient position.[3–6,8–11,18,19] If an exenteration is necessary, the prostatic fossa in the retropubic region can be treated through an abdominal (Figure 21.1b–d) incision. Tumor adherence to anterior pelvic structures, including the prostate or the base of the bladder, can produce a technical challenge, since a perineal approach for IOERT is usually necessary. Patients can be treated in either the prone or the supine position.

Since April 1989, both the operative procedure and delivery of IOERT at the Mayo Clinic at Rochester have been performed in a dedicated IORT suite within a hospital operating room,[2,8–11] and a similar facility became available at the MGH in June 1996.[10,18] The operating rooms were designed to allow complete OR capabilities as well as delivery of IOERT alone or plus dose modifiers. The linear accelerator at the Mayo Clinic is a refurbished Clinac 18 that provides variable electron energies from 6 to 18 MeV, while MGH uses the Siemens non-mobile dedicated IOERT linear accelerator with variable electron energies of 6–18 MeV.

The IOERT dose is calculated at the 90% isodose line, and the dose and electron energy are dependent on the amount of residual disease remaining after maximal resection and the amount of EBRT that has or can be delivered as a component of treatment. For patients in whom 45–50 Gy of fractionated EBRT is feasible, the following IOERT guidelines apply:

- negative margins or microscopic residual disease: 10–12.5 Gy;
- gross residual disease 2 cm or less in largest dimension: 15 Gy;
- unresected or gross residual disease 2 cm or larger: 17.5–20 Gy.

In retreatment situations where fractionated EBRT doses are restricted to 20–30 Gy, IOERT doses usually range from 15 to 20 Gy, but doses as high as 25 Gy may have to be considered. IOERT electron energies are chosen on the basis of maximum thickness of disease remaining after maximal resection, obliquity of the treatment field, and the ability to achieve complete hemostasis after surgical resection. The lower energies of 6, 9, and 12 MeV are used after gross total resection or with minimal residual disease. The 15–18 MeV energies and doses of 20 Gy are used more commonly in patients in whom gross residual or unresectable disease exists after attempts at resection.

IOERT versus HDR–IORT

Since 1992, IOERT has been performed at Ohio State University (OSU) using a dedicated Siemens linear accelerator with electron energies of 6–18 MeV, and sites that are non-accessible for IOERT have been treated intraoperatively using an HDR brachytherapy afterloader (HDR–IORT) that is transported to the shielded operating room from the radiation oncology department.[19] The Mayo Clinic achieved the availability of HDR–IORT in a dedicated OR setting in 2000 to complement the IOERT treatment that has been available in a dedicated OR setting since 1989. An expanded discussion of HDR–IORT techniques at OSU and the Memorial Sloan-Kettering Cancer Center (MSKCC) can be found elsewhere.[19,20]

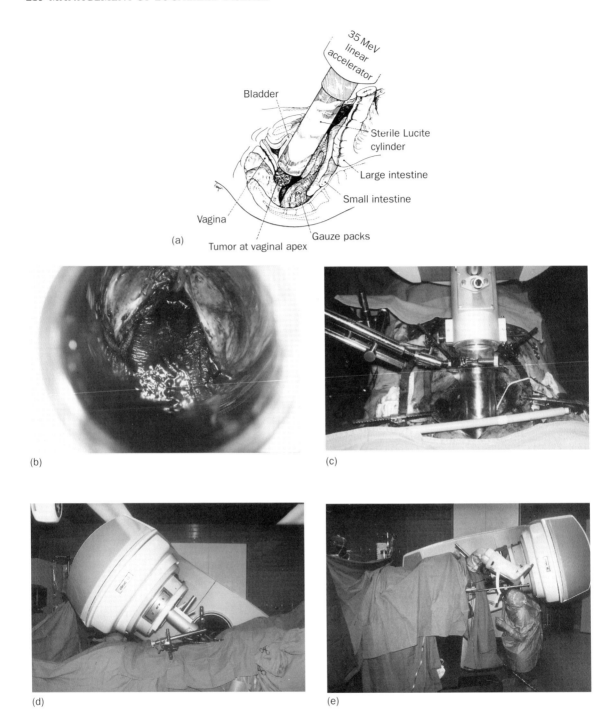

Figure 21.1 IOERT techniques. (a) Artists' idealized depiction of an IOERT applicator in position to include relapse at vaginal apex and pelvic floor. (b–d) The prostatic fossa in the retropubic region is included in the IOERT field (8.0 cm applicator with 30° bevel) after an exenterative procedure – gantry angle exceeds 45°. (e) Treatment of low-lying pelvic tumor or tumor bed via the perineal incision with the patient supine – the gantry angle approaches 90°. From Gunderson LL, Willett CG, Haddock MG et al, Recurrent colorectal – EBRT ± IOERT or HDR–IORT. In: *Intraoperative Irradiation – Techniques and Results* (Gunderson LL, Willett C, Harrison L, Calvo FC, eds). Totowa, NJ: Humana Press, 1999: 273–305.

RESULTS OF NON-IORT TREATMENT

Rationale for irradiation as a component of treatment

The rationale for using a combination of irradiation and chemotherapy as a component of treatment in locally advanced primary or locally recurrent colorectal cancers is based on the risks of both local and systemic relapse after surgery alone and evidence of radioresponsiveness in both preoperative and primary irradiation series for rectal cancers. With preoperative irradiation of clinically mobile rectal cancers, pathologic complete response rates of 10–20% have been reported, and with preoperative chemoirradiation, these rates have been as high as 30–35%.

Brierly et al[21] presented a series from Princess Margaret Hospital, Toronto (PMH) in which primary irradiation without concomitant chemotherapy was given to patients with tumor fixation (77 patients), partial fixation (37 patients), or clinically mobile lesions (97 patients). This final group of patients either were medically inoperable or had refused abdominoperineal resection. The most common irradiation dose was 45–50 Gy in 20 fractions of 2.25–2.5 Gy over 4 weeks. In the 97 patients with mobile lesions, complete clinical regression was achieved in 48 (50%), but 18 relapsed locally for an ultimate local control rate of 31% (30 of 97). The 5-year actuarial survival rate for those with mobile lesions was 48%. Surgical salvage was attempted in 25 patients with initially mobile lesions that persisted or relapsed, and was successful in 18. Although the PMH results are not competitive with combined-modality treatment that includes planned resection, they support the curative potential of irradiation as a single modality.

Results: external irradiation (with or without chemotherapy or resection)

In separate series from the PMH[21] and the Mayo Clinic[22] using EBRT alone or with immunotherapy for locally advanced primary or recurrent cancers, the local persistence or relapse rate was 90% or more in evaluable patients. In the PMH analysis by Brierly et al,[21] for the 77 patients with clinically fixed primary tumors who were treated with 45–50 Gy in 20 fractions over 4 weeks, the local control rate was only 3% and the 5-year survival rate only 4%.

As can be seen in Table 21.1, attempts to control locally recurrent cancers with EBRT alone or plus resection are usually palliative.[1–10,21–25] A recent Australian publication by Guiney et al[25] discussed results in 135 patients with pelvic relapse of rectal cancer who had no evidence of extrapelvic metastases. A select group of 39 patients were treated with radical intent (re-resection in 54% of patients and EBRT doses of 50–60 Gy in all 39) with a median survival of 18 months and a 5-year survival rate of 9% or less. In the non-radically treated patients, the 5-year survival rate was 0–4%.

Mayo analyses: EBRT alone or plus chemo- or immunotherapy

External irradiation has been used alone or in combination with chemotherapy, immunotherapy, surgical resection, or IOERT at the Mayo Clinic for locally advanced colorectal cancers. Earlier Mayo Clinic analyses did not analyze results separately as a function of locally recurrent versus locally advanced primary cancers. Two of the analyses that included patients with both locally advanced primary and recurrent lesions were small, single-institution randomized trials.[22,23]

In the first randomized trial, a group of 65 patients with locally unresectable or recurrent colorectal carcinoma was treated with 40 Gy in 2 Gy fractions over four weeks plus placebo or 5-FU (15 mg/kg on the first 3 days of EBRT).[22] The median survival was 10.5 months in the placebo group versus 16 months in those receiving 5-FU concomitant with EBRT ($p < 0.05$). The 2-year survival rate was 24% versus 38% and the 3-year survival rate 9% versus 19% (Table 21.1).

In a later trial, 44 patients with locally advanced rectal cancer (7 unresectable, 7 resected but residual, and 30 locally recurrent) received 50 Gy split-course pelvic irradiation with or without adjuvant immunotherapy.[23] The site of initial tumor progression could be evaluated in 31 patients, and local progression within the radiation field was diagnosed in 28 (90%). In 17 (55% of evaluable patients), it was the only site of disease. The median survival in both groups of patients was approximately 18 months. In this trial, 36 of 44 patients were experiencing significant pelvic or perineal pain prior to EBRT. Although 94% of patients experienced temporary improvement in pain following treatment, the median duration of pain relief was only 5 months.

Results: resection alone or plus adjuvant irradiation

Surgery alone: locally recurrent cancers
A majority of patients who develop local or regional

Table 21.1 Locally advanced primary or locally recurrent colorectal cancer survival and disease relapse with EBRT: various series

Disease category and treatment	No. of patients	Median survival (months)	Overall survival rate (%)			Disease relapse: actuarial 3-year rate	
			2-yr	3-yr	5-yr	Local	Distant
Primary: EBRT							
Princess Margaret Hospital – Brierly et al[21]	77	19[c]	36[c]	20[c]	4	3% (5-yr)	—
Recurrent plus primary: EBRT							
Mayo Clinic – Moertel et al[22]	65						
EBRT alone	—	10.5	24	9	—	—	—
EBRT + 5-FU	—	16	38	19	5	—	—
Recurrent: EBRT							
Netherlands – Lybeert et al[24]	76	14	25	13	5	43/63 (68%)	26/63 (41%)
EBRT < 50 Gy	—	12	20	6	0	—	—
EBRT ≥ 50 Gy	—	20	40	18	10	—	—
Australian – Guiney et al[25]	135	15	—	—	—	—	—
Low-dose palliative	16	9	13	6	—	94%	—
High-dose palliative[a]	80	15	26	12	4	94%	38%[b]
Radical (50–60 Gy in 2 Gy fractions)	39	18	31	28	≤9	82%	49%[b]

[a]High-dose palliative patients had 45 Gy/3 Gy Fx with a 1-week treatment break after 30 Gy in 10 fractions.
[b]The incidence of metastasis is underestimated, since patients were investigated as warranted by symptoms.
[c]Estimated from survival curves.

recurrence after curative resection of primary rectal or colon cancers are treated with palliative intent in most institutions in the USA and worldwide. Exceptions include patients with a true anastomotic relapse or female patients with a limited vaginal relapse in whom complete resection with negative margins may be feasible, and postoperative EBRT plus chemotherapy can be given as indicated. Patients with prior resection of rectal or sigmoid cancers often present with pelvic pain, which is a manifestation of local recurrence adjacent to or involving nerves in the presacrum or pelvic sidewalls. Presentation with pain usually indicates that a surgical approach will be unlikely to yield negative resection margins. Distal sacretomy with negative resection margins can occasionally be performed in patients with a central, distal pelvic relapse. If relapse develops after APR, male patients may also require a pelvic exenteration in view of bladder or prostate involvement. Most patients, however, either have no surgical resection or a subtotal resection with gross or microscopic residual disease in view of tumor fixation to presacrum, pelvic sidewalls, or both.

In a recent Mayo Clinic analysis of 106 patients with subtotal resection of a localized pelvic recurrence from rectal cancer, 12 patients were treated with surgery alone, and the remainder had some type of irradiation.[7] Of the 12 with no irradiation, the 3- and 5-year overall survival rates were 8% and 0%, respectively. If 8 patients who received EBRT with no planned spatial relationship to surgery are included, the 3-year survival rate increased to 15%, but the 5-year survival rate was still 0%.

Surgery plus adjuvant treatment (irradiation alone or plus chemotherapy)
Local relapse has been reduced in patients with locally advanced primary lesions by combining EBRT (alone or plus chemotherapy) with surgical resection.[2] External irradiation has been given either after

Table 21.2 Preoperative irradiation and resection of locally advanced primary rectal cancer

Series	No. of patients	Resectability rate for cure (%)	Local control rate of those resected (%)	5-year survival rate of those resected (%)
Tufts University[30]	28	50	—	41
Massachusetts General Hospital[31]	25	72	57	43[a]
University of Oregon[32]	72	39	68	10
University of Florida[33]	23	48	30	18

[a] The 6-year survival rate decreased sharply to only 26%.

subtotal resection of locally advanced lesions[26–29] (45–70 Gy in 1.8–2.0 Gy fractions) or before an attempt at resection for disease that is initially unresectable for cure[30–34] (45–60 Gy in 5–6.5 weeks preoperatively, followed by resection in 3–5 weeks). Long-term local control and survival can be obtained in a minority of patients, but the risk of local recurrence is still too high at 30–70% (Table 21.2).

Postoperative EBRT

Allee et al[26] reported the results of 31 patients with residual microscopic cancer after marginal gross total resection of rectal cancer treated at MGH with postoperative EBRT of 45 Gy in 25 fractions over 5 weeks followed by additional boost-field irradiation to as high as 60–70 Gy if small bowel could be excluded from the radiation field. The local control and 5-year disease-free survival rates were 70% and 45%, respectively. In contrast, these figures were 43% and 11% for 25 patients irradiated postoperatively for gross residual disease. A possible dose–response correlation was seen in patients with microscopic residual disease; the risk of subsequent local relapse was 11% (1 of 9) with doses of 60 Gy or greater versus 40% (8 of 20) if the boost dose was less than 60 Gy. There was no clear dose–response relationship in patients with gross residual disease after maximal resection.

Ghossein et al[27] treated patients at the Albert Einstein College of Medicine to 46 Gy in 1.8 Gy fractions followed by a field reduction to the area of persistent disease, which received 60 Gy. The incidences of subsequent local relapse and survival for rectal cancer patients treated with microscopic residual disease were 16% and 84%, respectively, whereas for patients with gross residual disease, these figures were 50% and 39%.

Of 17 Mayo Clinic patients receiving EBRT after subtotal resection of primary rectal cancers, Schild et al[28] observed that local control was achieved in 3 of 10 patients (30%) with microscopic residual cancer and 1 of 7 patients (14%) with gross residual cancer. The median survival was 18 months, and 4 of 17 patients (24%) have remained disease-free for more than 5 years.

Preoperative EBRT

For patients with primary rectal cancers that are unresectable for cure because of tumor fixation, the use of high-dose preoperative EBRT (45–50 Gy in 1.8–2.0 Gy fractions) has been used to reduce tumor size and facilitate resection[30–33] (Table 21.2). Emami et al[30] reported that the rate of resectability in 28 Tufts University patients after full-dose preoperative EBRT was 50%.

Dosoretz et al[31] reported MGH results in 25 patients with unresectable primary cancers in the rectum or rectosigmoid treated with 40–52 Gy preoperative EBRT. Of these 25 patients, 16 subsequently underwent potentially curative resection, and the 6-year survival rate was 26% (with 3 postoperative deaths). Pelvic relapse after resection occurred in 43% of resected patients (with local relapse in 5 of 13 (39%) with curative resection).

As reported by Stevens and Fletcher,[32] in a series from the University of Oregon, 28 of 72 patients (39%) with locally advanced primary carcinoma of the rectum or rectosigmoid who received 50–60 Gy preoperatively were resectable. However, tumor recurred locally in 9 of the 28 patients (32%), and the 5-year survival rate was only 10%.

Mendenhall et al[33] reviewed 23 patients with locally advanced primary rectal cancer who received 35–60 Gy of preoperative EBRT at the University of

Florida. Eleven patients were subsequently able to undergo complete resection, with a 5-year absolute survival rate of 18% and a local failure rate of 55%. The local relapse rate in all patients with resection after preoperative EBRT was about 70%.

There has been one randomized prospective study examining the merits of preoperative EBRT in patients with locally advanced primary rectal cancer. Under the auspices of the Northwest Rectal Cancer Group (Manchester, UK), 284 patients with tethered or fixed rectal cancer were entered into a prospective randomized trial between 1982 and 1986, assessing the effects of preoperative EBRT given 1 week before surgery:[34] 141 patients were randomized to surgery alone and 143 were randomized to receive 20 Gy in four fractions of 5 Gy given in the week before surgery. This study showed a marked reduction in local recurrences in the irradiated group (12.8%) compared with the surgery-alone group (36.5%). Although there was no significant difference in either overall survival or cancer-related mortality between the two treatment groups, subset analysis of the patients who underwent curative surgery reveals overall mortality rates of 53.3% for patients allocated to surgery alone and 44.9% for patients allocated to preoperative radiotherapy. This was a significant reduction in mortality.

In summary, following full-dose preoperative irradiation, most series report that one-half to two-thirds of patients with locally advanced rectal cancers will be converted to a resectable status. However, despite a complete resection and negative margins, the local failure rate depending on the degree of initial tumor fixation varies from 23% to 55%, and for all patients resected, the local relapse rate is as high as 70%.

Preoperative EBRT plus chemotherapy

Because of the efficacy of postoperative irradiation and 5-FU-based chemotherapy (concomitant alone or plus maintenance) in the adjuvant treatment of rectal cancer, there has been interest in examining this approach preoperatively.[35–37] These investigations have studied combinations of moderate- to full-dose preoperative irradiation (45–50.4 Gy) plus concomitant 5-FU-based chemotherapy for patients with clinical T3 and T4 rectal cancer.

In a report from the University of Texas MD Anderson Cancer Center (MDACC), 38 patients with locally advanced rectal cancer (T4 or tethered T3) received 45 Gy in 25 fractions of preoperative EBRT plus concomitant continuous-infusion 5-FU alone or plus cisplatin followed by surgery.[35] Of these 38 patients, 11 received an IOERT supplement to the site of adherence at time of resection. The 3-year survival and local recurrence rates were 82% and 3%, respectively. These results contrasted with 3-year survival and local recurrence rates of 62% and 33%, respectively, for 36 similarly staged patients undergoing preoperative EBRT without chemotherapy or IOERT at MDACC. There were no differences in rates of resectability or pathologic downstaging between the groups of MDACC patients receiving chemotherapy versus no chemotherapy. In contrast, a Swedish study reported an enhanced resectability rate in patients with initially unresectable rectal cancer who received preoperative EBRT plus 5-FU, methotrexate, and leucovorin rescue compared with 38 patients who received EBRT alone (71% versus 34%).[36]

In an analysis of 36 patients (30 primary and 6 recurrent) with locally advanced or unresectable disease who were treated with 50.4 Gy of pelvic irradiation and concurrent 5-FU and leucovorin at MSKCC, the resectability rate with negative margins was 97% and the total complete pathologic response rate was 25%.[37] In spite of these favorable findings, the 4-year actuarial rate of local relapse was 33%.

IORT RESULTS: PRIMARY UNRESECTABLE COLORECTAL CANCER

When intraoperative irradiation with electrons (IOERT) is combined with conventional treatment for locally advanced primary colorectal cancers, separate analyses from MGH and the Mayo Clinic suggest an improvement in both local control and survival.

MGH results (EBRT alone or plus 5-FU, resection, IOERT)

The IOERT program at MGH began in 1978, with locally advanced primary rectal cancer patients as one of the main target groups.[3,5,10] Sixty-four patients with locally advanced primary rectal cancer have undergone full-dose preoperative EBRT (alone or plus 5-FU) followed by resection and IOERT.[10] The 5-year actuarial local control and disease-specific survival rates for 40 patients undergoing complete resection plus IOERT were 91% and 63%, respectively (Table 21.3). For 24 patients undergoing partial resection, the local control and disease-specific survival rates correlated with the extent of residual cancer: 65% and 47%, respectively, for microscopic residual disease, and 57% and 14%, respectively, for gross residual disease.

Table 21.3 Primary colorectal IOERT series: 5-year actuarial disease control and survival rates by degree of resection – MGH (rectal), Mayo Clinic (colorectal)

Degree of resection, amount of residual disease	MGH (rectal)[a]			Mayo Clinic (colorectal)[a]			
	No. of patients[b]	LC (%)	DSS (%)	No. of patients	LC (%)	DF (%)	OS (%)
No tumor	—	—	—	2	100	0	100
Complete resection	40 (12)	91	63	18	93	54[c]	69
Partial resection	24 (5)	63	35				
Microscopic residual disease	17 (4)	65	47	19	86	50[c]	55
Macroscopic residual disease	7 (1)	57	14	16	73	83[c]	21
No resection	—	—	—	1	—	—	0
Total	64	—	—	56	84	59	46

[a]LC, local control rate; DSS, disease-specific survival rate; DF, distant failure rate; OS, overall survival rate.
[b]The numbers in parentheses indicate the numbers of MGH patients at risk at 5 years.
[c]There were 3-year actuarial distant failure rates of 43%, 38%, and 66% for complete resection, microscopic residual disease, and gross residual disease.

Local relapse versus disease extent after preoperative EBRT (no IOERT)

The incidence of local relapse as a function of disease extent after preoperative EBRT alone or plus concomitant 5-FU (no IOERT) has been evaluated in three separate MGH analyses. For 11 patients with locally advanced (T4) rectal cancer treated with preoperative EBRT and curative resection in the original MGH series, 5 of 8 patients (62.5%) who had persistent tumor extension grossly beyond the rectal wall relapsed in the pelvis, compared with none of three patients with tumor confined to the wall or only microscopic extrarectal extension.[31] In an analysis of 28 patients with tethered (T3) rectal cancers treated with preoperative EBRT and resection at MGH, the 5-year actuarial local relapse and disease-free survival rates were 24% and 66%, respectively.[38] No correlation between local control and post-treatment extent of tumor extension into or beyond the rectal wall and/or lymph node involvement was observed.

In the most recent MGH analysis, the outcome of 47 patients with locally advanced rectal cancer receiving 45–50.4 Gy preoperative EBRT and complete resection with clear resection margins by pathologic stage was evaluated.[10] These patients did not receive IOERT because it was judged not to be indicated, since the response to preoperative EBRT was favorable or IOERT was not technically feasible. For 24 patients with no residual tumor or tumor confined to the rectal wall after preoperative EBRT, the 5-year actuarial local relapse rate was only 13%. In contrast, the 5-year actuarial local relapse rate was 68% for 27 patients with persistent transmural tumor and/or lymph node metastases despite a favorable response to preoperative EBRT and no clearly defined indication for IOERT at surgery (i.e. no remaining tumor adherence or compromised soft tissue margins). Therefore, the extent of tumor regression after preoperative EBRT is no longer used as an absolute guide to the need for IOERT at MGH.

Mayo Clinic results (EBRT alone or plus 5-FU, resection, IOERT)

In a Mayo Clinic comparison of 17 non-IOERT[28] and 56 IOERT-plus-EBRT patients with locally advanced primary rectal or colon cancers,[4,8] the respective local control rates were 24% and 87%, median survivals 18 and 40 months, and 3-year survival rates 24% and 55% (Table 21.4). Prognostic factors that had a statistically positive impact on disease control and survival in IOERT patients (Table 21.5) included EBRT plus 5-FU versus EBRT alone (Figure 21.2a), treatment sequence of preoperative EBRT plus 5-FU versus postoperative EBRT plus 5-FU (Figure 21.2b),

Table 21.4 Locally advanced primary and recurrent colorectal cancer: EBRT alone or plus IOERT – Mayo Clinic analysis

Treatment	No. of patients at risk	Median survival (months)	Survival rate (%) 2-yr	3-yr	5-yr	Disease relapse: 3-year actuarial rate (%) Local	Distant
Primary disease							
EBRT[28,a]	17	18	35	24	24	76	59
EBRT + IOERT[8]	56	40	70	55	46	16	49
Localized recurrence							
Suzuki et al[7]							
No IOERT	64	17	26	18	7	93	54
IOERT ± EBRT	42	30	62	43	19	40	60
IOERT ± EBRT							
No prior EBRT[9]	123	28	62	39	20	25	64
Prior EBRT[17]	51	23	48	28	12	55	71

[a]All deaths within 30 months; local relapse range 3–15 months; distant relapse range 3–17 months.

colon versus rectal primary and microscopic or less residual disease after maximal resection (Figure 21.2c).

The impact of degree of resection and amount of residual disease on disease control and survival in the Mayo Clinic analysis is seen in Tables 21.3 and 21.5 and Figure 21.2(c). The 5-year survival rate for the entire group of 56 colorectal IOERT-plus-EBRT patients was 46%. Patients with microscopic or less residual disease fared better than those with gross residual disease, with a 5-year actuarial overall survival rate of 59% versus 21% ($p = 0.005$). Relapse within an irradiation field has occurred in 4 of 16 patients (25%) who presented with gross residual disease after partial resection, compared with 2 of 39 (5%) with microscopic or less residual disease after gross total resection ($p = 0.01$). Within the more favorable group, patients with negative margins or no residual tumor did somewhat better than those with positive margins with regard to local control and survival, but with no statistical significance.

A separate Mayo Clinic analysis was done regarding the use of EBRT (with or without chemotherapy) alone or plus IOERT as a supplement to maximal resection for 103 patients with locally advanced colon cancers.[29] The 5-year actuarial local relapse rates were 10% for patients with no residual disease, 54% for patients with microscopic residual disease, and 79% for patients with gross residual disease ($p < 0.0001$). For patients with residual disease, local relapse occurred in only 11% of patients receiving IOERT plus EBRT, compared with 82% of patients receiving only EBRT ($p = 0.02$). The 5-year actuarial survival rate was 66% for patients with no residual disease, 47% for patients with microscopic residual disease, and 23% for patients with gross residual disease ($p = 0.0009$). The 5-year survival rate in patients with residual disease was 76% for patients receiving IOERT plus EBRT and 26% for patients receiving EBRT alone ($p = 0.04$).

IORT RESULTS: LOCALLY RECURRENT COLORECTAL CANCER

Previously unirradiated patients: US IOERT results

For locally recurrent colorectal cancers, standard treatment with EBRT alone or plus chemotherapy results in excellent short-term palliation (usually <1 year), median survival of 10–18 months, but rare

Table 21.5 Primary colorectal IOERT: disease relapse and overall survival by prognostic factor – Mayo Clinic analysis[a]

Prognostic factor	No. of patients at risk	Local relapse (EBRT)			Distant relapse			Overall survival				
		No. of patients	3-yr rate (%)	p[b]	No. of patients	3-yr rate (%)	p[b]	Median (months)	2-yr rate (%)	3-yr rate (%)	5-yr rate (%)	p[b]
EBRT ± 5-FU (56 patients)												
EBRT	17	3 (18%)	24	—	13 (77%)	66	—	40	64	58	35	—
EBRT + 5-FU[c]	39	4 (10%)	11	0.54	14 (36%)	35	0.013	81	72	53	53	0.39
Treatment sequence (38 patients)												
Preop EBRT + 5-FU	29	4 (14%)	14	—	10 (35%)	32	0.18	81	77	62	62	0.003
Postop EBRT + 5-FU	9	0	0	0.37	4 (44%)	53	—	25	52	17	17	—
Amount of residual (56 patients)												
Gross	16[d]	4 (25%)	27	—	12 (75%)	66	—	22	49	28	21	—
Microscopic or less	39[d]	2 (5%)	9	0.01[d]	15 (39%)	37	0.008[d]	67	80	69	59	0.005
No resection	1	1	—	—	0	—	—	—	0	0	0	—
Site of primary (56 patients)												
Colon	18	1 (6%)	6	0.20	5 (28%)	29	0.03	81	77	63	63	0.10
Rectum	38	6 (16%)	21	—	22 (58%)	53	—	37	65	51	38	—
Grade[e] (56 patients)												
1, 2	27	2 (7%)	4	0.09	15 (56%)	43	0.83	67	73	60	54	0.28
3, 4	29	5 (17%)	32	—	12 (41%)	45	—	37	68	51	36	—
Nodal status (51 patients; 5 unknown)												
Negative	24	1 (4%)	4	0.11	12 (50%)	50	0.95	45	79	67	47	0.34
Positive	27	5 (19%)	23	—	14 (52%)	48	—	28	59	46	41	—
Total group	56	7 (13%)	16	—	27 (48%)	45	—	40	70	55	46	—

[a]Modified from Gunderson LL, Nelson H, Martenson J et al, Locally advanced primary colorectal cancer: intraoperative electron and external beam radiation ± 5FU. *Int J Radiat Oncol Biol Phys* 1997; **37**: 601–14.

[b]Log-rank p value.

[c]One of 39 had chemotherapy prior to but not concomitantly with EBRT.

[d]p value for comparison of two major variables (gross; microscopic or less); when all five variables are included (gross; microscopic or less; positive; negative margin, no tumor; no resection), p < 0.0001 for local control, <0.04 for distant control, <0.0001 for overall survival, and <0.008 for disease-free survival.

[e]Time to relapse by grade: for grade 2, local failure in EBRT field (LF) range 1.0–5.5 years and distant failure (DF) range 0.5–5.5 years; for grade 3, all LF by 3 years and DF by 1.5 years; for grade 4, all LF by 2 years and DF by 1.5 years.

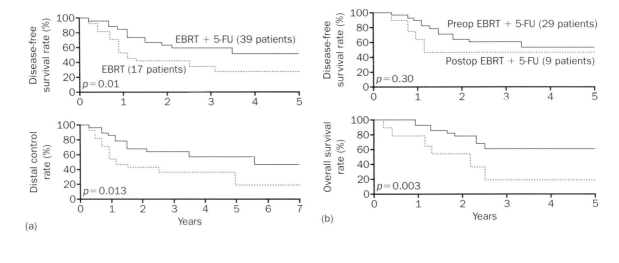

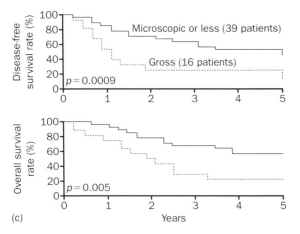

Figure 21.2 Impact of prognostic factors on distant control and survival: Mayo Clinic analysis of 56 patients with EBRT alone or plus 5-FU, resection, and IOERT for locally advanced primary colorectal cancer. (a) EBRT alone or plus 5-FU. (b) Treatment sequence of pre- versus postoperative EBRT in the 38 patients with EBRT plus concomitant 5-FU. (c) Amount of residual disease. Modified from Gunderson LL, Nelson H, Martenson J et al, Locally advanced primary colorectal cancer: intraoperative electron and external beam irradiation ± 5-FU. *Int J Radiat Oncol Biol Phys* 1997; **37:** 601–14.

long-term survival (0% to 7% at 5 years).[1–3,22–25] With the addition of IOERT supplements to standard treatment, 5-year survival rates of about 20% have been achieved in series from both MGH and the Mayo Clinic.[1–4,6,7,9,11,39]

MGH IOERT series

Willett et al[6] reported a 5-year actuarial survival rate of 19% in 32 patients who received EBRT (alone or with 5-FU), IOERT, and maximal resection at MGH for locally recurrent rectal lesions. Most of these patients had received no prior EBRT prior to diagnosis of a local relapse. Both 5-year actuarial local control (LC) and disease-free survival (DFS) were improved in MGH analyses if the surgeon was able to perform a gross total resection prior to IOERT. In the initial analysis of 32 patients by Willett et al,[6] the

5-year LC and DFS rates were 42% and 33%, respectively, with negative resection margins after gross total resection versus 11% and 6% with any degree of residual disease (microscopic or gross). In the most recent MGH analysis of 41 recurrent IOERT patients,[39] the 5-year actuarial LC and DFS rates were 47% and 21%, respectively, in the 27 patients with gross total resection with negative but narrow or microscopically positive margins versus 21% and 7% in the 14 patients with gross residual disease (Table 21.6). The 5-year DFS rate in all 41 patients was 16% and the 5-year overall survival rate 30% (5 of 41 received no or limited EBRT because of prior EBRT – 4 of 5 failed locally and died of disease). Data from Rush-Presbyterian Hospital,[40] the Radiation Therapy Oncology Group (RTOG),[41] and the University of Navarra[42] also support the correlation between local tumor control and amount of residual disease after resection (Table 21.6). Patients with gross total resection and only microscopic residual disease had better in-field disease control than those with unresected or gross residual disease.

Mayo EBRT alone or plus IOERT series

In a Mayo Clinic analysis by Suzuki et al,[7] of 106 patients with subtotal resection of a localized pelvic recurrence from rectal cancer, 42 received IOERT as a component of treatment (41 of the 42 received EBRT; $\geqslant$45 Gy in 38). EBRT was the only method of irradiation in 37 patients, and 29 of the 37 received the EBRT in close approximation to subtotal resection in a planned adjuvant role. The 3-year survival rate was only 18% in the 29 adjuvant EBRT patients versus 42.5% in patients with IOERT as a component of treatment, and the 5-year survival rate was 7% (EBRT only) versus 19% (IOERT plus EBRT) ($p = 0.005$ in a pairwise comparison). Disease control within irradiation fields also appeared to be better in IOERT patients. In previous Mayo Clinic EBRT analyses that included both locally advanced primary and recurrent lesions,[22,23] and in the Suzuki analysis,[7] local progression was documented in 90% of EBRT patients versus 40% in the 42 IOERT-plus-EBRT patients. Although differences seen from series to series may reflect selection bias in non-randomized series instead of treatment effect, it is

possible that improvements in control of the local regional component of disease with the addition of IOERT may translate into improved short-term, if not long-term, survival.

In the most recent Mayo Clinic analysis,[9] 123 colorectal patients with local or regional recurrence and no previous EBRT for their large-bowel cancer were treated with an aggressive multimodality approach including EBRT alone or plus 5-FU, maximal surgical resection, and IOERT (see Table 21.7). The median survival and 2-year survival rate appeared better than two prior Mayo Clinic EBRT trials that contained a large percentage of patients with recurrence[22,23] (IOERT median survival 28 months versus 16 months or 18 months with EBRT plus 5-FU or EBRT plus immunotherapy). Five-year actuarial survival was seen in 20% of patients in the most recent IOERT series versus 5%[22] to 7%[7] in earlier Mayo Clinic EBRT analyses that noted 5-year results.

The amount of residual disease after maximal resection had no statistically significant impact on either disease control or survival in the 123 Mayo IOERT patients (Table 21.7), although there were slight improvements in local control favoring the 57 patients with microscopic or less residual disease after maximal resection versus the 65 with gross residual disease.[24] Lack of difference in central control in the IOERT field is possibly accounted for by the differential IOERT dose used at the Mayo Clinic

Table 21.6 Colorectal IOERT: tumor failure in IOERT field (central failure, CF) or EBRT field (local failure, LF) versus amount of residual disease

Series	No. of patients	CF or LF rate (%)		Residual disease vs CF or LF rate (%)[a]		
		Primary	Recurrent	None	Res(m) or none	Unres or Res(g)
MGH (5-year actuarial						
Primary[5,10]	42	23	—	12	31	50
Recurrent[6,39]	41	—	70	—	53	79
Rush-Presbyterian[40]						
Primary	9	33	—	—	14	100
Recurrent	35	—	54	—	39	64
RTOG, recurrent[41]	37	—	62	—	33	89
Pamplona, recurrent[42]	27	—	74	—	50	84

[a]Res(m)(g), microscopic or gross residual disease; Unres, unresectable.

Rochester on the basis of amount of residual disease after maximal resection. Local relapse in the EBRT field, both absolute and actuarial, was slightly higher in patients with gross residual disease after resection, with absolute rates of 25% versus 14% and 3- and 5-year figures of 32% versus 16% and 40% versus 33% ($p = 0.30$). Overall survival in the 65 IOERT patients with gross residual disease versus the 57 with microscopic or less residual disease was similar, however, with a median of 28 months versus 30 months, and 3- and 5-year survival rates of 36% versus 41% and 18% versus 24%, respectively ($p = 0.56$). Disease-free survival curves were superimposable at 2, 3, and 5 years. IOERT results in patients with gross residual disease after maximal resection in the most recent Mayo Clinic series of 123 patients appear better than in other series. However, this may be a function of different patient selection, standard higher IOERT doses, and the ability to deliver EBRT doses of 45 Gy or more in 1.8 Gy fractions (or the TDF equivalent) in 119 of the 123 patients. In addition 91 of 123 patients received concomitant 5-FU with EBRT with trends for improvements in disease control and survival when compared to the 32 patients with no concomitant 5-FU (median survival 32 months versus 26 months; overall survival rates 43% versus 29% at 3 years and 22% versus 16% at 5 years, $p = 0.14$; disease-free survival rates 35% versus 27% at 3 years and 26% versus 18% at 5 years, $p = 0.22$).

Distant metastasis: implications for chemotherapy

Since the risk of subsequent distant metastases exceeds 50% in patients who present for IOERT at the time of local recurrence, effective systemic therapy will be needed as a component of aggressive treatment approaches including IOERT. In the most recent Mayo Clinic series,[24] 65 of 123 patients (53%) developed distant metastases, with a 3-year rate of 64%. Although 91 of the 123 patients (74%) received 5-FU-based chemotherapy simultaneously with EBRT, only 2 patients received maintenance chemotherapy after resection and IOERT. For patients who did or did not receive chemotherapy, the absolute rate of distant metastases was 45 of 91 (50%) versus 20 of 32 (63%), respectively ($p = 0.32$).

European results: IORT alone or plus EBRT

The current philosophy in Europe is closely related to the US concept, which utilizes IORT as a segment of a multidisciplinary approach in cancer management. A component of EBRT alone or plus 5-FU-based chemotherapy is always attempted, either before or after surgery, if no previous EBRT has been delivered. Maintenance 5-FU-based chemotherapy or new chemotherapeutic regimens (oxaliplatin or irinotecan) are also recommended, since local relapse is often the prelude of distant disease, even after thorough staging is performed. Published results from Pamplona[42] are in concordance with the experience from US institutions.

Pamplona experience

In a recent update of the Pamplona series,[12] 37 patients had been treated with IOERT for locally recurrent colorectal carcinoma with lesions fixed to the presacral space or pelvic sidewalls. In this set of patients, 12 were treated with IOERT alone, since they had received previous EBRT for their primary disease, and the remaining 25 were treated with EBRT plus IOERT (11 with postoperative EBRT and 14 with preoperative chemoradiation). In the preoperative approach, carboplatin (55 mg/m²) plus 5-FU (1000 mg/m², maximum tolerated dose of 1500 mg) were given as a continuous infusion for 3–5 days concurrently with the initiation and ending of the EBRT course. Doses of EBRT were in the range of 40–50 Gy, using standard techniques and fractionation schemes.

Results from the Pamplona update show local relapse in 50% of the 34 evaluable patients. The actuarial local control rate at 26 months was increased in patients treated with EBRT plus IOERT compared with IOERT alone, at 40% versus 0% ($p = 0.03$).

Long-term survival in the total group of patients was dismal, with a median survival time from initiation of treatment for patients treated with IORT alone of 15 months, compared with 22 months for those treated with EBRT plus IOERT ($p = 0.03$). In patients treated with adjuvant EBRT, the preoperative sequence seems to have better survival rates than postoperative EBRT, with median survivals of 23 months and 10 months, respectively ($p = 0.01$).

French IORT group

Similar findings have been observed by investigators from the French IORT group, as can be seen from Table 21.8.[43] In 30 patients treated with IORT alone, no long-term survivors were found after 42 months, compared with 70% for the 16 patients treated with IOERT plus EBRT. The actuarial local control rate was 60% for EBRT plus IORT versus 0% with IORT alone.

Eindhoven IOERT results

From 1994 to 1998, 37 patients with locally recurrent

Table 21.7 Colorectal IOERT: locally recurrent, no prior EBRT; disease relapse and overall survival by prognostic factor – Mayo Clinic analysis[a]

Prognostic factor	No. of patients at risk	Local relapse			Overall survival					
		No. of patients	3-yr (rate %)	p[b]	Median (months)	2-yr rate (%)	3-yr rate (%)	5-yr rate (%)	p[b]	
EBRT ± 5-FU										
EBRT	32	5 (16%)	16	0.46	25	55	29	16	—	
EBRT + 5-FU	91	19 (21%)	29	—	31	65	43	22	0.14	
Treatment sequence										
Preop EBRT + 5-FU	78[c]	17 (22%)	31	—	31	66	44	19	0.91	
Postop EBRT + 5-FU	13[c]	2 (15%)	17	0.43	28	56	38	28[d]	—	
Site of primary										
Colon	43	6 (14%)	20	0.51	27	59	26	21	—	
Rectum	80	18 (23%)	26	—	31	64	43	20	0.60	
Amount of residual disease										
Gross	65	16 (25%)	32	—	27	60	36	18	—	
Microscopic or less	57	8 (14%)	16	0.30	29	64	41	24	0.56	
No resection	1	0	—	—	—	100	—	—	—	
Total group	123	24 (20%)	25		28	62	39	20		

[a]Modified from Gunderson LL, Nelson H, Martenson J et al. Intraoperative electron and external beam irradiation with or without 5FU and maximal surgical resection for previously unirradiated locally recurrent colorectal cancer. *Dis Colon Rectum* 1996; **39**: 1380–96.
[b]Log-rank p-value.
[c]One patient in each group with EBRT dose <40 Gy.
[d]Survival rate decreased to 19% at 5.5 years.

rectal cancer (without distant metastasis) received IOERT as a component of treatment in Eindhoven.[44] Seventeen patients with no prior irradiation received preoperative EBRT of 16–60 Gy (1 received 16 Gy, 15 received 50.4 Gy, and 1 received 60 Gy) alone or with concomitant 5-FU-based chemotherapy (2 patients). The 20 patients who had received prior EBRT either had no further EBRT (15 patients) or in the latter part of the study were given 30 Gy in 2 Gy fractions (reported as well tolerated) (5 patients). Surgical resection was attempted 4–6 weeks following full-dose preoperative EBRT. Negative resection margins (R0) were achieved in 15 patients, gross total resection but microscopic residual disease (R1) in 8, and unresectable or gross residual disease (R2) in 14.

At 3 years, the local control (LC) rate was 60%, the disease-free survival (DFS) rate 32%, and the overall survival (OS) rate 58%. The ability to achieve a gross total resection with negative (R0) or microscopically positive margins (R1) impacted all three parameters when compared with R2 resection with regard to improvements in OS rate (74% for R0/R1 versus 35% for R2, $p < 0.05$), DFS rate 54% for R0/R1 versus 11% for R2, $p = 0.0008$), and LC rate ($p = 0.01$). The ability

to achieve a gross total resection was higher in patients who received preoperative EBRT (R0/R1 versus R2; $p = 0.001$). Patients who received preoperative EBRT had improved survival and disease control (OS, $p = 0.005$; DFS, $p = 0.001$; metastases, $p = 0.00007$; LC, $p = 0.08$). Patients who presented with symptomatic local recurrence had higher rates of R2 resection and worse prognosis ($p = 0.0005$).

Previously irradiated patients: IOERT alone or plus EBRT

Non-IORT salvage

There is little information in the literature regarding salvage therapy for patients with locally recurrent colorectal cancer who had previously received high- or moderate-dose irradiation. Previously irradiated patients who develop local relapse appear to have a worse prognosis than those with local relapse following surgical resection who have not received prior irradiation. In the series of Frykholm et al,[45] the 5-year survival rate following local relapse was 6% in patients treated initially with surgical resection alone

Table 21.8 Summarized European results with IORT alone or plus EBRT for locally recurrent colorectal cancer with regard to actuarial 3-year local control rates and survival

Institution	No. of patients	3-year local control rate (%)[a]	p	3-year survival rate (%)[a]	p
Pamplona:[11,42]					
IOERT + EBRT	25	30		38	
IOERT alone	12	0		12	
France:[43]					
IORT + EBRT	16	61		68	
IORT alone	30	0		24[b]	
Eindhoven:[44]	37	60		58	
EBRT + IORT	22	NS	0.08	NS	0.005
IORT alone	15	NS		NS	
R0/R1	23	79	0.01	74	<0.05
R2	14	21		35[c]	

[a]NS, not stated.

[b]No long-term survivors beyond 42 months.

[c]No disease-free survivors beyond 22 months.

versus 0% for previously irradiated patients. Nearly one-fourth (23%) of the previously irradiated patients died with local disease only, with no known distant metastases. In a randomized Swedish study[46] comparing preoperative radiation versus surgical resection alone for primary rectal cancers, 15% of irradiated patients suffered local recurrence, and had a median survival time of 11 months versus 15 months for locally recurrent patients treated initially on the surgery-alone arm ($p = 0.0002$). The 5-year survival rate was 0% among previously irradiated patients versus 5% in the previously unirradiated group.

Salvage IOERT without EBRT

Because of dose-limiting peripheral nerve toxicity, palliative resection plus IOERT without additional EBRT is unlikely to result in acceptable local control in previously irradiated patients. Wallace et al[39] treated 5 previously irradiated patients with IOERT and limited or no additional EBRT; 4 of these had subsequent local relapse. In the updated Pamplona series of 37 patients[12] discussed above, 12 previously irradiated patients received IOERT without additional EBRT. The reported local recurrence rate was 100%, with 3- and 5-year actuarial survival rates of 12% and 0%, respectively. Similar results were reported in the French analysis[44] in which 30 patients received IOERT alone because of prior EBRT (100% local relapse, and no long-term survivors beyond 42 months).

Medical College of Ohio series

Merrick et al[47] reported the Medical College of Ohio (MCO, Toledo) experience with 35 patients who were treated for locally recurrent rectal cancer with maximal surgical resection and IOERT, having received prior adjuvant EBRT for the primary lesion. All operations were performed with the intent of complete resection, but in 15 of the 35 cases, this could not be achieved because of extensive local disease.

The 3-year actuarial survival rate from the time of IOERT and surgical resection of local relapse was 20%. In the group of 20 patients in whom complete resection of gross disease was achieved, the 2-year survival rate was 45%, and the 3-year survival rate 30%; in the 15 patients with incomplete resection, the 2-year survival rate was only 27%. Of the 35 patients in this group, 10 (29%) again developed local relapse. Most patients reported at least partial pain relief.

Salvage IOERT alone or plus low-dose EBRT: Mayo analysis

IOERT following maximal surgical resection and selective EBRT has been utilized as attempted salvage therapy at the Mayo Clinic for patients with locally recurrent colorectal cancer following previous high- or moderate-dose irradiation.[17] In a series of 51 previously irradiated patients who received IOERT, additional EBRT alone or plus chemotherapy was delivered to 37 patients (75%). The median EBRT dose was 25.2 Gy (range 5–50.4 Gy), and care was taken not to exceed small-bowel tolerance.

Survival and disease control data in the Mayo Clinic IOERT series of previously irradiated patients are presented in Tables 21.4 and 21.9. The median survival was 23 months, with 3- and 5-year actuarial survival rates of 28% and 12%, respectively. Subsequent local relapse was noted in 18 patients (an absolute rate of 35% and a 3-year actuarial rate of 55%) and distant metastasis in 26 patients (an absolute rate of 51% and a 3-year actuarial rate of 71%). These results appear to be an improvement over the historically reported nearly uniform disease relapse and death reported in this group of patients.

Prognostic factors

Because of the limited number of previously irradiated patients who have been treated with IOERT as a component of salvage treatment, no clear prognostic factors for survival and disease control have been identified. In the Mayo Clinic analysis,[17] there was a non-statistically significant trend toward improved local control in the EBRT field and central control within the IOERT field when EBRT retreatment doses of 30 Gy or more could be safely used.

The amount of residual disease after surgical resection in previously irradiated patients may also be an important prognostic factor when IOERT is used as a component of salvage treatment. The median survival in the Mayo Clinic series was 34 months for patients with close but negative margins, 21 months for those with microscopically positive margins, and 16 months for those with gross residual disease.[17] There were no 5-year survivors in the Mayo Clinic patients with gross residual tumor at the time of IOERT. In the MCO analysis,[47] similar trends were seen, with an improvement in survival in the 20 patients with gross total resection versus the 15 patients with an incomplete resection (a 2-year survival rate of 45% versus 27%).

Distant relapse

Although aggressive local therapy with EBRT, surgery, and IOERT may control local disease in a

Table 21.9 Locally advanced recurrent colorectal cancer in previously irradiated patients: survival and disease control in Mayo Clinic IOERT series by prognostic factor[a]

| | | Survival | | | | Disease relapse: 3-year actuarial | | | | | |
| | | | Overall rate (%) | | | Local | | Central | | Distant | |
Prognostic factor	No. of patients at risk	Median (months)	2-yr	3-yr	5-yr	No.	3-yr rate (%)	No.	3-yr rate (%)	No.	3-yr rate (%)
EBRT dose											
<30 Gy	35	23	49	23	—	15 (43%)	61	10 (29%)	41	17 (49%)	76
≥30 Gy	16	18	43	34	17	3 (19%)	37	2 (13%)	25	9 (56%)	64
Residual disease											
Gross	17	16	42	21	—	4 (24%)	57	3 (18%)	54	8 (<7%)	—
Microscopic or less	34	27	52	27	17	14 (41%)	57	9 (26%)	36	18 (53%)	65
Positive margin	21	21	40	27	—	10 (48%)	65	7 (33%)	43	12 (57%)	62
Negative margin	13	34	73	25	25	4 (31%)	45	2 (15%)	24	6 (46%)	69
Grade											
1, 2	22	19	45	31	10	10 (45%)	55	8 (36%)	45	12 (55%)	60
3, 4	29	31	51	26	13	8 (28%)	55	4 (14%)	29	14 (<8%)	80
All patients	51	23	48	28	12	18 (35%)	55	12 (24%)	36	26 (51%)	71

[a]Modified from Haddock MG, Gunderson LL, Nelson H et al, Intraoperative irradiation for locally recurrent colorectal cancer in previously irradiated patients. *Int J Radiat Oncol Biol Phys* 2001; **49**: 1267–74.

significant number of patients who develop local relapse in spite of adjuvant treatment, long-term survival is limited by the high rate of distant relapse despite careful clinical staging at the time of local relapse in an attempt to detect occult distant disease. In the Mayo Clinic series of 51 patients,[17] the 3-year actuarial rate of distant relapse was 71%. Improvements in survival will require the addition of effective systemic therapy to aggressive local therapy.

Results with IOERT or HDR–IORT with or without EBRT

Ohio State experience: IOERT or HDR–IORT

Nag et al[12,48] reported the OSU IORT experience with 45 patients treated between March 1992 and November 1994. All but one had recurrent colorectal cancers. Of 45 cases, 26 had prior EBRT and 33 had received prior 5-FU-based chemotherapy.

The choice of IOERT versus HDR–IORT was based primarily on accessibility issues. If the target area was accessible to the IOERT applicator, a dedicated Siemens linear accelerator installed in a shielded operating room was used to deliver IOERT in 27 patients. HDR–IORT was used in 18 patients at OSU when the tumor bed was inaccessible to the IOERT applicator. Radiation doses delivered at the 90% isodose for IOERT or at 0.5 cm depth for HDR–IORT varied from 10 to 20 Gy, depending on the volume of residual disease and whether the patient had been previously irradiated. The 26 previously irradiated patients received an IORT dose of 10 Gy (3 patients), 15 Gy (15 patients), 17.5 Gy (3 patients), or 20 Gy (5 patients); the 19 previously unirradiated patients received IORT doses of 10 Gy (15 patients) or 15 Gy (4 patients). Eight previously unirradiated patients received postoperative EBRT, usually to 45 Gy in 25 fractions; one received 36 Gy to the periaortic region. Another 10 previously unirradiated patients did not receive the planned postoperative EBRT, because of patient refusal in 3 instances and poor medical condition in 7. Three previously irradiated patients received postoperative EBRT of 30–36 Gy. Two patients were subsequently retreated with IORT for re-recurrent disease.

The overall local control rate was 56%, with a mean follow-up time of 18.4 months. The overall median survival was 20 months, with 71%, 35%, and 17% actuarial survival rates at 12 months, 24 months, and 36 months, respectively. Patients with microscopic residual disease after maximal resection

appeared to have better local control (48%) than patients with gross residual disease (25%) ($p = 0.19$).

The OSU experience is unique in that, while most institutions deliver IORT to accessible sites using IOERT, the additional availability of HDR–IORT at OSU allows the delivery of IORT to sites that may be less accessible to IOERT (e.g. pelvic sidewall, retropubic areas). Ideally, both HDR–IORT and IOERT should be available for optimal management of patients with locally recurrent colorectal cancers.

Memorial Sloan-Kettering: HDR–IORT

The predominant initial experience in HDR–IORT at MSKCC has been in the management of locally advanced and/or locally recurrent colorectal adenocarcinoma.[20] From November 1992 through December 1996, 112 patients with rectal cancer were explored, and 68 were treated with HDR–IORT (22 primary unresectable; 46 locally recurrent, of whom results were reported in the 42 with adequate follow-up). Patients with primary, unresectable disease received preoperative EBRT to a total dose of 45–50 Gy over 5–5.5 weeks alone (2 patients) or plus concomitant 5-FU-based chemotherapy (usually 5-FU and leucovorin) (18 patients). Four to six weeks later, they underwent operation in the brachytherapy suite. If there was no evidence of metastatic disease, resection was performed, followed by HDR–IORT to a dose of 10–20 Gy (median 12 Gy) delivered at a depth of 5 mm from the surface of the HAM applicator. Patients with pelvic recurrence of a previously treated colorectal cancer had individualized management. For the 26 patients who had had prior radiation therapy, surgery was performed. If disease was limited to the pelvis, resection plus HDR–IORT was done. A total of 10–20 Gy (median 15 Gy) was delivered at a depth of 5 mm from the surface of the HAM applicator. If there was no prior radiation therapy (16 patients), preoperative chemoirradiation was given as for the primary unresectable patients, followed by maximal resection and HDR–IORT (range 10–20 Gy, median 12 Gy).

While follow-up in MSKCC patients receiving HDR–IORT as a component of treatment is too short to make durable assessment of local control or survival, early results are similar to results with IOERT series (Table 21.10). The actuarial local control rate at 2 years was 81% for primary unresectable and 63% for locally recurrent cases. Local control at 2 years was dependent on margin status after maximal resection in both groups of patients: for primary cases, the 2-year local control rate was 92% and 38% for negative and positive margins, respectively; for locally recurrent cases, it was 82% and 19% for negative and positive margins, respectively. The disease-free survival rate at 2 years was 69% and 47% for primary and recurrent cases, respectively, and was again related to margin status: for primary cases, the rate was 77% versus 38% for negative versus positive margins, respectively; for recurrent cases, it was 71% versus 0%. Results were best in previously unirradiated patients who could receive all components of treatment.

FUTURE POSSIBILITIES

Encouraging trends exist in colorectal IOERT analyses with regard to improvement in local control and possibly survival of patients with locally advanced primary and locally recurrent colorectal cancers when compared with non-IOERT series, and continued evaluation of IOERT approaches seems warranted. Disease persistence or relapse within the IOERT and EBRT fields is higher, however, when the surgeon is unable to accomplish a gross total resection. In the MGH analysis of locally recurrent rectal cancers, failure within irradiation fields was excessive even with gross total resections if margins were microscopically positive. Therefore, a protracted venous infusion of 5-FU (with or without other drugs) should consistently be considered during EBRT,[14] and dose modifiers should be evaluated in conjunction with IOERT. To maximize the percentage of patients who can technically receive an IORT component of treatment, it would be reasonable for large institutions to have both IOERT and HDR–IORT capability in an OR setting, since certain technical factors can result in inability to treat with either method (inaccessible location for IOERT, residual disease 1 cm or greater thickness for HDR–IORT).

Since the incidence of distant metastasis exceeds 50% in patients with either locally advanced primary or locally recurrent colorectal cancers, 4–6 months of systemic therapy should be evaluated as the systemic component of the aggressive treatment approaches discussed in this chapter. A number of randomized trials have revealed a significant advantage in tumor response rates for 5-FU plus leucovorin when compared with 5-FU alone in the treatment of advanced metastatic large-bowel cancer;[49] and in an adjuvant colon cancer setting, 5-FU plus leucovorin has demonstrated survival advantages over a surgery-alone control arm in a NCCTG coordinated intergroup study[50] and versus MOF (semustine, vincristine, and 5-FU) chemotherapy in an NSABP trial.[51] Finally, it would be reasonable to evaluate continuous-infusion 5-FU alone or combined with other agents as systemic therapy for locally recurrent colorectal cancers in view of its statistically significant impact on survival and distant metastasis in the Mayo Clinic NCCTG 86-47-51 randomized adjuvant rectal trial.[14]

In view of the extremely high rates of distant

Table 21.10 HDR–IORT for colorectal cancer: 2-year actuarial results by disease presentation and margin status – Memorial Sloan-Kettering Cancer Center[a]

Disease and margin status	No. of patients	2-year local control rate (%)	p	2-year disease-free survival rate (%)	p
Primary unresectable	22	81		69	
Negative margin	18	92	0.002	77	0.03
Positive margin	4	38		38	
Locally recurrent	42	63		47	
Negative margin	26	82	0.02	71	0.04
Positive margin	16	19		0	

[a]From Harrison L, Minsky B, White C et al, HDR–IORT for colorectal cancer: clinical experience. In: *Intraoperative Irradiation – Techniques and Results* (Gunderson LL, Willett CG, Harrison LB, Calvo FC, eds). Totowa, NJ: Humana Press, 1999: 307–14.

metastasis seen in these patients and the fact that many patients will have received adjuvant 5-FU-based chemotherapy, further 5-FU-based chemotherapy may be insufficient as the systemic modality of treatment. Irinotecan (CPT-11) is being evaluated in depth both as a single agent and in combination with other drugs.[52] On the basis of both laboratory and preliminary clinical data, interest exists in further evaluations of the use of antibodies as a component of treatment alone or in conjunction with chemotherapy. Monoclonal antibody therapy with 17-1a has demonstrated survival benefits in resected node-positive colon cancer patients similar to 5-FU/leucovorin and 5-FU/levamisole in one randomized European trial.[53] Most patients who present with recurrent colon cancer will have already received adjuvant 5-FU/leucovorin or 5-FU/levamisole. Those who present with local recurrence of rectal cancer after adjuvant EBRT will usually have received 5-FU-based chemotherapy both concomitantly with EBRT and as maintenance therapy. In such patients, the evaluation of alternative systemic agents, including antibody treatment, irinotecan, oxaliplatin, and additional agents discussed in other chapters of this book, will be of importance.

REFERENCES

1. Gunderson LL, Indications for and results of combined modality treatment of colorectal cancer. *Acta Oncol* 1999; **38:** 7–21.
2. Gunderson LL, Dozois RR, Intraoperative irradiation for locally advanced colorectal carcinomas. *Perspect Colon Rectal Surg* 1992; **5:** 1–23.
3. Gunderson LL, Cohen AM, Dosoretz DE et al, Residual, unresectable or recurrent colorectal cancer: external beam irradiation and intraoperative electron beam boost ± resection. *Int J Radiat Oncol Biol Phys* 1983; **9:** 1597–606.
4. Gunderson LL, Martin JK, Beart RW et al, External beam and intraoperative electron irradiation for locally advanced colorectal cancer. *Ann Surg* 1988; **207:** 52–60.
5. Willett CG, Shellito PC, Tepper JE et al, Intraoperative electron beam radiation therapy for primary locally advanced rectal and rectosigmoid carcinoma. *J Clin Oncol* 1991; **9:** 843–9.
6. Willett CG, Shellito PC, Tepper JE et al, Intraoperative electron beam radiation therapy for recurrent locally advanced rectal and rectosigmoid carcinoma. *Cancer* 1991; **67:** 1504–8.
7. Suzuki K, Gunderson LL, Devine RM et al, Intraoperative irradiation after palliative surgery for locally recurrent rectal cancer. *Cancer* 1995; **75:** 939–52.
8. Gunderson LL, Nelson H, Martenson J et al, Locally advanced primary colorectal cancer: intraoperative electron and external beam irradiation ± 5-FU. *Int J Radiat Oncol Biol Phys* 1997; **37:** 601–14.
9. Gunderson LL, Nelson H, Martenson J et al, Intraoperative electron and external beam irradiation with or without 5FU and maximal surgical resection for previously unirradiated locally recurrent colorectal cancer. *Dis Colon Rectum* 1996; **39:** 1380–96.
10. Willett C, Shellito PC, Gunderson LL, Primary colorectal – EBRT ± IOERT. In: *Intraoperative Irradiation – Techniques and Results* (Gunderson LL, Willett C, Harrison L, Calvo F, eds). Totowa, NJ: Humana Press, 1999: 249–72.
11. Gunderson LL, Willett CG, Haddock MG et al, Recurrent colorectal – EBRT ± IOERT or HDR–IORT. In: *Intraoperative Irradiation – Techniques and Results* (Gunderson LL, Willett C, Harrison L, Calvo F, eds). Totowa, NJ: Humana Press, 1999: 273–305.
12. Gastrointestinal Tumor Study Group, Prolongation of the disease-free interval in surgically resected rectal cancer. *N Engl J Med* 1985; **312:** 1465–72.
13. Krook JE, Moertel CG, Gunderson LL, Effective surgical adjuvant therapy for high risk rectal carcinoma. *N Engl J Med* 1991; **324:** 709–15.
14. O'Connell MJ, Martenson JA, Wieand HS et al, Improving adjuvant therapy for rectal cancer by combining protracted infusion fluorouracil with radiation therapy after curative surgery. *N Engl J Med* 1994; **331:** 502–7.
15. Moertel CG, Gunderson LL, Mailliard JA et al, Early evaluation of combined 5-FU and leucovorin as a radiation enhancer for locally unresectable, residual, or recurrent gastrointestinal cancer. *J Clin Oncol* 1994; **12:** 21–7.
16. Radice E, Nelson H, Mercill S et al, Primary myocutaneous flap closure following resection of locally advanced pelvic malignancies. *Br J Surg* 1999; **86:** 349–54.
17. Haddock MG, Gunderson LL, Nelson H et al, Intraoperative irradiation for locally recurrent colorectal cancer in previously irradiated patients. *Int J Radiat Oncol Biol Phys* 2001; **49:** 1267–74.
18. Willett C, Gunderson LL, Busse PM et al, IOERT treatment factors – technique, equipment. In: *Intraoperative Irradiation – Techniques and Results* (Gunderson LL, Willett C, Harrison L, Calvo F, eds). Totowa, NJ: Humana Press, 1999: 65–85.
19. Nag S, Gunderson LL, Willett CG et al, Intraoperative irradiation with electron beam or high dose rate brachytherapy: methodological comparisons. In: *Intraoperative Irradiation – Techniques and Results* (Gunderson LL, Willett C, Harrison L, Calvo F, eds). Totowa, NJ: Humana Press, 1999: 111–30.
20. Harrison L, Minsky B, White C et al, HDR–IORT for colorectal cancer: clinical experience. In: *Intraoperative Irradiation – Techniques and Results* (Gunderson LL, Willett CG, Harrison LB, Calvo F, eds). Totowa, NJ: Humana Press, 1999: 307–14.
21. Brierly JD, Cummings BJ, Wong CS et al, Adenocarcinoma of the rectum treated by radical external radiation therapy. *Int J Radiat Oncol Biol Phys* 1995; **31:** 255–9.
22. Moertel CG, Childs DS Jr, Reitemeier RJ et al, Combined 5-fluorouracil and supervoltage radiation therapy of locally unresectable gastrointestinal cancer. *Lancet* 1969; **ii:** 865–7.
23. O'Connell MJ, Childs DS, Moertel CG et al, A prospective controlled evaluation of combined pelvic radiotherapy and methanol extraction residue of BCG (MER) for locally unresectable or recurrent rectal carcinoma. *Int J Radiat Oncol Biol Phys* 1982; **8:** 1115–19.
24. Lybert MLM, Martijn H, DeNeve W et al, Radiotherapy for locoregional relapses of rectal carcinoma after initial radical surgery: definite but limited influence of relapse free survival and survival. *Int J Radiat Oncol Biol Phys* 1992; **24:** 241–6.
25. Guiney MJ, Smith JG, Worotniuk V et al, Radiotherapy treatment for isolated loco-regional recurrence of rectosigmoid cancer following definitive surgery: Peter MacCullum Cancer Institute experience, 1981–1990. *Int J Radiat Oncol Biol Phys* 1997; **38:** 1019–25.
26. Allee PE, Tepper JE, Gunderson LL et al, Postoperative radiation therapy for incompletely resected colorectal carcinoma. *Int J Radiat Oncol Biol Phys* 1989; **17:** 1171–6.
27. Ghossein NA, Samala EC, Alpert S et al, Elective postoperative radiotherapy after incomplete resection of colorectal cancer. *Dis Colon Rectum* 1981; **24:** 252–6.

28. Schild SE, Martenson JA, Gunderson LL, Dozois RR, Long-term survival and patterns of failure after postoperative radiation therapy for subtotally resected rectal adenocarcinoma. *Int J Radiat Oncol Biol Phys* 1989; **16**: 459–63.

29. Schild SE, Gunderson LL, Haddock MG et al, The treatment of locally advanced colon cancer. *Int J Radiat Oncol Biol Phys* 1997; **37**: 51–8.

30. Emami B, Pilepich M, Willett CG et al, Effect of preoperative irradiation on resectability of colorectal carcinomas. *Int J Radiat Oncol Biol Phys* 1982; **8**: 1295–9.

31. Dosoretz DE, Gunderson LL, Hedberg S et al, Preoperative irradiation for unresectable rectal and rectosigmoid carcinomas. *Cancer* 1983; **52**: 814–18.

32. Stevens KR, Fletcher WS, High dose preoperative pelvic irradiation for unresectable adenocarcinoma of the rectum or sigmoid. *Int J Radiat Oncol Biol Phys* 1983; **9**: 148.

33. Mendenhall WM, Bland KI, Pfaff WW et al, Initially unresectable rectal adenocarcinoma treated with preoperative irradiation and surgery. *Ann Surg* 1987; **205**: 41–4.

34. Marsh PJ, James RD, Scholfield PF, Adjuvant preoperative radiotherapy for locally advanced rectal carcinoma. *Dis Colon Rectum* 1994; **37**: 1205–14.

35. Weinstein GD, Rich TA, Shumate CR et al, Preoperative infusional chemoradiation and surgery with or without an electron beam intraoperative boost for advanced primary rectal cancer. *Int J Radiat Oncol Biol Phys* 1995; **32**: 197–204.

36. Frykolm G, Glimelius B, Pahlman L, Preoperative irradiation with and without chemotherapy (MFL) in the treatment of primary non-resectable adenocarcinoma of the rectum. Results from two consecutive studies. *Eur J Cancer Clin Oncol* 1989; **25**: 1535–41.

37. Minsky BD, Cohen AM, Enker WE et al, Preoperative 5-FU, low-dose leucovorin, and radiation therapy for locally advanced and unresectable rectal cancer. *Int J Radiat Oncol Biol Phys* 1997; **37**: 289–95.

38. Willett CG, Shellito PC, Rodkey GV, Wood WC, Preoperative irradiation for tethered rectal cancer. *Radiother Oncol* 1991; **21**: 141–2.

39. Wallace HJ, Willett CG, Shellito PC et al, Intraoperative radiation therapy for locally advanced recurrent rectal or rectosigmoid cancer. *J Surg Oncol* 1995; **60**: 122–7.

40. Kramer T, Share R, Kiel K, Rosman D, Intraoperative radiation therapy of colorectal cancer. In: *Intraoperative Radiation Therapy* (Abe M, ed). New York: Pergamon Press, 1991: 308–10.

41. Lanciano R, Calkins A, Wolkov H et al, A phase I, II study of intraoperative radiotherapy in advanced unresectable or recurrent carcinoma of the rectum: a RTOG study. In: *Intraoperative Radiation Therapy* (Abe M, ed). New York: Pergamon Press, 1991: 311–13.

42. Abuchaibe O, Calvo FA, Azinovic I et al, Intraoperative radiotherapy in locally advanced recurrent colorectal cancer. *Int J Radiol Oncol Biol Phys* 1993; **26**: 859–67.

43. Bussieres E, Gilly FN, Rouanet P et al, Recurrences of rectal cancers: results of a multimodal approach with intraoperative radiation therapy. *Int J Radiat Oncol Biol Phys* 1996; **34**: 49–56.

44. Mannaerts GHH, Martijn H, Crommelin MA et al, Intraoperative electron irradiation therapy for locally recurrent rectal carcinoma. *Int J Radiol Oncol Biol Phys* 1999; **45**: 297–308.

45. Frykholm GJ, Pahlman L, Glimelius B, Treatment of local recurrences of rectal carcinoma. *Radiother Oncol* 1995; **34**: 185–94.

46. Holm T, Cedermark B, Rutqvist LE, Local recurrence of rectal adenocarcinoma after 'curative' surgery with and without preoperative radiotherapy. *Br J Surg* 1994; **81**: 452–5.

47. Merrick HW, Crucitti A, Padgett BJ, Dobelbower RR Jr, IORT as a surgical adjuvant for pelvic recurrence of rectal cancer. In: *Intraoperative Radiation Therapy in the Treatment of Cancer* (Vaeth JM, ed). Frontiers in Radiation Therapy and Oncology, Vol 31. Basel: Karger, 1997: 234–7.

48. Nag S, Mills J, Martin E et al, IORT using high dose rate brachytherapy or electron beam for colorectal carcinoma. In: *Intraoperative Radiation Therapy in the Treatment of Cancer* (Vaeth JM, ed). Frontiers in Radiation Therapy and Oncology, Vol 31. Basel: Karger, 1997: 238–42.

49. International Multicentre Pooled Analysis of Colon Cancer Trials (IMPACT) investigators: efficacy of adjuvant fluorouracil and folinic acid in colon cancer. *Lancet* 1995; **345**: 939–44.

50. O'Connell MJ, Mailliard JA, Kahn MJ et al, Controlled trial of fluorouracil and low dose leucovorin given for six months as postoperative adjuvant therapy for colon cancer. *J Clin Oncol* 1997; **15**: 246–50.

51. Wolmark N, Rockette H, Fisher B et al, The benefit of leucovorin-modulated fluorouracil as postoperative adjuvant therapy for primary colon cancer: results from National Surgical Adjuvant Breast and Bowel Project Protocol C-03. *J Clin Oncol* 1993; **11**: 1879–87.

52. Pitot HC, Wender DB, O'Connell MJ et al, Phase 2 trial of irinotecan in patients with metastatic colorectal carcinoma. *J Clin Oncol* 1997; **15**: 2910–19.

53. Riethmuller G, Schneider-Gadicke E, Schlimok G et al, Randomized trial of monoclonal antibody for adjuvant therapy of resected Dukes' C colorectal carcinoma. *Lancet* 1994; **343**: 1177–83.

22

Radiotherapy for rectal cancer: The European approach

Lars Påhlman, Bengt Glimelius

INTRODUCTION

In the primary treatment for rectal cancer, surgery plays the most important role. The overall 5-year survival figures have slowly improved during recent decades, and today slightly more than 50% of all patients with rectal cancer will survive.[1,2] Between 20% and 30% of all newly diagnosed patients with rectal cancer have already developed distant metastases and/or have a locally inoperable tumour. Among those having undergone apparently curative surgery, the two main reasons for a fatal outcome are occult distant metastases not found at surgery and/or a locoregional recurrence. During the past 20 years or so, the average locoregional recurrence rate, as reported from all controlled trials worldwide, has been 29%.[3] In the light of the high morbidity and mortality from a local failure, this is an unacceptedly high figure. This is particularly so since the majority of local recurrences are probably due to inappropriate surgery. Recent data have demonstrated that a positive circumferential margin (i.e. microscopic tumour foci left behind laterally) is a very important prognostic marker for a local failure and for survival.[4,5] Adequate lateral clearance is also a good marker of good surgery. However, even if surgery is performed correctly, some areas with microscopic tumour foci will not always be resected, even with a total mesorectal excision (TME). It has been proposed that those areas should be resected using an even more aggressive surgical strategy.[6] This will substantially increase postoperative morbidity.[7] On the other hand, these deposits are usually small and therefore easily eradicated by radiotherapy. The rationale for combining surgery and radiotherapy is obvious, since radiotherapy will eradicate tumour cells in the periphery where surgery cannot be radical without causing too much morbidity. Surgery takes care of the tumour bulk, where radiotherapy will always fail owing to the presence of too many tumour cells. This requires that the additional radiotherapy can be given without significantly increasing morbidity.

This chapter will focus on how to use radiotherapy and chemo-radiotherapy in terms of local control and survival improvement. Moreover, the adverse effects (both acute and late) and the rationale for using radiotherapy provided that surgery is optimized will be discussed. It is of the utmost importance to distinguish whether the tumour is considered resectable (T1–T3) or non-resectable (T4). In patients with a T1–T3 tumour, the radiotherapy is an adjuvant treatment, and thus its use can always be questioned, whereas in patients with a T4 tumour, radiotherapy is essential (unless the overgrowth is towards an organ that can easily be removed), and it must be an integrated part of the treatment.

RADIOTHERAPY IN RESECTABLE RECTAL CANCER: ADJUVANT TREATMENT

The high local recurrence rate reported from numerous series worldwide has been the rationale for the use of radiotherapy additional to surgery. Recurrence rates have ranged from less than 10% to more than 50%.[8–12] This substantial variation is most likely multifactorial, and not always easy to explain, but factors such as patient selection, definition of local radical surgery, definition of a local recurrence, follow-up routines and surgeons' skill are well known. An estimation of the average recurrence rate after standard surgery can be found in the surgery-alone arm in the randomized trials using pre- or postoperative radiotherapy.[13–29] These trials, summarized in Table 22.1, have local recurrence rates rang-

Table 22.1 Pelvic recurrence after a combination of surgery and radiotherapy in rectal carcinoma (controlled trials with a surgery-alone group). Trials are compiled according to biological dose according to a linear–quadratic model

Study	Irradiation: dose (Gy)/ No. of fractions	LQ time (Gy)	Surgery alone: No. of local recurrences/total[a]	Surgery + radiotherapy: No. of local recurrences/total[a]	p value[b]	Percent reduction in local failure rates
Preoperative						
Rider et al[13]	5/1	7.5	–[c]			
Duncan et al[14]	5/1	7.5	–[d]			
	20/10	20.4	–[d]			
Goldberg et al[15]	15/3	22.5	51/210[e] (24)	31/185[e] (17)	NS	29
Roswit et al[16]	31.5/18	26.8	–[c]			
Horn et al[17]	31.5/18	26.8	31/131 (24)	24/138 (17)	NS	29
Higgins et al[18]	25/10	27.5	32/87[f] (37)	27/93[f] (22)	NS	22
Marsh et al[19]	20/4	30.0	58/141 (41)	26/143 (18)	**	63
Gérard et al[20]	34.5/15	35.2	49/175 (28)	24/166 (14)	**	50
MRC2[21,g]	40/20	36.0	50/132 (38)	41/129 (32)	NS	16
SRCSG[22]	25/5	37.5	120/425 (28)	61/424 (14)	**	50
SRCT[23]	25/5	37.5	131/557 (24)	51/553 (9)	***	61
Postoperative						
Bentzen et al[24]	50/25	35.4	57/250 (23)	46/244 (19)	NS	17
MRC3[25]	40/20	36.0	69/235 (29)	46/234 (20)	**	31
GITSG[26]	40–48/22	36.0	27/106 (25)	15/96 (16)	NS	36
Fisher et al[27]	46.5/26	39.3	45/184 (24)	30/184 (16)	NS	33
Arnaud et al[28]	46/23	40.8	30/88 (34)	25/84 (30)	NS	13
Treuniet et al[29]	50/25	43.8	28/84 (33)	21/88 (24)	NS	41

[a]Percentages in parentheses. [b]NS, $p > 0.05$; *, $p < 0.05$; **, $p < 0.01$; ***, $p < 0.001$. [c]Not reported. [d]Only actuarial data reported, with no difference between groups. [e]Outpatients only reported. [f]Autopsy series only reported. [g]Only tethered tumours.

ing from 23% to 41%. The average recurrence rate of 29% reflects the worldwide experience at centres interested in trials in rectal cancer, and thus probably interested in the treatment of this cancer. On a population level, this figure thus probably does not overestimate the real problem. Also, in the randomized preoperative trials, all patients with a resected cancer have been reported (R0, R1 and R2 resections), whereas in the postoperative trials, those who have undergone non-radical surgery have been excluded. In most reports with excellent results, often only patients with an R0 resection have been presented.[8,9,11,30]

Local recurrence rate

According to the data presented in Table 22.1, where all trials have been compiled according to the radiation dose intensity, a clear dose–response relation in the reduction of local recurrence rates can be seen. The reduction is greatest in trials where preoperative radiotherapy has been used. The dose level has varied considerably in the trials using preoperative radiotherapy, and in these trials, it can be seen that a higher dose will increase the reduction in local recurrence rates. It can also be seen that, at a comparable dose, preoperative radiotherapy is more effective than postoperative radiotherapy. This is further illustrated in Table 22.2. The question of the relative effi-

Table 22.2 Reduction in local failure rates grouped in pre- and postoperative radiotherapy trials according to biological dose (in the calculations, the α/β was assumed to be 10 Gy and the time factor γ/α to be 0.6 Gy/day)

		Surgery alone: No. of local recurrences/total[a]	Surgery + radiotherapy: No. of local recurrences/total[a]	Percent reduction in local failure rates
Preoperative				
LQ time (Gy)	0–20	–[b]	–[b]	0
	22.5–27.5	114/428 (27)	82/416 (20)	26
	30–37.5	408/1430 (29)	203/1415 (14)	52
Postoperative				
LQ time	35–44	256/947 (27)	183/930 (20)	26

[a]Percentages in parentheses. [b]Only actuarial data reported, with no difference between groups.

cacy of pre- and postoperative radiotherapy has been addressed in only one randomized trial, the Uppsala trial, where patients were randomly allocated to preoperative or postoperative radiotherapy.[31,32] In that trial, preoperative radiotherapy was superior to postoperative irradiation in reducing the local recurrence rates.

Thus preoperative radiotherapy is more dose-effective than postoperative. The reason for this is not clear, but two important factors could contribute to this difference. First, radiotherapy needs oxygen to work, and in a preoperative setting the tissue is well oxygenated. Secondly, the delay from surgery to postoperative radiotherapy is often more than 4 weeks. In fact, most patients do not start radiotherapy until after 6 weeks,[31] and this delay will probably enhance the repopulation of tumour cells, giving too big a tumour burden to allow eradication with a high probability.[33,34]

Survival

Radiotherapy to the pelvic region can hardly have any impact on occult distant metastases. Since local recurrence is often the first recurrence, and sometimes the only known one, it might be possible to improve survival if the local failure rate could be reduced to a great extent. The suggestion that better local control will in the end improve survival has been confirmed in a study where patients treated by surgeons having a low local recurrence rate had better survival than those treated by surgeons with a high local recurrence rate.[35] Consequently, if the recurrence rate could be lowered considerably with radiotherapy, a survival benefit might be achieved. No trial with postoperative radiotherapy alone has shown an effect on survival, probably because the reduction in local recurrence rate has not been high enough (26%, Table 22.2). After preoperative radiotherapy, on the other hand, an effect on cancer-specific survival has been shown in several trials using radiotherapy doses corresponding to an LQ time of above 30 Gy.[19,20,22,23,36,37] In the largest trial with preoperative radiotherapy (the Swedish Rectal Cancer Trial), not only was an effect on cancer specific survival seen but so was an effect on overall survival.[37] In that trial, a relative reduction in the local recurrence rate of 60% was found. The 5-year survival rate among patients having surgery alone was 48% compared with 58% ($p < 0.0035$) in the group of patients who received preoperative radiotherapy followed by surgery the next week.

Although postoperative radiotherapy alone does not have a demonstrable impact on survival, a combination of radiotherapy and chemotherapy in the postoperative setting has improved survival to the same extent as seen with preoperative radiotherapy alone.[26,38–40] If it is possible to extrapolate these data to the preoperative concept, an even better effect on survival might be achieved unless morbidity is increased such that it influences postoperative mortality. However, whether or not preoperative chemoradiotherapy will improve the results is still not proven, despite theoretical advantages,[41,42] since no trial has used preoperative radiotherapy and chemotherapy in combination. There is an ongoing trial by the European Organization for Research and Treatment of Cancer (EORTC) exploring this question. Combining radiotherapy and chemotherapy in a preoperative setting may increase toxicity,[43,44] although several single institution series have reported low complication rates.

TOXICITY TO RADIOTHERAPY

The adverse effects of radiotherapy can be seen both in the acute and subacute phases and as late toxicity. Acute and subacute toxicities have been relatively well studied in all the randomized trials. Unfortunately, this is not the situation with the late adverse effects, since their study requires long-term follow-up, which may impose logistic difficulties. However, it is very important to evaluate late toxicity, since the relative merits of pre- and postoperative radiotherapy cannot be judged until the full picture is known.

Acute toxicity

It is obvious that only preoperative radiotherapy could increase morbidity in the immediate postoperative period, and data from numerous trials have shown that there is an increase in perineal wound sepsis among patients who have had preoperative radiotherapy and have been operated upon with an abdominal perineal excision.[17,20–22,45] This negative effect has been seen both in trials using 'conventional' fraction sizes of about 2 Gy and in those using the high fraction of 5 Gy. Another important surgical consideration after rectal cancer surgery is anastomotic healing. Based upon experimental studies in dogs[46] and data from all the randomized trials,[17,20–22,45] no adverse effects regarding anastomotic healing have been shown, indicating that anastomotic integrity after a low anterior resection is not influenced by preoperative radiotherapy.

An essential factor when choosing the radiotherapy schedule is compliance and acute tolerability. The reports of the randomized trials indicate that preoperative radiotherapy is better tolerated than postoperative radiotherapy. A marked difference in acute toxicity was also noticed in the only trial where preoperative and postoperative radiotherapy were compared.[47] Data from the AXIS trial in the UK have recently been presented. In this trial, patients were randomly allocated to radiotherapy before surgery, but it was up to the discretion of the operating surgeon to choose pre- or postoperative radiotherapy.[48] Among the patients for whom preoperative radiotherapy was chosen, 96% received the intended treatment, compared with only 56% of patients for whom postoperative radiotherapy was chosen. An uneventful surgical outcome will influence the possibility for a patient to receive postoperative radiotherapy. In the postoperative chemo-radiotherapy trials, only those patients with an uneventful surgical outcome within a limited time period (about 6 weeks) have been eligible for inclusion. Obviously, if postoperative radiotherapy is chosen then several patients who would benefit from radiotherapy will not receive the treatment until after a prolonged time period because of postoperative fatigue or delayed wound healing.[31] Prolonging the start of the radiotherapy will decrease its efficacy owing to tumour cell proliferation.

Of great importance is the increased postoperative mortality found in two trials using preoperative radiotherapy.[15,22] In both trials, the radiation-treated volumes were large, and it was predominantly among elderly patients and those with generalized disease that an increase in in-hospital mortality was shown. The increase in postoperative mortality found in the Stockholm-Malmö trial[22] was actually the reason why the Swedish Rectal Cancer Trial was initiated, since in the other Swedish trial, the Uppsala trial, no increase in postoperative mortality was found, despite the same radiation dose.[31] The data from the Swedish Rectal Cancer Trial show that preoperative radiotherapy can be delivered without an increase in postoperative mortality.[45] This requires that the radiotherapy be optimized to cover only the tissue volumes at risk of containing tumour cells, i.e. the target volume.[49] Unfortunately, the Stockholm group simplified the radiation technique also in their second trial, which was part of the Swedish Rectal Cancer Trial.[50] Thus a tendency towards increased mortality within the first 60 days was seen also in the Stockholm II trial; the simplification through not using adequate shielding resulted in an increase in the volume irradiated outside the target volume. This tendency was not seen other than in the Stockholm part of the trial.

The Swedish concept using accelerated radiotherapy (5×5 Gy during 1 week) has been criticized by radiotherapists as causing more acute toxic reactions.

A very specific adverse effect of radiotherapy has been noticed from the Swedish trials. Acute neurogenic pain has been noticed as pain in the gluteal area and along the hamstrings, starting after the second or third fraction. In a very few patients, this radiotherapy-induced neuropathy has led to an inability to walk and persistent pain.[49] Although the effect has predominanty been seen after 5 Gy fractions, it can also be seen after 2 Gy fractions. The mechanism causing this pain is not at all clear, but it is important that the radiotherapy be optimized so that the nerve roots are shielded in areas where there is no risk of tumour cells being present. The dose used in the Swedish trials (5×5 Gy during 1 week) is radiobiologically considered to be suboptimal, since it results in a lower therapeutic index than the use of more conventional fraction sizes of 1.8–2 Gy. However, it is not only the fraction size that is important, but also the total dose. The total dose in the Swedish trials is kept low, at 25 Gy, compared with the 40–50 Gy when 1.8–2 Gy fractions are used. Thus, although the therapeutic index, particularly concerning late toxicity, is lowered, this may not be of any disadvantage, since the total dose may be below the dose causing significant late morbidity. Without question, it is cost-effective compared to other fractionation schedules, provided that it does not increase costs by increasing complications.

With the more anatomically precise type of surgery, more postoperative problems are encountered, and therefore there has been some scepticism among surgeons as to whether preoperative radiotherapy should be given to patients undergoing TME resection for rectal cancer. In the Dutch TME trial, where TME surgery is mandatory, the risk of an increase in adverse effects and particularly postoperative mortality has been considered. A recent interim report has shown no increase in postoperative mortality after TME surgery and preoperative radiotherapy (5×5 Gy), but (as has repeatedly been found earlier) there is an increased infection rate among irradiated patients.[51]

Data from the literature emphasize that the radiotherapy has to be optimized using three- or four-beam techniques with adequate shielding. A substantial risk of serious morbidity occurs if, for example, a two-beam technique is used, since the treated volume will then be substantially larger.[49] The Swedish Rectal Cancer Trial defined strictly how the radiotherapy should be given. As discussed above, this has not always been the case. However, the radiation technique defined in the Swedish Rectal Cancer Trial protocol was also simplified to allow it to be used at several hospitals with limited radiation

capacity. Technical developments during the last decade now allow a more appropriate coverage of the target volume, with less radiation burden outside the target than was the case in the trial initiated in the mid-1980s.

Late radiation-associated toxicity

It can be assumed the late toxicity can vary depending on whether pre- or postoperative radiotherapy has been used, and therefore it is regrettable that so few data have been published regarding late toxicity to radiotherapy in rectal cancer. Most of the literature has come from the Swedish trials where 25 Gy in 1 week has been used preoperatively. Institutions using a more conventional radiotherapy regimen (1.8–2 Gy fractions) given preoperatively or the more commonly used treatments in the USA (postoperative chemo-radiotherapy to a total dose of 45–50 Gy) have not examined and reported late toxicity to the same extent.

Intestinal obstruction

The cumulative risk of having a small-bowel obstruction after surgery for rectal cancer is estimated to be 5–10%. If preoperative radiotherapy, even at a high dose, is used with an optimized technique, this incidence is not increased.[32] However, if the treated volume is larger, as was, for example, the case in the Stockholm–Malmö trial[52] or if postoperative radiotherapy is used,[24,27,28,32] the risk is substantially increased. After postoperative radiotherapy, an increase in small-bowel obstruction can be explained by bowel loops becoming stuck in the lesser pelvis and thus within the irradiation volume.

Bowel function

Since parts of the small and large bowel may be irradiated both pre- and postoperatively, slight damage to the intestinal mucosa can occur, resulting in an increased risk of looser stools. Bowel function can particularly be affected in patients operated upon with an anterior resection and irradiated postoperatively, since the distal part of the rectum is irradiated as well as the large bowel, which is anastomosed down to the rectal stump or anal canal. There are reports where patients who have had postoperative radiotherapy have experienced a clear change in bowel function in the long term.[53,54] Recent data have also indicated that preoperative radiotherapy will have similar effects on bowel function,[55] despite the fact that the large bowel has not been irradiated. In a questionnaire study from the Swedish Rectal Cancer Trial, it was found that bowel function was impaired among the group of patients who received irradiation.[56] In the Swedish Rectal Cancer Trial, the target volume always included the sphincters. The adverse bowel function can be explained by fibrosis in the external sphincter, since the data reveal that the discrimination capacity was not altered.[56] Based upon those findings, it is important not to unnecessarily include the sphincters in the target.

Damage to the pelvic organs

With radiotherapy to the pelvic area, several organs are in danger of damage. Very little has been reported regarding damage to the genitourinary tract, but it appears that the risk of adverse bladder function after pre- or postoperative radiotherapy is rather small.[32,52] The Stockholm group has reported an increased risk of pelvic fractures and fractures of the femoral neck.[52] Since no appropriate shielding was used to decrease the radiation burden to the sacrum, this could be the explanation. A recent, still unpublished, register study on adverse effects in the Swedish Rectal Cancer Trial has not disclosed the same risk of fractures (M Dahlberg, personal communication).

IS IT NECESSARY TO USE RADIOTHERAPY IN THE TREATMENT OF RECTAL CANCER?

Recent data show that if a good surgical circumferential resection can be performed (often a TME), the local recurrence rate will be very low.[8,9] With this in mind, it is interesting to notice that all published trials with a surgery-alone arm have reported a local recurrence rate in the control group averaging 29% (Table 22.1), indicating that the surgical procedure has been suboptimal. Therefore it might be argued whether radiotherapy is actually necessary, provided that surgery can be optimized. In a nationwide study from Norway, it has been shown that it is possible to reduce the local recurrence rate from approximately 30% to just under 10% if surgery is optimized.[57] Similar results have also been reported from the Stockholm area[58] and from Uppsala.[59] All of these studies still have a limited follow-up period.

Only one trial has addressed this question of whether radiotherapy is worthwhile when surgery is

optimized – the Dutch TME trial, where all surgeons had 'accreditation' as TME surgeons before patients could be enrolled in the trial. The trial has not yet been completed, and no data are available. If preoperative radiotherapy (25 Gy in 1 week) is used together with optimized surgery, it is possible that the reduction in local recurrence rate is even higher, as has been seen in randomized trials with 'standard surgery'. In a population-based, but non-randomized, study from the Stockholm area, the overall local recurrence rate was 5.6% after the introduction of TME surgery. In patients who had had preoperative radiotherapy or surgery alone the figures were 1.7% and 10% respectively, after a follow-up of 2 years, indicating that radiotherapy will have an impact on local recurrence rates even if surgery is optimized.[58] Data from Uppsala also show that when TME surgery was combined with preoperative radiotherapy (25 Gy in 1 week), a recurrence rate of 2.6% was found after a follow-up of 2–10 years.[59] The area of concern here is the substantial overtreatment if adjuvant radiotherapy is used for all patients when optimized surgery is performed to obtain a locoregional control of 90% or above. The problem is how to find the risk groups.

HOW SHOULD RADIOTHERAPY BE USED?

Based on the fact that preoperative irradiation is more dose-effective than postoperative radiotherapy, many European centres use preoperative radiotherapy. An important question to address is whether the Swedish radiotherapy schedule, i.e. 5×5 Gy during 1 week with surgery the following week, is the optimal one. Although this treatment is cheap and quick, questions have been raised regarding the greater toxicity compared with the more conventional radiotherapy with 1.8–2 Gy fractions over a 5-week period and surgery after another 5-week period. So far, no trial has compared these two treatment schedules. It is not likely that the effect on local recurrence rates will be greatly different (although 25×2 Gy may be less effective), but it might be that the adverse effects can be more common using 5×5 Gy, although none of the analyses of the Uppsala trial[32] and the Swedish Rectal Cancer Trial[45] (also M Dahlberg et al, unpublished data) have been able to detect any relevant late toxicity provided that the irradiation technique was according to the protocol. This question is addressed in a new Swedish trial from the Stockholm group. The rationale for choosing the 1-week schedule instead of the 5-week treatment is more a matter of economics in terms of a less resource-demanding option, and it must be up to each centre to choose its own schedule. The Swedish experience using 5×5 Gy in 1 week is, however, very favourable.

The use of chemo-radiotherapy is another important question. The evidence that chemo-radiotherapy is superior to radiotherapy alone in the local control rates is limited. Postoperative chemo-radiotherapy is effective in slightly lowering local failure rates and improving survival.[38,39] The benefits may increase if chemotherapy is given concomitantly with radiotherapy.[43,44] Therefore the EORTC is currently testing this hypothesis in a trial where patients are randomly allocated to receive preoperative radiotherapy with conventional fractionation alone or the same irradiation with concomitant chemotherapy. Not only efficacy but also toxicity will be evaluated in this trial. Under no circumstances should the preoperative 5×5 Gy schedule be combined with concomitant chemotherapy, since this will most likely lead to a substantial increase in morbidity.

It has been claimed that the number of patients with preserved sphincter function will increase if prolonged preoperative chemo-radiotherapy is used.[60] The hypothesis is that combined treatment is more effective, and – provided that the interval from the end of the radiotherapy to surgery is prolonged – downstaging will increase the chance of preserving the sphincter. The question of using a prolonged period from radiotherapy to surgery has been studied in a recently published French trial.[61] In this trial, all patients received chemo-radiotherapy, but were randomized to have surgery immediately after irradiation or after 6 weeks. More patients had their sphincters preserved if surgery was delayed (76% versus 68% respectively). Moreover, the surgeons were asked before radiotherapy started whether or not they could preserve the sphincter function. The overall recurrence rate was 9%, but in the group of patients having an anterior resection where a sphincter-preserving operation did not seem possible initially, the local recurrence rate was 12%.[61] This trial was underpowered, but its data must be considered seriously. It might potentially be dangerous to rely on the downstaging effect after preoperative chemo-radiotherapy to preserve the sphincter. Also, the late effects of chemo-radiotherapy on sphincter function are largely unknown.

RADIOTHERAPY IN NON-RESECTABLE (T4) TUMOURS

This patient category must be discovered preoperatively. The rationale for radiotherapy in these patients is to achieve tumour shrinkage to such an

extent that curative surgery is possible. It is usually too late to notice at surgery that the tumour area should have had preoperative radiotherapy in order to become operable. If a tumour is considered non-resectable at diagnosis, preoperative radiotherapy to a dose of 50 Gy given with conventional fractionation (1.8–2.0 Gy fractions) is recommended. There is no real controversy about this type of treatment. Based upon experimental data, radiotherapy is often combined with chemotherapy in this patient category.[41,42] However, the evidence in support of this combined treatment is still limited, although theoretically it is tempting to combine chemotherapy and radiotherapy. An important observation is the increased toxicity noticed if radiotherapy is combined with chemotherapy in the preoperative setting.[43,44] Therefore there is an urgent need for trials exploring the hypothesis that combined chemo-radiotherapy is better than radiotherapy alone for locally inextirpable rectal cancers in terms of resectability and survival.

CONCLUSIONS

According to the collected worldwide experience, preoperative radiotherapy is more dose-effective than postoperative radiotherapy in reducing the local recurrence rate. Radiotherapy alone has influenced survival only if given preoperatively, but if postoperative radiotherapy is combined with chemotherapy, a similar effect on survival has been seen. The way in which adjuvant radiotherapy has been implemented in different countries is a balance between the attitudes of surgeons and radiotherapists, and has become a matter of national preferences and tradition. Irrational factors have probably also influenced the choice, and in the Scandinavian countries, in the UK and in many other countries in Europe, preoperative radiotherapy has become the predominant option, whereas the recommended treatment in the USA and Canada has been postoperative chemo-radiotherapy.[62] Several important questions still remain to be answered. One of these concerns late effects. Even if most patients are older than 70 years at diagnosis, several are below 60 years, which is why it is important to follow patients in the trials for 10 years or more. Another question concerns the type of radiotherapy, i.e. the Swedish concept with 5×5 Gy during 1 week, or a more traditional radiotherapy over a 5-week period with chemotherapy. Also, the use of chemotherapy given concomitantly with radiotherapy must be properly addressed. A most important and still unanswered question is whether radiotherapy should be used if surgery is optimized. Based upon ongoing trials, we might have an answer to whether or not there is a place for radiotherapy in most patients with rectal cancer or whether it should be used even more selectively.

REFERENCES

1. Stenbeck M, Rosén M, Holm L-E, Cancer survival in Sweden during three decades 1961–1991. *Acta Oncol* 1995; **34**: 881–91.
2. Dahlberg M, Påhlman L, Bergström R, Glimelius B, Improved survival in patients with rectal cancer: a population based register study. *Br J Surg* 1998; **85**: 515–20.
3. Glimelius B, Påhlman L, Perioperative radiotherapy in rectal cancer. *Acta Oncol* 1999; **38**: 23–32.
4. Adam IJ, Mohamdee MO, Martin IG et al, Role of circumferential margin involvement in the local recurrence of rectal cancer. *Lancet* 1994; **344**: 707–11.
5. Ny IOL, Luk ISC, Yuen ST et al, Surgical lateral clearance in resected rectal carcinomas, a multivariate analysis of clinicopathological features. *Cancer* 1993; **71**: 1972–6.
6. Moriya Y, Hojo K, Sawada T, Koyama Y, Significance of lateral node dissection for advanced rectal carcinoma at or below the peritoneal reflection. *Dis Colon Rectum* 1989; **32**: 307–15.
7. Hojo K, Sawada T, Moroija Y, An analysis of survival and voiding, sexual function after wide iliopelvic lymphadenectomy in patients with carcinoma of the rectum, compared with conventional lymphadenectomy. *Dis Colon Rectum* 1989; **32**: 128–33.
8. MacFarlane JK, Ryall RDH, Heald RJ, Mesorectal excision for rectal cancer. *Lancet* 1993; **341**: 457–60.
9. Enker WE, Total mesorectal excision – the new golden standard of surgery for rectal cancer. *Ann Med* 1997; **29**: 127–33.
10. Gunderson L, Sosin H, Areas of failure found at reoperation (second or symptomatic look) following 'curative surgery' for adenocarcinoma of the rectum. *Cancer* 1974; **34**: 1278–92.
11. Phillips RKS, Hittinger R, Blesovsky L et al, Local recurrence following 'curative' surgery for large bowel cancer: I. The overall picture. *Br J Surg* 1984; **71**: 12–16.
12. Påhlman L, Glimelius B, Local recurrences after surgical treatment for rectal carcinoma. *Acta Chir Scand* 1984; **150**: 331–5.
13. Rider WD, Palmer JA, Mahoney LJ, Robertson CT, Preoperative irradiation in operable cancer of the rectum: report of the Toronto trial. *Can J Surg* 1977; **20**: 335–8.
14. Duncan W, Smith AN, Freedman LS et al, The evaluation of low dose pre-operative X-ray therapy in the management of operable rectal cancer, results of a randomly controlled trial. *Br J Surg* 1984; **71**: 21–5.
15. Goldberg PA, Nicholls RJ, Porter NH et al, Long-term results of a randomised trial of short-course low-dose adjuvant pre-operative radiotherapy for rectal cancer: reduction in local treatment failure. *Eur J Cancer* 1994; **30A**: 1602–6.
16. Roswit B, Higgins G, Keehn R, Preoperative irradiation for carcinoma of the rectum and rectosigmoid colon: report of a National Veterans Administration randomized study. *Cancer* 1975; **35**: 1597–602.
17. Horn A, Halvorsen JF, Dahl O, Preoperative radiotherapy in operable rectal cancer. *Dis Colon Rectum* 1990; **33**: 823–38.
18. Higgins G, Humphrey E, Dwight R et al, Preoperative radiation and surgery for cancer of the rectum. VASOG Trial II. *Cancer* 1986; **58**: 352–9.
19. Marsh PH, James RD, Schofield PF, Adjuvant preoperative radiotherapy for locally advanced rectal carcinoma. Results of a prospective, randomized trial. *Dis Colon Rectum* 1994; **37**: 1205–14.
20. Gérard A, Buyse M, Nordlinger B et al, Preoperative radiotherapy as adjuvant treatment in rectal cancer. *Ann Surg* 1988; **208**: 606–14.
21. Medical Research Council Rectal Cancer Working Party, Randomised trial of surgery alone versus radiotherapy followed by surgery for potentially operable locally advanced rectal cancer. *Lancet* 1996; **348**: 1605–10.
22. Stockholm Rectal Cancer Study Group, Preoperative short-term radiation therapy in operable rectal carcinoma. A prospective randomized trial. *Cancer* 1990; **66**: 49–55.
23. Swedish Rectal Cancer Trial, Local recurrence rate in a randomized multicentre trial of preoperative radiotherapy compared to surgery alone in resectable rectal carcinoma. *Eur J Surg* 1996; **162**: 397–402.
24. Bentzen SM, Balslev I, Pedersen M et al, Time to loco-regional recurrence after resection of Dukes' B and C colorectal cancer with or without adjuvant postoperative radiotherapy. *Br J Cancer* 1992; **65**: 102–7.
25. Medical Research Council Rectal Cancer Working Party, Randomised trial of surgery alone versus surgery followed by radiotherapy for mobile cancer of the rectum. *Lancet* 1996; **348**: 1610–14.
26. Gastrointestinal Tumor Study Group, Prolongation of the disease-free interval in surgically treated rectal carcinoma. *N Engl J Med* 1985; **312**: 1464–72.
27. Fisher B, Wolmark N, Rockette H et al, Postoperative adjuvant chemotherapy or radiation therapy for rectal cancer: results from NSABP Protocol R-01. *J Natl Cancer Inst* 1988; **80**: 21–9.
28. Arnaud JP, Nordlinger B, Bosset JF et al, Radical surgery and postoperative radiotherapy as combined treatment in rectal cancer. Final results of a phase III study of the European Organization for Research and Treatment of Cancer. *Br J Surg* 1997; **84**: 352–7.
29. Treurniet-Donker AD, van Putten WLJ, Wereldsma JCJ et al, Postoperative radiation therapy for rectal cancer. *Cancer* 1991; **67**: 2042–8.
30. Bokey EL, Öjerskog B, Chapuis PH et al, Local recurrence after curative excision of the rectum for cancer without adjuvant therapy: role of total anatomical dissection. *Br J Surg* 1999; **86**: 1164–70.
31. Påhlman L, Glimelius B, Graffman S, Pre versus postoperative radiotherapy in rectal carcinoma: an interim report from a randomized multicentre trial. *Br J Surg* 1985; **72**: 961–6.
32. Frykholm G, Glimelius B, Påhlman L, Pre- or postoperative irradiation in adenocarcinoma of the rectum: final treatment results of randomized trial and evaluation of late secondary effects. *Dis Colon Rectum* 1993; **36**: 564–72.
33. Withers HR, Taylor JMG, Maciejewski B, The hazard of accelerated tumor clonogen repopulation during radiotherapy. *Acta Oncol* 1988; **27**: 131–46.
34. Glimelius B, Isacsson U, Jung B, Påhlman L, Radiotherapy in addition to radical surgery in rectal cancer – evidence for a dose–response effect favouring preoperative treatment. *Int J Radiat Oncol Biol Phys* 1997; **37**: 281–7.
35. Hermanek P, Wiebelt H, Staimmer D et al, Prognostic factors of rectum carcinoma – experience of the German multicentre study SGCRC. *Tumori* 1995; **81**(Suppl): 60–4.
36. Stockholm Colorectal Cancer Study Group, Randomized study on preoperative radiotherapy in rectal carcinoma. *Ann Surg Oncol* 1996; **3**: 423–30.
37. Swedish Rectal Cancer Trial, Improved survival with preoperative radiotherapy in resectable rectal cancer. *N Engl J Med* 1997; **336**: 980–7.
38. Krook JE, Moertel CG, Gunderson LL et al, Effective surgical

adjuvant therapy for high-risk rectal cancer. *N Engl J Med* 1991; **324:** 709–15.

39. Tveit KM, Gudvog I, Hagen S et al, Randomized controlled trial of postoperative radiotherapy and short-term time-scheduled 5-fluorouracil against surgery alone in the treatment of Dukes B and C rectal cancer. *Br J Surg* 1997; **84:** 1130–5.

40. Rockette H, Deutsch M, Petrelli N et al, Effect of postoperative radiation therapy (RTX) when used with adjuvant chemotherapy in Dukes' B and C rectal cancer: results from NSABP R-02. *Proc Am Soc Clin Oncol* 1994; **13:** 193.

41. Lawrence TS, Davis MA, Maybaum J, Dependence of 5-fluorouracil-mediated radiosensitization on DNA-directed effects. *Int J Radiat Oncol Biol Phys* 1994; **29:** 519–23.

42. Tannock F, Treatment of cancer with radiation and drugs. *J Clin Oncol* 1996; **14:** 3156–74.

43. Boulis-Wassif S, Ten years' experience with a multimodality treatment of advanced stages of rectal cancer. *Cancer* 1983; **45:** 2017–24.

44. Overgaard M, Bertelsen K, Dalmark M et al, A randomized feasibility study evaluating the effect of radiotherapy alone or combined with 5-fluorouracil in the treatment of locally or inoperable colorectal carcinoma. *Acta Oncol* 1993; **32:** 547–53.

45. Swedish Rectal Cancer Trial, Initial report from a Swedish multicentre study examining the role of preoperative irradiation in the treatment of patients with resectable rectal carcinoma. *Br J Surg* 1993; **80:** 1333–6.

46. Bubrik MP, Rolfmeyers ES, Schauer RM et al, Effects of high-dose and low-dose preoperative irradiation on low anterior anastomosis in dogs. *Dis Colon Rectum* 1982; **25:** 406–15.

47. Påhlman L, Glimelius B, Pre- or postoperative radiotherapy in rectal carcinoma: a report from a randomized multicenter trial. *Ann Surg* 1990; **211:** 187–95.

48. James R on behalf of the AXIS Collaborators MRC Clinical Trials Unit, UK et al, Perioperative radiotherapy (RT) and intraportal 5-fluorouracil (5-FU; PVI) in the adjuvant treatment of colorectal cancer. Adjuvant X-ray Infusion Study (AXIS) trial. *Dis Colon Rectum* 1999; **42:** A63.

49. Frykholm-Jansson G, Sintorn K, Montelius A et al, Acute lumbosacral plexopathy after preoperative radiotherapy in rectal carcinoma. *Radiother Oncol* 1996; **38:** 121–30.

50. Holm T, Rutqvist LE, Johansson H, Cedermark B, Postoperative mortality in rectal cancer treated with or without preoperative radiotherapy causes and risk factors. *Br J Surg* 1996; **83:** 964–8.

51. Kapiteijn E, Kranenberg EK, Steup WH et al, Total mesorectal excision (TME) with or without preoperative radiotherapy in the treatment of primary rectal cancer. *Eur J Surg* 1999; **165:** 410–22.

52. Holm T, Singnomklao T, Rutqvist L, Cedermark B, Adjuvant preoperative radiotherapy in patients with rectal carcinoma. Adverse effects during long term follow-up of two randomized trials. *Cancer* 1996; **78:** 968–76.

53. Lewis WG, Williamson MER, Stephenson BM et al, Potential disadvantages of postoperative adjuvant radiotherapy after anterior resection for rectal cancer: a pilot study of sphincter function, rectal capacity and clinical outcome. *Int J Colorectal Dis* 1995; **10:** 133–7.

54. Kollmorgen CF, Meagher AP, Wolf BG et al, The long-term effect of adjuvant postoperative chemoradiotherapy for rectal carcinoma on bowel function. *Ann Surg* 1994; **220:** 676–82.

55. Graf W, Ekström K, Glimelius B, Påhlman L, A pilot study of factors influencing bowel function after colorectal anastomosis. *Dis Colon Rectum* 1996; **39:** 593–600.

56. Dahlberg M, Glimelius B, Graf W, Påhlman L, Preoperative irradiation affects the functional results after surgery for rectal cancer: results from a randomized study. *Dis Colon Rectum* 1998; **41:** 543–51.

57. Wibe A, for the Norwegian Rectal Cancer Group, Total mesorectal excision (TME) in Norway – National Rectal Cancer Project. *Dis Colon Rectum* 1999; **42:** A26.

58. Lehander A, Holm T, Rutqvist LE et al, The impact of surgical training workshops on the outcome in rectal cancer in the population of Stockholm. *Eur J Cancer* 1999; **35**(Suppl 4): S67.

59. Dahlberg M, Glimelius B, Påhlman L, Changing strategy for rectal cancer is associated with improved outcome. *Br J Surg* 1999; **86:** 379–84.

60. Minsky BD, Cohen AM, Enker WE, Pary P, Sphincter preservation with preoperative radiation therapy and coloanal anastomosis. *Int J Radiat Oncol Biol Phys* 1995; **31:** 553–9.

61. Francois Y, Nemoz CJ, Baulieux J et al, Influence of the interval between preoperative radiation therapy and surgery on downstaging and on the rate of sphincter-sparing surgery for rectal cancer: the Lyon R90-01 randomized trial. *J Clin Oncol* 1999; **17:** 2396–402.

62. NCI Clinical Announcement: Adjuvant therapy of rectal cancer (14 March 1991).

23

Radiotherapy for rectal cancer: The US approach

Harvey Mamon, Christopher Willett

INTRODUCTION

Rectal cancer is a common health problem in the USA, with an estimated 34 700 cases and 8 700 deaths in 1999.[1] It spans a wide spectrum of presentations, from superficial, favorable disease that may be managed with limited procedures, through locally advanced and metastatic disease. While there may not be a clear 'standard of care' for the management of rectal cancer in the USA, this chapter will review common radiotherapeutic approaches used in this country for early-stage rectal cancers. The management of locally advanced and metastatic disease will not be included in this review.

FAVORABLE RECTAL CANCER

Favorable rectal cancers, i.e. those with less than transmural penetration of the bowel wall and no lymph-node metastases, have a high control rate with surgery alone. For proximal tumors, this may be accomplished with low anterior resection. Tumors located more distally in the rectum may be managed with abdominoperineal resection (APR), which offers a high probability of local control and survival. These benefits are associated with significant costs, however, including loss of anorectal function, with a permanent colostomy, and increased sexual and genitourinary dysfunction. There has thus been a great deal of interest in developing alternative surgical approaches, for example transanal, transsphincteric, or transsacral local excisions, for patients with favorable carcinomas of the distal rectum. The most appropriate patient selection criteria for these procedures, and the role of adjuvant chemotherapy and

radiation, are becoming increasingly well defined, though they remain areas of active investigation.

Tumors appropriate for local excision must be sufficiently small to permit excision and closure of the excision site without significant narrowing of the rectal lumen. They should also be confined to the rectal wall (T1 or T2), with a low probability of lymph-node metastases. Usual criteria for local excision thus include: tumor size less than 4 cm, location within 8 cm of the anal verge, well or moderately differentiated histology, mobile, not ulcerated, and without suspicion of perirectal or presacral adenopathy.[2]

Clinical and radiological evaluation

Despite advances in the radiographic staging of rectal cancer, digital rectal examination by an experienced practitioner remains among the most reliable methods of assessing the depth of penetration of the primary tumor, with accuracy rates reported to be approximately 80%.[3] As lymph-node metastases are seen only microscopically in a high percentage of cases, it is not surprising that the sensitivity of digital rectal examination for detecting lymph-node involvement is quite low.

Endoscopic ultrasound (EUS) may be used to assess both the depth of tumor penetration and lymph-node status.[3,4] With an experienced ultrasonographer, the correlation of T stage determined by EUS with pathological T stage generally ranges from 70% to 90%.[5] The importance of having an experienced operator was demonstrated in a study from the University of Minnesota, where the accuracy rate improved from 59% early in the study to 88% in the later phases.[6] Even in experienced hands, the accuracy of EUS is limited by its ability to visualize only macro-scopic changes, and it thus can never be as accurate as pathological staging.[7] The accuracy of EUS for assess-ing lymph-node status is less than for T stage, with reports in the 50–80% range.[4] Despite these limita-tions, EUS may be considered complementary to digi-tal rectal examination in the staging of rectal cancer, and more accurate than computed tomography (CT) or magnetic resonance imaging (MRI) scans.

CT and MRI, however, offer the advantages of offering a larger field of view than EUS, less operator dependence, and the ability to study stenotic tumors.[3,4] It is thus useful to obtain CT scans as well as EUS as part of the preoperative staging in patient selection for local excision. If any of the staging modalities offer convincing evidence of either trans-mural penetration or nodal involvement, radical resection is preferable to local excision, since the lat-ter is associated with a risk of tumor cut-through and inadequate removal of involved lymph nodes.

Surgery and pathological evaluation

Surgical technique is crucial in obtaining adequate control rates following local excision. Peranal and transsphincteric (York–Mason) excision, and excision via midline posterior proctotomy (Kraske), are rec-ommended, since these operations permit full-thick-ness excision of the bowel wall, with removal of the tumor and adjacent rectum in one piece without fragmentation of the tumor. This allows assessment of inked margins, histological differentiation, blood and lymphatic vessel invasion (LVI), and depth of penetration of the bowel wall. The pathologist should then carefully define the narrowest margin in fresh tissues and on slides using an inked margin, as well as other tumor features such as the degree of

differentiation. Use of fulguration or electrocoagula-tion is not recommended, since these procedures are associated with a high likelihood of residual disease, and inadequate pathological analysis of margin sta-tus and other histological features.

A key limitation of local procedures compared with APR is the inability to remove perirectal or mesenteric lymphatics for both diagnostic and thera-peutic purposes. The incidence of nodal involvement increases with the depth of penetration of the pri-mary tumor.[8–10] In a collective series, tumor penetra-tion to the submucosa, muscularis propria, and perirectal fat was associated with a 12%, 35%, and 44% incidence of nodal involvement, respectively.[2] Histological grade and LVI are also independent pre-dictors of nodal metastases. A series from Memorial Sloan-Kettering Cancer Center reported a 29–50% risk of perirectal lymph-node metastasis for patients with T1 and T2 tumors that were poorly differenti-ated or positive for LVI.[9] A summary of the risk of nodal metastasis by T stage and histological features is presented in Table 23.1.

Local excision alone would be inadequate treat-ment for those patients with T1–T2 tumors with pathological features that suggest a high risk of lymph-node metastases. Local failure in patients undergoing local excision has been correlated with histological features in the primary tumor suggesting a high risk of nodal involvement. A study from Erlangen, for example, reported a local failure rate of less than 10% in patients with 'low-risk' tumors, compared with 30% in patients with 'high-risk' tumors.[10] Many centers in the USA are investigating postoperative pelvic radiation with concurrent 5-flu-orouracil (5-FU) to improve the outcome after local excision of 'high-risk' patients. The results of several of these studies are summarized in Table 23.2.

Table 23.1 Risk of nodal involvement according to tumor histopathology			
Risk	**Low,** **<10%**	**Intermediate,** **10–20%**	**High,** **>30%**
Differentiation	Good	Moderate	Poor
Tumor invasion	Submucosa or inner muscularis propria	Muscularis propria	Muscularis propria or perirectal fat
LVI	–	–	+

Table 23.2 Outcome following local excision and postoperative radiation

Study	Local control (%)	Survival rate (%)
Princess Margaret Hospital[11]	76	80 (6-year median)
Fox Chase Cancer Center[12]	81	75 (5-year disease-free)
Memorial Sloan-Kettering Cancer Center[13]	73	70 (Overall)
CALGB Intergroup[14]	90	74 (Crude figures)
MGH/Emory University[15]	90	74

Treatment recommendations and results

Treatment recommendations are guided by the surgical and pathological findings of the local excision. Local excision appears to be sufficient treatment for patients with small tumors invading the mucosa and submucosa without adverse features. Several centers have reported local control and recurrence-free survival rates of 90% or greater following local excision of T1 tumors with favorable histology. Postoperative radiation is usually not advised unless there are concerning features such as compromised margins, poorly differentiated histology, or LVI.

For tumors with deeper invasion of the rectal wall, adjuvant radiation therapy and chemotherapy have been recommended following local excision. As patients with T2 tumors have a 20% risk of nodal involvement and local failure following local excision only, postoperative radiation with 5-FU-based chemotherapy is advised for these patients. Single-institution studies suggest excellent local control and survival following local excision and adjuvant radiation for T2 tumors. At the MD Anderson Cancer Center, for example, 15 patients with T2 tumors treated by local excision with postoperative radiation and 5-FU had a 93% rate of local control.[16] Similarly, the 5-year actuarial local control rate for 33 patients with T2 tumors treated by local excision and adjuvant radiation with or without 5-FU at the Massachusetts General Hospital was 85%.[15] A more recent report from Memorial Sloan-Kettering Cancer Institute, however, raises the concern that with longer follow-up there is a higher failure rate for T2 patients. In this series of 39 patients with 41-month median follow-up, 25 of whom had T2 tumors, the crude local failure rates for T1, T2, and T3 tumors were 0%, 24%, and 25%, respectively.[13] Five of the eight local failures were locally controlled with salvage APR.

An ongoing Cancer and Leukemia Group B (CALGB) Intergroup phase II study appears to support the use of local excision of T1 and T2 tumors, with appropriate selection of patients for adjuvant radiation and 5-FU.[14] Fifty-nine patients underwent local excision of T1 tumors without further therapy, and 51 patients with T2 tumors received radiation and 5-FU following local excision. There were four failures among the T1 patients, two of whom had local failures and remain without evidence of disease following salvage APR. Of nine failures among the T2 patients, three had distant metastases and died of disease without an attempt at salvage. Six underwent APR for local recurrence. Two had both local and distant disease, and subsequently died. Of the four with local-only recurrences, three remain free of disease at last follow-up; the fourth subsequently developed distant metastases and died of disease without local recurrence at the time of death.

Despite preoperative staging with DRE, EUS, and other techniques, pathology will nevertheless reveal T3 tumors following some local excisions. We recommend that these patients be brought back to the operating room for radical surgical resection (if feasible), since the limited available data for local excision with adjuvant chemotherapy and radiation for T3 tumors suggest unacceptably high local failure rates. The MD Anderson Cancer Center reports a 20% local failure rate among 15 patients with T3 tumors following local excision, radiation, and 5-FU,[16] whereas 75% of four similarly treated patients at the Massachusetts General Hospital failed locally.[17]

Techniques of chemo-radiotherapy

It is useful for radiation planning to place radio-opaque markers at the perimeter of the excision to identify the area at highest risk. Radiation is delivered at 1.8 Gy per fraction to 45 Gy in a three or four field technique, followed by a field reduction to 50.4 Gy with a lateral or three-field technique. If there is no small bowel in the field, a second field reduction may be added to 54 Gy directed at the 'marked' tumor bed. The field borders are the same as described in the following section on mobile rectal cancers. 5-FU may be given as a continuous infusion or as bolus injections during the first and last weeks of irradiation.

MOBILE RECTAL CANCERS

Practice patterns in the USA for resected stage II or III rectal cancer have been strongly influenced by a series of prospective randomized trials published in the 1980s and early 1990s. In protocol GI-7175, the Gastrointestinal Tumor Study Group (GITSG) randomized 227 patients with resected Dukes B2 and C rectal adenocarcinomas to one of four treatment arms.[18] These included observation, radiation alone to 40 or 48 Gy, chemotherapy alone with methyl-CCNU (semustine) and 5-FU, and combined-modality therapy consisting of radiation to 40 or 44 Gy with concurrent 5-FU and maintenance chemotherapy with 5-FU and methyl-CCNU. Patients treated with combined-modality therapy had a statistically significant improvement in outcome compared with surgery alone. Single-modality therapy with chemotherapy or radiation did not provide a statistically significant benefit. Local recurrence was 55% in the surgery-alone arm and 33% in the combined-modality arm. The increase in overall survival did not reach statistical significance in the initial report, but with longer follow-up a significant survival advantage to combined-modality therapy was seen.[19]

The National Surgical Adjuvant Breast and Bowel Project (NSABP) randomized patients with Dukes B and C rectal cancers to one of three arms in Protocol B-01.[20] Resected patients received no further treatment, adjuvant chemotherapy with methyl-CCNU, vincristine, and 5-FU, or adjuvant radiation to 46–47 Gy. There was no combined-modality therapy arm. Postoperative radiation improved local control, without a survival advantage, compared with surgery alone. Male patients receiving chemotherapy had improved survival relative to controls, with females receiving chemotherapy experiencing a lower survival rate than controls, though this gender difference has not been replicated in subsequent studies.

The Mayo/North Central Cancer Treatment Group (NCCTG) also carried out a prospective randomized trial for patients with resected rectal cancer. Two hundred and nine patients with T3–4 or node-positive tumors received either postoperative radiation to 50.4 Gy, or post-operative radiation to 50.4 Gy with concurrent 5-FU as well as pre- and postirradiation chemotherapy consisting of 5-FU and methyl-CCNU.[21] As in the GITSG study, there was a statistically significant improvement in local control and survival associated with combined-modality therapy. The addition of chemotherapy to radiation resulted in a 34% decrease in local recurrence, from 63% with radiation alone to 42% with combined-modality therapy ($p = 0.0016$), and a 29% decrease in the overall death rate ($p = 0.043$). The data from these prospective, randomized trials provide good evidence that postoperative pelvic radiotherapy combined with chemotherapy results in improved local control and survival compared with surgery alone or surgery plus radiation for transmural or node-positive tumors. Following publication of these trials, the National Cancer Institute Consensus Conference concluded that the standard of care for patients with resected T3–4 or node-positive rectal cancers without distant metastases should include adjuvant chemotherapy and pelvic radiotherapy.[22]

The above studies included methyl-CCNU as part of the chemotherapeutic regimens, which may predispose patients to treatment-related acute non-lymphocytic leukemia. An analysis of 3633 patients with gastrointestinal cancers treated in nine randomized clinical trials revealed 14 leukemic disorders among the 2067 patients receiving methyl-CCNU, versus one leukemic disorder among the 1566 patients who did not. The relative risk of developing leukemia attributed to methyl-CCNU was 12.4, with an incidence of 2.3 cases per 1000 persons per year.[23] Two randomized trials, one from the GITSG and one from NCCTG, have since demonstrated that methyl-CCNU does not provide any benefit beyond that achieved with 5-FU.[24,25] Methyl-CCNU has thus been omitted from subsequent chemotherapeutic regimens for colorectal cancer.

The above randomized studies clearly demonstrate a benefit to the combination of 5-FU-based chemotherapy and radiation in the management of rectal cancer. A remaining question, however, is how to optimize the combination of radiation and 5-FU.

In patients with metastatic disease, 5-FU given either with leucovorin or as a continuous infusion (225 mg/m^2/day) has produced a higher response rate than conventional bolus 5-FU. Continuous-infusion 5-FU has been compared with bolus 5-FU by the GI Intergroup.[25] In this study, 660 patients with resected stage II or III rectal cancer were randomized to pelvic radiotherapy (50.4–54 Gy), with either bolus 5-FU (500 mg/m^2 on three consecutive days during weeks 1 and 5 of radiation) or protracted-venous-infusion (PVI) 5-FU (225 mg/m^2 during the entire period of radiotherapy). Continuous-infusion 5-FU was associated with a decrease in overall tumor relapse from 47% to 37% ($p = 0.01$) and in distant metastases from 40% to 31% ($p = 0.03$), compared with bolus 5-FU (Table 23.3). In multivariate analysis, continuous-infusion 5-FU was significantly associated with an advantage in overall survival, 70% versus 60% at 4 years ($p = 0.005$). The toxicity profile was similar between the two treatments in terms of dermatitis, stomatitis, nausea, vomiting, and thrombocytopenia. More diarrhea was seen with continuous-infusion therapy; the incidence of leukopenia was higher with bolus 5-FU.

A GI Intergroup study has also compared 5-FU given with pelvic radiation versus 5-FU with fluorouracil modulators.[26] Almost 1700 patients with resected rectal cancer were treated with two cycles of bolus 5-FU chemotherapy before and after pelvic radiotherapy. The randomization involved four arms, which varied in the type of chemotherapy given concurrently with the pelvic radiation. These included 5-FU alone, 5-FU with leucovorin, 5-FU with levamisole, or 5-FU with leucovorin and levamisole. With a median follow-up of 48 months, none of the three multidrug arms demonstrated a statistically significant advantage over 5-FU alone. The analysis suggests that neither levamisole arm is likely to demonstrate a benefit even with longer follow-up, but that the 5-FU + leucovorin arm will require further analysis with additional follow-up to rule out a benefit compared with 5-FU alone.

Table 23.3 Randomized postoperative chemo-radiotherapy trials of rectal cancer

Study[a]	Local failure rate (%)	Distant failure rate (%)	Overall survival rate (%)
GITSG[18]			
RT + ChT	11	26	57
RT	20	30	43
ChT	27	27	43
Control	24	34	28
NSAPB[20]			
RT	16	31	50
ChT	21	24	58
Control	25	26	48
NCCTG/Mayo[21]			
RT + ChT	14	29	53
RT	25	46	38
GI Intergroup[25,b]			
RT + PVI 5-FU	NS[b]	31	70
RT + bolus 5-FU	NS	40	60

[a]RT, radiotherapy; ChT, chemotherapy; PVI, protracted venous infusion.
[b]The local recurrence rates were not stated. The paper does report that the difference in local control rates did not differ significantly according to the method of 5-FU administration ($p = 0.11$).

Additional studies are ongoing to determine the optimal method for combining radiation therapy and 5-FU, including testing of the newer oral agents. For patients treated off-protocol, many centers in the USA have adopted continuous-infusion 5-FU at 225 mg/m^2/day during pelvic radiotherapy as the current standard.

The improvements in local control and survival achieved with adjuvant chemotherapy and radiation have come at the expense of both acute and delayed treatment-related morbidity. Twenty-four percent of the patients receiving pelvic radiotherapy with concurrent continuous-infusion 5-FU in a recent Intergroup trial experienced severe or life-threatening diarrhea.[25] The incidence of late complications may be similar. A recent report of 306 rectal cancer patients receiving postoperative radiation at the Mayo Clinic from 1981 through 1990 found a 25% probability of developing chronic bowel injury at 10 years.[27] Approximately two-thirds of the patients received concurrent chemotherapy, which did not correlate with the risk of late enteritis. In addition to the commonly measured endpoints of acute and late bowel injury, there are also more subtle alterations in bowel function, which adversely impact on quality of life. A report from the Mayo Clinic found an increased rate of frequency, incontinence, pad requirements, and other measures of impaired bowel function in patients who received low anterior resection followed by postoperative chemo-radiotherapy compared with those undergoing low anterior resection alone.[28]

It is possible that administering radiotherapy preoperatively rather than postoperatively may reduce some of these treatment-related sequelae. In the preoperative setting, the small intestine is less likely to be fixed within the irradiated volume in the pelvis than after rectal surgery. The postoperative tumor bed may be hypoxic and relatively radioresistant.[29] In addition, for patients who require an APR rather than low anterior resection, the radiated field is considerably larger in the postoperative than in the preoperative setting, since the perineal scar must be included. The major disadvantage of neoadjuvant treatment is less accurate staging, with a potential for over-treatment of patients who are either T2N0 or have liver or other distant metastases too small to be appreciated by CT scan. In the USA, clinical research on rectal cancer has traditionally focused on adjuvant rather than neoadjuvant approaches. European studies, in contrast, have evaluated different schedules of preoperative radiation, with preoperative combined-modality approaches only recently gaining more acceptance in the USA.

The European preoperative radiation studies may be divided into three categories: low-dose, intermediate-dose, and the intensive short-course radiation utilized in Sweden (see Chapter 22). Of 11 modern randomized trials of preoperative radiotherapy, none of which used chemotherapy or conventional doses of radiation, one has shown a survival advantage. In this Swedish study, 1168 patients were randomized to surgery alone, or one week of radiation at 5 Gy per day to a total of 25 Gy, with surgery one week later.[30] The radiated patients had a 12% incidence of local failure, compared with 27% for the controls ($p = 0.001$), and the 5-year survival rate was improved from 48% to 58% ($p = 0.004$). The incidence of postoperative morbidity, however, was significantly higher in the radiated group: 44% versus 34%, $p = 0.001$. Other studies have also suggested a high risk of postoperative morbidity and mortality with preoperative radiation using this fractionation.[31,32] These complication rates are higher than those seen with preoperative radiation given with more conventional fractionation. Principally because of these concerns regarding late treatment-related morbidity, as well as the desire to integrate chemotherapy concurrently with preoperative radiation, the Swedish approach of preoperative radiation has not been widely adopted in the USA.

The demonstrated success of combining chemotherapy and radiation in the postoperative management of rectal cancer has generated interest in applying combined-modality therapy preoperatively. Many phase II studies have now demonstrated the safety of this approach, with local control and survival rates comparable to those expected in the adjuvant setting. Unfortunately, two prospective randomized trials of preoperative versus postoperative chemoradiation – one from the Intergroup and one from the NSABP – have closed owing to poor accrual. A preliminary analysis of the NSABP trial (R-03) suggested that preoperative treatment is as tolerable as postoperative.[33] As seen in Table 23.4, the phase II trials suggest a higher pathological complete response rate of 20–29%, compared with 6–12% seen following preoperative radiation without chemotherapy. Further maturation of these and other studies should help determine whether this increased response rate will lead to increases in local control and survival.

There is more variability in the schedule of

Table 23.4 Pathologic response rates to neoadjuvant chemo-radiotherapy

Study	No. of patients	Radiation dose (Gy)	Chemotherapy	Pathological complete response rate (%)
University of Florida[34]	132	30–50	None	11
Jewish Hospital[35]	208	40–50	None	6
MD Anderson[36]	77	45	5-FU infusion	29
Duke[37]	43	45	5-FU/cisplatin	27
Memorial Sloan-Kettering[38]	20	50.4	5-FU/leucovorin	20

chemotherapy utilized than in the radiation techniques among the neoadjuvant chemo-radiotherapy trials, all of which treat to 45–50.4 Gy in 1.8 Gy fractions utilizing a three- or four-field arrangement. The concurrent 5-FU has been given as a bolus for 3–4 consecutive days during the first and last weeks of radiation, or as a continuous infusion. Additional agents, including platinum and leucovorin, have been used as well. As the Intergroup trial has demonstrated the superiority of continuous-infusion over bolus 5-FU in the adjuvant setting, we have adopted this approach in the neoadjuvant setting as well. We have found that continuous-infusion 5-FU at 225 mg/m^2/day for 5 days per week with concurrent pelvic radiation to 45 Gy followed by a 5.4 Gy boost in 1.8 Gy fractions is well tolerated. Whether additional agents such as leucovorin, levamisole, or platinum will provide any additional benefit is currently under investigation.

Another potential benefit of neoadjuvant treatment is to increase the rate of sphincter preservation for distal rectal tumors that are too large or invasive to be managed with local excision. In the series listed in Table 23.5, patients were evaluated by their surgeon prior to initiating neoadjuvant therapy and declared to require an APR. In the majority of cases, sphincter preservation with coloanal anastomosis was possible after treatment, with the likelihood of sphincter preservation increasing with distance of the tumor from the sphincter.

TECHNICAL ASPECTS OF RADIOTHERAPY FOR RECTAL CANCER

Three- or four-field techniques are acceptable field arrangements for radiotherapy of rectal cancer (Figure 23.1). It is preferable to treat patients prone, which can help increase the separation between the rectum and the small intestine. Treatment with a full

Table 23.5 Sphincter preservation following neoadjuvant chemo-radiotherapy for distal rectal tumors

Study	No. of patients	Dose (Gy)	Sphincter preservation rate (%)	Local control rate (%)	Actuarial survival rate (%)	Bowel function
Minsky[39]	30	50.4	80	83 (4-year)	75 (4-year)	75% good to excellent
Rouanet[40]	27	60	78	93 (crude)	83 (2-year)	NA^a
Mohiuddin[41]	52	45–60	NA^a	86 (crude)	85 (5-year)	90% acceptable

^{a}Not available.

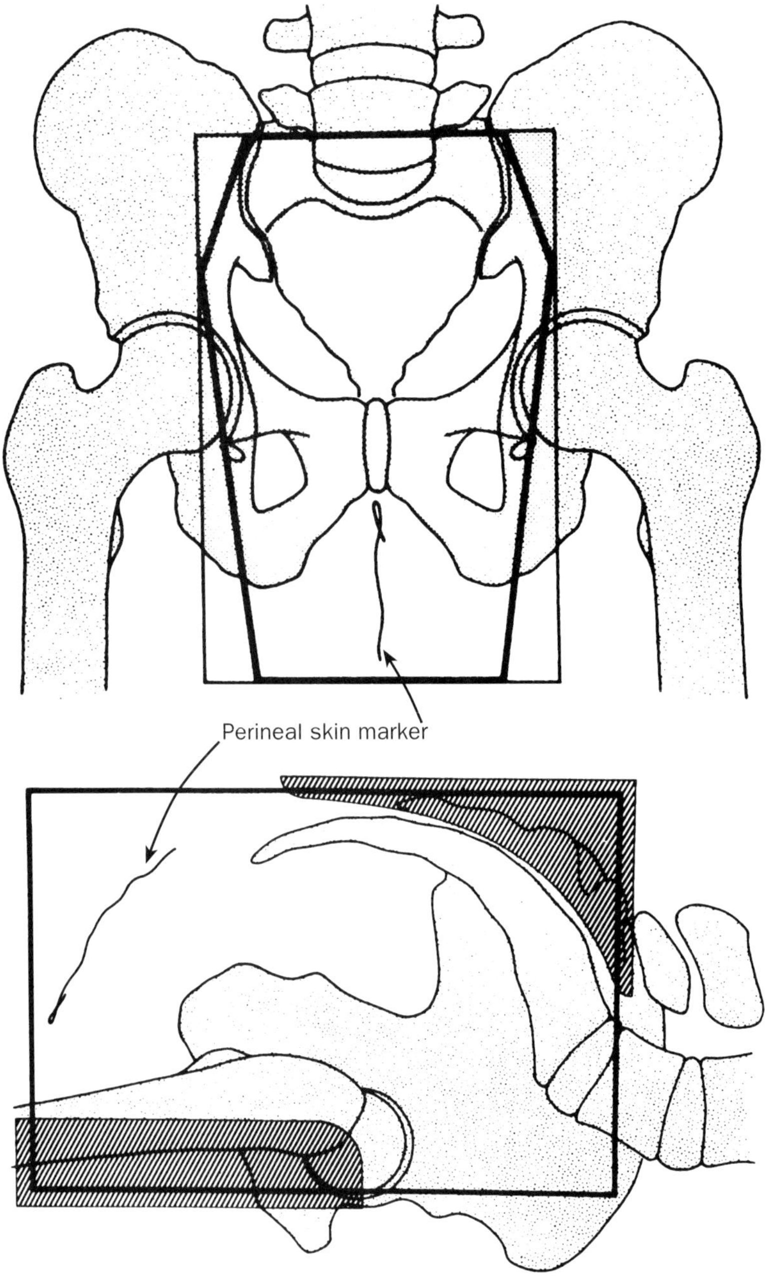

Figure 23.1 AP and lateral fields after abdominoperineal resection.

Perineal skin marker

bladder can also help to push the small intestine out of the radiation field. AP–PA fields are generally inappropriate, since anterior structures that are not at high risk for local failure, most notably small bowel, are treated to a high dose, resulting in increased toxicity from treatment. The superior border is at the inferior aspect of L5, and the inferior border is 4–5 cm below the anastomosis, or below the tumor in the case of preoperative treatment, including the entire sacrum. After APR, there is a substantial risk of recurrence in the perineum. The field must therefore include the perineum, which is best visualized by placing a wire over the perineal scar at the time of simulation. Bolus should be placed on the scar during treatment, and may be removed if there is an excessive skin reaction. The lateral borders of the AP and PA fields extend 1.5 cm beyond the bony pelvis so that the lateral pelvic soft tissues and internal iliac lymph nodes receive a full dose. Blocks may be used to reduce the dose to the femoral heads. The posterior border of the lateral fields is posterior to the sacrum, so that the presacral space (a common site of local failure) receives a full dose. The anterior border of the lateral fields should cover the original tumor volume with at least a 2 cm margin. In female patients, a vaginal marker placed at the time of simulation may be helpful in localizing the rectovaginal septum and defining the anterior border of the field.

The recommended treatment dose is 1.8 Gy/day, 5 days per week, to 45 Gy. The field size is then reduced and a boost is delivered to the tumor bed. The boost dose is determined by having the patient drink barium 30–60 minutes prior to simulation. This allows visualization of the location of the small bowel relative to the boost area. Ideally, the small-bowel dose will be limited to 45 Gy. If a significant amount of bowel is within the field, the boost should be limited to 5.4 Gy; otherwise the boost dose may be increased to 9 Gy, for a total of 54 Gy. It is helpful if the surgeon can exclude the small intestine from the pelvis at the time of surgery. Techniques to accomplish this include reperitonealizing the pelvic floor with a loop of omentum, retroverting the uterus, or placing an artificial mesh prosthesis. These measures are most important after APR, since remaining rectum and colon after low anterior resection may prevent some small bowel from being fixed in the pelvis.

CONCLUSIONS AND FUTURE DIRECTIONS

Radiation therapy for rectal cancer in the USA has been largely guided by multiple prospective randomized trials demonstrating a benefit to postoperative combined-modality therapy with concurrent 5-FU-based chemotherapy (Table 23.3). The focus on combined-modality therapy in the USA is in contrast to many European centers, which have focused on preoperative radiation without concurrent chemo-

therapy (see Chapter 22). Over recent years, preoperative combined-modality therapy has gained increasing acceptance in the USA. As the two trials designed to prospectively randomize patients to preoperative versus postoperative treatment have closed because of poor accrual, it is unlikely that the two approaches will be ever be compared in a randomized fashion in the USA. An ongoing prospective randomized trial of preoperative vs postoperative chemoradiation therapy for rectal cancer in Germany is nearing its accrual goal, and we would anticipate that the results of this trial will be very informative.[42] Future studies may help clarify the relative advantages and disadvantages of each approach, as well as introducing newer chemotherapeutic agents showing activity in colorectal cancer, particularly those with radiosensitizing properties.

For patients with the most favorable rectal cancers – that is, small T1 tumors with favorable histological features – the available data support the effectiveness of local excision without adjuvant treatment. The preponderance of currently available data support the use of local excision combined with adjuvant chemotherapy and radiation for many T2 tumors. Issues of patient selection, preoperative staging, and optimization of the combination of surgical, medical, and radiotherapeutic modalities continue to be areas of active investigation.

REFERENCES

1. Landis S, Murray T, Bolden S, Wingo P, Cancer statistics. *CA Cancer J Clin* 1999; **49:** 8–31.
2. Billingham RP, Conservative treatment of rectal cancer. Extending the indications. *Cancer* 1992; **70**(5 Suppl): 1355–63.
3. Nicholls RJ, Mason AY, Morson BC et al, The clinical staging of rectal cancer. *Br J Surg* 1982; **69:** 404–9.
4. Ng AK, Recht A, Busse PM, Sphincter preservation therapy for distal rectal carcinoma: a review. *Cancer* 1997; **79:** 671–83.
5. Alexander AA, The effect of endorectal ultrasound scanning on the preoperative staging of rectal cancer. *Surg Oncol Clin North Am* 1992; **1:** 39–56.
6. Orrom WJ, Wong WD, Rothenberger DA et al, Endorectal ultrasound in the preoperative staging of rectal tumors. A learning experience. *Dis Colon Rectum* 1990; **33:** 654–9.
7. Hulsmans FJ, Tio TL, Fockens P et al, Assessment of tumor infiltration depth in rectal cancer with transrectal sonography: caution is necessary. *Radiology* 1994; **190:** 715–20.
8. Minsky BD, Rich T, Recht A et al, Selection criteria for local excision with or without adjuvant radiation therapy for rectal cancer. *Cancer* 1989; **63:** 1421–9.
9. Brodsky JT, Richard GK, Cohen AM, Minsky BD, Variables correlated with the risk of lymph node metastasis in early rectal cancer. *Cancer* 1992; **69:** 322–6.

10. Gall FP, Hermanek P, Update of the German experience with local excision of rectal cancer. *Surg Oncol Clin North Am* 1992; **1:** 99–109.

11. Wong CS, Stern H, Cummings BJ, Local excision and post-operative radiation therapy for rectal carcinoma. *Int J Radiat Oncol Biol Phys* 1993; **25:** 669–75.

12. Fortunato L, Ahmad NR, Yeung RS et al, Long-term follow-up of local excision and radiation therapy for invasive rectal cancer. *Dis Colon Rectum* 1995; **38:** 1193–9.

13. Wagman R, Minsky BD, Cohen AM et al, Conservative management of rectal cancer with local excision and postoperative adjuvant therapy. *Int J Radiat Oncol Biol Phys* 1999; **44:** 841–6.

14. Steele GD, Tepper J, Herndon JE, Mayer R, Failure salvage after sphincter sparing treatment for distal rectal adenocarcinoma: a CALGB coordinated study. *Proc Soc Clin Oncol* 1999; **186:** 235a.

15. Chakravarti A, Compton CC, Shellito PC et al, Long-term follow-up of patients with rectal cancer managed by local excision with and without adjuvant irradiation. *Ann Surg* 1999; **230:** 49–54.

16. Ota DM, Skibber J, Rich TA, M.D. Anderson Cancer Center experience with local excision and multimodality therapy for rectal cancer. *Surg Oncol Clin North Am* 1992; **1:** 147–52.

17. Wood WC, Willett CG, Update of the Massachusetts General Hospital experience of combined local excision and radiotherapy for rectal cancer. *Surg Oncol Clin North Am* 1992; **1:** 131–6.

18. Prolongation of the disease-free interval in surgically treated rectal carcinoma. Gastrointestinal Tumor Study Group. *N Engl J Med* 1985; **312:** 1465–72.

19. Douglass HO Jr, Moertel CG, Mayer RJ et al, Survival after postoperative combination treatment of rectal cancer. *N Engl J Med* 1986; **315:** 1294–5.

20. Fisher B, Wolmark N, Rockette H et al, Postoperative adjuvant chemotherapy or radiation therapy for rectal cancer: results from NSABP Protocol R-01. *J Natl Cancer Inst* 1988; **80:** 21–9.

21. Krook JE, Moertel CG, Gunderson LL et al, Effective surgical adjuvant therapy for high-risk rectal carcinoma. *N Engl J Med* 1991; **324:** 709–15.

22. NIH Consensus Conference: Adjuvant therapy for patients with colon and rectal cancer. *JAMA* 1990; **264:** 1444–50.

23. Boice JD Jr, Greene MH, Killen JY Jr et al, Leukemia and preleukemia after adjuvant treatment of gastrointestinal cancer with semustine (methyl-CCNU). *N Engl J Med* 1983; **309:** 1079–84.

24. Radiation therapy and fluorouracil with or without semustine for the treatment of patients with surgical adjuvant adenocarcinoma of the rectum. Gastrointestinal Tumor Study Group. *J Clin Oncol* 1992; **10:** 549–57.

25. O'Connell MJ, Martenson JA, Wieand HS et al, Improving adjuvant therapy for rectal cancer by combining protracted-infusion fluorouracil with radiation therapy after curative surgery. *N Engl J Med* 1994; **331:** 502–7.

26. Tepper JE, O'Connell MJ, Petroni GR et al, Adjuvant postoperative fluorouracil-modulated chemotherapy combined with pelvic radiation therapy for rectal cancer: initial results of Intergroup 0114. *J Clin Oncol* 1997; **15:** 2030–9.

27. Miller AR, Martenson JA, Nelson H et al, The incidence and clinical consequences of treatment-related bowel injury. *Int J Radiat Oncol Biol Phys* 1999; **43:** 817–25.

28. Kollmorgen CF, Meagher AP, Wolff BG et al, The long-term effect of adjuvant postoperative chemoradiotherapy for rectal carcinoma on bowel function. *Ann Surg* 1994; **220:** 676–82.

29. Glimelius B, Isacsson U, Jung B, Påhlman L, Radiotherapy in addition to radical surgery in rectal cancer: evidence for a dose–response effect favoring preoperative treatment. *Int J Radiat Oncol Biol Phys* 1997; **37:** 281–7.

30. Swedish Rectal Cancer Trial, Improved survival with preoperative radiotherapy in resectable rectal cancer. *N Engl J Med* 1997; **336:** 980–7 [Erratum **336:** 1539].

31. Holm T, Singnomklao T, Rutqvist LE, Cedermark B, Adjuvant preoperative radiotherapy in patients with rectal carcinoma. Adverse effects during long term follow-up of two randomized trials. *Cancer* 1996; **78:** 968–76.

32. Holm T, Rutqvist LE, Johansson H, Cedermark B, Postoperative mortality in rectal cancer treated with or without preoperative radiotherapy: causes and risk factors. *Br J Surg* 1996; **83:** 964–8.

33. Hyams DM, Mamounas EP, Petrelli N et al, A clinical trial to evaluate the worth of preoperative multimodality therapy in patients with operable carcinoma of the rectum: a progress report of National Surgical Breast and Bowel Project Protocol R-03. *Dis Colon Rectum* 1997; **40:** 131–9.

34. Mendenhall WM, Bland KI, Copeland EM et al, Does preoperative radiation therapy enhance the probability of local control and survival in high-risk distal rectal cancer? *Ann Surg* 1992; **215:** 696–705; discussion 705–6.

35. Myerson RJ, Michalski JM, King ML et al, Adjuvant radiation therapy for rectal carcinoma: predictors of outcome. *Int J Radiat Oncol Biol Phys* 1995; **32:** 41–50.

36. Rich TA, Skibber JM, Ajani JA et al, Preoperative infusional chemoradiation therapy for stage T3 rectal cancer. *Int J Radiat Oncol Biol Phys* 1995; **32:** 1025–9.

37. Chari RS, Tyler DS, Anscher MS et al, Preoperative radiation and chemotherapy in the treatment of adenocarcinoma of the rectum. *Ann Surg* 1995; **221:** 778–86; discussion 786–7.

38. Minsky BD, Cohen AM, Kemeny N et al, Enhancement of radiation-induced downstaging of rectal cancer by fluorouracil and high-dose leucovorin chemotherapy. *J Clin Oncol* 1992; **10:** 79–84.

39. Wagman R, Minsky BD, Cohen AM et al, Sphincter preservation in rectal cancer with preoperative radiation therapy and coloanal anastomosis: long term follow-up. *Int J Radiat Oncol Biol Phys* 1998; **42:** 51–7.

40. Rouanet P, Fabre JM, Dubois JB et al, Conservative surgery for low rectal carcinoma after high-dose radiation. Functional and oncologic results. *Ann Surg* 1995; **221:** 67–73.

41. Mohiuddin M, Regine WF, Marks GJ, Marks JW, High-dose preoperative radiation and the challenge of sphincter-preservation surgery for cancer of the distal 2 cm of the rectum. *Int J Radiat Oncol Biol Phys* 1998; **40:** 569–74.

42. Sauer R, Fietkau R, Martus P et al, Adjuvant and neoadjuvant radiochemotherapy for advanced rectal cancer – first results of the German multicenter phase III trial. *Int J Radiat Oncol Biol Phys* 2000; **48**(3 Suppl): 119.

24

Radio-chemotherapy in rectal cancer: When and for which patients?

Jean-François Bosset, Georges Mantion, Philippe Maingon

INTRODUCTION

Over 30 years ago, Moertel et al[1] reported the results of a randomized clinical trial in which patients with locally advanced gastrointestinal tumours received either a moderate radiotherapy dose plus a placebo, or the same radiotherapy plus 5-fluorouracil (5-FU) delivered during the first 3 days of radiotherapy. A significant survival advantage was observed in the combined-modality treatment arm. These results prompted the development of combined-modality treatment in many studies for patients with digestive-tract cancers.

OBJECTIVES AND LIMITS OF RADIO-CHEMOTHERAPY

The main goal of radio-chemotherapy is to increase the local effect of ionizing radiation and therefore to enhance local control.[2] When the local effect is dramatically improved, a gain in survival can be expected as well.[3,4]

Radio-chemotherapy usually increases radiation-induced toxicities. Acute toxicity is due to the presence of tissues composed of rapidly dividing cell within the irradiated volume. The severity of toxicity is related to the irradiated volume, the radiotherapy technique and scheme (accelerated radiotherapy increases toxicity), the type of combined drug, and its delivery modality and dosage. When acute toxicity increases, this results in treatment modifications and poor compliance. It should be reported using the World Health Organization (WHO) recommendations.[5]

Late toxicity is expressed by tissues with a low rate of cell division, such as capillary endothelium, connective tissues, bone, muscle, and nervous tissues. It is related to the total dose of radiotherapy, the fractional dose (increased toxicity for dose greater than 2 Gy), and some types of concurrently delivered drugs such as bleomycin, methotrexate, and anthracyclines. Late toxicity can occur either a few months after treatment or several years later. It should be reported using the SOMA–LENT scale.[6]

The therapeutic index is the ratio between benefit and toxicity from a treatment, and is commonly used to assess overall results. An optimal radiotherapy technique and a proper selection of concurrently delivered drugs and dosages are both major factors increasing the therapeutic index. Finally, the consequences of radio-chemotherapy on residual organ functions and quality of life should be considered.[7]

THE PLACE OF RADIOTHERAPY ± CHEMOTHERAPY IN EARLY STAGES

The aim of treatment is cure and sphincter preservation. Low-risk T1 tumours can be managed with local excision alone, but such treatment has a 30–50% local failure rate in high-risk T1 or T2 tumours.[8] In this latter group, US workers are evaluating postoperative radio-chemotherapy after a R0 local excision. Among 51 patients, and after a 42-month median follow-up, 4 patients exhibited a local failure and 3 were salvaged with abdomino-perineal resection.[9]

Using intrarectal 50 kV contact X rays alone for T1 tumours, and in combination with interstitial brachytherapy for T2 tumours, Horiot et al[10] observed an ultimate local control rate of 94.5% and a sphincter preservation rate of 95% in 200 patients treated over 23 years.

Despite evidence of its efficacy, the application of intrarectal radiotherapy remains a rarity.

THE PLACE OF RADIOTHERAPY ± CHEMOTHERAPY IN LOCALLY RESECTABLE STAGES

Results with surgery alone

After a curative rectal resection for cancer, the 5-year survival rate is about 80% for stage I (T1–2N0M0), but drops rapidly if there is transmural and/or nodal involvement, indicating that surgery is appropriate for early-stage tumours only. In patients with stage II (T3–4N0M0) or stage III (TXN1–2M0) disease, local recurrence is observed in 25% and distant metastases in 25%.[11]

The local recurrence rate may vary from 5% in a few highly specialized centres to 16.3% and 28.6% for Dukes B and C tumours respectively in unselected centres.[12–14] Local recurrence is mainly related to inadequate surgical clearance of the radial margin[15] or to reduced distal margin.[16] In addition to these tumour-related factors, it also depends on the surgical technique, skill, and dedication of surgeons.[17,18]

Total mesorectal excision (TME) may reduce the local recurrence rate to about 10%. However, the safety and reproducibility of this technique has not yet been shown in standard practice.[19] Moreover, in European centres using TME, the local recurrence rate varies considerably, ranging from 5% in some to as high as 18% in others.[20]

Because local recurrences cause severe disabling symptoms and can be cured in less than 5% of cases, improving local control remains a major endpoint for treatment strategies in patients with rectal cancer.

Results with postoperative radio-chemotherapy

This approach has been developed in the USA. Its main advantage is the optimal selection of patients, allowing the exclusion of those with early-stage tumours and those who are discovered with metastases at surgery.

The treatment scheme was constructed in two sequences: one is concurrent radio-chemotherapy in which 5-FU-based chemotherapy is delivered during radiotherapy; the other is additional maintenance chemotherapy directed at microscopic distant disease.

In 1990, on the basis of early randomized trials that demonstrated improved survival with postoperative radio-chemotherapy in comparison with surgery alone or postoperative radiotherapy,[21–27] a US National Institutes of Health Consensus Conference recommended postoperative radio-chemotherapy and additional chemotherapy for stage II and III rectal cancer patients.[24] This recommendation is still valid in the USA.[25]

Since 1990, the efforts of US Intergroup trials have been directed at identifying the optimal radio-chemotherapy schemes and agents in the two treatment sequences.

The 86-47-41 four-arm trial demonstrated that delivering 5-FU as a continuous infusion during the radio-chemotherapy sequence produced a significant decrease in distant metastases and improved survival in comparison with a concurrent 5-FU bolus scheme.[26] This trial also demonstrated that a combination of 5-FU and semustine (methyl-CCNU) offered no advantage in comparison with 5-FU alone in the additional chemotherapy sequence.

The 0114 trial compared four different 5-FU-based additional chemotherapy sequences: 5-FU alone versus 5-FU plus leucovorin (LV) versus 5-FU plus levamisole (LEV) versus 5-FU plus LV plus LEV. The radio-chemotherapy sequences were identical in both arms, and used a 5-FU bolus scheme. After a 48-month follow-up, the modulated 5-FU regimens offered no advantage in comparison with the 5-FU-alone arm. Moreover, the three-drug arm appeared more toxic and less effective.[27]

The currently ongoing 0144 three-arm trial is comparing continuous-infusion 5-FU versus discontinuous 5-FU/LV in the concurrent sequence, and bolus 5-FU versus continuous-infusion 5-FU versus 5-FU/LV/LEV in the additional sequence.

Initially, the application of postoperative radio-chemotherapy resulted in increased acute haematological and small-bowel toxicity, resulting in decreased treatment compliance and a treatment-related death rate of about 5%.[28] Refinements in radiotherapy techniques, changes in the concurrent drug delivery, a reduction in the number of additional chemotherapy courses, and the introduction of quality control procedures[29] have increased treatment compliance to about 95% and have reduced the toxic death rate to about 0.5%.[26]

While acute small-bowel toxicity is increased by postoperative radio-chemotherapy, it does not translate into increased small-bowel obstruction, which remains at the same level as observed with surgery alone, at about 1–3%. However, postoperative radio-chemotherapy does result in impaired residual sphincter function, leading to decreased quality of life.[30]

Finally, the postoperative approach should be used cautiously, and needs to be learned from and audited by experienced teams, in order to provide the maximum efficacy and safety to patients with rectal cancer.

Results with preoperative radiotherapy ± chemotherapy

Preoperative radiotherapy has mainly been evaluated in Europe, and has demonstrated its ability to halve local recurrence rates and to improve survival in comparison with surgery alone.[28,31]

Two types of preoperative radiotherapy schemes have been developed:

- the Swedish scheme delivers 25 Gy in 5 fractions over 1 week, followed by surgery within 1 week;
- more standard schemes deliver 40–50 Gy in 20–25 fractions over 4–5 weeks, followed by surgery 3–4 weeks later.

With the short scheme, significant increased postoperative mortality was observed when the irradiated volume was extended to the para-aortic area or when the pelvis was treated with only two fields.[32,33] The postoperative mortality rate dropped to the level observed after surgery alone when the volume was reduced to the posterior part of the pelvis and a four-field technique was introduced.[34] However, as predicted by biological and clinical observations[35,36] the

Swedish scheme results in increased acute and late toxicities such as fistulae, veinous thrombosis, femoral/pelvic fractures, and deterioration of residual sphincter function.[37,38] These complications are not observed with a 45–50 Gy dose delivered using daily doses in the 2-Gy range and an appropriate technique. We therefore recommend a standard fractional radiotherapy scheme.

Preoperative radio-chemotherapy is an important topic of clinical research. It has already been tested in six phase II studies, which used radiotherapy doses from 37.8 Gy to 50.4 Gy.[39-44] The concurrent chemotherapy scheme was either continuous-infusion 5-FU or a bolus 5-FU-based scheme with LV, mitomycin C, or cisplatin. Among the 321 operated patients, there was only 1 postoperative death. The pathological complete response rate ranged from 9% to 29%. After follow-ups of 2–5 years, the local recurrence rate ranged from 4% to 10% (Table 24.1).

Preoperative radio-chemotherapy is currently under evaluation in two randomized trials. The four-arm EORTC 22921 trial is testing the value of preoperative radio-chemotherapy versus preoperative radiotherapy alone, and the value of additional chemotherapy (Figure 24.1). Patients with T3 or resectable T4 tumours, clinically defined or using endorectal ultrasonography, are selected for entry. In each arm, patients should receive a 45 Gy dose of preoperative radiotherapy over 5 weeks. In half of them, a 5-day concurrent 5-FU/LV chemotherapy course is delivered during the first and fifth weeks of radiotherapy. Surgery is planned after a 3-week minimal gap. After surgery, half of the patients should receive four additional chemotherapy courses. For each chemotherapy course, the respective daily doses

Table 24.1 Preoperative radio-chemotherapy in rectal cancer: results of phase II studies

Authors	No. of patients	Median follow-up (months)	Sterilization rate (%)	Local failure rate (%)
Grann et al[39]	32	24	9	—
Rich et al[40]	77	27	29	4
Stryker et al[41]	30	39	—	4
Chari et al[42]	43	25	27	5
Valentini et al[43]	83	38	9	10
Bosset et al[44]	66	54	15.6	4

for 5-FU and LV are 350 mg/m^2 and 20 mg/m^2.[45]

In March 1999, a progress report on 623 entered patients indicated the following treatment compliance rates: 97% for the two arms with radiotherapy, 94.6% for the two arms with radio-chemotherapy, and 70% for postoperative chemotherapy. A 1.2% treatment-related death rate was observed, including postoperative deaths.[46]

The German Rectal Cancer Study is currently comparing preoperative radio-chemotherapy versus postoperative radio-chemotherapy (Figure 24.2). Both arms use a conventional scheme delivering 50.4 Gy preoperatively and 50 Gy plus a boost dose of 5.4 Gy postoperatively. 5-FU is administered concurrently in the first and fifth weeks of radiation. Four additional cycles of 5-FU are delivered after postoperative radio-chemotherapy or after surgery. Surgery is total mesorectal excision. The primary endpoints are survival, and local and distant controls. By November 2000, 628 patients had been included, the target being 800 patients. A recent progress report indicates that the postoperative mortality and morbidity rates are equivalent in both arms.[47]

Recommendations for treatment selection

There are two typical situations:

- Surgery has not yet been performed. The tumour is located in the mid or lower rectum. Transmural involvement is seen on endorectal ultrasonography or the tumour is found to be tethered on digital rectal examination. We recommend preoperative radiotherapy delivering 45–50 Gy over 5 weeks with optimal technique and quality-assurance procedures.[34] Surgery is planned 3–4 weeks after radiotherapy. In this situation, preoperative radio-chemotherapy remains under evaluation.
- Surgery has already been performed. Pathological examination indicates transmural or nodal involvement (stage II or stage III). The radiotherapy scheme is a standard fractionation delivering 50 Gy over 5 weeks. The concurrent chemotherapy could be either continuous-infusion 5-FU alone or a 5-FU/LV course delivered in the first and fifth weeks of radiotherapy. Additional chemotherapy could be either 5-FU alone or a 5-FU/LV combination.

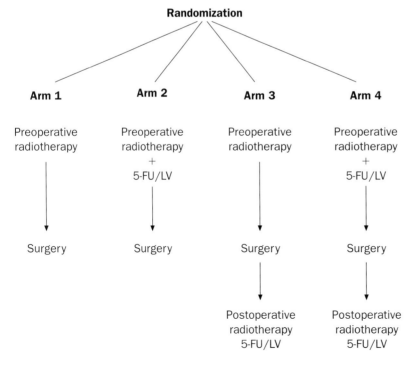

Figure 24.1 EORTC trial of preoperative radiation with or without chemotherapy (5-fluorouracil/leucovorin) for patients with clinically resectable T3/T4 rectal cancer

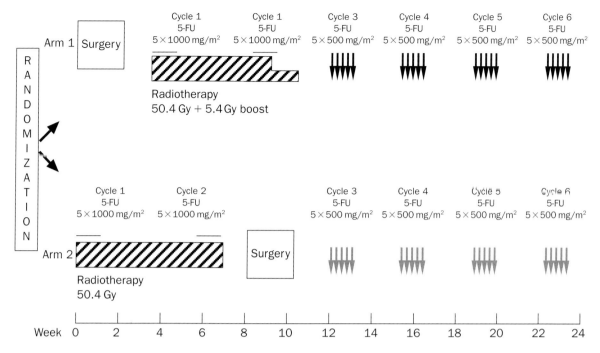

Figure 24.2 German trial of preoperative radio-chemotherapy versus postoperative radio-chemotherapy for patients with locally resectable T3/T4 rectal cancer.

Recommendations for improving the therapeutic index

The integration of radio-chemotherapy into the management of patients with rectal cancer requires a well-designed multidisciplinary action with well-trained physicians.

Radiotherapy recommendations

The target volume should be restricted to the close vicinity of the mesorectum. Its delineation is optimal with a computed tomography (CT)-based simulation technique (Figure 24.3). The anal sphincter could be spared if conservative surgery is planned. Treatment in a prone position with full bladder is appropriate in order to remove the small bowel from the pelvis. A multileaf collimator or customized shielding can be used to restrict the treatment to the target volume. A four-portal technique is recommended. Radiotherapy should be temporarily interrupted if grade 3 diarrhoea occurs.

Chemotherapy considerations

Schemes and dosages should be strictly applied.

During the radio-chemotherapy sequence, a complete blood count is obtained every week, and chemotherapy should be definitively stopped for this sequence if there is grade 2 haematological toxicity or grade ⩾3 diarrhoea.

Surgical considerations

After preoperative radiotherapy, a protective colostomy is not mandatory even if a coloanal anastomosis is planned. This decision depends upon the surgeon's practice. Postoperative management takes into account the possibility of increased risks of thromboembolism. When postoperative treatment is planned, pelvic reconstruction, reperitonization, and a pedicle omental flap are recommended in order to avoid small-bowel fixation in the pelvis.

Patient information

The patient should be asked to drink before each radiotherapy session, to exclude food that may cause diarrhoea, and to alert the radiation oncologist if any unusual symptoms occur.

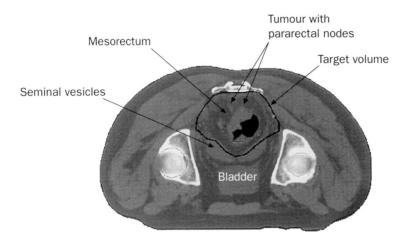

Figure 24.3 CT-based simulation technique: delineation of the target volume for radiotherapy.

Perspectives

Sphincter preservation is becoming an exciting new endpoint for preoperative strategies. The pertinent question here is the possibility for preoperative treatment to convert a planned abdominoperineal resection (APR) into a sphincter preservation procedure. There are four limited reported experiences from specialized centres in which patients declared by surgeons to require an APR received preoperative radiotherapy or radio-chemotherapy in order to save the sphincter. This strategy allowed a 70% sphincter preservation rate without any evident impairment in local control.[39,48–50] In this setting, the delay of surgery from the end of preoperative treatment could be critical in order to obtain an optimal tumour downstaging effect. In a randomized trial conducted in France, an increased sphincter preservation rate was observed in patients operated after a 6- to 8-week interval in comparison with patients operated after a 2-week interval.[51]

Whether radio-chemotherapy could work better in this situation than radiotherapy is an unanswered question. However, sphincter preservation is typically an area where improvements in radio-chemotherapy should be investigated by testing new combined drugs such as irinotecan.

These developments should be carefully conducted, and need precise evaluation of residual sphincter function, which is a major endpoint in the quality of life for patients with rectal cancer.[52]

Table 24.2 summarizes the role of radiotherapy and radio-chemotherapy in resectable rectal cancer.

CONCLUSIONS

Rectal cancer is a radiosensitive tumour. The addition of chemotherapy offers the chance to further increase the local effect of ionizing radiation. With early-stage tumours, intrarectal radiotherapy techniques can cure and preserve the sphincter. Whether the addition of chemotherapy could improve the overall results in this situation is unanswered.

In locally advanced stages, based on new techniques, the aim of surgery is now to lower the local recurrence rate to 10%. On the other hand, postoperative radio-chemotherapy and preoperative radiotherapy alone have already demonstrated their value in significantly reducing local recurrence and improving survival in patients undergoing conventional surgery.

The promising results obtained with preoperative radio-chemotherapy should lead surgeons and radiation oncologists to continue their collaboration to make eradication of local failure a realistic objective and to further increase the number of patients whose sphincters are spared.

ACKNOWLEDGEMENT

This work was supported in part by grants from le Ministère Français de la Santé, PHRC 1992.

Table 24.2 Role of radiotherapy ± chemotherapy in resectable rectal cancer

T stage	Tumour location within the rectum	Aim of treatment	Treatment option
T1 high-risk	Distal	Cure	Intrarectal radiotherapy techniques
T2		Sphincter preservation	Local excision + postoperative radio-chemotherapy is under evaluation
T3/resectable T4	Any	Local control, survival	Preoperative radiotherapy or postoperative radio-chemotherapy; preoperative radio-chemotherapy is under evaluation
T3	Distal	Sphincter preservation	Preoperative radiotherapy and radio-chemotherapy are both under evaluation

REFERENCES

1. Moertel C, Childs D, Reitemeier R et al, Combined 5-fluorouracil and supervoltage radiation therapy of locally unresectable gastrointestinal cancer. *Lancet* 1969; **ii:** 865–7.
2. Vokes EE, Combined modality therapy of solid tumours. *Lancet* 1997; **349:** 4–6.
3. Suit HD, Local control and patient survival. *Int J Radiat Oncol Biol Phys* 1992; **23:** 653–60.
4. Tubiana M, The role of local treatment in the cure of cancer. *Eur J Cancer* 1992; **28A:** 2061–9.
5. Miller AB, Hoogstraten B, Staquet M, Winkler A, Reporting results of cancer treatment. *Cancer* 1981; **47:** 207–14.
6. Pavy JJ, Denekamp J, Letschert J et al, EORTC late effects working group. Late effects toxicity scoring: the SOMA scale. *Int J Radiat Oncol Biol Phys* 1995; **31:** 1043–7.
7. Bosset JF, Marty M, Pavy JJ, Combinaisons radiothérapie et chimiothérapie. Applications aux radiochimiothérapies concomitantes. *Bull Cancer Radiother* 1993; **80:** 317–26.
8. Willet CG, Tepper JE, Donnelly S et al, Patterns of failure following local excision and local excision and postoperative radiation therapy for invasive rectal adenocarcinoma. *J Clin Oncol* 1989; **7:** 1003–8.
9. Steele G, Tepper J, Herndon J et al, Failure and salvage after sphincter sparing treatment for distal rectal adenocarcinoma – a CALGB Coordinated Intergroup study. *Proc Am Soc Clin Oncol* 1999; **18:** 235a.
10. Horiot JC, Gérard JP, Maingon P, Conservative and curative management of rectal adenocarcinomas by local radiotherapy alone. *Eur J Cancer* 1995; **31A:** 1340–2.
11. Galandiuk S, Wieand HS, Moertel CG et al, Patterns of recurrence after curative resection of carcinoma of the colon and rectum. *Surgery* 1992; **174:** 27–32.
12. MacFarlane JK, Ryall RDH, Heald RJ, Mesorectal excision for rectal cancer. *Lancet* 1993; **41:** 457–60.
13. Enker WE, Thaler HT, Cranor ML et al, Total mesorectal excision in the operative treatment of carcinoma of the rectum. *J Am Coll Surg* 1995; **181:** 335–46.
14. McCall JL, Cox MR, Wattchow DA, Analysis of local recurrence rates after surgery alone for rectal cancer. *Int J Colorectal Dis* 1995; **10:** 126–32.
15. Adam JJ, Mohamdee MO, Martin IG et al, Role of circumferential margin involvement in the local recurrence of rectal cancer. *Lancet* 1994; **344:** 707–11.
16. Schiessel R, Karner-Hanusch J, Herbst F et al, Intersphincter resection for low rectal tumours. *Br J Surg* 1994; **81:** 1376–8.
17. Hermanek P, Wiebelt H, Staimmer D et al, Prognostic factors of rectum carcinoma. Experience of the German Multicentre Study SGCRC. *Tumori* 1995; **81**(Suppl): 60–4.
18. Porter GA, Soskolne CL, Yakimets WW et al, Surgeon-related factors and outcome in rectal cancer. *Ann Surg* 1998; **227:** 157–67.
19. Carlsen E, Schlichting E, Guldvog I et al, Effect of the introduction of total mesorectal excision for the treatment of rectal cancer. *Br J Surg* 1998; **85:** 526–9.
20. Wiig JN, Carlsen E, Soreide O, Mesorectal excision for rectal cancer: a view from Europe. *Semin Surg Oncol* 1998; **15:** 78–86.
21. Gastrointestinal Tumor Study Group, Prolongation of the disease-free interval in surgically treated rectal carcinoma. *N Engl J Med* 1985; **312:** 1465–72.
22. Douglas HO, Moertel CG, on behalf of the Gastrointestinal Study Group, Survival after postoperative combination treatment of rectal cancer. *N Engl J Med* 1986; **315:** 1294.
23. Krook JE, Moertel CG, Gunderson LL et al, Effective surgical adjuvant therapy for high-risk rectal carcinoma. *N Engl J Med* 1991; **324:** 709–15.
24. NIH Consensus Conference, Adjuvant therapy for patients with colon and rectal cancer. *JAMA* 1990; **264:** 1444–9.
25. O'Connell MJ, Surgical adjuvant therapy of rectal cancer: chemotherapy considerations. In: *Educational Book, ASCO 34th Annual Meeting, Los Angeles, CA*, 1998: 419–24.
26. O'Connell MJ, Martenson JA, Wieand HS et al, Improving adjuvant therapy of rectal cancer by combining protracted-infusion fluorouracil with radiation therapy after curative surgery. *N Engl J Med* 1994; **331:** 502–7.
27. Tepper JE, O'Connell MJ, Petroni GR et al, Adjuvant postopera-

tive fluorouracil-modulated chemotherapy combined with pelvic radiation therapy for rectal cancer: initial results of Intergroup 0114. *J Clin Oncol* 1997; **15:** 2030–9.

28. Bosset JF, Horiot JC, Adjuvant treatment in the curative management of rectal cancer: a critical review of the results of clinical randomised trials. *Eur J Cancer* 1993; **29A:** 770–4.

29. Martenson JA, Urias R, Smalley M et al, Radiation therapy quality control in a clinical trial of adjuvant treatment for rectal cancer. *Int J Radiat Oncol Biol Phys* 1995; **32:** 51–5.

30. Kollmorgen CF, Meagher AP, Wolff BG et al, The long-term effects of adjuvant postoperative chemoradiotherapy for rectal carcinoma on bowel function. *Ann Surg* 1994; **220:** 676–82.

31. Swedish Rectal Cancer Trial, Improved survival with preoperative radiotherapy in resectable rectal cancer. *N Engl J Med* 1997; **336:** 980–7.

32. Goldberg PA, Nicholls RJ, Porter NH et al, Long-term results of a randomised trial of short-course low-dose adjuvant preoperative radiotherapy for rectal cancer: reduction in local treatment failure. *Eur J Cancer* 1994; **30A:** 1602–4.

33. Cedermark B, Johansson H, Rutqvist LE et al, The Stockholm I trial of preoperative short term radiotherapy in operable rectal carcinoma. A prospective randomised trial. *Cancer* 1995; **75:** 2269–75.

34. Horiot JC, Bosset JF, Pre-operative radiotherapy for rectal cancer: What benefit? Which technical parameters? *Eur J Cancer* 1994; **30A:** 1597–9.

35. Barendsen GW, Dose fractionation, dose rate and isoeffect relationships for normal tissue responses. *Int J Radiat Oncol Biol Phys* 1982; **8:** 1981–97.

36. Turesson I, Notter G, The influence of fraction size in radiotherapy on the late normal tissue responses. *Int J Radiat Oncol Biol Phys* 1984; **10:** 593–8.

37. Holm J, Singnomklao T, Rutqvist LE et al, Adjuvant preoperative radiotherapy in patients with rectal carcinoma. Adverse effects during long term follow-up of two randomised trials. *Cancer* 1996; **78:** 968–76.

38. Dahlberg M, Glimelius B, Graf W et al, Preoperative irradiation effects functional results after surgery for rectal cancer. Results from a randomised study. *Dis Colon Rectum* 1998; **41:** 543–51.

39. Grann A, Minsky BD, Cohen AM et al, Preliminary results of pre-operative 5-fluorouracil (5-FU), low dose leucovorin, and concurrent radiation therapy for resectable T3 rectal cancer. *Dis Colon Rectum* 1997; **40:** 515–22.

40. Rich TA, Skibber JM, Ajani JA et al, Preoperative infusional chemoradiation therapy for stage T3 rectal cancer. *Int J Radiat Oncol Biol Phys* 1995; **32:** 1025–9.

41. Stryker SJ, Kiel KD, Rademaker A et al, Preoperative 'chemora-

diation' for stage II and III rectal carcinoma. *Arch Surg* 1996; **131:** 514–19.

42. Chari RS, Tyler DS, Anscher MS et al, Preoperative radiation and chemotherapy in the treatment of adenocarcinoma of the rectum. *Ann Surg* 1995; **221:** 778–87.

43. Valentini V, Coco C, Cellini N et al, Preoperative chemoradiation for extraperitoneal T3 rectal cancer: acute toxicity, tumor response, sphincter preservation. *Int J Radiat Oncol Biol Phys* 1998; **40:** 1067–75.

44. Bosset JF, Magnin V, Maingon P et al, Preoperative radiochemotherapy in rectal cancer: long-term results of a phase II trial. *Int J Radiat Oncol Biol Phys* 2000; **46:** 323–7.

45. Bosset JF, Pavy JJ, Bolla M et al, Four arms phase III clinical trial for T3–T4 resectable rectal cancer comparing preoperative pelvic irradiation to preoperative irradiation combined with fluorouracil and leucovorin with or without postoperative adjuvant chemotherapy. EORTC Radiotherapy Cooperative Group. Protocol No. 22921. EORTC Data Center Brussels, 1992.

46. Bosset JF, Pierart M, Van Glabbeke M, Combined pre-operative radiochemotherapy versus pre-operative radiotherapy, with or without postoperative chemotherapy in patients with locally advanced resectable non-metastatic rectal cancers: EORTC 22921 phase III trial, progress report. EORTC–FFCD Meeting, Paris, June 1999.

47. Sauer R, Fietkau R, Wittekind C et al, Adjuvant versus neoadjuvant radiochemotherapy for locally advanced rectal cancer: a progress report of a phase III randomized trial (Protocol CAO/ARO/AIO-94). *Strahlenther Onkol* 2001; **177:** 173–81.

48. Rouanet P, Fabre JM, Dubois JB et al, Conservative surgery for low rectal carcinoma after high-dose radiation. Functional and oncologic results. *Ann Surg* 1995; **221:** 67–73.

49. Wagman R, Minsky BD, Cohen AM et al, Sphincter preservation with preoperative radiation therapy (RT) and coloanal anastomosis: long term follow-up. *Int J Radiat Oncology Biol Phys* 1997; **39:** 167.

50. Maaghfoor I, Wilkes J, Kuvshinoff B et al, Neoadjuvant chemoradiotherapy with sphincter-sparing surgery for low lying rectal cancer. *Proc Am Soc Clin Oncol* 1997; **16:** 274.

51. François Y, Nemoz CJ, Baulieux J et al, Influence of the interval between preoperative radiation therapy and surgery on downstaging and on the rate of sphincter-sparing surgery for rectal cancer: the Lyon R90-01 randomized trial. *J Clin Oncol* 1999; **17:** 2396–402.

52. Bosset JF, Mercier M, Pelissier EP, Pavy JJ, Validation of a patient's questionnaire testing the functional results after sphincter-sparing surgery for rectal cancer with correlation with the EORTC QLQ-c30. *Radiother Oncol* 1994; **32:** S133.

25

The future of radiotherapy in rectal carcinoma

Jean Bourhis, Antoine Lusinchi, François Eschwège

INTRODUCTION

Radiotherapy has been used for several decades in the management of patients with rectal adenocarcinoma, with the aim of decreasing the rate of local relapse and increasing sphincter preservation. Indeed, after surgery alone, 25–35% local failure is generally reported in patients with B2, C1–2 (Astler–Coller) rectal carcinoma.[1,2] The efficacy of radiotherapy in reducing the incidence of local relapse has been demonstrated in several randomized trials using total doses between 34.5 Gy and 45 Gy, as preoperative or postoperative treatment.[2,3–10] An overview of these randomized trials has been conducted by the Oxford and Institut Gustave Roussy meta-analysis groups, showing a significant (20%) reduction in the rate of locoregional relapse, which was more pronounced for pre- than for postoperative radiotherapy. A small but statistically significant difference in survival (5%) was also observed in favour of the use of radiotherapy compared with no treatment adjuvant to surgery (JP Pignon, personal communication). A direct comparison of preoperative versus postoperative radiotherapy has been performed by a Swedish group, showing that preoperative irradiation was more efficient in reducing local relapse and also was better tolerated.[3,11,12]

In summary, adjuvant radiotherapy has been shown to be effective in reducing the probability of locoregional relapse in rectal carcinoma, and this may ultimately lead to a survival benefit. Radiotherapy also plays an essential role in the management of fixed (T4) or recurrent rectal carcinomas.

The future of radiotherapy in rectal carcinoma depends upon the possibilities of improving its thera-peutic index and better integrating radiotherapy in combination with surgery and chemotherapy. New surgical techniques, including total mesorectal excision, have been developed in the past few years, with the aim of decreasing the rate of local relapse. In the view of some authors, the role of radiotherapy should be reconsidered, given the relatively low local relapse rate reported after this type of surgery.

Possible approaches to improving the therapeutic index of radiotherapy will be briefly presented in this chapter; the intention of these approaches is to increase the effect of radiotherapy on tumour cells, while minimizing toxicity to normal surrounding tissues. New protocols should take advantage of advances in radiation research in general, including new techniques to improve ballistics, combination with biological modifiers, and modified fractionation, among others.

INCREASING THE DIFFERENTIAL EFFECT BETWEEN TUMOUR AND NORMAL TISSUES

Increasing antitumour efficacy

Radio-chemotherapy combinations
The combination of radiotherapy with chemotherapy has been shown to be superior to radiotherapy alone in several types of carcinoma, including cervical, head and neck, bronchial, anal, and nasopharyngeal. Similarly, in rectal carcinoma, radio-chemotherapy combinations have been shown to be effective in improving disease-free survival, when given as adjuvant treatment to postoperative surgery. The Gastrointestinal Tumor Study Group (GITSG) ran-

domized trial showed, in a series of 202 patients with B2–C tumors, that the combination of postoperative pelvic irradiation with 5-fluorouracil (5-FU) and methyl-CCNU (semustine) was superior to postoperative radiotherapy alone, in terms of local control and distant metastases. The North Central Cancer Treatment Group (NCCTG) and Mayo Clinic also tested the value of combining radio- and chemotherapy in the postoperative setting, and showed comparable results.[5,7] Regarding the use of radio-chemotherapy combinations before surgery, the European Organization for Research and Treatment of Cancer (EORTC) is currently running a randomized trial (EORTC 22921), with over 700 patients included and 1000 expected, to determine whether the addition of 5-FU and low-dose leucovorin to preoperative pelvic irradiation (45 Gy/4.5 weeks) in resectable T3–4 tumours is superior to the same radiotherapy alone.

In order to optimize radio-chemotherapy combinations, the type of drug and the route of delivery could be of particular importance,[13] as suggested by the randomized trial conducted by O'Connell et al,[14] showing that continuous infusion of 5-FU during the course of radiation treatment led to a significant improvement in disease-free survival.

It remains to be studied whether radio-chemotherapy combinations could be optimized by integrating new effective drugs for colorectal carcinoma, such as irinotecan, gemcitabine and oxaliplatin.[15] Although most of these drugs are radiosensitizers, no information is available about their combination with irradiation in patients with rectal carcinoma. However, mucosal toxicity of the digestive tract could be a limiting factor for this type of combination, especially with drugs such as irinotecan, taxanes, gemcitabine and raltitrexed.[15–17] In contrast, oxaliplatin, which may induce less mucosal toxicity, could be more interesting to combine with irradiation in rectal cancer. In addition, the new generation of bioreductive drugs such as tirapazamine are essentially active against hypoxic cells, which are very radioresistant, and should be tested in rectal carcinoma.

Modified fractionation

In the past 10 years, considerable interest has arisen in non-conventional fractionation schemes in radiation therapy. Although most studies have been performed for carcinomas of the upper digestive tract and bronchus, this approach should be evaluated in other tumour types, including rectal carcinoma, given the promising and convergent results obtained in recently completed large-scale randomized trials. Hyperfractionation consists in decreasing the dose per fraction to minimize late radiation-induced toxicity, and by this means it is possible to increase the total dose, and hence the probability of tumour control. This hypothesis was demonstrated for head and neck cancer in the EORTC 22791 and Radiation Therapy Oncology Group (RTOG) 90-03 randomized trials,[18,19] in which the dose per fraction was 1.15–1.2 Gy (twice daily), and consequently the total dose could be raised to 80.5 Gy without increasing the probability of late toxicity. In addition to such pure hyperfractionated trials, accelerated radiotherapy has more recently been investigated, and it has been shown that high total doses of radiation can be delivered in overall treatment times much shorter than those of conventional radiotherapy. The rationale for accelerating radiotherapy is to minimize the repopulation of surviving tumour cells during the course of treatments.[20] The benefit of accelerated radiotherapy has been shown in head and neck and in bronchial carcinoma in recently completed randomized trials[20,21] (Danish Head and Neck Cancer Study (DAHANCA), J Overgaard, personal communication). Whether this approach could be beneficial in rectal carcinoma needs to be investigated. Preliminary results have been obtained by Coucke et al[22] in patients with operable rectal carcinoma, showing that accelerated pelvic irradiation is feasible, with 48 Gy being delivered in 3 weeks as a preoperative procedure.

Decreasing normal tissue reactions

Improvements in ballistics

The response of adenocarcinoma of the rectum to radiation probably depends on the possibility of applying a sufficiently high dose of radiation to the tumour without exceeding the limits of tolerance of the normal pelvic tissues. The concept of increasing probability of tumour control as the total dose of radiation increases has been illustrated by preoperative studies, showing complete pathological response at surgery in 2–5% of cases after 35 Gy, 10% after 45 Gy and 10–16% after 50 Gy.[23–25]

On the basis of these data, it is conceivable that a dose–effect relationship could also exist for higher doses: increasing the dose of radiation to the tumour while sparing normal tissues might help to improve the resectability of fixed and recurrent rectal carcinomas, and to increase the rate of sphincter preservation.

Several approaches can be proposed to increase the radiation dose selectively to the tumour, including perhaps intraoperative radiotherapy[26] and, more interestingly, three-dimensional (3D) conformal radiotherapy, which has recently been developed, and allows the delivery of high doses of radiation in volumes more accurately determined than with conventional radiotherapy. Recent developments in this area have shown that 3D conformal radiotherapy can be markedly improved by using intensity-modulated radiotherapy (IMRT), which allows the dose delivered to normal pelvic tissues to be kept within the limits of tolerance, while the dose to the tumour is increased. The value of these new radiotherapy techniques should be evaluated in rectal carcinoma, especially for fixed (T4) or recurrent carcinomas, and for tumours of the distal part of the rectum.[17,25] In this latter case, it has been reported that increasing the radiation dose could be an effective way to increase sphincter preservation,[27,28] suggesting that the evaluation of the IMRT technique should include a determination of whether optimization of the dose distribution could allow a greater degree of sphincter preservation.

Small-bowel exclusion

When postoperative pelvic radiotherapy is to be used, whenever possible irradiation of the small bowel should be avoided, for example by implanting a mammary prosthesis in the pelvis during the surgical procedure, which allows the small bowel to be spared.

Radioprotectors

Among various radioprotectors that could be tested in rectal carcinoma, amifostine is of particular interest. Amifostine (ethanethiol 2,3-aminopropylamino dihydrogen phosphate ester) is an aminothiol free-radical scavenger, known for more than 40 years as a radioprotector. Its potential interest in the context of radiotherapy of human tumours is based on the experimental observation, both in cell culture and in animals, of a protective effect that is greater for normal than for cancer cells.[29,30] The selective protection of normal tissues has been confirmed in patients in some recently completed randomized trials.[31] For rectal cancer, a randomized trial was performed some years ago in China, showing a significant protection against both acute and late radiation effects on normal tissues, without impairment of antitumour radiation efficacy.[32] These results strongly suggest that amifostine

should be further tested in rectal cancer in order to improve the therapeutic ratio of radiotherapy, especially in the framework of radio-chemotherapy combinations.

BIOLOGICAL MODIFIERS

It has been suggested that the results of radiotherapy might be improved if the treatment could be modified according to biological features known to be correlated with radiation resistance in experimental tumours. Among these biological parameters, tumour hypoxia[33] intrinsic radiosensitivity[34] and tumour cell kinetics[35,36] have been proposed to predict response to radiation. The identification of such parameters for each patient could be used to modulate radiotherapy individually, according to these biological findings. Indeed, accelerated radiotherapy could be used in cases of rapid tumour cell kinetics. Of these biological parameters, hypoxia is also likely to be important in influencing tumour response to radiotherapy. Changes in tumour oxygenation can be obtained by several means: oxygen partial pressure can increase dramatically with breathing of carbogen (95% O_2 5% CO_2).[37] The potential benefit associated with carbogen breathing is currently under investigation in patients with different tumour types, and should be tested in rectal carcinoma, depending on the results of these studies. New approaches should also be evaluated using compounds that are cytotoxic under hypoxic conditions, such as tirapazamine.

The potential for modern molecular biology to provide meaningful contributions to translational research and cancer therapeutics has to be highlighted. A particularly fertile area concerns growth factors and signal transduction inhibitors (e.g. inhibitors of protein kinase C (PKC), epidermal growth factor (EGF) and vascular endothelial growth factor (VEGF), especially when employed in combination with radiation and other cytotoxic agents. How valuable these growth factor and signal transduction inhibitors will ultimately prove to be in cancer therapy, especially in combination with irradiation, is under investigation. Other strategies to improve the efficacy of radiotherapy might include the transfer of genes known to have an impact on cellular response to radiation, such as the *p53* tumour suppressor gene.[38] Alteration (mutation or deletion) of the *p53* gene is a common genetic feature in colorectal carcinoma. Recently, a synergy between the transfer (via an adenoviral vector) of wild-type *p53* and irradiation has been shown in a xenograft model of a human colorectal carcinoma.[39] This study strongly suggests that there is a potentiation between low doses of ionizing radiation and wild-type *p53* in this type of cancer.

CONCLUSIONS

Several approaches, taking advantage of the progress in radiotherapy research in general, should be tested in order to determine whether the effectiveness of radiotherapy for rectal carcinoma can be improved without increasing toxicity to normal pelvic tissues. Ongoing and future clinical trials will determine the usefulness of these new methods.

REFERENCES

1. Adam I, Mohamdee M, Martin I, Role of circumferential margin in the local recurrence of rectal carcinoma. *Lancet* 1994; **344:** 707–10.
2. Bosset JF, Horiot JC, Adjuvant treatment in the curative management of rectal cancer; a critical review of the results of clinical randomized trials. *Eur J Cancer* 1993; **29:** 770–4.
3. Frikholm GJ, Glimelius B, Påhlman L, Preoperative or post-operative irradiation in adenocarcinoma of the rectum: final treatment results of a randomized trial and an evaluation of late secondary effects. *Dis Colon Rectum* 1993; **36:** 564–82.
4. Gerard JP, Buyse M, Nordlinger B, Pre-operative radiotherapy as adjuvant treatment in rectal cancer. Final results of a randomized study of the EORTC. *Ann Surg* 1988; **208:** 606–14.
5. GITSG, Prolongation of the disease-free interval in surgically treated rectal carcinoma. *N Engl J Med* 1985; **312:** 1465–70.
6. Higgins GA, Humphrey EW, Dwight RW, Preoperative radiation and surgery for cancer of the rectum. Veterans Administration Surgical Oncology Group Trial II. *Cancer* 1986; **58:** 352–9.
7. Krook JE, Moertel C, Gunderson L et al, Effective adjuvant therapy for high risk rectal carcinoma. *N Engl J Med* 1991; **324:** 709–15.
8. Minski BD, Cohen AM, Keeny N, Combined modality therapy of rectal cancer: decreased acute toxicity with the pre-operative approach. *J Clin Oncol* 1992; **10:** 1218–24.
9. MRC Working Party, The evaluation of low dose pre-operative X-ray therapy in the management of operable rectal cancer: results of a randomly controlled trial. *Br J Surg* 1984; **71:** 21–5.
10. Treumiet Donner A, Van Putten W, Wereldsma J, Postoperative radiation therapy for rectal cancer: an interim analysis of a prospective randomized multicentre trial in the Netherlands. *Cancer* 1991; **67:** 2042–8.
11. Påhlman L, Glimelius B, Pre- and post-operative radiotherapy in rectal and rectosigmoid carcinoma. Report from a random-
ized trial. *Ann Surg* 1990; **211:** 187–95.
12. Stockholm Rectal Cancer Study Group, Pre-operative short term radiation therapy in operable rectal carcinoma. A prospective randomized trial. *Cancer* 1990; **66:** 49–55.
13. Marsh R, Chu NC, Vauthey JN et al, Preoperative treatment of patients with locally advanced unresectable rectal adenocarcinoma utilizing continuous chronobiologically shaped 5-FU infusion and radiation therapy. *Cancer* 1996; **78:** 217–25.
14. O'Connell MJ, Martenson J, Wieland HS, Improving adjuvant therapy for rectal cancer by combining protracted-infusion 5-FU with radiation therapy after curative surgery. *N Engl J Med* 1994; **331:** 502–7.
15. Choy H, Taxanes in combined modality therapy for solid tumors. *Oncology* 1999; **13:** 23–38.
16. Backledge G, New developments in cancer treatment with the novel thymidilate synthetase inhibitor raltitrexed ('Tomudex'). *Br J Cancer* 1998; **77:** 29–37.
17. Teicher BA, Ara G, Chen YN et al, Interaction of Tomudex with radiation in vitro and in vivo. *Int J Oncol* 1998; **13:** 437–42.
18. Horiot JC, LeFur P, N'Guyen T et al, Hyperfractionated compared with conventional radiotherapy in oropharyngeal carcinoma an EORTC randomized trial. *Eur J Cancer* 1990; **26:** 779–80.
19. Fu K, Pajak TF, Trotti A et al, A Radiation Therapy Oncology Group (RTOG) phase III randomized study to compare hyperfraction and two variants of accelerated fractionation to standard fractionation radiotherapy for head and neck squamous cell carcinomas: first report of RTOG 9003. *Int J Radiat Oncol Biol Phys* 2000; **48:** 7–16.
20. Dische S, Saunders M, The rationale for continuous hyperfractionated accelerated radiotherapy (CHART). *Int J Radiat Oncol Biol Phys* 1990; **19:** 1317–20.
21. Horiot JC, Bontemps P, van den Bogaert W et al, Accelerated fractionation compared to conventional fractionation improves locoregional control in the radiotherapy of advanced head and neck cancer: results of the EORTC 22851 randomized trial. *Radiother Oncol* 1997; **44:** 39–46.
22. Coucke PA, Sartorelloi B, Cuttat JF et al, The rationale to switch from postoperative hyperfractionated radiotherapy to preoperative hyperfractionated accelerated radiotherapy in rectal cancer. *Int J Radiat Oncol Biol Phys* 1995; **32:** 181–8.
23. Horn A, Morild I, Dahl O, Tumor shrinkage and down staging after pre-operative radiation of rectal adenocarcinomas. *Radiother Oncol* 1990; **18:** 19–28.
24. Lusinchi A, Wibault P, Lasser P, Abdoperineal resection combined with pre- and post-operative radiation therapy in the treatment of low-lying rectal carcinoma. *Int J Radiat Oncol Biol Phys* 1997; **37:** 59–65.
25. Marks C, Mohiuddin M, Cludstein S, Sphincter preservation for cancer of the distal rectum using high dose pre-operative radiation. *Int J Radiat Oncol Biol Phys* 1988; **15:** 1065–8.
26. Willet CC, Shellito PC, Eliseo R, Intra-operative electron beam therapy for primary locally advanced rectal or rectosigmoid carcinoma. *Clin Oncol* 1991; **9:** 843–9.
27. Mohiuddin M, Marks J, Bannon J, High dose preoperative radiation and full thickness radical excision: a new option for selected T3 distal rectal cancer. *Int J Radiat Oncol Biol Phys* 1994; **30:** 845–9.
28. Rouanet P, Dravet F, Dubois JB et al, Proctectomie et anastomose colo anale après irradiation à haute dose descancers du tiers inférieur du rectum. *Ann Chir* 1994; **48:** 512–19.
29. Grdina D, Sigdestad C, Radiation protectors: the unexpected

benefit. *Drug Metab Rev* 1989; **20:** 13–42.

30. Travis E, Thames H, Tucker S, Protection of mouse jejunal crypt cells by WR-2721 after small doses of radiation. *Int J Radiat Oncol Biol Phys* 1986; **12:** 807–14.

31. Brizel D, Sauer R, Wannenmacher M et al, Randomized phase III trial of radiation +/− amifostine in patients with head and neck cancer. *Proc Am Soc Clin Oncol* 1998; **17:** 1487.

32. Liu T, Liu Y, Zhang Z, Kligerman M, Use of radiation with and without WR-22721 in advanced rectal cancer. *Cancer* 1992; **69:** 2280–5.

33. Lartigau E, Vitu L, Haie-Meder C, Measurements of oxygen tension in uterine cervix carcinoma: a feasibility study. *Eur J Cancer* 1992; **28:** 1354–7.

34. West C, Davidson S, Roberts S, Hunter R, Intrinsic radiosensitivity and prediction of patients' response to radiotherapy for carcinoma of the cervix. *Br J Cancer* 1993; **68:** 819–23.

35. Rew D, Wilson G, Taylor I, Proliferation characteristics of human colorectal carcinomas measured in vivo. *Br J Surg* 1991; **78:** 60–6.

36. Willet CC, Warland G, Coen J et al, Rectal cancer: the influence of tumor proliferation on response to pre-operative irradiation. *Int J Radiat Oncol Biol Phys* 1995; **32:** 57–61.

37. Martin L, Lartigau E, Weeger P, Changes in the oxygenation of head and neck tumors during carbogen breathing. *Radiother Oncol* 1993; **27:** 123–30.

38. Lee JM, Bernstein A, p53 mutations increase resistance to ionizing radiation. *Proc Natl Acad Sci USA* 1993; **90:** 5742–6.

39. Spitz FR, Nguyen D, Skibber J et al, Adenoviral mediated p53 gene therapy enhances radiation sensitivity of colorectal cancer cell lines. *Proc Am Assoc Cancer Res* 1996; **37:** 347.

Part 5

Follow-up of Colorectal Cancer

26

Which follow-up for colorectal cancer? Perhaps none

John MA Northover

INTRODUCTION

For most surgeons, postoperative follow-up is as much a part of colorectal cancer surgery as bowel preparation or closing the skin, but reliable evidence that this complex and costly process improves overall survival is lacking. Nevertheless, health systems around the world allow this to go on, despite tight resources and an increasing expectation of provable benefit from any health intervention. A recent US survey of different follow-up regimens showed a wide range of costs for five years of follow-up per patient;[1] the cheapest they found was $900, while the most expensive was nearly $27 000. With a million follow-up visits generated by each year's cohort of new US cases, this amounts to billions spent, but for what benefit? And the situation is similar in all industrialized countries.

HOW DID FOLLOW-UP START?

Follow-up was not routine a hundred years ago. Major surgery for this disease was unusual then, and cure even less common. Indeed, before Miles described the first 'Halstedian' rectal cancer resection in 1908, it is overwhelmingly likely that almost no patient survived the disease. And as surgery itself was so hazardous (Miles perioperative mortality was around 40%[2]) reoperative surgery for recurrence was a subtlety too far.

It appears that routine follow-up had its beginnings, not for the early detection and effective management of recurrence, but as a research tool to elucidate prognosis after surgery. Cuthbert Dukes and Percy Lockhart-Mummery, pathologist and surgeon respectively at St Mark's Hospital, London, began a programme of routine follow-up in the early 1920s aimed specifically at correlating clinical outcome with the pathological anatomy of the disease in resected specimens.[2] Thus the earliest and most palpable result of follow-up was the development of the prognostic Dukes staging system for rectal cancer.

In the middle years of the 20th century, routine follow-up became the norm at St Mark's Hospital, and in most other institutions dealing with this increasingly prevalent disease. In those days, it consisted of regular outpatient visits, and simple recording of clinical findings. It was only much later that technological advancement resulted in more complex and sensitive investigations, and with the assumption of utility rather than a questioning of the health gain secured by the process. By the 1960s and 1970s, the natural sense of follow-up was indelibly ingrained in surgical practice. For many surgeons, the utility of, and therefore the need for, follow-up were taken for granted. While conceding the existence of modern funding constraints, a recent review of this complex subject nevertheless clearly implies a perpetuation of this assumption:[3] 'Early detection of colorectal cancer recurrence can be a daunting and costly task in this era of budget cuts and cost containment, especially since the rewards are few when looked upon in the context of the vast number of patients treated for colorectal cancer every year. However, the rewards are real, and some patients can be cured as a result of diligent follow-up.' Such statements beg important questions. Do all patients benefit in some way? Might some benefit more if resources were targeted? In short, are the assumptions of the past acceptable today or in the future?

AIMS OF FOLLOW-UP

Traditionally, follow-up has had four main aims:[3,4]

1. *Early detection of recurrence or new primary tumour.* Following radical surgery for colorectal cancer, up to 50% of patients will develop local or distant recurrence of their cancer, and most will die as a direct result.[5] Moreover, up to 8% will develop a new (metachronous) primary malignancy,[6–8] and, in many more, premalignant adenomas will form. Therefore attempts to detect such lesions at the earliest stage should be made – or so runs the logic of follow-up aimed at their presymptomatic identification.

   But does a policy of regular, pro-active follow-up for all lead to more effective management of recurrence compared with investigation at symptom onset? If not, Charles Moertel's reflection on CEA monitoring, enunciated over 20 years ago, might be applied to the whole process of follow-up:[9] 'The only outcome for most patients [is] the needless anxiety produced by premature knowledge of the presence of a fatal disease.'

2. *Management of postsurgical complications.* Identifying wound problems, providing supportive stoma care, attending to difficulties with bowel function and neurological deficits after rectal cancer surgery – all these require postoperative outpatient supervision. Most such issues can be resolved, or helped to the limit of possibility, within one year of surgery. By themselves, these issues do not constitute a rationale for five years of regular visits.

3. *Reassuring patients.* Patients' reactions to the experience of having been diagnosed and treated for cancer vary widely, as all surgeons have witnessed. At one extreme, the patient becomes profoundly attached to the hospital and its staff, preoccupied by the fear of recurrence. Others simply want, indeed need, to put the whole experience behind them, to block out cancer and get on with their lives. Attitudes along the whole spectrum demand different approaches by the surgical team; and, in the absence of solid evidence of an oncological imperative for a particular follow-up regimen or individual tests, patients require different patterns of reassurance through postoperative patient/doctor contact. It is too simple, and perhaps paternalistic, to assume that all patients benefit from the 'reassurance' conferred by a uniform and rigid follow-up programme.

4. *Audit and quality control of surgical outcomes.* In a busy life with competing priorities, most surgeons have not seen the need to analyse the outcomes of their cancer surgery, but times and circumstances are changing in ways that may mandate follow-up in order that healthcare purchasers, potential patients, and, indeed, wider society can judge institutional or perhaps individual results. For the moment, however, few surgeons use follow-up data effectively to this end.

To this list should be added the process of deciding upon and delivering adjuvant therapy. As evidence for the efficacy of adjuvants in subgroups accumulates, this becomes a more widely applicable reason for continuing contact following surgery – though only initially with the surgeon. Further, as palliative chemotherapy and radiotherapy become more effective, particularly if evidence grows to suggest that treatment is more effective if given early in the natural history of recurrent disease, follow-up for early detection may have a more rational basis.

WHAT ARE THE KEY ELEMENTS OF THE FOLLOW-UP PROCESS?

Follow-up planning requires decisions to be made about the frequency of surveillance visits, and their clinical and investigative content. There is an enormous range of possible combinations of visit frequencies and investigations that could be included; Kievit and Bruinvels[10] recently computed that there are a mind-boggling $30\,000 \times 8^5$ different protocols that could be generated from these variables. The major elements are as follows.

Simple patient/doctor contact

This can range from symptom-prompted, or reactive, contact – with no planned, asymptomatic visits – through the more usual regular interview and physical examination, to frequent and expensive cycles of investigation. 'History and physical' may provide the first evidence in up to 50% of patients with recurrence.[11] Intervals between visits vary, depending on the time since surgery and the attitude of the clinician; as most recurrences manifest within two years,[12] most regimens concentrate on this period, with continuing though less frequent visits till five years after operation. Some argue that follow-up should continue indefinitely.[3] Each patient will make

12–15 visits over a five-year period.[10] However, most symptomatic recurrences become apparent to the patient *between* preplanned visits, leading either to unplanned urgent visits (making the planned programme irrelevant) or to unwarranted delay until the next planned visit – a delay that, of course, may or may not matter!

Simple outpatient contact includes symptomatic enquiry, and physical examination looking for abdominal signs – principally hepatomegaly – and sigmoidoscopic evidence of anastomotic recurrence in rectal cases. The use of various investigations may either be prompted by symptoms and signs, or be part of a planned surveillance programme; the discussion of investigative techniques in subsequent sections applies specifically to the latter.

Wangensteen gave us the most extreme form of doctor/patient contact after surgery, which predated any of the 'high-tech' investigative modalities to be discussed below, in the form of his programme of second-look surgery that he developed more than half a century ago.[13] His enthusiasm for early diagnosis and treatment of recurrence led him to submit his patients to a 'second-look' laparotomy six months after primary surgery – the ultimate physical examination! If he found recurrent cancer, he removed it if possible; additional operations were done at intervals of approximately six months until one operation was completed at which no more cancer was found. Ultimately it became apparent that the operative mortality outweighed patient benefit, so this extreme modality of follow-up was abandoned.

Serum tumour markers

Many surgeons worldwide use serum carcinoembryonic antigen (CEA) measurement in follow-up. Moertel et al[14] estimated that in the USA 500 000 patients are undergoing serial CEA monitoring at any one time, offering the prospect of recurrence detection on average six months before the onset of symptoms. There can be no doubt that this modality leads to earlier diagnosis and more second-look surgery,[15] but evidence that this approach improves the survivability of recurrent disease is very thin. This may be resolved when the results of the only randomized trial in the field are published in the near future.[16]

When CEA was discovered in 1965,[17] it was seen as *the* serum marker for colorectal cancer, with an anticipated role in mass population screening. It soon became apparent, however, that CEA might be raised in other cancers, in non-malignant bowel dis-

eases, and sometimes in otherwise-normal individuals. Moreover, serum CEA was normal in about 25% of patients with known bowel cancer. This lack of specificity and sensitivity ruled it out as a mass screening tool. CEA was seen to have a possible prognostic role when it was noted that recurrence within two years of primary surgery was twice as common in those with a preoperatively raised serum CEA level.[18] However, serum prognostic markers have not been found to improve upon the predictive accuracy of Dukes-based pathological staging systems.

Serial measurement of serum markers after primary surgery to predict recurrence, and hence to indicate those who might be candidates for second-look surgery, has been studied intensively; as already mentioned, it has been estimated that at any one time, 500 000 Americans are being sampled serially in order to predict recurrence prior to the onset of symptoms.[14] Whereas Dukes staging in Wangensteen's hands failed as the basis for a second-look program, there has been continuing advocacy of second-look surgery based on serum markers, CEA in particular.[19] So what is the evidence that serial CEA follow-up as an indicator for second-look surgery might alter prognosis favourably? Should such a policy be adopted universally – or should it go the way of Wangensteen's programme, and be consigned to the footnotes of surgical history?

Serum CEA rises in the majority of cases before the onset of symptoms and signs;[20] amongst more than 2000 cases described in series published in the early 1980s, 75% demonstrated a CEA rise as first indicator of recurrent disease.[21] In the mid 1970s, there were several reports that regular monitoring led to early diagnosis of recurrence, up to 30 months before symptoms occurred.[18,22–24] Using historical controls, it was suggested that early reoperation relying on CEA results as the sole indicator for surgery led to macroscopic clearance of recurrence in more patients (63% compared with 27% in a symptom-led second-look cohort).[15,19] Other non-randomized studies came to similar conclusions,[25–33] while others differed on its utility.[34–38] For many, it was taken as a 'matter of faith that better efforts would produce better results';[39] the Columbus group and others advocated monthly CEA testing to take maximal advantage of lead time.

CEA assay has deficiencies in sensitivity and specificity. Most CEA rises herald the discovery of unresectable hepatic recurrence,[40] while in 10–25% of patients the raised CEA is 'falsely' positive, i.e. is not due to recurrent cancer,[14,41–44] leading to negative laparotomy if acted upon. Conversely, a high proportion of patients have incurable disease at surgery.[44,45] Efforts to improve the efficacy of CEA monitoring led to its combination with other tumour markers, but without significantly improved clinical utility.[46]

Fletcher[39] pointed out that 'Americans have valued cure at almost any cost' – while suggesting that society could not be expected to pay for it. In the UK, a national screening policy in any field will be implemented only after development of convincing evidence of its clinical and economic utility. In the absence of prospective control data, it remained impossible to demonstrate any survival advantage from a policy of CEA-led second-look surgery. Fletcher suggested that the efficacy of a CEA-based second-look policy could only be demonstrated by a randomized trial, but that statistical difficulties precluded any such study.[14,39] Nevertheless, a trial (under the auspices of the UK Cancer Research Campaign, and initially funded by the US National Institutes of Health) was set up in the UK in the 1980s: its design optimized power and minimized sample size through the use of late randomization, at the time of CEA rise. Thus the therapeutic effect – if any – was more likely to be detected by excluding from randomization those individuals in whom no events occurred during follow-up.[16] In the trial, patients were registered with the trial centre after primary surgery, after obtaining fully informed consent for participation in the full protocol. Patients were offered monthly CEA assay as well as conventional clinical follow-up, and were told that their clinician would not be informed of routine, normal results. Clinical follow-up conformed with the broad norm used in the UK. Randomization was performed at the trial centre only after a significant CEA rise as defined by the trial CEA algorithm. Clinicians were only informed of the CEA rise if the patient was randomized to the 'aggressive' arm, leading to work-up towards second-look surgery. Patients in the 'conventional' arm continued to receive standard clinical follow-up, their clinicians remaining unaware of the CEA rise or the randomization. In any patient at any stage (including, of course, patients already randomized to the 'conventional' arm) in whom clinical evidence of recurrent disease became apparent, the clinician was at liberty to advise further surgery if it seemed appropriate. Using this efficient and powerful trial design, it was possible to seek evidence of a survival effect at a fixed time point after randomization as a result of the introduction of a single item of data into clinical management, namely a raised CEA level. The trial recruited almost 1500 patients, and closed in 1993. After an appropriate length of follow-up of all cases, data analysis is almost complete, so

that the results should be published shortly; it will provide the most powerful evidence yet on any therapeutic effect from a particular follow-up policy, in this case serial CEA estimation.

Other prognostic serum markers have been developed and used in the same way as CEA, including tissue polypeptide antigen (TPA), CA19-9 and CA50. There have been variable reports on their relative sensitivity and specificity compared with each other, with CEA, and with combinations of markers.[46,47] Comparisons are difficult, mainly owing to differences in quoted normal ranges, but by conversion of inverse distribution function values into specificity–sensitivity diagrams, comparison for equivalent specificities is possible. On this basis, Putzki and others[46] have shown no apparent advantage for other antigens or combinations, compared with CEA alone.

In summary, CEA and other serum markers are sensitive, presymptomatic indicators of recurrent disease, but unless more effective methods of treatment can be triggered by a raised marker level, their diagnostic ability offers no more to most patients and their attendants than protracted prior knowledge of a fatal outcome for most patients, as suggested a generation ago by Charles Moertel.[9]

Flexible endoscopy

Fibre-optic large-bowel endoscopy was first reported over 30 years ago,[48] ultimately leading to highly sensitive, minimally invasive diagnosis of primary and recurrent cancer, and to safe non-surgical removal of many adenomas. As a technique for follow-up in asymptomatic individuals, the superior sensitivity and therapeutic ability of colonoscopy has made barium enema practically redundant.

In theory, at least, flexible endoscopy can play a part in two aspects of follow-up: detection of metachronous neoplasia, both benign and malignant, and recognition of recurrent cancer.

Detection and removal of metachronous adenomas might cut the incidence and mortality of metachronous cancer,[49] which has been reported as having a better outlook than the initial malignancy.[50] Some have found high yields of adenomas, including the larger lesions more likely to progress to cancer, with lesions being found in up to 56% of cases in untargeted follow-up,[51,52] though the unselected rate is likely to be much less.[53] Metachronous cancer in the days before colonoscopic surveillance was reported in around 3–4% of postoperative cases.[54] Some modern series quote rates of only 0.2–3%,[53] perhaps resulting from a true decrease due to polypectomy during surveillance, though such comparisons are very difficult.

Since most recurrences begin outside the bowel lumen, endoscopy is relatively insensitive as a method for the detection of recurrent cancer.[1] Audisio's series indicated that colonoscopy yielded the first evidence of recurrence in less than 1% of cases,[12] though others have reported detection rates of up to 3–4%.[51,53,55,56]

The natural history of the adenoma–carcinoma sequence suggests that re-examination in less than three years after achievement of a 'clean colon' is unlikely to discover significant pathology. However, yearly examination in some hands has found adenomas in more than 14% of patients each year over a four-year period;[53] this probably reflects the reality of a follow-up programme, with lesions being missed at some examinations, rather than truly new pathology. Yearly colonoscopy is advocated by some,[56] perhaps tailored to the findings at each examination.[55] Nevertheless, the case for more frequent investigation than three-yearly in capable endoscopic hands was not accepted by the group providing guidance for the UK National Health Service (NHS),[57] who felt, however, that a strong case could be made for establishing a 'clean colon' colonoscopically either before surgery or within six months of primary treatment.

Scanning

Scanning modalities have become quite sensitive to small-volume recurrent disease in the past decade, and may be applied in follow-up to identify local or distant recurrence. As most local recurrences begin extraluminally, scanning is certainly more useful than endoscopy or luminal contrast studies.

Local recurrence

Ultrasound is more informative in, and close to, the bowel wall, while computed tomography (CT) and magnetic resonance imaging (MRI) are more sensitive to disease in the surrounding pelvic cavity. In two series comprising 168 patients in total, ultrasound was the sole indicator of recurrence in 6 of 23 cases.[58,59] The deeper focal length of endoluminal MRI may lead to its preferred use in this context.[60] A major difficulty with these three scanning modalities in the diagnosis of local recurrence is the differentiation of postsurgical changes from recurrent cancer; serial scanning, allowing recognition of increase in size and configuration of abnormal areas, may be more useful than 'one-off' examination.[61] The development of monoclonal antibody imaging (radio-immunoscintigraphy, RIS) and positron emission tomography (PET) scanning have allowed functional discrimination of malignant from scar tissue as a criterion in differential diagnosis.[62]

Liver metastasis

As well as being very considerably cheaper and more portable than CT and MRI, ultrasound is able to achieve sensitivity and specificity that compare well with the other modalities, detecting lesions of 1 cm diameter.[61] The technology is well developed, so the key question becomes clinical utility – in particular any benefit gained from presymptomatic diagnosis. This will be discussed below.

OUTCOME AND COSTS OF FOLLOW-UP PROGRAMMES

Kievet's and Bruinvels' four 'conditions of benefice' provided objectivity in trying to assess the usefulness of routine follow-up (Table 26.1).[10] They offer a realistic balance between trying to identify and help the curable few, a compassionate and sensible approach for the incurable majority, and a realistic eye on cost. However, it is extraordinarily difficult to dissect out the ability of individual tests, or various combinations in follow-up programmes, to live up to these stringent requirements.

There have been two broad approaches to this debate: the broadly descriptive review and the more focused randomized comparison. The former comprises the attempts to describe programmes in terms of their content, intensity, and cost, and to try to detect differences in outcome by inference. Virgo and her colleagues[1] made a recent attempt to collect, describe, and assess the relative merits of 11 surveillance strategies in use in the USA. Her main conclusion was that there is a wide range of cost without any indication that 'higher cost strategies increase survival or quality of life'. While cost is easy to compare between regimens (range $910–$26 717, a 28-fold difference), clinical outcome comparison is much more difficult owing to confounding variables. Perhaps the most reasonable inference is that clinical outcome varies less than the costs. Richard and McLeod[63] compiled a much larger list of studies and programmes by performing a Medline search spanning 30 years. They differentiated studied regimens according to their statistical and epidemiological quality, separating cohort studies from the few extant randomized trials. Their comprehensive and definitive exploration of this very difficult field led

Table 26.1 Kievit's and Bruinvels' four 'conditions of benefice'[10]

1. At least some recurrent disease should be localized and amenable to curative treatment.

   The process of recurrence development should involve two synchronous and counteractive mechanisms:

   undetectable → detectable preclinical → symptomatic . . .

   curable . . . → . . . palliatively resectable . . . → . . . irresectable

   (Present data suggest that curability of recurrent colorectal cancer is not usually a time-dependent process.)

2. Follow-up should be able to detect curable recurrence, *ideally without bringing forward the time of diagnosis of incurable disease.*

3. Overall, benefits of follow-up (increased quality-adjusted life expectancy, more curative resections) should outweigh non-monetary costs – early detection of incurability, reoperative morbidity and mortality, and false-positive tests.

4. Cost–benefit ratio should be sufficiently favourable to justify routine use.

them to the disappointing and inevitably vague judgement that 'there is inconclusive evidence either to support or to refute the value of follow-up surveillance programs to detect recurrence of colorectal cancer'. They point out importantly that existing data have not excluded an intensity-related effect of follow-up on cancer outcomes. These two large overviews, necessarily covering a very wide range of programmes, patient groups and clinical environments, both concluded that *large* randomized trials would be necessary to detect any realistic beneficial effect.

Four recent randomized trials have sought to compare the efficacy of different follow-up programmes, but have been similarly guarded in their conclusions.[64–67] We should examine these studies in some details before commenting on their contribution to the debate (Table 26.2). The problem with these trials is that none of them had sufficient statistical power to detect realistic differences in survival. As the authors of the Swedish trial pointed out, their study could not have detected any difference in overall mortality of less than 20%.[66] So, although the trials have not demonstrated an advantage for any particular approach – from no planned programme to the most intensive – nor have they excluded that possibility. As the likely maximum overall survival effect is no more than 5%,[68] the sample size calculations in these trials were unrealistic. Beart's group[69] tried to rectify this by performing a meta-analysis, but analysed three *non-randomized* studies together with two of the above-quoted randomized clinical trials (they did not have the Australian and Swedish data at the time of their

study). They demonstrated a 2.5-times excess of surgery for recurrence and a 1.16-times excess survival in the intensive follow-up group. Their effort to add power to the investigation of this issue is clearly well placed, but the inclusion of non-randomized data precludes definitive conclusions. Their assertion that targeting of follow-up to higher-risk groups 'will make follow-up a cost-effective endeavour' begs the inference that it is not cost-effective as presently applied to the mass of the postsurgical population.

WHAT FOLLOW-UP IS APPROPRIATE?

A recent review from New York described a follow-up regimen that many would adhere to, though the evidence for many of its elements is lacking (Table 26.3), as discussed earlier.

Unlike much government-generated advice, the UK NHS has been provided with sensible evidence-based conclusions on postoperative surveillance after surgery for colorectal cancer,[57] as described below. This advice carries an implication of 'guilt until proof of innocence', that, in the absence of evidence of efficacy, particular investigations or programmes should, in general, be omitted on the basis of known cost rather than included in patient management on the assumption of usefulness. The cases for perioperative colonoscopy and an 18-month postoperative liver ultrasound scan, while not proven, were apparently sufficiently attractive to gain tacit approval. The advice was as follows:

Table 26.2 Randomized trials of follow-up regimens

Trial	Total no. of patients randomized	Regimens[a]	Recurrence rate	'Curative' resections	5-year survival rate
Swedish[64]	107	HP, LFT, CEA, FOB, Σ, CXR, CT, C versus zero	33% versus 32%	5 versus 3 (10% versus 6%)	75% versus 67% ($p > 0.05$)
Finnish[65]	106	HP, FBC, CEA, CXR, Σ, BaE C, US, CT, flΣ versus HP, FBC, CEA, CXR, Σ, BaE	42% versus 39%	5 versus 3 (10% versus 6%)	59% versus 54% ($p = 0.5$)
Danish[66]	597	HP, LFT, FBC, CXR, C versus zero till 5 years	26% versus 26%	11 versus 3 (3% versus 1%)	76% versus 68% ($p = 0.48$)
Australian[67]	325	HP, FBC, LFT, CEA, FOB CXR, CT, C versus HP, FBC, LFT, CEA, FOB	33% versus 40%	13 versus 14 (8% versus 9%)	70% versus 70% ($p = 0.2$)

[a]BaE, barium enema; C, colonoscopy; CEA, serum carcinoembryonic antigen; CT, computed tomography; CXR, chest X-ray; FBC, full blood count; FOB, faecal occult blood; HP, history and physical examination; LFT, liver function tests; Σ, rigid sigmoidoscopy; flΣ, flexible sigmoidoscopy; US, ultrasound.

Table 26.3 A suggested follow-up programme from Parikh and Attiyeh[3]

Follow-up	Year 1	Year 2	Year 3	Year 4	>4 years
History and physical	3–4	3–4	2	2	1
Faecal occult blood	3–4	3–4	2	2	1
Sigmoidoscopy[a]	3–4	3–4	2	2	1
Plasma CEA	3–4	3–4	2	2	1
Colonoscopy or barium enema[b]	1	—	—	1	q3years
Chest X-ray	1	1	1	1	1
CT, MRI, ultrasound[c]	—	—	—	—	—

[a]For rectal and rectosigmoid cancer patients.
[b]If colon was not cleared preoperatively, then colonoscopy/barium enema should be performed within 6 months postoperatively. If cleared, then every 3 years is sufficient follow-up.
[c]These tests are only used if there is suspicion of recurrence.

Short-term follow-up

- Follow-up in the weeks after surgery for colorectal cancer should focus on postoperative problems, future planning (including possible use of adjuvant therapy), and stoma management. Patients' needs for emotional and/or practical support should be assessed and appropriate care provided.
- Patients who did not undergo complete

colonoscopy or barium enema before surgery should be offered colonoscopy within six months of discharge. If adenomatous polyps are found, repeat colonoscopy may be appropriate three years later. Colonoscopic examination should not be routinely carried out more than once every three years.

Longer-term follow-up

- There is insufficient reliable evidence on the value of follow-up intended to detect possible recurrence and progression of colorectal cancer after primary treatment. Multicentre clinical trials should therefore be conducted to assess the effectiveness and cost–effectiveness of various types and intensity of follow-up.

- Patients and their general practitioners should be given full information on symptoms that might signify cancer recurrence. They should have rapid access to the colorectal team if they become aware of such symptoms, so that treatment can be initiated as quickly as possible. They should be reassured that the risk of recurrence declines rapidly after the first two years after treatment, until, by year five, recurrence is very unlikely.

- It is thought by some that a yearly ultrasound scan, or an MRI or CT scan of the liver 18 months after surgery, may be appropriate for those patients who might be expected to benefit from early chemotherapy or surgery if they should develop metastatic disease. However, the effectiveness of this practice has not been fully evaluated.

CONCLUSIONS

Until evidence emerges to the contrary, in any healthcare system in which major decisions about funding are forced upon providers and consumers, the diffusion of improved primary surgical and colonoscopic techniques across the clinical community, and the application of population-based screening programmes, are the options most likely to produce cost-effective improvements in outcomes. In the absence of more effective treatment methods, follow-up programmes aimed at early identification of recurrence should continue to come below these and many other priorities aimed at minimizing the morbidity and mortality due to colorectal cancer. As an audit and research modality, and in the moral sup-

port of those who seek it, follow-up will continue to have a role.

REFERENCES

1. Virgo K, Vernava A, Longo W et al, Cost of patient follow-up after potentially curative colorectal cancer treatment. *JAMA* 1995; **273:** 1837–41.
2. Granshaw L, *St Mark's Hospital, London. A Social History of a Specialist Hospital.* London: King Edward's Hospital Fund for London, 1985.
3. Parikh S, Attiyeh F, Rationale for follow-up strategies. In: *Cancer of the Colon, Rectum and Anus* (Coehen A, Winawer S, eds). New York: McGraw-Hill, 1995: 713–24.
4. Cochrane J, Williams JT, Faber R et al, Value of outpatient follow-up after curative surgery for carcinoma of the large bowel. *BMJ* 1980; **280:** 593–5.
5. Attiyeh F, Guidelines for the follow-up of patients with carcinomas and adenomas of the colon and rectum. In: *Neoplasms of the Colon, Rectum and Anus* (Stearns M, ed). New York: Wiley, 1980: 93–7.
6. Reilly J, Rusin L, Theuerkauf FJ, Colonoscopy: its role in cancer of the colon and rectum. *Dis Colon Rectum* 1982; **25:** 532.
7. Ellis H, Recurrent cancer of the large bowel. *BMJ* 1983; **287:** 1741–2.
8. Bulow S, Svendsen L, Mellemgaard A, Metachronous colorectal carcinoma. *Br J Surg* 1990; **77:** 502–5.
9. Moertel C, Schutt A, Go V, Carcinoembryonic antigen test for recurrent colorectal cancer. *JAMA* 1978; **78:** 1065–6.
10. Kievit J, Bruinvels D, Detection of recurrence after surgery for colorectal cancer. *Eur J Cancer* 1995; **31A:** 1222–5.
11. Beart RJ, O'Connell M, Post-operative follow-up of patients with carcinoma of the colon. *Mayo Clin Proc* 1983; **58:** 361–3.
12. Audisio R, Setti-Carraro P, Segala M et al, Follow-up in colorectal cancer patients: a cost–benefit analysis. *Ann Surg Oncol* 1996; **3:** 349–57.
13. Wangensteen O, Lewis F, Arhelger S et al, An interim report upon the 'second look' procedure for cancer of the stomach, colon, and rectum and for 'limited intraperitoneal carcinosis'. *Surg Gynecol Obstet* 1954; **99:** 257–67.
14. Moertel C, Fleming T, Macdonald J et al, An evaluation of the carcinoembryonic antigen (CEA) test for monitoring patients with resected colon cancer. *JAMA* 1993; **270:** 943–7.
15. Martin E, Cooperman M, King G et al, A retrospective and prospective study of serial CEA determinations in the early detection of recurrent colon cancer. *Am J Surg* 1979; **137:** 167–9.
16. Northover J, Carcinoembryonic antigen and recurrent colorectal cancer. *Br J Surg* 1985; **72**(Suppl): S44–6.
17. Gold P, Freedman S, Demonstration of tumor-specific antigens in human colonic carcinomata by immunological tolerance and absorption techniques. *J Exp Med* 1965; **121:** 439–62.
18. Herrera M, Ming T, Holyoke E, Carcinoembryonic antigen (CEA) as a prognostic and monitoring test in clinically complete resection of colorectal carcinoma. *Ann Surg* 1976; **183:** 5–9.
19. Martin E, Cooperman M, Carey L, Minton J, Sixty second-look procedures indicated primarily by rise in serial carcinembryonic antigen. *J Surg Res* 1980; **28:** 389–94.
20. Tate H, Plasma CEA in the post-surgical monitoring of colorectal carcinoma. *Br J Cancer* 1982; **46:** 323–30.
21. Northover J, Carcinoembryonic antigen and recurrent colorectal cancer. *Gut* 1986; **27:** 117–22.
22. Mach JP, Jaeger P, Bertholet MM et al, Detection of recurrence of large bowel carcinoma by radioimmunoasssay of circulating carcinoembryonic antigen (CEA). *Lancet* 1974; **ii:** 535–40.
23. MacKay A, Patel S, Carter S et al, Role of serial plasma CEA

assays in detection of recurrent and metastatic colorectal carcinomas. *BMJ* 1974; **iv:** 382–5.

24. Sorokin J, Sugarbaker P, Zamcheck N et al, Serial carcinoembryonic antigen assays. *JAMA* 1974; **228:** 49–53.

25. Nicholson J, Aust J, Rising carcinoembryonic antigen titers in colorectal carcinoma: an indication for the second-look procedure. *Dis Colon Rectum* 1978; **21:** 163–4.

26. Liavag I, Detection and treatment of local recurrence. *Scand J Gastroenterol Suppl* 1988; **149:** 163–5.

27. Peters K, Grundmann R, The value of tumor markers in colorectal cancer. *Leber Magen Darm* 1989; **19:** 18–25.

28. Wanebo H, Llaneras M, Martin T, Kaiser D, Prospective monitoring trial for carcinoma of colon and rectum after surgical resection. *Surg Gynecol Obstet* 1989; **169:** 479–87.

29. Ovaska J, Jarvinen H, Mecklin J, The value of a follow up programme after radical surgery for colorectal carcinoma. *Scand J Gastroenterol* 1989; **24:** 416–22.

30. Jiang R, Clinical significance of serum CEA determination in the diagnosis of colorectal cancer. *Chung Hua Chung Liu Tsa Chih* 1989; **11:** 348–51.

31. Chu D, Erickson C, Russell M et al, Prognostic significance of carcinoembryonic antigen in colorectal carcinoma. Serum levels before and after resection and before recurrence. *Arch Surg* 1991; **126:** 314–16.

32. Pommier R, Woltering E, Follow up of patients after primary colorectal cancer resection. *Semin Surg Oncol* 1991; **7:** 129–32.

33. Himal H, Anastomotic recurrence of carcinoma of the colon and rectum. The value of endoscopy and serum CEA levels. *Am Surg* 1991; **57:** 334–7.

34. Fucini C, Tommasi M, Cardona G et al, Limitations of CEA monitoring as a guide to second-look surgery in colorectal cancer follow-up. *Tumori* 1983; **69:** 359–64.

35. Finlay I, McArdle C, Role of carcinoembryonic antigen in detection of asymptomatic disseminated disease in colorectal carcinoma. *BMJ* 1983; **286:** 1242.

36. Tagaki H, Morimoto T, Kato T et al, Diagnosis and operation for locally recurrent rectal cancer. *J Surg Oncol* 1985; **28:** 290–6.

37. Kagan A, Steckel R, Routine imaging studies for the post treatment surveillance of breast and colorectal carcinoma. *J Clin Oncol* 1991; **9:** 837–42.

38. Collopy B, The follow up of patients after resection for large bowel cancer, May 1992. Colorectal Surgical Society of Australia. *Med J Aust* 1992; **157:** 633–4.

39. Fletcher R, CEA monitoring after surgery for colorectal cancer. *JAMA* 1993; **270:** 987–8.

40. Hine K, Dykes P, Serum CEA testing in the post-operative surveillance of colorectal carcinoma. *Br J Cancer* 1984; **49:** 689–93.

41. Carlsson U, Stewenius J, Ekelund G et al, Is CEA analysis of value in screening for recurrences after surgery for colorectal carcinoma? *Dis Colon Rectum* 1983; **26:** 369–73.

42. Armitage N, Davidson A, Tsikos D, Wood C, A study of the reliability of carcinoembryonic antigen blood levels in following the course of colorectal cancer. *Clin Oncol* 1984; **10:** 141–7.

43. Minton J, Hoehn J, Gerber D et al, Results of a 400-patient carcinoembryonic antigen second-look colorectal cancer study. *Cancer* 1984; **55:** 1284–90.

44. Wilking N, Petrelli N, Herrera L et al, Abdominal exploration for suspected recurrent carcinoma of the colon and rectum based upon elevated carcinoembryonic antigen alone or in combination with other diagnostic methods. *Surg Gynecol Obstet* 1986; **162:** 465–4.

45. O'Dwyer P, Mojzisik C, McCabe D et al, Reoperation directed by carcinoembryonic antigen level: the importance of thorough preoperative evaluation. *Am J Surg* 1988; **155:** 227–31.

46. Putzki H, Student A, Jablonski M, Heymann H, Comparison of the tumor markers CEA, TPA, and CA 19-9 in colorectal carcinoma. *Cancer* 1987; **59:** 223–6.

47. Barillari P, Bolognese A, Chirletti P et al, Role of CEA, TPA, and Ca 19-9 in the early detection of localised and diffuse recurrent rectal cancer. *Dis Colon Rectum* 1992; **35:** 471–6.

48. Overholt B, Clinical experience with the fibersigmoidoscope. *Gastrointest Endosc* 1968; **15:** 27.

49. Neugut A, Lautenbach E, Abi-Rached B, Forde K, Incidence of adenomas after curative resection for colorectal cancer. *Am J Gastroenterol* 1996; **91:** 2096–8.

50. Bekdash B, Harris S, Broughton C et al, Outcome after multiple colorectal tumours. *Br J Surg* 1997; **84:** 1442–4.

51. Granqvist S, Karlsson T, Postoperative follow-up of patients with colorectal carcinoma by colonoscopy. *Eur J Surg* 1992; **158:** 307–12.

52. Chen F, Stuart M, Colonoscopic follow-up of colorectal carcinoma. *Dis Colon Rectum* 1994; **37:** 568–72.

53. Khoury D, Opelka F, Beck D et al, Colon surveillance after colorectal cancer surgery. *Dis Colon Rectum* 1996; **39:** 252–6.

54. Bussey H, Wallace M, Morson B, Metachronous carcinoma of the large intestine and intestinal polyps. *Proc R Soc Med* 1967; **60:** 208.

55. Brady P, Straker R, Goldsmid S, Surveillance colonoscopy after resection for colon carcinoma. *South Med J* 1990; **83:** 765–8.

56. Juhl G, Larson G, Mullins R et al, Six year results of annual colonoscopy after resection of colorectal cancer. *World J Surg* 1990; **14:** 255–60.

57. Haward R, *Improving Outcomes in Colorectal Cancer. The Manual.* London: NHS Executive, 1997.

58. Dresing K, Stock W, Ultrasonic endoluminal examination in the follow-up of colorectal cancer. Initial experience and results. *Int J Colorectal Dis* 1990; **5:** 188–94.

59. Rotondano G, Esposito P, Pellechia L et al, Early detection of locally recurrent rectal cancer by endosonography. *Br J Radiol* 1997; **70:** 567–71.

60. Hussain S, Stoker J, Schutte H, Lameris J, Imaging of the anorectal region. *Eur J Radiol* 1996; **22:** 116–22.

61. Theoni R, Colorectal cancer. Radiologic staging. *Radiol Clin North Am* 1997; **35:** 457–85.

62. Lunniss P, Skinner S, Britton K et al, Effect of radioimmunoscintigraphy on the management of recurrent colorectal cancer. *Br J Surg* 1999; **86:** 244–9.

63. Richard C, McLeod R, Follow-up of patients after resection for colorectal cancer: a position paper of the Canadian Society of Surgical Oncology and the Canadian Society of Colon and Rectal Surgeons. *Can J Surg* 1997; **40:** 90–100.

64. Ohlsson B, Breland U, Ekberg H et al, Follow-up after curative surgery for colorectal carcinoma. Randomised comparison with no follow-up. *Dis Colon Rectum* 1995; **38:** 219–26.

65. Makela J, Laitenen S, Kairoluoma M, Five-year follow-up after radical surgery for colorectal cancer. *Arch Surg* 1995; **130:** 1062–7.

66. Kjeldsen B, Kronborg O, Fenger C, Jorgensen O, A prospective randomized trial of follow-up after radical surgery for colorectal cancer. *Br J Surg* 1997; **84:** 666–9.

67. Schoemaker D, Black R, Giles L, Toouli J, Yearly colonoscopy, liver CT, and chest radiography do not influence 5-year survival of colorectal cancer patients. *Gastroenterology* 1998; **114:** 7–14.

68. August DA, Ottow RT, Sugarbaker PH, Clinical perspective of human colorectal cancer metastasis. *Cancer Metastasis Rev* 1984; **3:** 303–24.

69. Rosen M, Chan L, Beart R et al, Follow-up of colorectal cancer. A meta-analysis. *Dis Colon Rectum* 1998; **41:** 1116–26.

27

The case for CEA screening

John S Macdonald

INTRODUCTION

The role of plasma carcinoembryonic antigen (CEA) monitoring in patients with various stages of colorectal cancer has been debated almost from the time CEA was defined by Gold and Freedman[1] in 1965. There are several ways that plasma CEA monitoring could be of benefit in the management of colorectal cancer. For example, a truly sensitive plasma marker that becomes abnormal in patients with clinically asymptomatic disease who would have a high likelihood of cure with surgical resection would certainly be valuable as a tool in screening large populations for primary colon cancer. Another role for CEA monitoring might be in the patient with advanced colorectal cancer in whom changing levels of CEA in the plasma could direct therapy. In such a situation, ideally a CEA decrease would be a sensitive and specific indicator of response to chemotherapy. Likewise, an elevation of plasma CEA would be a reason to abandon the treatment being given and choose another form of regional or systemic therapy for the patient. Finally, in a patient with resected colorectal cancer, CEA elevation might be a means to detect recurrence. Periodic monitoring for CEA elevation postoperatively could be a valuable strategy if an increased CEA level detected recurrent disease at an early and highly treatable stage. This chapter will discuss the evidence for the use of CEA in the management of patients with colorectal cancer, and it will particularly explore the case for use of CEA monitoring in patients with resected colorectal cancer.

It is important to be aware that CEA is not a tumor-specific but rather a tumor-associated plasma marker. CEA is a glycoprotein that is expressed normally in the glycocalyx of gastrointestinal mucosal cells, particularly those of the colon and rectum. CEA appears to be particularly overexpressed in adenocarcinomas of the colon and rectum, but it may also be elevated in patients with other malignant neoplasms.[2] Generally, the upper limit of normal of plasma CEA varies with the particular assay being used, but almost always is in the range of 2.5–3.0 ng/ml. The CEA glycoprotein antigen appears to be increased in patients who are habitual smokers, and the upper limit of normal in this population is generally 5.0 ng/ml. Patients with liver function abnormalities may also have elevations of CEA, since plasma CEA is normally cleared by the liver.[3] CEA measurement is usually performed by radioimmunoassay, and clinicians and patients should be aware that the levels of CEA may vary according to the assay technique used. Therefore, it is advisable in following serial CEA levels in individual patients that the same assay technique be used throughout a patient's course.

As noted above, CEA elevations are not unique to colorectal cancer. Elevated circulating CEA levels may be present in a variety of tumors, including breast, pancreas, stomach, bladder, thyroid, and lung cancers. It also should be noted that in colorectal cancer, elevation of CEA correlates with the presence of relatively well-differentiated tumors. This may relate to the fact that CEA expression is an attribute of normal colonic mucosa, and poorly differentiated tumors may lose the ability to produce CEA as they dedifferentiate. In a study by Goslin et al[4] published in 1981, 85% of patients with poorly differentiated tumors had CEA levels below 2.5 ng/ml.

CEA MONITORING AFTER LARGE-BOWEL CANCER RESECTION WITH CURATIVE INTENT

In patients treated with surgical resection of large-bowel cancer with curative intent, relapse rates vary from approximately 25% (stage II) to 50–70% (stage III). Although adjuvant chemotherapy or combined-modality therapy may decrease the relapse rate in stage III patients by close to 20%, there is still substantial risk for relapse after curative resection. In general, patients who develop metastatic or recurrent colorectal cancer are not curable. An exception to this generalization is the group of patients who have resectable metastatic disease. This is particularly true for patients with liver metastasis.[6] It has been shown that approximately 25% of patients with up to three resectable liver metastases who undergo hepatic resection are long-term disease-free survivors.[7] Recent data reviewed the use of resection of metastatic disease in a group of 1247 patients treated on a national Intergroup adjuvant chemotherapy study.[5] This study has shown that 222 of 548 (41%) patients who recurred with colon cancer were considered candidates for attempted curative resection. In 109 of these patients (20%), curative intent surgery could be performed. Sites of resected metastasis included the liver, the lung, and local recurrence. Of note, the 5-year disease-free survival rate in all patients resected for cure, irrespective of the site of metastases, averaged 23%. The ability to dramatically improve survival and cure rate in 20–25% of patients with resectable metastatic disease suggests that monitoring for detection of recurrent cancer, if such monitoring increased the likelihood of finding resectable metastatic cancer, would be of great benefit to an important subset of patients.

The strategy of postoperative CEA monitoring has been evaluated in some controlled studies in patients with resected colorectal cancer. These studies suggest that elevation of CEA does appear to be an accurate means of detecting the presence of liver metastases. An example is the study reported by Arnaud et al[8] which evaluated 305 patients. The value of monitoring CEA levels was assessed in detecting liver metastasis. It was found that an elevated plasma CEA had a 94% sensitivity in detecting liver metastasis and a 96% specificity.

Although a high sensitivity and specificity in detecting metastatic disease is impressive, the most important information for clinicians with regard to CEA monitoring is whether detection of metastases by evaluating patients with elevated postoperative CEA levels results in improved survival and the potential for cure. A large meta-analysis including 3283 patients published in 1994 by Bruinvels et al[9] evaluated the usefulness of intensive follow-up including CEA monitoring for the 5-year survival of patients with resected colorectal cancer. Intensive follow-up frequently included CEA monitoring, but

also included physical examination, liver function tests, and endoscopic and radiographic examinations performed on a regular schedule. The results from the intensive follow-up group were compared with patient outcomes from studies included in the meta-analysis that did not mandate any routine protocol for follow-up. The results demonstrated that there was a 9% improvement in survival in patients undergoing intensive follow-up. When the detection of asymptomatic recurrences was evaluated, approximately 45% of patients found to recur on intensive follow-up protocols were asymptomatic, compared with only 8% in cases receiving less intensive follow-up. This meta-analysis also suggested that patients receiving intensive follow-up were more likely to be resected with curative intent than those in the less intensive follow-up group. Survival analysis showed that in the intensive follow-up group receiving regular CEA monitoring, survival was improved compared with the routine follow-up group.

A large non-randomized study assessing CEA monitoring was conducted by the Society of Surgical Oncology and reported in 1985.[10] Physicians participating in this study were encouraged to draw postoperative CEA samples every 1–2 months from their patients. In patients with close CEA monitoring developing metastatic disease, 54% were resectable for cure, compared with a maximum 30% resection rate for patients monitored with sporadic or less frequent CEA levels. Although CEA monitoring led to more resections, and some patients resected with curative intent were long-term survivors, the overall survival rate was not different between the CEA-monitored patients and patients who were resected with curative intent because of clinical evidence of recurrent disease. Although CEA monitoring alone as an independent variable did not improve survival, this study does show that resection with curative intent of metastatic colon cancer – no matter how resectable disease is detected – results in long-term disease-free survival in some patients.

Although there is no question that resection of metastatic disease may cure selected patients with recurrent colorectal cancer, there has been great concern expressed over the fact that only a small percentage of all patients will experience prolonged survival as a result of strategies to aggressively detect metastatic disease. There also is a concern over the cost–effectiveness of aggressive follow-up protocols that may yield very few long-term survivors. In a retrospective study published by Moertel et al[11] in 1993, the use of CEA monitoring and the impact of such monitoring on curative resection was reviewed in an Intergroup adjuvant study. It should be noted that in this study, postoperative CEA monitoring was not required by the protocol. Such monitoring was done at the discretion of the physician. The usefulness of detecting liver metastasis by CEA monitoring was reaffirmed by this study. In the patients receiving periodic CEA monitoring, most recurrences detected were in the liver, while in the group not undergoing CEA evaluation, most of the recurrences detected were local recurrences or pulmonary metastases. However, this study did not demonstrate an improvement in survival as a result of CEA monitoring, although, similarly to the study cited previously,[10] resection of recurrent cancer was essential, since the only patients with metastatic disease who experienced prolonged survival were those who were resected.

There also are small amounts of data from randomized studies of CEA monitoring. In a small randomized controlled trial,[12] 106 patients with resected colon cancer were randomized between regular CEA monitoring and a routine follow-up control group. The group receiving regular CEA monitoring had metastatic disease detected an average of 5 months earlier than the routine-monitoring group. However, there was no evidence that such early detection resulted in improvement in overall survival. Although this study confirms the finding that CEA monitoring resulted in early detection of recurrent disease, it also makes it clear that the ultimate clinical value of detecting recurrent disease early is critically dependent upon the ability to use the lead time in disease detection to successfully perform therapy with curative intent. If therapy with curative intent is not possible, early detection of incurable metastasis is hardly beneficial to the patient. A recent prospective randomized study from Italy[13] suggests benefits from monitoring of serum markers, including CEA, in patients with resected colorectal cancer. In this study, 315 patients with resected colon cancer were randomized between follow-up programs utilizing regular monitoring with CEA, CA19-9, and CA72-4 serum tumor markers, or routine follow-up without marker monitoring. The patients on this marker arm who recurred had a significantly earlier diagnosis of recurrence ($p \leqslant 0.0005$) than the control patients. Resection of metastases for cure was increased in the monitored patients (35%) compared with the control cases (26%). There was also an increase in survival in the monitored cases ($p \leqslant 0.02$) compared with the control cases. Kaplan–Meier survival analysis demonstrated significant overall improvement of survival for monitored cases ($p \leqslant 0.001$) compared with control cases. This randomized clinical trial suggests that monitoring of serum markers may result

not only in earlier detection but also in improved survival, because early detection leads to resection of metastatic disease.

Well-designed and appropriately statistically powered randomized studies of CEA monitoring, designed to test the endpoints of not only early detection of metastatic disease but also the impact of such detection upon survival, are not available. There has, however, been one study,[14] performed in an elegant fashion in the UK, which is now under final analysis.[15] This study was designed in a unique way (Figure 27.1), and its results will be of considerable value to clinicians managing patients with colorectal cancer. The design required that all patients with resected colorectal cancer have CEA blood samples drawn on a routine basis. These blood samples were sent to a central laboratory, where they were analyzed. The results of the analysis were blinded to the investigators and patients. Cases with rising CEA levels were randomized to either an aggressive or a conventional arm. The aggressive arm required that the clinician managing the patient with the rising CEA be informed of that elevation. The clinicians and patients in the conventional arm were not told of rising CEA levels. In the aggressive arm, work-up to detect occult recurrent cancer followed by therapy with curative intent with exploratory laparotomy could occur at the discretion of the clinician, who was made aware of a rising CEA. As noted previously, this study has not been fully analyzed, but over 1400 patients have been registered. This large randomized study with a unique design will certainly give an interesting and likely highly valuable result with regard to the clinical value of monitoring for plasma CEA elevation in patients with resected colorectal cancer.

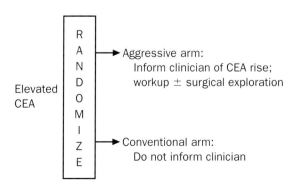

Figure 27.1 UK CEA follow-up study.

CONCLUSIONS

The value of the use of CEA monitoring postoperatively is still unclear, and certainly varies with the eye of the beholder. As described above, there is good evidence that in cases undergoing regular postoperative CEA monitoring, asymptomatic recurrence is detected earlier than in cases not receiving CEA monitoring. Given the fact that early detection is possible, the most important questions are: (1) does such detection result in curative therapy, and (2) is a CEA monitoring-based strategy of early detection cost-effective? The cost–effectiveness of follow-up protocols is a complex issue. Performing extensive and frequent follow-up procedures entailing physician visits, physical examinations, CEA monitoring, imaging studies, and endoscopic procedures is always expensive. The estimated yearly cost of intensive monitoring of all cases with resected colon cancer has been estimated to be as high as $27 000 per patient, with total costs per year of greater than $1 billion.[16] However, one must always remember that the only purpose of 'intensive follow-up' is to detect curable recurrent/metastatic cancer. The subset of cases with curable recurrence is undoubtedly a small, albeit critically important minority of patients. Therefore, if one chooses patients for aggressive follow-up who are likely to fall into the group of cases potentially curable if recurrent cancer develops, one narrows significantly the total group of patients to be monitored, and both significantly decreases the overall cost of follow-up and increases the likelihood of benefiting monitored cases.

In deciding whether to use routine CEA monitoring, the current (incomplete) data would suggest that clinicians should evaluate individual patients for the suitability of routine postoperative CEA monitoring. A reasonable, conceptual approach for the clinician to utilize in evaluating a patient with resected colorectal cancer is to first ask the question: is this patient a potential candidate for aggressive curative surgery if metastatic disease were to occur? If the managing clinician can answer 'yes' to that question, then it follows that a monitoring program aimed at detecting metastatic disease at its earliest, perhaps most resectable, point is reasonable. In such patients, monitoring CEA may be of benefit. Since it is known that resection of a single hepatic metastasis in a patient who has no extrahepatic metastatic disease results in a 2-year survival rate of at least 50% and a 6-year survival rate of 25–45%,[17] strategies aimed at detecting resectable metastatic disease are certainly appropriate to offer to patients in good general medical condition. One would, therefore, recommend the prudent use of postoperative CEA monitoring in patients who have a potential for undergoing resection of metastatic disease. A reasonable schema for CEA monitoring would be to evaluate CEA levels every 2 months for the first 2 years after colon resection. Such a selective CEA monitoring program in patients considered potential candidates for aggressive management of metastatic cancer was recommended as an appropriate standard of care by the ASCO Clinical Guidelines Committee.[18]

REFERENCES

1. Gold P, Freedman S, Demonstration of tumor specific antigens in human colonic carcinomata by immunologic tolerance and absorption techniques. *J Exp Med* 1965; **121:** 439–62.
2. American Society of Clinical Oncology, Clinical practice guidelines for the use of tumor markers in breast and colorectal cancer. *J Clin Oncol* 1996; **14:** 2843–77.
3. Fletcher RH, Carcinoembryonic antigen. *Ann Intern Med* 1986; **104:** 66–73.
4. Goslin R, O'Brien MJ, Steele G, Correlation of plasma CEA and CEA tissue staining in poorly differentiated colorectal cancer. *Am J Med* 1981; **71:** 246–9.
5. Goldberg RM, Fleming TR, Tangen CM et al, Surgery for recurrent colon cancer: Strategies for identifying resectable recurrence and success rates after resection. *Ann Intern Med* 1998; **129:** 27–35.
6. Alexander HR, Allegra CJ, Lawrence TS, Metastatic cancer to the liver. In: *Cancer: Principles and Practice of Oncology, 6th edn* (DeVita VT, Hellman S, Rosenberg SA, eds). Philadelphia: Lippincott, 2001: 2690–712.
7. Registry of Hepatic Metastases, Resection of the liver for colorectal carcinoma metastases: a multi-institutional study of indications for resection. *Surgery* 1988; **103:** 278–88.
8. Arnaud JP, Bergamaschi R, Casa C et al, The rationale for CEA dosage in the follow-up of patients operated for colorectal cancer. A prospective study on 800 cases. *Spec Int Col Mtg Surg Oncol* 1992; 25.
9. Bruinvels DJ, Stiggelbout AM, Kievit J et al, Follow up of patients with colorectal cancer. *Ann Surg* 1994; **219:** 174–82.
10. Minton JP, Hoehn JL, Gerber DM, Results of a 400 patient carcinoembryonic antigen second-look colorectal cancer study. *Cancer* 1985; **55:** 1284–90.
11. Moertel CG, Fleming TR, Macdonald JS et al, An evaluation for the carcinoembryonic antigen (CEA) test for monitoring patients with resected colon cancer. *JAMA* 1993; **270:** 943–7.
12. Makela JT, Laitinen SO, Kairaluoma MI, Five year follow up after radical surgery for colorectal cancer results of a prospective randomized trial. *Arch Surg* 1995; **130:** 1062–7.
13. Guadagni F, Roselli M, Mariotti S et al, Evaluation of the clinical impact of CEA, CA19-9, and CA72-4 serum tumor markers in colorectal cancer. A prospective longitudinal study. *Proc Am Soc Clin Oncol* 2000; **19:** 243a (Abst 940).
14. Northover J, Slack WW, A randomized controlled trial of CEA-prompted second look surgery in recurrent colorectal cancer. A preliminary report. *Dis Colon Rectum* 1984; **27:** 576.
15. Northover J, Prospective trial of serial CEA monitoring in patients with resected colon cancer. *Proceedings of European Association for Research in Oncology (AERO)*, Cannes, France, June 1998.
16. Virgo K, Vernova P, Longo W et al, Cost of patient follow up

after potentially curative colorectal cancer treatment. *JAMA* 1995; **273:** 1837–41.

17. Kemeny NE, Kemeny M, Lawrence TS, Liver metastases. In: *Clinical Oncology* (Abeloff MD, Armitage JO, Lichter AS, Niederhuber JE, eds). New York: Churchill Livingstone, 1995: 679–707.

18. ASCO Tumor Marker Panel, Clinical guidelines for the use of tumor markers in breast and colorectal cancer. *J Clin Oncol* 1996; **10:** 2843–77.

28

New methods for early detection of disease recurrence

Roland Hustinx, Frédéric Daenon, Robert F Dondelinger, Pierre Rigo

POSITRON-EMISSION TOMOGRAPHY

Positron-emission tomography (PET) imaging with
[18]F-fluorodeoxyglucose (FDG) has the unique capability of visualizing intracellular biochemical processes. Tumour cells display to some extent increased expression of glucose membrane transporters, enhanced glycolysis, or both. FDG is a glucose analogue, and cells take it up proportionally to the strength of these phenomena.[1] Unlike glucose, FDG is only phosphorylated by hexokinase and not further metabolized. It thus accumulates in glucose-avid tissues such as tumours. In recent years, PET has become a major tool for diagnosing and staging various neoplastic conditions, including colorectal carcinoma. The originality of the technique results from both the metabolic features of the signal and the technological improvements that have permitted its use in a clinical setting. Indeed, modern scanners now provide high-quality, fully corrected images of the whole body. These studies are performed in a time frame compatible with a clinical environment. In particular, image reconstruction using iterative algorithms and a more generalized utilization of attenuation correction have greatly improved the image quality and the clinical relevance of PET studies. An example of a normal study is shown in Figure 28.1.

In practice, the technique has some physical and biological limitations. Although spatial resolution is significantly improved as compared with single-photon imaging, it is usually admitted that most lesions smaller than 5 mm will not be visualized, and that the greatest sensitivity is obtained for lesions larger than 1 cm. Also, other tissues than tumours also show increased glucose metabolism and FDG uptake. Most benign tumours do not take up FDG, but many inflammatory, infectious, and granulomatous processes may be seen as foci of increased FDG uptake.[2] High physiological uptake is present in the brain and, in some circumstances, the heart, muscles, and bowel, among others. Knowledge of the pitfalls and appropriate patient preparation can greatly improve the performance of the test. Physiological uptake by the colon is reduced by giving patients spasmolytic drugs prior to the study, or by cleansing the bowel with an isosmotic solution.[3] Urinary artefacts are avoided in most cases by intravenous or oral hydration and administration of furosemide. Patient selection is also needed to increase the specificity of PET imaging. Ideally, patients with known active infectious processes should not be imaged until resolution of the episode. At the very least, the presence and extent of infectious or granulomatous processes must be well documented. Also, as a general rule, blood glucose levels should be measured before injecting the tracer, since abnormally high glycaemia lowers sensitivity when imaging several cancers, including colorectal.[4]

Metabolic and biochemical changes often precede structural modifications that can be visualized by 'conventional' imaging methods such as ultrasonography and computed tomography (CT). FDG-PET was therefore proposed for early diagnosis of colorectal cancer recurrence. In fact, there is now strong evidence in the literature demonstrating the additional value of the test. Initial reports suggested the particular value of FDG-PET for differentiating local recurrence of rectal cancer from scar tissue.[5,6] Presacral masses are usually visualized on CT, but

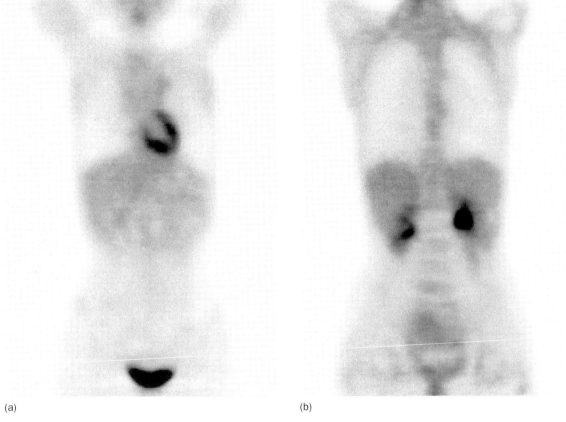

(a)   (b)

Figure 28.1 (a, b) Normal study of coronal slices at different levels: there is a high myocardial uptake, urinary excretion of the tracer, and mild liver, bowel, and bone marrow uptake.

determination of their nature is often difficult using conventional methods, even in conjunction with CT-guided biopsy. Further studies confirmed the critical role of PET in this indication.[7–12] In a study including 15 patients, FDG-PET and magnetic resonance imaging (MRI) provided comparable results, with 11 of 11 local recurrences detected with PET and 10 of 11 with MRI.[13] An example of locally recurrent rectal cancer is shown in Figure 28.2.

A major advantage of the technique is its ability to provide images of the entire body. A complete staging can thus be obtained through a single procedure, as reported by several authors.[10,12,14–16] Table 28.1 summarizes the results of the largest series published in the literature. In our experience, PET imaging is particularly useful for detecting local and loco-regional recurrences, both pelvic and abdominal, as well as retroperitoneal lymph nodes and liver metastases.[10] Few data are available regarding peritoneal involvement. CT is relatively insensitive in detecting

such lesions. In our series, both PET and CT performed poorly, but others have reported an additional value of PET.[17,18] Figures 28.3–28.5 illustrate the value of FDG-PET for whole-body staging.

Accurate staging of liver involvement is of particular importance in colorectal cancer. As discussed elsewhere in this book, prolonged survival can be obtained through surgery, in selected cases. Although CT angiography and MRI with liver-specific contrast agents are highly sensitive, they lack specificity and cannot stage the rest of the body. PET imaging has proven useful to select patients eligible for curative resection of liver metastases (Figure 28.6). Lai et al[19] studied 34 patients with suspected colorectal liver metastases. After conventional staging, 27 subjects were considered eligible for surgery. CT angiography or MRI assessed anatomical resectability. PET imaging disclosed additional extra-hepatic lesions in 32% of patients, modifying the management of 10 patients. Retroperitoneal nodes,

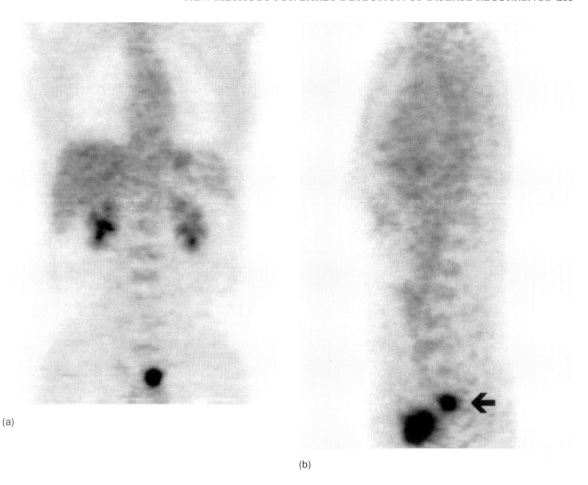

(a)

(b)

Figure 28.2 A patient with a previous history of carcinoma of the sigmoid colon treated by surgery and chemotherapy 14 months earlier. CA19.9 tumour marker levels are rising and the conventional work-up is negative. CT of the pelvis only shows scar tissue. PET clearly shows an intense focus of FDG uptake anterior to the sacrum (arrow) and posterior to the bladder: (a) coronal view; (b) sagittal view.

Table 28.1 Results of FDG-PET for diagnosing and staging recurrent colorectal carcinoma

Authors	Year	Patients	Sensitivity (%)	Specificity (%)
Schiepers et al[12]	1995	76	94	98
Delbeke et al[14]	1997	61	93	89
Ruhlmann et al[15]	1997	59	100	67
Valk et al[16]	1999	134	93	98
Hustinx et al[10]	1999	54	90	80

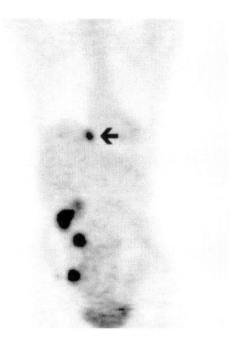

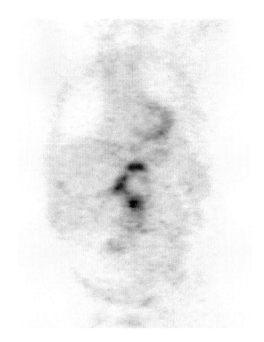

Figure 28.3 Multifocal recurrence of a left colon cancer treated by left hemicolectomy and adjuvant chemotherapy 27 months earlier. Several peritoneal lesions are easily seen, as well as a liver metastasis (arrow).

Figure 28.4 Nodal recurrence of a colon adenocarcinoma. CT showed several para-aortic lymph nodes, whose size was slightly increased. The lesions are clearly hypermetabolic on PET.

lung metastases, and locoregional recurrence were found in 6, 3, and 2 cases, respectively. The ability of PET to evaluate liver extension was further demonstrated by other groups.[20–22]

More generally, FDG-PET has a significant impact on patients' management, especially prior to surgery. Valk et al[16] performed FDG-PET in 78 patients where CT showed a single site of recurrence. Additional lesions were detected in 32% of cases, and recurrence was seen in 8%. Among the 42 patients who eventually went to surgery, 35 had a curative procedure. PET therefore had a great impact on therapeutic management. This should not only benefit the patient but also reduce the overall costs. In this study, the saving resulting from an accurate PET staging that demonstrated non-resectable disease was evaluated as $3003 per patient. Other groups have obtained similar results, with a clinical impact in 20–43% of patients studied by PET.[9,14,17,19,23]

Another clinical problem frequently encountered is the case of patients with increased tumour marker level (e.g. of carcinoembryonic antigen, CEA) and a negative conventional work-up. A large study has shown that with a threshold value set to 5 ng/dl,

CEA has only 59% sensitivity and 84% specificity.[24] Although CEA is widely used for surveillance, an increased level only indicates the presence of recurrent disease, without providing any clue regarding its localization. The clinician facing an increased CEA level with negative imaging studies has only two choices: repeat these studies a few months later or perform an exploratory laparotomy. PET imaging seems to be helpful in such a situation (Figure 28.7). Flanagan et al[25] studied 22 patients with abnormal CEA level and normal results of conventional methods. PET showed tumour foci in 17 of 22 patients. Recurrent disease was confirmed by pathology or follow-up in 15 of 17 patients, while PET was falsely positive in only 2 patients. The negative PET results were all confirmed. Therefore, in this limited series, PET provided the correct diagnosis in 20 of 22 patients (91%), with a significant clinical impact: 5 patients had curative surgery, 5 patients did not receive any treatment given the absence of disease, and 11 patients received chemotherapy for extensive disease.

As mentioned earlier, FDG-PET reflects tumour viability. Potentially, it could thus be employed as an

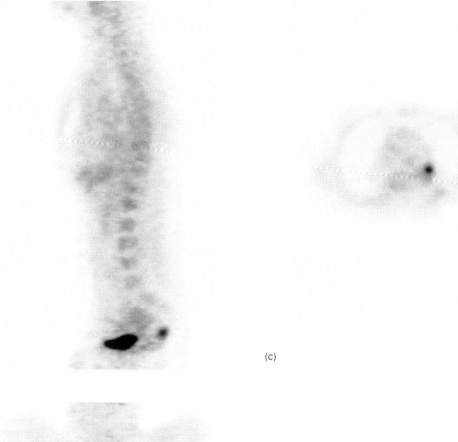

(a)

(c)

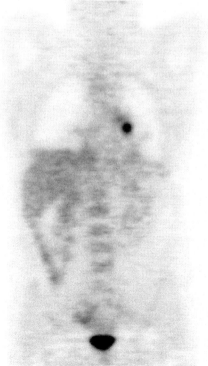

(b)

Figure 28.5 Patient with a rectal carcinoma previously
treated by surgery and chemotherapy. In addition to the
local recurrence ((a) sagittal view) already detected by CT,
PET also visualizes increased activity in a left mediastinal
lymph node ((b) coronal and (c) transaxial views).

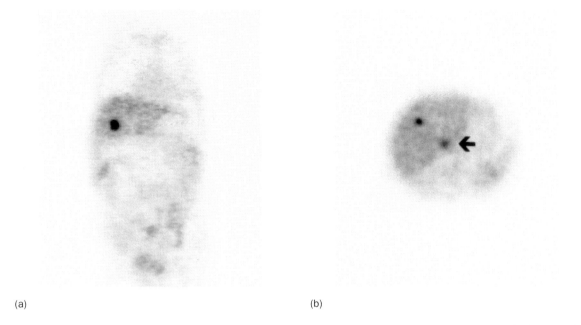

(a)   (b)

Figure 28.6 History of colon carcinoma treated by surgery and chemotherapy. A first liver recurrence was surgically removed, and this was followed by chemotherapy. On follow-up CT, a questionable 6 mm lesion is detected. PET demonstrates the hypermetabolic nature of the lesion ((a), coronal view), as well as an additional liver metastasis (arrow in (b) transaxial view).

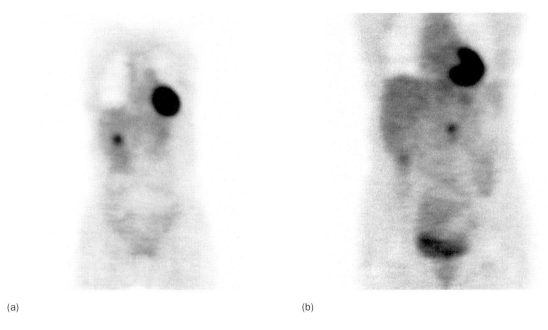

(a)   (b)

Figure 28.7 Colon cancer surgically treated 19 months earlier. The tumour marker level (CEA) is rising, but multiple conventional imaging studies are negative. PET discloses liver (a) and nodal (b) foci of increased activity, indicating multifocal recurrence. Note the very high cardiac uptake.

early marker of response to treatment. Few data are available so far, but preliminary results are encouraging. Bender et al[26] found a correlation between the final outcome and changes in glucose uptake measured by PET 72 hours after a single infusion of 5-fluorouracil (5-FU) in patients with unresectable liver metastases. Findlay et al[27] were also able to identify patients who would eventually respond to systemic chemotherapy by performing PET before and during the treatment. Similarly, chemoembolization of liver metastases was successfully monitored using FDG-PET.[28] After irradiation, however, inflammatory changes lead to an initial increase in FDG uptake. As a result, an early determination of the response to radiotherapy is usually not possible.[29,30]

Other works in progress utilize ^{18}F-labelled 5-FU to predict the outcome of therapy. Prior to treatment, a tracer dose of [^{18}F]5-FU is administered, and those patients with high uptake have a better chance to respond to subsequent 5-FU chemotherapy.[31]

In summary, FDG-PET now has several well-established indications in colorectal cancer patients. The biggest impact on management is obtained in three categories of patients:

- patients scheduled for curative surgery of recurrence;
- patients with inconclusive or conflicting results from conventional imaging methods;
- patients with confirmed elevated CEA level and negative conventional work-up.

Whether PET imaging can improve overall survival is very difficult to assess. The various surveillance strategies proposed so far have provided at best limited results in terms of survival. With its high sensitivity, FDG-PET has the potential to detect limited disease early on, so that surgery with curative intent could be attempted. An approach systematically using metabolic imaging as a first-line technique in selected patients with a high likelihood of recurrence has yet to be tested on a large scale.

RADIOIMMUNOSCINTIGRAPHY

Several tracers are currently either available for clinical use or under investigation. Two main molecular targets have been used for detecting recurrent colorectal cancers: TAG-72 and CEA. The tumour-associated glycoprotein TAG-72 is present in most colorectal adenocarcinomas. B72.3 (Oncoscint) is a whole antibody directed against TAG-72, and labelled with [111]In. Several studies have shown an additional value of this method as compared with CT for detecting extrahepatic lesions.[32] Non-specific accumulation of ^{111}In in the liver is, however, responsible for a low sensitivity in this organ. Arcitumomab (CEA-Scan) is a murine Fab' fragment whose target is CEA. The molecule is labelled with ^{99m}Tc, which ensures better imaging properties and a lower hepatic uptake. Improved sensitivity over conventional methods has also been reported.[33] In spite of an abundant literature suggesting a potentially large role of radioimmunoscintigraphy, the technique is not widely used, and seems to be reserved for selected cases.[34] In particular, its impact on patient management is not firmly established. Recently, however, radioimmunoscintigraphy has been proposed along with radioimmunoguided surgery. Intraoperative detection of monoclonal antibodies labelled with a variety of radiotracers, using a hand-held gamma probe, may significantly increase the accuracy of staging, thus modifying surgical plans and patient management.[35,36] Further studies are needed to clearly define the role of this emerging technique.

MORPHOLOGICAL IMAGING TECHNIQUES

Other 'morphological' imaging techniques, some already mentioned above, are currently used for surveillance of patients after curative surgery of colorectal carcinoma. They include barium studies, CT, transrectal ultrasound (TRUS), MRI, and transrectal MRI (TRMRI) using a specific probe or coil. Instrumental transluminal ultrasound or MRI examinations allow detailed imaging of the rectal wall and the perirectal environment. Endorectal techniques are not applicable after abdominoperineal amputation of the rectum or through a colostomy. Both transcutaneous and endoluminal imaging studies aim at the detection of cancer recurrence at the anastomotic site or in the operative bed on the basis of anatomical changes. CT and/or MRI are also able to detect remote metastases in lymph nodes, liver, and lung. Tumour recurrence may be evidenced by systematic screening despite the absence of abdominal symptoms and a negative colonoscopy.[37] However, a higher rate of detection of local recurrence does not necessarily result in prolonged survival.[38]

Barium studies

Barium studies are used as an alternative or together with colonoscopy to rule out a second colon cancer, which may occur in 5–8% of cases after surgery, or to survey Crohn's disease.[39,40] A median sensitivity of 94% was reported for screening of primary colon cancer, with similar results for single- and double-contrast techniques (90–95%).[41,42] Double-contrast barium enema is credited with a 20% higher sensitivity for detection of adenomatous polyps with a diameter of less than 1 cm, but this theoretical advantage is not relevant in elderly operated patients, since metachronous cancer requires 5–7 years to develop.[39,42–44] The rate of perianastomotic recurrence is higher for the rectum than for the colon. Intraluminal recurrence is best assessed by barium enema and colonoscopy, but occurs late, since most tumours predominantly develop in the perirectal space before invading the inner layers of the bowel wall.[45] Similar results are obtained by barium enema and colonoscopy for detection of recurrent carcinoma and polyps.[46] Both types of study evaluate the mucosal surface only, without giving information on bowel wall thickness and lymph nodes, which results in false negatives. False-positive findings on barium studies may be suggested by perianastomotic defects caused by postoperative fibrosis.[47,48] Barium studies are highly operator-dependent, and have the highest perception error rate compared with other imaging techniques. Nevertheless, single- or double-contrast barium enema, performed through the rectum or through a colostomy, is recommended after surgery, yearly for 2 years, then, if normal, every 3–4 years.

Computed tomography

Among the cross-sectional imaging techniques, sequential CT was initially recognized as the procedure of choice for preoperative staging of rectal cancer. Little has been published on colon cancer. Accuracies of 77–100% were initially reported, but later studies showed overall accuracy rates of 41–68%, which were not significantly improved by helical acquisition and thinner slices.[47,49–52] CT is relatively insensitive and unspecific for metastatic lymph nodes (22–73%), and microinvasion of pericolic fat is also frequently understaged. Therefore, CT does not accurately stage limited tumour, but does give acceptable results in advanced disease, or for recognition of distant metastases.[47,51] Furthermore, as local staging by CT influences the surgical approach only slightly, it is not recommended as a routine preoperative study. Conversely, in the postoperative period, CT is indicated for depicting local recurrence, which develops extrinsically to the anastomosis or in the fat of the posterior pelvis after abdominoperineal ampu-

tation of the rectum. A baseline CT examination should be obtained several months after surgery, when postoperative haemorrhage, inflammation, and oedema have largely resolved, to serve as a comparison for further studies. Recurrent tumour shows as a local soft tissue mass, typically with central hypodensities, after intravenous contrast injection. The mass has clear or ill-defined margins, and is located adjacent to the bowel wall or in the presacral space (Figure 28.8). It may invade the pelvic fat, or adjacent structures, and has an asymmetric distribution.[53] The following signs are highly suggestive of local recurrence: increase in size of a soft-tissue mass on subsequent CT examinations; invasion of cortical bone of the sacrum and coccyx (Figure 28.9) or of the obturator muscle or other pelvic structures (internal iliac vessels, prostate, seminal vesicles, urinary bladder, vagina and cervix, sacral plexus, ischiorectal fossa), presence of lymph nodes in addition to increase in CEA titres, and/or pelvic pain.[54,55] Differential diagnosis of a presacral space-occupying mass after amputation of the rectum includes fibrosis and normal anatomy (small-bowel loop, uterus, seminal vesicle). Inflammatory tissue is homogeneously enhanced after injection of intravenous contrast medium, and has a flat and symmetrical distribution in the posterior pelvis, without invasion (Figure 28.10). Strands extending into the surrounding fat are more suggestive of fibrosis than tumour infiltration (Figure 28.11). Radiation is responsible for pseudotumoral changes, including fibrotic masses and perianastomotic wall thickening. CT is not tissue-specific, and it might be difficult to differentiate local

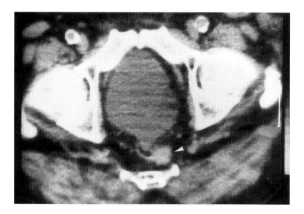

Figure 28.8 A 2 cm soft-tissue mass (arrowhead) with spiculated margins and surrounded by fat is seen on pelvic CT, 22 months after abdominoperineal rectal amputation. Biopsy-proven local recurrence.

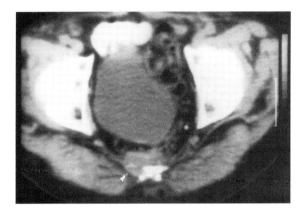

Figure 28.9 A 3 cm soft-tissue mass with central hypodensities is observed on pelvic CT in the presacral space 16 months after rectal amputation. Local invasion of the sacrum (arrowhead).

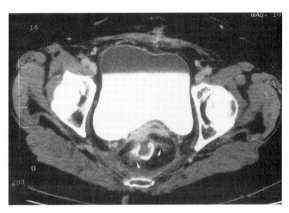

Figure 28.11 The same patient as in Figure 28.10. Strands (arrowheads) extending from the staple line into the posterior pelvis without a distinct mass are suggestive of postradiation fibrosis.

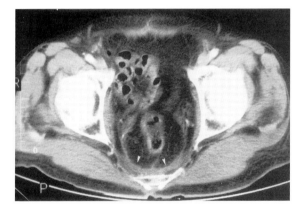

Figure 28.10 CT obtained after surgical resection and local radiotherapy for rectal cancer. Fibrosis shows as a flat and symmetrical opacity in contact with the sacrum (arrowheads).

recurrence from postoperative or postradiation changes. Percutaneous CT-guided needle biopsy by a transgluteal approach is indicated in selected patients, and has a high specificity and a low complication rate. Painful sampling is rather indicative of fibrosis.[56] As about 15–45% of all patients develop local recurrence, and 85% of recurrences occur within 30 months after surgery, particularly in patients with preoperative advanced disease, follow-up CT studies are recommended every 6 months following the baseline examination, during the first 3 years.[40] Proper examination technique is mandatory, which includes small-bowel opacification, distension

of the colon lumen with air, and intravenous contrast injection when a space-occupying lesion is evidenced. The same examination protocol should be used for all subsequent CT studies, and the upper abdomen and the base of the lung fields should be included in the same examination. Surveillance of local recurrence should be most intensive in patients who had invasion of adjacent structures at surgery – a 66% recurrence rate being reported for T3 and T4 tumours with positive lymph nodes.[52] Overall, CT is accurate in demonstrating local rectal cancer recurrence in 70–95% of cases.[54,57,58] CT is also the preferred imaging modality for assessing complications with an ileo-anal pouch following total colectomy.[52]

Ultrasonography

Transabdominal or transperineal ultrasound can be used for examination of the pelvis, but gives only limited information on the content of the posterior pelvis. Transrectal ultrasound (TRUS) has gained increasing popularity in the preoperative transmural staging of rectal carcinoma. The instruments used are the rigid, short probe and the endoscopic ultrasound probe using frequencies of 7.5–12 MHz. Both instruments provide high-resolution circumferential cross-sectional images with a penetration of less than 10 cm around the rectal or colon wall. Ultrasound obtained through the endoscope is capable of examining the entire colon, whereas the short probe is limited to the rectum. TRUS is more operator-dependent than CT or MRI. Five or seven wall layers, with distinctly alternating echoic interfaces, are described in

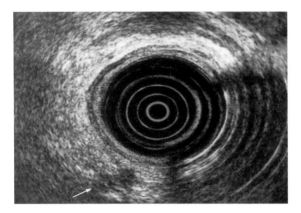

Figure 28.12 TRUS using a flexible endoscopic probe shows an irregular hypoechoic, limited mass (arrow) close to the rectal wall: proven local recurrence. Courtesy of Dr Gast.

the normal rectal wall, which has a thickness of 2–3 mm. The accuracy of TRUS in preoperative staging of rectal carcinoma is 80–90%.[59–62] CT fails to recognize minute changes in the perirectal fat owing to lack of resolution, and is more likely to understage T2 tumours, whereas endorectal ultrasound is more likely to visualize such limited abnormalities, but is also unable to differentiate inflammatory stromal reaction from tumour, leading to potential tumour overstaging.[59] Advanced disease with perirectal tumour extension is better staged with CT or MRI than with TRUS. On the other hand, perirectal adenopathies are evidenced with more confidence by endorectal ultrasound, but its specificity is low, based on lymph node-size criteria alone, thus accounting for accuracy rates of 70–80%.[60–63] Recurrent disease can be assessed in patients with sphincter-preserving surgery by transrectal introduction of the probe or endoscope. The anastomotic staple line is easily identified and does not degrade image quality by artefacts. Most perianastomotic recurrences are hypoechoic, but are not always differentiated from postoperative fibrosis (Figure 28.12). As for CT, serial examinations are necessary, particularly in patients in whom a high rate of local recurrence is expected.[63–65] Transmural biopsy can be performed with sonographic guidance when limited disease suspicious of tumour recurrence is evidenced.[65] In a prospective study, endorectal ultrasound did not show a significantly higher detection rate of local tumour recurrence than CT did.[38]

Magnetic resonance imaging

MRI offers better soft-tissue contrast than CT in the display of normal pelvic anatomy and in separation between tumour and adjacent structures. Contrast is further increased by intravenous administration of gadolinium. Local staging of rectal cancer is more accurately displayed by image acquisition in the frontal and sagittal planes, owing to the orientation of the levator ani muscle. The relationship of the muscle and tumour is more precisely depicted than on axial images. T_{1w} images are most helpful for the assessment of tumour extension beyond the rectal wall, owing to the high contrast difference between the hyperintense pelvic fat and the tumour, which shows moderate intensity similar to that of pelvic muscles. On T_{2w} images, the difference in signal between fat and tumour decreases, owing to the long T_2 relaxation times of both structures, but contrast between uterus and muscle increases, and advanced disease with visceral extension may thus be better shown. Overall, despite the increased contrast given by MRI, its accuracy in staging rectal carcinoma is similar to that of CT.[66] Endorectal probes have been developed to improve on the results obtained with the body coil. A 70–90% accuracy is reported with endorectal MRI in the preoperative staging of rectal carcinoma. Gadolinium injection did not significantly modify these results.[67] Invasion of cortical bone, nerve plexus, and muscles appear to be more precisely shown with MRI than with CT,[52] but MRI does not increase specificity in the diagnosis of metastatic adenopathies. In fact, MRI has similar limitations to CT, both methods being unable to confirm limited local infiltration of the perirectal fat and to diagnose metastatic spread to normal-sized lymph nodes.[68] MRI has a tendency to overstage tumours staged T2, by evidencing unspecific changes, whereas CT understages these tumours owing to failure in recognition. The use of short acquisition sequences such as in echoplanar imaging, prone patient positioning, oral or rectal administration of endoluminal paramagnetic contrast agents, and the use of dedicated surface coils or endorectal coils have the potential to improve the results of MRI in the assessment of postsurgical tumour recurrence. In postoperative follow-up, the quality of MR images is degraded by surgical clips at the anastomotic site. MRI does not separate with confidence tumour recurrence from fibrosis on the basis of high T_2 contrast, which is typical of tumour but not specific.[69–71] In fact, florid granulation tissue also exhibits high signal intensity on T_{2w} MR images, and high T_2 signal may persist in postradiation fibrosis for up to 1 year[52] (Figures 28.13–28.15).

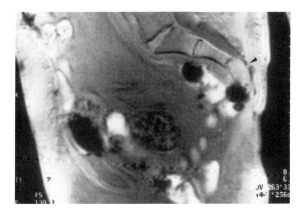

Figure 28.13 MRI obtained 6 months following rectal amputation and partial resection of the sacrum. On this sagittal T_{1w} image, a mass (arrowhead) with intermediate signal intensity is located adjacent to the sacrum.

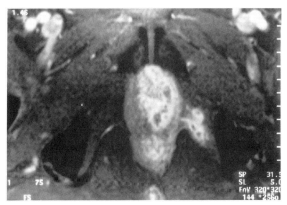

Figure 28.15 MRI obtained 2 years after resection of rectal carcinoma following radiotherapy and chemotherapy. Normal CEA level. On this T_{1w} gadolinium-enhanced image, a mass is situated posterior to the pelvic symphysis, with mixed intensities and peripheral enhancement, suggestive of tumour recurrence, surrounded by hypodense fibrosis that is best seen to the right. Similar small lesions are seen in the surrounding pelvic fat: local recurrence.

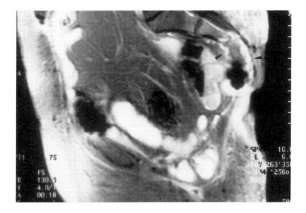

Figure 28.14 The same patient as in Figure 28.13. After intravenous gadolinium injection, there is better delineation of local recurrence by peripheral enhancement of the mass (arrowheads).

REFERENCES

1. Pauwels EK, McCready VR, Stoot JH, van Deurzen DF, The mechanism of accumulation of tumour-localising radiopharmaceuticals. *Eur J Nucl Med* 1998; **25**: 277–305.

2. Strauss LG, Fluorine-18 deoxyglucose and false-positive results; a major problem in the diagnostics of oncological patients. *Eur J Nucl Med* 1996; **23**: 1409–15.

3. Vesselle HJ, Miraldi FD, FDG PET of the retroperitoneum: normal anatomy, variants, pathologic conditions, and strategies to avoid diagnostic pitfalls. *Radiographics* 1998; **18**: 805–23; discussion 823–4.

4. Crippa F, Gavazzi C, Bozzetti F et al, The influence of blood glucose levels on [¹⁸F]fluorodeoxyglucose (FDG) uptake in cancer: a PET study in liver metastases from colorectal carcinomas. *Tumori* 1997; **83**: 748–52.

5. Strauss LG, Clorius JH, Schlag P et al, Recurrence of colorectal tumors: PET evaluation. *Radiology* 1989; **170**: 329–32.

6. Schlag P, Lehner B, Strauss LG et al, Scar or recurrent rectal cancer. Positron emission tomography is more helpful for diagnosis than immunoscintigraphy. *Arch Surg* 1989; **124**: 197–200.

7. Keogan MT, Lowe VJ, Baker ME et al, Local recurrence of rectal cancer: evaluation with F-18 fluorodeoxyglucose PET imaging. *Abdom Imag* 1997; **22**: 332–7.

8. Takeuchi O, Saito N, Koda K et al, Clinical assessment of positron emission tomography for the diagnosis of local recurrence in colorectal cancer. *Br J Surg* 1999; **86**: 932–7.

9. Ogunbiyi OA, Flanagan FL, Dehdashti F et al, Detection of recurrent and metastatic colorectal cancer: comparison of positron emission tomography and computed tomography. *Ann Surg Oncol* 1997; **4**: 613–20.

10. Hustinx R, Paulus P, Daenen F et al, Clinical value of positron emission tomography in the detection and staging of recurrent colorectal cancer (in French). *Gastroenterol Clin Biol* 1999; **23**: 323–9.

11. Gupta N, Bradfield H, Role of positron emission tomography scanning in evaluating gastrointestinal neoplasms. *Semin Nucl Med* 1996; **26**: 65–73.

12. Schiepers C, Penninckx F, De Vadder N et al, Contribution of PET in the diagnosis of recurrent colorectal cancer: comparison with conventional imaging. *Eur J Surg Oncol* 1995; **21**: 517–22.

13. Ito K, Kato T, Tadokoro M et al, Recurrent rectal cancer and scar: differentiation with PET and MR imaging. *Radiology* 1992; **182**: 549–52.

14. Delbeke D, Vitola JV, Sandler MP et al, Staging recurrent metastatic colorectal carcinoma with PET. *J Nucl Med* 1997; **38**: 1196–201.

15. Ruhlmann J, Schomburg A, Bender H et al, Fluoprodeoxyglucose whole-body positron emission tomography in colorectal cancer patients studied in routine daily practice. *Dis Colon Rectum* 1997; **40**: 1195–204.

16. Valk PE, Abella-Columna E, Haseman MK et al, Whole-body

PET imaging with [^{18}F]fluorodeoxyglucose in management of recurrent colorectal cancer. *Arch Surg* 1999; **134:** 503–11; discussion 511–13.

17. Flamen P, Stroobants S, Van Cutsem E et al, Additional value of whole-body positron emission tomography with fluorine-18–2-fluoro-2-deoxy-D-glucose in recurrent colorectal cancer. *J Clin Oncol* 1999; **17:** 894–901.

18. Yasuda S, Makuuchi H, Sadahiro S et al, Peritoneal recurrence of colon cancer detected by positron emission tomography: report of a case. *Surg Today* 1999; **29:** 633–6.

19. Lai DT, Fulham M, Stephen MS et al, The role of whole-body positron emission tomography with [^{18}F]fluorodeoxyglucose in identifying operable colorectal cancer metastases to the liver. *Arch Surg* 1996; **131:** 703–7.

20. Vitola J, Delbeke D, Sandler MP et al, Positron emission tomography to stage suspected metastatic colorectal carcinoma to the liver. *Am J Surg* 1996; **171:** 21–6.

21. Delbeke D, Martin WH, Sandler MP et al, Evaluation of benign vs malignant hepatic lesions with positron emission tomography. *Arch Surg* 1998; **133:** 510–15; discussion 515–16.

22. Hustinx R, Paulus P, Jacquet N et al, Clinical evaluation of whole-body ^{18}F-fluorodeoxyglucose positron emission tomography in the detection of liver metastases. *Ann Oncol* 1998; **9:** 397–401.

23. Beets G, Penninckx F, Schiepers C et al, Clinical value of whole-body positron emission tomography with [^{18}F]fluorodeoxyglucose in recurrent colorectal cancer. *Br J Surg* 1994; **81:** 1666–70.

24. Moertel CG, Fleming TR, Macdonald JS et al, An evaluation of the carcinoembryonic antigen (CEA) test for monitoring patients with resected colon cancer. *JAMA* 1993; **270:** 943–7.

25. Flanagan FL, Dehdashti F, Ogunbiyi OA et al, Utility of FDG-PET for investigating unexplained plasma CEA elevation in patients with colorectal cancer. *Ann Surg* 1998; **227:** 319–23.

26. Bender H, Bangard N, Metten N et al, Possible role of FDG-PET in the early prediction of therapy outcome in liver metastases of colorectal cancer. *Hybridoma* 1999; **18:** 87–91.

27. Findlay M, Young H, Cunningham D et al, Noninvasive monitoring of tumor metabolism using fluorodeoxyglucose and positron emission tomography in colorectal cancer liver metastases: correlation with tumor response to fluorouracil. *J Clin Oncol* 1996; **14:** 700–8.

28. Vitola JV, Delbeke D, Meranze SG et al, Positron emission tomography with F-18-fluorodeoxyglucose to evaluate the results of hepatic chemoembolization. *Cancer* 1996; **78:** 2216–22.

29. Haberkorn U, Strauss LG, Dimitrakopoulou A et al, PET studies of fluorodeoxyglucose metabolism in patients with recurrent colorectal tumors receiving radiotherapy. *J Nucl Med* 1991; **32:** 1485–90.

30. Engenhart R, Kimmig BN, Strauss LG et al, Therapy monitoring of presacral recurrences after high-dose irradiation: value of PET, CT, CEA and pain score. *Strahlenther Onkol* 1992; **168:** 203–12.

31. Moehler M, Dimitrakopoulou-Strauss A, Gutzler F et al, ^{18}F-labeled fluorouracil positron emission tomography and the prognoses of colorectal carcinoma patients with metastases to the liver treated with 5-fluorouracil. *Cancer* 1998; **83:** 245–53.

32. Pinkas L, Robins PD, Forstrom LA et al, Clinical experience with radiolabelled monoclonal antibodies in the detection of colorectal and ovarian carcinoma recurrence and review of the literature. *Nucl Med Commun* 1999; **20:** 689–96.

33. Moffat FL Jr, Gulec SA, Serafini AN et al, A thousand points of light or just dim bulbs? Radiolabeled antibodies and colorectal cancer imaging. *Cancer Invest* 1999; **17:** 322–34.

34. Stocchi L, Nelson H, Diagnostic and therapeutic applications of monoclonal antibodies in colorectal cancer. *Dis Colon Rectum* 1998; **41:** 232–50.

35. Bakalakos EA, Young DC, Martin EW Jr, Radioimmunoguided surgery for patients with liver metastases secondary to colorectal cancer. *Ann Surg Oncol* 1998; **5:** 590–4.

36. Bertoglio S, Benevento A, Percivale P et al, Radioimmunoguided surgery benefits in carcinoembryonic antigen-directed second-look surgery in the asymptomatic patient after curative resection of colorectal cancer. *Semin Surg Oncol* 1998; **15:** 263–7.

37. Meyenberg C, Huch Boni RA, Bertschinger P et al, Endoscopic ultrasound and endorectal magnetic resonance imaging: a prospective, comparative study for preoperative staging and follow-up of rectal cancer. *Endoscopy* 1995; **27:** 469–75.

38. Romano G, Esercizio L, Santangelo M et al, Impact of computed tomography vs intrarectal ultrasound on the diagnosis, resectability and prognosis of locally recurrent rectal cancer. *Dis Colon Rectum* 1993; **36:** 261–5.

39. Cali RL, Pitsch RM, Thorson AG, Cumulative incidence of metachronous colorectal cancer. *Dis Colon Rectum* 1993; **36:** 388–93.

40. Smith C, Colorectal cancer, radiological diagnosis. *Radiol Clin North Am* 1997; **35:** 439–56.

41. Gelfand DW, Ott DJ, The economic implications of radiologic screening for colonic cancer. *AJR* 1991; **156:** 939–43.

42. Fork FT, Double-contrast enema and colonoscopy in polyps detection. *Gut* 1981; **22:** 971–7.

43. Ott DJ, Chen YM, Gelfand DW, Single-contrast vs double-contrast barium enema in the detection of colonic polyps. *AJR* 1986; **146:** 993–6.

44. Gelfand DW, Colorectal cancer: screening strategies. *Radiol Clin North Am* 1997; **35:** 431–8.

45. Ott DJ, Wolfman NT, Integrated imaging in colorectal cancer. *Semin Roentgenol* 1996; **31:** 166–9.

46. Ott DJ, Barium enema: colorectal polyps and carcinoma. *Semin Roentgenol* 1996; **31:** 125–41.

47. Thoeni RF, Moss AA, Schnyder P, Detection and staging of primary rectal and rectosigmoid cancer by computed tomography. *Radiology* 1981; **141:** 135–8.

48. Beynon J, Mortensen NJM, Foy DMA, The detection and evaluation of locally recurrent rectal cancer with rectal endoscopy. *Dis Colon Rectum* 1989; **32:** 509–17.

49. Balthazar EJ, Megibow AJ, Hulnick D, Carcinoma of the colon: detection and preoperative staging by CT. *AJR* 1988; **150:** 301–6.

50. Grabbe E, Lierse W, Winkler R, The perirectal fascia: morphology and use in staging of rectal carcinoma. *Radiology* 1983; **149:** 241–6.

51. Hamlin DJ, Burgener FA, Sischy B, New techniques to stage early rectal carcinoma by computed tomography. *Radiology* 1981; **141:** 539–40.

52. Thozni RF, Colorectal cancer: radiologic staging. *Radiol Clin North Am* 1997; **35:** 457–85.

53. Lee JKT, Stanley RJ, Sagel SS, CT appearances of the pelvis after abdominoperineal resection for rectal carcinoma. *Radiology* 1981; **141:** 737–41.

54. Freeny PC, Marks WM, Ryan JA, Colorectal carcinoma evaluation with CT: preoperative staging and detection of postoperative recurrence. *Radiology* 1986; **158:** 347–53.

55. Kelvin FM, Maglinte DT, Colorectal carcinoma: a radiologic and clinical review. *Radiology* 1987; **164:** 1–8.

56. Butch RJ, Wittenberg J, Mueller PR, Presacral masses after abdominoperineal resection for colorectal carcinoma: the need for needle biopsy. *AJR* 1985; **144:** 309–12.

57. Pema PJ, Bennet WF, Bova JG, CT vs MRI in diagnosis of recurrent rectosigmoid carcinoma. *J Comput Assist Tomogr* 1994; **18:** 256–61.

58. Romano G, Esercizio L, Santangelo M, Impact of computed tomography vs intrarectal ultrasound on the locally recurrent rectal cancer. *Dis Colon Rectum* 1993; **36:** 261–5.

59. Hulsmans FJH, Thiot L, Flockens P, Assessment of tumor infiltration depth in rectal cancer with transrectal sonography: caution is necessary. *Radiology* 1994; **190:** 715–20.

60. Katsura Y, Yamada K, Ishizawa T, Endorectal ultrasonography for the assessment of wall invasion and lymph node metastasis in rectal cancer. *Dis Colon Rectum* 1992; **35:** 362–8.

61. Hildebrandt T, Schuder G, Feifel G, Preoperative staging of rectal and colonic cancer. *Endoscopy* 1994; **26:** 810–12.

62. Herzog U, Von Flue M, Tondelli P, How accurate is endorectal ultrasound in the preoperative staging of rectal cancer? *Dis Colon Rectum* 1993; **36:** 127–34.

63. Wolfman NT, Ott DJ, Endoscopic ultrasonography. *Semin Roentgenol* 1996; **31:** 154–61.

64. Ramirez JM, Mortensen NJM, Takeuchi NJM, Endoluminal ultra-sonography in the follow up of patients with rectal cancer. *Br J Surg* 1994; **81:** 692–4.

65. Nielsen MB, Pedersen JF, Hald J, Recurrent extraluminal rectal carcinoma: transrectal biopsy under sonographic guidance. *AJR* 1992; **158:** 1025–7.

66. Bachmann G, Pfeiffer T, Bauer T, MRT and dynamic CT in the diagnosis of recurrence of rectal carcinoma. *ROFO* 1994; **161:** 214–19.

67. Zagoria RJ, Wolfman NT, Magnetic resonance imaging of colorectal cancer. *Semin Roentgenol* 1996; **31:** 162–5.

68. Onodera H, Maetani S, Nishikawa T, The reappraisal of prognostic classifications for colorectal cancer. *Dis Colon Rectum* 1989; **32:** 609–14.

69. Ebner F, Kressel HY, Mintz MC, Tumor recurrence versus fibrosis in the female pelvis: differentiation with MR imaging at 1.5 T. *Radiology* 1988; **166:** 333–40.

70. Thoeni RF, Colorectal cancer, cross-sectional imaging for staging of primary tumor and detection of local recurrence. *AJR* 1991; **159:** 909–14.

71. Blomquist L, Franson P, Hindmarsh T, The pelvis after surgery and radiochemotherapy for rectal cancer studied with Gd-DTPA enhanced fast dynamic MR imaging. *Eur Radiol* 1998; **8:** 781–7.

Part 6
Treatment of Other Sites

29

Cancer of the appendix and pseudomyxoma peritonei syndrome

Paul H Sugarbaker

INTRODUCTION

Malignancies of the appendix are a diverse group of rare gastrointestinal tumors. They constitute approximately 0.4% of all intestinal neoplasms. About 1% of all large-bowel cancers arise from the appendix. Despite the diminutive size of this organ and the infrequent occurrence of such tumors, the histopathology of appendiceal malignancy has been confusing and the approach to therapy is complex. Unfortunately, a majority of the appendiceal tumors have perforated at the time of definitive surgical treatment. In these patients, carcinomatosis is present at the time of initial surgery, although liver metastases and lymph node metastases are seldom present. To improve salvage of patients with perforated tumors and those with documented distant spread within the abdominal cavity, a new and curative approach to this previously uniformly lethal condition (the spread of tumor on peritoneal surfaces) is presented.

PATHOLOGY OF APPENDICEAL MALIGNANT TUMORS

The two most common malignant tumors of the appendix are carcinoid and adenocarcinoma. Approximately two-thirds of appendiceal malignancies are carcinoid. The other one-third are variations of adenocarcinoma (Table 29.1).

Carcinoid tumors

By far the most common tumor within the appendix is the carcinoid. This lesion is usually found incidentally during the removal of an asymptomatic appen-dix. A small, hard tumor mass is found in the distal portion of the appendix. The appendix is the site of 45% of all gastrointestinal carcinoid tumors. Their incidence in females is higher than in males, probably because of the greater number of incidental appendectomies performed in women undergoing hysterectomies and cholecystectomies.

Although 90% of appendiceal carcinoids are incidental findings, approximately 10% result in acute appendicitis. Rarely is the carcinoid syndrome the presenting feature. If the patient has the carcinoid syndrome, distant spread of tumor to the liver is inevitably present.

The selection of treatment options for carcinoid tumor depends on the size of the malignancy, and, in large tumors, on the extent of local spread. It is extremely important to determine these clinical features at the time of exploration, since the histopathology of aggressive tumors and those with no malignant potential is essentially the same. If the malignancy is 2 cm or larger, a right colectomy with ileocolic lymph-node dissection is recommended because of the propensity for lymphatic dissemination.

Adenocarcinoid tumors of the appendix (goblet cell carcinoid)

A small percentage of carcinoid tumors have malignant epithelial cells scattered among the carcinoid tumor cells. More often, these tumors are diffusely infiltrating the wall of the appendix, rather than occurring at the tip of the organ. More frequently than with carcinoid tumors, these tumors present as acute appendicitis. The 5-year survival rate of such patients is much less than that of those with carcinoid because of the high incidence of diffuse

Table 29.1 Survey of appendiceal tumors

	Carcinoid	Pseudomyxoma peritonei[a]	Adenocarcinoma[a]	Adenocarcinoid	Signet ring[a]
Incidence	66%	20%	10%	Rare	Rare
Location	Tip of appendix	Middle to tip of appendix	Base of appendix	Diffuse along appendix	Diffuse along appendix
Major symptom	Incidental finding	Expanding abdomen, ovarian mass, hernia, appendicitis	Appendicitis	Expanding abdomen, ovarian mass	Appendicitis
Prognosis	<1 cm: 100% cure >2 cm: 50% cure	Localized: 100% cure Adenomucinosis: 90% cure at 5 years	Follows Dukes stages: A: 80% cure B: 50% cure C: 20% cure	84% cure at 5 years if unperforated; 0% cure at 5 years if perforated	Poor
Clinical syndromes	Carcinoid	Pseudomyxoma peritonei	Peritoneal carcinomatosis	Mucinous peritoneal carcinomatosis	Mucinous peritoneal carcinomatosis
Treatment	<1 cm: appendectomy only >2 cm: right colectomy plus cytoreductive surgery	Appendectomy plus cytoreductive surgery plus intraperitoneal chemotherapy	Right colectomy or cytoreductive surgery plus intraperitoneal chemotherapy if peritoneal implants	Appendectomy only or cytoreductive surgery plus intraperitoneal chemotherapy	Radical surgery plus intraperitoneal chemotherapy

[a] In separating pseudomyxoma peritonei, adenocarcinoma, and signet ring cancer, it must be remembered that these represent a spectrum of disease and are probably not distinct clinical entities. Benign mucocele is not included as an appendiceal tumor but is rather a cystic process. A perforated mucocele usually develops into pseudomyxoma peritonei.

peritoneal dissemination. Patients with peritoneal carcinomatosis from adenocarcinoid have a grim prognosis despite aggressive treatments.

Adenocarcinoma of the appendix

The most common variety of epithelial malignancy within the appendix is a mucinous one.[1] The mucinous tumors are at least three times as common as the intestinal type of adenocarcinoma. In contrast, only approximately 15% of colonic adenocarcinomas are of the mucinous variety. The preponderance of mucinous tumors is probably related to the high proportion of goblet cells within the appendiceal epithelium (Table 29.2) and an early perforation of the appendiceal wall because of the tiny appendix lumen and copious mucus production.

On gross examination, it may be difficult or impossible to distinguish a mucinous tumor of the appendix from a benign mucocele (Figure 29.1). Both benign and malignant tumors of the appendix are likely to cause appendicitis, and there may be mucin collections within the right lower quadrant or throughout the abdominopelvic space.

Two histologic features should be determined that will histopathologically separate tumors as inconsequential with complete removal from those capable of causing death from progressive cystadenocarcinoma (malignant):

1. Is there invasion through the appendiceal wall by neoplastic glands?
2. Are atypical epithelial cells found within the extra-appendiceal mucin collection?

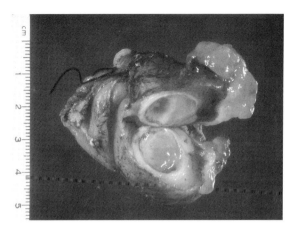

Figure 29.1 The distal appendix has ruptured from mucin within the mucocele. Adenomatous epithelial cells are widely distributed on peritoneal surfaces.

If either of these clinical features occurs, special follow-up and aggressive treatments are required.

The most common epithelial appendiceal tumor is pseudomyxoma peritonei. This clinical entity has the perforated appendiceal adenoma as its primary site. Hyperplastic polyps, adenomatous polyps, and villous polyps within the appendix that have resulted in an appendiceal 'blow-out' have been implicated in the pseudomyxoma peritonei syndrome. The mucus accumulations are distributed in a characteristic fashion around the peritoneal surfaces. Histologically, epithelial cells in single layers are surrounded by lakes of mucin. These epithelial cells show little atypia, and absent mitosis, and result in mucinous

Table 29.2 Comparison of colorectal and appendiceal malignant tumors

Incidence	Colon	Appendix
Adenocarcinoma	85%	10%
Carcinoid	<1%	70%
Mucinous adenocarcinoma	10–15%	20%
Signet ring adenocarcinoma	1/1000	1/10
Adenocarcinoid	Not reported	Rare
Differentiation of adenocarcinoma	20% well	60% adenomucinosis
	60% moderate	20% intermediate
	20% poor	20% mucinous adenocarcinoma
Associated malignancy	Unusual	Common

tumor accumulations that follow the flow of peritoneal fluid within the abdomen and pelvis. These accumulations of mucinous tumor in the abdominal cavity and on peritoneal surfaces are referred to as adenomucinosis.[2]

A second less common variant of appendiceal adenocarcinoma is the intestinal type of tumor, which appears similar to a colon cancer by light microscopy. This cancer is usually located at the base of the appendix, and resembles intestinal-type adenocarcinoma in its histopathologic appearance and natural history.

A third type of appendiceal adenocarcinoma is the signet ring tumor. This rare tumor tends to involve the appendix diffusely, and is associated with widespread invasive mucinous peritoneal carcinomatosis. It has an extremely poor prognosis, as might be expected from comparisons with other signet ring tumors found in the stomach, colon, or rectum.

DIAGNOSIS OF APPENDICEAL MALIGNANT TUMORS

As mentioned earlier, 90% of carcinoid tumors are found as incidental findings upon removal of an otherwise-normal appendix. Approximately 10% of patients with carcinoid have appendicitis, and only an unusual patient presents with the carcinoid syndrome. In patients with the malignant carcinoid syndrome, elevated urine levels of 5-hydroxyindoleacetic acid are routinely found. Also, elevated serum serotonin assays can be obtained. These patients present with liver metastases.

The preoperative diagnosis in patients with adenocarcinoma of the appendix is usually appendicitis, a right lower quadrant abscess, or tumor mass (Table 29.3). Mucinous appendiceal cancer has usually perforated prior to diagnosis. This results in tumor spread bilaterally to the ovary. Although ovarian

Table 29.3 Preoperative diagnosis of appendix cancer at the time of initial laparotomy in 296 case reports[a]

Diagnosis	No. of patients	Percentage
Acute appendicitis	139	47
Ruptured appendix with/without abscess	53	18
Intra-abdominal cancer or right lower quadrant mass	30	10
Inguinal hernia or chronic appendicitis	17	5
Incidental operations except for cholecystitis[b]	14	—
Cholecystitis (acute and chronic)[c]	10	—
Ovarian tumor or cyst	10	—
Small-bowel obstruction	8	—
Right-sided groin mass or fistula	6	—
Acute abdomen	4	—
Appendiceal carcinoma	3	—
Hydronephrosis	2	—
Total	296	
Autopsy finding[d]	10	

[a] Modified from Lyss AP, Appendiceal malignancies. *Semin Oncol* 1988; **15:** 129–37.
[b] Preoperative diagnoses include gynecologic cases (eight) and one each of incisional hernia, gastric, esophageal, and sigmoid cancer, duodenal ulcer, and torsion of the small bowel.
[c] Not listed as incidental, since the present symptom complex may have been related to appendiceal disease in some cases.
[d] Some patients died with postmortem diagnosis of metastatic malignancy.

involvement occurs in nearly all women with appendiceal tumors, it occurs in only about 50% of women with colon cancer. In addition, the tumor may present as peritoneal carcinomatosis within a hernia sac. An aggressive mucinous adenocarcinoma may invade the retroperitoneum and appear as a mucus accumulation in the buttock or thigh. Also, abdominal wall invasion with an enterocutaneous fistula may occur. Obstruction of the right ureter by a mucus-containing mass or invasion into the urinary bladder has also occurred.

PSEUDOMYXOMA PERITONEI SYNDROME

These minimally invasive appendiceal tumors have a high propensity for spread to peritoneal surfaces, but are unlikely to metastasize through lymphatic channels into lymph nodes, or through venules into the liver. After the appendiceal mucocele ruptures from pressure, adenomucinosis may progress for months or even years within the abdomen and pelvis without causing other symptoms. When this occurs, the clinical syndrome termed pseudomyxoma peritonei

occurs. The peritoneal cavity becomes filled in a characteristic pattern with mucinous tumor and mucinous ascites. The greater omentum is greatly thickened (omental cake) and extensively infiltrated by tumor. All dependent parts of the abdomen that tend to entrap malignant cells are also filled by tumor (Figure 29.2a). This involves the undersurface of the right and left hemidiaphragms, the right subhepatic space, the splenic hilus, the right and left abdominal gutters, and especially the pelvis and cul-de-sac. An important clinical feature of pseudomyxoma peritonei is the relative sparing of the small bowel by this process (Figure 29.2b). Because the small bowel is free of tumor involvement, meticulous cytoreductive surgery combined with intraperitoneal chemotherapy may provide long-term disease-free survival in over 60% of patients.

Preoperative diagnosis of pseudomyxoma peritonei is quite different from that of appendiceal adenocarcinoma. The most common symptom in both men and women with pseudomyxoma peritonei syndrome is a gradually increasing abdominal girth. In women, the second most common symptom is an ovarian mass, usually on the right side and fre-

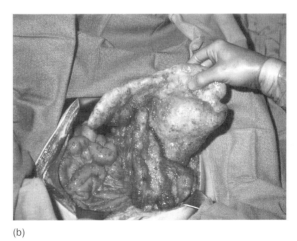

(b)

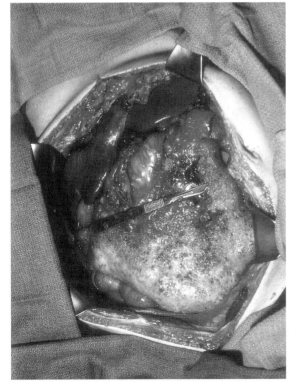

(a)

Figure 29.2 (a) 'Omental cake' characteristically present in patients with pseudomyxoma peritonei. (b) When the omentum is elevated, there is a sparing of small bowel by this tumor.

quently diagnosed at the time of a routine gyneco-logic examination. In men, the second most common symptom is a hernia. The hernia sac is found to be filled by mucinous tumor. In both males and females, the third most common presenting feature is appendicitis. This is the clinical manifestation of rupture of an appendiceal mucocele.[3]

There is one caveat that should be mentioned. If a mucocele of the appendix is found at the time of a planned laparoscopic appendectomy, then open appendectomy should be performed. Laparoscopic resection of a mucocele is likely to cause rupture of that structure, and pseudomyxoma peritonei syndrome will then result within a few months or years. Resection of the appendiceal mass without trauma and without tumor spillage results in a complete eradication of the disease process.

When a patient presents with increasing abdominal girth as a result of presumed malignant ascites, a paracentesis or laparoscopy with biopsy is usually performed in order to establish a diagnosis. In about one-half of these patients, an ovarian neoplasm will be found. In approximately one-quarter, a perforated adenocarcinoma from the gastrointestinal tract will be found. The remainder of these patients will have a rare peritoneal surface malignancy such as pseudomyxoma peritonei, peritoneal mesothelioma, papillary serous tumor, or peritoneal adenocarcinoma (formerly referred to as adenocarcinoma of unknown site). In all instances, paracentesis or laparoscopy with biopsy should be performed directly within the midline and through the linea alba. These sites can be excised as part of a midline abdominal incision. No lateral puncture sites or port sites should be used, because these will seed the abdominal wall with tumor and greatly interfere with disease eradication. Cytoreductive surgery and intraperitoneal chemotherapy are not effective for tumors within the abdominal wall.

TREATMENT AND PROGNOSIS OF APPENDICEAL MALIGNANT TUMORS

With appendiceal cancer, as with almost all gastrointestinal cancers, the prognosis of the tumor depends on the stage at which it is diagnosed and definitively treated. Fortunately, for 90% of carcinoid tumors, the disease is in an asymptomatic state, and cure is expected in nearly 100% of cases (Figure 29.3). In those patients with symptomatic carcinoid tumors, the prognosis depends on the size of the lesion and its demonstrated capacity to invade locally. In patients with tumors 1 cm or less in size, simple

appendectomy is all that is required. In this situation, the prognosis is extremely good, with nearly all patients surviving free of disease. In patients with tumors 2 cm or larger, there is a greater likelihood for dissemination through lymph channels into lymph nodes or portal venules into the liver. If the tumor is over 2 cm in size, if there are involved lymph nodes, or if the tumor has invaded outside of the appendix into the mesoappendix or nearby small bowel, an en bloc right hemicolectomy is advised. Sometimes there is extensive spread of the tumor into the ileocolic mesentery. Even in this situation, a vigorous attempt is made to excise radically all tumor and involved adjacent organs en bloc.

In patients with the carcinoid syndrome, hepatic metastases are present in addition to an invasive local tumor process. If the local tumor can be excised even with minimal margins of resection, one should undertake removal of hepatic metastases. Occasionally, several repeat hepatic resections may be required. A segmental approach or a metastasectomy procedure is preferred over a right or left hepatectomy. Whatever liver surgery is required to remove all visible deposits of tumor, it should be completed in order to gain maximal long-term palliation.

In patients with adenocarcinoma of the appendix, a right hemicolectomy has been shown to result in nearly twice the survival rate as occurs following routine appendectomy.[4] Therefore, all patients with invasive appendiceal adenocarcinoma, whether or not lymph nodes are involved, should receive a right hemicolectomy either during the same surgical procedure in which the appendectomy is performed or in a subsequent procedure. Certainly, when the surgeon performing an appendectomy finds that the appendix is infiltrated by a malignant process, emergency cryostat sectioning should be performed. If there is adequate bowel preparation and if a diagnosis of adenocarcinoma can be made definitively, one should proceed without hesitation with a standard right hemicolectomy procedure.

A majority of patients with mucinous tumors of the appendix show perforation of the appendix at the time of exploration. In most of these patients, peritoneal carcinomatosis or pseudomyxoma peritonei is found at the time of appendectomy. In the past, this was a lethal condition without exception. Recently, peritonectomy procedures combined with intraperitoneal chemotherapy have been employed for the treatment of pseudomyxoma peritonei and peritoneal carcinomatosis. The essential features of this approach are shown in Figure 29.4. The surgeon is responsible for doing as much as possible to remove

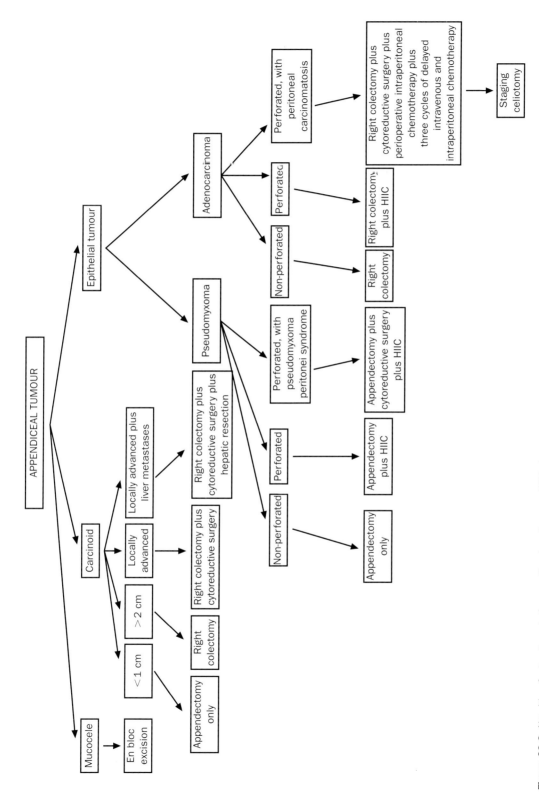

Figure 29.3 Algorithm for treatment of appendiceal malignancy (HIIC, heated intraoperative intraperitoneal chemotherapy).

all tumor on peritoneal surfaces. This is done by a cytoreductive procedure in patients who have gross spread of tumor around the peritoneal cavity. This involves a greater and lesser omentectomy and splenectomy. This is followed by peritonectomy procedures to strip tumor from the abdominal gutters, pelvis, right subhepatic space, and right and left subphrenic spaces.[5,6]

After the resection, and with the abdomen open, the peritoneal space is extensively washed by the surgeon's hand using heated mitomycin C chemotherapy (Figure 29.5). If the tumor is aggressive, a window of time exists in which all intraperitoneal surfaces are available for intraperitoneal chemotherapy utilizing 5-fluorouracil (5-FU). Uniformity of treatment with intraperitoneal chemotherapy to all peritoneal surfaces, including those surfaces dissected by the surgeon, can be achieved if the intraperitoneal chemotherapy is used during the first postoperative week. As the chemotherapy is dwelling, distribution is facilitated by turning patients alternately onto their right and left sides as well as into the prone position.[5,6]

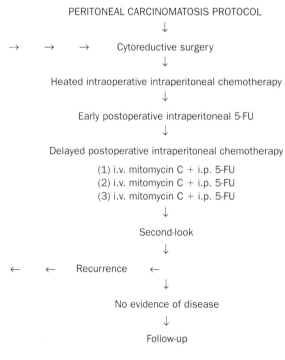

PERITONEAL CARCINOMATOSIS PROTOCOL
↓
→   →   →   Cytoreductive surgery
↓
Heated intraoperative intraperitoneal chemotherapy
↓
Early postoperative intraperitoneal 5-FU
↓
Delayed postoperative intraperitoneal chemotherapy

(1) i.v. mitomycin C + i.p. 5-FU
(2) i.v. mitomycin C + i.p. 5-FU
(3) i.v. mitomycin C + i.p. 5-FU
↓
Second-look
↓
←   ←   Recurrence   ←
↓
No evidence of disease
↓
Follow-up

Figure 29.4 Approach to the treatment of peritoneal carcinomatosis from appendix cancer (i.v., intravenous; i.p., intraperitoneal; 5-FU, 5-fluorouracil).

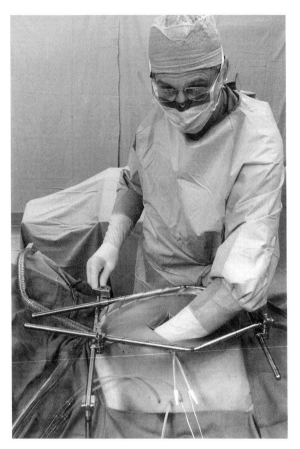

Figure 29.5 Coliseum technique for intraoperative chemotherapy. The skin edges are suspended on a self-retaining retractor. Warm (41–42°C) chemotherapy solution is perfused while being manually distributed throughout the abdomen and pelvis.

This perioperative intraperitoneal chemotherapy (combination of heated intraoperative mitomycin C and early postoperative 5-FU) has been utilized in over 250 patients, and has not been associated with an increased incidence of anastomotic disruptions. In patients who have had extensive cytoreductive procedures, there is an increased incidence of postoperative bowel perforation. This is presumably a result of the combined effects of heat necrosis of small bowel from electrosurgical dissection (seromuscular damage) and systemic effects of intraperitoneal chemotherapy on the intestine (mucosa and submucosa damage). In those patients who have intermediate- or high-grade appendiceal mucinous peritoneal carcinomatosis, three additional cycles of combined intravenous and intraperitoneal chemotherapy are recommended. This chemotherapy is given once a month.

Approximately 9 months after the completion of the intraperitoneal chemotherapy, a staging celiotomy is recommended. If at the staging celiotomy small tumor foci are found in 'nooks and crannies' of the abdomen, a final intraperitoneal chemotherapy treatment is performed.

It is important that definitive treatment of peritoneal carcinomatosis be instituted in a timely fashion. Each subsequent surgical procedure makes cytoreductive surgery more difficult. The relative sparing of the small bowel is only seen early on in the natural history of peritoneal carcinomatosis and pseudomyxoma peritonei. After several surgical procedures have been performed, the fibrous adhesions that inevitably result are infiltrated by tumor. This leads to extensive involvement of the small bowel by the malignant process. Eventually, it becomes impossible to cytoreduce the tumor safely, and the effects of the intraperitoneal chemotherapy by itself are not adequate to keep the patient disease-free.

The results of these treatments for peritoneal surface dissemination of appendiceal malignancies are unexpectedly good. Recently, the results of treatment of 385 patients with prolonged follow-up have been reported.[7]

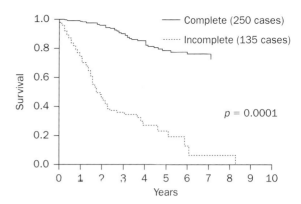

Figure 29.6 Survival according to cytoreduction (modified from ref. 7).

SURVIVAL ACCORDING TO COMPLETENESS OF CYTOREDUCTION

The mean follow-up of this group of 385 appendix malignancies was 37.6 months. After the completion of the cytoreductive surgery, all these patients had the abdomen inspected for the presence or absence of residual disease. A completeness-of-cytoreduction (CC) score was obtained for all patients. The CC score was based on the size of individual tumor nodules remaining unresected.[6] A CC-0 score indicated that there was no visible tumor remaining after surgery. CC-1 indicated the presence of tumor nodules smaller than 2.5 mm. CC-2 indicated the presence of tumor nodules between 2.5 mm and 2.5 cm. CC-3 indicated the presence of tumor nodules larger than 2.5 cm or a confluence of implants at any site. In Figure 29.6, the survival of patients who had a complete cytoreduction (CC-0 and CC-1) is compared with the survival of those with an incomplete cytoreduction (CC-2 and CC-3). Survival differences were significant with a p value of less than 0.0001. Patients who left the operating room after cytoreductive surgery with tumor nodules less than 2.5 mm in diameter remaining (CC-1) were much more likely to survive in the long term than were those with an incomplete cytoreduction. There were no significant

differences in survival between patients with CC-2 and CC-3 cytoreductions.

SURVIVAL ACCORDING TO HISTOLOGY

At the time of cytoreductive surgery and whenever possible from a review of the primary appendiceal malignancy, a histologic assessment was made. The designations of adenomucinosis, hybrid, and mucinous adenocarcinoma have been described.[2] Adenomucinosis included minimally aggressive peritoneal tumors that produced large volumes of mucous ascites. The primary appendiceal tumor was described as cystadenoma. Hybrid malignancies showed adenomucinosis combined with mucinous adenocarcinomas. Mucinous adenocarcinoma showed the signet ring morphology and was poorly differentiated.

Figure 29.7 shows the survival of these appendix malignancy patients according to histology. The survival differences between patients with adenomucinosis and those with hybrid or mucinous adenocarcinoma were significant, with a p value of less than 0.0001. A non-invasive histopathology is extremely important in selecting patients who are most likely to benefit from this treatment strategy. There were no significant differences between patients with hybrid and mucinous adenocarcinoma histologies.

SURVIVAL ACCORDING TO PREVIOUS SURGICAL SCORE

When the previous operative notes on these patients were reviewed, a judgement was made regarding the

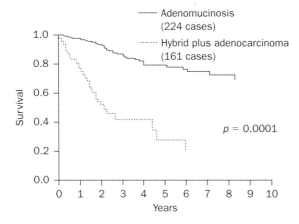

Figure 29.7 Survival according to histology (modified from ref. 7).

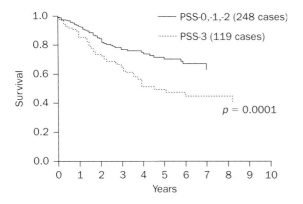

Figure 29.8 Survival according to previous surgical score (PSS) (modified from ref. 7).

anatomic sites of previous surgical dissections. The summation of these dissections was recorded on a diagram of the abdominopelvic regions.[7] This allowed an assessment of the anatomic locations in which previous surgery had been performed. In patients with a previous surgical score (PSS) of 0, diagnosis of peritoneal carcinomatosis was obtained through biopsy only, or by laparoscopy plus biopsy. PSS-1 indicated only a previous exploratory laparotomy. PSS-2 indicated exploratory laparotomy with some resections. Usually this was a greater omentectomy or greater omentectomy plus a right colectomy. With PSS-3, patients had an attempt at a complete cytoreduction. This was usually greater omentectomy, right colectomy, hysterectomy, and bilateral salpingo-oophorectomy, with the possibility of other resections from both abdominal organs or parietal

peritoneal regions. The survival according to previous surgical score is shown in Figure 29.8. Patients with PSS scores of 0–2 had an improved survival compared with those with PSS-3. The p value was 0.001. Extensive surgery without intraperitoneal chemotherapy resulted in a diminished prognosis.

SURVIVAL ANALYSIS ACCORDING TO COX SEMIPARAMETRIC MODEL

All of the significant clinical features were investigated to determine their dependent versus independent status. The independent variables were determined to be complete versus incomplete cytoreduction. All the other clinical features investigated were found to have no independent predictive value. Complete versus incomplete cytoreduction had a risk ratio for death of 9.98. The 95% confidence limits were 4.23 to 23.09.

MORBIDITY AND MORTALITY OF 155 CONSECUTIVE PATIENTS TREATED IN 1998 AND 1999

The extensive cytoreductive surgery combined with early postoperative intraperitoneal chemotherapy presents a major physiologic insult to these patients. Nevertheless, the mortality rate remains at 2% in this group of patients. Pancreatitis (7.1%) and fistula formation (4.7%) are the major complications. Anastomotic leaks were no more common in this group of patients than in a routine general surgical setting (2.4%). The overall grade 3/4 morbidity was 27%. There was no mortality associated with the adjuvant chemotherapy administration. Stoma construction was rarely required in patients with adenomucinosis. Seven percent of patients with hybrid or mucinous adenocarcinoma required a permanent ileostomy.

In this treatment strategy for patients with peritoneal carcinomatosis from appendiceal malignancy, there were several distinct changes in the use of both surgery and chemotherapy (Table 29.4). Surgery was more extensive and more meticulous than in other cytoreductive protocols. Because of the very limited penetration of tumor nodules by chemotherapy, the cytoreduction attempted to reduce the cancer within the abdomen and pelvis to its smallest volume. This involved the use of peritoneal stripping procedures, now commonly referred to as peritonectomy procedures. These procedures often required many hours in the operating room. Frequently, they left the

Table 29.4 Suggested changes in the use of chemotherapy for gastrointestinal cancer (modified from ref. 7)

Chemotherapy methodology	Change suggested
1. Route	Intraperitoneal or intraperitoneal plus intravenous
2. Timing	Perioperative not delayed adjuvant treatment
3. Patient selection	Minimal peritoneal surface not systemic disease
4. Target	Intraperitoneal spread not metastases to lymph node or liver
5. Surgical approach	Peritonectomies not debulking
6. Results	Benefit versus prior failure

abdomen without peritoneal surfaces except that which was found on the small bowel. This approach represents a departure from the previous conservative surgical approach to peritoneal carcinomatosis.

Several changes occurred in the use of chemotherapy in this patient population. First, the route of chemotherapy administration was changed from intravenous to intraperitoneal. Maximal doses of perioperative intraperitoneal mitomycin C and intraperitoneal 5-FU were used for the first five postoperative days. This chemotherapy was instilled during this time period to allow it to contact all the abdominal and pelvic surfaces before the onset of wound healing. Once fibrinous deposits became organized, the chemotherapy would be unable to reach the residual tumors, and local recurrence would occur where the surfaces were adherent.

The timing of chemotherapy administration was also changed. Chemotherapy was used in the perioperative period rather than 4–6 weeks after surgery in an adjuvant setting.

Also, the selection of patients for treatment was changed. Patients with minimal peritoneal surface residual disease were treated more successfully. Patients with large-volume residual disease in the abdomen did not achieve a complete response. The targets of these therapies were not metastases present at distant sites such as the liver, bone marrow, or lungs; rather, these therapies were directed at tumor dissemination on both the parietal and visceral surfaces. Patients with metastases that could not be resected with the cytoreductive surgery were excluded from these treatments.

Finally, it is hoped that with these changes in chemotherapy and changes in surgical approach, patients with peritoneal carcinomatosis can benefit from these aggressive treatment strategies. Hopefully, the previous failures of palliative chemotherapy can be converted to success with perioperative intraperitoneal chemotherapy.

REFERENCES

1. Higa E, Rosai J, Pizzimbono CA, Wise L, Mucosal hyperplasia, mucinous cystadenoma and mucinous cystadenocarcinoma of the appendix. Cancer 1973; 32: 1525–41.
2. Ronnett BM, Shmookler BM, Sugarbaker PH, Kurman RJ, Pseudomyxoma peritonei: new concepts in diagnosis, origin, nomenclature, and relationship to mucinous borderline (low malignant potential) tumors of the ovary. In: Anatomic Pathology. Chicago: ASCP Press, 1997: 197–226.
3. Esquivel J, Sugarbaker PH, Clinical presentation of the pseudomyxoma peritonei syndrome. Br J Surg 2000; 87: 1414–18.
4. Hesketh KT, The management of primary adenocarcinoma of the vermiform appendix. Gut 1963; 4: 158–68.
5. Sugarbaker PH, Ronnett BM, Ancher A et al, Management of pseudomyxoma peritonei of appendiceal origin. Adv Surg 1997; 30: 233–80.
6. Sugarbaker PH, Management of Peritoneal Surface Malignancy Using Intraperitoneal Chemotherapy and Cytoreductive Surgery: A Manual for Physicians and Nurses, 3rd edn. Grand Rapids, MI: Ludann, 1998.
7. Sugarbaker PH, Chang D, Results of treatment of 385 patients with peritoneal surface spread of appendiceal malignancy. Ann Surg Oncol 1999; 6: 727–31.

30

Treatment of anal canal carcinoma

Didier Peiffert

INTRODUCTION

The main goal of cancer treatment is to cure patients. The ideal treatment is one that achieves a cure with preservation of normal function. Radiation-based treatment protocols now make it possible to offer this hope of cure with preservation to patients who present small as well as locally advanced epidermoid carcinomas of the anal canal. Over a few decades, surgical treatment has given way to conservative treatment as standard treatment in most cases.

NATURAL HISTORY AND STAGING

Anal canal carcinoma is an uncommon malignancy, accounting for only a small percentage (4–6%) of all cancers of the lower intestinal tract, reaching a standardized incidence of 1/100 000. It develops predominantly in females, with most patients being 65 years old or more. The suggested risk factors are male homosexuality, human papilloma virus pelvic infection, and tobacco smoking, and this can explain the recent increase in incidence as well as the modification of the sex ratio.[1,2]

The anal canal is anatomically defined as the terminal part of the intestinal tract, extending from the rectum to the perianal skin. It measures 3–4 cm in height. The pectineal line is at the midline of the canal. Tumours of the anal margin, classified with skin tumours, extend below the anal verge and involve the perianal hair-bearing skin.[3]

Ninety-five percent of all primary cancers of the anus are squamous cell (epidermoid) carcinomas, including large keratinized cell type, non-keratinizing type (transitional or cloacogenic), and well-differentiated basaloid type. Adenocarcinomas, small cell carcinomas, undifferentiated carcinomas, sarcomas, lymphomas, and melanomas are exceptional cases, and are not treated on the same basis as squamous cell carcinomas.

The TNM (tumour, node, metastasis) classification of the International Union against Cancer (UICC) was modified in its 4th edition (1987),[3] and was adapted by the American Joint Committee on Cancer (AJCC). It was based on clinical pretreatment evaluation of tumours increasingly treated by non-surgical methods.

FROM SURGERY TO SPHINCTER-SPARING CONSERVATIVE RADIATION

Until the 1980s, abdominoperineal resection (APR) was recommended as the standard treatment, but pelvic nodal dissection and en bloc removal were not systematic. At that time, the locoregional failure rate was high, ranging from 27% to 60%, and the overall survival rate was poor, from 37% to 71%. Some selected less advanced cases were treated by local excision, but with poor results. Later, two approaches were envisaged.

Low-dose radiation and concomitant chemotherapy

In the USA, Nigro et al[4] prescribed preoperative low-dose combined radio-chemotherapy. The aim of this association was to improve the resectability of tumours, and to reduce the locoregional failure rate after APR. An intermediate dose of irradiation (30 Gy in 15 fractions over 3 weeks) was chosen in order not to compromise postoperative perineal wound healing. 5-Fluorouracil (5-FU) was chosen as radiosensitizer, initially administered as a continuous infusion (1 g/m^2) during 5 days, although this was later reduced at 4 days to decrease observed acute toxicity. A similar cycle was delivered in the

5th week, after completion of irradiation. Mitomycin C (MMC) was delivered as a single intravenous bolus of $15 \, mg/m^2$ on day 1; it was chosen on the basis of experimental demonstration of its activity in epidermoid carcinoma and in hypoxic conditions. Nigro et al observed 5 sterilized samples after APR of the first 6 patients, and then recommended that in the case of objective complete response, only the scar should be excised. Out of a series of 104 consecutive patients, there were 97 complete responses. Nevertheless, 24 received APR, and no residual disease was observed on histological examination of the samples. The scars were excised in 62 patients, and were histologically negative in 61 of them. Surgery was refused by 11 patients, and 9 were long-term survivors. At 5 years, 81 patients were disease-free. These results allowed mutilation to be avoided and a conservative treatment to be offered for clinically and biopsy-proven complete responders. On the basis of the initial experience of Nigro et al, low-dose radio-chemotherapy (5-FU–MMC) became the treatment of choice, radical surgery being reserved for incomplete histological responders. Several retrospective series or phase II trials have confirmed the high rate of local control (Table 30.1).[5–13]

High-dose radiation alone

In Europe (mainly in France), Papillon and Montbarbon[14] tested high-dose radiation alone with a split-course scheme, including a brachytherapy boost. From a series of 207 patients treated by 30 Gy delivered by a perineal cobalt field (30 Gy in 10 fractions and 18 days), and boosted by iridium implant (20 Gy) 2 months later, 80% were cured, in 90% of whom a functional sphincter was conserved. Several series using a similar split-course schedule, with a conventional or hypofractionated first course, and a boost delivered by brachytherapy or external-beam radiation, showed comparable results (Table 30.2).[14–20] On the basis of high local control and sphincter preservation rates, and the low rate of late complications, this was considered as an alternative to surgery as standard treatment. Prognostic factors after radiotherapy alone have been described (Table 30.3).[6,14–17,19–22] T stage has been reported to influence outcome, in terms of both local control and survival. Synchronous metastasis to inguinal lymph nodes has also been considered as an indicator of poor prognosis for survival, but in most series, multifactorial analysis indicates that T stage is more significant. Different cut-points of the size of the primary have been analysed, from 2 cm (T1 versus T2, T3, or T4) to 4 cm. Several authors have shown that the high value

Table 30.1 Selected series of patients treated with low doses of radiation (≤50 Gy) and concomitant (5-FU–MMC) chemotherapy

Authors	No. of patients	Tumour control rate (%)	Grade 4 complications[a]	5-year survival rate (%)[b]
Nigro et al[5]	104	90	—	78
Sischy et al[6]	79	61	1 stenosis	73
Michaelson et al[7]	37	81	None	80
Cummings et al[8]	69	90	5 APR	sp. 76
Flam et al[9]	30	85	1 stenosis	90
Habr-Gramma et al[10]	30	87	None	80
Hugue et al[11]	25	T1–3: 78	1 death	—
		T4: 33	—	—
Marti and Pipard[12]	52	≤4 cm: 96	3 APR	≤4 cm: 100
		>4 cm: 85		>4 cm 80
Tanum et al[13]	106	Histological response: 84	14 (2 deaths)	70

[a]APR, abdominoperineal resection.
[b]sp., specific survival.

Table 30.2 Selected series of patients treated with high doses of radiation (>60 Gy) alone

Authors	No. of patients	Relapse rate (%)	5-year survival rate (%)
Salmon et al[15]	183	34	58
Eschwege et al[16]	64	19	46
Papillon and Montbarbon[14,a]	159	12	65 (crude)
Touboul et al[17]	270	20	74
Allal et al[18,a]	125	20	65
Wagner et al[19,a]	108	17	64
Peiffert et al[20,a]	118	20	60

[a]Brachytherapy boost.

Table 30.3 Prognostic factors for survival in series studying radiotherapy alone[a]

Authors	Histology	Nodal involvement	Size of primary
Bedenne et al[21]		−[b]	− (T1, T2, T3 vs T4)[c]
Schlienger et al[22]	−	−[b]	+[c]
Sischy et al[6]		+	+ (<3 cm)
Touboul et al[17]	+[b]	−	+[c]
Salmon et al[15]	−	+	+
Papillon and Montbarbon[14]	+	+	+ (<4 cm)
Wagner et al[19]	−	−	+ (T1, T2 vs T3, T4)
Eschwege et al[16]	−	+	+ (T1, T2 vs T3, T4)
Peiffert et al[20]	−	+[c]	+ (<4 cm)[c]

[a]+, significant; −, not significant.
[b]Univariate analysis.
[c]Multivariate analysis.

of 4 cm discriminates those patients who need an intensification of treatment.[6,16,20]

In the 1980s, the consensus became that conservative radiation-based treatment should be used in place of surgery, but the radiation dose and the association with and planning for chemotherapy remained to be defined. On the one hand, some authors[12,13] pointed out the poor prognosis of large tumours compared with small tumours, and considered a high-dose radiotherapy approach, combined with chemotherapy. On the other hand, late grade 4 complications observed in long-term survivors in combined radio-chemotherapy series raised the question of the usefulness of mitomycin C, considered as radiosensitizer for cutaneomucous tissues. Nevertheless, the poor prognosis of tumours larger than 4 cm or with nodal involvement raised the question of treatment intensification.

Treatment intensification

In a selected group of patients with a tumour of 4 cm or larger, Papillon[23] employed low doses of

5-FU–MMC during the first course of radiation. The tolerance was good, and the local control rate seemed higher, rising from 70% to 90% in a historical comparative series. At the same time, Cummings et al[8] obtained similar results, delivering 50 Gy in one or two courses, combined with 5-FU–MMC chemotherapy in one group (including T1, T2).[8] Once again, the local control rate seemed higher in the group treated with chemotherapy (56% versus 90%), although the survival was not improved.[24] Later, two randomized trials were designed to confirm these results.[24,25]

RANDOMIZED TRIALS OF COMBINED RADIO-CHEMOTHERAPY

In the 1990s, three phase III trials were conducted in North America and Europe after confirmation of the good results of conservative treatments. However, the goals of these trials were rather contradictory. While the Radiation Therapy Oncology Group/Gastrointestinal Tumor Study Group (RTOG/GITSG)[26] trial was intended to test the potential deleterious effect of mitomycin C, the two European trials[24,25] were designed to demonstrate the benefit of concomitant radio-chemotherapy.

The RTOG/GITSG trial addressed the need for mitomycin C as part of the concomitant chemotherapy regimen.[26] In this study, 291 evaluable patients were randomly assigned to receive radiation and 5-FU with or without mitomycin C. Toxicity was increased in the mitomycin C arm for grade 4 complications, including lethalities (1 versus 4 deaths from toxicity respectively). There was no significant difference in overall survival rate at 4 years (71% without mitomycin C and 78% with it; (p = NS)), but there was a highly significant advantage to the mitomycin C-containing arm with regard to colostomy-free survival rate (59% without mitomycin C versus 73% with it; p = 0.016) and disease-free survival rate (51% versus 73%; p = 0.0003). The complete response rate was not significantly different (89% versus 92%), except for tumours of 5 cm or larger. It was concluded that the two-drug combination was better than monochemotherapy.

In the European Organization for Research and Treatment of Cancer (EORTC) trial, chemotherapy plus radiation was compared with radiation alone.[24] In this trial, 108 patients with T3–4 tumours or with positive lymph nodes were randomly assigned to receive radiation (45 Gy in 5 weeks) with or without concurrent 5-FU (1 g/m^2 intravenously on days 1–5 and 28–33) and mitomycin C (15 mg/m^2 on day 1).

After a 6-week gap, good responders (complete or partial response) received a 20 Gy boost by an external-beam or interstitial technique. Early and late toxicities of the combined-modality approach were not significantly greater than those observed with radiation alone. The colostomy-free survival rate and local control rate at 5 years were higher (72% and 68% respectively) for patients receiving combined therapy than for patients receiving only radiation (40% and 55% respectively). The overall survival rate was not different (57% versus 55%).

The United Kingdom Co-ordinating Committee on Cancer Research (UKCCCR) trial addressed the same issue of the addition of chemotherapy to radiation, on 585 patients, with T1–4 and N0–3 tumours, randomized to radiation with and without 5-FU and mitomycin C (at the same doses as the EORTC trial).[25] At 3 years, the relative risk of local failure was 0.54 in the combined arm, compared with radiation alone. No difference in overall survival was detected, but the tumour-specific survival rate was higher in the group receiving the combined treatment compared with radiation alone (72% versus 61%; p = 0.02, RR = 0.71).

Taken together, these phase III trials support the use of combined therapy using both 5-FU and mitomycin C as the standard of care for most patients with anal canal cancer, particularly for locally advanced disease (T3–4 or N1–3). The best chemotherapy–radiation regimen and the most appropriate radiation dose to use in patients with anal canal tumours limited to the primary site have not yet been defined. Local recurrence remains the main site of treatment failure, especially if the radiation dose is low. 5-FU probably acts as a radiosensitizer, although there is some disagreement about this, but mitomycin C is poorly or not synergistic. Other doses of irradiation and other drugs are to be investigated, with long-term follow-up.

RECENT PHASE II TRIALS AND CLINICAL EXPERIENCE

The best chemotherapy and radiotherapy regimens and the most appropriate radiation dose to use for patients with anal canal tumours limited to the primary site have not yet been defined. Distant failure is not the major clinical problem in these patients – local recurrence is more common.

Recently, a number of combinations of drugs have been tested, as well as different times of administration. Several doses of radiation have been tested as well. Long-term follow-up is now available for most of these trials.

Concomitant radio-chemotherapy with new drugs

The concomitant use of bleomycin (5 mg/day, intramuscularly, before 15–18 fractions of irradiation) has been reported in a series of 159 patients.[27] The acute toxicity was high. The 5-year tumour-specific survival and preservation rates were 72% and 64% respectively. Bleomycin did not appear to have any effect on treatment.

Cisplatin is considered to be less toxic than mitomycin C and to be among the most active drugs in squamous cell carcinoma as well as one of the most strongly radiosensitizing agents.[28] It is used in several treatments of epidermoid malignancies in combination with 5-FU, which is synergistic. The 5-FU–cisplatin association gave partial or complete responses in advanced or metastatic anal canal tumours,[29,30] and was tested on early stages as part of combined radio-chemotherapy in place of 5-FU–MMC, with the cisplatin being delivered in each cycle.

At the University of Texas MD Anderson Cancer Center, 58 patients were treated with low-dose continuous 5-FU infusion (300 mg/m^2/day, reduced to 250 mg for acute toxicity), with and without cisplatin (4 mg/m^2/day) and radiation doses of 54–55 Gy (in 1.8 Gy/fraction).[31] In 18 patients receiving 5-FU plus cisplatin, the 2-year local control and survival rates of 85% and 92% respectively, coupled with the absence of late morbidity, seem to show benefit compared with a series treated with radiotherapy alone. The benefit of cisplatin itself was not clearly stated.

Doci et al[32] designed a phase II study of 5-FU (750 mg/m^2 intravenously on days 1–4 and 21–24) and cisplatin (100 mg/m^2 intravenously on day 1), combined with radiotherapy, including 35 patients (9 T1, 21 T2, and 5 T3; 26 N0 and 9 N1–3). A first course of 36–38 Gy delivered in 4 weeks (1.8 Gy/fraction) by anteroposterior/posteroanterior fields (AP/PA), including the inguinal nodes, was followed by a localized boost of 18–24 Gy. Leukopenia was the prime toxicity (31%). Complete response was assessed in 31 patients; the two partial responders were out of the five T3 cases. After a median follow-up of 37 months, 94% of the patients were alive without evidence of disease and 86% were colostomy-free. The toxicity did not exceed that of 5-FU–MMC association, but the total dose, ranging from 54 Gy to 62 Gy, seemed low to control T3 tumours.

An Eastern Cooperative Oncology Group (ECOG) phase II study combined 5-FU (1 g/m^2/day intravenously on days 1–4) and cisplatin (75 mg/m^2 intravenously on day 1) with radiotherapy (59.4 Gy in 33 fractions by AP/PA fields, including a 2-week interval after 36 Gy).[33] One cycle of chemotherapy was started on day 1 of each of the two courses of radiotherapy. Nineteen patients were entered in the study: 68% had a complete response, 26% a partial response, and 1 stable disease. A grade 4 toxicity was observed in six patients, and a grade 5 toxicity in one patient (postantibiotic therapy *Clostridium difficile* pseudomembranous colitis). With 12 T1–2 N0 patients out of the 19, these results seemed comparable to radiation alone for local control, with increased toxicity.

Induction chemotherapy

Induction chemotherapy in combination with radiotherapy was evaluated for locoregionally advanced disease.[34] Cisplatin (100 mg/m^2 intravenously on day 1) and 5-FU (1 g/m^2 intravenously on days 2–6), delivered during three cycles (every 21 days) to 19 patients with locally advanced disease (T1–2 N0 excluded), yielded 92% objective responses. A 45 Gy irradiation delivered in 5 weeks and a boost of 20 Gy by brachytherapy achieved 90% local control. With a 26-month follow-up, the overall survival rate was 90%, the specific survival rate 100%, and sphincter preservation rate 88%.

Gérard et al[35] published a series of 95 patients (all stages), treated with 5-FU (1 g/m^2/day intravenously on days 1–4) and cisplatin (25 mg/m^2/day intravenously on days 1–4) concomitantly with high-dose radiation (>60 Gy). Seven patients received one course of 5-FU–cisplatin before starting irradiation. Six of these 7 patients had a partial response after a single course. The overall tumour response of the whole series was complete plus very good response in 90%, partial response in 8%, and stable disease in one patient. The toxicity was low. The 5-year overall survival and colostomy-free survival rates were 84% and 71% respectively. Among 78 patients who benefited from anus preservation, the anal sphincter function was excellent or good in 72 (92%).

A French cancer centre's phase II trial associated induction chemotherapy (5-FU 800 mg/m^2 intravenously on days 1–4 and cisplatin 80 mg/m^2 on day 1) for two cycles with a 4-week interval, followed by concomitant radio-chemotherapy (45 Gy pelvic irradiation in 5 weeks, with 5-FU–cisplatin started on days 1 and 28) for locally advanced tumours.[36] After a 4- to 6-week gap, a 20 Gy boost was delivered on the anal canal. Out of the first 30 patients (1 T1, 16 T2, 8 T3, and 5 T4; 10 N1, 1 N2, and 8 N3), 1 died of a pulmonary embolism on day 4, but the remaining 29 received the entire treatment. 5-FU doses were reduced in 11 patients owing to acute toxicity, and the radiation boost was delayed for 1 patient (aplasia). The complete and partial responses rates were respectively 11% and 61% after induction chemotherapy and 59% and 31% after concomitant radio-chemotherapy. An APR was performed in 4 non-responding patients. After completion of the treatment, a 96% complete response rate was observed. The 2-year analysis pointed out a high rate of local control and sphincter preservation.[37]

The Cancer and Leukemia Group B (CALGB) conducted a phase II study for poor-prognosis patients in which 45 patients presenting locally advanced disease were treated with induction 5-FU (1 g/m²/ day intravenously on days 1–5) plus cisplatin (100 mg/m² intravenously on day 1) in weeks 1 and 5.[38] A 45 Gy irradiation was started in week 9 (with 19 days' break after 30.6 Gy), with concurrent 5-FU (1 g/m²/day intravenously on days 1–4) plus mitomycin C (10 mg/m² on day 1) in the first week of the two cycles of radiation. If residual disease persisted, an additional 9 Gy was given in week 19 with concomitant 5-FU–cisplatin. Induction chemotherapy led to 8 complete responses, 21 partial responses, 13 cases of stable disease, 1 case of progressive disease, and 1 treatment-related death (pneumonia). After combined-modality treatment, there were 36 complete and 5 partial responses, 2 cases of stable disease and 1 of progressive disease, and 1 death. Ten patients required colostomies: 4 for persistent disease and 6 for recurrent disease. Most toxicity was haematological. After a median follow-up of 21 months, 78% remain alive, 67% are disease-free, and 56% are colostomy- and disease-free.

Induction carboplatin (300–375 mg/m² intravenously on day 1) and 5-FU (1 g/m²/day intravenously on days 1–5) were delivered during three courses in 31 patients (tumour size ≥ 4 cm or T4 or node-positive), followed by external-beam radiation (46–50 Gy completed to 64–68 Gy for good responders, after a 2- to 3-week gap).[39] The toxicity of the chemotherapy was low. The objective response (complete plus partial) was 45% after induction chemotherapy. After the primary therapy, 29 patients were tumour-free. The 5-year overall survival, recurrence-free, and sphincter preservation rates were 67%, 80%, and 69% respectively.

Doses and schedule of irradiation

Anal canal carcinoma is mostly a local or locoregional disease, and distant metastases are rare. The best way to deliver the radiation, which is the most effective part of the treatment, has been questioned for early as well as for advanced disease, with higher doses having a benefit with regard to local control, but also having the potential adverse effects, with late mucous and sphincter complications. The total dose and the time factor have been analysed. Radiotherapy alone with 60–65 Gy doses, rather lower than for other squamous cell carcinomas, yields high local control rates with a low rate of late complications, mainly in T1–2 N0 tumours.[14,18–20,35] Conversely, 30 Gy delivered with concomitant chemotherapy has given high rates of local control.[4] This demonstrates the high sensitivity of this rare tumour both to radiation alone and to combined treatments.

Concerning series investigating radiation alone, a significant dose–effect relationship has been described in retrospective studies. Schlienger et al[22] observed a benefit for higher doses in multivariate analysis, for a series of 236 patients treated with total doses of radiation ranging from 55 Gy to 65 Gy. Eschwege and Lusinchi[40] described complete response rates after 45 Gy radiation of 75%, 54%, and 24% for T1, T2, and T3–4 tumours respectively. After a 20 Gy boost delivered 4–6 weeks later, these rates reached 100%, 85%, and 76%. A dose effect for low-dose radiation with combined chemotherapy has also been described. An 85% local control rate was observed for patients treated with doses higher than 55 Gy.[31] Myerson et al[41] reported colostomy-free and disease-free rates of 50% for a dose of 30 Gy and 83% for 40–50 Gy (p = 0.03).

The split technique was initially designed for accelerated perineal irradiation. The gap of 8 weeks after 30 Gy delivered in 18 days was justified by the need to observe the delayed tumour shrinkage, to allow recovery from acute reactions, and to boost the minimal volume by an interstitial technique.[14] At present, fractions of 1.8–2 Gy are delivered to the pelvis to 45–50 Gy, over 5 weeks to minimize late toxicity. Tumour shrinkage is observed earlier after the end of irradiation, acute reactions are lower, and the primary can be boosted earlier. Some authors have stressed the impact of the total time of irradiation (≥75 days versus 75 days) on local control.[18,42] A 2- to 3-week gap is now recommended for radiation alone, and its tolerance has been evaluated in radio-chemotherapy series.[43]

The RTOG 8704 phase III trial explored the effectiveness of a salvage boost by radio-chemotherapy on 25 out of 28 patients with histological confirmation of residual primary disease after 45.6 Gy.[26] An additional 9 Gy was delivered with concomitant chemotherapy with 5-FU–cisplatin. Out of 22 post-salvage biopsies, 12 were negative (55%). The toxicity of the salvage regimen was limited. The 4-year follow-up of the 12 patients successfully salvaged showed that 4 remained free of disease, 4 had a subsequent APR (and were later free of disease), and 4 had died (3 with recurrent disease and 1 free of disease). Additional radio-chemotherapy was able to salvage without colostomy one-third of assessable patients who failed to respond to initial standard radio-chemotherapy. Overall, 50% of these patients were alive without disease at 4 years. This study opened a new era in North America, with the possibility of intensifying treatment by dose escalation for incomplete responders or poor-prognosis patients.

The EORTC 22953 phase II trial tested the feasibility of reducing the interval from 6 weeks to 2 weeks while delivering continuous 5-FU (200 mg/m^2/day) during all treatment sequences and mitomycin C (10 mg/m^2) at the beginning of each sequence. The first sequence delivered 36 Gy in 26 days, and, after a 16-day gap duration, the second sequence delivered 23.4 Gy in 17 days. Thirty-four patients are evaluable (7 T2, 20 T3, and 7 T4; 18 N0, 9 N1, 3 N2, and 4 N2). Treatment was stopped only once during the second sequence. There were no toxic deaths or acute grade 4 toxicities. The overall tumour response rate 8 weeks after treatment was 95%.[43]

Future prospects for obtaining the best therapeutic index for patients have to be studied in prospective trials. For early stages (T1–2 N0), the total dose and overall timing of radiation have to be explored, as well as the boost technique. Concomitant chemotherapy remains an option. For locally advanced stages, the upper limit of the high doses must be determined, considering the potential adverse effects. Concomitant chemotherapy must be adapted to this high risk of late complications and the important functional role of the anal canal. The high chemosensitivity and radiosensitivity of these tumours, compared with head and neck carcinomas, opens the possibility of considering induction chemotherapy, and studies are running at the present time.

FUTURE PROSPECTS AND ONGOING PHASE III TRIALS

In 1998 and 1999, three phase III trials were designed in North America and Europe, to test different policies of treatment intensification.

The second UKCCCR Anal Cancer Trial (ACT-II) began with a phase II study of a three-drug schedule. The objective was to evaluate the toxicity of a new regimen, to be used in a randomized trial. The three drugs, 5-FU (750 mg/m^2/day intravenously on days 1–5), mitomycin C (10 mg/m^2 intravenous bolus on day 1), and cisplatin (60 mg/m^2 intravenously on day 1), were administered in the first week of radiotherapy, and 5-FU only was administered during the last week of radiotherapy. The radiotherapy delivered 40–45 Gy in 4–5 weeks, followed 3 weeks later by a boost with an iridium implant (25 Gy) or perineal field (15 Gy). Three courses of adjuvant chemotherapy using the three drugs (except for mitomycin C on course number 2) ended the treatment, delivered every 21 days. Nineteen patients were included, and results are to be published. The decision to open a phase III trial will be taken in the near future. The phase III trial aims at determining (1) whether a three-drug regimen (5-FU–MMC–cisplatin) offers any benefit in terms of local control and survival compared with that obtained with the standard two-drug regimen (5-FU–MMC) used in the previous trial (ACT–I), and (2) whether adjuvant chemotherapy (three courses of the two or three drugs used as primary therapy) impacts on the development of metastatic disease or prolongs survival.

A phase III randomized intergroup study is being conducted by the RTOG (9811), ECOG, CLGB, and the Southwest Oncology Group (SWOG). The objectives are (1) to compare the initial and total local and distant failure rates in patients with anal canal cancer treated either with 5-FU–MMC concurrently with radiotherapy or with 5-FU–cisplatin followed by 5-FU–cisplatin concurrently with radiotherapy, (2) to identify any differences in local control and colostomy rates at 2 years in the patients randomized into the two arms, and (3) to determine any difference in colostomy-free, disease-free, or overall survival in these patients in these two arms. Eligibility criteria are T2–4, any N, M0 (stages II or III), and all ages over 18. Radiotherapy is administered daily, 5 days a week for 5–6.5 weeks (45–59.4 Gy). In November 1999 45 patients were included, for a total of 650 patients accrued over 5 years.

A French intergroup phase III trial of therapeutic intensification for locally advanced anal canal carcinomas was opened for inclusions in March 1999. The objectives are (1) to compare the efficacy of concurrent chemotherapy and radiotherapy with or without induction chemotherapy, (2) to compare two levels of radiation dose, in patients with stages II or III (M1 and T1N0 or T2N0 with tumour smaller than 4 cm excluded). Sphincter preservation is the main endpoint, but local control, survival, and quality of life will also be analysed. Chemotherapy doses per cycle are 5-FU (800 mg/m²/day intravenously on days 1–4), and cisplatin (80 mg/m²/day intravenously on day 1). Radiotherapy delivers 45 Gy over 5 weeks in a first course, followed, after a 2- to 3-week gap, by 15 Gy in two arms and 20–25 Gy in two arms, by an interstitial technique or external-beam irradiation. In May 2001, 101 patients were included, for a total of 350 accrued over 4 years.

PRESERVATION OF STRUCTURE AND FUNCTION

The acceptance of radiation alone or combined with chemotherapy as primary treatment of early-stage or locally advanced anal cancer has led to the cure of many patients without the need to sacrifice anorectal function. Nevertheless, the measurement and reporting of functional results are generally confined to subjective parameters less precise than tumour control or survival. The local tumour recurrence-free rate measures preservation of structure, but this does not include the integrity of function (fistulas or colostomies). The colostomy-free rate measures preservation of function, but does not consider a local relapse managed by means other than colostomy. It is therefore difficult to compare techniques using these results, although this remains the main goal of most of the prospective trials.

As early as the first publications on conservative treatment, results clearly showed a difference in the rate of patients locally controlled and the rate of patients locally controlled who retained normal anal function.[8,14] An analysis by the Princess Margaret Hospital in Toronto, Canada, on functional results is in progress.[44]

Functional disability can probably be reduced by paying attention to the technical aspects of the irradiation, the selection of the patients, and the skill of the radiation oncologist. Results of series of patients treated using the same technique are presented in Table 30.4 for series of combined radiotherapy and brachytherapy; differences are probably linked to the staging of patients[19,35] or to improvements in the technique and skill of the team during the time period under study.[20]

Recent publications have stressed the quality of life in long-term colostomy-free survivors after curative treatment for anal carcinomas.

The Gastrointestinal Quality of Life Index (GIQLI) questionnaire[45] was completed by 32 patients, 16 of whom were explored by anorectal manometry.[46] The sphincter length, resting pressure, and maximum squeeze pressure were lower in anal carcinoma patients than in healthy volunteers. However, complete continence was found in 56% of patients.

The EORTC QLQ-C30 cancer-specific questionnaire and QLQ-CR38 site-specific module were completed by 41 evaluable patients treated with radiotherapy with or without chemotherapy.[47] In patients treated with sphincter preservation, the long-term quality of life appears to be acceptable, with the exception of diarrhoea (a threefold increase)

Table 30.4 Series of combined radiotherapy and brachytherapy

Authors	No. of patients	Overall survival rate (%)	Specific survival rate (%)	Sphincter conservation rate (%)	Rate of locoregional recurrences after conservation (%)	Rate of APR or colostomy for complications (%)
Papillon and Montbarbon[14]	159	65	82	89	20	2.2
Wagner et al[19]	108	64	72	85	17	9
Allal et al[18]	125	65.5	77		30	6
Peiffert et al[20]	119	60	77	75 (84[a])	20	15 (5[a])
Gérard et al[35]	95	84	75	71 (50 for T3)	15	7

[a]The rate of sphincter conservation has improved in the patients treated since 1989, and at the same time the rate of late complications has decreased, owing to modifications of doses and the volumes treated.

and perhaps sexual functions. The subset of patients who presented with severe complications and/or anal dysfunctions showed poorer scores in most scales. In response to an additional question about the decision to have conservative treatment, 71% of patients expressed a high satisfaction with their present anorectal function, and only 7% even considered the possibility that APR might have been a preferable approach.

An unvalidated questionnaire was evaluated in 39 patients.[48] The full sphincter function of 77% of patients in whom the anal sphincter had been preserved was maintained in 93% of the cases.

Clinical and manometric effects of external beam and interstitial irradiation evaluated in 8 patients described perfect continence in 4 patients and incontinence for gas and urgencies in the case of liquid stools in 4 patients.[49]

It is obviously unfair to impose a functionally invasive investigational technique upon all the patients treated successfully with conservative schedules for anal cancer. On the other hand, the questionnaires recently developed and validated offer a useful tool to evaluate both patient satisfaction and physician's evaluation of the treatment. These questionnaires should be included in all future studies, to make it possible to obtain objective results regarding patients' functional results, which could be among the criteria for deciding the best treatment to offer to patients.

NODAL MANAGEMENT

At the time when APR was the standard treatment of anal cancer, bilateral inguinal lymph-node dissection was performed in patients undergoing radical surgical resection of their primary tumour, until it was shown at the Memorial Sloan-Kettering Cancer Center that prophylactic inguinal lymph node dissections were beneficial in only 6% of patients.[50] The high morbidity with little gain led others to quickly condemn the use of the procedure. The interpretation that all patients with grossly positive inguinal lymph nodes synchronous with the primary tumour were incurable has now been abandoned. Current recommendations are for limited surgical sampling, and combined chemotherapy and radiotherapy with boost doses to the involved groin. In series of patients treated by radiation therapy with or without chemotherapy, half of the patients with concomitant inguinal node involvement were cured at 5 years.[20]

Multimodality therapy controls over 90% of inguinal nodal disease.[17,20,35]

METASTATIC DISEASE

Because of its rarity, there are few data on the treatment of patients with metastatic disease. Nevertheless, anal canal carcinoma is a chemosensitive tumour, and 5-FU–MMC or 5-FU–cisplatin combinations can be delivered as first-line chemotherapy.[29,30] Complete remissions have been described, but relapse is the rule. Doxorubicin and bleomycin have been reported to have activity. Good palliation of symptoms can be achieved with concomitant or sequential local or locoregional irradiation. Surgery is useful in cases of no control or local recurrence.

SALVAGE TREATMENT

In patients treated with low-dose radiation and chemotherapy, and presenting a small clinical residual disease or histologically positive biopsies at the end of the schedule, salvage radio-chemotherapy achieves a 50% rate of local success with sphincter preservation.[26] Local relapses occurring after high-dose radiation can be successfully salvaged by APR in 50% of cases.[51,52]

Metachronous isolated inguinal recurrences can be salvaged by combined radio-chemotherapy if no treatment was previously delivered to these areas, or by surgical salvage with a formal groin dissection followed by chemotherapy if prophylactic or curative radiation was delivered. Half of the patients can be cured if the inguinal node areas were not prophylactically treated at first presentation.

TREATMENT OPTIONS

Treatment options of squamous cell carcinomas of the anal canal depend on the TNM stage, the possibility of obtaining a continent sphincter after preservation, and patients' general condition, including the HIV status in some patients.[53,54]

T1N0M0 anal canal cancer

High-dose radiotherapy alone or low-dose radiation combined with concomitant chemotherapy are suitable. For T1 less than 1 cm, chemotherapy can be avoided. Interstitial iridium implants after external-beam radiation are well adapted to deliver the radiation boost to the residual disease. Inguinal prophylactic treatment is not considered.

T2N0M0 anal canal cancer

Treatment options depend on the size of the tumour. Tumours less than 4 cm are treated with the same schedules as T1N0 tumours. Tumours of 4 cm or more are usually treated like T3, with combined radio-chemotherapy.

T1–2 N1–3 M0, T3–4 any N M0

Combined radio-chemotherapy is the recommended treatment for most patients. Chemotherapy with 5-FU–MMC combined with primary radiotherapy appears to be more effective than radiotherapy alone. The optimal dose of radiation is under evaluation. Alternative combinations of chemotherapy using cis-platin or carboplatin in place of mitomycin C or using three drugs are under evaluation. The impacts of induction chemotherapy and adjuvant chemotherapy are under evaluation. Prophylactic irradiation of bilateral inguinal areas is recommended for all these patients with locally advanced tumours.

In cases of synchronous nodal involvement, the treatment can include lymph-node sampling followed by radio-chemotherapy including inguinal fields, or radio-chemotherapy alone.

Metastatic disease

Palliation of symptoms can be obtained by chemotherapy combined with radiotherapy, depending on sensitive normal tissues surrounding the tumour. 5-FU–MMC or 5-FU–cisplatin can be delivered as first-line treatment.

CONCLUSIONS

At present, combined radio-chemotherapy is considered as the primary therapy in epidermoid carcinoma of the anal canal. The usefulness of chemotherapy, delivered concomitantly with high-dose radiation, has been confirmed in terms of specific survival, local tumour control, and functional results in locally advanced tumours. In early stages exclusive high-dose radiotherapy gives a high rate of cure, similar to low-dose radiation combined with chemotherapy. The optimal radiation dose is to be determined according to tumour stage and associated chemotherapy. Radiation techniques should be studied in terms of volumes, fractionation, and duration. Functional results are of outstanding impor-

tance, and should be expressed in terms of measurable data, to allow comparison of treatments.

Induction chemotherapy, justified by functional endpoints, is under evaluation in prospective studies. Other treatment schedules should be explored.

The prime improvements over the last two decades with regard to this rare disease have prompted the inclusion of patients in ongoing and future prospective studies.

REFERENCES

1. Melbye M, Cote TR, Kessler L et al, High incidence of anal cancer among AIDS patients. *Lancet* 1994; **343**: 636–9.
2. Rabbin CS, Biggar RJ, Melbye M, Curtis RE, Second primary cancers following anal and cervical carcinoma. Evidence of shared etiologic factors. *Am J Epidemiol* 1992; **136**: 54–8.
3. UICC, *TNM Classification of Malignant Tumors*, 4th edn (Hermaneck P, Sobin LM, eds). Berlin: Springer-Verlag, 1987: 50–2.
4. Nigro ND, Vaitkevicius VK, Considine B, Combined therapy for cancer of the anal canal. *Colon Rectum* 1974; **27**: 763–6.
5. Nigro ND, Vaitkevicius VK, Herskovic AM, Preservation of function in the treatment of cancer of the anus. In: *Important Advances in Oncology* (DeVita VT, ed). Philadelphia: Lippincott, 1989: 161–77.
6. Sischy B, Dogget RLS, Krall JM et al, Definitive irradiation and chemotherapy for radiosensitization in management of anal carcinoma: interim report on Radiation Therapy Oncology Group Study No. 8314. *J Natl Cancer Inst* 1989; **81**: 850–6.
7. Michaelson RA, Magill G, Quan SHQ et al, Preoperative chemotherapy and radiation therapy in the management of anal epidermoid carcinoma. *Cancer* 1983; **51**: 390–5.
8. Cummings BJ, Keane TJ, O'Sullivan B et al, Epidermoid anal cancer: treatment by radiation alone or by radiation and 5-fluorouracil with and without mitomycin C. *Int J Radiat Oncol Biol Phys* 1991; **21**: 1115–25.
9. Flam M, John MJ, Mowry PA et al, Definitive combined modality therapy of carcinoma of the anus. *Dis Colon Rectum* 1987; **30**: 495–502.
10. Habr-Gramma A, Da Silva E, Sousa AH et al, Epidermoid carcinoma of the anal canal. Results of treatment by combined chemotherapy and radiation therapy. *Dis Colon Rectum* 1989; **32**: 773–7.
11. Hughes LL, Rich TA, Delclos L et al, Radiotherapy for anal cancer. Experience from 1979–1987. *Int J Radiat Oncol Biol Phys* 1989; **17**: 1153–60.
12. Marti MC, Pipard G, Epidermoid carcinoma of the anal canal. Value of a multidisciplinary approach. *Chirurgie* 1989; **115**: 715–22.
13. Tanum G, Tveit K, Karlsen KO, Hauer-Jensen M, Chemotherapy and radiation therapy for anal carcinoma. *Cancer* 1991; **67**: 2462–6.
14. Papillon J, Montbarbon JF, Epidermoid carcinoma of the anal canal. A series of 276 cases. *Dis Colon Rectum* 1987; **30**: 324–33.
15. Salmon RJ, Fenton J, Asselain B et al, Treatment of epidermoid anal cancer. *Am J Surg* 1984; **147**: 43–8.
16. Eschwege F, Lasser P, Chavy A et al, Squamous cell carcinoma of the anal canal: treatment by external beam irradiation. *Radiother Oncol* 1985; **4**: 145–50.
17. Touboul E, Schlienger M, Buffat L et al, Epidermoid carcinoma of the anal canal. Results of curative-intent therapy in a series of 270 patients. *Cancer* 1994; **73**: 1569–79.
18. Allal AS, Mermillod B, Kurtz JM et al, The impact of treatment factors on local control in T2–T3 anal carcinomas treated by radi-

ation with or without chemotherapy. *Cancer* 1997; **79:** 2329–35.

19. Wagner JP, Mahe MA, Romestaing P et al, Radiation therapy in the conservative treatment of carcinoma of the anal canal. *Int J Radiat Oncol Biol Phys* 1994; **29:** 17–23.

20. Peiffert D, Bey P, Pernot M et al, Conservative treatment by irradiation of epidermoid cancers of the anal canal: prognostic factors of tumoral control and complications. *Int J Radiat Oncol Biol Phys* 1997; **37:** 313–24.

21. Bedenne L, Janoray I, Arveux P et al, Le cancer épidermoïde du canal anal dans le département de la Côte d'Or. *Gastroenterol Clin Biol* 1989; **15:** 130–6.

22. Schlienger M, Touboul E, Mauban S et al, Résultats du traitement de 286 cas de cancers épidermoïdes du canal anal dont 236 par irradiation à visée conservatrice. *Lyon Chir* 1991; **87:** 61–9.

23. Papillon J, Effectiveness of combined radio-chemotherapy in the management of epidermoid carcinoma of the anal canal. *Int J Radiat Oncol Biol Phys* 1990; **19:** 1217–18.

24. Bartelink H, Roelofsen F, Eschwege F et al, Concomitant radiotherapy and chemotherapy is superior to radiotherapy alone in the treatment of locally advanced anal cancer: results of a phase III randomized trial of the European Organization for Research and Treatment of Cancer Radiotherapy and Gastrointestinal Cooperative Groups. *J Clin Oncol* 1997; **15:** 2040–9.

25. UKCCCR Anal Cancer Trial Working Party, Epidermoid anal cancer: results from the UKCCCR randomised trial of radiotherapy alone versus radiotherapy, 5-fluorouracil, and mitomycin. *Lancet* 1996; **348:** 1049–54.

26. Flam M, John M, Pajak TH et al, Role of mitomycin in combination with fluorouracil and radiotherapy, and of salvage chemoradiation in the definitive nonsurgical treatment of epidermoid carcinoma of the anal canal: results of a phase III randomized intergroup study. *J Clin Oncol* 1996; **14:** 2527–39.

27. Friberg B, Svensson C, Goldman S, Glimelius B, The Swedish national care program of anal carcinoma. *Acta Oncol* 1998; **37:** 25–32.

28. Dewit L, Combined treatment of radiation and *cis*-diamminedichloroplatinum(ɪɪ): a review on experimental and clinical data. *Int J Radiat Oncol Biol Phys* 1987; **13:** 403–26.

29. Ajani JA, Carrasco CH, Jakson DE et al, Combination of cisplatin plus fluoropyrimidine chemotherapy effective against liver metastases from carcinoma of the anal canal. *Am J Med* 1989; **87:** 221–4.

30. Mahjoubi M, Sadek H, François E et al, Epidermoid anal canal carcinoma (EACC): activity of cisplatin (P) and continuous 5 fluorouracil (5 FU) in metastatic (M) and/or local recurrent (LR) disease. *Proc Am Soc Clin Oncol* 1990; **9:** 114.

31. Rich TA, Ajani JA, Morrison WH et al, Chemoradiation therapy for anal cancer: radiation plus continuous infusion of 5 fluorouracil with or without cisplatin. *Radiat Oncol* 1993; **27:** 207–15.

32. Doci R, Zucali R, La Monica G et al, Primary chemoradiation therapy with fluorouracil and cisplatin for cancer of the anal: results in 35 consecutive patients. *J Clin Oncol* 1996; **14:** 3121–5.

33. Martenson JA, Lipsitz SR, Wagner H et al, Initial results of a phase II trial of high dose radiation therapy, 5-fluorouracil, and cisplatin for patients with anal cancer (E4292): an Eastern Cooperative Oncology Group study. *Int J Radiat Oncol Biol Phys* 1996; **35:** 745–9.

34. Brunet R, Sadek H, Vignoud J et al, Cisplatin (P) and 5 fluorouracil (5 FU) for the neoadjuvant treatment (Tt) of epidermoïd anal canal carcinoma (EACC). *Proc Am Soc Clin Oncol* 1990; **9:** 104.

35. Gérard JP, Ayzac L, Hun D et al, Treatment of anal canal carcinoma with high dose radiation therapy and concomitant fluorouracil–cisplatinum. Long-term results in 95 patients. *Radiother Oncol* 1998; **46:** 249–56.

36. Peiffert D, Seitz JF, Rougier P et al, Preliminary results of a phase II study of a high-dose radiation therapy and neoadjuvant plus concomitant 5-fluorouracil with CDDP chemotherapy for patients with anal canal cancer: a French cooperative study. *Ann Oncol* 1997; **8:** 575–81.

37. Peiffert D, Giovannini M, Ducreux M et al, High-dose radiation therapy and neoadjuvant plus concomitant chemotherapy with 5-fluorouracil and cisplatin in patients with locally advanced squamous-cell anal canal cancer: final results of a phase II study. *Ann Oncol* 2001; **12:** 397–404.

38. Meropol NJ, Niedzwieck D, Shank B et al, Combined-modality therapy of poor risk anal carcinoma: a phase II study of the Cancer and Leukemia Group B (CALGB). *Proc Am Soc Clin Oncol* 1999; **18:** 237 (Abst 909).

39. Svensson C, Goldmann S, Friberg B et al, Induction chemotherapy and radiotherapy in loco-regionally advanced epidermoid carcinoma of the anal canal. *Int J Radiat Oncol Biol Phys* 1998; **41:** 863–7.

40. Eschwege F, Lusinchi A, Combined radiotherapy and chemotherapy in the treatment of anal cancer. In: *Progress in Anti-Cancer Chemotherapy*, Vol II (Hortobagyi GN, Khayat D, eds). Boston: Blackwell Science, 1999: 270–86.

41. Myerson RB, Shapiro SJ, Lacey D et al, Carcinoma of the anal canal. *Am J Clin Oncol* 1998; **18:** 32–9.

42. Constantinou EC, Daly W, Fung CT et al, Dose–time considerations in the treatment of anal cancer. *Int J Radiat Oncol Biol Phys* 1996; **36:** 295 (abst).

43. Bosset JF, Roelofsen F, Morgan D et al, Radiochemotherapy in locally advanced anal carcinoma. First results of the EORTC 22953 phase II trial. In: *Abstract Book of the EORTC–FFCD Joint Meeting, June 23–26, 1999, Paris, France.*

44. Cummings BJ, Preservation of structure and function in epidermoid cancer of the anal canal. In: *Infusion Chemotherapy – Irradiation Interactions* (Rosenthal CJ, Rotman M, eds). North Holland: Elsevier Science, 1998: 165–71.

45. Eypasch E, Williams JI, Wood-Dauphinee S et al, Gastrointestinal Quality of Life Index: development, validation and application of a new instrument. *Br J Surg* 1995; **82:** 216–22.

46. Vordermark D, Sailer M, Flentje M et al, Curative-intent radiation therapy in anal carcinoma: quality of life and sphincter function. *Radiother Oncol* 1999; **52:** 239–43.

47. Allal AS, Sprangers MAG, Laurence F et al, Assessment of long-term quality of life in patients with anal carcinomas treated by radiotherapy with or without chemotherapy. *Br J Cancer* 1999; **80:** 1588–94.

48. Kapp KS, Geyer E, Gebhart FH et al, Evaluation of sphincter function after external beam irradiation and Ir-192 high-dose-rate (HDR) brachytherapy ± chemotherapy in patients with carcinoma of the anal canal. *Int J Radiat Oncol Biol Phys* 1999; **45**(Suppl 3)**:** 339.

49. Broens P, Van Limbergen E, Penninckx F, Kerremans R, Clinical and manometric effects of combined external beam irradiation and brachytherapy for anal cancer. *Int J Colorectal Dis* 1998; **13:** 68–72.

50. Greenall MJ, Quah SHQ, De Cosse J et al, Epidermoid cancer of the anus margin. *Br J Surg* 1985; **72:** S97.

51. Touboul E, Schlienger M, Buffat L et al, A conservative vs. non conservative treatment of epidermoid carcinoma of the anal canal for tumors longer than or equal to 5 centimeters. A retrospective comparison. *Cancer* 1995; **75:** 786–93.

52. Allal AS, Laurencet FM, Reymond MA et al, Effectiveness of surgical salvage therapy for patients with locally uncontrolled anal carcinoma after sphincter conserving treatment. *Cancer* 1999; **86:** 405–9.

53. Holland JM, Swift PS, Tolerance of patients with human immunodeficiency virus and anal carcinoma to treatment with combined chemotherapy and radiation therapy. *Radiology* 1994; **193:** 251–4.

54. Peddada AV, Smith DE, Rao AR et al, Chemotherapy and low-dose radiotherapy in the treatment of HIV-infected patients with carcinoma of the anal canal. *Int J Radiat Oncol Biol Phys* 1997; **37:** 1101–5.

Part 7
Management of Metastatic Disease

31

Resection of liver metastases

Matthias Lorenz, Stefan Heinrich

INTRODUCTION

The only curative treatment for liver metastases from colorectal cancer is hepatic resection, and even if a total cure cannot be achieved, this approach can lead to long-term survival. This is confirmed by several retrospective analyses of major liver centres and multicentre evaluations, demonstrating a median survival time of 25–40 months and a 5-year survival rate of 25–50%.[1-3] These convincing results can be achieved with an acceptable morbidity and lethality rate of less than 5%. For these reasons, liver resection is the optimal treatment in cases of resectable liver metastases, and should therefore be performed in all eligible patients.

Surgical research has been focused on strategies to increase the rate of resectability and to prevent intra- and extrahepatic recurrence. Careful patient selection before surgery is required, since a technically successful resection is not always associated with a survival benefit to the patient. Therefore sound knowledge of the natural history and prognostic factors of this disease as well as detailed information about the extent of the disease are mandatory for the liver surgeon.

This chapter presents and discusses general guidelines for the optimal perioperative management of patients with colorectal cancer metastatic to the liver. It includes eligibility criteria, the required preoperative diagnostic work-up, technical aspects of hepatic resection, the value of second and third liver resections, and the potential improvements that can be obtained with the use of (neo)adjuvant treatment.

NATURAL HISTORY

The historical median survival of untreated patients with colorectal cancer metastatic to the liver is 4.5

months.[4] This prognosis is significantly dependent on the presence of an unresectable primary tumour or local recurrences, as well as the extent of hepatic infiltration and extrahepatic disease.[5] A more recent evaluation has demonstrated that patients in a poor general condition or elevated alkaline phosphatase serum levels have a worse prognosis; a median survival of 11 months can be expected in the remaining patients.[6]

The natural history of patients with potentially resectable hepatic metastases has only been documented in a few publications. Patients with solitary metastases exhibited a median survival time of 24 months, but none survived more than 5 years, in contrast to patients with curative hepatic resection, who exhibit a 25% survival rate.[7]

PREOPERATIVE DIAGNOSTICS

A complete tumour staging – in addition to evaluation of the location and extent of hepatic involvement – concerning the radicality of the resection of the primary tumour, as well as exclusion of local recurrence and extrahepatic disease, is necessary before planning a curative resection: a colonoscopy is required in all colorectal cancer patients. In patients who had surgery for rectal carcinoma, an additional endoluminal ultrasound of the neorectum and computed tomography (CT) of the pelvis are mandatory. The routine chest X ray must be supplemented by CT of the thorax in the case of abnormal findings. The standard examination for the detection and localization of hepatic metastases with the highest sensitivity and specificity is a biphasic CT of the abdomen. An improvement in accuracy has only been achieved by magnetic resonance imaging (MRI) using unspecific (gadolinium) or specific (e.g. ferric oxide) contrast media.[8] The formerly performed CT portography resulted in more false-positive results, and therefore no longer has any indication in the diagnosis of hepatic metastases.[9]

The advantage of positron emission tomography (PET) with ^{18}F-fluorodeoxyglucose (FDG) is the specific detection of additional intrahepatic as well as extrahepatic disease, with its additional value of differentiating between benign and malignant disease by the specific uptake.[10] Further studies, however, are needed to define its role in preoperative work-up.

Since the risk of liver failure increases with resections of more than half of the functional hepatic parenchyma, CT volumetry can help by determination of the partial hepatic resection rate (PHRR) in order to calculate the remaining functional liver volume.[11]

Preoperative liver function is an important factor defining the risk of liver failure after hepatic resection. Apart from small wedge resections or monosegmentectomies, resection should not be performed in Child B or C patients. However, Yamanaka et al[12] tried to develop a reliable prediction system with a large number of hepatocellular carcinoma patients. They demonstrated that biochemical tests and nutritional parameters do not influence the postoperative outcome of patients with non-cirrhotic livers. Only the PHRR, the preoperative prothrombin activity (Quick test) and γ-glutamyltranspeptidase levels predicted significantly for postoperative liver failure in a recently published multivariant analysis. Particular liver function tests, such as the aminopyrine test, were of no help in the selection of patients.[13]

INCLUSION AND EXCLUSION CRITERIA

Resectability

As already mentioned above, patients with a reduced liver function (Child B/C) or severe cardiopulmonal diseases are not eligible for liver resections.

The resectability (i.e. whether a resection is technically possible or not) is determined by the degree of liver involvement and the localization of the metastases. This can be ascertained by segmentectomies, hemihepatectomy, or a combination of anatomical and wedge resections in the case of bilobal disease (Figure 31.1).

Resection margin

In contrast to more recent trials, tumour-free margins of at least 1 cm were demanded in the past.[14] Since a curative resection has recently been demonstrated to be any resection with tumour-free margins, more functional liver parenchyma can be preserved in properly unresectable patients: while Fong et al[1] did not demonstrate any superiority in terms of survival of patients with tumour-free margins of more than 1 cm compared with those with less than 1 cm, the Pittsburgh series showed a slightly better 5-year survival rate (42% versus 32%) and 5-year disease-free survival (29 months versus 25 months) in 95 patients with tumour-free margins of more than 1 cm compared with 92 patients with a margin up to 1 cm.[15] In our own analysis, the long-term results were not statistically different in patients with resection margins of less than 4 mm compared with those with larger than 4 mm margins (Figure 31.2). Very similar results were reported by Elias et al,[16] Nakamora et al,[17] and Scheele and Altendorf-Hofmann.[3] Scheele et al[18] documented 38 long-term survivors with a resection margin of 0–4 mm.

However, only R0 resections, as defined by the removal of all microscopically intra- and extrahepatically detectable disease and microscopically tumour-free margins, should be performed. Debulking or palliative resections did not result in a benefit for the affected patients: the survival in these patients was not improved compared with that in patients with palliative treatment only.[19] The prognosis of these incompletely resected (so-called R1-resected) patients was significantly inferior compared with those with clear resection margins.[1]

The liver resection can also be combined with thermoablative, intraoperative techniques such as radiofrequency therapy or cryotherapy to extend the resectability in cases with bilobal disease.[20] The thermal necrosis during and after radiofrequency therapy can be monitored by intraoperative ultrasound.

Number of metastases

In earlier reports, the main prognostic parameter was the number of metastases.[21] The median survival of patients with 3 or 4 metastases was significantly inferior to that of patients with a single tumour in the liver. For this reason, 3–6 metastases as well as bilobal disease were regarded as a contraindication for liver resections.[14] Today, even the prognostic significance of multiple metastases is a matter of controversy. A critical number of liver metastases does not

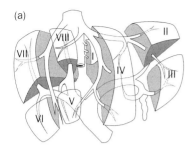

(a)

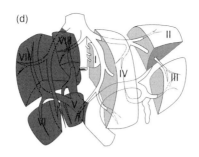

(d)

Figure 31.1 (a) Segmental anatomy of the liver and possible standard major hepatic resections. A cholecystectomy is always performed with resection of segment IV and/or V. (b) Left hemihepatectomy. (c) Extended left hemihepatectomy. (d) Right hemihepatectomy. (e) Extended right hemihepatectomy.

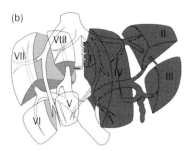

(b)

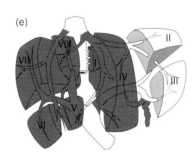

(e)

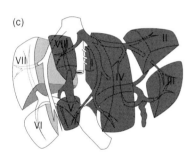

(c)

exist.[3] In 1986, Iwatsuki et al[22] reported that none of seven patients with 4 metastases survived for more than 3 years, whereas Nordlinger et al,[2] Scheele et al,[23] Doci et al,[24] and Fegiz et al[25] did not find such a relationship. Nordlinger et al[2] described 14 patients in whom 5 or more metastases were removed: the survival was identical to that of a group with a resection of 2, 3, or 4 metastases. Scheele et al[2] described 15 long-term survivors in 35 patients with 4 or more metastases, 14 of whom were recurrence-free after 5 years. Therefore, despite a certain influence on prognosis, most authors now do not exclude patients with 4 or more lesions from resection. However, patients in whom a curative resection requires the removal of more than 70% are excluded from surgery.

If a hemihepatectomy would result in curative resection but the remaining lobe appears to be too small, an embolization of the portal vein of the metastatic lobe can induce hypertrophy of the remaining lobe.[8,26] On the other hand, intrahepatic tumour growth can also be induced by the increase in growth factors.[27]

Extrahepatic disease

The presence of resectable extrahepatic disease, either as local recurrence of the primary tumour or as lung metastases, is no longer regarded as a contraindication for a liver resection: in patients with one or two lung metastases, long-term survivors

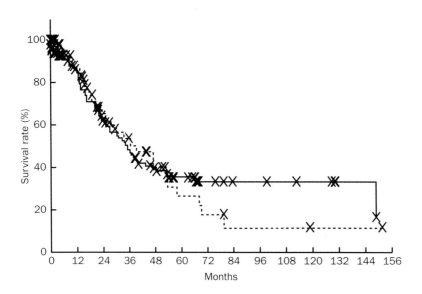

Figure 31.2 Long-term results after hepatic resection with resection margins of less than 4 mm (_____) and greater than 4 mm (_ _ _). The difference is not statistically significant (authors' own unpublished data).

were observed to have a 5-year survival rate of at least 25% after simultanous or sequential lung and liver resections.[28] In contrast to resectable lung metastases, Adson and co-workers[29] reported in 1984 that none of their patients with unresectable extra-hepatic metastases survived 5 years and that the 2- and 3-year survival rates were reduced to 36% and 11% respectively. In series of larger liver registries, patients with extrahepatic disease demonstrated a 5-year survival rate of 15–20%.[2,21] However, only 5% of these patients survived without relapse; poor results were reported in cases of lymph node metastases in the hepatoduodenal ligament and coeliac trunk[19,30,31] (Figure 31.3). August et al[32] stated that tumour spread to hepatic coeliac lymph nodes occurs retro-gradely because of lymphatic re-metastasis from the known liver tumours. For this reason, many centres exclude patients with visibly enlarged lymph nodes from hepatic resection. Some, however, state that in these cases, hepatic resection should be performed and combined with lymph node dissection to pre-vent early occurrence of obstructive jaundice.[33]

OPTIMAL TIME FOR LIVER RESECTION

Today, liver resections are usually performed close to the diagnosis of the metastases, no matter whether they occur syn- or metachronously. Most authors are currently of the opinion that this may prevent lym-phatic or further haematogenous spread to other organs. In contrast to this, a recent report[34] has revealed that the prognosis of patients is not nega-tively influenced if a CT control is performed after 2–6 months and the resection is only performed in those patients who do not develop additional metas-tases. However, initially large metastases may become unresectable during this interval as a result of invading important vascular structures or sur-rounding tissues. For this reason, large tumours (>4 cm) should be resected immediately after diag-nosis, whereas small metastases (<1 cm), particu-larly if they are located in several segments of the liver and require a major hepatic resection, should be planned for resection after a CT control 3 months later. Disseminated metastasis with a consecutive minor outcome can be excluded during this period.

Whether a liver resection should be performed synchronously with the resection of the primary tumour or in a second operation depends on the localization of the primary tumour and the metas-tases: segmentectomies or bisegmentectomies of seg-ments II, III, V and VI can be performed safely together with a colonic resection. However, deep anterior rectal resections should never be combined with any liver resection except for wedge excisions. Major hepatic resections should not be combined with any colonic resection.[3]

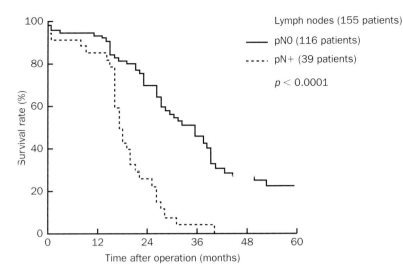

INTRAOPERATIVE APPROACH

Principles of liver surgery for resection of hepatic metastases

The aim of a hepatic resection for liver metastases is the radical removal of all detectable tumour with minimal mortality. The evaluation and recognition of the segmental structure of the liver anatomy has led to the develpoment of segment-oriented resection techniques.

Intraoperative ultrasound (IUS) of the liver has become a standard diagnostic technique before the resection. Up to 20% of hepatic lesions that have not been detected preoperatively or by intraoperative palpation are detected by IUS.[35–37] In addition, IUS helps to identify the segmental borders and the relationship of the tumour to the surrounding vessels, which allows for adequate margins during parenchymal dissection.

From the oncological view, segment-oriented resection reduces the risk of tumour recurrence caused by infiltrated margins or by intersegmental microscopic tumour growth. In contrast to the classic hemihepatectomy, the tumour-free parenchyma can be preserved by the segment-oriented resection, resulting in a reduced risk of postoperative liver failure. DeMatteo et al[38] were not able to demonstrate any differences in blood loss, operative time, and complications on comparing segment-oriented resections and wedge resections. However, the rate of positive resection margins was significantly reduced

from 16% to 2% in patients with segment-oriented resections, and the median survival time increased from 38 to 53 months.

Techniques of parenchymal dissection

A preoperative positive end expiratory pressure (PEEP) of below 2 mmHg is required to reduce intraoperative blood loss.[39] After complete luxation out of its bed and palpation of the liver, the parenchymal dissection is performed either by an ultrasonic dissector or water-jet dissector. The finger-fracture technique, which was commonly used in the past, results in severe parenchymal damage, since the tissue is crushed between two fingers, and is no longer used in hepatic surgery. However, several surgeons dissect the liver parenchyma manually using Kelly forceps, and report similar results to those achieved using an ultrasonic dissector.

Possible resections, excluding segmentectomies, are illustrated in Figure 31.1. Segment-oriented resections can only be performed by different methods of in- and outflow occlusion during parenchymal dissection. An inflow occlusion only is used in the majority of resections by means of portal triad clamping (Pringle manoeuvre) or selective vascular clamping (preliminary ligation) of the Glisson's capsule of the segment.[40] Even in cases where the need for a Pringle manoeuvre appears to be unlikely, it should always be prepared before starting the resection. The Pringle manoeuvre significantly reduces intraoperative blood loss, and is well tolerated for 90 minutes by a non-cirrhotic liver. This period can be extended if preconditioning of the vascular occlusion is used: the tourniquet is closed for 10 minutes; after a reopening phase of a further 10 minutes, the tourniquet is closed for as long as is required.[13]

In addition, total vascular exclusion (TVE) has become widely accepted when operating on lesions infiltrating the vena cava or those that are located close to the junction of the hepatic veins and the vena cava: two vascular clamps are placed tangentially on the vena cava from cranial and caudal.[41] In addition to the reduced backflow into the liver, the flow to the heart is also decreased: severe haemodynamic changes are reported to occur in about 15% of cases due to the caval clamping. An alternative technique is TVE with preservation of the caval flow by selective clamping of the hepatic veins.[42]

In very rare cases, when the confluences of the hepatic veins, the portal vein, or the vena cava are infiltrated by tumour and therefore have to be resected, a veno-venous bypass with veins or prosthetic grafts must be used. In these cases, when the hepatic confluence is infiltrated, or the tumour is localized at a critical site, ex situ liver resection with consecutive autotransplantation has been shown to be feasible. However, this technique has been associated with a high rate of perioperative morbidity and mortality. For this reason, ex situ liver resection should only be performed in otherwise technically unresectable tumours, and it is questionable whether colorectal hepatic metastases are an indication for ex situ liver resections.[43]

The parenchymal dissection itself can be performed using an ultrasonic- or water-jet dissector. These techniques produce minimal damage to the parenchyma because of the sharp resection margin: the desired area of parenchyma is destroyed while the structure of the vessels and bile ducts remains intact. Vessels and bile ducts are coagulated or are ligated with sutures and clips. Major branches of vessels and bile ducts should be selectively ligated. After the removal of the resected segments, the resection surface is checked for bleeding and bile leakage. Major bleeding and bile leakage have to be stopped by sutures. Definite haemostasis of the entire resection surface is achieved by coagulation: the depth of coagulation when using monopolar high-frequency or infrared coagulation is up to 2–7 mm, which can possibly cause secondary bleeding and bile leakage due to necrosis. Argon-beam plasma coagulation provides a contact-free coagulation with a depth of 0.5 mm, and is therefore preferably performed. Finally, we usually seal the resection surface with fibrin tissue adhesive or an additional collagen sponge.

COMPLICATIONS OF HEPATIC RESECTIONS

Hepatic resection is a safe procedure in patients with a preoperatively unimpaired liver function, and can be performed with a low mortality and morbidity rate (Table 31.1).[44] The most important intraoperative complication is bleeding from the liver surface during and after the resection. Several techniques have been developed to prevent intraoperative haemorrhage and to reduce blood loss.

The most common postoperative complications are summarized in Table 31.1. Besides the minor complications (e.g. pleural effusion, biloma, and wound infection), major complications are secondary haemorrhage and postoperative hepatic failure. Depending upon the extent of resection, the remaining liver does not provide sufficient function, resulting in fibrinolysis and a decrease in coagulation factors, reflecting the decreased synthesis by the liver. The plasma concentrations of the vitamin-K-dependent factors (II, VII, IX, and X) are more commonly and severely reduced than non-vitamin-K-dependent factors, resulting in a decrease in thromboplastin-time and partial thromboplastin-time activity.[45] In addition, the serum levels of protein C inhibitors and the anticoagulants antithrombin III (AT III), protein C, and protein S decrease.[45]

These changes in haemostasis can lead to postoperative bleeding. Freshly frozen plasma (FFP) is the appropriate agent in cases of postoperative haemorrhage due to hepatic insufficiency. A dose of 10 ml/kg body weight FFP results in an increase in the serum concentration of 15–20%, and should be applied at 6- to 12-hour intervals because of the short half-life of factor VII (6 hours). Substitution with AT III is indicated in cases of consumption coagulopathy to prevent or treat disseminated intravascular coagulopathy (DIC). When it is necessary to avoid infusion of large volumes of FFP because of renal failure or for other reasons, prothrombin complex concentrates (PPSB) can be applied as an alternative to FFP after the infusion of AT III.

In those cases when the conservative treatment of secondary haemorrhage fails or a surgical haemorrhage has occurred, a surgical approach becomes necessary: haemostasis is achieved by sutures or, if this is not possible owing to diffuse bleeding, by a tamponade with abdominal pads for 2–3 days.

Table 31.1 Rates of complications of hepatic resection for colorectal metastases[a]

Authors	No. of patients	Perioperative mortality (%)	Haemorrhage (%)	Bilioma (%)	Bile fistula (%)	Abscess (%)	Liver failure[b] (%)	Wound infection (%)	Systemic infection (%)	Pleural effusion (%)	Pneumonia (%)	Others (%)
Doci et al[24] (1995)	208	2.4	2	—	4	6.2	1	—	—	—	—	5
Rees et al[44] (1996)	143	0.7	<1	—	2	—	4	—	—	—	2	11
Fong et al[1] (1997)	456	2.8	1	2	1	1	1	3	1	—	3	10
Cady and Stone[14] (1998)	244	3.6	1	—	2	1	1	2	2	2	1	5
Authors' own data	180	3.3	1	4.4	4	3.3	5	6	3	11	2	5

[a] —, not listed in original publication.

[b] Temporary and definite hepatic failure.

Table 31.2 Results of hepatic resection for colorectal metastases

Authors	No. of patients	Perioperative mortality (%)	Median survival (months)	Disease-free survival (months)	1-year survival rate (%)	3-year survival rate (%)	5-year survival rate (%)
Gayowski et al[15] (1994)	204	0	33	62.5	91	43	32
Fong et al[46] (1999)	1001	2.8	42	19	89	57	37
Scheele et al[23] (1995)	182[a]	4.3[a,b]	36	22	64	39	30
	168[b]		42	28	70	44	37

[a]Male
[b]Female

RESULTS OF LIVER RESECTION

The benefit of liver resections, with 5-year survival rates ranging from 20% to 45%, has been demonstrated by several retrospective analyses of patient collections of more than 100 patients (Table 31.2). The results from these retrospective analyses are confirmed by data from registries including nearly 3000 patients. Fong et al[46] reported on 1001 consecutive patients, and concluded that for ethical reasons, randomized trials on the efficacy of surgical resection versus no resection must not be performed.

Despite this success, the tumour recurrence rates range between 59% and 81%. Detailed information about this pattern of recurrence is available from the pooled data of American, French, and German registries and publications. Tumour relapse usually occurs after a median interval of 9–19 months from the initial liver resection. The recurrence is located in the resected liver in 41–92% of patients; the liver is the only site of recurrence in 50–60% of patients. A minority of patients (20–30%) develop only extrahepatic recurrence.[47]

PROGNOSTIC FACTORS AND SCORING SYSTEMS

As already mentioned, the majority of patients will suffer tumour relapse after hepatic resection. Several investigations have been performed by means of uni- and multivariate analyses to evaluate factors that predict for the risk of recurrence, enabling preoperative patient selection. A study by the French Surgical Association collected data from 1568 patients undergoing hepatic surgery for colorectal metastases: the most important factors were found to be the number of metastases and the diameter of the largest metastasis, as well as the stage of the primary tumour and the date of occurrence of the metastases. Six prognostic factors were identified, and led to the development of a scoring system that predicts for patients' survival (Table 31.3).[2] The most important aspect of this scoring system is that it allows an estimation of the risk for an intrahepatic recurrence before resection. Patients with a point score of 2 or less had a low risk of recurrence, associated with a 2-year survival rate of 79%. The relapse rate increased with the

Table 31.3 Nordlinger score for the preoperative estimation of the risk of local recurrence in the liver

Prognostic factors[a]	Points
• Infiltration into the serosa	1
• Lymphatic spread	1
• Delay from primary tumour operation of 2 years or less	1
• More than 3 metastases	1
• Preoperative CEA level: 5–30 µg/l	1
> 30 µg/l	2
• Resection margin of the liver resection > 1 cm	1

[a]CEA, carcinoembryonic antigen.

number of factors in this evaluation; 5-year survival was rare and the value of surgery was limited in the group of patients with a score of 5 or more. The age of the patients influenced the median survival, as reported in the literature.

After applying this scoring system to the data from a prospective German multicentre study of 226 patients, it was found that the estimation of prognosis was much more reliable than with the use of a single factor (e.g. the number of metastases): patients with a score of five or more had a 2-year survival rate of 35% (Figures 31.4 and 31.5).

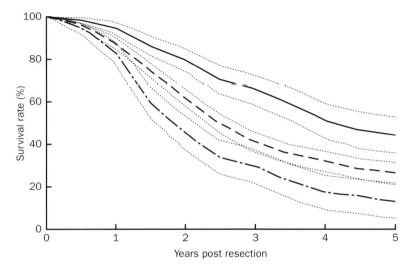

Figure 31.4 Retrospective analysis of 1273 patients following hepatic resection for colorectal metastases, depending on the Nordlinger score.[2]

Nordlinger score	Number of patients					
0–2 (——)	305	222	138	88	51	33
3–4 (— —)	738	512	276	133	76	46
5–7 (—·—)	230	149	55	22	9	5

The dotted lines indicate 95% confidence intervals

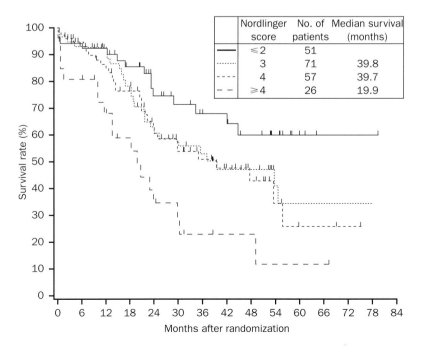

Nordlinger score	No. of patients	Median survival (months)
—— ≤2	51	
·········· 3	71	39.8
- - - - 4	57	39.7
– – ≥4	26	19.9

Figure 31.5 Retrospective analysis at the University of Frankfurt of 205 patients following hepatic resection for colorectal metastases, depending on the Nordlinger score.

Comparable scoring systems have recently been published by Fong et al[46] and Iwatsuki et al.[48] The Iwatsuki score also includes extrahepatic metastasis.

RE-RESECTION

In the majority of patients, the recurrences are diffuse and unresectable. However, in about 10–20% of these patients, the recurrent metastases appear to be technically resectable. A second liver resection should be considered in these patients, if the liver is the only site of metastasis.[19,49] Eligibility criteria are the same as those for the first resection.

Despite the growing experience with re-resections, much of the available data in the literature is derived from small series of about 10 patients, and none has exceeded 65 patients, except for multicentre registries. Two-thirds of the re-resections have been performed in the contralateral lobe of the primary resected liver, and have even been shown to be possible in cases with previously performed hemihepatectomy. However, most patients had undergone previous restricted resections.

Re-resection has been proven to be safe, with a mortality rate of 0.9% in the series of 116 patients of the French Surgical Association survey, with the complication rate being similar to or even less than that after the first hepatic resection. The reported morbidity ranged from 11% to 52%.[50] Adam and co-workers[51] reported a 3-year survival rate of 60% and a 5-year survival rate of 41% after second resection. This is comparable to the results from the French multicentre registry (a 3-year survival rate of 57%). Inferior results were demonstrated after synchronous hepatic re-resection and resection of extrahepatic disease (mean survival 16 months). For this reason, a close follow-up after hepatectomy should have the aim of detecting resectable recurrences.

In some patients, even third and fourth resections were performed, if technically feasible. However, the number of reported third resections was too small for any conclusion to be drawn about long-term results.[52]

ADJUVANT TREATMENT

The success of adjuvant systemic chemotherapy after curative resection of the primary tumour has rekindled interest in its use after resection of hepatic metastases, since recurrences usually occur early after resection and the benefit is limited by risk-prone surgical interventions. Occult metastases in the remaining liver as well as isolated tumour cell nests are responsible for recurrences after liver resection. The release of growth factors by the regenerating liver stimulates intrahepatic mitosis of tumour cells as well as normal cells: in animal experiments, growth factors led to tumour growth following partial hepatectomy.[53,54] Various attempts have been undertaken using adjuvant intra-arterial, portal vein, intraperitoneal, or systemic chemo- or immunotherapy to reduce the relapse rate after hepatic resection. At least four randomized multicentre trials were initiated comparing systemic (intravenous) or hepatic arterial infusion (HAI) with 5-fluorouracil (5-FU)/folinic acid (FA, leucovorin) or intra-arterial 5-fluoro-2-deoxyuridine (FUDR, floxuridine) versus a control group undergoing systemic 5-FU treatment.[55] A randomized trial of the German cooperative group on liver metastases (Arbeitsgruppe Lebermetastasen, ALM) investigated the effect of HAI after liver resection: 226 patients were randomized either to receive 5-FU (1000 mg/m^2/day/5 days) plus FA (200 mg/m^2/day/5 days) or no further chemotherapy.[56] The recurrence rates in the liver were 33% and 37% with and without adjuvant treatment, respectively ($p = 0.715$). This first interim analysis demonstrated a median survival of 35 months after adjuvant treatment versus 41 months without postoperative HAI ($p = 0.15$). The study was closed because the relative risk of death was reduced by at best 15% and at worst doubled by the application of adjuvant treatment.

Two randomized adjuvant HAI studies in the USA have completed their recruitment, and data indicate a benefit in using HAI – in contrast to the above-mentioned study. In both of these studies, HAI FUDR for 1 or 2 weeks was combined with a systemic (intravenous) 5-FU (monotherapy) treatment or an FA-modulated 5-FU treatment.[57,58] A significant reduction of the hepatic recurrence rate was reported after 2 years. The rate of recurrence-free survival was 90% in the HAI FUDR plus 5-FU/FA group, versus 60% in a group that was treated with intravenous 5-FU/FA. However, a significant effect on median survival was not demonstrated. For this reason, the optimal postoperative treatment is uncertain.[59]

NEOADJUVANT TREATMENT

Similar to other organs, preoperative treatment has been investigated in patients with liver metastases to improve the resectability rate and the median survival. Results of the first study on this approach were reported by Patt et al[60] in 1987: two cycles of preoperative HAI were administered using an angiographically placed catheter, and liver resection was performed after a break of 3–4 weeks. Postoperative chemotherapy was administered only in patients without curative resection who had responded to the neoadjuvant treatment, resulting in a median survival of 51 months, which was on a par with that of the R0-resected patients.

Bismuth et al[61] and Adam et al[62] reported the positive effect of chronomodulated therapy with 5-FU/FA and oxaliplatin in 701 primarily unresectable patients. Of these patients, 95 became resectable; the overall survival rate was 35% at 5 years. After a mean follow-up of 42 months, 66% of these patients relapsed.[61] This promising approach will be tested by a phase III European Intergroup trial in resectable patients with up to four metastases.

CONCLUSIONS

At present, liver resection is the only curative option in the treatment of colorectal liver metastases. Resection of liver metastases is a safe procedure associated with a low mortality rate in specialized centres; even if the patient is not cured by the resection, the quality of life is generally high. Scoring systems, which include simple preoperatively measurable prognostic factors, can be used for the prediction of patients' prognosis and postoperative risk of relapse. Long-term survival has been proven for 5 and also for 10 years, but has never been reported from untreated patients.

Combined treatment strategies have not yet improved prognosis. However, the use of new and more effective systemic chemotherapy regimens, either neoadjuvant or adjuvant, seems to be a promising approach requiring further investigation in prospective studies – a neoadjuvant European study has already been initiated.

REFERENCES

1. Fong Y, Cohen A, Fortner J et al, Liver resection for colorectal metastases. *J Clin Oncol* 1997; **15:** 938–46.
2. Nordlinger B, Guiguet M, Vaillant JC et al, Surgical resection of colorectal carcinoma metastases to the liver. A prognostic scoring system to improve case selection, based on 1568 patients. Association Française de Chirurgie. *Cancer* 1996; **77:** 1254–62.
3. Scheele J, Altendorf-Hofmann A, Resection of colorectal liver metastases. *Langenbeck's Arch Surg* 1999; **384:** 313–27.
4. Bengtsson G, Carlsson G, Hafström L et al, Natural history of patients with untreated liver metastases from colorectal cancer. *Am J Surg* 1981; **141:** 586–9.
5. Stangl R, Altendorf-Hofmann A, Charnley RM et al, Factors influencing the natural history of colorectal liver metastases. *Lancet* 1994; **343:** 1405–10.
6. Rougier P, Milan C, Lazorthes F et al, Prospective study of prognostic factors in patients with unresected hepatic metastases from colorectal cancer. Fondation Française de Cancérologie Digestive. *Br J Surg* 1995; **82:** 1397–400.
7. Wagner JS, Adson MA, Van Heerden JA et al, The natural history of hepatic metastases from colorectal cancer. A comparison with resective treatment. *Ann Surg* 1984; **199:** 502–8.
8. Robinson P, Imaging liver metastases: current limitations and future prospects. *Br J Radiol* 2000; **73:** 234–41.
9. Valls C, Lopez E, Guma A et al, Helical CT versus arterial portography in the detection of hepatic metastases of colorectal carcinoma. *Am J Radiol* 1998; **170:** 1341–7.
10. Fong Y, Saldinger PF, Akhurst T et al, Utility of ^{18}F-FDG positron emission tomography scanning on selection of patients for resection of hepatic colorectal metastases. *Am J Surg* 1999; **178:** 282–7.
11. Blobitza G, Lamade W, Demiris AM et al, Virtual planning of liver resections: image processing, visualization and volumetric evaluation. *Int J Med Inf* 1999; **53:** 225–37.
12. Yamanaka N, Okamoto E, Oriyama T et al, A prediction scoring system to select the surgical treatment of liver cancer. Further refinement based on 10 years of use. *Ann Surg* 1994; **219:** 342–6.
13. Rau H, Schauer R, Helmberger T et al, Impact of virtual reality imaging on hepatic liver tumor resection: calculation of risk. *Langenbecks Arch Surg* 2000; **385:** 162–70.
14. Cady B, Stone MD, The role of surgical resection of liver metastases in colorectal carcinoma. *Semin Oncol* 1991; **18:** 399–406.
15. Gayowski T, Iwatsuki S, Madariaga J et al, Experience in hepatic resection for metastatic colorectal cancer: analysis of clinical and pathologic risk factors. *Surgery* 1994; **116:** 703–10.
16. Elias D, Cavalcanti A, Sabourin J et al, Resection of liver metastases from colorectal cancer: the real impact of the surgical margin. *Eur J Surg Oncol* 1998; **24:** 174–9.
17. Nakamura S, Suzuki S, Baba S, Resection of metastases of colorectal carcinoma. *World J Surg* 1997; **21:** 741–7.
18. Scheele J, Altendorf-Hofmann A, Stangl R et al, Surgical resection of colorectal liver metastases: gold standard for solitary and radically resectable lesions. *Swiss Surg* 1996; Suppl 4: 4–17.
19. Geoghegan J, Scheele J, Treatment of colorectal liver metastases. *Br J Surg* 1999; **86:** 158–69.
20. Elias D, Debaere T, Muttillo I et al, Intraoperative use of radiofrequency treatment allows an increase in the rate of curative liver resections. *J Surg Oncol* 1998; **67:** 190–1.
21. Hughes K, Simons R, Songhorabodi S et al, Resection of the liver for colorectal carcinoma metastases: a multi-institutional study of indications for resection. *Surgery* 1988; **103:** 278–88.
22. Iwatsuki S, Esquivel CO, Gordon RD, Starzl TE, Liver resection for metastatic colorectal cancer. *Surgery* 1986; **100:** 804–10.
23. Scheele J, Stangl R, Altendorf-Hofmann A et al, Resection of colorectal liver metastases. *World J Surg* 1995; **19:** 59–71.
24. Doci R, Gennari L, Bignami P et al, Morbidity and mortality of hepatic resection of metastases from colorectal cancer. *Br J Surg* 1995; **82:** 377–81.
25. Fegiz G, Ramacciato G, Gennari L et al, Hepatic resection for colorectal metastases: the Italian multicenter experience. *J Surg Oncol* 1991; **2:** 144–54.
26. Imamura H, Shimada R, Kubota M et al, Preoperative portal vein embolization: an audit of 84 patients. *Hepatology* 1999; **29:** 1099–105.
27. Elias D, De Baere T, Roche A et al, During liver regeneration following right portal embolization the growth rate of liver metastases is more rapid than that of the liver parenchyma. *Br J Surg* 1999; **86:** 784–8.

28. Lehnert T, Knaebel HP, Duck M et al, Sequential hepatic and pulmonary resections for metastatic colorectal cancer. *Br J Surg* 1999; **86:** 241–3.

29. Adson M, van Heerden J, Adson M et al, Resection of hepatic metastases from colorectal cancer. *Arch Surg* 1984; **119:** 647–51.

30. Rosen C, Nagorney D, Taswell H et al, Perioperative blood transfusion and determinants of survival after resection for metastatic colorectal carcinoma. *Ann Surg* 1992; **216:** 493–504.

31. Harms J, Obst T, Thorban S et al, The role of surgery in the treatment of liver metastases for colorectal cancer patients. *Hepatogastroenterology* 1999; **46:** 2321–8.

32. August DA, Ottow RT, Sugarbaker PH, Clinical perspective of human colorectal cancer metastasis. *Cancer Metastasis Rev* 1984; **3:** 303–24.

33. Yasui K, Hirai T, Kato T et al, Major anatomic hepatic resection with regional lymph node dissection for liver metastases from colorectal cancer. *J Hepatobiliary Pancreat Surg* 1995; **2:** 103–6.

34. Lambert A, Colacchio T, Barth R, Interval hepatic resection of colorectal metastases improves patient selection. *Arch Surg* 2000; **135:** 473–80.

35. Machi J, Isomoto H, Kurohiji T et al, Accuracy of intraoperative ultrasonography in diagnosing liver metastasis from colorectal cancer: evaluation with postoperative follow-up results. *World J Surg* 1991; **15:** 551–7.

36. Luck A, Maddern G, Intraoperative abdominal ultrasonography. *Br J Surg* 1999; **86:** 5–16.

37. Benson M, Gandhi M, Ultrasound of the hepatobiliary–pancreatic system. *World J Surg* 2000; **24:** 166–70.

38. DeMatteo R, Palese C, Jarnagin W et al, Anatomic segmental hepatic resection is superior to wedge resection as an oncologic operation for colorectal liver metastases. *J Gastrointest Surg* 2000; **4:** 178–84.

39. Mendelez J, Arslan V, Fischer M et al, Perioperative outcomes of major hepatic resections under low central venous pressure anaesthesia: blood loss, blood transfusion, and the risk of postoperative renal dysfunction. *J Am Coll Surg* 1998; **187:** 620–5.

40. Launois B, Jamieson GG, The importance of Glisson's capsule and its sheaths in the intrahepatic approach to resection of the liver. *Surg Gyn Obstet* 1992; **174:** 7–10.

41. Grazi GL, Mazziotti A, Jovine E et al, Total vascular exclusion of the liver during hepatic surgery. *Arch Surg* 1997; **132:** 1104–9.

42. Cherqui D, Malassagne B, Colau P et al, Hepatic vascular exclusion with preservation of the caval flow for liver resections. *Ann Surg* 1999; **230:** 24–30.

43. Oldhafer K, Lang H, Schlitt H et al, Long-term experience after ex situ liver surgery. *Surgery* 2000; **127:** 520–7.

44. Rees M, Plant G, Wells J et al, One hundred and fifty hepatic resections: evolution of technique towards bloodless surgery. *Br J Surg* 1996; **83:** 1526–9.

45. Joist J, Hemostatic abnormalities in liver disease. In: *Hemostasis and Thrombosis: Basic Principles and Clinical Practice*, 3rd edn (Colman R, Hirsh J, Marder V, Salzman E, eds). Philadelphia: JB Lippincott, 1994: 906–20.

46. Fong Y, Fortner J, Sun R et al, Clinical score for predicting recurrence after hepatic resection for metastatic colorectal cancer. Analysis of 1001 consecutive cases. *Ann Surg* 1999; **230:** 309–21.

47. Köhne H, Lorenz M, Herrmann R, Colorectal cancer liver metastasis: local treatment for a systemic disease. *Ann Oncol* 1998; **9:** 967–71.

48. Iwatsuki S, Dvorchik I, Madariaga J et al, Hepatic resection for metastatic colorectal adenocarcinoma: a proposal of a prognostic scoring system. *J Am Coll Surg* 1999; **189:** 291–9.

49. Sugarbaker P, Repeat hepatectomy for colorectal metastases. *J Hepatobiliary Pancreat Surg* 1999; **6:** 30–8.

50. Nordlinger B, Vaillant JC, Guiguet M et al, Survival benefit of repeat liver resections for recurrent colorectal metastases: 143 cases. Association Française de Chirurgie. *J Clin Oncol* 1994; **12:** 1491–6.

51. Adam R, Bismuth H, Castaing D et al, Repeat hepatectomy for colorectal liver metastases. *Ann Surg* 1997; 51–60.

52. Sugarbaker P, Repeat hepatectomy for colorectal metastases. *J Hepatobiliary Pancreat Surg* 1999; **6:** 30–8.

53. Rashidi B, An Z, Sun F et al, Minimal liver resection strongly stimulates the growth of human colon cancer in the liver of nude mice. *Clin Exp Metastasis* 1999; **17:** 497–500.

54. Picardo A, Karpoff H, Ng B et al, Partial hepatectomy accelerates local tumor growth: potential roles of local cytokine activation. *Surgery* 1998; **124:** 57–64.

55. Lorenz M, Müller H, Staib-Sebler E et al, Relevance of neoadjuvant and adjuvant treatment for patients with resectable liver metastases of colorectal carcinoma. *Langenbeck's Arch Surg* 1999; **384:** 328–38.

56. Lorenz M, Müller H, Schramm H et al, Randomized trial of surgery versus surgery followed by adjuvant hepatic arterial infusion with 5-fluorouracil and folinic acid for liver metastases of colorectal cancer. *Ann Surg* 1998; **228:** 756–62.

57. Kemeny N, Conti J, Blumgart L et al, Hepatic arterial infusion of floxuridine (FUDR), dexamethasone (Dex) and high-dose mitomycin C (Mit C): comparable responses to FUDR/leucovorin/dex but with greater toxicity. *Proc Am Soc Clin Oncol* 1995; **14:** 201–9.

58. Kemeny N, Huang Y, Cohen A et al, Hepatic arterial infusion of chemotherapy after resection of hepatic metastases from colorectal cancer. *N Engl J Med* 1999; **341:** 2039–48.

59. Lorenz M, Müller H. Letter to the editor. *N Engl J Med* 2000; **342:** 1524–7.

60. Patt Y, McBride C, Ames F et al, Adjuvant perioperative hepatic arterial mitomycin C and floxuridine combined with surgical resection of metastatic colorectal cancer in the liver. *Cancer* 1987; **59:** 867–73.

61. Bismuth H, Adam R, Levi F et al, Resection of nonresectable liver metastases from colorectal cancer after neoadjuvant chemotherapy. *Ann Surg* 1996; **224:** 509–20.

62. Adam R, Avisar E, Ariche A et al, Five-year survival following hepatic resection after neoadjuvant therapy for nonresectable colorectal liver metastases. *Ann Surg Oncol* 2001; **8:** 374–83.

32

Surgery of lung and brain metastases

Christophe Penna, Robert Malafosse, Bernard Nordlinger

INTRODUCTION

Distant metastases, particularly liver deposits, represent the major cause of death of patients treated for colorectal adenocarcinoma. Depending on the stage of the primary tumour, liver metastases occur in 20–70% of patients and lung metastases in 10–20%. Brain and adrenal metastases are less frequent. Unlike many other types of cancer, in colorectal cancer, the presence of distant metastases does not preclude curative treatment. Surgical resection remains the only treatment that can ensure long-term survival in some patients. However, selection criteria for surgical resection of metastases should be strict, and less than 10% of liver metastases and 4% of lung metastases are suitable for surgery. We shall discuss the preoperative assessment, surgical techniques, and results of surgical resection for lung metastases, and shall also give some information on the few available data on the surgical treatment of brain metastases. Resection of liver metastases is discussed in Chapter 31.

LUNG METASTASES

Although lung metastases are less frequent than liver metastases, the indications for their resection are similar. After complete resection, there are significant improvements in survival, and long-term survivors can be observed. Indications for surgery have increased in the last decade, and resection is now proposed not only for patients with solitary deposits but also for some with multiple metastases or in whom liver metastases have been resected previously.

Selection criteria

As for liver metastases, the primary tumour should be totally resected, with no evidence of local recurrence or other extrapulmonary disease. However, in selected cases, combined resection of liver and lung metastases can be discussed. In a recent series, among 239 patients operated upon for pulmonary metastases of colorectal cancer, 43 (18%) had synchronous liver metastases surgically resected previously. There was no postoperative mortality, 7 patients (16%) underwent subsequent pulmonary resection for recurrences, and the median survival from pulmonary resection was 19 months.[1] Similar results were reported by the Metastatic Lung Tumour Study Group of Japan, with 47 patients who underwent pulmonary and hepatic resection, with 3-, 5-, and 8-year survival rates of 36%, 31%, and 23% respectively.[2]

Surgery can be considered only when complete removal of all pulmonary metastases is possible. Preoperative evaluation should include a computed tomography (CT) scan to detect small lesions less than 5 mm in size and a bronchoscopy to visualize any endobronchic lesion that would preclude a simple metastastectomy and indicate a segmental resection. Pulmonary function (gasometry and spirometric tests) as well as general status (ASA score) should be assessed.

Only 2–4% of patients with lung metastases are amenable to surgical resection.[3,4]

Surgical aspects

The incision is usually a posterolateral thoracotomy in the fifth intercostal space. In cases of bilateral metastases, the choice is between a median sternotomy, allowing the treatment of all lesions in one session with less detrimental effects on pulmonary function,[5] or two thoracotomies at 7–12 days' interval, allowing a better exploration of each lung.[6] Recent studies have shown the feasibility of video-assisted thoracic surgery (VATS) to perform wedge resections for peripheral lung lesions, with a significantly decreased amount of postoperative pain and functional morbidity compared with thoracotomy or sternotomy.[7,8] The results of VATS for lung metastases, mostly of colorectal origin, have been assessed in few studies.[9,10] A large retrospective study has recently reported the results obtained after VATS wedge excision of metastases in 177 patients, of whom 78 had diagnostic resection and 99 curative resection.[11] Inclusion criteria for the VATS metastatectomy included: (1) control of the primary tumour, (2) no evidence of extrapulmonary or disseminated metastatic disease, (3) cardiopulmonary reserve to tolerate the operation, (4) localization of the lesion in the outer third of the lung parenchyma, and (5) tumour less than 3 cm in diameter. VATS was successfully performed in all cases, there were no postoperative deaths, and the mean hospital stay was 5 days. After a mean follow-up of 37 months, 37% of patients were free of disease. The mean survival of patients operated on with curative intent was 28 months. VATS for metastases necessitates few precautions. Because of the inability to bimanually palpate the lung and the usually close gross surgical margins obtained with wedge excision, the staple line must be confirmed to be free of disease by frozen section. The stapling device must be carefully applied to avoid crushing or dividing the lesion. A retrieval device should be routinely used, since pulling the lung specimen directly through the intercostal opening has been implicated in tumour recurrence at the intercostal access site.

In contrast to the liver, there is no regeneration after pulmonary resection. Therefore surgery should be more conservative whenever possible,[6,12–14] and wedge resections are preferred in most cases. Anatomical resections (lobectomy, bi-lobectomy, or pneumonectomy) may, however, be mandatory in the case of a large lesion, endobronchic involvement, or resectable lymph-node metastases. In published series, wedge resections were performed in 50–68% of cases, lobectomies in 40–45%, and pneumonectomies in 6–8%, and the total number of metastases resected in a single patient reached 12.[3,4,15–17]

Results

The postoperative mortality rate is low, ranging from 0% to 5%,[3,17] and the postoperative morbidity rate varies from 2% to 12%, depending on the preoperative status of the patient and the type of resection performed.[3,4,15]

Surgical resection of lung metastases significantly prolongs survival; the 5-year survival rates observed in the principal reported series are given in Table 32.1.

Prognostic factors are similar to those associated with resection of liver metastases. Age, sex, and type of resection have no impact on survival.[3,4,15–17] In the series of McAfee et al,[15] the outcome was related to the number of lesions, the 5-year survival rate being 36.5% for solitary nodules (98 patients), 19.3% for two deposits (28 patients), and 7.7% when three or more lesions were resected (13 patients). Others reported 5-year survival rates ranging from 22% to 35% after resection of multiple metastases.[3,17] The delay between the treatment of the primary tumour and the lung metastases had no prognostic value in

---

Table 32.1 The 5-year survival rates following pulmonary resections for lung metastases from colorectal cancer

Authors	No. of patients	5-year survival rate (%)
Cahan et al[22]	31	30
Wilkins et al[23]	34	28
Mountain et al[12]	28	28
McCormack et al[13]	35	22
Goya et al[4]	65	41
McCormack et al[3]	144	44
McAfee et al[15]	139	30.5

most series.[3,4,15–17] The size of the largest metastasis had no impact on survival in some studies,[16,17] but lesions of more than 3 cm were associated with a worse outcome in others.[4] Patients who had had previous resection of liver metastases before lung metastases had similar survival, with 5-year actuarial survival rates of 30.5–68%.[15,16] A preoperative plasma carcinoembryonic antigen (CEA) level greater than 5 ng/ml was associated with a poor outcome, with a 5-year survival rate of 16% compared with 46.8% for those with normal CEA values. Complete removal of all metastatic disease appears to be the main prognostic factor in all series.

Following resection, the lung is the first site of recurrence in 50–70% of cases, followed by locoregional recurrences at the site of the primary, and brain and liver metastases.[15,16,18] Repeat lung resections can be discussed in some cases, since 5-year actuarial survival rates of 30% have been reported.[15]

BRAIN METASTASES

Brain metastases from colorectal cancer are rare, and are associated with disseminated disease in most cases. The available data on the surgical management of brain metastases from colorectal cancer are scarce. Their prognosis is even worse than those of other metastases. The brain is infrequently the sole site of the disease, and only 10–30% of patients with brain metastases die from strictly neurological causes. Treatment of brain metastases is based on steroids, radiotherapy, and surgery. In a controlled trial including patients with brain metastases of various origins, it was shown that for solitary lesions, resection improved local control rates, overall survival, and functional independence as compared with radiation. On the other hand, combined treatments increased survival and disease-free survival, and reduced the rate of recurrences at the original site.[19] In a series of 19 patients with brain metastases of colorectal origin, the mean survival was 4.9 months after resection (5 patients) and 2.6 months after radiation therapy (14 patients). The 6-month survival rates were 40% and 25% respectively, but there were no survivors at 1 year.[20] Others reported more encouraging results, with a mean survival of 8.3 months in a series of 73 patients who had a resection for brain metastases from colorectal cancer. The 1- and 2-year survival rates were 31.5% and 5.5% respectively, and 5 patients were alive at 19, 39, 40, 60, and 126 months. Prognosis was better for supratentorial than for cerebellar localization. At the time of brain metastases, 36 (49%) patients had liver metastases and 53 (73%) lung metastases, and 28 metastases at both sites. Of the 36 patients who had recurrences, 15 were reoperated upon, and the mean survival was 11.4 months.[21]

Surgical excision can be proposed for a very limited number of patients, especially in cases of a solitary lesion and control of the metastatic disease at other sites.

REFFRENCES

1. Regnard JF, Grunenwald D, Spaggiari L et al, Surgical treatment of hepatic and pulmonary metastases from colorectal cancers. *Ann Thorac Surg* 1998; **66**: 214–18.
2. Kobayashi K, Kawamura M, Ishihara T, Surgical treatment for both pulmonary and hepatic metastases from colorectal cancer. *J Thorac Cardiovasc Surg* 1999; **118**: 1090–6.
3. McCormack PM, Burt ME, Bains MS et al, Lung resection for colorectal metastases. 10-year results. *Arch Surg* 1992; **127**: 1403–6.
4. Goya T, Miyazawa N, Kondo H et al, Surgical resection of pulmonary metastases from colorectal cancer. Ten-year follow-up. *Cancer* 1989; **64**: 1418–21.
5. Johnson MR, Median sternotomy for resection of pulmonary metastasis. *J Thorac Cardiovasc Surg* 1983; **85**: 516–21.
6. Regnard JF, Marzelle J, Cerrina J et al, Chirurgie des metastases pulmonaires. *Chirurgie* 1985; **111**: 512–22.
7. Kirby TJ, Mack MJ, Landreneau RJ et al, Video-assisted thoracic surgery versus muscle-sparing thoracotomy. A randomized trial. *J Thorac Cardiovasc Surg* 1995; **109**: 997–1002.
8. Landeneau RJ, Hazelrigg SR, Mack MJ et al, Postoperative pain-related morbidity: video-assisted thoracic surgery versus thoracotomy. *Ann Thorac Surg* 1993; **56**: 1285–9.
9. Dowling RD, Landreneau RJ, Miller DL, Video-assisted thoracoscopic surgery for resection of lung metastases. *Chest* 1998; **113**: 2–5.
10. McCormack PM, Bains MS, Begg CB et al, Role of video-assisted thoracic surgery in the treatment of pulmonary metastases: results of a postoperative trial. *Ann Thorac Surg* 1996; **62**: 213–17.
11. Lin JC, Wiechmann RJ, Szwerc MF et al, Diagnostic and therapeutic video-assisted thoracic surgery resection of pulmonary metastases. *Surgery* 1999; **126**: 636–41.
12. Mountain CF, McCurtrey MJ, Hermes KE, Surgery for pulmonary metastasis: a twenty year experience. *Ann Thorac Surg* 1984; **38**: 323–30.
13. McCormack PM, Martini N, The changing role of surgery for pulmonary metastases. *Ann Thorac Surg* 1979; **28**: 139–45.
14. Takita H, Edgerton F, Karakousis C, Surgical management of metastases to the lung. *Surg Gynecol Obstet* 1981; **152**: 751–4.
15. McAfee MK, Allen MS, Trastek VF et al, Colorectal lung metastases: results of surgical excision. *Ann Thorac Surg* 1992; **53**: 780–6.
16. Yano T, Hara N, Ichinose Y et al, Results of pulmonary resection of metastatic colorectal cancer and its application. *J Thorac Cardiovac Surg* 1993; **106**: 875–9.
17. Mori M, Tomoda H, Ishida T et al, Surgical resection of pulmonary metastases from colorectal adenocarcinoma. Special reference to repeated pulmonary resections. *Arch Surg* 1991; **126**: 1279–301.
18. Foster JH, Berman MM, Solid liver tumours. *Major Probl Clin Surg* 1977; **22**: 242.
19. Patchell RA, Tibbs PA, Walsh JW et al, A randomized trial of surgery in the treatment of single metastases to the brain. *N Engl J Med* 1990; **322**: 494–500.

20. Alden TD, Gianino JW, Saclarides TJ, Brain metastases from colorectal cancer. *Dis Colon Rectum* 1996; **39:** 541–5.

21. Wronski M, Arbit E, Bilsky M, Galicich JH, Resection of brain metastases from colorectal cancer. *Dis Colon Rectum* 1996; **39:** A33.

22. Cahan WG, Castro EB, Hajdu SI, The significance of a solitary lung shadow in patients with colon carcinoma. *Cancer* 1974; **33:** 414–21.

23. Wilkins EW Jr, Head JM, Burke JF, Pulmonary resection for metastatic neoplasms in the lung. *Am J Surg* 1978; **135:** 480–3.

33

Ablative technique for liver metastases

Steven N Hochwald, Yuman Fong

INTRODUCTION

Treatment of primary colorectal cancer with surgical resection, combined with chemotherapy or radiation therapy in certain cases, is frequently curative. However, 25% of patients present with metastases to the liver at the time of diagnosis.[1] Also, following potentially curative resection of the primary, 50% of patients will have tumor recurrence in the liver within five years.[2] In appropriate patients, liver resection for colorectal metastases must be considered the standard of care, since surgical resection of metastatic disease isolated to the liver can result in cure in approximately one-third of patients.[3] However, the majority of patients with metastatic disease due to primary colorectal cancers are not candidates for surgical resection because of either anatomic considerations or extrahepatic disease. In fact, only 5–10% of these patients will have surgically resectable disease. Therefore, other ablative therapies are being investigated to eradicate colorectal metastases in the liver in patients for whom resection is not feasible, or who have recurred following resection. These therapies are also undergoing evaluation to determine if an alternative to resection that is less invasive can be utilized to provide cure for metastatic liver deposits.

Unlike surgical resection, regional therapies for liver metastases attempt to destroy tumors in situ. Generally, these therapies can be described as involving freezing, hyperthermia, use of tissue-destroying reagents, or reduction of blood supply to the tumor. An advantage of these techniques is that tumor killing can be performed with less destruction of non-neoplastic liver parenchyma than with formal liver resection. This may be useful in the treatment of hepatocellular carcinoma, when there often is coexistent cirrhosis and hepatic reserve is poor. However,

the advantages are less clear for hepatic colorectal metastases, where resection of up to 80% of the liver is associated with low operative mortality and a potential for cure.[3] Despite the development of new ablative devices and improvements in the application of older ablative techniques, direct comparisons of ablative therapies with surgical resection for colorectal metastases have not been performed. Therefore, at this time, there still is no role for ablative therapy when tumors are completely resectable, except for their evaluation in the context of clinical trials. Physicians interested in utilizing ablative therapies for colorectal metastases should be experienced in standard surgical resection, so that patients are not denied a chance at potential cure. At present, ablative procedures appear to be best suited for non-resectable disease or when there are medical contraindications to standard resection.

RADIOFREQUENCY ABLATION

Background

The technique of radiofrequency ablation (RFA) involves the placement of needle electrodes in the tumor to be ablated. These electrodes emit alternating current in the radiofrequency range which causes thermal injury. Schematically, a closed-loop circuit is created by placing a generator, a large dispersive electrode (ground pad), a patient, and a needle electrode in series. The patient is the resistor, while both the dispersive and needle electrodes are active electrodes. Between the electrodes in the tissue to be ablated, the alternating current causes agitation of numerous ions (Figure 33.1). Friction and thus heat are created from the ionic agitation. The needle itself is not hot. Rather, the marked discrepancy between

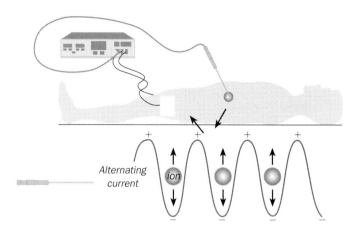

Figure 33.1 Schematic illustrating the method of action of radiofrequency ablation. Between the electrodes, alternating current causes agitation of numerous ions, leading to heat production.

the surface areas of the needle electrode and the dispersive electrode causes the generated heat to be tightly concentrated around the needle electrode. The heat is rapidly dissipated with increasing distance from the needle electrode.[4]

In RFA, the alternating electric current is administered in such a manner as to cause desiccation of tissue by evaporating or drying the intracellular water and producing coagulation necrosis. Cauterization of tissue and subsequent char formation from rapid heating is avoided. This is important because buildup of char around electrodes leads to increased resistance and limits the size of the thermal injury. Even in the absence of charring, however, this technique is limited by the small area of ablation, since the impedance rises as treated tissue dries out, leading to interruption of the electrical circuit. Consequently, only tumors less than 3–4 cm in size can be ablated with confidence with a single application.

Equipment and technique

The equipment consists of a low-wattage and low-voltage alternating electric current generator and needle electrodes. The most common design of the electrodes consists of 15-gauge needles with retractable curved prongs (Figure 33.2). Each prong is hollow, and contains a thermocouple that is used to register the temperature of the treated tissue. RFA can be performed using a percutaneous, open, or laparoscopic approach. Under sonographic guidance, the needle electrode is advanced into the target tumor. At the appropriate point, the electrode prongs are deployed, extending into the tumor and adjacent hepatic parenchyma (Figure 33.3). Ablation is initi-

ated at a generator power of 20–25 W. The power is gradually increased until the temperatures of at least three of the four prongs exceed 90°C, and this temperature is held for at least 6 minutes. To destroy a large tumor, overlapping ablations may be necessary. The larger the lesion, the more ablations that will be needed to treat the entire tumor.

The radiologic technique most commonly utilized to guide RFA is ultrasound. Each ablation creates numerous small bubbles in the heated tissue, which increases the echogenicity of the tissue. This is detected by ultrasound, and is a useful marker in small tumors for estimating whether the entire tumor has been treated. With a larger lesion, the echogenicity from the bubbles may make detection of the needle tip difficult and obscure untreated areas of the tumor. Large lesions must be treated in a systematic fashion so that all areas of the lesion are ablated.

Because of the charcoal effect created by tissue destruction from the radiofrequency electrodes, ultrasound is not useful in the immediate post-procedure period in determining if a tumor has been completely ablated.[4,5] In addition, the post-procedure interpretation of the effectiveness of the treatment according to the size of tumors on computed tomography (CT) images is misleading. The peritumoral hyperemia from the ablative process is impossible to distinguish from enhancing residual tumor around the margin of the lesion. The final interpretation of the completeness of the ablative process is probably best made at least one month after treatment. At this point, the inflammatory hyperemia will have resolved and residual hypervascular tumor will show enhancement on contrast-enhanced three-phase spiral CT (Figure 33.4). Others feel that visceral angiography may be useful to demonstrate the

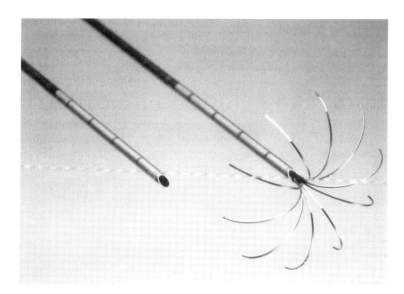

Figure 33.2 Needles utilized for radiofrequency ablation. Prongs can be deployed through the needle into the target tissue.

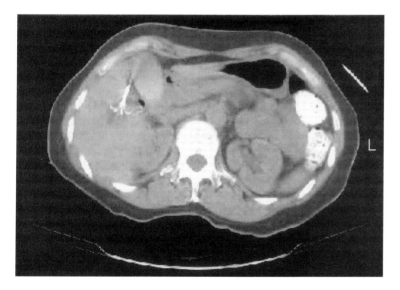

Figure 33.3 Deployed electrodes in a metastatic colorectal deposit in the liver.

result of RFA in the immediate time period following treatment.[6] There may be a role for positron-emission tomography (PET) scanning to determine if residual abnormalities seen on CT scan are biologically active.

Results

The reported experience of RFA for the treatment of colorectal metastases to the liver is limited. One of the first series utilizing RFA was published in 1996.[7] In general, studies suffer from small numbers and lack of follow-up (Table 33.1). Solbiati et al[5] percutaneously treated 16 patients with liver metastases: 9 colorectal carcinomas, 3 gastric carcinomas, 2 leiomyosarcomas, 1 ampullary carcinoma and 1 pancreatic cystic and papillary carcinoma. There were a total of 31 lesions, which measured 1.2–7.5 cm in diameter. Two or three treatment sessions were employed in the majority of patients. Of the 16 patients in the study, 3 were treated while under general anesthesia and 13 were treated using only conscious intravenous sedation. Four patients underwent surgical resection 15–60 days after

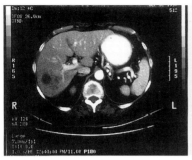 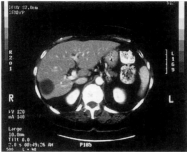 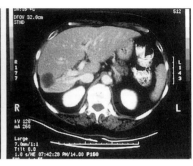

Figure 33.4 Radiofrequency ablation of a malignant tumor in the right lobe of the liver. Follow-up scans are shown at 6 months (middle panel) and 1 year (right panel) after treatment. Note the residual defect seen in the liver at the site of ablation.

RFA. Residual, viable tumor was seen in all of these patients. The remaining 12 patients were followed up for 9–29 months (mean 18.1 months). In these patients, 18 of 27 (67%) lesions remained stable or decreased in size and showed no enhancement at CT or magnetic resonance imaging (MRI) for at least 9 months. Disease-free survival was achieved in 8 of these 12 patients, with a minimum follow-up of 12 months. Only one complication, self-remitting peritoneal hemorrhage, was observed at CT on day 3 after ablation.

In a recent report, investigators combined RFA with the Pringle maneuver (temporary occlusion of blood flow to the liver) to treat 61 patients with hepatic colorectal metastases through either a percutaneous or an open method.[8] Patients with only one or two small (diameter < 3.0 cm) cancers located peripherally in the liver were considered for percutaneous ultrasound-guided RFA. All other patients were treated surgically during an open operative procedure. The median number of tumors treated was 1 and the median size was 3.4 cm. There were no treatment-related deaths and the complication rate was 2.4%. With a median follow-up of 15 months, tumor has recurred in 3 of 169 treated lesions (1.8%). This series is notable because of the large numbers of patients evaluated and the low local recurrence rate (1.8%). For comparative purposes, the local recurrence rates of other previously published RFA series in which a similar endpoint was used were 50% or greater.[5,8,9] Some parameters that are different in this study when compared with other RFA studies include the large proportion of patients who had RFA performed intraoperatively rather than percutaneously, and the use of the Pringle maneuver.

The advantages of intraoperative RFA may be that the tumor can be better seen with intraoperative ultrasound when compared with percutaneous ultrasound owing to lack of an intervening body wall. This should result in more precise localization of tumors and increased sensitivity for lesion detection. It may be that RFA generators currently in use may not produce enough thermal energy to overcome the cooling effect of intrahepatic blood flow when used without a Pringle maneuver. Combining RFA with a Pringle maneuver may lead to a decrease in the amount of heat that is lost from the tumor, which allows a larger zone of tissue ablation. However, utilizing RFA during an open surgical procedure rather than via the percutaneous route negates many of the advantages of the technology.

LASER THERMAL ABLATION

Background

High-intensity light can be used to heat by tissue absorption of energy. As the amount of energy delivered to tissues increases, intracellular and interstitial water is vaporized. This leads to tissue contraction. All cellular material is vaporized at higher energy levels and a void is created in the treated tissue. Lasers with energy outputs that are suitable for thermal ablation of tissue are the argon ion laser, the carbon dioxide laser, and the neodymium : yttrium aluminum garnet (Nd : YAG) laser. Most clinical information is available for the Nd : YAG laser, which appears to be most appropriate for deep tumor ablation.

Interstitial hyperthermia of tumors induced by light-conducting quartz fibers attached to laser

Table 33.1 Experience with radiofrequency ablation for colorectal metastases to the liver

Study	No. of patients	Method	Median no. of lesions[a]	Median site[a] (cm)	Mean or median follow-up[a] (months)	Response or survival rates[b]	Complications
Rossi et al (1996)[7]	6	Percutaneous	1 (1–1)	3.5 (1.8–3.5)	11 (3–27)	DFS 33%	None
Nagata et al (1997)[44]	20	Percutaneous	—	—	—	1-year survival 33% DFS 5 mo[c]	Fat necrosis (12%) Gastric ulcer (2%)
Livraghi et al (1997)[45]	12	Percutaneous	2	3.1 (1.2–4.5)	—	CR 52% PR 48%	Pleural effusion (2 patients)
Solbiati et al (1997)[5]	9	Percutaneous	1 (1–6)	— (1.2–7.5)	18 (9–29)	No growth progression 67% CR 11%	None
Jiao et al (1999)[6]	17	Percutaneous open	Solitary 1 Multiple 12	>3.0	5.1	Stable disease 10 (59%) Progression 7 (41%) DOD 4 (23%)	—
Bilchik et al (1999)[46]	13	Percutaneous, open	2.2	—	—	DFS 92%	—
Kainuma et al (1999)[47]	9	Open[d]	6.0 (2–13)	2.1 (0.5–4.8)	15.2	2-year survival 33%; LR 56%	Pneumothorax
Cuschieri et al (1999)[48]	8	Laparoscopic	4.0 (3–18)	1.5 (0.5–3.5)	13 (6–20)	DFS 75%	None
Curley et al (1999)[8]	61	Percutaneous, open	1 (1–5)	3.4 (0.5–12.0)	15	LR 1.8%	Minimal bleeding

[a] Range in parentheses.
[b] CR, complete response; PR, partial response; LR, local recurrence; DFS, disease-free survival; DOD, died of disease.
[c] Median survival.
[d] Intra-arterial infusion chemotherapy also utilized.

generators has been available for about 15 years. Studies have shown that areas of thermal necrosis of predictable extent could be produced in the livers of rats using the Nd : YAG laser.[10] Energy is delivered via fiberoptics placed interstitially under ultrasound guidance. The procedure may be monitored with ultrasound or MRI, and the area of necrosis can be seen with various radiologic modalities. This technology was first utilized in patients with metastatic colorectal cancer to the liver in 1989.[11]

Technique and results

An 18-gauge needle is inserted into the tumor to be treated. Next, a laser fiber needle is inserted through the access needle. Microthermocouple needles are placed around the margins of the tumor and are used to monitor the temperature of the treated tissue. Energy is delivered from the laser until the heated tissues reach 60°C.

Nolsoe et al[12] performed interstitial hyperthermia with the Nd : YAG laser on 11 patients with 16 colorectal liver metastases. The range of tumor size was 1–4 cm in diameter. Follow-up fine-needle aspiration biopsy was performed in 11 of 16 laser-treated metastases. In 9 of these cases, the specimen showed necrotic material, while in 2 cases, viable tumor tissue was present. Four cases that had recurrences had original tumors that were on average 3.4 cm in size. This appeared to be larger than tumors that were considered completely destroyed (mean size 2.4 cm). Another study of interstitial laser therapy in 21 patients with 55 liver metastases showed that necrosis of tumor volume was more than 50% in 82% of the tumors, and 100% necrosis was achieved in 38%.[13] Metastases smaller than 4 cm in diameter were treated more effectively and required fewer treatment sessions than did those larger than 4 cm. Complications were minor, and included severe pain, asymptomatic subcapsular hematoma, and pleural effusion.

Vogl et al[14] have used MRI-guided interstitial laser therapy of liver metastases in 20 patients with 33 metastases from colorectal carcinoma (75%) or other primary tumors (25%). In 69% of lesions 2 cm in diameter or smaller, contrast-enhanced MRI depicted substantial necrosis, with a local tumor control rate of 69% after 6 months and 44% after 12 months. Among lesions larger than 2 cm, necrosis was frequently incomplete, with a local control rate of only 41% after 6 months and 27% after 12 months. In metastatic colorectal cancer, there are few 2 cm lesions residing away from major vessels that are not resectable. Even though this technique is capable of ablating small tumors, a clinical role for interstitial laser therapy has yet to be found.

MICROWAVE THERMAL ABLATION

Mechanism and technique

Microwaves are electromagnetic waves that are capable of inducing hyperthermia. The mechanism is through the displacement of free electrons and ions and the relaxation of electric dipoles, which generates kinetic energy that causes an increase in temperature in the treated tissue. Thermal coagulation is induced by local heat production.[15]

Microwave ablation is usually accomplished percutaneously. Under local anesthesia, a large-gauge access needle is inserted into the tumor under ultrasound guidance. A microwave electrode is inserted through the access needle and the tip is positioned within the tumor. The electrode is connected to the microwave generator by coaxial cables. Microwaves at a frequency of 2450 MHz are produced for a fixed length of time. A small amount of tissue (1.6–2.4 cm in diameter) around the microwave electrode is coagulated. Therefore, lesions which are less than 2 cm in diameter can be ablated in 1 or 2 sessions. Multiple treatment sessions may be necessary for tumors greater than 2 cm in diameter.[16]

There are sparse clinical data on the use of microwave therapy for colorectal metastases to the liver. Shibata et al[17] reported a 60% rate of tumor ablation with the use of microwave therapy during laparotomy in 10 patients with 67 metastatic lesions. In addition, microwave therapy was utilized via a percutaneous approach in 22 patients with ablation of tumor. Matsukawa et al[18] reported their experience with 7 metastatic tumors (3 colon carcinomas) to the liver. On follow-up, one lesion disappeared, 3 were reduced, and 3 were enlarged. Based mainly on their experience with hepatomas, the authors felt that this therapy was most effective in tumors less than or equal to 3 cm in diameter.

Microwave therapy is best for small tumors, and lesions greater than 2 cm in size require multiple sessions.[16] When used during laparotomy, microwave ablation is no less invasive than more established ablative techniques such as cryoablation. The main advantage of microwave ablation is that it can be performed percutaneously. Comparative trials are needed to determine the relative efficacy of microwave ablation and other ablative modalities that are performed through a percutaneous approach.

CRYOABLATION

Background

Of all ablative techniques for treating malignant liver tumors, cryosurgery is perhaps the current standard with which others should be compared. Cryoablation of both primary and metastatic hepatic cancer has been extensively reported. Hepatic cryosurgery involves the freezing and thawing of liver tumors by means of a cryoprobe inserted into the tumor. Cryoprobes are insulated probes that have flowing and recirculating very cold liquid. Studies have demonstrated that malignant tumors show less susceptibility to cooling than normal liver tissue.[19] Therefore, very low temperatures (less than $-40°C$) may be necessary in the tumor to maximize tissue destruction. For this reason, liquid nitrogen at $-196°C$ is utilized in the cryoprobes.

The primary effects of cryosurgery on tissues are both direct cellular damage from altered physiologic environment and indirect cell damage as a result of loss of structural integrity and vascular channels.[20] As cooling proceeds, ice forms in the intracellular and extracellular compartments, leading to tissue shrinkage, damage to the cell membrane, and protein denaturation. Further damage to tissue occurs during the thawing process from recrystallization of ice, grinding of cells, and the sudden increase in cell volume. Therefore, warming should be slow and passive. Any viable cells may be destroyed by a second freeze–thaw process. Thrombosis and destruction of tissue microvasculature further propagates cell death by hypoxia. The major determinants of cellular injury are the rate of cooling, the lowest temperature reached within the tissue, the period of time for which such a temperature is maintained, and the number of freeze–thaw cycles.

Equipment and technique

Several cryosurgical systems are currently available. Units are now available that can accommodate several probes simultaneously and therefore reduce procedure time and cost. Also, it is important to have cryoprobes of different sizes available, since the probe size will determine the size of the freeze zone that can be created. Ultrasound equipment (e.g. transabdominal, laparoscopic, or intraoperative) is essential for localizing the tumor and probe position and for following the 'ice ball' that is created. Cryoablation of metastatic lesions in the liver may be performed via a percutaneous, laparoscopic, or open approach. Depending on the depth of the lesion, direct introduction of the cryoprobe into the tumor or the needle-guided J-wire Seldinger-type technique may be used. To minimize tumor spillage, the cryoprobe should be inserted through normal liver parenchyma before entering the tumor. Care is taken to avoid major blood vessels or bile ducts. Probes should be placed to completely encompass the tumor by freeze ball. A freeze front appears on ultrasound as an advancing hyperechoic rim with acoustic shadowing. Freezing is continued until a 1 cm freeze zone beyond the tumor is achieved. Each cycle consists of a freeze phase of 15 minutes once the maximum freeze ball is reached, followed by a passive thaw over 10–20 minutes. Certainly, the peripheral 1 cm of the freeze ball should be thawed before refreezing is begun. The second freeze–thaw is completed using the same technique. To allow disengagement of the probe from the ice ball, after the second freeze is complete, the probe is actively warmed and removed. Any bleeding from the probe tract is controlled with hemostatic packing and manual pressure.

Indications and results

Indications for hepatic cryotherapy of colorectal metastases are similar to those for other ablative techniques. It is generally reserved for patients in whom one or more lesions are not surgically resectable, except for patients enrolled in formal clinical trials designed to compare resection with cryoablation. Patients should have disease limited to the liver, although this technique has been utilized in the liver in selected patients with resectable metastases in the lungs.

Important criteria for patient selection for cryoablation include number and size of lesions as well as proximity to major blood vessels (Figure 33.5). Most surgeons will not freeze more than five lesions. On average, it takes 30 minutes to freeze each lesion; therefore, there is a limit to the number of lesions that can be treated based on time restraints. Lesions that are 5 cm or smaller can be ablated with more confidence than lesions larger than 5 cm. Lesion location is an important determinant of the safety and effectiveness of cryoablation. Major blood vessels may serve as heat sinks and prevent adequate freezing of adjacent tumor. According to a collective review of the literature on hepatic cryosurgery, recurrence of tumor adjacent to large blood vessels remains a problem.[21] Others disagree that it is more dangerous or significantly more difficult to freeze

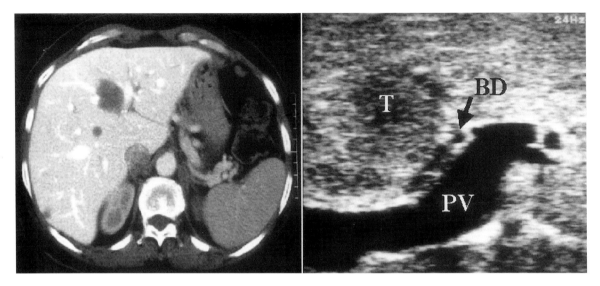

Figure 33.5 In the left panel, a metastatic colorectal lesion is seen in the left lobe of the liver near the left portal vein. On ultrasound (right panel) the lesion (T) is demonstrated in close proximity to the left hepatic duct (BD), which lies superior to the left portal vein (PV).

tumors near major vascular structures. They argue that the freezing process does not have to be modified except for the placement of more probes. In addition, they feel that blood vessels are quite resistant to damage from freezing, even when completely frozen.[22]

Published studies utilizing hepatic cryosurgery for colorectal metastases suffer from small numbers, lack of long-term follow-up and varied reported treatment endpoints (Table 33.2). Most studies report the use of cryosurgery during laparotomy and less often during laparoscopy. However, there is a recent report that describes a limited preliminary experience with percutaneous cryotherapy for liver metastases (6 patients) and hepatocellular carcinoma (2 patients).[23] Onik et al[24] treated 58 patients with metastatic colorectal disease with cryotherapy during laparotomy. Some patients had concomitant liver resection. A mean of 4.6 lesions were treated per patient. With an 18-month mean follow-up, the disease-free survival rate was 27%. Local recurrence rates were not reported. Weaver et al[25] treated 47 patients (median 3 lesions per patient) with metastatic colorectal disease to the liver with cryotherapy, some undergoing liver resection as well. With a median follow-up of 26 months, the median survival was 26 months. There were no documented recurrences at the site of cryosurgery in 22 patients who were alive at the end of the study. However, the

recurrence rate at the cryosurgery site was not reported in the patients who expired. At a mean follow-up of 16 months, Adam et al[26] identified a 44% local recurrence rate in 25 patients undergoing cryoablation of hepatic colorectal metastases. Seifert and Morris,[27] at a median follow-up of 22 months, identified a 33% local recurrence rate at the cryosite in 85 patients undergoing cryotherapy for unresectable liver metastases. Cryotreated metastases larger than 3 cm were associated with a shorter disease-free interval at the cryosite. The largest reported experience with cryotherapy for hepatic colorectal metastases is from Australia.[28] In 121 cases with a mean follow-up of 36 months, the median survival was 800 days. No information regarding rates of local recurrence was reported in this study.

A comprehensive description of complications associated with cryotherapy of malignant liver tumors has been recently published. Seifert et al[21] surveyed a large number of clinical centers throughout the world, and obtained data regarding complications on 2173 patients undergoing hepatic cryotherapy. The total mortality was 33 of 2173 patients (1.5%). Cryoshock was responsible for a high proportion (18%) of all mortality following hepatic cryotherapy. The syndrome of multiorgan failure, severe coagulopathy, and disseminated intravascular coagulation similar to septic shock but without evidence of any systemic sepsis has been

Table 33.2 Experience with hepatic cryosurgery for colorectal metastases

Study	No. of patients	Method	Median no. of lesions[a]	Median site[a] (cm)	Mean or median follow-up[a] (months)	Response or survival rates[b]	Major complications
Ravikumar et al (1991)[49]	24	Open	—	—	24 (5–60)	Actuarial survival 39%[c]	Subphrenic abscess (1)
Charnley et al (1991)[30]	11	Open	5.2 (2–12)	4.5 (2–12)	6 (2–17)	DOD 2 Alive 9	—
Onik et al (1993)[24]	58	Open: ± liver resection	4.6 (1–16)	—	18 (6–87)	27% DPS	Renal failure (3), hemorrhage (1), hepatic failure (2), bile fistula (1), abscess (1)
Preketes et al (1995)[50]	38	Open: ± HAC[c]	4.9	4.5	—	Median survival 570 days	—
Weaver et al (1995)[25]	47	Open: ± hepatic resection	3.0 (1–12)	—	26 (24–57)	Median survival 26 mo	MSOF[d] (2), bile fistula (5)
Cuschieri et al (1995)[51]	15	Open and laparoscopic	2.0 (1–4)	3.0 (1.0–6.5)	—	1-year survival 48%	None
Shafir et al (1996)[52]	25	Open	4.8 (1–30)	—	14	2-year survival 65%	Overall 9% renal failure, skin or lung burns, coagulopathy
Morris and Ross (1996)[28]	121	Open	—	—	36	Median survival 800 days	Renal failure (2), abscess (1)
Adam et al (1997)[26]	25	Open	>3.0	—	16	2-year survival 52% DFS 20%	Biloma (1), bile fistula (1)
Seifert and Morris (1999)[27]	85	Open	3.4 (1–9)	3.4 (1–13)	22 (0–64)	LR 33%; 2-year DFS 16%	—

[a] Range in parentheses.
[b] CR, complete response; PR, partial response; LR, local recurrence; DFS, disease-free survival; DOD, died of disease.
[c] Hepatic artery chemotherapy.
[d] Multisystem organ failure.

described in cryotherapy, and is referred to as the cryoshock phenomenon. This is thought to be related to the volume of tumor/liver frozen and to the number of freeze–thaw cycles, and is thought to be due to cytokine release. Release of interleukin-6 (IL-6) and tumor necrosis factor α (TNF-α) has been demonstrated in an animal model following large-volume double freezing of the liver.[29] In addition, it was determined in this survey that more than 20% of patients who died following hepatic cryotherapy had an acute myocardial infarction. This may be because often patients with severe comorbidity are selected for cryotherapy since they are considered medically unfit for a liver resection. Severe intraoperative arrhythmias have been described during hepatic cryotherapy, and may be related to the cold blood returning from the liver when freezing close to the inferior vena cava or to transient hyperkalemia from lysed cells.[21] Other morbidity included cracking of the iceball, with major hemorrhage (6 patients), rebleeding (5 patients), subcapsular hematoma (2 patients), hepatic sequestration of the cryolesion (2 patients), hepatic abscess (12 patients), bile fistula or biloma (10 patients), biliary stricture (1 patient), and wound infection (4 patients).

Hepatic cryotherapy of malignant tumors has been one of the most popular and widely used ablative techniques, and, clearly, lessons learned from studying patterns of complications from its use can be applied to other ablative liver tumor techniques. Careful patient and lesion selection has decreased the risk of hepatic cryosurgery, and complications after this procedure are now unusual.

After cryoablation, most centers follow lesions sequentially with radiologic studies and serum tumor markers.[27,30] Within 1–2 weeks, evidence of necrosis is present on CT. The ablated region evolves to become a fibrous scar, which does not enhance with contrast injection. The lesion may either remain stable in size or show a gradual decrease over several months. Follow-up contrast-enhanced CT scans are usually performed to examine the liver for either local recurrence or the presence of new liver lesions. If carcinoembryonic antigen (CEA) levels are elevated prior to cryoablation, they should fall following treatment. A subsequent rise in CEA warrants further investigation. Other imaging modalities, such as whole-body PET after ^{18}F-FDG ([^{18}F]fluorodeoxyglucose) injection or functional MRI, may yet provide even more sensitive methods for evaluating treatment results (Figure 33.6). Repeat hepatic cryotherapy for recurrent or new hepatic colorectal metastases has also been shown to be safe, well tolerated, and associated with occasional prolonged disease-free survival.[31]

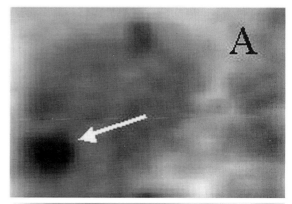

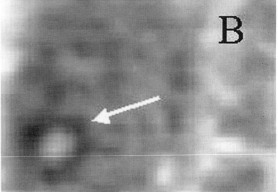

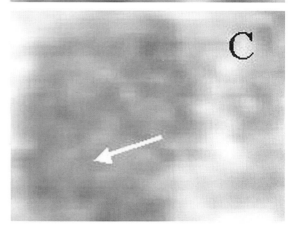

Figure 33.6 (A) PET scan shows activity at area of colorectal metastases in the liver prior to treatment. (B) PET scan of lesions following cryotherapy. There is still residual activity indicating residual tumor. (C) Following chemotherapy, residual activity has disappeared.

The advantages of cryoablation are that it is a low-morbidity technique and that it can produce larger areas of tumor destruction than can be accomplished with thermal ablation techniques. There is quite wide experience with this technique owing to its ease of use. The zone of freezing can be easily identified by the surgeon as a hyperechoic rim on ultrasound. Local recurrence rates are not well documented in the literature, but it is clear that this therapy provides a local cure in very carefully selected patients.

The disadvantage of hepatic cryoablation is that it is best performed via laparotomy or laparoscopy. There is limited experience with the percutaneous route, although reports are beginning to appear in the literature. Morbidity rates, which may have been considered high in earlier reports of hepatic cryoablation, should be low at present. This is because, as lessons learned from this and other hepatic ablative techniques become more widespread, there will be better selection of patients suitable for hepatic cryoablation.

TISSUE-DESTROYING AGENTS

Ethanol injection

Percutaneous ethanol injection (PEI) has an unclear role in the treatment of metastatic colorectal disease in the liver.[32,33] In a model of PEI of implanted tumor nodules in the liver of rabbits, tumors failed to hold sufficient ethanol for successful ablation. Following PEI of the tumor, CT images revealed that extratumoral tracking of ethanol occurred into normal parenchyma and the hepatic capsule. Histologic analysis confirmed incomplete tumor necrosis.[34] This observation is consistent with expectations, since metastases are usually harder than the surrounding liver.

Large series have established the efficacy of PEI in the treatment of hepatocellular carcinoma.[35] However, data are sparse regarding the use of PEI in metastatic liver disease. Livraghi and colleagues reported on 14 patients with 21 liver metastases 1.0–3.8 cm in diameter. Complete responses were obtained in 11 lesions (52%), 9 of which were less than 2 cm in diameter. Long-term survival data were not available in this series. Others have had less encouraging results. Amin et al[36] treated 22 metastatic colorectal cancers to the liver by PEI. None of the tumors had complete necrosis.

Unlike hepatocellular carcinoma, liver metastases are usually hypovascular, which limits the impact of ethanol-mediated endothelial damage. In addition, the lack of hepatic cirrhosis and the absence of a tumor capsule lead to failure to confine injected ethanol within the tumor. This results in decreased alcohol–tumor contact time and rapid dilution of injected ethanol. Therefore, currently, we do not recommend PEI for metastatic colorectal lesions in the liver.

The technique of hot saline injection is similar to that of PEI. A potential advantage of hot saline is its decreased toxicity as compared with ethanol. No data on the use of this modality in the treatment of metastatic colorectal cancer have been published to date.

HEPATIC ARTERY LIGATION

Hepatic artery ligation has been advocated for the treatment of liver metastases, and is based on the fact that metastases derive their principal blood supply from the hepatic artery. Many reports dating back over 25 years have retrospectively described experience with this technique.[37,38] Its effect on survival has been difficult to demonstrate because of the inability to compare groups in various studies. Following arterial ligation, revascularization is rapid from branches of the portal vein and peritoneal arteries. Therefore, the duration of the treatment effect is short-lived, and failure is frequent. This technique cannot be routinely recommended in the therapy of colorectal hepatic metastases.

HEPATIC TUMOR IRRADIATION

Ablation of hepatic metastases with high-dose interstitial irradiation has been reported. Through needles inserted into the tumor at laparotomy, 22 patients with unresectable colorectal hepatic metastases were treated with high-dose-rate iridium-192. The median actuarial local control at irradiated sites was 8 months, with a 26% actuarial local control at 26 months. Two patients had a biopsy-proven complete pathologic response.[39]

Selective internal radiation therapy with radiolabeled microspheres has undergone limited evaluation in the treatment of colorectal metastases in the liver. Gray et al[40] performed laparotomy, insertion of a catheter into the hepatic artery and embolization of yttrium-90 microspheres into unresectable colorectal liver metastases of 29 patients. In 18 of 22 evaluable patients, CT-measured tumor volumes decreased following internal radiation. In 48% of patients (10 of 22), the decrease in tumor volume was more than

Table 33.3 Comparison of ablative therapies for colorectal metastases to the liver

Parameter	Cryotherapy	Radiofrequency	Laser	Microwave
Size of lesion treatable	Moderate	Small–moderate	Moderate	Moderate
Precision of treatment	High	Moderate	Moderate	Moderate
Ease of performance	Moderate	Easy–moderate	Moderate	Moderate
Personnel	Surgeon	Surgeon/radiologist	Surgeon/radiologist	Surgeon/radiologist
Discomfort	High	Moderate	Moderate	Moderate
Anesthesia	General	Local/general	Local/general	Local/general
Cost of equipment	Moderate	Low	High	Moderate
Ease of repeat treatment	Poor	High	Poor	Moderate

50%. With this technique, calculated tumor doses of 50–100 Gy can be delivered. This initial modest response rate has also been observed in other studies.[41] There is little information available on the duration of the treatment response and whether complete responses are achieved with this technique.

A monoclonal antibody developed against CEA and labeled with iodine-131 has been evaluated in patients with colorectal hepatic metastases. Responses were not impressive, and the tumor concentration of radioactivity was not different from that of normal liver parenchyma.[42] Antibodies against other antigens and new isotopes are being evaluated further, and may prove to be of interest in the future.

CHEMOEMBOLIZATION OF HEPATIC MALIGNANCIES

A review by Tellez et al[43] summarized 19 trials evaluating chemoembolization in the treatment of patients with metastatic colorectal carcinoma. Studies have utilized lipid particles, Gelfoam, or collagen in combination with multiple chemotherapy regimens. Radiologic and biologic criteria were used to assess response. Response rates have ranged between 25% and 100%, depending on the criteria used for measurement. However, follow-up time is short in most studies and median survival is between 7 and 23 months. Chemoembolization may be useful in colorectal hepatic metastases when disease is refractory to other systemic modalities. Clinical trials comparing this therapy with other regional treatment modalities are necessary.

SUMMARY

Surgical resection remains the treatment of choice for hepatic colorectal metastases. For patients who are not candidates for surgical resection, local ablative techniques may offer alternative strategies for therapy. Several ablative techniques exist, each with its advantages and disadvantages. Most recently, radiofrequency ablation has been undergoing evaluation for treatment of hepatic malignancies. Ablative techniques can focally treat the tumor while conserving normal liver parenchyma, and therefore may increase the number of patients who are candidates for therapy.

The role of each ablative technique has yet to be defined, and a comparison of parameters involved in the utilization of each modality is listed in Table 33.3. For unresectable patients with hepatic colorectal metastases, prospective randomized trials comparing the efficacy of ablative modalities in improving local recurrence rates and survival are necessary. Individual centers lack the patient populations necessary to conduct randomized studies of sufficient power in this disease. Therefore, multicenter randomized trials need to be performed. Despite any advances in local control achieved with ablative therapies to the liver, these treatments will have to be evaluated in combination with regional and systemic treatments to give the greatest chance of improving patient survival. Continued evaluation of imaging modalities for guiding and monitoring ablative therapy requires study. Developments in PET and functional MRI may advance our ability to determine results from therapy, and may be utilized routinely in the near future.

REFERENCES

1. Fong Y, Blumgart LH, Cohen AE, Surgical resection of colorectal metastases. *CA Cancer J Clin* 1995; **45**: 50–62.

2. Kavolius J, Fong Y, Blumgart LH, Surgical resection of metastatic liver tumors. *Surg Oncol Clin North Am* 1996; **5**: 337–51.

3. Fong Y, Cohen AM, Fortner JG et al, Liver resection for colorectal metastases. *J Clin Oncol* 1997; **15**: 938–46.

4. Organ LW, Electrophysiologic principles of radiofrequency lesion making. *Appl Neurophysiol* 1976; **39**: 69–76.

5. Solbiati L, Ierace T, Goldberg SN et al, Percutaneous US-guided radio-frequency tissue ablation of liver metastases: treatment and follow up in 16 patients. *Radiology* 1997; **202**: 195–203.

6. Jiao LR, Hansen PD, Havlik R et al, Clinical short-term results of radiofrequency ablation in primary and secondary liver tumors. *Am J Surg* 1999; **177**: 303–6.

7. Rossi S, Di Stasi M, Buscarini E et al, Percutaneous RF interstitial thermal ablation in the treatment of hepatic cancer. *AJR* 1996; **167**: 759–68.

8. Curley SA, Izzo F, Delrio P et al, Radiofrequency ablation of unresectable primary and metastatic hepatic malignancies. *Ann Surg* 1999; **230**: 1–8.

9. Mazziotti A, Grazi GL, Gardini A et al, An appraisal of percutaneous treatment of liver metastases. *Liver Transplant Surg* 1998; **4**: 271–5.

10. Matthewson K, Coleridge-Smith P, O'Sullivan JP et al, Biological effects of intrahepatic neodymium: yttrium-aluminum-garnet laser photocoagulation in rats. *Gastroenterology* 1987; **93**: 550–7.

11. Steger AC, Lees WR, Walmsley K, Bown SG, Interstitial laser hyperthermia: a new approach to local destruction of tumours. *BMJ* 1989; **299**: 362–5.

12. Nolsoe CP, Torp-Pedersen S, Burcharth F et al, Interstitial hyperthermia of colorectal liver metastases with a US-guided Nd-YAG laser with a diffuser tip: a pilot clinical study. *Radiology* 1993; **187**: 333–7.

13. Amin Z, Donald JJ, Masters A et al, Hepatic metastases: interstitial laser photocoagulation with real-time US monitoring and dynamic CT evaluation of treatment. *Radiology* 1993; **187**: 339–47.

14. Vogl TJ, Muller PK, Hammerstingl R et al, Malignant liver tumors treated with MR imaging-guided laser-induced thermotherapy: technique and prospective results. *Radiology* 1995; **196**: 257–65.

15. Coughlin CT, Douple EB, Strohbehn JW et al, Interstitial hyperthermia in combination with brachytherapy. *Radiology* 1983; **148**: 285–8.

16. Seki T, Wakabayashi M, Nakagawa T et al, Ultrasonically guided percutaneous microwave coagulation therapy for small hepatocellular carcinoma. *Cancer* 1994; **74**: 817–25.

17. Shibata T, Takami M, Fujimoto T et al, Microwave tumor coagulation (MTC) in liver tumor: indication and percutaneous approach. *Gan to Kagaku Ryoho* [*Jpn J Cancer Chem*] 1994; **21**: 2128–31 (in Japanese).

18. Matsukawa T, Yamashita Y, Arakawa A et al, Percutaneous microwave coagulation therapy in liver tumors. *Acta Radiol* 1997; **38**: 410–15.

19. Bischoff J, Christov K, Rubinsky B, A morphological study of cooling rate response in normal and neoplastic human liver tissue: cryosurgical implications. *Cryobiology* 1993; **30**: 482–92.

20. Ravikumar TS, Interstitial therapies for liver tumors. *Surg Oncol Clin North Am* 1996; **5**: 365–77.

21. Seifert JK, Junginger T, Morris DL, A collective review of the world literature on hepatic cryosurgery. *J R Coll Surg Edin* 1998; **43**: 141–54.

22. Mahvi DM, Lee FT Jr, Radiofrequency ablation of hepatic malignancies: is heat better than cold? *Ann Surg* 1999; **230**: 9–11.

23. Schuder G, Pistorius G, Schneider G, Feifel G, Preliminary experience with percutaneous cryotherapy of liver tumours. *Br J Surg* 1998; **85**: 1210–11.

24. Onik GM, Atkinson D, Zemel R, Weaver ML, Cryosurgery of liver cancer. *Semin Surg Oncol* 1993; **9**: 309–17.

25. Weaver ML, Atkinson D, Zemel R, Hepatic cryosurgery in treating colorectal metastases. *Cancer* 1995; **76**: 210–14.

26. Adam R, Akpinar E, Johann M et al, Place of cryosurgery in the treatment of malignant liver tumors. *Ann Surg* 1997; **225**: 39–50.

27. Seifert JK, Morris DL, Indicators of recurrence following cryotherapy for hepatic metastases from colorectal cancer. *Br J Surg* 1999; **86**: 234–40.

28. Morris DL, Ross WD, Australian experience of cryoablation of liver tumors. *Surg Oncol Clin North Am* 1996; **5**: 391–7.

29. Seifert JK, Finlay I, Armstrong N, Morris DL, Thrombocytopenia and cytokine release following hepatic cryosurgery. *Aust NZ J Surg* 1998; **68**: 526 (abst).

30. Charnley RM, Thomas M, Morris DL, Effect of hepatic cryotherapy on serum CEA concentration in patients with multiple inoperable hepatic metastases from colorectal cancer. *Aust NZ J Surg* 1991; **61**: 55–8.

31. Seifert JK, Morris DL, Repeat hepatic cryotherapy for recurrent metastases from colorectal cancer. *Surgery* 1999; **125**: 233–5.

32. Livraghi T, Vettori C, Lazzaroni S, Liver metastases: results of percutaneous ethanol injection in 14 patients. *Radiology* 1991; **179**: 709–12.

33. Redvanly RD, Chezmar JL, Strauss RM et al, Malignant hepatic tumors: safety of high-dose percutaneous ethanol ablation therapy. *Radiology* 1993; **188**: 283–5.

34. Hahn PF, Gazelle GS, Jiang DY et al, Liver tumor ablation: real-time monitoring with dynamic CT. *Acad Radiol* 1997; **4**: 634–8.

35. Livraghi T, Bolondi L, Buscarini L et al, No treatment, resection and ethanol injection in hepatocellular carcinoma: a retrospective analysis of survival in 391 patients with cirrhosis. *J Hepatol* 1995; **22**: 522–6.

36. Amin Z, Bown SG, Lees WR, Local treatment of colorectal liver metastases: a comparison of interstitial laser photocoagulation (ILP) and percutaneous alcohol injection (PAI). *Clin Radiol* 1993; **48**: 166–71.

37. Petrelli NJ, Barcewicz PA, Evans JT et al, Hepatic artery ligation for liver metastasis in colorectal carcinoma. *Cancer* 1984; **53**: 1347–53.

38. Fortner JG, Mulcare RJ, Solis A et al, Treatment of primary and secondary liver cancer by hepatic artery ligation and infusion chemotherapy. *Ann Surg* 1973; **178**: 162–72.

39. Thomas DS, Nauta RJ, Rodgers JE et al, Intraoperative high-dose rate interstitial irradiation of hepatic metastases from colorectal carcinoma. Results of a phase I–II trial. *Cancer* 1993; **71**: 1977–81.

40. Gray BN, Anderson JE, Burton MA et al, Regression of liver metastases following treatment with yttrium-90 microspheres. *Aust NZ J Surg* 1992; **62**: 105–10.

41. Herba MJ, Illescas FF, Thirlwell MP et al, Hepatic malignancies: improved treatment with intraarterial Y-90. *Radiology* 1988; **169**: 311–14.

42. Order SE, Klein JL, Leichner PK et al, Radiolabeled antibody treatment of primary and metastatic liver malignancies. *Recent Dev Cancer Res* 1986; **100**: 307–14.

43. Tellez C, Benson AB, Lyster MT et al, Phase II trial of chemoembolization for the treatment of metastatic colorectal carcinoma to the liver and review of the literature. *Cancer* 1998; **82**: 1250–9.

44. Nagata Y, Hiraoka M, Nishimura Y et al, Clinical results of radiofrequency hyperthermia for malignant liver tumors. *Int J Radiat Oncol Biol Phys* 1997; **38**: 359–65.

45. Livraghi T, Goldberg N, Monti F et al, Saline-enhanced radio-frequency tissue ablation in the treatment of liver metastases. *Radiology* 1997; **202:** 205–10.

46. Bilchik A, Rose M, Bostick P et al, Radiofrequency ablation: A novel, minimally invasive technique with multiple applications. *Cancer J* 1999; **2:** 118 (abst).

47. Kainuma O, Asano T, Aoyama H et al, Combined therapy with radiofrequency thermal ablation and intra-arterial infusion chemotherapy for hepatic metastases from colorectal cancer. *Hepatogastroenterology* 1999; **46:** 1071–7.

48. Cuschieri A, Bracken J, Boni L, Initial experience with laparoscopic ultrasound-guided radiofrequency thermal ablation of hepatic tumours. *Endoscopy* 1999; **31:** 318–21.

49. Ravikumar TS, Kane R, Cady B et al, A 5-year study of cryosurgery in the treatment of liver tumors. *Arch Surg* 1991; **126:** 1520–4.

50. Preketes AP, Caplehorn JRM, King J et al, Effect of hepatic artery chemotherapy on survival of patients with hepatic metastases from colorectal carcinoma treated with cryotherapy. *World J Surg* 1995; **19:** 768–71.

51. Cuschieri A, Crosthwaite G, Shimi S et al, Hepatic cryotherapy for liver tumors. *Surg Endosc* 1995; **9:** 483–9.

52. Shafir M, Shapiro R, Sung M et al, Cryoablation of unresectable malignant liver tumors. *Am J Surg* 1996; **171:** 27–31.

34

Neoadjuvant treatment of colorectal liver metastases allowing resection

René Adam, Eli Avisar, Arie Ariche, Sylvie Giachetti, Daniel Azoulay, Denis Castaing, Marian Delgado, François Guinet, Francis Kunstlinger, Francis Lévi, Henri Bismuth

INTRODUCTION

The major advance in the treatment of metastatic colorectal cancer in recent years has been the increase in efficiency of chemotherapy regimens and the consequent possible change in resectability of hepatic metastases, offering a possibility of cure through a multidisciplinary approach. It is estimated that 15–20% of colorectal cancer patients present with synchronous liver metastases[1] and approximately half of the patients with colorectal tumors will experience liver failure at some point during the course of their disease.[2] In almost one-third of cases, the liver is shown at autopsy to be the only site of cancer spread.[3] This is in accordance with the 20–45% 5-year survival rate obtained with surgical resection of hepatic metastases.[4–9] Unfortunately, however, only 10–20% of patients presenting with liver metastases are amenable to curative resection.[10–12] Palliative and symptomatic treatment is commonly offered to the remaining patients, and the median survival does not exceed 15–18 months. Over the past 8 years, we have managed these patients in a protocol of neoadjuvant chemotherapy. Using a multidisciplinary approach, liver resection has been routinely reconsidered in all cases of objective response to the treatment. This chapter summarizes our experience with this approach.

PATIENTS AND METHODS

Treatment

All the patients with colorectal liver metastases who presented to Paul Brousse Hospital, Villejuif from February 1988 to September 1996 were entered into a prospective non-randomized study. Upon initial evaluation, the patients were divided in two groups according to the resectability of the liver disease. Patients with resectable disease were scheduled for surgery. The non-resectable group were treated with a neoadjuvant chemotherapy protocol. As previously described,[10] we classified the non-resectable lesions into four categories, namely, large size, poor location, multinodularity, and extrahepatic disease. The great majority of those patients were treated with intravenous chronomodulated chemotherapy with 5-fluorouracil (5-FU: 700–1200 mg/m^2/day), folinic acid (leucovorin: 300 mg/m^2/day), and oxaliplatin (25 mg/m^2/day). Each course lasted 4–5 days, with intervals of 2–3 weeks between courses. The treatment was administered in an ambulatory setting via a time/dose multichannel pump (Intelliject, Aguettant, Lyon). The rationale for this technique, which has been described elsewhere,[13] is to optimize dose intensities and tolerance of the drugs by a treatment that is modulated in a sinusoidal fashion with a 24-hour period with peak flow rates at 04.00 hours for 5-FU and folinic acid and at 16.00 hours for oxaliplatin (Figure 34.1). Evaluation for objective response was performed with ultrasound and abdominal computed tomography (CT) scan every three treatments, by the same radiology team. Biochemical criteria of response included decreased carcinoembryonic antigen (CEA) and CA19-9 levels. Reconsideration for resection followed each evaluation. The criteria for surgery consisted of the feasibility of a curative resection (be it in one or two stages), coupled with a plateau in the response to chemotherapy. Different surgical techniques were used to enable the resection. These techniques included portal vein embolization to hypertrophy the remaining liver, as described elsewhere,[14] two-stage hepatectomies when all the lesions could not be resected by a single

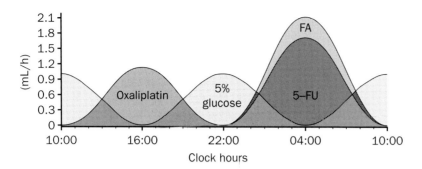

Figure 34.1 Chronomodulated infusion of 5-fluorouracil (5-FU), folinic acid (leucovorin, FA), and oxaliplatin.

procedure, and cryotherapy, usually combined with surgery, to allow for a complete treatment of tumours, in patients otherwise unresectable. All the patients treated surgically after neoadjuvant chemotherapy received additional chemotherapy according to the same protocol for 6 months after the resection. The treatment was then discontinued in stable patients with no evidence of disease. Follow-up was performed every 3 months, with physical examination, ultrasound, CEA, and CA19-9. In addition, a CT scan of the chest and abdomen was performed every 6 months. Recurrent disease was treated according to the same protocol again, with reoperation (when feasible) or chemotherapy. All the demographic, clinical, surgical, radiological, and biochemical patient information was entered in a database that served to assess the results of our treatment.

Survival analysis

Survival rates from surgery were calculated according to the Kaplan–Meier actuarial survival technique. Also, the true 5-year survival rate was calculated from the onset of chemotherapy, to maintain uniformity with the oncological literature, for those patients who completed 5 years of follow-up.

RESULTS

Resectability rate

This study enrolled 872 patients. Of these, 171 (20%) had a curative resection, while the remaining 701 were considered non-resectable and were treated with our protocol of neoadjuvant chemotherapy. Of these latter patients, 95 (14%) achieved a measurable response sufficiently important to allow subsequent, and potentially curative, resection (Figure 34.2). Thus

neoadjuvant chemotherapy was able to increase the tumour resectability rate from 20% (171/872) to 30% (266/872). The main cause of initial non-resectability was multinodularity of liver metastases (48 patients), followed by concomitant extrahepatic tumours (26 patients), large tumours (10 patients) or poorly located liver tumours (9 patients).

Duration and effects of neoadjuvant chemotherapy

The patients who became resectable received 3–29 courses of chemotherapy (mean 10 courses), over

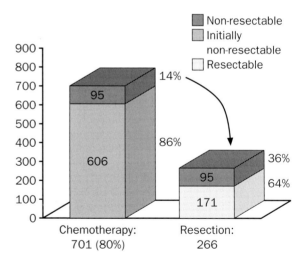

Figure 34.2 Resectability of colorectal liver metastases following neoadjuvant chemotherapy at the Paul Brousse Hospital (1988–1996). Of 872 patients, 171 were initially resectable, and had a curative resection; of the 701 initially non-resectable patients, 95 became resectable following neoadjuvant treatment and underwent a potentially curative resection.

3–29 months (mean 10.6 months). An objective reduction in tumour size following chemotherapy was observed in all patients who subsequently underwent liver resection. A significant reduction in tumour markers was also demonstrated: mean CEA levels fell from 190 (range 1–4225) to 47 (range 1–1243) ng/ml and CA19-9 levels from 4477 (range 22–228 000) to 219 (range 2–5900) IU/ml.

Perioperative procedures used to allow resection or radicality

Portal vein embolization or ligation was performed in 9 patients (9%). Cryotherapy combined with liver resection was used in 11 patients. All visible extra-hepatic disease was resected at the same time or during a second operation. Accordingly, 12 patients had concomitant resection of tumour localizations in the abdominal cavity (omentum, peritoneum, lymph nodes, primary recurrence), and 20 underwent resection of pulmonary metastases diagnosed either at the time of hepatic metastases or thereafter. Five patients had a two-stage resection (5%).

Mortality and morbidity

There was no perioperative mortality during the first 30 days after surgery. Twenty-two (23%) complications were recorded: 2 postoperative hemorrhages requiring a laparotomy, 4 infected and 8 sterile fluid collections treated non-operatively, 4 transient biliary fistulas, and 4 systemic complications (Table 34.1).

Table 34.1 Complications of surgery: 22 out of 95 cases (23%)

- 4 biliary leaks
- 2 reoperations for bleeding
- 4 infected collections (percutaneous drainage)
- 8 fluid collections (spontaneous resolution)
- 4 systemic complications

Survival

The actuarial 5-year survival rate for the overall group is 34%, from the time of liver resection (Figure 34.3). When divided into the different categories of non-resectability, the 5-year survival rate is 60% for large lesions, 49% for poorly located tumours, 34% for multinodular disease, and 18% for extrahepatic disease.

Eighty-seven patients have completed 5 years of follow-up. Thirty-four patients (39%) are alive 5 years after the onset of chemotherapy (Figure 34.4), of whom 19 have no evidence of disease (22%).

With regard to extrahepatic disease at the time of liver metastases, a marked difference in survival was found for different extrahepatic locations. While solid-organ (liver, lung, adrenal glands, ovary) resectable disease is associated with a 5-year survival rate of 36%, lymph-node disease carries a dismal prognosis (Table 34.2).

A complete pathological response was found in 6 of 95 patients (6%). Five of these patients (83%) are alive at a mean follow-up of 5.7 years (range 4.7–7.9

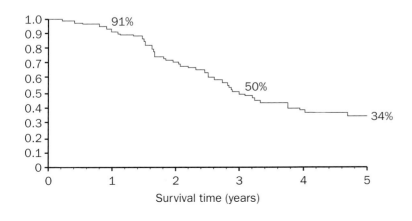

Figure 34.3 Actuarial survival of resection of initially non-resectable liver metastases after neoadjuvant chemotherapy for all 95 patients.

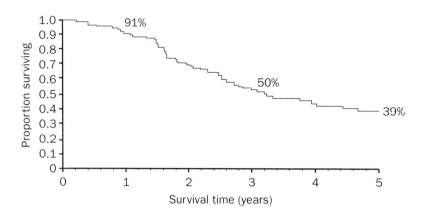

Figure 34.4 Survival of resection of initially non-resectable liver metastases after neoadjuvant chemotherapy for the 87 patients who have completed 5 years of follow-up.

Table 34.2 Extrahepatic disease by site

Site	No. of cases	5-year survival rate (%)
Lungs	10	30
Peritoneum	6	33
Lymph nodes	3	0
Ovaries	2	50
Adrenal	1	100
Multiple	9	33

Table 34.3 Complete pathological response: 6 out of 95 patients (6.3%)

• Mean follow-up	5.7 years
• Overall survival	5/6 (83%)
• Disease-free survival	3/6 (50%)

years). Three patients (50%) have no evidence of disease (Table 34.3).

DISCUSSION

Surgical resection is the only effective treatment for hepatic metastases of colorectal cancer. However, this option is available only to a minority of patients. For the majority, where surgery is not a curative option, only palliative therapy is available, resulting in no long-term survivors. The reasons for unre-

sectability can be divided into two categories, diffuse extrahepatic disease that would not be controlled by treatment of the liver disease and intrahepatic disease that would endanger the patient's life if resected. In the vast majority of cases, no available form of systemic therapy can effectively eradicate diffuse metastatic disease, but a partial response to chemotherapy could be used to downstage the liver disease, which would then be amenable to a surgical resection. This approach has been used in a limited number of patients after either systemic[15] or intra-arterial hepatic chemotherapy.[16] In a selected number of cases, the same logic can be applied to a limited amount of extrahepatic disease, which could also be resected after initial chemotherapy. The combination of 5-FU, folinic acid, and oxaliplatin has recently been shown to have a response rate of 59%.[17] Oxaliplatin is a recently developed platinum derivative with no nephrotoxicity and good activity against colorectal tumours.[18] Chronomodulation of the therapy enables the delivery of higher concentrations of these agents, with a higher tolerance rate and fewer complications.[19–21] The most significant decrease in complications concerns severe stomatitis, which was shown in a randomized trial to drop from 89% to 18%.[22] In another recent multicentre trial, chronotherapy reduced fivefold the rate of severe mucosal toxicity, halved the incidence of functional impairment from peripheral sensory neuropathy, and increased the response rate from 29% to 51%.[23]

Our results with neoadjuvant chemotherapy for colorectal liver metastases were previously published for a smaller number of patients and a shorter follow-up.[10] In this series, we have shown a 14% rate of conversion from unresectability to resectability with a curative potential. If calculated for the whole group of 872 patients, neoadjuvant chemotherapy was able to increase the tumour resectability rate from 20% to 30%. This increased number of curative resections was accompanied by a 'reasonable' complication rate and a 5-year survival rate of 34%, which is in the range of the survival rates with initially resectable lesions. It is noteworthy that surgery in these patients aims at a real strategy of tumour eradication, should metastases be located in the liver or at extrahepatic sites.

In this study, we also included patients who failed first-line chemotherapy and entered the protocol as a second or third line of treatment. Such patients have a more limited chance of their tumours becoming resectable after neoadjuvant treatment. It seems logical to assume that the resectability rate after treatment would have been higher had only patients treated for the first time been included.

As expected from the nature of the disease, patients with multinodular lesions had a worse prognosis, and were more likely to require more than one operation and additional procedures such as portal vein embolization or cryotherapy. Almost 30% of the patients in this series required a repeated liver resection.

The actuarial survival rates after surgery (34%) and the true survival rates from the onset of chemotherapy (39%) are very similar, despite an average of 10 months of neoadjuvant treatment. This is in agreement with the flattening of the survival curves after 3–4 years, indicating a plateau pattern in long-term survival.

Extrahepatic disease has commonly been a reason for a nihilistic approach. Some reports, however, were able to demonstrate a reasonable 5-year survival for concomitant hepatic and pulmonary involvement, provided that the disease is resectable.[24,25] Our results concur with these findings, showing a survival rate of 36% in those patients with resectable extrahepatic disease in solid organs (lung, ovary, adrenal glands). The use of neoadjuvant therapy may help to define those tumours that will benefit from an attempt to eradicate the disease. On the other hand, the survival rate is only 18% when extrahepatic disease is the main cause of non-resectability, and our findings do not support an aggressive approach in trying to resect lymphatic disease.

This series suffers from the limitations of a non-randomized prospective study; however, it would have been unethical to exclude the potential benefit of surgery combined with chemotherapy from a control arm.

Only six patients were found to have a pathological complete response, but those patients had an excellent survival. The assessment of clinical response by ultrasound was not able to accurately predict the pathological responders because of residual scarring and fibrosis at the site of the lesions, which is not echographically different than viable tumour. On the other hand, complete ultrasound resolution of the lesions, when it did (rarely) occur, did not correlate with disappearance of viable cancer cells. All this explains why it is reasonable to propose a liver resection to all patients who become technically resectable, even when the residual hepatic disease seems limited and possibly non-active.

In conclusion, hepatic resection after tumour response to chemotherapy can provide a significant hope for long-term survival. The survival pattern is very similar to that of primarily resected patients. Further analysis is required to better define the subset of patients who are most likely to benefit from this approach.

REFERENCES

1. Fong Y, Kemeny N, Paty P et al, Treatment of colorectal cancer hepatic metastasis. *Semin Surg Oncol* 1996; **12:** 219–52.
2. Steele G Jr, Ravikumar TS, Resection of hepatic metastases from colorectal cancer; biologic perspectives. *Ann Surg* 1989; **210:** 127–38.
3. Weiss L, Grundmann E, Torhorst J et al, Hematogenous metastatic patterns in colonic carcinoma: an analysis of 1541 necropsies. *J Pathol* 1986; **150:** 195–203.
4. Fortner JG, Silva JS, Golbey RB et al, Multi-variate analysis of a personal series of 247 consecutive patients with liver metastases from colorectal cancer. *Ann Surg* 1984; **199:** 306–16.
5. Adson MA, Van Heerden JA, Adson MH et al, Resection of hepatic metastases from colorectal cancer. *Arch Surg* 1984; **119:** 647–51.
6. Hughes KS, Simon R, Songhorabodi S et al, Resection of the liver for colorectal carcinoma metastases: a multi-institutional study of indications for resection. *Surgery* 1988; **103:** 278–88.
7. Nordlinger B, Jaeck D, Guiguet M et al, *Traitement des Metastases Hepatiques des Cancers Colorectaux.* Monographies de l'Association Francaise de Chirurgie (AFC). Paris: Springer-Verlag, 1992: 129–46.
8. Scheele J, Stang R, Altendorf-Hofmann A et al, Resection of colorectal liver metastases. *World J Surg* 1995; **19:** 59–71.
9. Fong Y, Cohen A, Fortner JG et al, Liver resection for colorectal metastases. *J Clin Oncol* 1997; **15:** 938–46.
10. Bismuth H, Adam R, Levi F et al, Resection of nonresectable liver metastases from colorectal cancer after neoadjuvant chemotherapy. *Ann Surg* 1996; **224:** 509–22.
11. Adson MA, Resection of liver metastases. When is it worthwhile? *World J Surg* 1987; **11:** 511–20.
12. Doci R, Gennari L, Bignami P et al, One hundred patients with hepatic metastases from colorectal cancer treated by resection: analysis of prognostic determinants. *Br J Surg* 1991; **78:** 797–801.
13. Lévi F, Misset JL, Brienza S et al, A chronopharmacologic phase II clinical trial with 5-fluorouracil, folinic acid and oxaloplatin using an ambulatory multichannel programmable pump. *Cancer* 1992; **69:** 893–900.
14. Azoulay D, Raccuia JS, Castaing D et al, Right portal vein embolization in preparation for major hepatic resection. *J Am*

Coll Surg 1995; **181:** 267–9.

15. Fowler WC, Eisenberg BL, Hofflan JP, Hepatic resection following systemic chemotherapy for metastatic colorectal carcinoma. *J Surg Oncol* 1992; **51:** 122–5.

16. Elias D, Lasser Ph, Rougier Ph et al, Frequency, technical aspects, resultants, and indications of major hepatectomy after prolonged intra-arterial hepatic chemotherapy for initially unresectable hepatic tumors. *J Am Coll Surg* 1995; **180:** 213–19.

17. Giachetti S, Itzhaki M, Gruia G et al, Long term survival of patients with unresectable colorectal cancer liver metastases following infusional chemotherapy with 5-fluorouracil, leucovorin, oxaliplatin and surgery. *Ann Oncol* 1999; **10:** 663–9.

18. Becouarn Y, Ychou M, Ducreux M et al, Oxaloplatin (L-OHP) as first line chemotherapy in metastatic colorectal cancer (MRC) patients: preliminary activity/toxicity report. *Proc Am Soc Clin Oncol* 1997; **6:** 299A (Abst 804).

19. Lévi F, Giacchetti S, Adam R et al, Chronomodulation of chemotherapy against metastatic colorectal cancer. *Eur J Cancer* 1995; **31A:** 1264–70.

20. Lévi F, Zidani R, Brienza S et al, A multicenter evaluation of intensified ambulatory chronomodulated chemotherapy with oxaliplatin, 5-fluorouracil and leucovorin as initial treatment of patients with metastatic colorectal carcinoma. *Cancer* 1999; **85:** 2532–40.

21. Bertheault-Cvitkovic F, Jami A, Ithzaki M et al, Bi weekly intensified ambulatory chronomodulated chemotherapy with oxaloplatin, 5-fluorouracil and folinic acid in patients with metastatic colorectal cancer. *J Clin Oncol* 1996; **14:** 2950–8.

22. Lévi F, Zidani R, Vannetzel JM et al, Chronomodulated versus fixed-infusion-rate delivery of ambulatory chemotherapy with oxaliplatin, fluorouracil and folinic acid (leucovorin) in patients with colorectal cancer metastases: a randomized multi-institutional trial. *J Natl Cancer Inst* 1994; **86:** 1608–17.

23. Lévi F, Zidani R, Misset JL et al, Randomised multicentre trial of chronotherapy with oxaliplatin, fluorouracil, and folinic acid in metastatic colorectal cancer. *Lancet* 1997; **350:** 681–6.

24. Murata S, Moriya Y, Akasu T et al, Resection of both hepatic and pulmonary metastases in patients with colorectal carcinoma. *Cancer* 1998; **83:** 1086–93.

25. Regnard JF, Grunenwald D, Spaggiari L et al, Surgical treatment of hepatic and pulmonary metastases from colorectal cancers. *Ann Thorac Surg* 1998; **66:** 214–19.

35

Adjuvant chemotherapy after hepatic resection for metastatic colorectal carcinoma

Nancy Kemeny, Don S Dizon

INTRODUCTION

Colorectal cancer is the second leading cause of cancer-related deaths in the USA and Europe. Sixty percent of patients diagnosed with colorectal cancer go on to develop hepatic metastases.[1] In as many as 30%, the liver will be the only site of disease. In general, the liver is a frequent site of metastatic involvement by a variety of tumors, including breast, colon, lung, stomach, and pancreas. In the cases of colorectal cancer, drainage of the gastrointestinal tract by the portal system to the liver provides a physiologic rationale for hepatic metastasis.

Traditionally, the average survival for patients with untreated hepatic metastases from colorectal cancer has been approximately 4–9 months.[5] In one series, less than 3% were alive at 3 years.[2] Systemic chemotherapy with fluoropyrimidines achieves a response rate between 15% and 30%, but median survival is approximately 1 year. Combination of new agents such as irinotecan (CPT-11) or oxaliplatin with 5-fluorouracil (5-FU) has produced higher response rates, but generally less than 20% of patients are alive at 2 years.[3–8] Overall, the median survival time for patients with hepatic metastases is between 6 and 12 months, and, in the presence of significant involvement, it drops to less than 6 months, with no reported 5-year survivors.[9–14] Given these rather poor response rates, other modalities of therapy have been investigated, including the role of liver resection and regional therapy.

For patients undergoing liver resection, poor prognostic factors have been investigated in two large trials.[15,16] These include: (1) four or more liver metastases; (2) large liver lesions, 5 cm or greater; (3) age of 60 years or more; (4) invasion of serosa by the primary tumor; and (5) early recurrence in the liver, defined as less than 2 years between primary resection and hepatic recurrence. In the presence of three or four factors, the overall survival rate at 2 years is 60%, and with five or six factors, it drops to 43%.[16] This may be due to the presence of micrometastatic disease at the time of resection. In one report, approximately 35% of liver specimens examined after resection had micrometastases.[17]

The refinement of surgical technique and the delineation of the segmental anatomy of the liver have made liver resection much more effective and safer. Through the use of stringent criteria for patient selection, it has proven to be the most effective means for long-term survival in the setting of hepatic metastasis from a colon or rectal primary. Multiple studies have consistently reported a median survival of 24 months following resection.[18–22] The 3-year survival rate following resection approximates 40% and the 5-year survival rate ranges between 25% and 40%. In addition, as many as 20% of patients achieve 10-year survival.[23–25] Thus, for patients with liver metastases amenable to resection, this is the most appropriate treatment. Still, 75% of patients who undergo hepatic resection experience recurrent metastases within 2 years, and approximately half recur in the liver.[3,25–28]

The utility of systemic chemotherapy in the adjuvant setting following hepatic resection of metastatic colorectal cancer has never been subjected to a randomized trial. Thus, the role of this modality remains unclear. In the chemotherapy-naive patient, fluoropyrimidine-based regimens are considered the standard of care. Otherwise, expectant observation has been recommended and further chemotherapy has usually not been offered.

RATIONALE FOR HEPATIC ARTERIAL INFUSION IN THE ADJUVANT SETTING

Colorectal cancers metastasize to the liver via the portal circulation. However, their blood supply evolves and changes as they grow.[29,30] Initially, they are dependent on surrounding vessels, relying on diffusion from these surrounding vessels to survive. Once they grow beyond 3 mm angiogenesis enables them to form their own system for the supply of blood, which they draw from the arterial circulation. This contrasts sharply to normal hepatocytes, which continue to receive blood flow via the portal circulation. With hepatic resection of liver metastases, residual disease, if present, may be 2–3 mm in diameter, and therefore derive its predominant blood supply from the hepatic artery. By direct infusion of chemotherapy into the hepatic artery (hepatic arterial infusion, HAI), a larger concentration of drug would then be targeted to any residual tumor.

INTRA-ARTERIAL PUMP PLACEMENT

Historically HAI was administered via hepatic arterial pump. Although this was shown to be effective, catheter-associated problems, including clotting, hepatic artery thrombosis, and duodenal ulcers, led physicians to abandon the procedure. Totally implantable pump devices have made infusion much safer. In addition to providing long-term access to the hepatic arterial flow, patency has been well maintained and the incidence of infection reduced. Yasuda et al[31] reported on the patency of catheters and the ability to administer chemotherapy in three different styles: by surgically placed arterial catheters, by percutaneously placed catheters, and by reservoir placement done surgically. They reported that implantation of the reservoir afforded the most chemotherapy administered, with 115 days, as opposed to 31 days for the surgical catheter and 25 days for the percutaneously placed catheters.

MEDICATIONS

The ideal agent for HAI is one that is extracted in significant concentration by the liver. In addition, a short half-life and high total-body clearance are important in order to diminish entry of significant drug concentrations into the systemic circulation. Based on work done by Ensminger and colleagues, floxuridine (5-fluoro-2′-deoxyuridine, FUDR) would be an ideal agent since it has a 94–99% extraction rate

by the liver during the first-pass effect.[32] This contrasts well with 5-FU, where only between 19% and 55% of the drug is extracted. Other chemotherapeutic agents studied are reviewed in Chapter 38.

Dexamethasone was used to decrease periportal inflammation in order to decrease the incidence of hepatic toxicity. A randomized trial of FUDR plus dexamethasone versus FUDR alone conducted by Kemeny et al[33] revealed a trend towards lower bilirubin levels in the patients treated with FUDR plus dexamethasone compared with those receiving FUDR alone: 9% versus 30%, respectively ($p = 0.07$). Interestingly, the response rate was improved in the group receiving FUDR plus dexamethasone over the group treated with FUDR alone: 71% versus 43%, respectively ($p = 0.03$). In addition, survival was improved in the FUDR-plus-dexamethasone group: 23 months versus 15 months. These results support the use of FUDR and dexamethasone in hepatic arterial infusion.

TRIALS

There have been eight randomized trials looking at the use of HAI of chemotherapy in colorectal cancer with non-resectable liver metastases. Response rates with HAI ranged from 42% to 62%, compared with systemic therapy, which achieved response rates between 10% and 21%.[34–41] A recent meta-analysis[42] confirmed that the response rate with HAI FUDR was statistically increased over that with systemic 5-FU: 41% versus 14%, respectively. In addition, despite crossover in many of these trials, an increase in survival was seen: 16 months in the HAI FUDR group versus 13 months in the systemic group.

Although hepatic resection for liver metastases is the standard of care, nearly two-thirds of patients who undergo resection will recur within a year. In approximately 50%, the relapse will be in the remaining liver due to microscopic residual disease undetected at the time of resection. Given the benefit gained with HAI therapy in the metastatic setting, the use of HAI as adjuvant therapy is appropriate.

Single-arm studies have reported on the feasibility of adjuvant therapy administered via HAI. Moriya et al[43] studied the use of intra-arterial 5-FU and mitomycin C and oral 1-hexylcarbamoyl-5-fluorouracil (HCFU) after hepatic resection for colorectal metastasis in 16 patients. The recurrence rate was 31%. In patients with solitary hepatic lesions, no recurrence was seen; in patients with multiple hepatic lesions, the recurrence rate was 45%. The incidence of chemical sclerosing cholangitis was reported to be 19%. Curley et al[44] treated 20 consecutive patients after curative hepatic resection with weekly bolus 5-FU via HAI ports. At a median of 33 months, 50% had recurrence, with 17% developing isolated hepatic recurrence. In the half of evaluable patients without recurrence, the median survival was 39 months. Eight patients had therapy stopped early because of 5-FU toxicity (4 patients), hepatic arterial thrombosis (1 patient), and irreversible port or catheter occlusion (3 patients). Comparing these results with historic controls, an apparent survival advantage was suggested. In a Japanese study, 31 of 57 patients who underwent hepatic resection were treated with HAI of 5-FU, mitomycin C, and either doxorubicin or epirubicin.[45] The 3- and 5-year survival rates were 57% and 57%, with an improved 5-year survival rate compared with the cohort treated with hepatectomy alone (23%).

RANDOMIZED TRIALS

Memorial Sloan-Kettering Cancer Center

Kemeny et al[46] reported the results of a randomized trial of HAI FUDR plus dexamethasone and systemic administration of 5-FU with or without leucovorin (LV), compared with systemic chemotherapy alone after the resection of hepatic metastases. The endpoints of the study were overall survival, survival free of hepatic progression, and overall progression-free survival at 2 years. This study enrolled 156 patients, 27% of whom had more than four hepatic lesions. Treatment in the HAI plus systemic therapy ('HAI + systemic') arm consisted of 5-FU 320 mg/m^2 and LV 200 mg/m^2 followed by HAI FUDR and dexamethasone, initiated 2 weeks after systemic therapy. Patients received pump infusion for 14 days, after which the pump was emptied and the patient given 1 week of rest before the re-initiation of systemic therapy. In the systemic-therapy ('systemic') arm 5-FU was administered at 375 mg/m^2 with the same dose of LV for 5 days every 4 weeks. A total of six cycles were scheduled for each group. In patients previously treated with 5-FU and LV, 5-FU was administered as a continuous infusion at a dose of 850 mg/m^2 in the HAI group and 1000 mg/m^2 in the systemic group.

Patients were stratified according to the number of liver metastases (1, 2–4, or >4) and type of chemotherapy (none, 5-FU with or without levamisole, or 5-FU with or without LV). Numerous other parameters were compared as well, as summarized in Table 35.1.

The actuarial survival rate at 2 years was signifi-

cantly increased with combined-modality therapy (86% versus 72%, $p = 0.03$). Univariate analysis showed an unadjusted risk ratio of 2.13 for death in the systemic group compared with the HAI + systemic group. Additionally, increased survival was seen with the HAI + systemic group: 72.2 months, as opposed to 59.3 months in the systemic group. After adjustment for location of the primary tumor and lesions 5 cm or larger, the risk ratio for death in the systemic group compared with the HAI + systemic group was statistically significant, at 2.34 ($p = 0.027$). Hepatic recurrence was also much decreased in the patients treated with HAI plus systemic therapy. Comparing the HAI + systemic arm with the systemic arm, the actuarial rates of survival free from hepatic recurrence at 2 years were 90% and 60%, respectively. Median time free from hepatic recurrence has not been reached in the HAI + systemic arm, but was reported at 42.7 months in the systemic arm. The overall progression-free survival rate at 2 years was 57% in the HAI + systemic group and 42% in the systemic group. While equivalent numbers of patients in each group progressed in the lungs (15 patients in the HAI + systemic group versus 17 patients in the systemic group), 7 patients and 30 patients, respectively, progressed in the liver. Hepatic recurrence was documented in 4 patients in the HAI + systemic arm and 1 patient in the systemic arm.

The numbers of deaths were similar: 5 deaths were reported prior to initiation of therapy, 2 in the HAI + systemic group and 3 in the systemic group. During treatment, 3 deaths occurred: one in the HAI + systemic group and two in the systemic group during treatment.

More patients in the HAI + systemic group compared with the systemic group experienced diarrhea (29% versus 14%) and nausea (10% and 5%). Twenty-nine patients required hospitalization in the HAI + systemic arm, compared with 18 patients in the systemic arm.

Hepatic enzyme elevations occurred in the following: 29% had a doubling of the serum alkaline phosphatase, 65% had a tripling of the aspartate aminotransferase levels, and 18% had increases in their serum bilirubin to more than 3.0 mg/dl.[37] Biliary abnormalities returned to normal in all but four patients who required biliary stents. Two patients in the systemic group required biliary stents.

City of Hope, Los Angeles, CA

This was a small series of 100 patients undergoing potential hepatic resection for colorectal metastases.[47]

Table 35.1 Baseline characteristics of patients from the Kemeny trial[37]

Characteristic	Combined-therapy group (74 patients)	Monotherapy group (82 patients)
Age: median (range)	59 years (28–79 years)	59 years (30–77 years)
Sex: male/female	44 (59%)/30 (41%)	47 (57%)/35 (43%)
Karnofsky score: median (range)	90 (70–100)	90 (70–100)
% liver involvement: median (range)	20 (5–50)	20 (10–60)
Lactate dehydrogenase (LDH): median (range)	182 U/l (105–1104 U/l)	197 U/l (110–1398 U/l)
Serum aspartate aminotransferase (AST, SGOT): median (range)	84 U/l (42–238 U/l)	86 U/l (31–276 U/l)
Serum total bilirubin: median (range)	0.5 mg/dl (0.2–4.0 mg/dl)	0.6 mg/dl (0.2–4.0 mg/dl)
No. of liver metastases:		
1	27 (36%)	33 (40%)
2–4	33 (45%)	34 (41%)
>4	14 (19%)	15 (18%)
Type of disease:		
Synchronous	23 (31%)	27 (33%)
Metachronous	51 (69%)	55 (67%)
Positive surgical margins	10 (14%)	11 (13%)
Prior treatment:		
None	35 (47%)	37 (45%)
Adjuvant chemotherapy	29 (39%)	33 (40%)
Chemotherapy for metastases	10 (14%)	12 (15%)
5-FU and leucovorin	16 (22%)	19 (23%)

Patients were divided into three groups based on their degree of hepatic involvement. Group A comprised 8 patients with solitary liver lesions: 5 patients were treated with adjuvant HAI; the other 3 were observed after hepatic resection. In group B, patients with multiple resectable hepatic metastases were randomized to hepatic resection and HAI (10 patients) versus HAI alone (12 patients). In group C, non-resectable patients with positive portal lymph nodes were treated with HAI. In group D, patients with unresectable disease were randomized to either HAI of FUDR or systemic 5-FU. It was found that partial responses were achievable with HAI FUDR, even in the presence of unresectable disease. In this small trial, 52% of patients with unresectable disease had at least a partial response.

An update of the study revealed that in group A, the time to treatment failure was significantly increased in the group receiving HAI following resection (A1) compared with the group who underwent resection only (A2): 31 months versus 9 months, respectively ($p < 0.003$).[48] In group B, the 5-year survival rate also favored adjuvant therapy over resection alone (30% versus 7%, respectively). Therefore, HAI following resection seemed to improve results after hepatic resection. However, the effect on overall survival was not reported.

German Cooperative on Liver Metastases

The German Cooperative on Liver Metastases performed a multicenter randomized trial of hepatic resection versus hepatic resection and adjuvant HAI with 5-FU and LV.[49] Patients were enrolled in 26 centers in Germany and Switzerland. All patients were stratified according to number of liver metastases (1–2 or 3–6) and the site of the primary tumor (colon or upper rectum, or mid or lower rectum). Each group comprised 113 patients.

Despite the initial randomization, 24 patients (21%) in the HAI arm and 18 patients (16%) in the control group did not receive the assigned treatment. In the group randomized to adjuvant treatment, it was not performed for the following reasons: anatomic variants, documentation of extrahepatic disease at time of surgery, technical complications with port placement, and patient refusal after randomization. In the group randomized to resection alone, reasons for not following the randomized assignment were unresectable disease, microscopic residual disease, and extrahepatic disease. In the control group, 3 patients received HAI 5-FU/LV and 10 received palliative systemic chemotherapy. Therefore, at the start of the trial, 87 (77%) were actually treated in the group receiving HAI and systemic therapy and 114 patients in the control group.

At the 18-month interim analysis, the relapse rate was 33% in patients receiving adjuvant therapy and 36.7% in patients treated with resection alone. No survival advantage was seen, and the median survival time was reported as 34.5 months in the HAI group versus 40.8 months in the control group ($p = 0.1519$). In addition, an increased risk of death by intention to treat with HAI was observed.

In the secondary analysis comparing the group who actually received treatment (87 patients) with the group receiving no adjuvant therapy (114 patients), the median survival was lengthened: 44.8 months versus 39.7 months, respectively. The median survival time to liver progression doubled in the group receiving HAI 5-FU/LV as compared with the control group: 44.8 months versus 23.3 months. Finally, the median time to progression of disease or death was increased in the group receiving adjuvant HAI 5-FU/LV: 20 months versus 12.6 months.

The results of this randomized trial must be interpreted with caution. Of the 113 patients randomized, 73 (64.6%) had chemotherapy data available, and only 34 (30%) patients completed the assigned protocol. This suggests that the power to detect a difference, even with an intention-to-treat analysis, was not adequate, given that the majority of patients did not receive their assigned treatment.

Eastern Cooperative Oncology Group/Southwest Oncology Group

The Eastern Cooperative Oncology Group (ECOG) and Southwest Oncology Group (SWOG) conducted a prospective randomized multicenter trial of hepatic resection alone versus resection followed by four cycles of HAI with FUDR and 12 cycles of systemic infusional 5-FU.[50] Only patients with three or less hepatic metastases from colorectal cancer were enrolled. One hundred and ten patients were randomized preoperatively. A trend towards increased survival was seen, with a 63% 5-year survival rate with HAI plus systemic therapy versus 32% in the control group. The 3-year recurrence-free rate was significantly greater with combined-modality therapy compared with resection alone: 58% and 34%, respectively ($p = 0.039$). In addition, less involvement of the liver with hepatic recurrence was noted in the group receiving HAI plus systemic therapy (8 cases) compared with the control group (24 cases) ($p = 0.035$). The overall median survival was not significantly different in the group treated with HAI and systemic therapy (47.5 months) from that in the group that underwent resection alone (34.2 months). However, 11 of 56 patients (19.6%) in the control group and 21 of 54 patients (38.8%) in the HAI plus systemic treatment group ultimately were withdrawn from the study owing to operative findings of more than three liver metastases, extrahepatic disease, or no evidence of liver metastases. The authors concluded that although no overall survival benefit had yet been demonstrated in the interim analysis, a trend towards increased survival was already apparent in the chemotherapy-treated patients.

NEOADJUVANT CHEMOTHERAPY

A fairly new concept in the treatment of unresectable liver metastases from colorectal cancer is to administer chemotherapy in the neoadjuvant setting. The intent is to downsize the tumor with chemotherapy and proceed with hepatic resection. This has not been tested in a randomized prospective trial, but the results of a retrospective analysis have been presented and the results appear promising.

Giacchetti et al[51] retrospectively reviewed 389 patients with metastatic colorectal cancer treated with 5-FU, LV, and oxaliplatin, a new platinum compound that lacks renal toxicity and has been shown to be active against colon cancer. Of these, 151 patients met criteria for unresectable liver-only metastases. The criteria used to define unresectability were: (1) more than four liver metastases (30%); (2) a single tumor larger than 5 cm (34%); (3) tumor in both hepatic lobes; (4) invasion of the intrahepatic vascular structures; (5) a high percentage of liver involvement (over 25% liver involvement in 48%). Of the 151 patients, 77 (51%) became resectable, with 58 able to undergo complete resections.

For the 77 resectable patients, the median survival was 48 months. The 58 patients undergoing complete resections have not reached median survival; the 5- and 7-year survival rates are 58% and 50%, respectively. The progression-free survival was 17 months for the 77 resectable patients. Of the completely resected patients, 72% had relapsed within a median of 12 months and 35 (60%) had extrahepatic recurrence. For those patients who remained unresectable, 25% were alive at 2 years. Multivariate regression analysis showed that number of metastases (four or less) and the interval between chemotherapy onset and surgery (6 months or less) impacted on the achievement of a complete remission.

Although encouraging, these results were obtained through a retrospective analysis using criteria for unresectability that are not universally accepted. Therefore, a prospective trial is needed to determine whether or not this is an acceptable form of therapy. Such a trial is underway at the Mayo Clinic, enrolling patients considered unresectable owing to: (1) involvement of all three major hepatic veins, the portal vein bifurcation, or the retrohepatic vena cava; (2) involvement of the main right or main left portal vein and the main hepatic vein of the opposite lobe; (3) disease requiring more than a right or left trisegmentectomy; or (4) six or more metastatic lesions distributed diffusely in both lobes of the liver. In the presence of any of the above, the patients will be treated with 5-FU, LV, and oxaliplatin. They will be reevaluated for resectability if they respond.

Given that no other prospective data are available regarding neoadjuvant therapy, such an approach should be considered investigational and only undertaken in the context of a clinical trial.

CONCLUSIONS

Hepatic arterial infusion after hepatic resection has been shown to be a successful modality to achieve disease control. In addition, on the basis of the collected experience of hepatic arterial infusion in the treatment of hepatic metastases from colorectal cancer, the placement of hepatic arterial pumps can be done safely with low operative mortality. By being aware of the potential side-effects of pump therapy, including those of cholangitis, pump pocket infections, and thrombosis, pump infusions can be used safely.

Neoadjuvant chemotherapy in patients with unresectable liver metastases is a promising approach to downsize these tumors in order to proceed with resection. Further work is needed to define its role in the management of these patients.

Additional work is needed to investigate the role of other systemic chemotherapeutic agents in the treatment of advanced colorectal cancer in association with HAI FUDR. Of particular interest are irinotecan, a camptothecin derivative, or oxaliplatin, a new platinum compound. Both of these agents have been shown to be active in advanced colorectal cancer when combined with 5-FU. Through these means, better extrahepatic control would hopefully be gained while continuing to provide the liver with high concentrations of active drug to maintain hepatic control.

REFERENCES

1. Landis SH, Murray T, Bolden S, Wingo PA, Cancer statistics, 1999. *CA Cancer J Clin* 1999; **49:** 8–31.
2. Wagner JS, Adson MA, Van Heerden JA et al, The natural history of hepatic metastases from colorectal cancer. *Ann Surg* 1984; **199:** 502–7.
3. Baker LH, Tulley RW, Blumgart LH, A retrospective study of the natural history of patients with liver metastases from colorectal cancer. *Clin Oncol* 1976; **2:** 285–8.
4. Grage TB, Vassiolopoulos IP, Shingleton WW et al, Results of a prospective randomized study of hepatic artery infusion with 5-fluorouracil versus intravenous 5-fluorouracil in patients with hepatic metastases from colorectal cancer: a Central Oncology Group study. *Surgery* 1970; **86:** 550–5.
5. Macdonald JS, Kimer DF, Smythe T et al, 5-Fluorouracil (5-FU), methyl-CCNU, and vincristine in the treatment of advanced colorectal cancer phase II study utilizing weekly 5-FU. *Cancer Treat Rep* 1976; **60:** 1597–600.
6. Burgker T, Kim PN, Grappe C et al, 5-FU infusion with mitomycin-C versus 5-FU infusion with methyl-CCNU in the treatment of advanced colon cancer. *Cancer* 1978; **42:** 1228–33.
7. Kemeny N, Yeynes A, Selter K et al, Interferon-alpha-2a and 5-fluorouracil for advanced colorectal carcinoma. *Cancer* 1990; **66:** 2470–5.
8. Erlichman C, Fine S, Wong A, Elhakim T, A randomized trial of

fluorouracil and folinic acid in patients with metastatic colorectal carcinoma. *J Clin Oncol* 1988; **6:** 469–75.

9. Jaffe BM, Donegan W, Watson F, Factors influencing survival in patients with untreated hepatic metastases. *Surg Gynecol Obst* 1968; **127:** 1–11.

10. Bengmark S, Hafstrom L, The natural history of primary and secondary malignant tumors of the liver. The prognosis for patients with hepatic metastases from colonic and rectal carcinoma at laparotomy. *Cancer* 1969; **23:** 198–202.

11. Goslin R, Steele G, Zamcheck N et al, Factors influencing survival in patients with hepatic metastases from adenocarcinoma of the colon and rectum. *Dis Colon Rectum* 1982; **25:** 749–54.

12. Bengtsson G, Carlsson G, Hafstrom L, Natural history of patients with untreated liver metastases from colorectal cancer. *Am J Surg* 1981; **141:** 586–9.

13. Finan P, Marshall R, Cooper E et al, Factors affecting survival in patients presenting with synchronous hepatic metastases from colorectal cancer: a clinical and computer analysis. *Br J Surg* 1985; **72:** 373–7.

14. DeBrauw L, DeVelde C, Bouwhuis-Hoogerwerf M, Diagnostic evaluation and survival analysis of colorectal cancer patients with liver metastases. *J Surg Oncol* 1987; **34:** 81–6.

15. Fong Y, Fortner J, Sun RL et al, Clinical score for predicting recurrence after hepatic resection for metastatic colorectal cancer: analysis of 1001 consecutive cases. *Ann Surg* 1999; **230:** 309–21.

16. Nordlinger B, Guiguet M, Vaillant JC et al, Surgical resection of colorectal carcinoma metastases to the liver: a prognostic scoring system to improve case selection, based on 1568 patients. *Cancer* 1996; **77:** 1254–62.

17. Ambiru S, Miyakazi M, Ito H et al, Adjuvant regional chemotherapy after hepatic resection for colorectal metastases. *Br J Surg* 1999; **86:** 1025–31.

18. Doci R, Gennari L, Bignami P et al, One hundred patients with hepatic metastases from colorectal cancer treated by resection: analysis of prognostic determinants. *Br J Surg* 1991; **78:** 797–801.

19. Iwatsuki S, Esquivel C, Gordon RD, Starzi TE, Liver resection for metastatic colorectal cancer. *Surgery* 1986; **100:** 804–10.

20. Scheole J, Liver resection for colorectal metastases. *World J Surg* 1995; **19:** 59–71.

21. Fong Y, Cohen AM, Fortner JG et al, Liver resection for colorectal metastases. *J Clin Oncol* 1997; **15:** 938–46.

22. Jamison RL, Donohue JH, Negomey DM et al, Hepatic resection for metastatic colorectal cancer results in cure for some patients. *Arch Surg* 1997; **132:** 505–10.

23. Nordlinger B, Fare J, Delya E et al, Hepatic resection for colorectal liver metastases. *Ann Surg* 1987; **205:** 256–63.

24. Coppa GF, Eng K, Rason JH et al, Hepatic resection for metastatic colon and rectal cancer. An evaluation of preoperative and postoperative factors. *Ann Surg* 1985; **202:** 203–8.

25. Scheele J, Stangl R, Altendorf-Hoffman A, Fall FP, Indicators of prognosis after hepatic resection for colorectal secondaries. *Surgery* 1991; **110:** 13–29.

26. van Ooijen B, Wiggers T, Meijer S et al, Hepatic resections for colorectal metastases in the Netherlands: a multiinstitutional 10-year study. *Cancer* 1992; **70:** 28–34.

27. Fegiz F, Ramacciato G, Genari L et al, Hepatic resections for colorectal metastases: the Italian multicenter experience. *J Surg Oncol* 1991; **2**(Suppl): 1444–54.

28. Cady B, Stone MD, McDermontt WV Jr et al, Technical and biologic factors in disease-free survival after hepatic resection for colorectal cancer metastases. *Arch Surg* 1992; **126:** 561–9.

29. Ackerman NB, The blood supply of experimental liver metastases. I. The distribution of hepatic artery and portal vein blood to 'small' and 'large' tumors. *Surgery* 1969; **66:** 1067–72.

30. Ackerman NB, The blood supply of experimental liver metas-

tases. IV. Changes in vascularity with increasing tumor growth. *Surgery* 1974; **75:** 589–96.

31. Yasuda S, Noto T, Ikeda M et al, Hepatic arterial infusion chemotherapy using implantable reservoir in colorectal liver metastases. *Gan to Kagaku Ryoho* 1990; **8:** 1815–19.

32. Ensminger WD, Gyves JW, Clinical pharmacology of hepatic arterial chemotherapy. *Semin Oncol* 1983; **10:** 176–83.

33. Kemeny N, Seiter K, Niedzwiecki D et al, A randomized trial of intrahepatic infusion of floxuridine (FUDR) with dexamethasone versus FUDR alone in the treatment of metastatic colorectal cancer. *Cancer* 1992; **69:** 327–34.

34. Kemeny N, Daly J, Oderman P et al, Randomized study of intrahepatic versus systemic infusion of flurodeoxyuridine in patients with liver metastases from colorectal carcinoma. *Ann Intern Med* 1987; **107:** 159–65.

35. Chang AE, Schneider PD, Sugarbaker PH, A prospective randomized trial of regional versus systemic continuous 5-fluorodeoxyuridine chemotherapy in the treatment of colorectal liver metastases. *Ann Surg* 1987; **206:** 685–93.

36. Hohn D, Stagg R, Friedman M et al, A randomized trial of continuous versus hepatic intra-arterial floxuridine in patients with colorectal cancer metastases to the liver: the Northern California Oncology Group trial. *J Clin Oncol* 1989; **7:** 1646–54.

37. Martin JK, O'Connell J, Wieland H et al, Intra-arterial floxuridine vs. systemic fluorouracil for hepatic metastases from colorectal cancer. A randomized trial. *Arch Surg* 1990; **125:** 1022–7.

38. Wagman L, Kemeny M, Leong L et al, A prospective randomized evaluation of the treatment of colorectal cancer metastases to the liver. *J Clin Oncol* 1990; **8:** 1885–93.

39. Rougier P, LaPlanche A, Huguier M et al, Hepatic arterial infusion of floxuridine in patients with liver metastases from colorectal carcinoma: long term results of a prospective randomized trial. *J Clin Oncol* 1992; **10:** 1112–18.

40. Allen-Mersh TG, Earlam S, Fordy C et al, Quality of life and survival with continuous hepatic artery floxuridine infusion for colorectal liver metastases. *Lancet* 1994; **344:** 1255–60.

41. Lorenz M, Muller H, Randomized, multicenter trial of fluorouracil plus leucovorin administered either via hepatic arterial or intravenous infusion versus fluorodeoxyuridine administered via hepatic arterial infusion in patients with nonresectable liver metastases from colorectal cancer. *J Clin Oncol* 2000; **18:** 243–54.

42. Meta-Analysis Group in Cancer, Reappraisal of hepatic arterial infusion in the treatment of nonresectable liver metastases from colorectal cancer. *J Natl Cancer Inst* 1996; **88:** 252–8.

43. Moriya Y, Sugihara K, Hojo K, Makuchi M, Adjuvant hepatic intra-arterial chemotherapy after potentially curative resection of colorectal liver metastases. *Eur J Surg Oncol* 1991; **17:** 519–25.

44. Curley SA, Roh MS, Chase JL, Hohn DC, Adjuvant hepatic artery infusion chemotherapy after curative resection of colorectal liver metastases. *Am J Surg* 1993; **166:** 743–8.

45. Nonami T, Takaguchi Y, Yasui M et al, Regional adjuvant chemotherapy after partial hepatectomy for mesenteric colorectal carcinoma. *Semin Oncol* 1997; **24:** 130–4.

46. Kemeny N, Huang Y, Cohen AM et al, Hepatic arterial infusion of chemotherapy after resection of hepatic metastases from colorectal cancer. *N Engl J Med* 1999; **341:** 2039–48.

47. Kemeny MM, Goldberg D, Beatty JD et al, Results of a prospective randomized trial of continuous regional chemotherapy and hepatic resection as treatment of hepatic metastases from colorectal primaries. *Cancer* 1986; **57:** 492–8.

48. Wagman LD, Kemeny MM, Leong L et al, Prospective randomized evaluation of the treatment of colorectal cancer metastatic to the liver. *J Clin Oncol* 1990; **8:** 1885–93.

49. Lorenz M, Muller H, Schramm H et al, Randomized trial of surgery versus surgery followed by adjuvant hepatic arterial

infusion with 5-fluorouracil and folinic acid for liver metastases of colorectal cancer. *Ann Surg* 1998; **228:** 756–62.

50. Kemeny MM, Adak S, Lipsitz B et al, Results of the intergroup [Eastern Cooperative Oncology Group (ECOG) and Southwest Oncology Group (SWOG)] prospective randomized study of surgery alone versus continuous systemic infusion of 5FU after hepatic resection for colorectal liver metastases. *Proc Am Soc Clin Oncol* 1999; **18:** 264a.

51. Giacchetti S, Itzhaki M, Grula G et al, Long-term survival of patients with unresectable colorectal cancer liver metastases following infusional chemotherapy with 5-fluorouracil, leucovorin, oxaliplatin, and surgery. *Ann Oncol* 1999; **10:** 663–9.

36

Locoregional chemotherapy for metastatic colorectal cancer to the liver

Don S Dizon, Nancy Kemeny

INTRODUCTION

One-third of patients with colorectal cancer will be diagnosed with hepatic involvement during the course of their disease. In many of them, it will be the only site of metastatic spread. The degree of hepatic involvement is known to be a prognostic factor. In a retrospective study by Wood et al,[1] the 1-year survival rate was 60% in the presence of solitary liver lesions, and dropped to 5.7% in the presence of widespread hepatic disease. The primary treatment for liver metastases is surgery.[2,3] The 3-year survival rate is over 40%, and in series with long follow-up, the 10-year survival rate approximates 20%.[4–8] While surgical resection remains the standard of care in the treatment of isolated metastatic disease to the liver from colorectal cancer, over 90% of patients will be ineligible for resection. For these patients, systemic chemotherapy with 5-fluorouracil (5-FU) and leucovorin (LV) has been the standard treatment, with 2-year survival rates of less than 20%. Although better responses may be seen with newer agents such as oxaliplatin or irinotecan (CPT-11) in combination with 5-FU and LV, the majority of patients treated with systemic chemotherapy are not alive at 2 years. Given this poor response to standard chemotherapy, alternative options for locoregional control have been investigated. The most promising of these options is hepatic arterial infusion (HAI).

BACKGROUND

The rationale for HAI can be justified both anatomically and pharmacologically.

1. Hepatic metastases usually arrive in the liver from the portal system. However, once they grow beyond 3 mm, they are fed by the hepatic artery, while normal hepatocytes are fed by the portal vein.[9] With HAI, selective drug delivery to the tumor can be obtained while sparing the normal liver parenchyma from such high doses of chemotherapy.

2. The model of a stepwise pattern of metastatic progression is that initially the liver becomes involved by metastatic spread through the portal vein; then there is spread to the lung, and then systemically. Therefore, by targeting the liver early, and interfering with this progression, theoretic cure in metastatic disease should be possible.

3. By using agents that are taken up by the liver via the first-pass effect, significant concentrations within the intrahepatic circulation can be obtained while minimizing systemic toxicity.

4. Using agents with high total-body clearance, maximum effect can be achieved in the liver and the systemic circulation can be spared.

5. If drugs with a steep dose–response curve are chosen, then, with HAI, large amounts can be delivered regionally.

Work by Ensminger et al[10] documented that between 94% and 99% of 5-fluoro-2'-deoxyuridine (FUDR, floxuridine) is extracted in the liver during the first-pass effect, providing an estimated 100- to 400-fold increase in hepatic exposure with HAI.[10] This represents a 10-fold increase in drug concentration in the liver compared with 5-FU. Table 36.1 lists the percentage increased exposure of other agents if delivered by HAI.

Table 36.1 Drugs used for hepatic arterial infusion[a]

Drug	Estimated increased exposure by hepatic arterial infusion (-fold)
5-Fluorouracil (5-FU)	5–10
5-Fluoro-2'-deoxyuridine (FUDR, floxuridine)	100–400
Bischlorocthylnitrosurea (BCNU, carmustine)	6–7
Mitomycin C	6–8
Cisplatin	4–7
Doxorubicin	2

[a] Data derived from Ensminger and Gyves.[10]

EVALUATION OF PATIENTS PRIOR TO PUMP PLACEMENT

Patients undergoing locoregional therapy need to be given a thorough preoperative evaluation to rule out the presence of extrahepatic disease. This should include a chest X-ray, computed tomography (CT) of the abdomen and pelvis, and colonoscopy. In addition, definitive arterial anatomy by angiography should be delineated. This is done to visualize the arterial anatomy to both the liver and adjacent structures and to ensure the patency of the portal vein. This is important, since pump placement in the presence of portal vein thrombosis carries a high risk of hepatic failure. Finally, prior to pump placement, a laparoscopic examination should be performed and biopsy done on any suspicious lesions.

Once done, perfusion of the entire liver without evidence of involvement into the adjacent structures should be checked. Radionuclide studies prior to the initial use of the HAI perfusion pump need to be performed. A technetium sulfur colloid scan followed by injection of technetium microaggregated albumin (MAA) through the side port allows full imaging of the pump perfusion; ideally, the entire bilobar architecture is perfused. In this way, if there is perfusion of the adjacent structures, one can attempt to correct this prior to the administration of HAI therapy.

COMPLICATIONS OF PORT PLACEMENT

Complications from the pump placement can be seen in the immediate postoperative period or later on. Early events include hepatic arterial thrombosis, usually due to hepatic arterial injury, incomplete perfusion of the liver with or without misperfusion to the

stomach or duodenum, pump pocket hematomas, or infections.[11] Late complications tend to be more common, including pump pocket infections, catheter thrombosis, and peptic ulceration.

A review of the pump placement at the Memorial Sloan-Kettering Cancer Center (MSKCC) over an 8-year period showed that of 303 infusion pumps placed, there were only 2 deaths during the first 30 days: 1 from a myocardial infarction and 1 from disease progression.[11] Fourteen patients experienced arterial thrombosis (4.7%) and six patients had evidence of extrahepatic infusion (3%). Five patients did not have adequate liver perfusion (1.7%). The remaining complications were quite rare, but included gastric ulceration, pneumonia, hemorrhage, pocket infection, and pump failure. The overall morbidity rate was 11.8%.

RANDOMIZED TRIALS

Eight randomized trials have been performed looking at the use of HAI infusion of chemotherapy in the treatment of unresectable hepatic metastases from colorectal cancer. Most of them stratified patients in terms of percentage liver involvement, performance status, and lactate dehydrogenase (LDH) level, all of which are accepted parameters that influence outcome. The results of these trials are summarized in Table 36.2.

At MSKCC, 162 patients were randomized to FUDR delivered systemically versus delivery by HAI.[12] All patients underwent surgical exploration to confirm the absence of extrahepatic disease. Treatment consisted of a 14-day infusion of FUDR in both groups, although a lower dose was used in the systemic arm because of excessive toxicity at the

Table 36.2 Randomized trials of hepatic arterial infusion (HAI) versus systemic chemotherapy for hepatic metastases from colorectal cancer

Authors	No. of patients	Agents	Response rate (%)	Survival (months)
Kemeny et al[12]	162	HAI FUDR vs	52	17
		i.v. FUDR	20	12
Chang et al[13]	64	HAI FUDR vs	62	22
		i.v. FUDR	17	12
Hohn et al[14]	143	HAI FUDR vs	42	16
		i.v. FUDR	10	15
Martin et al[15]	69	HAI FUDR vs	48	12.6
		i.v. 5-FU/LV	21	10.5
Wagman et al[16]	41	HAI FUDR vs	55	13.8
		i.v. 5-FU	20	11.6
Rougier et al[17]	163	HAI 5-FU vs	49	15
		i.v. 5-FU	14	10
Allen-Mersch et al[18]	100	HAI 5-FU vs	50	13.1
		i.v. 5-FU/palliation	0	7.3
Lorenz et al[19]	168	HAI 5-FU/LV vs	45	18.7
		HAI FUDR vs	43	12.7
		i.v. 5-FU	19.7	17.6

higher dose. A response rate of 52% was seen with HAI, while a rate of only 20% was reported with systemic administration. Of note, 60% of patients crossed over into the HAI arm. The survival based on the initial randomization was 17 months in patients in the HAI arm and 12 months in the systemic FUDR arm. In patients who crossed over, a median survival of 18 months was seen in those who received HAI versus 8 months in those who did not.

At the US National Cancer Institute (NCI), 64 patients, including patients with positive portal lymph nodes, were randomized to HAI FUDR versus systemic FUDR.[13] Response rates were 62% in the HAI arm and 17% in the systemic arm. The actuarial 2-year survival rates were 34% and 17%, respectively, but this was not statistically significant. However, in a subset analysis excluding patients with portal lymph node involvement, the 2-year survival rate was significantly better in patients treated with HAI as opposed to systemic chemotherapy: 47% versus 13%.

The Northern California Oncology group performed a similar study of systemic FUDR versus HAI FUDR in 143 patients.[14] Patients with positive hepatic lymph nodes were included. In this trial, a partial response rate of 42% was reported with HAI FUDR and a rate of 10% with systemic FUDR. Although the median time to progression was increased in patients treated with HAI as opposed to systemic FUDR (503 and 484 days, respectively), no increase in overall survival was seen. Crossover was allowed in those patients who did not respond to systemic therapy, and those who did had a doubling of survival compared with those who did not.

A randomized trial at the Mayo Clinic enrolled 69 patients to HAI FUDR versus 5-FU/LV given as a systemic bolus for 5 days.[15] Comparing the HAI and systemic-treatment arms, 48% and 21% had an objective response, respectively. In addition, a significant increase in time to hepatic progression was noted with HAI therapy: 15.7 months, as opposed to 6 months with systemic therapy. Despite these results, however, survival was not significantly improved (12.6 months versus 10.5 months). Again, these results need to be treated with caution, since almost 50% of patients randomized to the HAI arm did not receive treatment for reasons including pump failure and extrahepatic disease.

At the City of Hope National Medical Center, Duarte, CA, 41 patients with non-resectable liver metastases received HAI versus systemic chemotherapy.[16] In the group receiving HAI FUDR, the response rate was 55%, with a median survival duration of 13.8 months. These results compared favorably with those obtained with systemic chemotherapy, where a 20% response rate was seen and the median survival was 11.6 months.

A French trial randomized 163 patients to bolus 5-FU given systemically versus FUDR given intrahepatically.[17] Comparing the two groups, the patients treated with HAI FUDR had a 49% response rate, which compared favorably against the systemic group, where a 14% response rate was seen. The median times to hepatic progression were 15 and 6 months, respectively. The 2-year survival rate was 22% in the HAI FUDR arm and 10% in the systemic FUDR arm, which was statistically significant ($p < 0.02$). The median survival was 14 months in the HAI group and 10 months in the systemic group; however, patients in the systemic group were sometimes treated only when they became symptomatic.

A trial from the UK randomized 100 patients to HAI FUDR versus conventional therapy, and looked at the endpoints of quality of life and overall survival in patients with liver metastases.[18] Conventional therapy was aimed at palliation, and included systemic chemotherapy, although in a significant group chemotherapy was delayed until patients were symptomatic. A significant improvement in survival was seen in the HAI group compared with the control arm: 405 days versus 226 days. In addition, the quality of life of patients receiving HAI FUDR was significantly prolonged in terms of normal-quality survival for physical symptoms, anxiety, and depression. However, only 22% in the conventional-treatment arm were advised or received systemic chemotherapy. The authors concluded that in addition to the survival benefit with HAI, it is well tolerated, leading to a better and longer sustained performance status.

The German Cooperative Group on Liver Metastases recently published the results of a multi-center trial with 168 patients randomized to HAI FUDR versus 5-FU/LV administered by either HAI or systemic intravenous (i.v.) infusion.[19] An intention-to-treat analysis was used, although only 40 of 57 (70%) patients randomized to HAI 5-FU/LV and 37 of 54

(68.5%) randomized to HAI FUDR were treated as assigned; 24.6% more patients than randomized to i.v. 5-FU/LV received this treatment. This calls into question the validity of their results, since a large number of patients did not start their assigned treatment. The median time to progression was 5.9 months in patients treated with HAI FUDR, 9.2 months in patients treated with HAI 5-FU/LV, and 6.6 months in patients treated with i.v. 5-FU/LV, none of which were statistically significant. The median survival times for HAI FUDR and HAI 5-FU/LV were 12.7 and 18.7 months, respectively. Survival in the i.v. 5-FU/LV group was 17.6 months, which is well above the median survival reported with i.v. 5-FU/LV of 7–12 months. The tumor response rates with HAI FUDR, HAI 5-FU/LV, and i.v. 5-FU/LV were 43.2%, 45%, and 19.7%, respectively. There was development of extrahepatic disease in the HAI FUDR, HAI 5-FU/LV, and i.v. 5-FU arms in 40.5%, 12.5%, and 18.3% of cases, respectively. Toxicity data indicate that 5-FU/LV therapy was much more toxic than FUDR. Stomatitis occurred in 75% of cycles of HAI 5-FU/LV and 64.6% in the i.v. 5-FU/LV group, compared with 8% of the HAI FUDR cycles. No grade 3–4 diarrhea was reported in the group treated with HAI FUDR. In both groups receiving 5-FU/LV, the incidence of severe diarrhea was 11%. The authors report that roughly two-thirds of patients treated with 5-FU/LV, whether it be HAI or intravenously, experienced severe grade 3–4 side-effects, compared with only one-third in the group treated with FUDR. It is difficult to interpret the results of the HAI group, because very little information was given about their treatment, such as how many cycles the patients received and further information regarding the complications experienced, such as catheters clotting. Finally, dose adjustment was very crude, i.e. doses were decreased after two cycles, not based on standard guidelines.

A meta-analysis combining the results of seven trials supports the use of HAI FUDR in the treatment of non-resectable liver metastases from colorectal cancer.[20] A significantly better local response rate of 41% was achieved with HAI FUDR, compared with a 14% response rate with systemic 5-FU. In addition, median increased survival time was increased in patients treated with HAI FUDR compared with the group treated with systemic 5-FU: 16 months versus 13 months.

TOXICITY

Unlike systemic chemotherapy, HAI is well tolerated. The myelosuppressive side-effects are not seen with HAI administration of FUDR, and occur to a lesser degree with HAI administration of mitomycin C or carmustine than with systemic therapy. With regard to gastrointestinal side-effects, HAI is well tolerated, and is rarely complicated by significant nausea and vomiting. However, occasional gastritis or ulcer disease can be seen. Ulceration is usually due to aberrant perfusion from small collaterals to the stomach and duodenum originating from the hepatic artery. If it is associated with significant diarrhea, shunting to the bowel needs to be ruled out.

HAI therapy is associated with hepatic toxicity. The physiologic basis of this toxicity is not clear. Some believe it to be due to a hepatitis-like reaction, evidenced by the necrosis and cholestasis seen on biopsies. Others feel that it is due to a pericholangitic process and fibrosis stemming from biliary radicals. These changes resolve early on if the drug is withdrawn and the patient is given a treatment holiday. However, in later stages, it can be permanent. In those who develop permanent biliary toxicity, endoscopic retrograde cholangiopancreatography (ERCP) reveals findings similar to idiopathic sclerosing cholangitis.[21] If the patient develops jaundice that does not resolve with cessation of therapy, ERCP may also reveal fibrosis of the main biliary radical, which may be amenable to stenting.

In one autopsy series in patients who have had HAI therapy, damage of the biliary tree associated with small vessel necrosis was uniformly documented.[22] The selective destruction of the biliary system is likely due to its blood supply, which is drawn from the hepatic artery. With HAI, these structures are exposed to a significant concentration of drug.

Given the hepatotoxicity, liver function tests must be monitored very carefully. A method to decrease the dosing of chemotherapy or for ceasing treatment is included in Table 36.3. Serum bilirubin levels exceeding 3 mg/dl necessitate treatment holidays until normalization occurs to prevent sclerosing complications.

An additional toxicity reported in prior studies is the development of cholecystitis. In one series, the reported incidence was 33%.[21] However, this problem has been resolved with the standard procedure of cholecystectomy during pump placement.

Addressing hepatic toxicity

In order to decrease hepatic toxicity, three strategies have been tested. The use of dexamethasone has been evaluated in order to decrease inflammation associated with biliary toxicity. In 1992, a randomized trial of dexamethasone and FUDR versus HAI

FUDR was performed by Kemeny et al.[23] A trend towards decreased bilirubin elevations was seen in the group receiving additional dexamethasone, 9% versus 30% ($p = 0.07$). Interestingly, there was an increased response rate: 71% for FUDR plus dexamethasone and 43% in patients treated with FUDR alone. Survival was also better in patients treated with FUDR: 23 months in patients treated with FUDR plus dexamethasone and 15 months in those treated with FUDR.

Another method of decreasing hepatic toxicity has been to administer HAI FUDR by circadian modulation. Day-cycling of chemotherapy has been shown to be less toxic in animal models.[24,25] In addition, it has been shown that chronomodulation enables higher doses of FUDR to be infused without an increase in toxicity.[26] However, to date, no randomized controlled trial has been completed to address this modality as an alternative to bolus or continuous infusion in metastatic colorectal cancer.

The use of alternating drug regimens has also been investigated as a means to decrease hepatotoxicity from HAI FUDR. Stagg et al[27] enrolled 68 patients in a phase II study utilizing HAI FUDR on days 1–8 followed by hepatic arterial bolus of 5-FU on days 14, 21 and 28 via the side port, every 35 days. Fifty percent of patients achieved a major response, and the median survival from pump implantation was 22.4 months. There were no treatment terminations with this regimen. Davidson and colleagues[28] treated 57 patients with a similar regimen. A response rate of 54% was seen. Biliary sclerosis occurred in 3.5% of patients. Metzger et al[29] treated 30 patients with metastatic colorectal cancer confined to the liver with an alternating regimen of HAI 5-FU on days 1–5 and mitomycin C every 6 hours on day 6. Treatment cycles were given every 6 weeks. No hepatic toxicity was reported, although 7% of patients developed severe mucositis.

Addressing extrahepatic recurrence

One of the main criticisms of HAI therapy is the occurrence of extrahepatic disease. While relapse within the liver is significantly reduced, 40–70% of patients will develop metastases outside of the liver. Therefore, combination systemic chemotherapy and HAI has been attempted to reduce the rate of extrahepatic recurrence. In one trial, HAI FUDR was compared with concurrent HAI FUDR and intravenous FUDR.[30] Both were given as 14-day infusions every 4 weeks. While both groups achieved a response rate of 60%, the rate of extrahepatic disease was significantly

Table 36.3 FUDR dose-modification schedule[a]

Serum aspartate aminotransferase (AST, SGOT)

Reference values:[b]	≤50 U/l	>50 U/l	FUDR dose
Level:[c]	0–<3 × ref	0–<2 × ref	100%
	3–<4 × ref	2–<3 × ref	80%
	4–<5 × ref	3–<4 × ref	50%
	≥5 × ref	≥4 × ref	Hold

Alkaline phosphatase

Reference values:[b]	≤90 U/l	>90 U/l	FUDR dose
Level:[c]	0–<1.5 × ref	0–<1.2 × ref	100%
	1.5–<2.0 × ref	1.2–<1.5 × ref	50%
	≥2.0 × ref	≥1.5 × ref	Hold

Total bilirubin

Reference values:[b]	≤1.2 mg/dl	>1.2 mg/dl	FUDR dose
Level:[c]	0–<1.5 × ref	0–<1.2 × ref	100%
	1.5–<2.0 × ref	1.2–<1.5 × ref	50%
	≥2.0 × ref	≥1.5 × ref	Hold

[a] Reproduced from Kemeny N, Atiq OT, Intrahepatic chemotherapy for metastatic colorectal cancer. In: *Regional Chemotherapy: Clinical Research and Practice* (Markham M, ed), Totowa, NJ: Humana Press, 2000.
[b] Reference values are defined as the values obtained on the day of the last dose of FUDR.
[c] To determine if dose modification is necessary, compare the value obtained on the day the pump is emptied or the day it is to be filled – whichever is the higher.

Recommendations on restarting treatment
- If due to an abnormal AST, only restart when level has fallen to 4 × reference value (if reference ≤ 50 U/l) or within 3 × reference value (if reference > 50 U/l). If started, we recommend re-initiation at 50% of the last FUDR dose given.
- If due to an abnormal alkaline phosphatase, restart once level has fallen to 1.5 × reference value (if reference ≤ 90 U/l) or 1.2 × reference value (if reference > 90 U/l). If started, recommence at 25% of last FUDR dose given.
- If due to an abnormal bilirubin, restart once level has fallen to 1.5 × reference value (if reference ≤ 1.2 mg/dl) or within 1.2 × reference value (if reference > 1.2 mg/dl). Restart chemotherapy at 25% of last FUDR dose. However, if a marked abnormality of the bilirubin compared with reference exceeding 2 × reference value (in patients with reference value ≤ 1.2 mg/dl) or 1.5 × reference value (in patients with reference value > 1.2 mg/dl) occur, then the next cycle should not be administered. Instead, levels should be re-checked at 14 days. If the bilirubin continues to be normal, FUDR can be restarted at 25% of the usual dose.

less in the group treated with intravenous and HAI FUDR than in the group treated with HAI alone: 56% versus 79%. In another study, 40 patients with colon cancer who had unresectable hepatic metastases were treated with HAI FUDR for 14 days and systemic 5-FU/LV for 5 days delivered 1 week after the start of HAI FUDR.[31] The response rate was 62%, with 3% of patients progression-free at 24 months. The median time to progression was 9 months and the median survival duration was 18 months. The incidence of extrahepatic progression was 45%. In another study, at MSKCC, Ron et al[32] combined systemic irinotecan with HAI FUDR plus dexamethasone in 18 patients with unresectable hepatic metastases from colorectal cancer. All of them had been treated with intravenous 5-FU/LV, and 4 had been treated with irinotecan. Partial responses were seen in 12 of 15 patients analyzed.

COST

An economic analysis was performed by the Meta-Analysis Group in Cancer to determine the cost–effectiveness of HAI treatment.[33] Medical and hospital costs were computed for HAI FUDR and a control group (intravenous chemotherapy or symptom palliation) using individual patient data from the seven clinical trials used in the original meta-analysis of HAI in the treatment of colorectal cancer reported in 1996. Total costs encompassed the cost of the pump, procedure and hospitalization, chemotherapy, follow-up costs, and toxic effect costs. In France, the total costs of HAI and the control group were estimated at $29 562 and $9926, respectively. In the USA, the total costs were estimated at $25 208 and $5928, respectively. However, considering the annual cost of hemodialysis in France, which is estimated at between $70 000 and $90 000, the cost of HAI compares quite favorably. In addition, it is in line with the costs of newer chemotherapeutic regimens including irinotecan, which on average costs $54 000 for 1 year of treatment, including the cost of drug and drug administration, in the USA.[34] Therefore, when compared to the costs of treatment for other severe medical illnesses, and other regimens for colorectal cancer, HAI falls within the range of accepted therapies.

CONCLUSIONS

Metastatic colorectal cancer continues to be a difficult problem to manage. Newer chemotherapeutic agents such as irinotecan and oxaliplatin have improved survival over standard treatment, but a majority of patients still succumb to their disease within 2 years. The work summarized here brings other options in the locoregional management of metastatic colorectal cancer.

Hepatic arterial infusion of FUDR plus dexamethasone has been shown to be a viable treatment option in patients with metastatic colorectal cancer to the liver. Multiple studies have demonstrated an increased response rate in the liver that is three times higher than the responses attainable with systemic chemotherapy. The toxicity can be managed effectively by ensuring proper technique with pump placement and the use of dexamethasone in order to decrease portal inflammation. In addition, HAI is an economically viable option, especially when compared with other therapies for severe conditions.

The impact of HAI on survival has been difficult to ascertain. Many trials allowed crossover in those patents who progressed. Systemic failure has been an ongoing dilemma in patients treated with HAI. Further clinical trials will need to be done incorporating systemic chemotherapy and HAI in the treatment of advanced colorectal cancer. An ongoing trial conducted by the Cancer and Leukemia Group B (CALGB) will attempt to address whether or not this therapy influences survival by not allowing crossover in its design. Quality-of-life measures, molecular markers, including thymidylate synthase, and a cost–effectiveness analysis will also be examined.

REFERENCES

1. Wood C, Gillis C, Blumgart L, A retrospective study of the natural history of patients with liver metastases from colorectal cancer. *Clin Oncol* 1976; **2**: 285–8.
2. Hughes K, Scheele J, Sugarbaker P, Surgery for colorectal cancer metastatic to the liver. *Surg Clin North Am* 1989; **69**: 340–59.
3. Steele G, Ravinkumar T, Resection of hepatic metastases from colorectal cancer. *Am Surg* 1989; **210**: 127–38.
4. Iwatsuki S, Esquiviel CC, Gordon RD, Starzl TE, Liver resection for metastatic colorectal cancer. *Surgery* 1986; **100**: 804–10.
5. Nordlinger B, Faro J, Delva E et al, Hepatic resection for colorectal liver metastases. *Ann Surg* 1987; **205**: 256–63.
6. Scheele J, Stang R, Altendorf-Hoffman A, Paul M, Resection of colorectal liver metastases. *World J Surg* 1995; **19**: 59–71.
7. Jamison RL, Donohue JH, Nagorney DM et al, Hepatic resection for metastatic colorectal cancer results in cure for some patients. *Arch Surg* 1997; **132**: 505–11.
8. Fong Y, Fortner JG, Sun RL et al, Clinical score for predicting recurrence after hepatic resection for metastatic colorectal cancer: analysis of 1001 consecutive cases. *Ann Surg* 1999; **230**: 309–21.
9. Breedis C, Young C, Blood supply of neoplasms in the liver. *Am J Pathol* 1954; **30**: 969.
10. Ensminger WD, Gyves JW, Clinical pharmacology of hepatic arterial chemotherapy. *Sem Onc* 1983; **10**: 176–82.
11. Kemeny N, Sigurdon E, Intra-arterial chemotherapy for liver tumors. In: *Surgery of the Liver and Biliary Tract*, 2nd edn (Blumgart L, ed). New York: Churchill Livingstone, 1994: 1458–91.
12. Kemeny N, Daly J, Oderman P et al, Randomized study of intrahepatic versus systemic infusion of fluorodeoxyuridine in patients with liver metastases from colorectal carcinoma. *Ann Intern Med* 1987; **107**: 459–65.
13. Chang AE, Schneider PD, Sugarbaker PH, A prospective randomized trial of regional versus systemic continuous 5-fluoroxyuridine chemotherapy in the treatment of colorectal liver metastases. *Ann Surg* 1987; **206**: 685–93.
14. Hohn D, Stagg R, Friedman M et al, A randomized trial of continuous versus hepatic intra-arterial floxuridine in patients with colorectal cancer metastases to the liver: the Northern California Oncology Group trial. *J Clin Oncol* 1989; **7**: 1646–54.
15. Martin JJ, O'Connell J, Wieland H et al, Intra-arterial floxuridine vs. systemic fluorouracil for hepatic metastases from colorectal cancer. A randomized trial. *Arch Surg* 1990; **125**: 1022–7.
16. Wagman L, Kemeny M, Leong L et al, A prospective randomized evaluation of the treatment of colorectal cancer metastatic to the liver. *J Clin Oncol* 1990; **8**: 1885–93.
17. Rougier P, LaPlanche A, Huguier M et al, Hepatic arterial infu-

sion of floxuridine in patients with liver metastases from colorectal carcinoma: Long term results of a prospective randomized trial. *J Clin Oncol* 1992; **10:** 1112–18.

18. Allen-Mersch TG, Earlam S, Fordy C et al, Quality of life and survival with continuous hepatic artery floxuridine infusion for colorectal liver metastases. *Lancet* 1994; **344:** 1255–60.

19. Lorenz M, Muller H, Randomized, multicenter trial of fluorouracil plus leucovorin administered either via hepatic arterial or intravenous infusion versus fluorodeoxyuridine administered via hepatic arterial infusion in patients with nonresectable liver metastases from colorectal cancer. *J Clin Oncol* 2000; **18:** 243–54.

20. Meta-Analysis Group in Cancer, Reappraisal of hepatic arterial infusion in the treatment of nonresectable liver metastases from colorectal cancer. *J Natl Cancer Inst* 1996; **88:** 252–8.

21. Kemeny M, Battifora H, Flayney D et al, Sclerosing cholangitis after continuous hepatic artery infusion of FUDR. *Ann Surg* 1985; **202:** 176–81.

22. Pettavel J, Gardiol D, Bergier N et al, Necrosis of main bile ducts caused by hepatic artery infusion of 5-fluoro-2-deoxyuridine. *Reg Cancer Treat* 1988; **1:** 83–92.

23. Kemeny N, Seiter K, Diedzweikei D et al, A randomized trial of intrahepatic infusion of floxuridine (FUDR) with dexamethasone vs. FUDR alone in the treatment of metastatic colorectal cancer. *Cancer* 1992; **69:** 327–34.

24. Kemeny MM, Alava G, Oliver JM, Smith FB, The effects on toxicity of circadian patterning of continuous hepatic artery infusion. *Hepatobil Surg* 1992; **5:** 185–93.

25. Kemeny MM, Alava G, Oliver JM, The effects on liver metastases of circadian patterned continuous hepatic artery infusion of FUDR. *Hepatobil Surg* 1994; **7:** 219–24.

26. Von Roemeling R, Hrushesky WJ, Circadian patterning of continuous floxuridine infusion reduces toxicity and allows higher dose intensity in patients with widespread cancer. *J Clin Oncol* 1989; **11:** 1710–19.

27. Stagg RJ, Venook AP, Chase JL et al, Alternating hepatic intra-arterial floxuridine and fluorouracil: a less toxic regimen for treatment of liver metastases from colorectal cancer. *J Natl Cancer Inst* 1991; **83:** 423–8.

28. Davidson BS, Izzo F, Chase JL et al, Alternating floxuridine and 5-fluorouracil hepatic arterial chemotherapy for colorectal cancer liver metastases minimizes biliary toxicity. *Am J Surg* 1996; **172:** 244–7.

29. Metzger U, Weder W, Rothlin M, Largiader F, Phase II study of intra-arterial fluorouracil and mitomycin-C for liver metastases of colorectal cancer. *Rec Results Cancer Res* 1991; **121:** 198–204.

30. Safi F, Bittner R, Roscher R et al, Regional chemotherapy for hepatic metastases from colorectal carcinoma (continuous intra-arterial versus continuous intra-arterial/intravenous therapy). *Cancer* 1989; **64:** 379–87.

31. O'Connell M, Nagorney D, Barmath A et al, Sequential intrahepatic fluorodeoxyuridine and systemic fluorouracil plus leucovorin for the treatment of metastatic colorectal cancer confined to the liver. *J Clin Oncol* 1998; **16:** 2528–33.

32. Ron IG, Kemeny N, Tong B et al, Phase I/II study of escalating doses of systemic irinotecan (CPT-11) with hepatic arterial infusion of floxuridine (FUDR) and dexamethasone (D), with or without cryosurgery for patients with unresectable hepatic metastases from colorectal cancer. *Proc Am Soc Clin Oncol* 1999; **18:** 236a.

33. Durand-Zaleski I, Roche B, Buyse M et al, Economic implications of hepatic arterial infusion chemotherapy in treatment of nonresectable colorectal liver metastases. *J Natl Cancer Inst* 1997; **89:** 790–5.

34. Kemeny N, Ron IG, Hepatic arterial chemotherapy in metastatic colorectal patients. *Semin Oncol* 1999; **26:** 524–35.

37

Predictive markers in the treatment of colorectal cancer

Cynthia Gail Leichman

INTRODUCTION

In the earliest part of the new century, there have been promising new developments in the treatment of colorectal cancer. After 40 years of therapeutic utilization and clinical investigations of 5-fluorouracil (5-FU) in colorectal cancer, there is also strong evidence that we now have available rational means of deciding appropriate use of this rationally designed drug. Moreover, for the first time, a 5-FU-based combination therapy for colorectal cancer has demonstrated an improvement in survival compared with single-agent therapy for disseminated disease.[1,2] The advent of irinotecan as only the second chemotherapeutic agent with demonstrable cytotoxic activity in this cancer *appears* to represents a major step forward in the treatment of this prevalent disease. If 5-FU and irinotecan are found to improve survival after potentially curative surgery, the promise of a useful combination chemotherapy for colorectal cancer patients will be realized.

The new century also brings diverse types of new anticancer agents targeting specific molecular targets that have previously not been exploited. These include antiangiogenics, matrix metalloproteinase inhibitors, signal transduction inhibitors, monoclonal antibodies, tumor vaccines, and antisense oligonucleotides. For clinical and basic investigators, the most pressing questions are which of the new agents and molecular targets should be tested first and how these trials should be conducted. Experience indicates that if we persist in adding one new compound on top of another and another, it could take another 40 years before the next breakthrough in colorectal cancer. If tradition is not broken, each new trial will require hundreds of patients per treatment arm, will take years to complete,

and will run the risk of failed accrual due to unsustained interest as new developments and questions supervene. The untreated patient resource becomes increasingly thinly spread in the competition amongst industry and academia, with numerous trials for unproven agents, and the private medical sector, with an expanded armamentarium of standard agents.

Fortunately, the rapid expansion of information regarding the human genome and the molecular genetics of cancer – mechanisms of carcinogenesis, invasion, metastasis, and resistance – as well as the technology to study these events and characteristics in real time and in small amounts of tumor tissue, afford the possibility of assessing treatment efficacy in specifically targeted tumor cohorts. Such selection should allow the detection of activity more specifically in shorter time periods, and should enhance response rates for selected subsets of cancer patients. If new measures of therapeutic activity for promising rationally designed agents are to be defined, careful selection of therapies and targeted molecular markers to be prospectively tested in 'proof of principle' trials is mandatory.

This chapter will review a number of molecular markers of prognosis and therapeutic response that have been investigated as they relate to colorectal cancer. An attempt is made to define where sufficient data exist to sustain current use, in what settings the use of these markers is appropriate, and areas where new molecular parameters are – or should be – examined.

TUMOR SUPPRESSION: *p53*

The *p53* tumor suppressor gene is the most common genetic abnormality found, and one of the most heavily investigated, in human tumors.[3] The role of mutation of this gene as a late event in the pathogenesis of colorectal cancer was postulated by Vogelstein in the late 1980s, and its prognostic significance in gastrointestinal malignancies has been the subject of numerous investigations.[4,5] Point mutation of the *p53* gene occurs in approximately 50% of colorectal carcinomas. *p53* mutations have been shown to be strongly associated with lymphatic invasion, with poorer prognosis across stages I–III.[6]

Since accepted theories of the action of chemotherapeutic agents include their role as inducers of apoptosis or programmed cell death, this mechanism of action may intersect with the *p53*-mediated apoptotic pathway. Whether this is a positive or negative interaction remains under active investigation, since there are contradictory reports regarding the impact of *p53* mutation or deletion upon chemosensitivity.[7,8] Furthermore, the impact of *p53* status on chemotherapy response may differ depending upon the molecular target of the drug, and may exist in balance with the status of other genes such as *p21*, *hMLH1*, *bcl-2/bax*, and *MDR1*.[9–11]

The interaction of *p53*, a determinant of cell-cycle activity, and thymidylate synthase (TS), an important cell-cycle enzyme and target for fluorinated-pyrimidine anticancer therapy (see below), has been of great interest for colorectal cancer investigators. In an analysis of untreated stage II colon cancer cases, Lenz et al[12] demonstrated that *p53* status and TS expression are associated and are predictive of tumor recurrence. Likewise, in a disseminated colon cancer cohort, for whom TS results are cited below, wild-type (WT) *p53* is closely associated with low TS expression and higher response rates, while high TS, mutated *p53*, and non-responsiveness segregated together.[13] Therefore, *p53* status may influence TS expression, and thus may become important to future therapeutic strategies.

18q DELETION

As with *p53*, the role of 18q, the locus of the tumor suppressor gene *DCC* ('deleted in colon cancer'), has been extensively investigated as a prognostic factor since it was identified by Vogelstein as being associated with tumor progression in the development of colorectal cancer. Unlike *p53*, loss of heterozygosity (LOH) at 18q has not been associated with sensitivity to available fluoropyrimidine therapy. The impor-

tance of the 18q deletion in clinical practice was first noted by Jen et al[14] in 1994. These investigators found that allelic LOH at 18q significantly discriminated for poorer outcome in both stage II and stage III colon cancer. The difference was most dramatic in stage II, where, in 65 untreated patients, a 93% 5-year survival rate was observed for patients with no allelic loss, as opposed to a 54% survival rate for those with allelic loss.

Using immunohistochemistry, Shibata et al[15] confirmed Jen's findings by demonstrating a dichotomization for stage II colon cancer into those with survival identical to stage I (no allelic loss) and those whose survival mimicked stage III (18q deletion) (Figure 37.1). A number of subsequent studies have confirmed these findings, using both microsatellite markers and immunohistochemical methodologies, although doubt was raised by Carethers et al, whose study was unable to confirm the negative survival impact of allelic loss at this site.[16–18]

Although a prospective intergroup trial in the USA (Cancer and Leukemia Group B (CALGB) 9581) is investigating the role of LOH at 18q, as part of a panel of molecular markers, in conjunction with randomization to monoclonal antibody therapy versus control for stage II colon cancer patients, there is need for a prospective trial of LOH at 18q as a prognostic marker for chemotherapy for stage II patients. Indeed, as stage II colon cancer patients with LOH at 18q have a prognosis similar to untreated stage III patients, the goal of such a trial would be to identify whether therapy with 5-FU and leucovorin offers a similar benefit to these patients as it does for all stage III patients. Until such a trial is completed, it is not safe or reasonable to assume that treatment of these patients is worthwhile.

THYMIDYLATE SYNTHASE (TS)

TS, the target enzyme of 5-FU, the first rationally designed chemotherapy agent, is the most widely analyzed molecular marker of both response and prognosis of the past decade. Although its synthesis by Heidelberger took place over 40 years ago, 5-FU was, until recently, the only effective agent for disseminated colorectal cancer. As 5-FU has been widely used in combination therapies for all other gastrointestinal as well as many non-gastrointestinal cancers in disseminated disease, and in adjuvant and

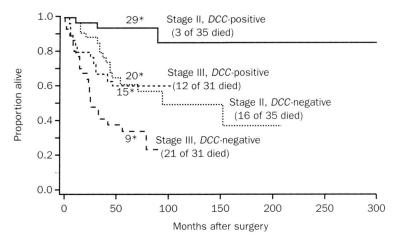

Figure 37.1 Kaplan–Meier life-table analysis of the overall survival of patients with colorectal cancer, according to TNM stage and the expression of *DCC*. Patients with stage II disease whose tumors were *DCC*-positive had a significantly better prognosis than patients with stage II disease whose tumors were *DCC*-negative ($p < 0.001$). Similarly, in stage III disease, patients with *DCC*-positive tumors had a significantly better overall survival rate than patients with *DCC*-negative tumors ($p = 0.03$). The numbers of patients who died of colorectal cancer during the entire study are shown in parentheses. The asterisks indicate the numbers of patients at risk at 60 months.

definitive therapies, it is not surprising that a great deal of interest has been focused on improving its efficacy. Since more patients have tumors that are resistant rather than sensitive to 5-FU, with new agents now available against colorectal cancer, it is imperative to use this drug as efficiently as possible. This is especially important since 5-FU remains a part of *all* of the new therapies in colorectal cancer. Quantitation of intratumoral markers that can predict relative sensitivity and/or absolute resistance to 5-FU will greatly aid the clinicians' efficiency and will, undoubtedly, save the patient the stress of an additional, but useless, cytotoxic agent.

Biochemical modulation of 5-FU in the clinical setting, and translational studies that have sought to define tumor resistance and sensitivity, have focused on the inhibition of TS or on the catabolic or metabolic enzymes necessary for 5-FU activity and breakdown.

As the target enzyme for fluoropyrimidines, TS is a catalyst for the reaction converting 2-deoxyuridylate (dUMP) to thymidylate (dTMP). Thus by inhibiting the de novo synthesis of thymidylate, 5-FU affects DNA synthesis. Although resistance to fluoropyrimidines may occur through a

variety of mechanisms, several investigators have demonstrated that intratumoral levels of TS have a demonstrable effect on drug response in cell culture systems.[19] Overproduction of TS (possibly as a result of gene amplification) can lead to tumor resistance to 5-FU.[20]

Although the mechanism of action of 5-FU had been widely accepted, understanding the role of TS in resistance or sensitivity to treatment had been limited by the ability to accurately quantitate the enzyme in tumor tissue. The development of the polymerase chain reaction (PCR), a highly sensitive and efficient method of amplifying specific DNA segments present at low concentrations, provides an approach for estimating the relative amounts of enzymes in tumors from very small amounts of tissue. By amplifying cDNA reverse-transcribed from RNA, the PCR can be used to quantitatively measure the expression of specific genes in tumor cells, i.e. mRNA quantitation. Danenberg and co-workers[21] developed an alternative PCR quantitation strategy for quantitating TS gene expressions (TS mRNA) in tumors using a housekeeping gene, β-actin, as a comparative internal standard. Comparison of TS mRNA expression with TS protein expression from tumors of patients confirmed that TS gene expression and TS protein expression are closely associated.[22]

TS EXPRESSION AS PREDICTOR OF RESPONSE

Directed by the hypothesis that TS mRNA within a disseminated colorectal cancer has an inverse relationship to 5-FU response, a clinical trial was conducted for patients with measurable disseminated colorectal cancer to test this relationship. Measurable tumors had to be available for pretreatment biopsy for TS mRNA quantitation. After biopsy of a measurable metastatic lesion for determination of TS mRNA level, patients were then treated with continuous-infusion 5-FU, 200 mg/m^2/day, with weekly leucovorin 20 mg/m^2 given as an intravenous bolus for two 3-week cycles separated by a 1-week rest. Tumor assessments were repeated after two treatment cycles. Patients who had been previously treated with 5-FU by bolus administration were eligible for this protocol.

Of 46 patients entered in the trial, TS/β-actin ratios were successfully obtained for 42 patients (91%). TS/β-actin ratios ranged from 0.3×10^{-3} to 18.2×10^{-3} (median 3.5×10^{-3}). The standard definition of partial response was used, namely a decrease by 50% or more in the sum of the products of the perpendicular diameters of the measurable lesion(s). Until the patient was fully evaluated after eight weeks of therapy, the TS mRNA levels were blinded to the clinicians and the responses were blinded to the basic scientists who conducted the assay for TS mRNA levels.

Consistent with expectations for a trial of this nature, 12 patients (26%) responded to treatment

(median TS/β-actin ratio 1.7×10^{-3}). Thirty-four patients did not respond (median TS/β-actin ratio 5.6×10^{-3}). No patient with a TS mRNA level greater than 4.1×10^{-3} responded, whereas 53% of patients with TS levels of 4.1×10^{-3} or less demonstrated a partial response to treatment. The median TS/β-actin ratio (3.5×10^{-3}) significantly segregated responders from non-responders ($p = 0.001$)[23] (Table 37.1).

TS levels were not affected by the patient's gender; however, younger age was associated with higher TS levels, and site of metastatic disease also suggested an association with TS levels. It is probable that, with current trials, the cut-point will be further refined. Furthermore, if larger trials confirm initial results, a subset of patients (with relatively low TS levels in their disseminated colorectal cancer) who will have an enhanced survival when treated with 5-FU-based therapy can be defined.

Significantly, responding patients who consented to re-biopsy at the time of disease progression were found to have intratumoral TS expression levels that were markedly higher than their pretreatment levels. One patient electively stopped treatment at the point of maximal response to therapy; a repeat biopsy at the time of tumor progression demonstrated a TS level unchanged from pretreatment levels, and the patient again responded to the same treatment regimen (Table 37.2).

TS EXPRESSION AS PREDICTOR OF SURVIVAL

As a prognostic indicator of survival in the adjuvant setting, TS was initially examined by immunohisto-

Table 37.1 Response and resistance to protracted-infusion 5-FU in relation to TS mRNA level (TS/β-actin mRNA ratio): range (0.3–22.6) $\times$ 10^{-3} (median 3.5 $\times$ 10^{-3})

TS level	Number of patients	Number of responders	Response rate (%)
$(0.3–18.2) \times 10^{-3}$	42	12	29
$\leq 3.5 \times 10^{-3}$ [a]	21	11	52
$\leq 4.1 \times 10^{-3}$	23	12	53
$> 4.1 \times 10^{-3}$	19	0	0

[a]The median TS level (3.5×10^{-3}) significantly distinguishes responders and non-responders based on a maximal chi-square ($p = 0.001$).

Table 37.2 TS variation from response to resistance

Patient demographic	Pretreatment TS/β-actin ratio	Posttreatment TS/β-actin ratio[a]
67 y.o. woman (liver)	0.5×10^{-3}	12.5×10^{-3} (12 months therapy)
56 y.o. man (liver)	1.1×10^{-3}	4.0×10^{-3} (8 months therapy)
72 y.o. man (liver)	1.5×10^{-3}	4.5×10^{-3} (13 months therapy)
69 y.o. woman (liver)	1.0×10^{-3}	7.7×10^{-3} (6 months therapy)
66 y.o. man (L supraclavicular node)	3.5×10^{-3}	39.1×10^{-3} (9 months therapy)
56 y.o. man[b] (liver)	2.2×10^{-3}	2.4×10^{-3} (14 months therapy)

[a]Time to resistance in parentheses.
[b]This patient interrupted therapy while in response. When tumor regrowth was noted, another biopsy was performed for TS.

chemistry in tumor blocks of primary rectal cancer obtained from patients entered on the National Surgical Adjuvant Breast and Bowel Project (NSABP) trial R-01. The three-arm clinical trial for Dukes stage B and C rectal cancer, reported in 1988, demonstrated a survival advantage for patients treated with chemotherapy consisting of 5-FU, vincristine, and semustine (MOF) compared with pelvic radiation or no postoperative therapy. Low TS expression was significantly associated with prolonged disease-free survival (DFS) and overall survival (OS) compared with high TS expression as measured by immunohistochemistry (Figure 37.2). While tumor TS expression increased with increasing stage, the prognostic value of high versus low TS expression for DFS and OS remained, independently of tumor stage. Patients with high-TS-expressing tumors who received adjuvant chemotherapy enjoyed a significant improvement in DFS and OS compared with those having no postoperative therapy (Figure 37.3). The differential impact of adjuvant chemotherapy on DFS and OS for those patients with low-TS-expressing tumors was not statistically significant.[24]

While it appears somewhat counterintuitive that primary rectal cancers with high TS expression would derive benefit from 5-FU-based chemother-

apy, when in disseminated bowel cancer this group is resistant to such treatment, the inclusion of other chemotherapy drugs in the treatment regimen may have impacted on this finding. The fact that low TS expressors were not seen to derive benefit may have been a function of the number of patients included, since only slightly over half of the cohort eligible by treatment group had tumor specimens available for analysis. It should also be noted that the improved survival of the chemotherapy-treated high TS expressors brought them to the survival level equivalent to that of the low-TS cohort. Lack of precision of the immunohistochemical methodology may have affected this outcome, as well as lack of differential benefit for treatment in the low-TS-expressing group.

In the University of Southern California (USC) trial that found a strong association between TS mRNA levels and response for patients with disseminated large-bowel cancer, among the stated objectives was the correlation of a quantitative cut-point for TS gene expression with response to 5-FU and demonstration of an increased TS gene expression associated with development of resistance to 5-FU; survival parameters were not an initial goal. When response data were analyzed, however, it was clear that survival was also associated with TS gene

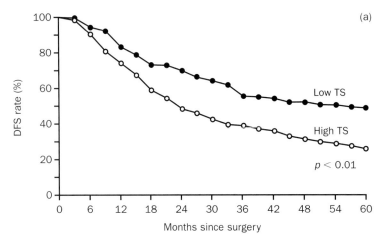

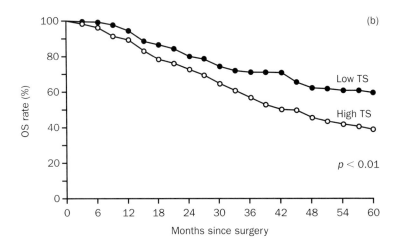

Figure 37.2 The correlation of the TS level with disease-free survival (a) and survival (b) in patients with rectal cancer. The TS staining intensity was compared with the percentage of patients who are disease-free or surviving 5 years (DFS (a) and OS (b), respectively). The log-rank test adjusted for Dukes stage and treatment group was used to test the difference between life-table distributions.

expression level, and that this association was statistically significant. Median survival for patients with TS/β-actin ratios of 3.5×10^{-3} or less was 13.6 months; for patients with TS/β-actin ratios of more than 3.5×10^{-3}, it was 8.2 months ($p = 0.02$).[23]

Following the NSABP rectal cancer study and the USC disseminated colorectal cancer trial, a number of investigators conducted retrospective analyses of primary tumor TS gene expression in colorectal cancer as it related to survival, with or without adjuvant chemotherapy. Confirmations of inverse correlation of tumor tissue TS expression and response to 5-FU therapy have been published by several groups in the USA, Europe and Japan.[25–28] TS analyses in these reports have been performed by immunohistochemical methods using monoclonal antibodies and

tumor blocks from the primary cancer resection in cohorts of patients treated with a consistent protocol. Predictive value of TS expression was shown for infusional delivery of systemic 5-FU,[29] for 5-FU with leucovorin[26] or methotrexate[27] modulation, and for intra-arterial floxuridine (5-FUdR).[30] Differential TS expression by metastatic site was observed, with lung and peritoneal metastases generally producing higher TS expression than liver metastases, and correspondingly demonstrating less frequent responses.[26,31] The only trial that failed to demonstrate a correlation of intratumoral TS expression with response used a polyclonal antibody against TS on primary tumors compared with response in metastases.[32]

Subsequent analyses have also confirmed the

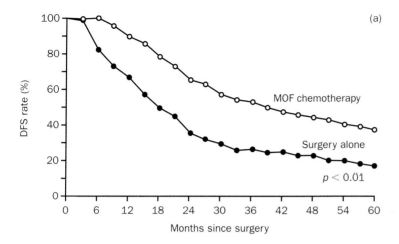

(a)

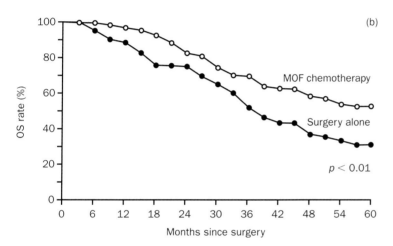

(b)

Figure 37.3 The effect of MOF chemotherapy on disease-free survival (DFS (a)) and overall survival (OS (b)) in patients with high TS levels. The curves are significantly different when the log-rank test is adjusted for Dukes stage and when it is unadjusted for Dukes stage.

independent value of intratumoral TS as a prognostic indicator of survival in colorectal cancer.[27,33] These reports additionally demonstrated significance of other molecular co-predictors of survival – thymidine phosphorylase and vascular endothelial growth factor – discussed below. The one group that failed to demonstrate a correlation of low TS expression with survival advantage used a protein expression assay as their methodology.[34]

All of the above reports involved small patient numbers – between 40 and 100. With the exception of the prospective USC trial[23] and the German hepatic artery infusion trial,[30] all used an analysis of tumor TS expression from the primary tumor and correlated the data with response in metastatic disease.

These considerations leave open the questions of whether TS expression in primary and metastasis are similar enough to allow the former to predict for response in the latter, and whether immunohisto-chemical methodology, with interobserver variability and inability to quantitate cut-points, will be accurate enough for prospective use in deciding which patients should not receive 5-FU-based chemotherapy.

THYMIDINE PHOSPHORYLASE (TP)

Thymidine phosphorylase (TP) catalyzes the reversible phosphorylation of thymidine to thymine.

It plays two major roles in the promotion and suppression of cancers. It has been identified as being identical to platelet-derived endothelial cell growth factor (PD-ECGF): in this setting its enzymatic functions promote both angiogenic and cell-motility functions necessary to growth and progression of malignancy.[35] Its role in phosphorylation promotes the transformation of pyrimidine antimetabolite drugs to active cytotoxic metabolites.[36] As levels of TP are generally found to be higher in tumor cells than in normal tissue, a potential selective cytotoxicity can be mediated by this enzyme.[37] In vitro and in vivo studies have demonstrated that tumor cells either with endogenously high levels of TP expression or transfected with the TP cDNA are more sensitive to 5-FU, floxuridine, and tegafur than cells with lower levels of TP activity.[38] This differential has been exploited in the design of one of the new oral fluoropyrimidine prodrugs, capecitabine, for which the final metabolic step toward activation is by TP, thus potentially enhancing drug exposure to the tumor while limiting toxicity in normal tissue.[39]

While the metabolic effect of TP may be beneficial in terms of tumor response to fluoropyrimidine therapy, its angiogenic effects imply that elevated levels of TP may be a harbinger of poorer prognosis.[40] Elevated TP has been associated with advanced tumors, node positivity, and microvessel count, all of which have been correlated with unfavorable outcome in a variety of solid tumors. As an optimal quantitative expression of TP for enhancement of fluoropyrimidine activity is not known, there may be a range for favorable versus unfavorable effects of this enzyme. Furthermore, the level of expression of TP is probably dependent upon the intratumoral status of other tumor suppressor genes.[41] Finally, the benefit seen from enhanced activity of fluorinated pyrimidines with elevated expression of TP may exist in balance with intratumoral expression of catalytic enzymes (e.g. dihydropyrimidine dehydrogenase, DPD[42]).

TP mRNA expression can also be measured as its ratio to β-actin (TP mRNA level) by PCR, and was determined for 38 of the patients described above in the USC trial examining the role of TS in disseminated colon cancer. There were approximately 200-fold differences in the TP mRNA levels measured in these tumors: TP mRNA ranged from 0.4×10^{-3} to 82.6×10^{-3}, with a median value of 9.8×10^{-3}. The median TP level for the 11 responders was 8.8×10^{-3}, with a range of $(1.3–16.3) \times 10^{-3}$. All

responders, who by definition had TS mRNA levels of 4.1×10^{-3} or less, had TP/β-actin ratios below 18×10^{-3} (Figure 37.4). Survival for patients with TS/β-actin ratios below 4.1×10^{-3} and TP/β-actin ratios below 18×10^{-3} was significantly longer than for those patients with both TS/β-actin ratios above 4.1×10^{-3} and TP/β-actin ratios above 18×10^{-3} (7 months versus 18 months, $p = 0.002$). For those patients with TS/β-actin ratios of 4.1×10^{-3} or less, no differences could be determined for TP/β-actin ratios either above or below 18×10^{-3} with the small numbers in this cohort.[43]

DIHYDROPYRIMIDINE DEHYDROGENASE (DPD)

While the above results have shown that tumor TS expression above a certain level reliably predicts for resistance to 5-FU-based therapy, a significant fraction of tumors with low TS expression also fail to respond. In these tumors, other response determinants apparently supersede the otherwise favorable prognostic value of a low TS level. One such determinant may be the tumor's catabolic potential. Compared with the anabolic pathway by which the active metabolite FdUMP is formed, the catabolic pathway had been relatively neglected; however, observations of severe 5-FU toxicity in the presence of DPD deficiency have demonstrated the profound

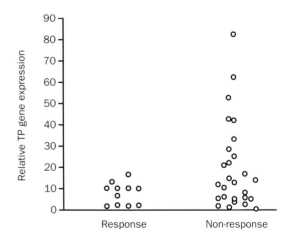

Figure 37.4 Comparison of relative TP gene expressions in 38 colorectal tumors grouped according to response (>50% tumor shrinkage) or non-response (<50% tumor shrinkage).

effect of this pathway on the therapeutic index of fluorinated pyrimidines, and have led to considerable investigation in this area.[44,45]

DPD is the rate-limiting enzyme of the 5-FU catabolism pathway. DPD activity has been measured in various human tissues and in human tumor xenografts, demonstrating high activity in human liver and variable activity in tumors.[46] In cell lines, low activity of both TS and DPD demonstrated significantly more sensitivity to 5-FU than was seen in cell lines with high activity of either or both enzymes.[47] Recent analysis of DPD in tumor, normal tissue, and peripheral blood mononuclear cells demonstrated both wide variability of levels, and non-correspondence of tumor with normal tissue levels.[48] These findings suggest that activity in tumor tissue itself must be analyzed for accurate prediction of therapeutic impact.

Studies using DPD inhibitors in vivo together with 5-FU have provided further evidence for the potential importance of the 5-FU metabolic pathway in chemotherapy. The most potent inhibitor of DPD activity developed to date is 5-ethynyluracil (EU, 776C85), which is a mechanism-based irreversible inhibitor of this enzyme.[49] Thus, if high activity of DPD is found to be a significant predictor of tumor resistance to 5-FU in spite of low TS expression, EU offers a rational approach to overcoming resistance. Moreover, combining EU with 5-FU may alter the range of TS expression for which efficacy can be expected in the treatment of disseminated colorectal cancer.

Based on the known coding sequence of the DPD gene, PCR methodology has been developed to measure gene expression of DPD. Thirty-three patients on the USC phase II trial had adequate tumor specimen remaining to allow for PCR analysis of DPD mRNA expression. As with the TS assay, results are expressed as a ratio to β-actin. In this cohort, the DPD/β-actin ratio (DPD mRNA levels) varied over an 80-fold range. For the 11 responders in this group, the DPD mRNA levels did not exceed 2.5×10^{-3}, while for the 22 non-responders, the maximum ratio was 16×10^{-3} ($p = 0.005$). For those patients whose tumors' DPD mRNA level was 2.5×10^{-3} or less, median survival was 10 months, while for those whose DPD mRNA level was greater than 2.5×10^{-3}, the median survival was 5 months ($p = 0.0015$) (Figure 37.5a). All responders had low expression of both TS and DPD, whereas 21 of 22 non-responders had high expression of either or both of these molecular markers[50] (Table 37.3).

IMPACT OF TS, TP, AND DPD

Data for all three of these parameters are available for 33 patients from the original cohort. Of these patients, 11 were responders, for a 29% response rate to protracted-infusion 5-FU. For the 19 patients having a TS level of 4.1×10^{-3} or less, the response rate was 57%. For the 14 patients with low TS and a TP level below 18×10^{-3}, the response rate was 79%. For the 12 patients with low TS and low DPD, the response rate was 92% (Table 37.4). Furthermore, patients whose tumors expressed low levels of all three markers had significantly improved survival compared with patients whose tumors demonstrated a high expression of any one of the three (Figure 37.5b).[50]

In a cohort of 32 untreated colorectal cancer patients, van Triest et al[51] also confirmed that both TS and TP were of prognostic significance for survival. They further identified that TP immunostaining correlated with vascular endothelial growth factor (VEGF) expression – a finding of potential significance for selection of chemotherapy agents and for combinations including anti-VEGF antibodies.[51]

The patient numbers presented here are too small to allow definitive statistical conclusions to be drawn. Also, the values for DPD and TP are arbitrarily defined within a population selected prospectively for determination of TS only. Undoubtedly, the numerical values will be altered in a larger patient population; nonetheless, the trend suggests that the use of these parameters could define a cohort of patients expected to benefit from treatment with fluoropyrimidine therapy. The trends also suggest that within a favorable molecular category, resistance may be defined as a function of association with a less favorable value for another molecular parameter. Understanding the relative values and interactions may allow us to modulate one or more of these parameters to enhance the likelihood of therapeutic response.

VASCULAR ENDOTHELIAL GROWTH FACTOR (VEGF)

Over the past decade, a considerable body of anticancer research has been directed toward strategies targeting tumor stroma, separately, or in conjunction with more traditional cytotoxics targeting the cancer cell. In directing therapy against tumor stroma,

Table 37.3 Summary of response data for tumors with different expressions of DPD and TS genes

Gene expression status	Number of responding patients	Number of non-responding patients	p-value[a]
DPD $< 2.5 \times 10^{-3}$ ($n = 22$)	11	11	0.005
DPD $> 2.5 \times 10^{-3}$ ($n = 11$)	0	11	
DPD $< 2.5 \times 10^{-3}$, TS $< 4.1 \times 10^{-3}$ and TP $< 18 \times 10^{-3}$ ($n = 11$)	11	0	0.0001
DPD $> 2.5 \times 10^{-3}$ or TS $> 4.1 \times 10^{-3}$ or TP $> 18 \times 10^{-3}$ ($n = 22$)	0	22	

[a]Based on Fisher's two-tailed exact test.

Table 37.4 Molecular determinants of response to protracted-infusion 5-FU in advanced colon cancer: effect of TS, TP and DPD

	Responders/patients	Response rate (%)	p-value[a]
All patients	11/38	29	
TS $\leq 4.1 \times 10^{-3}$	11/19	57	<0.001
TS $\leq 4.1 \times 10^{-3}$ TP $< 18 \times 10^{-3}$	11/14	79	0.011
TS $\leq 4.1 \times 10^{-3}$ DPD $< 2.9 \times 10^{-3}$	11/12	92	0.005
TS $\leq 4.1 \times 10^{-3}$ TP $< 18 \times 10^{-3}$ DPD $< 2.9 \times 10^{-3}$	11/11	100	

[a]Based on Fisher's two-tailed exact test.

agents designed to inhibit or destroy tumor microvasculature, i.e. antiangiogenics, have been of particular interest. Elucidating mechanisms by which antiangiogenic and cytotoxic agents influence response and/or resistance in human tumors is of considerable interest.[52]

Colorectal cancer has been demonstrated to express elevated levels of the angiogenic factor VEGF, the biologic effects of which include regulation of pathologic angiogenesis through enhanced endothelial cell mitogenesis, migration and remodeling of the extracellular matrix, and increasing vascular permeability.[53] The net result of these effects in the presence of cancer is stimulation of growth of both primary and metastatic disease, as well as promotion of the development of metastases. Indeed, human colorectal cancer cell lines are among those for which inhibition of growth has been demonstrated in the presence of an anti-VEGF antibody.[54] Further, combination of the antibody with chemotherapy has now been demonstrated to enhance antitumor activity compared with either single agent in a clinical trial setting where the addition of rhuMAb VEGF (recombinant humanized murine anti-VEGF monoclonal antibody) to bolus 5-FU and leucovorin produced a higher response rate and longer time to disease progression than with the cytotoxic alone.[55] rhuMAb VEGF alone produced tumor response in a small percentage of 5-FU-treated patients. VEGF has also been correlated with TP

expression in colorectal cancer.[51] This may prove important both as a prognostic discriminant and as a means of selecting therapies, such as capecitabine (which takes advantage of differential expression of TP in normal versus tumor tissue in its metabolic activation), for single-agent use or for combination with rhuMAb VEGF.

THE ROLE OF MISMATCH REPAIR

Up to 15% of newly diagnosed colon cancers will be diagnosed in the setting of hereditary disease. The most common of these that we are currently able to identify is hereditary non-polyposis colon cancer (HNPCC), which is represented by a phenotype identified as microsatellite instability (MSI). Individuals with this syndrome demonstrate widespread alterations of repetitive nucleotide sequences in their genomic DNA, secondary to defective mismatch repair due to methylation-induced post-transcriptional silencing of the *hMLH1* repair gene (among others of this repair gene class). Colon cancers with this phenotype have been considered to have a better prognosis, even though the genotypic setting in which they occur produces multiple cancers with an early age of onset.

For the past decade, it has been accepted that adjuvant therapy for stage III (Dukes C) colon cancer is the standard of care, since randomized trials in the

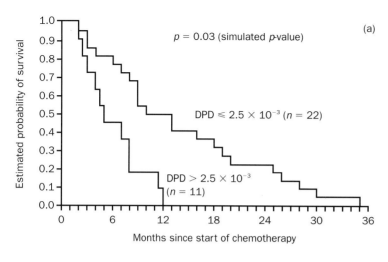

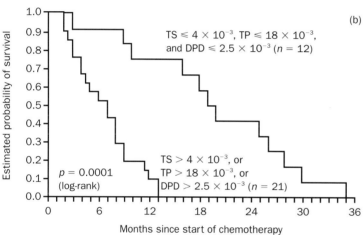

Figure 37.5 Survival (Kaplan–Meier) plots indicating probability of survival: (a) for patients with DPD expressions above or below the non-response cut-off (DPD/β-actin ratio = 2.5×10^{-3}); (b) for patients with DPD, TS, and TP expressions either above or below their respective non-response cut-off values (DPD/β-actin ratio = 2.5×10^{-3}; TS/β-actin ratio = 4.1×10^{-3}; TP/β-actin ratio = 18×10^{-3}).

1980s demonstrated a significant survival advantage for 5-FU-based therapy in this setting. A provocative, recently published study from Australia has challenged this assumption based on a predictive molecular parameter, MSI, in addition to site of tumor origin and sex.[56] Consistent with prior observations in the setting of HNPCC, which is characterized by right-sided colon cancers, right-sided tumors were more frequently MSI-positive than left-sided tumors in this 656-patient cohort. A survival advantage for adjuvant chemotherapy was seen for patients with right-sided tumors, for women, and for patients with MSI-positive cancers (Figure 37.6). Men with right-sided cancers received benefit from therapy, whereas men with left-sided cancers did not. These data sug-

gest that, rather than investing large patient, investigator, and financial resources in new phase III trials aimed at incremental increases in survival advantage, we need to re-analyze our trial-based assumptions in the light of molecular predictors to select patients who will receive benefit from known therapies, and focus future investigations on those who will not be aided.

CONCLUSIONS AND FUTURE DIRECTIONS

The sphere of research in predictive molecular markers for solid tumors is relatively young. The geometric increase in our knowledge of cancer genetics,

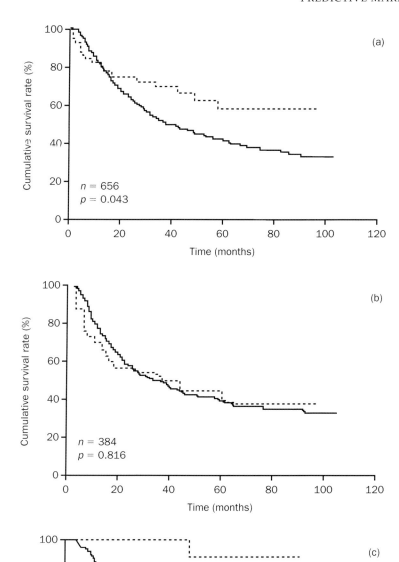

Figure 37.6 Kaplan–Meier survival curves for patients with (dashed lines) and without (solid lines) microsatellite instability: (a) overall; (b) without chemotherapy; (c) with chemotherapy.

signal transduction mechanisms, and the role of tumor stroma, with new agents to target treatment in all of these areas, provides exciting new prospects as well as significant strategic obstacles. Future clinical research needs to be focused on research questions that define appropriate patient and tumor environments. By addressing treatment questions in populations defined by molecular parameters, smaller trials could more quickly answer questions, leaving appropriate patients eligible as new candidate targets or agents are available for study. Trials of specifically targeted agents need to be designed with appropriate molecular markers built in initially, so as not to miss potential specific activity.

In colorectal cancer, the predictive molecular marker for which we have the most data at present is intratumoral TS. The data presented above clearly suggest that gene expressions such as the TP gene, the DPD gene, *p53*, and *DCC* can give additive prognostic and therapeutic information for chemotherapy treatment decisions. Additional tumor analysis for VEGF along with TP may indicate where additive therapies will have potential. At the host level, selection of patients for specific therapy should include considerations of sex, tumor site, and germline or tumor mismatch-repair status. Data are beginning to accrue regarding the *ERCC* repair gene family in the context of radiation as a possible treatment option, as in rectal cancer, and regarding *bax/bcl* in balance with *p53* status as measures of apoptotic response to treatment.

None of the small cohorts presented above are by themselves sufficient to establish prospective use of the predictive marker in question for treatment selection. The data are, however, sufficient to demand inclusion of molecular markers in all future clinical trials. The multinational contribution to these data suggests that the oncology community is able to accomplish this goal. The tools are available to enhance treatment efficacy and survival by tailoring individual cancer treatments, putting an end to 'one size fits all'.

REFERENCES

1. Douillard JY, Cunningham D, Rothe AD et al, Irinotecan combined with fluorouracil alone as first-line treatment for metastatic colorectal cancer: a multicentre randomised trial. *Lancet* 2000; **355:** 1041–7.
2. Saltz LB, Locker PK, Pirotta N et al, Weekly irinotecan (CPT-11), leucovorin (LV), and fluorouracil (FU) is superior to daily ×5 LV/FU in patients (PTS) with previously untreated metastatic colorectal cancer (CRC). *Proc Am Soc Clin Oncol* 1999; **18:** 898.
3. Greenblatt MS, Bennett WP, Hollstein M, Harris CC, Mutations in the p53 tumor suppressor gene: clues to cancer etiology and molecular pathogenesis. *Cancer Res* 1994; **54:** 4855–78.
4. Vogelstein B, Fearon ER, Hamilton SR et al, Genetic alteration during colorectal-tumor development. *N Engl J Med* 1998; **319:** 525–32.
5. Yamaguchi A, Kurosaka Y, Fuyshida S et al, Expression of p53 protein in colorectal cancer and its relationship to short-term prognosis. *Cancer* 1992; **70:** 2778–84.
6. Goh HS, Chan CS, Khine K, Smithe DR, p53 and the behaviour of colorectal cancer. *Lancet* 1994; **344:** 233–4.
7. Pocard M, Bras-Goncalves R, Hamelin R et al, Response to 5-fluorouracil of orthotopically xenografted human colon cancers with a microsatellite instability: influence of p53 status. *Anticancer Res* 2000; **20**(1A): 85–90.
8. Benhatter J, Cerottini JP, Saraga E et al, p53 mutations as a possible predictor of response to chemotherapy in metastatic colorectal cancer. *Int J Cancer* 1996; **69:** 190–2.
9. Nita ME, Nagawa H, Tominaga O et al, 5-Fluorouracil induces apoptosis in human colon cancer cell lines with modulation of Bcl-2 family proteins. *Br J Cancer* 1998; **78:** 986–92.
10. Vikhanskaya F, Colella G, Valenti M et al, Cooperation between p53 and hMLH1 in a human colocarcinoma cell line in response to DNA damage. *Clin Cancer Res* 1999; **5:** 937–41.
11. Thottassery JV, Zambetti GP, Arimori K et al, p53-dependent regulation of MDR1 gene expression causes selective resistance to chemotherapeutic agents. *Proc Natl Acad Sci USA* 1997; **94:** 11037–42.
12. Lenz HJ, Danenberg K, Leichman CG et al, p53 status and thymidylate synthase (TS) expression are associated and predict for tumor recurrence in patients with stage II colon cancer. *Clin Cancer Res* 1998; **4:** 1227–34.
13. Lenz HJ, Hayashi K, Salonga D et al, p53 point mutations and thymidylate synthase messenger RNA levels in disseminated colorectal cancer: an analysis of response and survival. *Clin Cancer Res* 1998; **4:** 1243–50.
14. Jen J, Kim H, Piantadosi S et al, Allelic loss of chromosome 18q and prognosis in colorectal cancer. *N Engl J Med* 1994; **331:** 213–21.
15. Shibata D, Reale MA, Lavin P et al, The DCC protein and prognosis in colorectal cancer. *N Engl J Med* 1996; **335:** 1727–32.
16. Lanza G, Matteuzzi M, Gafa R et al, Chromosome 18q allelic loss and prognosis in stage II and III colon cancer. *Int J Cancer* 1998; **79:** 390–5.
17. Reymond MA, Dworak O, Remke S et al, DCC protein as a predictor of distant metastases after curative surgery for rectal cancer. *Dis Colon Rectum* 1998; **41:** 755–60.
18. Carethers JM, Hawn MT, Greenson JK et al, Prognostic significance of allelic loss at chromosome 18q21 for stage II colorectal cancer. *Gastroenterology* 1998; **114:** 1188–95.
19. Washtien WL, Thymidylate synthetase levels as a factor in 5-fluorodeoxyuridine and methotrexate cytotoxicity. *Mol Pharmacol* 1982; **21:** 723–8.
20. Berger SH, Jenh CH, Johnson LF, Berger FG, Thymidylate synthase overproduction and gene amplification in fluorodeoxyuridine-resistant human cells. *Mol Pharmacol* 1985; **28:** 461–7.
21. Horikoshi T, Danenberg KD, Stadlbauer THW et al, Quantitation of thymidylate synthase, dihydrofolate reductase, and DT-diaphorase gene expression in human tumors using the polymerase chain reaction. *Cancer Res* 1992; **52:** 108–16.

22. Johnston PG, Lenz HJ, Leichman CG et al, Thymidylate synthase and protein expression correlate and are associated with response to 5-fluorouracil in human colorectal and gastric tumors. *Cancer Res* 1995; **55:** 1407–12.

23. Leichman CG, Lenz HJ, Leichman L et al, Quantitation of intratumoral thymidylate synthase expression predicts for disseminated colorectal cancer response and resistance to protracted infusion 5-fluorouracil and weekly leucovorin. *J Clin Oncol* 1997; **15:** 3223–9.

24. Johnston PG, Fisher ER, Rockette HE et al, The role of thymidylate synthase expression in prognosis and outcome of adjuvant chemotherapy in patients with rectal cancer. *J Clin Oncol* 1994; **12:** 2640–7.

25. Bathe OF, Franceschi D, Livingstone AS et al, Increased thymidylate synthase gene expression in liver metastases from colorectal carcinoma: implications for chemotherapeutic options and survival. *Cancer J Sci Am* 1999; **5:** 34–40.

26. Cascinu S, Aschele C, Barni S et al, Thymidylate synthase protein expression in advanced colon cancer: correlation with the site of metastasis and the clinical response to leucovorin-modulated bolus 5-fluorouracil. *Clin Cancer Res* 1999; **5:** 1996–9.

27. Paradiso A, Simone G, Petroni S et al, Thymidylate synthase and p53 primary tumor expression as predictive factors for advanced colorectal cancer patients. *Br J Cancer* 2000; **82:** 560–7.

28. Yamachika T, Nakanishi H, Inada K et al, A new prognostic factor for colorectal carcinoma, thymidylate synthase, and its therapeutic significance. *Cancer* 1998; **82:** 70–7.

29. Aschele C, Debernardis D, Casazza S et al, Immunohistochemical quantitation of thymidylate synthase expression in colorectal cancer metastases predicts for clinical outcome to fluorouracil-based chemotherapy. *J Clin Oncol* 1999; **17:** 1760–70.

30. Kornmann M, Link KH, Lenz HJ et al, Thymidylate synthase is a predictor for response and resistance in hepatic arterial infusion therapy. *Cancer Lett* 1997; **118:** 29–35.

31. Gorelick R, Metzger R, Danenberg KD et al, Higher levels of thymidylate synthase gene expression are observed in pulmonary as compared with hepatic metastases of colorectal adenocarcinoma. *J Clin Oncol* 1998; **16:** 1465–9.

32. Findlay MP, Cunningham D, Morgan G et al, Lack of correlation between thymidylate synthase levels in primary colorectal tumours and subsequent response to chemotherapy. *Br J Cancer* 1997; **75:** 903–9.

33. Edler D, Kressner U, Ragnhammar P et al, Immunohistochemically detected thymidylate synthase in colorectal cancer: an independent prognostic factor of survival. *Clin Cancer Res* 2000; **6:** 488–92.

34. Sanguedolce R, Vultaggio G, Sanguedolce F et al, The role of thymidylate synthase levels in the prognosis and the treatment of patients with colorectal cancers. *Anticancer Res* 1998; **18:** 1515–20.

35. Takebayashi Y, Akiyama S, Akiba S et al, Clinicopathologic and prognostic significance of an angiogenic factor, thymidine phosphorylase, in human colorectal carcinoma. *J Natl Cancer Inst* 1996; **88:** 1110–17.

36. Kato Y, Matsukawa S, Muraoka R, Tanigawa N, Enhancement of drug sensitivity and a bystander effect in PC-9 cells transfected with platelet-derived endothelial cell growth factor thymidine phosphorylase cDNA. *Br J Cancer* 1997; **75:** 506–11.

37. Luccioni C, Beaumatin J, Bardot V, Lefrancois D, Pyrimidine nucleotide metabolism in human colon carcinomas: comparison of normal tissues, primary tumors and xenografts. *Int J Cancer* 1994; **58:** 517–22.

38. Evrard A, Robert B, Cuq P et al, Enhancement of 5-fluorouracil cytotoxicity by human thymidine phosphorylase expression in cancer cells: in vitro and in vivo study. *Proc Am Assoc Cancer Res* 1998; **39:** 3538.

39. Schuller J, Cassidy J, Reigner BG et al, Tumor selectivity of Xeloda™ in colorectal cancer patients. *Proc Am Soc Clin Oncol* 1997; **16:** 797.

40. Moghaddam A, Zhang HT, Fan TP et al, Thymidine phosphorylase is angiogenic and promotes tumor growth. *Proc Natl Acad Sci USA* 1995; **92:** 998–1002.

41. Bicknell R, Harris AL, Mechanisms and therapeutic implications of angiogenesis. *Curr Opin Oncol* 1996; **8:** 60–5.

42. Ishikawa T, Sekiguchi F, Fukase Y et al, Positive correlation between the efficacy of capecitabine and doxifluridine and the ratio of thymidine phosphorylase to dihydropyrimidine dehydrogenase activities in human cancer xenografts. *Cancer Res* 1998; **58:** 685–90.

43. Metzger R, Danenberg K, Leichman CG et al, High base level gene expression of thymidine phosphorylase (platelet-derived endothelial cell growth factor) in colorectal tumors is associated with nonresponse to 5-fluorouracil. *Clin Cancer Res* 1998; **4:** 2371–6.

44. Lyss AP, Lilenbaum RC, Harris BE, Diasio RB, Severe 5-fluorouracil toxicity in a patient with decreased dihydropyrimidine dehydrogenase activity. *Cancer Invest* 1993; **11:** 239–40.

45. Van Kuilenburg AB, van Lenthe H, Blom MJ et al, Profound variation in dihydropyrimidine dehydrogenase activity in human blood cells: major implications for the detection of partly deficient patients. *Br J Cancer* 1999; **79:** 620–6.

46. Naguib FNM, El Kouni AM, Cha S, Enzymes of uracil catabolism in normal and neoplastic human tissues. *Cancer Res* 1985; **45:** 5405–12.

47. Porter DJT, Harrington JA, Almond MR et al, Inactivation of dihydropyrimidine dehydrogenase in vivo. *Biochem Pharmacol* 1994; **47:** 1165–71.

48. McLeod HL, Sludden J, Murray GI et al, Characterization of dihydropyrimidine dehydrogenase in human colorectal tumours. *Br J Cancer* 1998; **77:** 461–5.

49. Hohnecker JA, Clinical development of Eniluracil: current status. *Oncology* 1998; **12:** 52–6.

50. Salonga D, Danenberg KD, Johnson M et al, Colorectal tumors responding to 5-fluorouracil have low gene expression levels of dihydropyrimidine dehydrogenase, thymidylate synthase, and thymidine phosphorylase. *Clin Cancer Res* 2000; **6:** 1322–7.

51. Van Triest B, Pinedo HM, Blaauwgeers JL et al, Prognostic role of thymidylate synthase, thymidine phosphorylase/platelet-derived endothelial growth factor, and proliferation markers in colorectal cancer. *Clin Cancer Res* 2000; **6:** 1063–72.

52. Klagsbrun M, Angiogenesis and Cancer: AACR Special Conference in Cancer Research. *Cancer Res* 1999; **59:** 487–90.

53. Takahashi Y, Kitadai Y, Bucana CD et al, Expression of vascular endothelial growth factor and its receptor, KDR, correlates with vascularity, metastasis and proliferation of human colon cancer. *Cancer Res* 1995; **55:** 3964–8.

54. Kondo S, Asano M, Suzuki H, Significance of vascular endothelial growth factor/vascular permeability factor for solid tumor growth, and its inhibition by the antibody. *Biochem Biophys Res Comm* 1993; **194:** 1234–41.

55. Bergsland E, Hurwitz H, Fehrenbacher L et al, A randomized phase II trial comparing rhuMAb VEGF (recombinant humanized monoclonal antibody to vascular endothelial cell growth factor) plus 5-fluorouracil/leucovorin (FU/LV) to FU/LV alone in patients with metastatic colorectal cancer. *Proc Am Soc Clin Oncol* 2000; **19:** 939.

56. Elsaleh H, Joseph D, Grieu F et al, Association of tumor site and sex with survival benefit from adjuvant chemotherapy in colorectal cancer. *Lancet* 2000; **355:** 1745–50.

38

Mechanism of action of 5-fluorouracil in colorectal cancer treatment

Alberto F Sobrero

INTRODUCTION

The demonstrated activity of irinotecan, oxaliplatin, raltitrexed, and the oral 5-fluorouracil (5-FU) pro-drugs (discussed in detail elsewhere in this book) has shifted much attention from the field of biochemical modulation of 5-FU to that of combination chemo-therapy for colorectal cancer in the last few years. This general paradigm appears justified on the basis of clinical reports[1,2] suggesting higher response rates, longer progression-free survival, and in some cases prolonged survival for the combinations compared with 5-FU alone. Nevertheless, most of the positive combination studies have used complex scheduling of modulated 5-FU as backbone for the combination. In addition, combination regimens with the new agents are more toxic than modulated 5-FU alone, and the overall improvement of efficacy parameters remains limited. Furthermore, it must be remem-bered that, although appealing for their convenient administration route, the new oral fluoropyrimidines require conversion to 5-FU to exert their cytotoxic effects. These three reasons, coupled with the strong and active interest in determining the molecular fac-tors predictive for response to 5-FU, have maintained and renewed interest in the pharmacology of the fluoropyrimidines.

DEVELOPMENT OF 5-FU

5-FU represents one of the few examples of 'rational drug design': it was developed after the observation that cancer cells utilize uracil more avidly than nor-mal cells.[3] Uracil metabolism was thus perceived as a possible target for selective antineoplastic drug development. The hydrogen atom in position 5 was substituted with a fluorine atom. This halogen was chosen for two reasons: its similarity in size to hydrogen and its profound effects on the properties of the resulting compounds. To better understand this point, it helps to compare acetic acid, which is a normal component of our metabolism, with fluo-roacetic acid, which is extremely toxic because of its action in inhibiting one of the steps in the citric acid cycle and thus blocking normal cellular metabolism. Similarly, the fluorine atom was expected to convert uracil into a cytotoxic agent for those cells that pref-erentially utilize uracil. This was found to be the case, and 5-FU gained a wide spectrum of antineo-plastic activity.

THE THREE MECHANISMS OF ACTION

5-FU by itself is inactive. It requires metabolic activa-tion.[4] The similarity between the fluorine atom and the hydrogen is such that 5-FU utilizes the same transport system and activation pathways as uracil, but, once activated, it may alter cellular function, resulting in cell death. Figure 38.1 illustrates the metabolic pathways of 5-FU activation and degrada-tion. There are three key active metabolites.

- 5-fluoro-2'-deoxyuridine 5'-monophosphate (FdUMP), which inhibits the enzyme involved in the rate-limiting step in DNA synthesis, thymidylate synthase (TS);
- 5-fluorouridine 5'-triphosphate (FUTP), which becomes incorporated into RNA, causing crucial alterations in its processing and function;
- 5-fluoro-2'-deoxyuridine 5'-triphosphate (FdUTP), which may be incorporated into DNA in place of the normal substrate for DNA poly-merase, namely deoxythymidine triphosphate

(dTTP), which is depleted owing to the inhibition of TS; in addition, the inhibition of TS leads to an accumulation of deoxyuridine triphosphate (dUTP), which may also be incorporated into DNA in place of dTTP.

The first two mechanisms predominate in the great majority of experimental tumour systems, while the third seems to operate only in a few others. In addition it has long been postulated, and demonstrated in animal tumour models, that the antitumour activity of 5-FU depends upon its 'anti-DNA effect', while its toxicity is caused by the anti-RNA mechanism. However, the relative contribution to cytotoxicity of the three mechanisms of action is not so well understood. In fact, it is surprising how little clinical evidence is available to support this notion. This is particularly true considering that the strategies for the development of many TS inhibitors, oral fluoropyrimidines, and novel antifolates are based upon different interpretations of these different patterns of activation and cytotoxicity.

RELEVANCE OF SCHEDULING TO THE MECHANISM OF ACTION

The existence of a relationship between the schedule of 5-FU administration and a specific mechanism of action is suggested by several observations.

1. Plasma levels above the threshold for cytotoxic effects (1 μM) following conventional intravenous bolus doses are maintained for only a few hours.[5] TS inhibition is strictly S-phase-dependent. It is thus unlikely that this enzyme represents a major site of action under conditions of short-term, high-dose exposure. Rather, continuous exposure is likely to affect this mechanism. Conversely, the relative independence of 5-FU incorporation into RNA from a specific cell-cycle phase is compatible with significant cytotoxicity, even under conditions of short-term administration. 5-FU peak concentration, rather than duration of exposure, may be the key factor for incorporation into RNA.[6]
2. Prolonged low-dose 5-FU produces cytotoxicity that is prevented by thymidine, whereas, in general, short-term, high-dose 5-FU administration

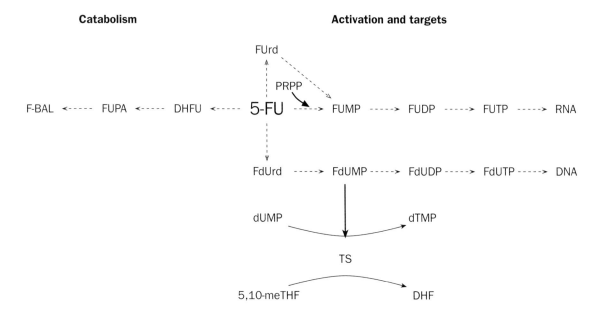

Figure 38.1 The mechanism of action of 5-FU. *Abbreviations:* FUrd, 5-fluorouridine; FUMP/FUDP/FUTP, 5-fluorouracil 5′-mono-/di-/triphosphate; PRPP, 5-phosphoribosyl 1-pyrophosphate; FdUrd, 5-fluoro-2′-deoxyuridine (floxuridine); FdUMP/FdUDP/FdUTP, 5-fluoro-2′-deoxyuridine 5′-mono-/di-/triphosphate; dUMP, deoxyuridine monophosphate; dTMP, deoxythymidine monophosphate; TS, thymidylate synthase; 5,10-meTHF, N^5,N^{10}-methylenetetrahydrofolate; DHF, dihydrofolate; DHFU, dihydro-5-fluorouracil; FUPA, α-fluoro-β-ureidopropionate (N-carbamoyl-α-fluoro-β-alanine); F-BAL, α-fluoro-β-alanine.

results in growth inhibition refractory to thymidine protection.[7]

3. Finally, long-term, low-dose repeated exposures to 5-FU result in resistance due to impaired stability of TS inhibition, while short-term, high-dose exposures are associated with resistance due to decreased incorporation into RNA.[8] And cells resistant to pulse 5-FU still retain sensitivity to a prolonged exposure to the fluoropyrimidine.[9]

These observations support the contention that 5-FU may be considered as two different drugs, depending on the dose and schedule of administration.[10] As we shall see later in this chapter, this may have important consequences on how to best modulate this drug. In addition, the de Gramont schedule derives its rationale from these concepts in that it is a combination of bolus and infusional 5-FU (see Chapter 44).

DETERMINANTS OF 5-FU ACTIVITY

Table 38.1 summarizes the determinants of sensitivity and resistance to fluoropyrimidines:[4] the complexity is such that it can easily be understood why it is so difficult to predict the sensitivity and the toxicity of 5-FU in individual patients' tumours. The biochemical determinants are subdivided into those contributing to the anti-DNA effects of 5-FU (TS inhibition), those contributing to the anti-RNA effects, and those responsible for the incorporation of 'fraudulent' nucleotides (FdUTP or dUTP) into DNA. The best known of these is the level of the target enzyme TS – the higher its activity, the lower the chances of a patient's tumour to respond to 5-FU chemotherapy.[11]

But this is only one facet. There are at least three other levels on which to approach this problem:

1. One can look at pharmacokinetic parameters (including the intratumoral distribution of 5-FU and its metabolites) that may be dependent upon serum dihydropyrimidine dehydrogenase activity.[12]

2. One can study the expression and regulation of key enzymes such as TS, dihydrofolate reductase (DHFR), ribonucleotide reductase, and thymidine kinase. The expression of these enzymes is regulated by molecular determinants such as E2F, which in turn depends upon the status of phosphorylation of the retinoblastoma protein (Rb).[13]

3. One can look at the so-called 'downstream

Table 38.1 Determinants of sensitivity to 5-FU

1. TS-related mechanism
  (A) Enzyme-related
    (a) Baseline activity of enzyme
    (b) Affinity of TS for FdUMP
    (c) Upregulation of TS expression following 5-FU exposure
  (B) Substrate-related
    (a) Baseline dUMP concentration
    (b) dUMP expansion following 5-FU exposure
  (C) Cofactor-related
    (a) Concentration of 5,10-meTHF
    (b) Polyglutamylation of 5,10-meTHF
  (D) Inhibitor-related (FdUMP)
    (a) Concentration of FdUMP following 5-FU exposure
      • Cellular entry
      • Activity of anabolic and catabolic enzymes
      • Availability of substrates and cofactors
    (b) Duration of FdUMP levels above cytotoxic concentration
  (E) Product-related (dTTP)
    (a) Capacity to salvage endogenous thymidine

2. RNA-incorporation-related mechanism
  (A) FUTP-related
    (a) Concentration of FUTP following 5-FU exposure
      • Cellular entry
      • Activity of anabolic and catabolic enzymes
      • Availability of substrates and cofactors
    (b) Extent of FUTP incorporation into RNA
  (B) UTP-related
    (a) Concentration of uridine triphosphate (UTP) and cytidine triphosphate (CTP)
    (b) Capacity to salvage endogenous uridine

3. DNA-damage-related mechanism
  (A) 'Fraudulent' nucleotide-related
    (a) Extent of FdUTP incorporation into DNA
    (b) Extent of dUTP incorporation into DNA
  (B) DNA-repair-related
    (a) dUTP hydrolase activity
    (b) Uracil DNA glycosylase activity

events' taking place after 5-FU-induced metabolic perturbations, and leading to apoptosis, mitotic cell death, cell-cycle arrest, or differentiation.[14]

GENERAL RATIONALE FOR BIOCHEMICAL MODULATION

The mechanism of action of 5-FU is very complex and the number of biochemical determinants of its cytotoxicity very high. It is therefore reasonable to look for strategies that may favour the activation of 5-FU towards this or that active metabolite in order to increase its activity or decrease its toxicity. For example, if it is true that TS inhibition accounts for the antitumour effect, while the anti-RNA effect is only responsible for toxicity, then optimizing the conditions for prolonged and complete TS inhibition should enhance the efficacy of 5-FU. This could be obtained by the use of exogenous leucovorin (5-formyltetrahydrofolate, folinic acid) (LV) or by decreasing the rise in deoxyuridine monophosphate (dUMP) that follows exposure to 5-FU. However, we still do not know if the rationale behind this example holds for every case; it is very likely that some colorectal cancers are more sensitive to TS inhibition, while others may be more sensitive to the consequences of FUTP incorporation into RNA. What may be an effective strategy against one patient's cancer may be deleterious for the next patient. Predictive tests would be essential for biochemical modulation, but the number of determinants, the complexity of the assays, and the ethical problems connected with sampling limit the results of these studies.

Finally, if it is true that the mechanism of action of 5-FU depends upon the schedule of administration, its biochemical modulation should be schedule-specific.[10,15] In particular, enhancement of 5-FU cytotoxicity with LV might be greater when the 5-FU is administered as a continuous infusion, while channeling 5-FU into RNA using methotrexate (MTX), trimetrexate, or N-phosphonoacetyl-L-aspartate (PALA) might improve results when high-dose short-term administration is used. These factors have not been taken into account in most clinical trials. Indeed, an alternating regimen consisting of 5-FU bolus modulated by MTX and continuous-infusion 5-FU modulated by LV (called schedule-specific biochemical modulation) is among the most active 5-FU regimens available today without the added toxicity of the new agents, as demonstrated in a recently reported randomized trial.[16]

ENHANCED CYTOTOXICITY VERSUS REDUCED HOST TOXICITY

In general, biochemical modulation can be divided into strategies that enhance antitumour cytotoxicity and strategies that decrease toxicity.

An example of the latter approach is delayed uridine rescue from RNA-directed toxicity of 5-FU.[17] But the intrinsic toxicity of the rescue nucleoside and the risk of interfering with the antitumour activity of 5-FU has limited its use. Similarly, allopurinol may antagonize 5-FU by inhibiting its activation to FUMP.[18] Therefore, in general, attempts to reduce toxicity are not so popular.

Another important consideration in this respect is the low clinical activity of unmodulated 5-FU (with a response rate of only 10%): it makes little sense to reduce the toxicity of an agent that is so weakly active on its own and that is rarely used unmodulated anyway. Thus, higher antitumour activity at the cost of the same toxicity must be reached first. Pursuing strategies to reduce toxicity will then make much more sense. In this connection, the use of interleukin-15 (IL-15) may be promising: in a preclinical animal model, this cytokine has recently been shown to protect rats from enteric damage induced by 5-FU plus LV or by irinotecan, without compromising the antitumour activity of these agents, both of which have diarrhoea as their limiting toxicity.[19]

5-FU PLUS LV

This is the most popular of all modulations. Inhibition of TS is considered the most important mechanism of cytotoxicity of 5-FU. This enzyme catalyses the last step in the de novo synthesis of deoxythymidine monophosphate (dTMP), and it is the rate-limiting step for DNA synthesis.

In the absence of inhibitors, this enzyme binds the substrate, deoxyuridine monophosphate (dUMP), and adds a methyl group to it, producing dTMP. This is phosphorylated to dTTP and incorporated into DNA. In this reaction, the source of the methyl group is the reduced folate cofactor N^5,N^{10}-methylenetetrahydrofolate (5,10-meTHF). After binding dUMP, TS binds 5,10-meTHF and transfers the methyl group to dUMP. This is made possible by the elimination of the hydrogen attached to the C-5 position of uracil.[4]

Following exposure to 5-FU, and formation of a sufficient amount of FdUMP, the methyl transfer does not take place, because the fluorine atom in the

C-5 position of FdUMP is much more tightly bound than hydrogen. The enzyme is then trapped in a slowly reversible ternary complex. The presence of 5,10-meTHF (or its polyglutamates) is essential for tight binding of FdUMP to TS. The longer the excess 5,10-meTHF is around, the longer TS is blocked, and the more likely it is that the cell will die. Conversely, if insufficient 5,10-meTHF is present, the extent and particularly the duration of TS inhibition will be limited, and the cell may survive. Since endogenous reduced folate levels are suboptimal, supplementation with exogenous folates should enhance TS inhibition. Besides the biochemical determinants listed in Table 38.1, there are three pharmacological variables affecting the outcome of this combination: the schedule of 5-FU employed, the dose of reduced folates, and the length of exposure to excess exogenous reduced folates.

The importance of the schedule of 5-FU has already been addressed and specifically investigated in experimental[20] and clinical studies.[15,21]

The dose of reduced folate is important in that concentrations of LV below 1 μM are insufficient to expand intracellular folate pools, and 10 μM is usually considered the target concentration. However, the duration of exposure to LV is also crucial. In fact, prolonged exposure to reduced folates allows extensive polyglutamylation of 5,10-meTHF, and the 5,10-meTHF polyglutamates promote ternary complex formation much more efficiently than 5,10-meTHF itself.[22]

5-FU PLUS INHIBITORS OF DE NOVO PYRIMIDINE SYNTHESIS

dUMP accumulation that occurs following exposure to 5-FU may reverse the cytotoxic effects of the fluoropyrimidine via competition with FdUMP binding to TS. In addition, uridine triphosphate (UTP) may compete with FUTP for binding to RNA polymerase, thereby limiting the anti-RNA effects of 5-FU. Inhibitors of pyrimidine biosynthesis might be used to enhance 5-FU activity by depleting the natural uridine nucleotide pools (dUMP and UTP) and promoting the utilization of 'fraudulent' pyrimidine nucleotides, such as FdUMP and FUTP.

The de novo synthesis of pyrimidines begins from simple components and proceeds to UMP through six reactions. A number of compounds are available to inhibit each of these reactions. PALA has been pursued most actively in the clinic. Two features are particularly appealing in the biochemical modulation of 5-FU with this drug. First, non-cytotoxic doses of

PALA are sufficient to lower ribonucleotide pools, and, second, these changes appear to spare normal tissues. Therefore low, non-toxic doses of PALA might successfully modulate 5-FU activity, allowing the use of maximally tolerated doses of 5-FU.[23] Despite this strong rationale, the clinical relevance of this combination is limited by its modest clinical activity.

5-FU PLUS INHIBITORS OF DE NOVO PURINE SYNTHESIS

The conversion of 5-FU to FUMP by orotate phosphoribosyltransferase (OPRT) requires 5-phosphoribosyl 1-pyrophosphate (PRPP) as a cofactor. Its level is an important determinant of 5-FU cytotoxicity, and depends on the activity of the enzyme PRPP synthetase as well as on its rate of utilization in reactions of nucleotide biosynthesis. 6-Methylmercaptopurine ribonucleoside (MMPR) is an inhibitor of the first enzyme of the de novo pathway of purine biosynthesis,[24] leading to an increased availability of PRPP.

5-FU PLUS ANTIFOLATES

All three major mechanisms of 5-FU cytotoxicity may be implicated in this complex schedule-dependent synergistic interaction.

1. When TS is not blocked, it consumes 5,10-meTHF; inhibition of DHFR by antifolates therefore results in progressive depletion of 5,10-meTHF. The whole reduced folate pool decreases, including N^{10}-formyltetrahydrofolate, a required substrate for purine synthesis (Figure 38.2). In addition, dihydrofolate increases, and this cofactor inhibits purine biosynthesis by itself. Because of this antipurine effect, the PRPP pool expands, thereby enhancing 5-FU anabolism to FUMP and its RNA-directed cytotoxicity.[25] This occurs only if antifolates are given before fluoropyrimidines.

   Conversely, antagonism occurs[26] when antifolates are given after fluoropyrimidines, because the inhibition of TS by FdUMP prevents the consumption of 5,10-meTHF, preserving the tetrahydrofolate pool for purine and protein synthesis, and therefore antagonizing the effects of MTX on both of these pathways.

   The sequence of administration of the two agents is thus critical.

2. Enhanced TS inhibition has also been implicated

in the synergism: this may result as a consequence of marked increase in the activity of ribonucleotide reductase[27] (triggered by MTX-induced lower dTTP pools), an enzyme that converts FUDP into FdUDP; alternatively,[28] dihydrofolate polyglutamates, accumulating as a consequence of MTX inhibition of DHFR, may tighten the binding of FdUMP to TS, enhancing ternary complex stability. MTX and, in particular, its polyglutamate derivatives may also enhance the binding of FdUMP to TS, by substituting for 5,10-meTHF.[29] However, the fact that trimetrexate[30] (an antifolate with the same mechanism of action as MTX, but incapable of polyglutamylation) still synergizes with fluoropyrimidines in the same sequence-dependent manner renders this last mechanism unlikely.

3. Finally, the reduced dTTP levels, as a consequence of TS inhibition by MTX,[31] may promote FdUTP or dUTP incorporation into DNA and contribute to the synergism.

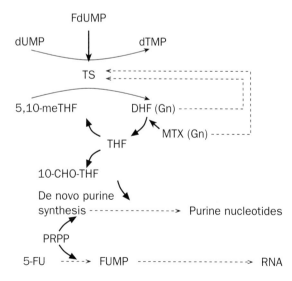

Figure 38.2 The interactions between 5-FU and methotrexate (MTX). *Abbreviations:* THF, tetrahydrofolate; 10-CHO-THF, N^{10}-formyltetrahydrofolate; Gn, n glutamyl residues; other abbreviations are as in Figure 38.1.

OTHER FLUOROPYRIMIDINES

5-Fluorouridine and 5-fluoro-2′-deoxyuridine (floxuridine) are the ribonucleoside and deoxyribonucleoside derivatives of 5-FU, respectively. The rationale for their development may be found in their different metabolic activation pathways. Following phosphorylation, 5-fluorouridine is incorporated into RNA, while floxuridine inhibits TS. Phosphorylases, however, may convert these nucleosides back to 5-FU, therefore limiting this approach to selectively targeting one or the other major mechanisms of fluoropyrimidine action.

5-Fluorouridine has long been dropped from clinical use owing to its toxicity. Floxuridine is much more efficiently metabolized by the liver than 5-FU is. This is why its major clinical use is in hepatic arterial administration for colorectal cancer with metastases limited to the liver.[32]

Tegafur (ftorafur) is a prodrug of 5-FU. It is a highly lipophilic molecule (a furan nucleoside), and this property accounts for its nearly complete oral bioavailability.[33] In addition, conversion to 5-FU is slow (via a two-step enzymic reaction that takes place mainly in the liver) and the plasma half-life is very long (around 10 hours). As a consequence of these properties, repeated oral administrations of tegafur should simulate continuous infusion of 5-FU, without the inconvenience of catheter implantation and the cost of infusion pumps.

Doxifluridine (5-fluoro-5′-deoxyuridine) cannot be converted as such into fluorinated nucleotides because (in contrast to floxuridine) it has the deoxy structure in position 5′, which is where phosphorylation occurs.[34] In order to become active, this compound must be converted into 5-FU by the enzyme pyrimidine nucleoside phosphorylase. The rationale for its development is the postulate that the activating enzyme is principally located in tumour tissues and in the intestinal tract, whereas normal proliferating tissues have only low activity.[35] The oral administration of doxifluridine results in 5-FU within the intestinal tract. This is why the major dose-limiting toxicity of this agent is diarrhoea.

In an attempt to overcome this limitation, capecitabine was developed:[36] this orally active compound is designed to pass the intestinal barrier as the intact molecule. Much less diarrhoea occurs. Once in the liver, it is converted to doxifluridine by two enzymes and hence into 5-FU.

For further discussions of tegafur (in combination with uracil as UFT) and capecitabine, see Chapter 47 on oral fluoropyrimidines.

ACKNOWLEDGEMENTS

This work was supported in part by a grant of the AIRC 1999 and CNR Biotechnology 1999.

REFERENCES

1. Douillard JY, Cunningham D, Roth AD et al, Irinotecan combined with fluorouracil compared with fluorouracil alone as first line treatment for metastatic colorectal cancer: a multicenter randomized trial. *Lancet* 2000; **355:** 1041–7.

2. Lévi F, Zidani R, Misset JL, Randomised multicentre trial of chronotherapy with oxaliplatin, fluorouracil, and folinic acid in metastatic colorectal cancer. *Lancet* 1997; **350:** 681–6.

3. Heidelberger C, Chauduari NK, Danenberg P et al, Fluorinated pyrimidines. A new class of tumor inhibitory compounds. *Nature* 1957; **179:** 663–4.

4. Grem J, 5-Fluoropyrimidines. In: *Cancer Chemotherapy and Biotherapy: Principles and Practice* (Chabner BA, Longo D, eds). Philadelphia: Lippincott-Raven, 1996: 149–211.

5. Fraile RJ, Baker LH, Buroker TR et al, Pharmacokinetics of 5-fluorouracil administered orally, by rapid intravenous and by slow infusion. *Cancer Res* 1980; **40:** 2223–8.

6. Nord LD, Stolfi RL, Martin DS, Biochemical modulation of 5-fluorouracil with leucovorin or delayed uridine rescue: correlation of antitumor activity with dosage and FUra incorporation into RNA. *Biochem Pharmacol* 1992; **43:** 2543–9.

7. Evans RM, Laskin JD, Hakala MT, Assessment of growth-limiting events caused by 5-fluorouracil in mouse cells and in human cells. *Cancer Res* 1980; **40:** 4113–22.

8. Aschele C, Sobrero A, Faderan MA et al, Novel mechanism(s) of resistance to 5-fluorouracil in human colon cancer (HCT-8) sublines following exposure to two different clinically relevant dose schedules. *Cancer Res* 1992; **52:** 1855–64.

9. Sobrero A, Aschele C, Guglielmi A et al, Synergism and lack of cross-resistance between short-term and continuous exposure to fluorouracil in human colon adenocarcinoma cells. *J Natl Cancer Inst* 1993; **85:** 1937–44.

10. Sobrero A, Aschele C, Bertino J, Fluorouracil in colorectal cancer. A tale of two drugs: implications for biochemical modulation. *J Clin Oncol* 1997; **15:** 368–81.

11. Aschele C, Debernardis D, Casazza S et al, Immuno-histochemical quantitation of thymidylate synthase expression in colorectal cancer metastases predicts for clinical outcome to fluorouracil-based chemotherapy. *J Clin Oncol* 1999; **17:** 1760–70.

12. Etienne MC, Lagrange JL, Dassonville O et al, A population study of dihydropyrimidine dehydrogenase in cancer patients. *J Clin Oncol* 1994; **12:** 2248–53.

13. Bertino JR, pRB–E2F and drug resistance. *Proc Am Assoc Cancer Res* 1999; **40:** 771.

14. Pritchard DM, Watson AJM, Potten CS et al, Inhibition by uridine but not thymidine of p53-dependent intestinal apoptosis initiated by 5-fluorouracil: evidence for the involvement of RNA perturbation. *Proc Natl Acad Sci USA* 1997; **94:** 1795–9.

15. Sobrero AF, Aschele C, Guglielmi A et al, Schedule-selective biochemical modulation of 5-fluorouracil: a phase II study in advanced colorectal cancer. *Clin Cancer Res* 1995; **1:** 955–60.

16. Sobrero A, Zaniboni A, Frassineti GL et al, Schedule specific biochemical modulation of 5-fluorouracil in advanced colorectal cancer: a randomized study. *Ann Oncol* 2000; **11:** 1413–20.

17. Leyva A, Van Groeningen CJ, Kraal I, Phase I and pharmacokinetic studies of high dose uridine intended for rescue from 5-FU toxicity. *Cancer Res* 1984; **44:** 5928–33.

18. Wooley P, Ayoob M, Smith FP, A controlled trial of the effect of 4-hydroxypyrazolopyrimidine (allopurinol) on the toxicity of a single bolus dose of 5-fluorouracil. *J Clin Oncol* 1985; **3:** 103–9.

19. Cao S, Black JD, Troutt AB et al, Interleukin 15 offers protection from drug induced intestinal toxicity in a preclinical animal model. In: *Chemotherapeutic Strategies for Treatment of Colorectal Cancer.* Amsterdam: 1999: 57.

20. Moran RG, Scanlon KL, Schedule-dependent enhancement of the cytotoxicity of fluoropyrimidines to human carcinoma cells in the presence of folinic acid. *Cancer Res* 1991; **51:** 4618–23.

21. Leichman CG, Leichman L, Spears CP et al, Prolonged infusion of fluorouracil with weekly bolus leucovorin: a phase II study in patients with disseminated colorectal cancer. *J Natl Cancer Inst* 1993; **85:** 41–4.

22. Nadal JC, Van Groeningen CJ, Pinedo HM et al, In vivo potentiation of 5-fluorouracil by leucovorin in murine colon carcinoma. *Biomed Pharmacother* 1988; **42:** 387–93.

23. Martin DS, Stolfi LR, Sawyer RC et al, Therapeutic utility of utilizing low doses of *N*-(phosphonacetyl)-L-aspartic acid in combination with 5-fluorouracil: a murine study with clinical relevance. *Cancer Res* 1983; **43:** 2317–21.

24. Paterson ARP, Wang MC, Mechanism of the growth inhibition potentiation arising from combination of 6-mercaptopurine with 6-(methylmercapto)purine ribonucleoside. *Cancer Res* 1970; **30:** 2379–87.

25. Cadman E, Heimer R, Davis L, Enhanced 5-fluorouracil nucleotide formation after methotrexate administration: explanation for drug synergism. *Science* 1979; **205:** 1135–7.

26. Bowen D, Folsch E, Guernsey LA, Fluoropyrimidine-induced antagonism to free and tightly bound methotrexate: suppression of ^{14}C formate incorporation into RNA and protein. *Eur J Cancer* 1980; **16:** 893–9.

27. Elford HC, Bonner EL, Kerr BH et al, Effect of methotrexate and 5-fluorodeoxyuridine on ribonucleotide reductase activity in mammalian cells. *Cancer Res* 1977; **37:** 4389–94.

28. Fernandes DJ, Bertino JR, 5-Fluorouracil–methotrexate synergy. Enhancement of 5-fluorodeoxyuridine binding to thymidylate synthetase by dihydropteroylpolyglutamates. *Proc Natl Acad Sci USA* 1980; **77:** 5663–7.

29. Santi DV, McHenry CS, Sommer H, Mechanism of interaction of thymidylate synthetase with 5-fluorodeoxyuridylate. *Biochemistry* 1974; **13:** 471–81.

30. Romanini A, Li WW, Colofiore JR, Bertino JR, Leucovorin enhances cytotoxicity of trimetrexate/fluorouracil, but not methotrexate/fluorouracil, in CCRF–CEM cells. *J Natl Cancer Inst* 1992; **84:** 1033–8.

31. Goulian M, Bleile B, Tseng BY, The effects of methotrexate on levels of dUTP in animal cells. *J Biol Chem* 1980; **225:** 10630–7.

32. Kemeny N, Daly J, Reichman B et al, Intrahepatic or systemic infusion of fluorodeoxyuridine in patients with liver metastases from colorectal carcinoma. *Ann Intern Med* 1987; **107:** 459–65.

33. Au J, Wu AT, Friedman MA, Sadee W, Pharmacokinetics and metabolism of ftorafur in man. *Cancer Treat Rep* 1979; **63:** 343–50.

34. Geng YM, Gheuens E, De Bruijn EA, Activation and cytotoxicity of 5′-deoxy-5-fluorouridine in c-Ha-ras transfected NIH 3T3 cells. *Biochem Pharmacol* 1991; **41:** 301–7.

35. Suzuky S, Hongu Y, Fukazawa H et al, Tissue distribution of 5′-deoxy-5-fluorouridine and derived 5-fluorouracil in tumor bearing mice and rats. *Gann* 1980; **71:** 238–45.

36. Twelwes C, Budman DR, Creaven PJ et al, Pharmacokinetics and pharmacodynamics of capecitabine in two phase I studies. *Proc Am Soc Clin Oncol* 1996; **15:** 1509.

39

From the laboratory to the clinic: The limitations of rationally designed fluoropyrimidine-based therapy and the problem of apoptosis-impaired cancer cells

Jean L Grem

INTRODUCTION

5-Fluorouracil (5-FU) has been used in the treatment of colorectal cancer for over 40 years, and traditionally has been given by the intravenous route owing to its poor oral bioavailability. Appreciation of the pharmacology of 5-FU has led to the development of diverse, clinically useful schedules. Insights into its cellular pharmacology have led to the combination of 5-FU with modulatory agents to enhance its metabolism, prolong its intracellular retention, or augment its cytotoxic effects.[1] 5-FU has also been used to potentiate the activity of other antineoplastic agents or modalities such as cisplatin and ionizing radiation. Despite the preclinical rationale, not all strategies have demonstrated clinical utility, for many reasons. While a detailed discussion of the experimental and clinical data is beyond the scope of this chapter, some problems and pitfalls associated with translating preclinical strategies into the clinical setting will be discussed. The activities of irinotecan and oxaliplatin allow therapy aimed at different molecular targets, and combination therapy is an area of active clinical research (reviewed in other chapters of this book). A major obstacle in the therapy of colorectal cancer is its intrinsic insensitivity to a variety of

cytotoxic agents. A challenge will be to develop approaches to treating cancers with deranged apoptotic pathways.

5-FLUOROPYRIMIDINE-BASED THERAPY FOR COLORECTAL CANCER: AN EVOLVING STRATEGY

Therapeutic strategies for colorectal cancer have evolved over the past four decades. Early empirical approaches included the identification of drugs with single-agent activity. Two or more drugs were then combined in the hope that the multidrug regimen would be more effective than the individual agents given alone. 5-FU emerged as the most useful agent for colorectal cancer, although nitrosourea compounds and mitomycin C also had modest activity. Initial studies involving a combination of semustine, vincristine, and 5-FU seemed promising in advanced disease (with response rates of about 40%). Semustine plus 5-FU (with or without vincristine) were subsequently evaluated in the adjuvant therapy of colorectal cancer. Many years elapsed before two definitive randomized trials refuted the benefit of adding semustine to 5-FU. Because both mitomycin C and nitrosoureas have the potential for chronic hematologic, pulmonary, and renal toxicity, they are now infrequently used to treat colorectal cancer.

In concert with empirical approaches, laboratory studies unveiled information concerning mecha-

Note This manuscript has been written outside the capacity of my official duties as a US federal government employee. The views expressed herein reflect my personal viewpoint.

nisms of resistance to 5-FU. The traditional in vitro models focused on cell lines selected for resistance. A single mechanism of resistance was usually identified, and strategies were then designed to circumvent the specific resistance mechanism. However, this model of 5-FU resistance is too simplistic. Different mechanisms of resistance are elicited when cancer cells are subjected to mutagenic stimuli prior to selection, continuously exposed to gradually increasing concentrations of drug, or exposed intermittently to high drug concentrations.[2] Studies evaluating colorectal cancer cells that have not been subjected to selection pressure suggest a multifactorial basis for intrinsic resistance to antimetabolites.[3,4] Thus, strategies designed to circumvent a single mechanism of resistance may be unsuccessful.

Biochemical modulation focused on using pharmacologic means to enhance the metabolism of 5-FU and/or increase the inhibition of thymidylate synthase (TS). The interaction of 5-FU and a second agent was assessed in vitro to identify possible synergism, to elucidate the underlying mechanisms of interaction, and to define a biochemical or molecular target that might correlate with tumor response. If available, data from in vivo models strengthened the rationale. A major tenet was the importance of defining the optimal dose of the modulatory agent rather than the maximally tolerated dose. Clinical pharmacology studies documented whether the achievable plasma levels of the modulatory agent were relevant with respect to the preclinical model, and the toxicity profile of modulator plus 5-FU was a crucial factor.

The impetus for testing pharmacologic doses of leucovorin (LV, folinic acid) as a biochemical modulator of 5-FU stemmed from appreciation of the importance of 5,10-methylenetetrahydrofolate mono- and polyglutamate on the formation and stability of the TS ternary complex.[1] Preclinical models showed that LV increased the intracellular pools of reduced folates and the duration of TS inhibition. A meta-analysis of nine randomized trials (1381 patients) comparing single-agent intravenous bolus 5-FU with LV-modulated 5-FU revealed a highly significant increase in the response rate (22.5% versus 11.1%; $p < 10^{-7}$).[5]

Another successful strategy involves sequential methotrexate (MTX)/5-FU. Sequential exposure establishes dihydrofolate reductase inhibition, which in turn results in inhibition of purine synthesis.[1] Consequently, phosphoribosyl pyrophosphate pools increase, thus promoting the anabolism of 5-FU to fluorouridine monophosphate (FUMP). In contrast, establishing TS inhibition prior to MTX antagonizes its antipurine effects. Preclinical models showed

improved antitumor activity with MTX given about 24 hours prior to bolus 5-FU, accompanied by increased formation of 5-FU ribonucleotides and 5-FU–RNA incorporation. One randomized trial in colorectal cancer demonstrated superiority of a 24-hour versus 1-hour interval between MTX and 5-FU.[6] In contrast, a trial involving MTX/5-FU/LV in head and neck cancer patients showed no advantage for an 18-hour interval compared with concurrent administration.[7] The most common MTX/5-FU-containing regimens developed empirically for breast cancer use simultaneous administration. The ability of MTX to modulate 5-FU toxicity and the optimal time of administration may thus depend on the tissue type. Meta-analysis of eight randomized trials in advanced colorectal cancer (1178 patients) comparing sequential MTX/5-FU with single-agent bolus 5-FU showed a significantly higher response rate: 19% versus 10% ($p < 0.0001$).[8] Many of these trials employed higher than standard doses of MTX, and delayed LV rescue was used to protect the patient, leading to speculation that the improved activity of these regimens may be due to LV modulation.

Monitoring the biochemical or molecular effects of the modulator is an important caveat. Ideally, tumor tissue should be sampled, but this requires tissue procurement prior to and following treatment. Host tissues are more easily procured. Although the surrogate tissue may not reflect the tumor milieu, establishment of a correlation between a biochemical/molecular effect in the host tissue and clinical endpoints would provide a rationale for monitoring the effects in tumor tissue in subsequent trials. Another problem is the selection of the appropriate surrogate tissue. Different host tissues respond differently to a drug, leading to contrary conclusions concerning the lowest active biochemical dose. For example, in a clinical trial evaluating escalating doses of N-phosphonacetyl-L-aspartic acid (PALA), two surrogate endpoints were used. Appreciable decreases in plasma uridine levels, which largely reflect drug effect on hepatic aspartate carbamoyltransferase activity, was seen with the lowest dose tested ($250 \, mg/m^2$), while significant inhibition of enzyme activity in peripheral blood mononuclear cells required a fivefold higher dose.[9] Another study evaluating the effect of PALA in tumor tissue suggested that doses of $3000 \, mg/m^2$ or more were needed to inhibit target enzyme activity.[10] Some biochemical or radiochemical assays are relatively insensitive, and require larger tumor specimens; distinguishing a true negative from an inadequate sample can also be problematic. Newer techniques include determination of protein expression by immunohistochemistry, Western immunoblot or flow cytometry, quantitative measurement of mRNA expression by reverse-transcriptase polymerase chain reaction (RT-PCR) techniques, and global assessment of gene expression by microchip array technology. These emerging technologies are poised to revolutionize the field of translational research.

Modulation of 5-FU by interferons represents another failed clinical strategy despite a compelling preclinical rationale. A variety of laboratory studies documented augmentation of 5-FU cytotoxicity by interferons. The basis for the enhanced cytotoxicity varied among different cell lines, and included increased anabolism to fluorodeoxyuridine monophosphate (FdUMP), increased activity of thymidine phosphorylase, increased inhibition of TS, repression of 5-FU-associated increases in TS protein content, marked deoxyadenosine triphosphate/deoxythymidine triphosphate (dATP/dTTP) imbalance, and increased nascent and parental DNA damage.[1] A variety of clinical regimens were developed. Since the preclinical data suggested optimal results with prolonged exposure to interferons, we designed a regimen in which patients received 5 MU/m² interferon-α (IFN-α) subcutaneously on days 1–7, and LV 500 mg/m² given intravenously over 30 minutes followed 1 hour later by bolus 5-FU 370 mg/m² intravenously on days 2–6. This schedule of IFN-α produced a relevant pharmacologic effect (a decrease in 5-FU clearance associated with inhibition of 5-FU catabolism by dihydropyrimidine dehydrogenase).[11] In a phase II trial, 54% of 44 colorectal cancer patients responded.[12] The worth of IFN-α as a modulator of 5-FU/LV was then evaluated in a large adjuvant colon cancer trial in which 2129 patients were randomized to receive six monthly cycles of LV 500 mg/m² plus 5-FU 370 mg/m² intravenously on days 1–5, or the same 5-FU/LV regimen given on days 2–6 with IFN-α 5 MU/m² subcutaneously on days 1–7. No significant improvement was seen in the 4-year disease-free rate (69% versus 70%) or overall survival rate (80% versus 81%) with the addition of interferon.[13] In contrast, the interferon arm was significantly more toxic; three times as many patients stopped therapy prematurely (22% versus 6%). The clinical data indicate that normal host tissues are very susceptible to interferon modulation of 5-FU/LV toxicity, and the non-selective modulation of 5-FU toxicity may account for the disappointing clinical results.

THE MOLECULAR BASIS OF INHERENT CHEMO-INSENSITIVITY OF COLORECTAL CANCER

The chemotherapeutic paradigms for human cancers were initially guided by the activity of combination chemotherapy in patients with lymphoma, acute leukemia, and germ cell neoplasms. Persuasive evidence suggests that these models of curable cancers may not be applicable to malignancies arising from many epithelial and mesenchymal tissues.

Preclinical studies have shown marked differences in fluoropyrimidine sensitivity despite comparable TS inhibition, implying that adequate TS inhibition may be insufficient to induce cell death. DNA fragmentation plays an integral role in mediating cytotoxicity resulting from thymidylate depletion.[1] The pattern and extent of DNA damage induced by fluoropyrimidines in human colorectal cancer cells varies, and may be affected by the activity of enzymes involved in DNA repair.[14,15] Recent studies indicate that factors operating downstream from TS influence sensitivity to fluoropyrimidines. Overexpression of the *Bcl-2* oncogene, homozygous mutations in the *p53* gene, and increased activity of deoxyuridine triphosphatase are associated with insensitivity to 5-FU-mediated cell death.[15–17]

Thus, genotoxic stress resulting from events such as TS inhibition is necessary, but not sufficient, for lethality. While growth inhibition may result, additional downstream pathways are required to implement cellular destruction. Improved understanding of how cell death pathways are initiated in response to genotoxic events such as TS inhibition and the cellular factors that influence the ability of cells to undergo apoptosis will be crucial to decipher the molecular basis of intrinsic insensitivity to cytotoxic agents.

DEFECTS IN CELL-CYCLE CHECKPOINTS

Three major classes of genes appear to predispose to cancer: oncogenes that positively regulate cell growth; tumor suppressor genes that negatively regulate cell growth; and DNA repair genes (such as aberrant nucleotide mismatch DNA repair), which indirectly control proliferation by limiting the rate of mutations in growth-controlling genes.

Mutations in the genes encoding cell-cycle-related proteins are a common genetic change in cancer cells.[18–20] The cancer cell's ability to grow and divide under conditions where non-cancer cells do not may result from such diverse factors as independence from external signals that are normally required for cell-cycle progression (mitogenic signals, cell-type-specific cytokines, cell–cell or cell–substratum interactions), faster cycling time, and insensitivity to metabolic or genotoxic insults that would halt the growth of normal cells. Gain or loss of function of proteins that constitute the cell-cycle machinery may largely explain the dysregulated growth of cancer cells.

Disruption of normal cell-cycle controls enhances genetic instability and promotes progression to a more aggressive, malignant phenotype. Several stages in the cell cycle are regulated in response to DNA damage, apparently to prevent propagation of genetic changes and loss of genetic material.[18–22] These cell-cycle transitions serve as 'checkpoints' that delay cell-cycle progression to allow DNA damage repair before entering S phase, to ensure that DNA synthesis is complete and to prevent mitosis until the mitotic spindles are properly assembled and aligned.

The cyclin-dependent kinases (CDKs) are a group of serine/threonine protein kinases that stimulate cell proliferation by phosphorylating specific substrates, such as the retinoblastoma protein (Rb), p53,

centromeric proteins, and lamins, in a cell-cycle-dependent fashion.[18–22] CDK subunits associate with a regulatory cyclin subunit to form a heterodimeric molecule (Figure 39.1). While the CDK proteins are expressed at relatively constant levels throughout the cell cycle, their enzymatic activity is regulated by phosphorylation and dephosphorylation at specific points. Mammalian CDK-activating kinase (CAK), composed of the polypeptide subunits CDK7 and cyclin H, is involved in controlling multiple cell-cycle transitions by phosphorylating specific threonine residues (Thr 160 and Thr 161) in the CDKs. The CDC25 (cell-division control) family of protein phosphatases activate the cyclin B–CDK1 and cyclin A–CDK1 complexes by removing inhibitory phosphate residues (from Thr 14 and Thr 15). Once fully activated, the CDK–cyclin complexes in turn phosphorylate and thereby activate a set of proteins necessary for transition through the appropriate phase of the cell cycle. The D-type cyclins (D1, D2, and D3) and cyclin E are the primary G_1-phase cyclins in mammalian cells, while cyclins A and B are necessary for the transition through S and G_2/M phases (Table 39.1).

A group of CDK inhibitors negatively regulate the

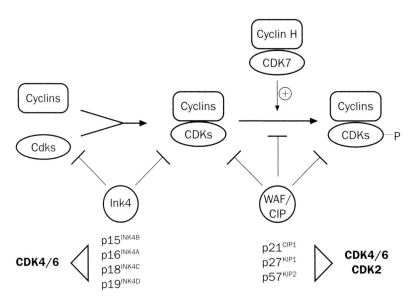

Figure 39.1 Activation and inhibition of the cyclin-dependent kinases (CDKs). This cartoon presents a simplified scheme for the steps involved in activation of the CDKs. Association of the CDKs with specific cyclin proteins causes conformational changes leading to partial activation. The CDKs are further activated by phosphorylation of specific threonine residues (residues 160 or 161) by the cyclin H–CDK7 complex. The INK family of proteins preferentially interact with the cyclin-D-dependent kinases, and interfere with both the assembly of CDK4–cyclin D complexes and the catalytic activity of any preformed complexes. The CIP family of proteins interact with both CDK4/6– and CDK2–cyclin complexes. The CDK inhibitors are responsive to distinct sets of growth-regulatory signals.

Table 39.1 Primary cyclins and cyclin-dependent kinases (CDKs) involved in cell-cycle control

Cell-cycle phase	Predominant cyclin	Predominant CDKs
G_1	D cyclins (D1, D2, D3)	CDK4, CDK6
Late G_1	cyclin E	CDK2
S	cyclin A	CDK2
Late S	cyclin A	CDK1
G_2M	cyclin B	CDK1

Cyclins are synthesized and degraded in a carefully orchestrated manner coinciding with specific points in the cell cycle. The levels of each cyclin are regulated at both the levels of transcription and degradation. While the protein content of the CDKs is relatively constant, their enzymatic activity is regulated by phosphorylation (by the action of CDK7/cyclin H complex) and dephosphorylation (by the action of the CDC25 family of phosphatases).

transition through each cell cycle phase by forming stable complexes with the CDK proteins and inactivating the catalytically operative unit.[23,24] The expression of these inhibitors is under the control of different pro- and anti-mitogenic signals. One class of CDK inhibitors, the KIP/CIP family (kinase inhibitory proteins/CDK interacting proteins), consists of three structurally related proteins (p21, p27, and p57) that bind to and inhibit several cyclin–CDK complexes. The expression of the KIP/CIP family of inhibitors is under the control of different upstream signals. For example, p21 is induced by p53 in response to DNA damage, while p27 is induced by other signals, including contact inhibition.[23–25] The ratio of p21 to cyclin–CKD4 governs whether the p21–cyclin–CDK complex is active or inactive.

The second class of CDK inhibitors (INK4 proteins, inhibitors of CDK4) consists of four related molecules, p16, p15, p18, and p19, that are specific inhibitors of CDK4/6.[23,24] The INK4 proteins bind to monomeric CDK subunits to form independent binary complexes, thus inhibiting the formation of cyclin D–CDK4/6 complexes. The INK4 proteins also inhibit the catalytic activity of assembled cyclin–CDK4 complexes. The gene for p16 is referred to as the multiple tumor suppressor gene 1 (*MTS1*), because it is homozygously deleted or translocated from chromosome 9p21 at high frequency in cell lines derived from a wide range of solid tumors.[26] The INK4 family members also respond to different upstream signals: for example, p16, senescence, p15, and transforming growth factor β (TGF-β).

Proteins such as the cyclins that drive the cell cycle forward are frequently overexpressed in primary tumors, while proteins such as p16 and Rb that restrain cell-cycle progression are frequently inacti-

vated.[18–24,26] The Rb family proteins include Rb, p107, and p130. Rb protein in its underphosphorylated form binds to and sequesters specific proteins necessary for cell-cycle progression, including members of the E2F family of transcription factors (E2F1 … E2F6). The E2F proteins contain a DNA-binding domain in the central part of the molecule, and an Rb-binding domain at the carboxy-terminal portion. E2F proteins are required for the expression of many genes that encode proteins involved in DNA replication such as DNA polymerase α, proliferating cell nuclear antigen (PCNA, an accessory subunit of DNA polymerase), thymidine kinase, dihydrofolate reductase, thymidylate synthase, CDK1 and C-Myc. DP1 and DP2 (differentiation-regulated transcription factor polypeptides) belong to another protein family, are constitutively expressed throughout the cell cycle, and interact with E2F to form a specific DNA-binding heterodimer. Binding of E2F–DP1 to Rb converts it to a transcriptional repressor. During mid-G_1 phase, Rb undergoes phosphorylation (Figure 39.2). The levels of cyclin E increase dramatically at the end of G_1 phase, and cyclin E–CDK2 complexes also contribute to Rb phosphorylation. These events release E2F–DP1 from Rb, and transcription of E2F-responsive genes ensues, allowing progression into S phase. The cyclin E–CDK2 complex has histone H1 kinase activity, and phosphorylation of key substrates is thought to regulate a key transition point for the initiation of DNA synthesis and entry into S phase.

The underphosphorylated form of Rb is sequestered by binding to certain proteins of DNA tumor viruses (SV40 large T antigen, adenovirus E1A, and human papilloma virus (HPV) E7). Many tumor suppressor genes are inactivated by intragenic mutations in one allele, accompanied by the loss of a

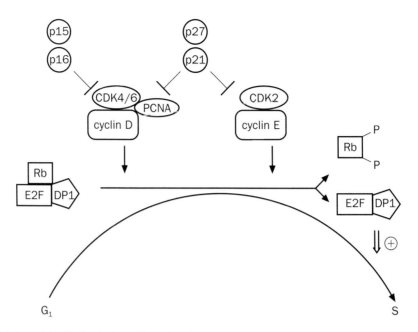

Figure 39.2 Regulation of the G_1 checkpoint of the cell cycle. (Abbreviations: CDK, cyclin-dependent kinase; PCNA, proliferating cell nuclear antigen; Rb, retinoblastoma protein.) E2F is a family of transcription factors that regulate cell-cycle activity. DP1 contains a dimerization domain allowing it to complex with E2F to form an E2F site-specific DNA-binding heterodimer. p21 and p27 are members of the CIP family of CDK inhibitors, while p16 and p15 belong to the INK4 family of CDK inhibitors. The underphosphorylated form of Rb binds to and inhibits the transcriptional activity of E2F–DP1. Phosphorylation of Rb by cyclin–CDK complexes releases E2F–DP1, which is then capable of activating cellular genes needed for DNA synthesis.

chromosome region containing the other allele (loss of heterozygosity). Mutational inactivation of the tumor suppressor gene *Rb* occurs frequently in certain tumor types. These phenomena result in the loss of the antiproliferative control normally imposed by Rb. Inactivation or co-deletion of the *p15/p16* genes also occurs frequently in solid tumors, leading to unopposed, constitutive activation of the cyclin D complexes.

Timed destruction of key proteins including the cyclins by a process called ubiquitination also plays a critical role in regulating the cell cycle.[18–24] A dramatic fall in the levels of specific cyclins at precise times during the cell cycle causes CDKs to stop functioning. A specific short amino acid sequence on a cyclin directs the attachment of ubiquitin, which in turn targets the cyclin for destruction by proteolysis.[27] Mutations in this portion of the cyclin protein prevent its destruction. Amplification of cyclins has been identified in various solid tumors: of cyclin D1 in squamous cell cancers arising in the head, neck, and esophagus; of cyclin D2 in human colorectal cancers; and of cyclins E, A, and B in breast cancer.[23,28,29]

Loss of p27 occurs frequently in human tumors, apparently due to alterations in the proteolytic pathways that lead to its degradation.[29]

The protein product of the *p53* tumor suppressor gene (on chromosome 17p13) plays a pivotal role in the regulation of gene expression through both transcriptional activation and repression, cell-cycle progression, and induction of apoptosis after DNA damage.[30,31] p53, a nuclear phosphoprotein of $M_r \approx 53$ kDa, binds to specific DNA sequences within the promoter regions of a number of specific target genes, resulting in their transcriptional activation. The p53-responsive element is composed of a 20 bp consensus-binding site. Several functional domains of p53 have been identified: an amino-terminal transcriptional activation domain, a central DNA-binding domain, and a carboxy-terminal regulatory domain that contains an oligomerization region as well as sequences that influence DNA binding. The amino-terminal activation domain stimulates transcription by interacting with components of a basal transcription factor TFIID in the RNA polymerase II transcriptional apparatus.[32] p53 tends to oligomerize, and also interacts with various proteins. In this regard, a polyproline-rich region of p53 contains binding motifs typical of those that mediate protein–protein interactions. Wild-type p53 protein also downregulates the expression of a variety of genes that lack the p53-responsive element (such as c-*fos*, *β-actin*, and *hsc70*), presumably through a distinct inhibitory domain.[33,34]

p53 protein levels are highly regulated by post-translational mechanisms.[30,31] Degradation may involve ubiquitin-dependent proteolysis, and regulated changes in p53 degradation permit rapid increases in p53 protein levels in response to specific stimuli. Levels of p53 protein and its transcriptional activity rise dramatically after DNA damage.[25] The gene that codes for p21 was initially called *WAF1* (wild-type p53-activated fragment 1) because of its activation by p53. p21-mediated inhibition of cyclin D–CDK4 and cyclin E–CDK2 complexes prevents phosphorylation of the Rb protein, leading to G1 arrest.[35] Through a functionally distinct domain, p21 binds to and inhibits PCNA, thereby preventing acti-

vation of DNA polymerase ϵ and δ. The cell cycle is thus halted in mid-cycle (G_1 arrest) before the cell is committed to divide, and DNA replication is blocked. p53 also stimulates DNA repair machinery by transcriptionally activating the *GADD45* gene (growth arrest and DNA damage-inducible), which codes for an enzyme involved in excision repair of damaged DNA. p53 is thought to upregulate the activity of ERCC3 (excision repair cross-complementing), a nucleotide excision-repair enzyme that recognizes and removes damaged DNA segments. The p53-dependent G_1 checkpoint prevents entry of cells into S phase if the genome contains damaged DNA, affording time to repair this damage. Another cell-cycle control gene activated by p53 is *14-3-3σ*, whose protein product inhibits CDC25C; this in turn prevents activation of cyclin B–CDK1 complexes, and blocks cells in G_2 phase.

If the degree of DNA damage is too severe for repair, however, p53 transcriptionally activates a different spectrum of target genes that promote programmed cell death (Table 39.2).[31,36,37] Several protein

---

Table 39.2 Mechanisms of regulation of apoptosis by p53

Transcriptional activation of pro-apoptotic genes	Representative proteins thought to be upregulated: • Bax: a pro-apoptotic member of the Bcl-2 family • IGF-BP3 (insulin-like growth factor 1 binding protein 3): binds to and prevents anti-apoptotic signaling of IGF-1 • PAG608: a nuclear zinc finger protein that induces apoptosis • Fas and DR5: cell death receptors • p85: regulates phosphatidyl-3-OH-kinase that is induced by oxidative stress • PIG3 (p53-induced gene) proteins: quinone oxidoreductase homologs that induce oxidative stress • cathepsin D: a serine protease involved in macrophage-mediated apoptosis • caveolins: the major membrane proteins of caveolae (small vesicular invaginations of the cell membrane that are enriched in glycosphingolipids and cholesterol) involved in the dynamic cholesterol-dependent regulation of specific signal transduction pathways
Transcriptional repression of pro-survival genes	• Bcl-2 • IGF-1 receptor • MAP4 (microtubule-associated protein 4): stabilizes polymerized microtubules
Non-transcriptional mechanisms	Direct protein–protein interactions implicated in induction of apoptosis: • xeroderma pigmentosa groups B and D helicases: components of basal transcription/DNA repair TFIIH complex • protein 53BP2: p53 competes with Bcl-2 for binding to this protein • translocation of intracellular Fas to the cell surface

kinases, including ATM kinase (ataxia telangiectasia mutated), ATR kinase (ataxia telangiectasia related) and DNA-PK (DNA-dependent protein kinase), appear to be involved in the cellular response to DNA damage, including activation of p53 through phosphorylation at its N-terminus, and activation of the CHK1 protein kinase (which plays a role in the G_2–M checkpoint pathway). Non-transcriptional mechanisms may also contribute to p53-mediated apoptosis. Defects either in the ability of cancer cells to sense DNA damage or in the machinery that implements responses to the genotoxic stress may contribute to the malignant phenotype.

Point mutations or allelic loss of *p53* are found commonly in many human cancers. Mutations occur at nearly every position of *p53*, but preferentially occur in regions encoding the DNA-binding motif.[38] Point mutations that disrupt the complex conformation of p53 remove its ability to recognize or bind to its specific DNA motif, thereby crippling p53's transactivating function. Because p53 contains several modular-type domains, certain mutations might prevent DNA binding yet permit oligomerization. Binding of mutant p53 to wild-type p53 protein may prevent the normal association of wild-type p53 with its constituents, resulting in a functional inactivation of wild-type p53 protein partners.[39] Thus, some *p53* gene mutations function as dominant-negative mutations. Various p53 mutant proteins may upregulate the expression of certain genes that do not rely on the wild-type p53-binding site for transcriptional activation.

Mutations of *p53* have been associated with an increased rate of aneuploidy and gene amplification. Germline *p53* mutations are associated with a high propensity for tumor formation in animals and humans. Tumors with mutated *p53* are resistant to both ionizing radiation and various cytotoxic agents.[40,41] Even if certain drugs induce genotoxic stress and growth inhibition in cancer cells, the *p53*-mutant cells are resistant to dying. Following relief from the genotoxic stress, the apoptosis-impaired cancer cell may then recover and resume replication. This aberrant process allows the accumulation of genomic errors that would normally have resulted in either cell-cycle arrest and DNA repair, or induction of cell death. Indeed, colorectal cancer patients whose tumor tissue contains point mutations in *p53* have a much worse prognosis.[42,43]

Functional inactivation of wild-type p53 can occur through binding of p53 to proteins from DNA tumor viruses (SV40 T antigen, adenovirus E1B, and HPV E6) or to cellular oncoproteins such as MDM2, and by cytoplasmic sequestration.[30,31,44] HPV E6 protein, which promotes ubiquitin-mediated degradation of p53, is linked with cervical and anogenital carcinomas. MDM2 binds to p53 and negatively regulates its transcriptional activating function by preventing its sequence-specific binding to DNA. MDM2 also interacts with the E2F1–DP1 complex and stimulates its transcriptional activation of target genes necessary for the transition to S phase. MDM2 also binds to underphosphorylated Rb–E2F complexes and promotes the release of E2F.[45,46] Induction of p53 increases MDM2 transcription, thus establishing a feedback loop. MDM2 is a target for DNA-PK in the DNA-damage response. MDM2 is thought to play a critical role in keeping p53 at low levels in non-damaged cells by promoting p53 degradation, and its overexpression leads to p53 inactivation.[47] A second protein produced by the *p16^INK4A* tumor suppressor gene, p14^ARF (alternative reading frame), interacts with and blocks the ability of MDM2 to degrade p53. The frequent deletion of this gene in human cancers thus has two consequences that dysregulate the cell cycle.

KEY COMPONENTS OF PROGRAMMED CELL DEATH MACHINERY

Several groups of molecules that participate in programmed cell death have been conserved throughout evolution (Table 39.3).[48] The caspase family of cysteine proteases, mammalian homologs of the *Caenorhabditis elegans* gene product CED-3, are involved in mediating cellular self-destruction.[49] The first identified family was interleukin-1β-converting enzyme (ICE, or caspase-1). There are presently 13 known members, which can be grouped into the 'ICE-like' caspases (caspases-1, -4, and -5), and the 'CED-3'-like caspases (caspases-3, -6, -7, -9, and -10). These enzymes have similarities in amino acid sequence, structure, and substrate specificity (cleavage at specific aspartic acid residues). They are synthesized as inactive proenzymes, and are activated by proteolytic cleavage at caspase consensus sites by another protease or by autocatalysis (triggered by binding of a cofactor or removal of an inhibitor). Proteolytic processing releases the prodomain, following which a heterodimer forms between a large and small subunit; two heterodimers then form a tetramer. The proteolytic cascade has both upstream initiator caspases (caspases-8 and -9) and downstream effector caspases (caspases-3, -6, and -7).

At least two pathways are known to lead to activation of downstream effector caspases: a mitochondria-dependent pathway governed by the Bcl-2

Table 39.3 Key molecules participating in programmed cell death

Protein family (C. elegans homolog)	Characteristics and function	Potential resistance mechanisms
caspases (*CED-3*)	• Family of cysteine proteinases that cleave substrates after aspartic acid residues • Synthesized as inactive proenzymes • Activated by proteolytic cleavage at two conserved aspartate residues • Proteolytic cascade: upstream initiator caspases and downstream effector caspases • Irreversible cleavage of specific protein substrates accounts for biochemical and morphologic features of apoptosis • Mediate cellular self-destruction	• Loss of expression of caspases • Mutational inactivation of caspase genes
IAP: inhibitors of apoptosis	• Family of proteins that function as inhibitors of apoptosis • Bind to and inhibit 'effector' caspase family members, including caspases-3, -7, and -9	• The IAP protein survivin is overexpressed in many human cancers
Apaf-1: apoptotic protease activating factor-1 (*CED-4*)	• Contains an ATP-binding P loop • N-terminal domain homologous to prodomains of caspases-2 and -9; 'caspase recruitment domain' (CARD) • C-terminal region flanked by 12 tandem copies of a WD-40 domain[a] that functions to keep Apaf-1 inactive • Requires an activation step (cytochrome c binding) to interact with caspases	• Cells from Apaf-1 knockout mice are resistant to many apoptosis-inducing agents, but remain sensitive to Fas-mediated cell death • Gene-transfer-mediated overexpression of Apaf-1 in vitro increases sensitivity to apoptosis-inducing agents • ARC (apoptosis repressor with caspase recruitment domain) is a decoy protein that contains a CARD, but does not activate the caspase

[a] The WD-40 domain refers to a regulatory domain on proteins containing multiple repeats of tryptophan and aspartate residues.

Table 39.3 continued

Protein family (*C. elegans* homolog)	Characteristics and function	Potential resistance mechanisms

Bcl-2 (*CED-9*)	• Family of proteins involved in regulation of apoptosis (17 members identified)
	
	• Dimerization with other family members may inhibit or promote apoptosis
	
	• Three main families:
	  1. Bcl-2 subfamily – suppress apoptosis: Bcl-2, Bcl-x$_L$, Bcl-w, Mcl-1, A1/Bfl-1, Boo/Diva, NR-13
	  2. Bax subfamily – promote apoptosis: Bax, Bak, Bok/Mtd, Bcl-x$_S$ (bind to Bcl-2 but also can autonomously activate apoptosis)
	  3. BH3 subfamily – promote apoptosis: Bid, Bad, Bik/NBK, Blk, Bim/Bod, Hrk, Nip3, Nix/Bnip3
	
	• Have structural similarity to pore-opening domains of some bacterial toxins
	
	• Bcl-2 typically resides on cytoplasmic face of outer mitochondrial membrane, endoplasmic reticulum, and nuclear envelope
	
	• May play a role in ion channel formation through membranes
		• Structural alterations in genes:
		  – t(14;18) chromosome translocations that activate Bcl-2
		  – single-nucleotide substitution and frameshift mutations that inactivate Bax
		  – retrovirus gene insertions that activate the *bcl-x$_L$* gene (murine leukemia)
		
		• Changes in transcriptional and post-transcriptional regulation networks
		
		• Overexpression of anti-apoptotic Bcl-2 family proteins confers a clinically relevant chemoresistant phenotype
		
		• Reduced expression of pro-apoptotic Bcl-2 family proteins also associated with chemoresistance

family proteins, and a parallel pathway involving activation of upstream caspases such as those involved in cell death receptor signaling.[50-54] The various initiator caspases transmit distinct signals: caspase-8 initiates apoptosis associated with ligand binding to death receptors, while caspase-9 initiates apoptosis associated with DNA-damaging agents. At the onset of apoptosis, caspase-mediated proteolytic cleavage of specific protein 'death' substrates accounts for the biochemical and morphologic features of apoptosis (chromatin condensation, cell shrinkage, loss of the nuclear envelope, and DNA fragmentation). The proteins destroyed by the caspases include those that protect cells from apoptosis, are involved in maintaining structural integrity of the cell, or are responsible for DNA repair, DNA replication, and mRNA splicing (Table 39.4).

A family of proteins called inhibitors of apoptosis (IAPs) inhibit the caspase family, through either direct binding of IAPs to specific caspases and/or prevention of proenzyme activation.[48,49] One member of the IAP family, survivin, is expressed in the G_2/M phase of the cell cycle and appears to inhibit downstream effector caspases.[50] Interestingly, survivin is expressed in a variety of solid tumors, but not in the normal tissue counterpart. Activation of initiator caspases requires binding to specific cofactors through one of at least two distinct structural domains present in both the procaspase and the cofactor. Apaf-1 (apoptotic protease activating factor 1) is an essential component of the cell death machinery in response to genotoxic stress. In concert with cytochrome c and dATP, Apaf-1 interacts with procaspase-9 through a caspase recruitment domain (CARD). The latter is a homophilic interaction site found in several procaspases (procaspases-2, -8, and -9). Binding of Apaf-1 is thought to change the conformation of the procaspase either directly or by removing an inhibitor. Similarly, activation of procaspase-8 requires association with its cofactor FADD (Fas-associated protein with death domain) through a death-effector domain (DED, a specific type of CARD).

The Bcl-2 family of proteins, homologous to the CED-9 protein in *C. elegans*, are involved in the regulation of apoptosis.[30,31,51-53] At least 17 members have been identified to date. Bcl-2 contains four homology domains termed BH1, . . . , BH4. The Bcl-2 subfamily (Table 39.3) display anti-apoptotic (or pro-survival) properties, and generally contain both the BH1 and BH2 domains; some members have all four domains. There are two anti-apoptotic subfamilies: Bax and BH3. The Bax subfamily has domains BH1, . . . , BH3, and resembles Bcl-2. The BH3 subfamily has only a central short residue in common with Bcl-2.

Bcl-2 family members interact with each other to form homodimers or heterodimers. Bcl-2–Bcl-2 homodimers prevent cell death, while Bax–Bax homodimers stimulate cell death. The ratio of the Bcl-2-related inhibitors and promoters of apoptosis is thought to influence whether a cell death signal invokes programmed cell death. Although heterodimerization may not be required for pro-survival functions of the Bcl-2 subfamily, heterodimerization of BH3-domain subfamily members is essential for pro-apoptotic activity. Bax subfamily members also form heterodimers, but also appear to have autonomous ability to activate apoptosis.

The Bcl-2 protein contains a highly hydrophobic α-helical region and appears to be anchored in the outer mitochondrial membrane by its carboxy terminus; the bulk of the protein protrudes into the cytoplasm. Bcl-2 also resides in the endoplasmic reticulum and perinuclear membrane. Other Bcl-2 family proteins (but not all) reside in the outer membrane of the mitochondria. Bcl-x_L has structural similarity to pore-opening domains of some bacterial toxins, and Bcl-2, Bcl-x_L, and Bax can form ion channels in vitro when added to synthetic membranes, suggesting a possible role in ion-channel formation. A variety of adverse mitochondrial events induced by chemicals that either inhibit the ATPase proton pump (located on the inner membrane) or poison oxidative phosphorylation can be opposed by the Bcl-2 subfamily. Cytochrome c release from the mitochondria, a necessary prerequisite for activation of caspase-9, is inhibited by Bcl-2. Bcl-2 and Bcl-x_L also prevent mitochondrial changes associated with drug-induced cell death through caspase-independent mechanisms (such as with oxidant and hypoxia-induced cell death). Bcl-x_L binds directly to procaspase-8, suggesting a possible mechanism of interference with caspase-8 recruitment to the death receptor–ligand complex. Further, Bax can induce deleterious mitochondrial changes without involving caspases. p53 transcriptionally activates the *bax* gene, and may suppress expression of the *bcl-2* gene.[55] Caspases indirectly control the mitochondrial commitment step that leads to programmed cell death by activating pro-apoptotic Bcl-2 family proteins and/or by inactivating pro-survival Bcl-2 family proteins.

APOPTOSIS TRIGGERED BY CELL DEATH RECEPTORS

Some cells have death receptors on their surface that belong to the tumor necrosis factor (TNF) receptor

Table 39.4 Caspase-mediated proteolysis of specific substrates

Inactivate proteins that protect cells from apoptosis

I^{CAD}/DFF45:
- I^{CAD} = inhibitor of caspase-activated deoxyribonuclease
- DFF45 = DNA fragmentation factor 45 kDa subunit

Bcl-2 subfamily

Retinoblastoma protein

Disassembly of cell structures

Lamin:
- member of the intermediate filament family of proteins
- component of the nuclear lamina localized to the inner nuclear membrane
- lamin meshwork provides a skeletal framework and attachment sites for chromatin
- provides mechanical continuity between the cytoskeleton and nuclear interior

Alpha-fodrin (alpha-II spectrin):
- cytoskeletal actin-binding protein

Gelsolin:
- calcium-activated multifunctional actin-regulatory protein involved in remodeling the actin cytoskeleton

Focal adhesion kinase:
- co-localizes with integrin receptor in cellular focal adhesions
- involved in transducing signals from integrin–extracellular matrix interactions

p21-activated kinase 2 (PAK-2)
- family of serine/threonine kinases that are targets for GTP-binding proteins
- involved in signaling pathways that influence gene expression and the cytoskeleton

Deregulate/inactivate proteins involved in DNA synthesis, repair or mRNA splicing

Poly-ADP-ribosylpolymerase

DNA protein kinase:
- serine/threonine protein kinase involved in repair of DNA double-strand breaks

DNA replication factor C:
- adapter protein that cooperates with PCNA to form a moving platform that serves to facilitate interaction of DNA polymerases ϵ and δ with DNA.

U1 snRNPs (small nuclear ribonucleoproteins)

gene superfamily (Table 39.5), which are characterized by a cysteine-rich extracellular domain and a conserved cytosolic domain (the death domain, DD).[36,48,54] The DD recruits adapter proteins, which contain a homologous DD, to the receptor complex after ligand binding (Figure 39.3). The adapter proteins also have a distinct domain that functions as a DED. One of the best-characterized death receptors is CD95 (Fas/Apo-1). The Fas ligand (Fas-L) is a homotrimeric molecule, a common feature of TNF protein family members. Fas-L plays an important role in mediating physiologic apoptosis in the immune system. Many tumor cell lines, including colon cancer, also produce Fas-L, and shed and/or sequester Fas. Binding of Fas-L to its receptor leads to clustering of the receptor's death domains; the adapter protein FADD then binds to Fas through its own DD. The DED of FADD binds to a homologous domain present on procaspase-8; caspase-8 oligomerization then drives its own activation through self-cleavage. The activated caspase-8 in turn activates downstream effector caspases. A cellular protein called c-FLIP contains a DED that is similar to the corresponding domain in FADD and procaspase-8,

---

Table 39.5 Tumor necrosis factor receptor gene superfamily

Death receptors that transduce apoptotic signals from extracellular environment

Initiation of apoptosis is independent of p53:

Receptor	Ligand
• TNF-RI (CD 120a)	TNF-α, TNF-β
• CD95 (Fas, Apo-1)	CD95L (Fas ligand)
• DR3 (Wsl-1, TRAMP)	Apo-3 ligand (TWEAK)
• DR4 (TRAIL-R1)	Apo-2 ligand (TRAIL)
• DR5 (TRAIL-R2)	Apo-2 ligand (TRAIL)
• CAR-1	unknown

Cysteine-rich extracellular domain

Conserved cytosolic domain (death domain):
- recruits adapter proteins to receptor complex after ligand binding
- adapter proteins contain a death domain (DD) and a death effector domain (DED):
    FADD/Mort-1
    Daxx
    TRADD
- binds caspases-8 and -10, which contain homologous DEDs within their prodomains: oligomerization of caspases within the death receptor complex results in transprocessing of the zymogens, and removal of the DED-containing prodomain of caspase releases the activated protease into the cytosol

Mechanisms of tumor cell resistance to apoptosis:
- downregulation of death receptors
- mutations of genes encoding the receptors – 'decoy' receptors that bind ligand, but do not transduce signal
- defects in the apoptotic signaling pathway – antiapoptotic DED-containing protein inhibitors:
    - bind to the proforms of certain upstream caspases or their adapter proteins, which prevents activation
    - FLIPs (FADD-like ICE inhibitory proteins)
    - c-FLIP is a homolog of caspases-8 and -10 that lacks proteolytic activity
    - compete with caspases for binding to FADD/Mort-1
    - overexpression of FLIP associated with Fas resistance

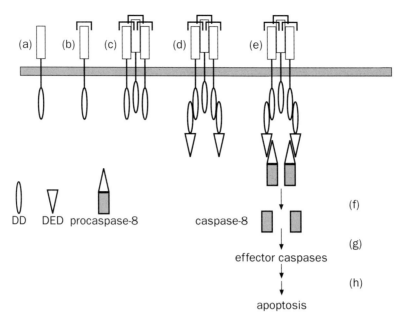

Figure 39.3 A simplified schema for death receptor signaling and modulation. This cartoon presents the steps involved in signaling by a cell death receptor using Fas (CD95) as an example. (a) unbound Fas receptor; (b) Fas-L binds to the Fas receptor; (c) Fas-L binding leads to clustering of the receptor's death domains (DDs); (d) an adapter protein (in this case, FADD) binds through a homologous DD to the DDs of the clustered receptors; (e) the death effector domain (DED) of the adapter protein recruits an inactive form of an upstream initiator caspase (in this case, procaspase-8) by interacting with an analogous DED on the zymogen; (f) binding of the procaspase to the adapter protein leads to activation of the caspase by autocatalysis; (g) the initiator caspase in turn stimulates a cascade that leads to activation of downstream effector caspases; (h) cleavage of specific protein substrates leads to the biochemical and morphologic features of apoptosis. Binding of other adapter proteins can activate different death pathways.

but does not result in caspase activation; the precise role of c-FLIP is unclear. Other proteins in the cytoplasm can bind to Fas after the ligand is bound. One such example is Daxx, which activates a FADD-independent pathway involving the stress-activated c-Jun amino terminal kinase.

Although these cell death receptors are thought to mediate apoptosis through p53-independent mechanisms, there is considerable 'crosstalk' between the p53-genotoxic stress and death receptor signaling pathways. The development of therapeutic strategies aimed at exploiting expression of the various death receptors on tumor cells is an active area of investigation.[56] Examples include G-3139 (Genta), an 18-mer all-phosphorothioate Bcl-2 antisense oligonucleotide, which binds to Bcl-2 mRNA and prevents protein translation. Antagonists of death-receptor signaling such as c-FLIP and survivin are additional targets for antisense therapy. Recombinant TRAIL (Apo-2L) hold the promise as a therapeutic agent because of the differential sensitivity of human cancer cell lines compared to normal cell types. Preclinical studies with active-site mimetic peptide ketones of caspase that inhibit caspase function have shown promising results in limiting apoptotic cell death in various animal models, including ischemia-reperfusion injury, status epilepticus, and Parkinson's disease. Several pharmaceutical companies are developing potent specific caspase inhibitors that are capable of crossing the cell membrane.

NEWER THERAPEUTIC AGENTS

Identification of new molecular targets is one approach to improving therapy for patients with advanced disease. Representative investigational agents that are currently being evaluated are listed in Table 39.6 by therapeutic target. Detailed discussion of each of these agents is beyond the scope of this chapter, but many interfere with signal transduction pathways.

Agents targeted against the extracellular matrix (ECM) or that are direct inhibitors of angiogenesis are listed in Table 39.7. Members of the matrix metalloproteinase (MMP) family are either membrane-bound or secreted zinc endopeptidases that degrade the various components of the extracellular matrix.[57] The members differ in their substrate specificity. MMP-1, -8, and -13 target fibrillar collagens; MMP-2 and -9 interact with collagen type IV in the basement membrane; MMP-7, -9, and -12 catalyze the conversion of plasminogen to angiostatin. MMP activity promotes tumor cell invasion and metastasis by several distinct mechanisms: degradation of macromolecular components of the ECM that otherwise serve as physical barriers; effects on cell–matrix and cell–cell attachments; catalytic release of biologically active molecules.

Several approaches are capable of interfering with tumor angiogenesis.[58] One strategy is to block the interaction of vascular endothelial growth factor (VEGF) with its receptors through the use of either antibodies, soluble VEFG receptors, or peptides that interact with the receptor and block its binding site. Fibroblast growth factor (FGF) exists as either an acidic form (FGF1) or a basic form (FGF2); the latter comprises a family of four transmembrane receptor tyrosine kinases. Investigational approaches that target FGF include synthetic molecules that block the FGF receptor, or agents that induce secondary messengers that in turn interfere with FGF signaling. Integrins are heterodimeric transmembrane proteins comprising α and β subunits that control cell motility, differentiation, and proliferation through interactions with the extracellular matrix. Two members of this family that are upregulated in proliferating endothelial cells are integrins $\alpha_v\beta_3$ and $\alpha_v\beta_5$. Inhibition of integrin $\alpha_v\beta_3$ through the use of humanized monoclonal antibodies and synthetic peptide antagonists is also being explored in the clinic. Endostatin and angiostatin are two 'endogenous'

inhibitors of tumor angiogenesis. Other agents specifically target endothelial cells.

CONCLUSIONS

It is well known from retrospective analyses of clinical trials that patient selection influences the efficacy of various chemotherapeutic agents, including 5-FU. In the past, these selection factors were primarily based on clinical features, such as performance status, number/sites of metastatic disease, etc. Innovative biochemical and molecular biology techniques will permit comparison of the phenotype of colorectal tumors with clinical outcome in both the adjuvant and the advanced disease settings. This approach offers great promise in identifying patients at greatest risk of relapse following primary therapy, and the likelihood of patients with advanced disease responding to available anticancer therapies. This molecular profiling may one day permit rational selection of therapy according to the individual characteristics of the tumor, and also to spare patients from the toxicity of agents that are unlikely to be beneficial. A major problem in improving the effectiveness of our chemotherapeutic armamentarium is the intrinsic resistance of many colorectal cancers, which are either indifferent to genotoxic stress and/or have impaired apoptotic pathways. Hopefully, further elucidation of the signal transduction pathways involved in both p53-dependent and p53-independent apoptosis, and their interplay, may unveil new therapeutic strategies to activate cell death programs in cancer cells.

If the majority of colorectal adenocarcinomas are intrinsically resistant to many different anticancer drugs through multiple mechanisms, then systemic treatment with curative intent may not be a realistic goal in the near future. In addition, a shift towards containment of metastatic disease has generated therapeutic paradigms aimed at inducing cytostasis.

Table 39.6 Novel targets of investigational anticancer agents in clinical trials

Target	Agent(s)
3-Hydroxy-3-methylglutaryl-coenzyme A reductase	Apomine (SR-450023A)
Proteosome inhibitor	PS-341
Phospholipase	Perifosine
CDK1, -2, -4, and -7	Flavopiridol
P-glycoprotein (PgP) and multidrug-resistance associated protein (MRP)	MS209 XR9576
Type II ribosome-inactivating proteins	Galactoside-specific lectin
Glycoprotein processing	KRN 5500
Dual inhibition of topoisomerases I and II	Intoplicine (RP 60475) F 11782 TAS 103
Microtubule depolymerization; stabilization of preformed microtubules	Epothilone A and B
Topoisomerase II α and β	Chloroquinoxaline sulfonamide (NSC 33904)
RIα-subunit of cAMP-dependent protein kinase A	GEM 231
Induction of a variety of cytokines, including STAT, NFκB, and TNF-α; inhibition of DT diaphorase (NAD(P)H quinone acceptor reductase)	DMXAA
Tubulin binder: interferes with microtubule assembly in endothelial cells	Combrestatin A4-phosphate
DNA-binding agents:	
DNA intercalater, novel topoisomerase II inhibitor	Rebeccamycin analog (NSC 655649)
Minor-groove alkylating agents (target AT tracts)	Bizelesin and adozelesin
Protein kinase C	UCN-01 CGP 41251
Farnesyl transferase	BMS-214662 R115777
Epidermal growth factor tyrosine kinase inhibitor	ZD1839 (Iressa)

Table 39.7 Antiangiogenic and antimetastatic agents undergoing clinical evaluation		
Target	**Drug names**	**Pharmaceutical sponsor**
Matrix metalloproteinases (MMPs)	Synthetic inhibitors of various MMPs:	
	Marimastat	British Biotech
	AG3340 (prinomastat)	Agouron
	Metastat (COL-3)	Collagenex
	Neovastat	Aeterna Laboratories
	BMS-275291	Bristol-Myers Squibb
	Bay 12-9566	Bayer
	CGS 27023A 02 (oral)	Novartis
Vascular endothelial growth factor (VEGF)	Monoclonal antibody to VEGF	Genentech
	Su5416 (blocks VEGFR-2 signaling)	Sugen
	PTK787 (blocks VEGFR signaling)	Novartis
Fibroblast growth factor (FGF)	SU6668 (synthetic molecule that blocks FGFRs, PDGFR and VEGFR-2)	SuGen
	Interleukin-12 (induces IFN-γ and IP-10, which blocks FGF2 activity)	Genetics Institute
Integrins	EMD 121974 (cyclic peptide antagonist of integrin $\alpha_v\beta_3$	Merck
	Vitaxin (humanized antibody against integrin $\alpha_v\beta_3$)	Ixsys
Endogenous inhibitors	Endostatin (20 kDa fragment of collagen XVIII)	EntreMed
	Angiostatin (38 kDa fragment of plasminogen)	
Endothelial cells and miscellaneous	TNP-470	TAP Pharmaceuticals
	Thalidomide	EntreMed
	ZD0101 (bacterially derived polysaccharide toxin)	AstraZeneca
	IM862 (naturally occurring peptide)	Cytran
	ZD6126	AstraZeneca
	ZD6474	AstraZeneca

REFERENCES

1. Grem JL, 5-Fluorinated pyrimidines. In: *Cancer Chemotherapy and Biotherapy. Principles and Practice* (Chabner BA, Longo DL, eds). Philadelphia: Lippincott-Raven, 1966: 149–210.

2. Sobrero AF, Aschele C, Guglielmi AP et al, Synergism and lack of cross-resistance between short-term and continuous exposure to fluorouracil in human colon adenocarcinoma cells. *J Natl Cancer Inst* 1993; **85:** 1937–44.

3. Grem JL, Voeller DM, Geoffroy F et al, Determinants of trimetrexate lethality in human colon cancer cells. *Br J Cancer* 1994; **70:** 1075–84.

4. Grem JL, Geoffroy F, Politi PM et al, Determinants of sensitivity to 1-β-D-arabinofuranosylcytosine in HCT 116 and NCI-H630 human colon carcinoma cells. *Mol Pharmacol* 1995; **48:** 305–15.

5. The Advanced Colorectal Cancer Meta-Analysis Project, Modulation of fluorouracil by leucovorin in patients with advanced colorectal cancer: evidence in terms of response rate. *J Clin Oncol* 1992; **10:** 896–903.

6. Marsh JC, Bertino RJ, Katz KH et al, The influence of drug interval on the effect of methotrexate and fluorouracil in the treatment of advanced colorectal cancer. *J Clin Oncol* 1991; **9:** 371–80.

7. Browman GP, Levine MN, Goodyear MD et al, Methotrexate/fluorouracil scheduling influences normal tissue toxicity by non antitumor effects in patients with squamous cell head and neck cancer. Results from a randomized trial. *J Clin Oncol* 1988; **6:** 963–8.

8. The Advanced Colorectal Cancer Meta-analysis Project, Meta-analysis of randomized trials testing the biochemical modulation of fluorouracil by methotrexate in metastatic colorectal cancer. *J Clin Oncol* 1994; **12:** 960–9.

9. Grem JL, McAtee N, Steinberg SM et al, A phase I study of continuous infusion 5-fluorouracil plus calcium leucovorin in combination with N-(phosphonacetyl)-L-aspartate in metastatic gastrointestinal adenocarcinoma. *Cancer Res* 1993; **53:** 4828–36.

10. Moore EC, Friedman J, Valdivieso M et al, Aspartate carbamoyl-transferase activity, drug concentrations, and pyrimidine nucleotides in tissues from patients treated with N-(phosphonacetyl)-L-aspartate. *Biochem Pharmacol* 1982; **31:** 3317–21.

11. Grem JL, Chu E, Boarman D et al, Biochemical modulation of 5-fluorouracil with leucovorin and interferon: preclinical and clinical investigations. *Semin Oncol* 1992; **19**(Suppl 3): 36–55.

12. Grem JL, Jordan E, Robson ME et al, Phase II study of fluorouracil, leucovorin, and interferon alfa-2a in metastatic colorectal carcinoma. *J Clin Oncol* 1993; **9:** 1737–45.

13. Wolmark N, Bryant J, Smith R et al, Adjuvant 5-fluorouracil and leucovorin with or without interferon alfa-2a in colon carcinoma. National Surgical Adjuvant Breast and Bowel Project Protocol C-05. *J Natl Cancer Inst* 1998; **90:** 1810–16.

14. Canman CE, Tang H-Y, Normolle DP et al, Variations in patterns of DNA damage induced in human colorectal tumor cells by 5-fluorodeoxyuridine: implications for mechanisms of resistance and cytotoxicity. *Proc Natl Acad Sci USA* 1992; **89:** 10474–8.

15. Canman CE, Lawrence TS, Shewach DS et al, Resistance to fluorodeoxyuridine-induced DNA damage and cytotoxicity correlates with an elevation of deoxyuridine triphosphatase activity and failure to accumulate deoxyuridine triphosphate. *Cancer Res* 1993; **53:** 5219–24.

16. Fisher TC, Milner AE, Gregory CD et al, Bcl-2 modulation of apoptosis induced by anticancer drugs: resistance to thymidylate stress is independent of classical resistance pathways. *Cancer Res* 1993; **53:** 3321–6.

17. Lowe SW, Ruley HE, Jacks T, Housman DE, p53-dependent apoptosis modulates the cytotoxicity of anticancer agents. *Cell* 1993; **74:** 957–67.

18. Hartwell LH, Kastan MB, Cell cycle control and cancer. *Science* 1994; **266:** 1821–8.

19. Clurman BE, Roberts JM, Cell cycle and cancer. *J Natl Cancer Inst* 1995; **87:** 1499–501.

20. Lundberg AS, Weinberg RA, Control of the cell cycle and apoptosis. *Eur J Cancer* 1999; **35:** 531–9.

21. Elledge SJ, Cell cycle checkpoints: preventing an identity crisis. *Science* 1996; **274:** 1664–72.

22. Nurse P, Checkpoint pathways come of age. *Cell* 1997; **91:** 865–7.

23. Hirama T, Koeffler HP, Role of the cyclin-dependent kinase inhibitors in the development of cancer. *Blood* 1995; **86:** 841–54.

24. Sherr CJ, Roberts JM, CDK inhibitors: positive and negative regulators of G1-phase progression. *Genes Dev* 1999; **13:** 1501–12.

25. El-Deiry WS, Harper JW, O'Connor PM et al, WAF1/Cip1 is induced in p53-mediated G1 arrest and apoptosis. *Cancer Res* 1994; **54:** 1169–71.

26. Okamato A, Demetrick DJ, Spillare EA et al, Mutations and altered expression of p16INK4 in human cancer. *Proc Natl Acad Sci USA* 1994; **91:** 11045–9.

27. King RW, Jackson PK, Kirschner MW, Mitosis in transition. *Cell* 1994; **79:** 563–71.

28. Leach FS, Elledge SJ, Sherr CJ et al, Amplification of cyclin genes in colorectal carcinomas. *Cancer Res* 1993; **53:** 1986–9.

29. Tsihlias J, Kapusta L, Slingerland J, The prognostic significance of altered cyclin-dependent kinase inhibitors in human cancer. *Annu Rev Med* 1999; **50:** 401–23.

30. Shimamura A, Fisher DE, p53 in life and death. *Clin Cancer Res* 1996; **2:** 435–40.

31. Bennet MR, Mechanisms of p53-induced apoptosis. *Biochem Pharmacol* 1999; **58:** 1089–95.

32. Lu H, Levine AJ, Human TAF$_{II}$31 protein is a transcriptional coactivator of p53 protein. *Proc Natl Acad Sci USA* 1995; **92:** 5154–8.

33. Seto E, Usheva A, Zambetti GP, Al E, Wild-type p53 binds to the TATA-binding protein and represses transcription. *Proc Natl Acad Sci USA* 1992; **89:** 12028–32.

34. Mack DH, Vartikar J, Pipas JM, Laimins LA, Specific repression of TATA-mediated but not initiator-mediated transcription by wild-type p53. *Nature* 1993; **363:** 281–3.

35. Waldman T, Kinzler KW, Vogelstein B, p21 is necessary for the p53-mediated G1 arrest in human cancer cells. *Cancer Res* 1995; **44:** 5187–90.

36. Evan G, Littlewood T, A matter of life and death. *Science* 1998; **281:** 1317–22.

37. Yu JY, Zhang L, Hwang PM et al, Identification and classification of p53-regulated genes. *Proc Natl Acad Sci USA* 1999; **96:** 14517–22.

38. Hollstein M, Sidransky D, Vogelstein B, Harris CC, p53 mutations in human cancers. *Science* 1991; **253:** 49–53.

39. Kern SE, Pietenpol JA, Thiagalngam S et al, Oncogenic forms of p53 inhibit p53-regulated gene expression. *Science* 1992; **256:** 827–30.

40. Lowe SW, Bodis S, McClatchey A et al, p53 status and the efficacy of cancer therapy in vivo. *Science* 1994; **266:** 807–10.

41. Bunz F, Hwang PM, Torrance C et al, Disruption of p53 in human cancer cells alters the responses to therapeutic agents. *J Clin Invest* 1999; **104:** 263–9.

42. Goh H-S, Yao J, Smith DR, p53 point mutation and survival in colorectal cancer patients. *Cancer Res* 1995; **55:** 5217–21.

43. Lenz HJ, Danenberg KD, Leichman CG et al, p53 and thymidylate synthase expression in untreated stage II colon cancer: associations with recurrence, survival, and site. *Clin Cancer Res* 1998; **4:** 1227–34.

44. Kaelin WG Jr, The emerging p53 gene family. *J Natl Cancer Inst* 1999; **91:** 594–8.

45. Martin K, Trouche D, Hagemeier C et al, Stimulation of E2F1/DP1 transcriptional activity by MDM2 oncoprotein. *Nature* 1995; **375:** 691–4.

46. Xiao Z-H, Chen J, Levine AJ et al, Interaction between the retinoblastoma protein and the oncoprotein MDM2. *Nature* 1995; **375:** 694–8.

47. Haupt Y, Maya R, Kazaz A, Oren M, Mdm2 promotes the rapid degradation of p53. *Nature* 1997; **387:** 296–9.

48. Reed JC, Dysregulation of apoptosis. *J Clin Oncol* 1999; **17:** 2941–53.

49. Thornberry NA, Lazebnik Y, Caspases: enemies within. *Science* 1998; **281:** 1312–16.

50. Escuín D, Rosell R, The anti-apoptosis survivin gene and its role in human cancer: an overview. *Clin Lung Cancer* 1999; **1:** 138–43.

51. Green DR, Reed JC, Mitochondria and apoptosis. *Science* 1998; **281:** 1309–12.

52. Adams JM, Cory S, The Bcl-2 protein family: arbiters of survival. *Science* 1998; **281:** 1322–6.

53. Gross A, McDonnell JM, Korsmeyer SJ, BCL-2 family members and the mitochondria in apoptosis. *Genes Dev* 1999; **13:** 1899–911.

54. Ashkenazi A, Dixit VM, Death receptors: signaling and modulation. *Science* 1998; **281:** 1305–8.

55. Miyashita R, Reed JC, Tumor suppressor p53 is a direct transcriptional activator of the human bax gene. *Cell* 1995; **80:** 293–9.

56. Nicholson DW, From bench to clinic with apoptosis-based therapeutic agents. *Nature* 2000; **407:** 810–16.

57. Kleiner DE, Stettler-Stevenson EG, Matrix metalloproteinases and metastasis. *Cancer Chemother Pharmacol* 1999; **43**(Suppl): S42–51.

58. Hagedorn M, Bikfalvi A, Target molecules for anti-angiogenic therapy: from basic research to clinical trials. *Crit Rev Oncol Hematol* 2000; **34:** 89–110.

40

Pharmacogenetics of colorectal cancer chemotherapy drugs: Implications for the pharmacokinetic adjustment of chemotherapy

Erick Gamelin, Michèle Boisdron-Celle

INTRODUCTION

Although new anticancer drug families, such as camptothecin and platinum derivatives, are of great interest in the treatment of colorectal cancer, their therapeutic index (i.e. the ratio of the theoretical minimum effective dose to the maximum tolerated dose) remains narrow compared with that of older drugs. The antitumour specificity of chemotherapy drugs is far from complete, and toxic side-effects are often observed – even in conventional regimens. Moreover, efficacy remains limited because of the wide panel of resistance mechanisms that can be displayed by colorectal cancer cells. On the other hand, retrospective analyses have strongly suggested a relationship between drug dose and tumour response, and have emphasized the impact of dose intensity on the response rate.[1–5] Up to now, dose-limiting haematological and non-haematological toxicities have hindered the development of intensive dose strategies.

In addition to narrow therapeutic index, chemoresistance, and problems associated with dose intensity, there is a marked variability in drug handling (i.e. pharmacokinetic parameters) among patients. For instance, for a given standard dose, systemic clearance and volume of diffusion of many drugs exhibit wide interpatient variability.[6] This contributes to variability in the pharmacodynamic effects of a given dose of that drug. Consequently, some interpatient differences, in terms of toxicity and efficacy, can be expected from this variability in systemic exposure. Therefore an identical dose of a drug given to three different patients may result in a therapeutic response with acceptable toxicity in one patient, unacceptable and possibly life-threatening toxicity in the second, and no response and no toxicity in the third.

Body surface area (BSA) is most often used for drug dosage calculation, but, for many drugs, it is obsolete and can itself generate errors,[7,8] although it is useful in preclinical trials, even in phase I studies.[9] It must be emphasized that BSA is not calculated but rather is estimated from a chart set up in 1916 with 9 patients! Despite its great limitations, the use of BSA was extended in the 1950s to drug dose calculation in routine practice.[10] BSA takes into account neither the pharmacogenetics of metabolism of a drug nor the fact that it can require activation. For anthracyclines, cyclophosphamide, carboplatin and 5-fluorouracil, clear arguments have been given against the use of BSA for dose calculation.[11–15]

Before the introduction of the concept of dose intensity in colorectal cancer – the increasing risk of both haematological and non-haematological side-effects with dose and the wide interpatient variability of systemic clearance – many studies were carried out with the purpose of defining new methods of dose calculation, such as drug monitoring through pharmacokinetic follow-up.[16] Pharmacokinetic and pharmacodynamic (PK–PD) studies analyse, on the one hand, what happens to the drug in the body, and, on the other hand, the effects of the drug, both on the body and on the disease. Such investigations have taken advantage of recent progress in techniques such as chromatography and mass spectrometry, and in computer software. Dose adjustment with pharmacokinetic follow-up requires some conditions to be satisfied for it to be useful. The therapeutic index must be determined. The drug kinetics in plasma must be such that the pharmacokinetic parameters of the drug, such as clearance and the area under the curve, can be determined from a limited number of blood samples.[17] This is usually achieved either by multiple linear regression or with a Bayesian approach.

The possibility of a significant link between systemic drug exposure and the risk of drug-related toxicities must be assessed. The next step is to analyse the link between systemic exposure and treatment efficacy, even though the weak relationship between extratumoral and intratumoral drug concentrations and sometimes the need for intracellular drug activation can lead to difficulties in demonstrating such a pharmacodyamic relationship.

The major pharmacokinetic parameter for quantifying the systemic exposure in the pharmacodynamic study of a drug is the *area under the curve (AUC)*. This takes in account both the plasma concentration of the drug and the time of exposure to it. It is better correlated with the intensity of pharmacodynamic effects than the absolute dose, which is subject to variabilities in physiological parameters and genetic characteristics that influence the effects of the drug.

Definition of the relationship between pharmacokinetic parameters and pharmacodynamic endpoints – both toxicity and tumour response – can allow the administration of the optimum drug dosage.[18,19] The goal is to maximize the likelihood of response and simultaneously minimize the likelihood of toxicity. For some drugs, such as carboplatin, the optimum dosage can be defined for an individual patient from measurable physiological variables, such as renal function.[14] For other drugs, the problem is more complex – the determination of the dosage will require pharmacokinetic data obtained from an initial and often from subsequent doses of a given drug.

In this chapter, we shall develop the concept of dose intensity in colorectal cancer – the analysis of the link between drug exposure and both the toxicity and the efficacy of the treatment. We shall focus on the pharmacokinetic and pharmacodynamic relationships of the three most important drugs in colorectal cancer: 5-fluorouracil (5-FU), irinotecan, and oxaliplatin. Then, we shall describe the different approaches for individual dosage adjustment.

5-FLUOROURACIL

Concept of 5-FU dose intensity

A clear relationship between 5-FU dose and response in metastatic colorectal cancer has been strongly suggested by retrospective meta-analyses,[1,3] but, up to now, dose-limiting haematological and mucosal toxicities have hindered both the application and the development of intensive dose strategies. Hryniuk et al[1] in 1987 and then Arbuck[2] in 1989, in meta-analyses, showed a clear relationship between 5-FU dose, in mg/m²/week, and response. Brohee,[3] in a multivariate analysis of the response rates in studies, found that the most important variables delineated were 5-FU cumulative dose, weekly schedule, and use of folinic acid (leucovorin).

Variability in metabolism and pharmacokinetics

The pharmacokinetics of 5-FU have been extensively studied, and display wide interpatient variability.[20] 5-FU disappears quickly from plasma, and its half-life is 10–20 minutes. Its total-body clearance varies according to the administration schedule: 0.5–1.5 l/min with intravenous bolus, it reaches 5–58 l/min with continuous infusion.[20,21] The elevated plasma clearance of 5-FU with continuous infusion is due to the addition of sites of catabolism other than the liver, such as lung and kidney. This explains why continuous infusion allows the administration of higher doses of 5-FU than bolus schedules – and also why it is possible to compare dose intensities between continuous and bolus administrations.

5-FU is metabolized to 5-fluoro-5,6-dihydrouracil by dihydropyrimidine dehydrogenase (DPD), the key enzyme of pyrimidine catabolism, which is widespread in the organism – mainly in liver, lung, kidney, and lymphocytes (Figure 40.1). A wide range of degrees of DPD activity, measured by radioenzymatic assay in lymphocytes, has been found among a population of patients, with a Gaussian distribution.[22,23] Complete deficiencies seem to be rather exceptional, but are responsible for the occurrence of an extremely severe polyvisceral toxicity of 5-FU, frequently lethal in patients as early as the first course of treatment.[24] Extremely high and prolonged levels of 5-FU were measured after a low dose of drug. Several families with this complete DPD deficiency have been described, and an autosomal dominant transmission has been described.[25] This deficiency is

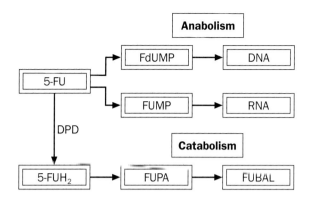

Figure 40.1 Anabolic and catabolic pathways of 5-fluorouracil (5-FU). Dihydropyrimidine dehydrogenase (DPD) displays a genetic polymorphism that interferes with 5-FU pharmacokinetics.
DPD, dihydropyrimidine dehydrogenase; 5-FUH$_2$, 5-fluoro-5,6-dihydrouracil; FUPA, fluoro-β-ureidopropionic acid; FUBAL, fluoro-β-alanine; FdUMP, 5-fluoro-2'-deoxyuridine 5'-monophosphate; FUMP, 5-fluorouridine 5'-monophosphate.

also known as 'familial pyrimidinuria or uraciluria', because uracil and thymine, which are not hydrogenated by DPD, are excreted directly in urine and can be found there although they should not normally be detected.[26] Familial pyrimidinuria is usually asymptomatic. Partial deficiencies are responsible for the toxic events encountered in the population of patients treated with 5-FU, which are related precisely to 5-FU steady-state plasma levels.[23] On the other side of the Gaussian distribution, some patients had a high degree of DPD activity. These patients are potentially underdosed with standard doses in conventional regimens.

The genetic polymorphism of 5-FU metabolism and the link between 5-FU plasma levels and both toxicity and response to treatment, shown by different authors, pose two different and independent problems: (1) the detection of patients with DPD deficiency, and (2) individual adjustment of 5-FU dose. The first concerns the avoidance of severe toxicities, while the second concerns how the 5-FU dose should be adapted to the metabolism of each patient, in order to improve results in terms of efficacy and tolerance.

Detection of 5-FU metabolism deficiency

Detection of DPD deficiency has become of major interest, since high doses of 5-FU are now being used and 5-FU indications are being extended to adjuvant

therapy, for patients who are potentially already cured.

Several authors have developed a method for the determination of DPD activity in lymphocytes before treatment, using radioenzymatic techniques with radiolabelled substrates. This method is accurate and is the reference one.[27,28] Fleming et al[27] found a significant linear correlation between DPD activity in peripheral blood mononuclear cells (PBMC) and 5-FU plasma clearance, but the correlation coefficient was weak ($p = 0.31$).[28] Thus DPD activity level cannot explain the high variability in 5-FU kinetics, and although DPD determination before treatment remains helpful for detecting patients with severe DPD deficiency (so that initial treatment can be with markedly decreased 5-FU doses or even with an alternative chemotherapy regimen), it is not a useful indicator for improving 5-FU dose-adaptation strategy. Moreover, difficulties arise when dealing with large populations, owing to the complex procedures used for measuring enzyme activity.[29] It requires significant quantities of blood, and a Ficoll separation of lymphocytes, and must be performed in specialized laboratories with facilities for radiochemicals.

The measurement of pyrimidines (uracil or thymine) in urine by liquid chromatography can be performed relatively easily.[30–32] Normal DPD activity is sufficient for pyrimidine metabolism, and only traces should be detected in urine.[31,32] Methods have been described for the measurement of uracil, thymine, and their metabolites in urine.[30–33] However, none of them reported the normal values of thymine and uracil excretion in healthy populations, and no reference values were given for the ratios of dihydrometabolites to original pyrimidines in urine. Moreover, to the best of our knowledge, no correlation between the degree of DPD deficiency and the urine level of pyrimidines has been sought. This approach warrants further study.

Another approach is the measurement of uracil and its dihydro derivative in plasma and the determination of their ratio.[34] In a population of 47 healthy volunteers, the ratio of dihydrouracil to uracil (UH$_2$: U) followed a Gaussian curve that can be compared to that of DPD activity, as reported previously by Etienne et al.[29] The purpose of this method is to determine the global fate of uracil before 5-FU administration and thus to detect complete or partial DPD deficiency, but it also takes into account other parameters that can interfere with 5-FU kinetics in plasma, such as the anabolic pathway and the fate of dihydrouracil. The coefficient of correlation between the UH$_2$: U ratio and 5-FU plasma clearance was 0.64.[35] Stringent precautions should be taken in the case of a ratio less than 2. Thus pretreatment determination of the $UH_2 : U$ ratio can detect DPD-deficient patients and help in determining the best 5-FU dose range very quickly. This method does not need radioactively labelled material, and can be performed in any laboratory with liquid chromatography apparatus. It remains to be assessed in different 5-FU regimens, such as 5-day continuous infusions, combined or not with platinum derivatives.

Limited sampling strategy

5-FU concentrations can be predicted in the case of continuous infusion, which is an excellent model for the study of anticancer drug pharmacodynamics, especially if the duration of the infusion is long enough to approximate a steady-state plasma concentration C_{ss}. Either C_{ss} or AUC can be used for pharmacodynamic modelling. Spicer et al,[36] Erlichman et al,[21] Milano et al,[37] and Thyss et al[38] found a linear correlation between the dose of 5-FU and the plasma concentration at steady state for patients treated with very prolonged continuous infusion of 300–500 mg/m² 5-FU,[36] or with 5-day continuous-infusion schedules at 1.25–2.25 g/m²/day, and concluded that under these conditions, 5-FU concentrations proportionally followed 5-FU dose modifications.[21,37,38] Equivalent results were found with a weekly 8-hour infusion, and a dose adjustment chart was established, to reach within three weekly cycles the optimal therapeutic range previously determined.[39] The predictability of 5-FU concentrations was reliable and very efficient.

Relationship between toxicity and 5-FU plasma levels (Table 40.1)

A close relationship has been described between exposure to 5-FU and haematological toxicity for different regimens and indications. Yoshida et al[40] and Au et al[41] noted that for patients with colorectal cancer treated with continuous-infusion 5-FU, the 5-FU concentrations at steady state and the AUC over 72 hours were higher in the group with toxicity than in the group with no toxicity, for the same 5-FU dosage according to body area. A threshold of 1.5 µmol/l for 5-FU steady-state plasma concentrations was associated with a high risk of leukopenia. Trump et al[42] reported equivalent results for patients treated with a 3-day continuous infusion of 5-FU, showing a close

relationship between steady-state 5-FU plasma concentrations and the risk of leukopenia and mucositis.

Similar relationships have been found for non-haematological toxicities. In spite of quite different 5-FU schedules, the same AUC toxic threshold was found in several studies.[39–42] The toxicity profile, however, does depend on the 5-FU schedule: leukopenia is more frequent with bolus administration, mucositis and diarrhoea with 5-day infusion, and hand–foot syndrome and diarrhoea with weekly 8- or 48-hour administration. Thyss et al[38] have demonstrated a relationship between an elevated AUC of 5-FU over 30 mg·h/l and the frequency of cycles with leukopenia, mucositis, and diarrhoea for patients with head and neck cancer, treated with chemotherapy combining cisplatin and a 5-day continuous infusion of 5-FU. Milano et al[37] found the same AUC threshold value for patients with metastatic colorectal cancer treated with a 5-day continuous infusion of 5-FU without cisplatin.

Equivalent results were reported for a 5-FU weekly 8-hour administration plus folinic acid in metastatic colorectal cancer.[39] There was a close link between both hand–foot syndrome and diarrhoea and steady-state 5-FU plasma levels above 3 mg/l. This toxic threshold corresponded to a value of AUC of over 25 mg·h/l, which is very close to the above-mentioned value of 30 mg·h/l, in spite of a very different administration schedule.[37,38] The slightly lower value of AUC that we found in this regimen could be explained by the addition of folinic acid, which is known to potentiate 5-FU toxicity.

Relationship between tumour response and 5-FU plasma levels (Table 40.1)

The next step in defining the therapeutic index is the determination of the therapeutic threshold. The relationship between 5-FU pharmacokinetics and treatment response has been less extensively explored than that between pharmacokinetics and toxicity. Other mechanisms, such as intrinsic cellular resistance and tumour kinetics, can be involved in treatment failure. Hillcoat et al[43] were the first to show that for patients with digestive tract cancer treated with 5-day continuous-infusion 5-FU, AUC values were significantly higher when objective response or stabilization were observed. Seitz et al[44] reported equivalent results with 5-FU bolus in colorectal cancer. More recently, a close link has been found between 5-FU concentrations in plasma and therapeutic outcome in the above-mentioned phase I

Table 40.1 Studies of the relationships between haematological and non-haematological toxicities and response and pharmacokinetics of 5-FU for different schedules of administration

Pharmacokinetic variable threshold[a]	Toxicity	Administration schedule; tumour[b]	Study
Relationship between haematological toxicity and pharmacokinetic variables			
$C_{ss} > 1.5$ µmol/l	Leukopenia	5-day CVI; CRC	Au et al (1982)[41]
C_{ss}	Leukopenia	3-day CVI; CRC	Trump et al (1991)[42]
AUC	Leukopenia	5-day CVI; CRC	Yoshida et al (1990)[40]
AUC	Leukopenia	Weekly IVB; CRC	Van Groeningen et al (1988)[71]
AUC > 30 mg·h/l	Leukopenia	5-day; HNC	Thyss et al (1986)[38]
Relationship between non-haematological toxicity and pharmacokinetic variables			
AUC > 30 mg·h/l	Stomatitis, diarrhoea	5-day CVI + CP; HNC	Thyss et al (1986)[38]
AUC > 30 mg·h/l	Stomatitis, diarrhoea	5-day CVI; CRC	Milano et al (1988)[37]
AUC > 30 mg·h/l	Stomatitis, diarrhoea	5-day CVI; HNC	Santini et al (1989)[45]
AUC	Stomatitis	Weekly IVB; CRC	Van Groeningen et al (1988)[71]
C_{ss}	Stomatitis	3-day CVI; CRC	Trump et al (1991)[42]
AUC > 24 mg·h/l, $C_{ss} > 3$ mg/l	Diarrhoea, hand–foot syndrome	Weekly 8-hour CVI + LV	Gamelin et al (1996)[39]
Relationship between response and pharmacokinetic variables			
AUC		5-day CVI; DTC	Hillcoat et al (1978)[43]
AUC		Weekly IVB	Seitz et al (1989)[44]
AUC > 16 mg·h/l, $C_{ss} > 2$ mg/l		Weekly 8-hour CVI	Gamelin et al (1996)[39]

[a]C_{ss}, steady-state concentration; AUC, area under the curve.
[b]CVI, continuous venous infusion; IVB, intravenous bolus; CRC, colorectal cancer; HNC, head and neck cancer; DTC, digestive tract cancer.

study carried out in 40 patients treated for advanced colorectal cancer.[39] The patients who experienced an objective response had significantly higher levels, whatever the dose, than patients whose tumours failed to respond. The therapeutic threshold was 2.5 mg/l. The overall survival at 1 year and later was better for patients who had plasma levels over 2.5 mg/l, but the difference was not significant ($p < 0.2$). The lack of statistical difference may be due in part to the small number of patients.

Individual 5-FU dose adjustment

Dose adjustment has been poorly investigated in advanced colorectal cancer, despite the concept of dose intensity, the polymorphism of 5-FU metabo-

lism, and the link between 5-FU plasma levels and both toxicity and response to the treatment. Moreover, 5-FU kinetics permits dose prediction.

The method of the test dose appears difficult to put in practice, since the plasma kinetics of 5-FU are complex. Pretreatment determination of DPD activity using a radioenzymatic technique would be an elegant solution. A relationship between DPD activity in lymphocytes and 5-FU plasma levels has been reported in certain studies,[27,28] but it is insufficient for the prediction of 5-FU plasma concentrations in practice, since the correlation coefficient between PBMC DPD activity and 5-FU plasma clearance is only 0.31. Other sites of catabolism are involved, and modifications of 5-FU metabolism can occur during prolonged treatment. Thus the determination of DPD activity cannot be a useful indicator for improving

5-FU dose-adaptation strategy.[27,28] Individual dose adjustment with a pharmacokinetic follow-up appears to be actually more interesting and practicable.

Some studies have been carried out on head and neck tumours, and some authors have attempted to adjust 5-FU dose individually, principally to reduce the incidence of toxicity.[45,46] They controlled the AUC at the middle of a 5-day infusion, and then adjusted the 5-FU dose with a nomogram to maintain the total AUC below the toxic value. It was shown that pharmacologically guided dosing was feasible and provided an improved haematological tolerance.

With the aim of dose intensification with control of the risk of toxicity, a large prospective multicentre phase II study has been carried out in 152 patients treated for metastatic colorectal cancer by first-line weekly 8-hour 5-FU infusion, plus leucovorin, with individual dose adjustment and pharmacokinetic follow-up.[47] The 5-FU dose was adjusted weekly according to steady-state 5-FU plasma concentrations and a dose adjustment chart (AUC optimal range 20–25 mg·h/l).[39] Fifty-six percent objective responses (17% complete responses) were observed. These results were better than, or at least equivalent to, those previously reported with weekly high-dose 5-FU in much more toxic schedules. The incidence of toxicity was less than 5% of all the courses (mean duration of treatment 1 year), and the toxicity was mild (grade II or less); none of the toxic events was life-threatening or led to a total interruption of the treatment. The mean weekly 5-FU dose was 1800 mg/m², which is higher than that usually administered with a conventional regimen, and a little lower than those reported by Ardalan et al[48] for a 24-hour weekly regimen. However, the latter authors reported a very high incidence of toxicity, which required treatment interruption every 6 weeks. In contrast, in the trial discussed here, patients were treated every week, with no interruption. The 5-FU optimal dose differed greatly within the population of patients for identical therapeutic plasma range. For a mean optimal total dose of 1800 mg/week, the range was 750–3500 mg/m². Five patients who presented a DPD deficiency were in the toxic zone with the first dose, and, without dose adjustment, they would have been at high risk of toxicity with a conventional regimen. The overall and event-free survival rates were respectively 68% and 46.6% at 1 year and 38% and 17.5% at 2 years. The median survival was 16 months.

The promise of individual 5-FU dose adjustment was confirmed later in a multicentre randomized study.[49] Two hundred patients were treated for metastatic colorectal cancer with first-line weekly 8-hour 5-FU infusion, plus folinic acid, using either a dose calculated from the body surface area, or a dose individually adjusted by pharmacokinetic follow-up. The mean 5-FU dose was 1200 mg/m² in the first group and 1800 mg/m² in the second, with a wide range (700–3600 mg/m²). The objective response rate was 18% in the first group and 38% in the second ($p < 0.0004$). Survival was higher in the second group, but the difference was not significant, probably because of the small number of patients. This trial proved that individual dose adjustment permits 5-FU dose intensification and objective response rate improvement, compared with calculation of the dose from the body surface area.

IRINOTECAN

Irinotecan (CPT-11) is a semisynthetic derivative of camptothecin that has been recently approved for the treatment of metastatic colorectal cancer in combination with 5-FU and folinic acid in first-line chemotherapy[50] (for further details, see Chapters 49 and 52–54). Its cytotoxic activity is mediated through the action of its active metabolite SN38, whose inhibitory action against the nuclear enzyme topoisomerase I is 100–1000 times stronger in vitro than that of irinotecan itself. The principal dose-limiting toxicities are delayed diarrhoea and neutropenia, which are non-cumulative, reversible, and dose-related.

Dose-intensity relationships

The activity and tolerability of high doses of irinotecan have been investigated in phase I studies.[4,5] The best tumour response rates were observed at higher doses, and thus these results indicated a dose-dependent activity of this drug. This strongly suggests that high-dose irinotecan is more likely to produce an antitumour effect through greater exposure to SN38.

Variability of metabolism and pharmacokinetics

Irinotecan is extensively metabolized in the human liver through different pathways (Figure 40.2). The anabolic pathway is mediated by carboxylesterase and leads to the active metabolite SN38.[51,52] This enzymatic step is not saturated at high doses, since the SN38 AUC increases proportionally with the

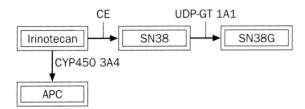

Figure 40.2 Anabolic and catabolic pathways of irinotecan. Carboxylesterase (CE), the UDP-glucuronyltransferase 1A1 isoform (UDP-GT 1A1), and cytochrome P450 3A4 (CYP450 3A4) display polymorphism of expression.

dose. SN38 is further converted into inactive and non-toxic SN38 glucuronide by hepatic UDP-glucuronyltransferase. The other major metabolite is APC, produced in the liver through the activity of cytochrome P450 3A4 (CYP450 3A4).[53]

Many studies have been carried out to characterize the inter- and intrapatient pharmacokinetic variability. Prior exposure to irinotecan did not modify the drug's pharmacokinetic parameters, and there was no induction or inhibition and no intrapatient variability.[54] The influence of several patient characteristics on irinotecan clearance and metabolic ratio (SN38 AUC/irinotecan AUC) was examined. Age, body weight, body surface area, gender, renal function, course number, and race had no influence on those parameters.[55,56] There was, however, wide interpatient pharmacokinetic variability.[55,56] Canal et al[54] reported coefficients of variations reaching 27% for irinotecan clearance, 51.6% for the SN38 AUC/irinotecan AUC ratio, and 87% for the glucuronidation ratio (SN38G AUC/SN38). Two factors can interfere with irinotecan and SN38 pharmacokinetics and metabolism. First, SN38 glucuronidation is mediated through the action of the UDP-glucuronyltransferase 1A1 isoform.[57] This isoenzyme is involved in bilirubin conjugation. Iyer et al[57,58] reported wide interpatient variability of glucuronidation in hepatic microsomes (coefficient of variation 69%) and a significant correlation between SN38 and bilirubin glucuronidation ($r = 0.89$). Genetic variation in the bilirubin UDP-glucuronosyltransferase gene promoter has been shown to exist, and severe toxicities have been reported in patients with Gilbert's syndrome (i.e. patients who are partially deficient in bilirubin glucuronidation).[59,60] More recently, Ando et al[61] assessed the influence of UDP-glucuronyltransferase 1A1 deficiency on SN38 and SN38G pharmacokinetics. They recommend that the plasma concentration of free bilirubin be determined before treatment in order to prevent irinotecan delayed toxicity. However, this determination remains insufficient, since a rise in γ-glutamyl transpeptidase is also a risk factor for haematological and/or digestive tract toxicity.[62]

The other route for irinotecan metabolism, the CYP450 3A4 pathway, is also subject to wide interpatient variability. Moreover, many drugs (e.g. loperamide) can interfere with enzymatic activity and behave as competitive inhibitors.[55]

Pharmacokinetic and pharmacodynamic (PK–PD) relationships

PK–PD studies must be carried out on a large number of patients, and thus require a number of blood samples (as limited as possible). Several groups have already proposed limited sampling strategies allowing the determination of the pharmacokinetic parameters of irinotecan from a minimum number of blood samples. This was achieved either by multiple linear regression or with a Bayesian approach. The difficulty is that studies should combine precision of the estimation of the kinetics of the drug and the number of species simultaneously studied, i.e. irinotecan, SN38, and even SN38G. Therefore the selected sampling times should be optimal for all the products.

Estimation of the population pharmacokinetics was first developed in Japan, and took into account only irinotecan. Yamamoto et al[63] determined two sampling times, 1 and 8 hours post infusion, for determination of irinotecan AUC with a precision (root mean square error percentage) of 3.2%. Chabot[64] predicted the AUCs of irinotecan and SN38 using three blood samples at 0.5, 1, and 6 hours after the start of infusion. The precision was around 13% for irinotecan and 35% for SN38. Sasaki et al[65] proposed a two-point limited sampling strategy using blood samples at 2.5 and 13.5 hours after administration. The precision was 12.7% for irinotecan and 6% for SN38. Mick et al[66] attempted to determine simultaneously the AUCs of irinotecan, SN38, and SN38G, but optimal times for blood sampling did not allow the selection of two time points. Three points, at 3, 9.5, and 11.5 hours, permitted the determination of the biliary index, which has a predictive value for late-onset diarrhoea.

Relationships between pharmacokinetic parameters and clinical effects, such as haematological and gastrointestinal toxicities and response to treatment, have been evaluated in phase I and II studies. In most studies, there was a significant correlation between the AUC of irinotecan and that of SN38 and the percentage decrease in neutrophil number.[54,56] The correlation between the severity of diarrhoea and the pharmacokinetic parameters was better with the AUC and C_{max} of SN38 than with the AUC of irinotecan. The authors concluded that the rate of metabolism of irinotecan to SN38 probably plays an important role in the genesis of diarrhoea. Rather than only SN38 AUC, Gupta et al[67] focused on the glucuronidation of SN38 and on its role in limiting intestinal toxic effects. They defined a biliary index of SN38 that is the product of the relative AUC ratio SN38/SN38G and the AUC of irinotecan. They proposed that index as a predictor of the occurrence and severity of late-onset diarrhoea. For instance, a patient with a low rate of glucuronidation has higher concentrations of SN38 in plasma, but also in the bile and in the bowel, and his or her biliary index is high. Such a patient is at higher risk for severe diarrhoea. In two successive studies, Gupta et al showed that 90% of patients with grade 3–4 diarrhoea had a biliary index greater than 4000, whereas all the patients with grade 0–2 diarrhoea had a biliary index less than 4000.

To the best of our knowledge, no clinical trial has compared irinotecan dosage based on body surface area with a pharmacokinetically based dosage adjustment. This would, however, probably be useful, taking into account the wide individual variability and the genetic polymorphism of both metabolic pathways – via CYP450 3A4 and via UDP-glucoronyltransferase.

OXALIPLATIN

Oxaliplatin is a novel platinum derivative, recently approved in Europe, Asia, and Latin America for the treatment of metastatic colorectal cancer in combination with 5-FU (see also Chapters 50, 52, and 54). Clinically, the safety and efficacy of a variety of dosing regimens with 5-FU and folinic acid have been investigated. Their combination has shown a marked antitumour efficacy against colorectal cancer, with a relatively favourable toxicity profile, essentially marked by acute and chronic neurotoxicity, thrombopenia, and anaemia.[68]

Although oxaliplatin has been used for almost 15 years in the treatment of colorectal cancer, clinical and pharmacokinetic data are recent, and pharmacodynamic studies are still lacking.

Concept of dose intensity

There has been no study permitting assessment of the superiority of high doses of oxaliplatin. Although 100 mg/m^2 every 2 weeks could be more efficient in terms of tumour response rate than 85 mg/m^2, this intensified schedule is marked by more severe neurotoxicity.

Pharmacokinetic studies

Despite a long terminal half-life of 10 days, oxaliplatin does not accumulate in plasma after 130 mg/m^2 every 3 weeks or after 85 mg/m^2 every 2 weeks.[69] Interpatient variability in platinum exposure is about 55%. Urinary excretion is the predominant route of platinum elimination. Renal clearance of platinum significantly correlated with glomerular filtration rate, indicating that glomerular filtration is the principal mechanism of platinum elimination by the kidneys. Clearance of ultrafilterable platinum is lower in patients with mild renal impairment, but the drug's toxicity is moderately increased.[70] Little is known about the impact of severe renal impairment on platinum clearance and toxicity.

To the best of our knowledge, no PK–PD data are available and no limited sampling model has been established. Oxaliplatin dosage monitoring would be interesting, however – at least for managing the neurotoxic side-effects, which can severely affect patients' quality of life.

CONCLUSIONS

The goal of pharmacokinetic and pharmacodynamic studies is to optimize the therapeutic index of cytotoxic agents that exhibit substantial pharmacokinetic variability and have a narrow therapeutic index, such as 5-FU, irinotecan, and oxaliplatin. Therapeutic drug monitoring would be of value in maintaining a precise level of systemic exposure while avoiding overtreatment.

The challenge in practice is how to manage these drugs to optimize therapy on an individual basis. Already for 5-FU and irinotecan, a clear relationship has been shown between drug plasma levels and toxicity. Data on the correlation between drug plasma concentrations and tumour response are available for 5-FU, but are still lacking for irinotecan. The therapeutic index, close to the maximum tolerated AUC, should be reached to improve response rate and hopefully survival. Individual dose adjustment can help to intensify treatment and improve outcome, and a pharmacokinetic follow-up with plasma measurement appears to be the best method currently available. This helps to detect metabolic deficiencies and prevent toxicity. On the other hand, it also permits increases in dose for patients with high metabolic activity (which can lead to underdosage). Compared with clinical dose adjustment, pharmacokinetically guided dose adjustment enables therapeutic 5-FU plasma levels to be reached much more quickly and safely. Moreover, it allows the 5-FU dose to be adapted throughout prolonged treatments, and could help to prolong remission duration. A controlled randomized trial has already proved its significance for 5-FU in terms of tumour response rate. Its impact on overall and disease-free survival remains to be proven, a fortiori, for irinotecan. Once developed and validated, limited sampling strategies will have to be easily accessible to busy practising clinicians. Simple formulae have already been set up. With such a goal in mind, the benefit of pharmacodynamic research will reach the level of common practice.

REFERENCES

1. Hryniuk WM, Figueredo A, Goodyear M, Applications of dose intensity to problems in chemotherapy of breast and colorectal cancer. *Semin Oncol* 1987; **14:** 3–11.

2. Arbuck SG, Overview of clinical trials using 5-fluorouracil and leucovorin for the treatment of colorectal cancer. *Cancer* 1989; **63:** 1036–44.

3. Brohee D, 5-Fluorouracil with or without folinic acid in human colorectal cancer? Multivariate meta-analysis of the literature. *Med Oncol Tumor Pharmacother* 1991; **8:** 271–80.

4. Armand JP, Extra JM, Catimel G et al, Rationale for the dosage and schedules of CPT11 selected for phase II studies, as determined by European phase I studies. *Ann Oncol* 1996; **7:** 837–42.

5. Merrouche Y, Extra JM, Abiberges D et al, High dose intensity of irinotecan administered every three weeks in advanced cancer patients: a feasibility study. *J Clin Oncol* 1997; **15:** 1080–6.

6. Pinedo HM, Peters GFJ, Fluorouracil: biochemistry and pharmacology. *J Clin Oncol* 1988; **6:** 1653–64.

7. Gilles E, Is dose adjustment for body surface area valid? *Proc Am Assoc Cancer Res* 1992; **33:** 3164.

8. Grochow LB, Baraldi C, Noe D, Is dose normalization to weight or body surface area useful in adults? *J Natl Cancer Inst* 1990; **82:** 323–5.

9. Freireich EJ, Gehan EA, Rall DP, Quantitative comparison of toxicity of anticancer agents in mouse, rat, hamster, dog, monkey, and man. *Cancer Chemother Rep* 1996; **50:** 219–44.

10. Crawford JD, Terry ME, Rourke GM, Simplification of drug dosage calculation by application of the surface area principle. *Pediatrics* 1950; **5:** 783–89.

11. Dodds NA, Twelves CJ, What is the effect of adjusting epirubicin doses for body surface area? *Br J Cancer* 1998; **78:** 662–6.

12. Gurney HP, Ackland S, Gebski V, Farrell G, Factors affecting epirubicin pharmacokinetics and toxicity: evidence against using body surface area for dose calculation. *J Clin Oncol* 1998;

16: 2299–304.

13. Powis G, Reece P, Ahman DL, Effect of body weight on the pharmacokinetics of cyclophosphamide in breast cancer patients. *Cancer Chemother Pharmacol* 1987; **20:** 219–22.

14. Calvert AH, Newell DR, Gumbrell LA et al, Carboplatin dosage: prospective evaluation of a simple formula based on renal function. *J Clin Oncol* 1989; **7:** 1748–56.

15. Gamelin E, Boisdron-Celle M, Guérin-Meyer V et al, Correlation between uracil and dihydrouracil plasma ratio, and 5-fluorouracil pharmacokinetic parameters and tolerance in patients with advanced colorectal cancer. A potential interest for predicting 5-FU toxicity and for determining optimal 5-FU dosage. *J Clin Oncol* 1999; **17:** 1105.

16. Canal P, Gamelin E, Vassal G, Robert J, Benefits of pharmacological knowledge in the design and monitoring of cancer chemotherapy. *Pathol Oncol Res* 1998; **4:** 171–8.

17. Ratain MJ, Schilsky RLR, Conley BA et al, Pharmacodynamics in cancer therapy. *J Clin Oncol* 1990; **8:** 1739–53.

18. Jusko WJ, A pharmacodynamic model for cell-cycle-specific chemotherapeutic agents. *J Pharmacokinetics Biopharmacol* 1973; **1:** 175–200.

19. Sheiner LB, Population pharmacokinetics/pharmacodynamics. *Annu Rev Pharmacol Toxicol* 1993; **32:** 185–200.

20. Wagner JG, Gyves JW, Stetson PL et al, Steady state non linear pharmacokinetics of 5-fluorouracil during hepatic arterial and intravenous infusions in cancer patients. *Cancer Res* 1986; **46:** 1499–506.

21. Erlichman C, Fine S, Elhakim T, Plasma pharmacokinetic of 5FU given by continuous infusion with allopurinol. *Cancer Treat Rep* 1986; **70:** 903–4.

22. Lu Z, Zhang R, Diasio RB, Dihydropyrimidine dehydrogenase activity in human peripheral blood mononuclear cells and liver: population characteristics, newly identified deficient patients, and clinical implication in 5-fluorouracil chemotherapy. *Cancer Res* 1993; **53:** 5433–8.

23. Harris BE, Carpenter JT, Diasio RB, Severe 5-fluorouracil toxicity secondary to dihydropyrimidine dehydrogenase deficiency: a potentially more common pharmacogenetic syndrome. *Cancer* 1991; **68:** 499–501.

24. Tuchman M, Stoeckler JS, Kiang DT et al, Familial pyrimidinemia and pyrimidinuria associated with severe fluorouracil toxicity. *N Engl J Med* 1985; **313:** 245–9.

25. Diasio RB, Beavers TL, Carpenter JT, Familial deficiency of dihydropyrimidine dehydrogenase. Biochemical basis for familial pyrimidinemia and severe 5-fluorouracil-induced toxicity. *J Clin Invest* 1988; **81:** 47–51.

26. Berger R, Stoker-de Vries SA, Wadman SK et al, Dihydropyrimidine dehydrogenase deficiency leading to thymine–uraciluria. An inborn error of pyrimidine metabolism. *Clin Chim Acta* 1984; **141:** 227–34.

27. Fleming R, Milano G, Thyss A et al, Correlation between dihydropyrimidine dehydrogenase activity in peripheral mononuclear cells and systemic clearance of fluorouracil in cancer patients. *Cancer Res* 1992; **52:** 2899–902.

28. Harris BE, Song R, Soong SJ, Diasio RB, Relationship between dihydropyrimidine dehydrogenase activity and plasma 5-fluorouracil levels with evidence for circadian variation of enzyme activity and plasma drug levels in cancer patients receiving 5-fluorouracil by protracted continuous infusion. *Cancer Res* 1990; **50:** 197–201.

29. Etienne MC, Lagrange JL, Dassonville O et al, Population study of dihydro pyrimidine dehydrogenase in cancer patients. *J Clin Oncol* 1994; **12:** 2248–53.

30. Voelter W, Determination of selected pyrimidines, purines and their metabolites in serum and urine by reversed-phase ion-pair chromatography. *J Chromatogr* 1980; **199:** 345–54.

31. Van Gennip AH, Van Bree-Blom EJ, Wadman SK et al, HPLC of urinary pyrimidines for the evaluation of primary and secondary abnormalities of pyrimidine metabolism. In: *Biological and Biomedical Applications of Liquid Chromatography, III* (Hawk GL, ed). New York: Marcel Dekker, 1982: 285–96.

32. Bakkeren JAJM, De Abreu RA, Sengers RCA et al, Elevated urine and cerebrospinal fluid levels of uracil and thymine in a child with dihydrothymine dehydrogenase deficiency. *Clin Chim Acta* 1984; **140:** 247–56.

33. Hayashi K, Kidouchi K, Sumi S, Possible prediction of adverse reactions to pyrimidine chemotherapy from urinary pyrimidine levels and a case of asymptomatic adult dihydropyrimidinuria. *Clin Cancer Res* 1996; **2:** 1937–41.

34. Gamelin E, Boisdron-Celle M, Larra F, Robert J, Simple chromatographic method for the analysis of pyrimidines and their dihydrogenated metabolites. *J Liq Chromatogr Rel Technol* 1997; **20:** 3155–72.

35. Gamelin E, Boisdron-Celle M, Guérin-Meyer V et al, Correlation between uracil and dihydrouracil plasma ratio, and 5-fluorouracil pharmacokinetic parameters and tolerance in patients with advanced colorectal cancer. A potential interest for predicting 5-FU toxicity and for determining optimal 5-FU dosage. *J Clin Oncol* 1999; **17:** 1105–10.

36. Spicer DV, Ardalan B, Daniels JR et al, Reevaluation of the maximum tolerated dose of continuous venous infusion of 5-fluorouracil with pharmacokinetics. *Cancer Res* 1998; **48:** 459–61.

37. Milano G, Roman P, Khater P et al, Dose versus pharmacokinetics for predicting tolerance to 5-day continuous infusion of 5-FU. *Int J Cancer* 1988; **41:** 537–41.

38. Thyss A, Milano G, Renee N et al, Clinical pharmacokinetic study of 5-FU in continuous 5-day infusions for head and neck cancer. *Cancer Chemother Pharmacol* 1986; **16:** 64–6.

39. Gamelin EC, Danquechin-Dorval EM, Dumesnil Y et al, Relationship between 5-fluorouracil dose intensity and therapeutic response in patients with advanced colorectal cancer receiving 5-FU containing infusional therapy. *Cancer* 1996; **77:** 441–51.

40. Yoshida T, Araki E, Ligo M et al, Clinical significance of monitoring serum levels of 5-fluorouracil by continuous infusion in patients with advanced colonic cancer. *Cancer Chemother Pharmacol* 1990; **26:** 352–4.

41. Au JLS, Rustum YM, Lederma EJ et al, Clinical pharmacological studies of concurrent infusion of 5-fluorouracil and thymidine in the treatment of colorectal carcinoma. *Cancer Res* 1982; **42:** 2903–37.

42. Trump DL, Egorin MJ, Forrest A et al, Pharmacokinetic and pharmacodynamic analysis of fluorouracil during 72-hour continuous infusion with and without dipyridamole. *J Clin Oncol* 1991; **9:** 2027–35.

43. Hillcoat BL, McCulloch PB, Figueredo AT et al, Clinical response and plasma levels of 5-fluorouracil in patients with colonic cancer treated by drug infusion. *Br J Cancer* 1978; **38:** 719–24.

44. Seitz JF, Cano JP, Rigault JP et al, Chimiothérapie des cancers digestifs étendus par le 5-fluorouracile: relations entre la réponse clinique et la clairance plasmatique du médicament. *Gastroentérol Clin Biol* 1989; **7:** 374–80.

45. Santini J, Milano G, Thyss A et al, 5-FU therapeutic monitoring with dose adjustment leads to an improved therapeutic index in head and neck cancer. *Br J Cancer* 1989; **59:** 287–90.

46. Milano G, Etienne MC, Renee N et al, Relationship between fluorouracil systemic exposure and tumor response and patient survival. *J Clin Oncol* 1994; **12:** 1291–5.

47. Gamelin E, Boisdron-Celle M, Delva R et al, Long-term weekly treatment of colorectal metastatic cancer with fluorouracil and leucovorin: results of a multicentric prospective trial of fluorouracil dosage optimization by pharmacokinetic monitoring in

152 patients. *J Clin Oncol* 1998; **16:** 1470–8.

48. Ardalan B, Chua L, Tian E et al, A phase II study of weekly 24 hour infusion with high dose fluorouracil with leucovorin in colorectal carcinoma. *J Clin Oncol* 1991; **9:** 625–30.

49. Gamelin E, Jacob J, Danquechin-Dorval E et al, Multicentric randomized trial comparing weekly treatment of advanced colorectal cancer with intensified 5-fluorouracil and folinic acid with 5-FU pharmacokinetic monitoring to a constant dose calculated with body surface area. *Proc Am Soc Clin Oncol* 1998; **17:** 1039.

50. Douillard JY, Cunningham D, Roth AD et al, Irinotecan combined with fluorouracil alone as first-line treatment for metastatic colorectal cancer: a multicentre randomised trial. *Lancet* 2000; **355:** 1041–7.

51. Rivory LP, Bowles MR, Robert J, Pond SM, Conversion of irinotecan to its active metabolite SN-38 by human liver carboxylesterase. *Biochem Pharmacol* 1996; **52:** 1103–11.

52. Kawato Y, Aonuma M, Hirota Y et al, Intracellular roles of SN-38, a metabolite of a camptothecin derivative CPT-11, in the antitumor effect of CPT-11. *Cancer Res* 1991; **51:** 4187–91.

53. Haaz MC, Rivory L, Riche C et al, Metabolism of irinotecan by human hepatic microsomes: participation of cytochrome P-450 and drug interactions. *Cancer Res* 1998; **58:** 468–72.

54. Canal P, Gay C, Dezeuze A et al, Pharmacokinetics and pharmacodynamics of irinotecan during a phase II clinical trial in colorectal cancer. *J Clin Oncol* 1996; **14:** 2688–95.

55. Chabot GG, Clinical pharmacokinetics of irinotecan. *Clin Pharm* 1997; **33:** 245–59.

56. Gupta E, Mick R, Ramirez J et al, Pharmacokinetic and pharmacodynamic evaluation of the topoisomerase inhibitor irinotecan in cancer patients. *J Clin Oncol* 1997; **15:** 1502–10.

57. Iyer L, King CD, Whitington PF et al, Genetic predisposition to the metabolism of irinotecan. *J Clin Invest* 1998; **101:** 847–54.

58. Iyer L, Hall D, Das S et al, Phenotype–genotype correlation of in vitro SN-38 (active metabolite of irinotecan) and bilirubin glucuronidation in human liver tissue with UGT1A1 promoter polymorphism. *Clin Pharm Ther* 1999; **65:** 576–82.

59. Monhagan G, Ryan M, Seddon R et al, Genetic variation in bilirubin UDP-glucuronosyltransferase gene promoter and Gilbert's syndrome. *Lancet* 1996; **347:** 578–81.

60. Wasserman E, Myara A, Lokiec F et al, Severe CPT-11 toxicity in patients with Gilbert's syndrome: two case reports. *Ann Oncol* 1997; **8:** 1049–51.

61. Ando Y, Saka H, Asai G et al, UGT1A1 genotypes and glucuronidation of SN-38, the active metabolite of irinotecan. *Ann Oncol* 1998; **9:** 845–7.

62. Van Groeningen CJ, Van der Vijgh WJF, Baars JJ et al, Altered pharmacokinetics and metabolism of CPT-11 in liver dysfunction: a need for guidelines. *Clin Cancer Res* 2000; **6:** 1342–6.

63. Yamamoto N, Tamura T, Nishiwaki Y et al, Limited sampling models for area under the concentration time curve of irinotecan and its application to a multicentric phase II trial. *Clin Cancer Res* 1997; **3:** 1087–92.

64. Chabot GG, Limited sampling models for simultaneous estimation of the pharmacokinetics of irinotecan and its active metabolite SN-38. *Cancer Chemother Pharmacol* 1995; **36:** 463–72.

65. Sasaki Y, Misuno S, Fuji H et al, A limited sampling model for estimating pharmacokinetics of CPT11 and its metabolite SN-38. *Jpn J Cancer Res* 1995; **86:** 117–23.

66. Mick R, Gupta E, Vokes EE, Ratain MJ, Limited sampling models for irinotecan pharmacokinetics–pharmacodynamics: prediction of biliary index and intestinal toxicity. *J Clin Oncol* 1996; **14:** 2012–19.

67. Gupta E, Lestingi TM, Mick R et al, Metabolic fate of irinotecan in humans: correlation of glucuronidation with diarrhea. *Cancer Res* 1994; **54:** 3723–5.

68. Bleiberg H, de Gramont A, Oxaliplatin plus 5-fluorouracil: clini-

cal experience in patients with advanced colorectal cancer. *Semin Oncol* 1998; **25:** 32–9.

69. Gamelin E, Le Bouil A, Boisdron-Celle M et al, Cumulative pharmacokinetic study of oxaliplatin administered every three weeks combined with 5-fluorouracil in colorectal cancer patients. *Clin Cancer Res* 1997; **3:** 891–9.

70. Massari C, Brienza S, Rotarski M et al, Pharmacokinetics of

oxaliplatin in patients with normal versus impaired renal function. *Cancer Chemother Pharmacol* 2000; **45:** 157–64.

71. Van Groeningen CJ, Pinedo HM, Heddes J et al, Pharmacokinetics of 5-fluorouracil assessed with a sensitive mass spectrometric method in patients on a dose escalation schedule. *Cancer Res* 1988; **48:** 6956–61.

41

The Mayo Clinic/ NCCTG (North Central Cancer Treatment Group) regimen of 5-fluorouracil and leucovorin: Origins, activity, toxicity, and future applications

Richard M Goldberg, Daniel J Sargent

INTRODUCTION

Hundreds of articles in the medical literature explore the activity of fluorinated pyrimidines in the treatment of colorectal and other cancers. As a result, the background data regarding the mechanisms of action are well known to oncologists, and will be reviewed here only briefly to provide historical context. Fluorinated pyrimidines, of which 5-fluorouracil (5-FU) is the most ubiquitous, exert their antineoplastic effect at least in part by inhibiting the activity of the enzyme thymidylate synthase (TS). TS inhibition interferes with DNA synthesis in dividing cells, preventing successful mitosis, and often causing lethal damage to the parent cell. A number of different fluorinated pyrimidines have been administered as single agents and as part of combinations with other cytotoxic drugs. Often fluorinated pyrimidines are combined with agents designed to improve their therapeutic index by preferentially sensitizing tumor but not host cells to the agent(s). The latter drugs, which are not cytotoxic themselves, are commonly referred to as biochemical modulators. Leucovorin is one of the most commonly employed biochemical modulators, and is principally used with fluorinated pyrimidines. The Mayo Clinic/North Central Cancer Treatment Group (NCCTG) regimen of 5-FU and leucovorin is one example of biochemical modulation of a fluorinated pyrimidine that is in common use.

During the 1960s, 1970s, and early 1980s, 5-FU was mainly administered as a single agent with pre-dictable but limited activity and moderate toxicity. Oncologists in clinical practice at that time recall the rarity with which tumor shrinkage was observed when patients with metastatic colorectal cancer were treated with bolus or infusion schedules of single-agent 5-FU. Only approximately 11% of patients with metastatic colorectal cancer had measurable tumor shrinkage, and responses were short-lived, lasting on average a few months.[1]

PRECLINICAL BACKGROUND STUDIES

In the 1970s, laboratory investigators observed that leucovorin (also known as folinic acid, citrovorum factor, or 5-formyltetrahydrofolate) potentiated the cytotoxicity of 5-FU in vitro and in human tumor xenografts.[2–5] When leucovorin was added to cell culture with 5-FU, the two agents enhanced binding to and inhibition of thymidylate synthase (TS) as compared with the binding noted when 5-FU was used alone. Leucovorin modulation led to the formation of stable, covalently bound, ternary complexes of TS–FdUMP–5,10-methylenetetrahydrofolate (where FdUMP is 5-fluoro-2'-deoxyuridine-5'-5'-monophosphate, the active metabolite of 5-FU). In contrast, in the absence of sufficient folate, the ternary complexes were weak and unstable, leading to only transient TS inhibition. More effective inhibition of TS in turn more efficiently inhibited DNA synthesis, resulting in enhanced tumor shrinkage. In model tumor systems, the optimal concentrations of leucovorin ranged from 1 mmol/l to 20 mmol/l.[6–9] These studies support clinical leucovorin doses ranging from 10 to 600 mg/m^2 to modulate 5-FU in order to achieve tissue concentrations ranging from 1 to 20 mmol/l in patients.

A number of experiments were designed to determine the optimum dose, schedule of administration, and intracellular concentration of leucovorin when administered with 5-FU. These studies indicated that the interplay between 5-FU, leucovorin, and cellular replicative machinery depended, at least in part, on the cell lines employed in the experiments. For example, in H630 colon carcinoma cells, the highest concentrations of the ternary complex were noted when leucovorin preceded administration of 5-FU by 18 hours.[10] In contrast, the optimal conditions for ternary complex formation occurred with 5-FU administration 4 hours after leucovorin exposure in the MCF-7 breast adenocarcinoma model.

In a study done in Ward colorectal carcinomas, 5-FU was administered with or without leucovorin in three different schedules at different leucovorin doses in a factorial design.[9] The three leucovorin doses were high (200 mg/m^2), low (20 mg/m^2), and none; the three administration schedules were: (1) a 96-hour infusion of 5-FU with leucovorin given daily over 2 hours, (2) a daily 5-FU bolus for 4 consecutive days given midway through a 2-hour leucovorin infusion, and (3) three consecutive weekly bolus injections of 5-FU given midway through a 2-hour infusion of leucovorin. The administration of high-dose leucovorin induced more complete tumor responses in this experiment than did low-dose or no leucovorin, regardless of schedule.

While this study provided information on the leucovorin modulation of 5-FU in this cell line, the general applicability of these results to humans with colorectal cancer remains speculative. People with colorectal cancer clearly exhibit clinically significant variability in their response to treatment, just as cell lines do. The sequence of 5-FU and leucovorin, the concentration of leucovorin, the interval between the administration of the 5-FU and the leucovorin, and the length of exposure of tumor cells to leucovorin are all variables that affect tumor inhibition. Therefore, it is unlikely that any single fixed-dose schedule of the two agents is optimal for all tumors.[11]

ORIGINS OF THE MAYO/NCCTG REGIMEN

David Machover and colleagues were among the early investigators who popularized the biochemical modulation of 5-FU with leucovorin in the treatment of colorectal and gastric cancers.[12,13] The Machover regimen consists of high-dose leucovorin at a dose of 200 mg/m^2/day administered prior to 5-FU at a dose of 370 mg/m^2/day. Both drugs are given for 5 consecutive days. This dose of leucovorin is associated with blood levels of 10–20 µmol/l.[14] The Mayo/NCCTG regimen was originally devised to replace the high-dose leucovorin with a lower dose of 20 mg/m^2/day as the biochemical modulator of 5-FU. The 5-FU dose and schedule were identical to those used in the Machover regimen, namely 370 mg/m^2/day for 5 consecutive days. The scientific rationale for this treatment program was to test whether a low-dose leucovorin regimen projected to achieve systemic leucovorin concentrations of 1–2 µmol/l would provide sufficient biochemical modulation of 5-FU to augment the response rate and survival of patients with metastatic colorectal cancer compared with 5-FU alone. One advantage of the low-dose leucovorin regimen was its lower cost.

In the initial study of this regimen, patients with advanced unresectable colorectal cancer were randomized to one of six chemotherapy regimens.[15] Only three of the treatment arms will be considered in this discussion:

(1) 5-FU alone administered at a dose of 500 mg/m^2/day by intravenous bolus for 5 consecutive days every 5 weeks;
(2) 5-FU and high-dose leucovorin administered for 5 consecutive days (the Machover regimen), repeated at 4 weeks, 8 weeks, and every 5 weeks thereafter:
(3) 5-FU and low-dose leucovorin given for 5 consecutive days (the Mayo/NCCTG regimen), repeated at 4 weeks, 8 weeks, and every 5 weeks thereafter.

A 5-week interval between courses after the third set of treatments was adopted in recognition of the cumulative nature of the toxicity observed. The initial 4-week interval allowed initial dose-intensive treatment, with the dose intensity then being reduced for patients with stable or responsive disease over time.

Upon analysis of the toxicity patterns of the first 100 patients, the starting dose of 5-FU for the low-dose leucovorin (Mayo) regimen was increased to 425 mg/m^2/day per protocol specification.[16] Dose escalation of 5-FU on all treatment arms was called for in this study if no significant myelosuppression or non-hematologic toxicity was observed during the previous treatment course. The protocol change was made upon observation that, in this trial, the majority of patients treated with the Mayo/NCCTG regimen were dose-escalating per protocol. The original low-dose leucovorin regimen with 370 mg/m^2/day of 5-FU for 5 consecutive days was an empiric one – no formal phase I trial of this regimen had been performed. The dosage adjustment to 425 mg/m^2/day was made to produce definite but tolerable toxicity that was of similar magnitude in each of the six treatment programs.

At the conclusion of the protocol, 208 eligible patients had been entered on the three study arms of interest here. The overall response rates were 10% for 5-FU alone, 26% for the high-dose leucovorin (Machover) regimen, and 43% for the low-dose leucovorin (Mayo/NCCTG) regimen. With regard to response rate, the two leucovorin-modulated regimens were significantly better than 5-FU alone ($p = 0.04$ and 0.001 respectively). Survival was also significantly longer for the two leucovorin-modulated regimens, at 12.2 months (high-dose leucovorin) and 12.0 months (low-dose leucovorin) as compared with 7.7 months for single-agent 5-FU ($p = 0.037$ and 0.05, respectively).

MAYO/NCCTG REGIMEN: ACTIVITY

Advanced disease

Investigators from Roswell Park Memorial Cancer Institute (RPMI) devised a weekly high-dose regimen of leucovorin 500 mg/m^2/day with 5-FU 600 mg/m^2/day given for 6 consecutive weeks followed by a 2-week rest period.[17] This RPMI regimen has also been shown to significantly improve the response rate when compared with single-agent 5-FU, with a response rate of 30% for the RPMI regimen versus 12% for 5-FU alone ($p < 0.01$). Based on these results, the RPMI and Mayo/NCCTG regimens were compared in a randomized trial of 366 patients performed by the NCCTG.[18] The observed objective tumor response rates were similar (35% for the Mayo/NCCTG regimen and 31% for the RPMI regimen), and no survival difference between regimens was observed.

It should be noted that, consistent with the NCCTG policy at that time, in these early studies[15,18] tumor shrinkage at only a single point in time was sufficient to be categorized as a complete or partial response. More recent studies have specified that tumor shrinkage be sustained for 4 or more weeks in order to be classified as a response, resulting in variable response rates between series, depending upon the response criteria specified.

The Mayo/NCCTG regimen in the adjuvant setting

The observed activity of leucovorin-modulated 5-FU naturally led to the evaluation of the various regimens in the treatment of patients with stage II and III colon cancer. The initial report on the Mayo/NCCTG regimen in this setting was published in 1997.[19] In this trial, patients with resected stage II or III colon cancer were randomized to the Mayo/NCCTG 5-FU-plus-leucovorin regimen for 6 months or to a no-treatment control arm. The study was suspended after accrual of 317 patients when the results of the GI Intergroup trial of 5-FU plus levamisole were released, establishing that effective treatment was available in this setting.[20] In the 317 patients enrolled before suspension, the 5-year survival rate for treated patients was 74%, compared with 63% in the control group ($p = 0.02$). This 1997 trial clearly established the efficacy of the Mayo/NCCTG 5-FU-plus-leucovorin regimen in the adjuvant setting.

Subsequently, a large trial sponsored by the GI Intergroup (INT-0089) randomized 3759 stage II and III colon cancer patients to one of four 5-FU and leucovorin and/or levamisole programs. The regimens included the Mayo/NCCTG 5-FU-plus-leucovorin regimen for 6 months, 5-FU plus levamisole for 12 months, 5-FU with high-dose leucovorin (the RPMI regimen) for 8 months, or 5-FU plus leucovorin plus levamisole for 12 months. The results have been presented only in abstract form to date.[21] However, outcomes were similar for the Mayo/NCCTG regimen, the RPMI 5-FU-plus-leucovorin program, and the regimen with 5-FU plus both leucovorin and levamisole. These three regimens resulted in a 5-year overall survival rate of 65–67%. With essentially identical activity profiles at present, the choice between the Mayo/NCCTG and RPMI 5-FU-plus-leucovorin regimens relates to schedule (some patients prefer weekly therapy over 5 consecutive days of treatment), cost, toxicity profile, and the clinician's preference.

MAYO/NCCTG REGIMEN: TOXICITY

Early experience in advanced disease

A substantial amount of data exists regarding the rate of adverse events associated with the Mayo/NCCTG regimen. Summary toxicity data from several of the initial trials of this regimen[15,18,22] are shown in Table 41.1. The rates of severe (grade $\geq$ 3) toxicity were consistent in the early studies, with diarrhea rates of 10–18%, nausea/vomiting rates of 5–10%, and leukopenia rates of 17–29%, while thrombocytopenia was rarely observed. In all of these trials, stomatitis was common, with rates ranging from 12% to 26% grade $\geqslant 3$. However, Mahood et al[23] reported that holding ice chips in the mouth during 5-FU treatment significantly reduced the incidence of stomatitis with the Mayo/NCCTG regimen. The prophylactic use of ice chips has since been standard practice for patients enrolled on Mayo/NCCTG clinical trials and also those treated off study at the Mayo Clinic with the Mayo/ NCCTG regimen. In many comparative trials done by other investigators, this supportive-care measure is not standard practice.

The studies in Table 41.1 were conducted before routine collection of neutropenia data. The use of data from Poon et al[15] and Buroker et al,[18] and a conservative assumption that every patient with fever or infection was also neutropenic, allows the calculation of an upper boundary on the rate of febrile neutropenia in these trials. Of 343 patients with advanced disease treated with the Mayo/NCCTG regimen on these trials, 13 patients had grade $\geqslant 3$ fever or infection, resulting in a worse-case rate of febrile neutropenia of 3.8%.

Table 41.1 Toxicity of the Mayo/NCCTG regimen: initial studies (the numbers shown are the percentages with each toxicity)			
Toxicity	Poon et al[15] (68 patients)	Buroker et al[18] (183 patients)	Leichman et al[22] (85 patients)
Diarrhea:			
Any	64	64	48
Severe	14	18	10
Stomatitis:			
Any	80	71	49
Severe	26	24	12
Vomiting:			
Any	46	43	31
Severe	9	8	5
Nausea:			
Any	76	60	
Severe	10	9	
Leukopenia:			
<4000/µl	83	78	51
<2000/µl	21	29	17
Granulocytopenia:			
<2000/µl			54
<1000/µl			40
Thrombocytopenia:			
<LLN[a]		21	12
<50 000/µl		3	2

[a]LLN, lower limit of normal.

As previously mentioned, the Buroker study[18] randomized patients between the Mayo/ NCCTG and Roswell Park regimens, allowing a direct toxicity comparison in advanced disease. In that study, stomatitis was significantly worse on the Mayo/NCCTG regimen (24% versus 2% for grade ≥ 3), while diarrhea was significantly worse on the Roswell Park regimen (32% versus 18% for grade ≥ 3). Leukopenia was more common on the Mayo/NCCTG regimen, but was rarely accompanied by fever or infection. Other toxicities were similar between the two arms. In this study, significantly more patients on the RPMI regimen required hospitalization than on the Mayo/NCCTG regimen (31% versus 21%, respectively; $p = 0.02$). The number of toxic deaths did not differ between the two arms (5 deaths on the Mayo/NCCTG regimen and 2 on the RPMI regimen; $p = 0.26$).

Recent experience in advanced disease

The toxicity profile of the Mayo/NCCTG regimen in the advanced-disease setting was documented in the abstracts from five large randomized trials reported at the 1999 American Society of Clinical Oncology meeting. Four of these trials[24–27] compared the Mayo/NCCTG regimen with an oral 5-FU-based regimen using an equivalence trial design. Comparative toxicity was thus a primary focus of the trials. The remaining trial[28] compared the Mayo/NCCTG regimen with a three-drug regimen containing 5-FU, leucovorin, and irinotecan (CPT-11), and was designed with response rate and overall survival as the primary endpoints. Toxicity data from three of the abstracts are summarized in Table 41.2. These data are similar to those shown in Table 41.1, with the exception of the high frequency of neutropenia. As mentioned, only leukopenia (not neutropenia) data were collected in the early trials using the Mayo/NCCTG regimen, so a direct comparison is not possible.

It should be noted that in four of these five trials,[24,25,27,28] a variation of the Mayo/NCCTG regimen was used. In these studies, a 4-week cycle was used throughout the course of the study, rather than a schedule prescribing treatment every 4 weeks for the first two cycles followed by every 5 weeks thereafter. The use of ice chips in an attempt to reduce stomatitis was also not apparently standard in these studies. Therefore, caution is required when interpreting these toxicity data relative to the classic Mayo/NCCTG regimen.

Toxicity in the adjuvant setting

Representative toxicity data of the Mayo/NCCTG regimen in the adjuvant setting for the two studies mentioned above[19,21] (toxicity data for INT-0089 kindly provided by Dr Dan Haller, PI) are summarized in Table 41.3. No toxic deaths were observed in the O'Connell study,[19] while 5 of 984 patients (0.5%) expired due to treatment-related causes on the Mayo/NCCTG regimen INT-0089.[21] These rates are consistent with those shown in Table 41.1 in the advanced-disease setting. In addition, while explicit data on febrile neutropenia are not available in INT-0089, the rate of grade ≥ 3 infection was 2%, and that of grade ≥ 3 fever without infection was less than 1%; therefore, the rate of febrile neutropenia is 3% or less.

IS THE MAYO/ NCCTG REGIMEN STILL STANDARD?

This is a controversial issue at the time of this writing, and one in which regional preferences are relevant. It is likely that the answer to this question is in transition. There have been several randomized trials conducted in Europe in which infusion-based 5-FU regimens or regimens that combine 5-FU and irinotecan or oxaliplatin have resulted in higher response rates than those seen with the Mayo/NCCTG regimen. Several examples will be discussed. Few studies in the advanced-disease setting, and none in the adjuvant setting, have indicated any survival advantage over that seen with the Mayo/NCCTG regimen.

A number of trials have examined the potential utility of administering 5-FU with leucovorin by infusion. Perhaps the most relevant of these is a French randomized phase III trial of infusion versus bolus 5-FU administration.[29] In this study, the Mayo/NCCTG program was compared with a bimonthly program of two consecutive days of high-dose leucovorin (200 mg/m²) followed by bolus 5-FU (400 mg/m²) followed by a 22-hour 5-FU infusion (600 mg/m²). The response rate in 348 randomized patients with measurable disease was 14% for the Mayo/NCCTG regimen versus 33% for the infusion regimen ($p = 0.0004$); however, the median survivals were not statistically significantly different: 57 weeks versus 62 weeks ($p = 0.07$).

In Germany, the Association of Medical Oncology of the German Cancer Society (AIO) has developed a regimen of high-dose leucovorin at 500 mg/m² followed by a 24-hour infusion of 2600 mg/m² of 5-FU administered weekly for 6 of every 8 weeks. Although this regimen has not been compared in a

Table 41.2 Toxicity of the Mayo/NCCTG regimen: recent reports (the numbers shown are the percentages with each toxicity)

Toxicity	Carmichael et al[26] (190 patients)	Pazdur et al[24] (408 patients)	Saltz et al[28] (221 patients)
Diarrhea:			
Any	60	76	
Severe	11	16	13
Stomatitis/mucositis:			
Any	55	75	
Severe	16	20	10
Nausea/vomiting:			
Any	58	75	
Severe	9	10	4
Neutropenia:			
Any	67	77	
Severe	31	56	37
Neutropenic fever:			
Any			
Severe			13
Thrombocytopenia:			
Any	28	31	
Severe	2	2	
Anemia:			
Any	89	87	
Severe	4	7	

randomized trial directly with the Mayo/NCCTG regimen, its activity is well documented. In a randomized study, the response rate was 44%, with a median survival of 16 months.[30]

In order to address the question whether the Mayo/NCCTG regimen is still the standard, we must consider all of the available evidence. As described briefly in the toxicity section of this chapter, preliminary results are available from several randomized trials in which patients received either oxaliplatin or irinotecan in addition to 5-FU with leucovorin. These studies have been presented at international meetings, but have only been reported in abstract form to date. Two phase III trials of irinote-

can plus 5-FU/leucovorin have been reported. The trial by Saltz et al[28] randomly assigned 221 patients to the Mayo/NCCTG regimen as the control arm. In the experimental arm of this study, the RPMI regimen was empirically modified by decreasing the dose of leucovorin to $20 \, \text{mg/m}^2/\text{day}$ and adding irinotecan administered at $125 \, \text{mg/m}^2/\text{day}$. The response rate to the Mayo/NCCTG regimen was 27%, compared with the three-drug regimen's response rate of 49% ($p < 0.001$). There was no significant difference in survival among patients randomized to the two regimens; the median survivals in the two groups were 12.2 months and 14.4 months, respectively.

Table 41.3 Toxicity of the Mayo/NCCTG regimen: adjuvant setting (the numbers shown are the percentages with each toxicity)

Toxicity	O'Connell et al[19] (158 patients)	Haller et al[21] (984 patients)
Diarrhea:		
Any	73	—
Severe	21	21
Stomatitis/mucositis:		
Any	75	—
Severe	34	18
Vomiting:		
Any	31	—
Severe	6	3
Nausea:		
Any	56	—
Severe	8	4
Leukopenia:		
Any	69	—
Severe	14	12
Thrombocytopenia:		
Any	13	—
Severe	0	1
Granulocytopenia:		
Any		—
Severe		25

Another study randomized 387 previously untreated patients to either the de Gramont or the AIO 5-FU leucovorin regimens described above, or to one of those regimens plus irinotecan.[31] Response rates were 31% for the pooled control regimens versus 49% for the pooled experimental arms of the trial ($p < 0.001$). There was a small but statistically significant difference in survival between the control and experimental regimens, with median survivals of 14 versus 16.8 months, respectively ($p = 0.03$).

A randomized trial reported by de Gramont et al[32] compared treatment with the infusion regimen described above[29] compared with that regimen plus oxaliplatin. This 420-patient trial was presented at the 1998 ASCO meeting, and published in abstract form. Observed response rates were 26% in the two-drug regimen and 57% in the three-drug regimen ($p < 0.05$). The median survivals for patients entered in the two study arms were 14.7 months and 16.2 months, respectively ($p = 0.11$).

Clearly, these trials suggest that triple-drug therapy significantly improves the response rate compared with that seen with 5-FU/leucovorin, with a suggestion of a small survival improvement due to the addition of irinotecan or oxaliplatin. However, in all three of these studies, the addition of the third agent altered the toxicity profile, and in two of the three studies,[31,32] it clearly lead to increased toxicity. Therefore, in the absence of a definitive survival advantage, it is unclear at this time whether the triple-drug combinations should become the standard of care.

An important consideration when evaluating studies in which two-drug regimens are compared with three-drug regimens is whether a lack of a significant survival advantage for the three-drug regimen is due to the fact that patients randomized to the control arms often cross over to other agents upon progression. This then raises the issue of whether sequential therapy is as good a strategy as is initial treatment with three or even four agents combined.

There are two practical considerations that suggest a positive answer to the question of whether the Mayo/NCCTG regimen is still standard – at least in the setting of advanced disease. In the USA, new drugs that have shown equivalence to the Mayo/NCCTG regimen in phase III trials (e.g. capecitabine) have been approved by the Food and Drug Administration (FDA), while those that have not shown equivalence (e.g. raltitrexed) have been turned down (see Chapter 56). Secondly, Protocol N9741, the current GI Intergroup trial for advanced disease in the USA, employs as its control arm the Mayo/NCCTG regimen. The members of the GI Intergroup committee have discussed the appropriateness of this control regimen extensively. If triple-drug therapy provides an advantage in quality of life or survival, this 1800-patient trial should definitively identify those advantages.

In the USA, many still consider either the Mayo/NCCTG regimen or the RPMI regimen to be the standard initial treatment for patients with advanced colorectal cancer. In Europe, it is probably more common for the de Gramont or AIO regimens to be considered standard in this setting (see Chapters 52, 57 and 58). On both sides of the Atlantic, adjuvant therapy with 5-FU plus leucovorin remains the standard of practice. We are hopeful that in the next five years, new regimens in the adjuvant and advanced-disease settings will supplant those considered standard today.

REFERENCES

1. Advanced Cancer Meta-Analysis Project, Modulation of fluorouracil by leucovorin in patients with advanced colorectal cancer: evidence in terms of response rate. *J Clin Oncol* 1992; **10:** 896–903.

2. Ullman B, Lee M, Martin DW Jr, Santi DV, Cytotoxicity of 5-fluoro-2-deoxyuridine: requirement for reduced folate co-factors and antagonism by methotrexate. *Proc Natl Acad Sci USA* 1978; **75:** 980–3.

3. Evans RM, Laskin JD, Hakala MT, Effect of excess folates and deoxyinosine on the activity and site of action of 5-fluorouracil. *Cancer Res* 1981; **41:** 3288–95.

4. Waxman S, Bruckner H, The enhancement of 5-fluorouracil antimetabolic activity by leucovorin, menadione, and alpha-tocopherol. *Eur J Cancer Clin Oncol* 1982; **18:** 685–92.

5. Keyomarsi K, Moran RG, Folinic augmentation of the effects of fluoropyrimidines on murine and human leukemic cells. *Cancer Res* 1986; **46:** 5229–35.

6. Houghton JA, Williams LG, Loftin SK et al, Relationship between the dose rate of [6*RS*]leucovorin administration, plasma concentrations of reduced folates, and pools of 5,10-methylenetetrahydrofolates and tetrahydrofolates in human colon adenocarcinoma xenografts. *Cancer Res* 1990; **50:** 3493–502.

7. Houghton JA, Williams LG, Loftin SK et al, Factors that influence the therapeutic activity of 5-fluorouracil–[6*RS*]leucovorin combinations in colon adenocarcinoma xenografts. *Cancer Chemother Pharmacol* 1992; **30:** 423–32.

8. Houghton JA, Williams LG, Cheshire PJ et al, Influence of the dose of [6*RS*]leucovorin on reduced folate pools and 5-fluorouracil-mediated thymidylate synthase inhibition in human colon adenocarcinoma xenografts. *Cancer Res* 1990; **50:** 3940–6.

9. Cao S, Frank C, Rustum YM, Role of fluoropyrimidine scheduling and (6*R,S*)leucovorin dose in a preclinical animal model of colorectal carcinoma. *J Natl Cancer Inst* 1996; **88:** 430–6.

10. Drake JC, Voeller DM, Allegra CJ et al, The effect of dose and interval between 5-fluorouracil and leucovorin on the formation of thymidylate synthase ternary complex in human cancer cells. *Br J Cancer* 1990; **71:** 1145–50.

11. Machover D, A comprehensive review of 5-fluorouracil and leucovorin in patients with metastatic colorectal carcinoma. *Cancer* 1997; **80:** 1179–87.

12. Machover D, Goldschmidt E, Chollet P et al, Treatment of advanced colorectal and gastric adenocarcinomas with 5-fluorouracil and high-dose folinic acid. *J Clin Oncol* 1986; **4:** 685–96.

13. Machover D, Schwartenberg L, Goldschmidt E et al, Treatment of advanced colorectal and gastric adenocarcinomas with 5-FU combined with high-dose folinic acid: a pilot study. *Cancer Treat Rep* 1982; **66:** 1803–7.

14. Rustum YM, Trave F, Zakrzewski SF et al, Biochemical and pharmacologic basis for potentiation of 5-fluorouracil action by leucovorin. *NCI Monogr* 1987; **5:** 165–70.

15. Poon MA, O'Connell MJ, Moertel CG et al, Biochemical modulation of fluorouracil: evidence of significant improvement in survival and quality of life in patients with advanced colorectal carcinoma. *J Clin Oncol* 1989; **7:** 1407–18.

16. O'Connell MJ, A phase III trial of 5-fluorouracil and leucovorin in the treatment of advanced colorectal cancer: a Mayo Clinic/North Central Cancer Treatment Group study. *Cancer* 1989; **63:** 1026–30.

17. Petrelli N, Herrara L, Rustum Y et al, A prospective randomized trial of 5-fluorouracil vs. 5-fluorouracil and high dose leucovorin + 5-fluorouracil and methotrexate in previously untreated patients with advanced colorectal carcinoma. *J Clin Oncol* 1987; **5:** 1559–65.

18. Buroker TR, O'Connell MJ, Wieand HS et al, Randomized comparison of two schedules of fluorouracil and leucovorin in the treatment of advanced colorectal cancer. *J Clin Oncol* 1994; **12:** 14–20.

19. O'Connell MJ, Mailliard JA, Kahn MJ et al, Controlled clinical trial of fluorouracil and low-dose leucovorin given for 6 months as postoperative adjuvant therapy for colon cancer. *J Clin Oncol* 1997; **15:** 246–50.

20. Moertel CG, Fleming TR, Macdonald JS et al, Levamisole and

fluorouracil for adjuvant therapy of resected colon carcinoma. *N Engl J Med* 1990; **322:** 352–8.

21. Haller DG, Catalano PJ, Macdonald JS et al, Fluorouracil (FU), leucovorin (LV), and levamisole (LEV) adjuvant therapy for colon cancer: five-year final report of INT-0089. *Proc Am Soc Clin Oncol* 1998; **17:** 256a.

22. Leichman CG, Fleming TR, Muggia FM et al, Phase II study of fluorouracil and its modulation in advanced colorectal cancer: a Southwest Oncology Group Study. *J Clin Oncol* 1995; **13:** 1303–11.

23. Mahood DJ, Dose AM, Loprinzi CL et al, Inhibition of fluorouracil-induced stomatitis by oral cryotherapy. *J Clin Oncol* 1991; **9:** 449–52.

24. Pazdur R, Douillard J-Y, Skillings JR et al, Multicenter phase III study of 5-fluorouracil (5-FU) or UFT® in combination with leucovorin (LV) in patients with metastatic colorectal cancer. *Proc Am Soc Clin Oncol* 1999; **18:** 263a.

25. Twelves C, Haper P, Van Cutsem E et al, A phase III trial (S014796) of Xeloda® (Capecitabine) in previously untreated advanced/metastatic colorectal cancer. *Proc Am Soc Clin Oncol* 1999; **18:** 263a.

26. Carmichael J, Popiela T, Radstone D et al, Randomized comparative study of ORZEL® (oral uracil/tegafur (UFT®) plus leucovorin (LV) versus parenteral 5-fluorouracil (5-FU) plus LV in patients with metastatic colorectal cancer. *Proc Am Soc Clin Oncol* 1999; **18:** 264a.

27. Cox JV, Pazdur R, Thibault A et al, A phase III trial of Xeloda™ (capecitabine) in previously untreated advanced/malignant colorectal cancer. *Proc Am Soc Clin Oncol* 1999; **18:** 265a.

28. Saltz LB, Locker PK, Pirotta N et al, Weekly irinotecan (CPT-11), leucovorin (LV), and fluorouracil (FU) is superior to daily × 5 LV/FU in patients with previously untreated metastatic colorectal cancer (CRC). *Proc Am Soc Clin Oncol* 1998; **19:** 233a.

29. de Gramont A, Bosset J-F, Milan C et al, Randomized trial comparing monthly low-dose leucovorin and fluorouracil bolus with bimonthly high-dose continuous infusion for advanced colorectal cancer: a French Intergroup study. *J Clin Oncol* 1997; **15:** 808–15.

30. Kohne C-H, Schoffski P, Wilke H et al, Effective biomodulation by leucovorin of high-dose infusion fluorouracil given as a weekly 24-hour infusion: results of a randomized trial in patients with advanced colorectal cancer. *J Clin Oncol* 1998; **16:** 418–26.

31. Douillard JY, Cunningham D, Roth AD et al, A randomized phase III trial comparing irinotecan (IRI) + 5FU/folinic acid (FA) to the same schedule of 5FU/FA in patients (pts) with metastatic colorectal cancer (MCRC) as front line chemotherapy (CT). *Proc Am Soc Clin Oncol* 1998; **18:** 233a.

32. de Gramont A, Figer A, Seymour M et al, A randomized trial of leucovorin (LV) and 5-fluorouracil (5FU) with or without oxaliplatin in advanced colorectal cancer (CRC). *Proc Am Soc Clin Oncol* 1998; **17:** 257a.

42

The Roswell Park regimen: Weekly 5-FU and high-dose leucovorin for colon cancer

Peter C Enzinger, Robert J Mayer

INTRODUCTION

By the early 1950s, a number of nucleic acid analogues were under development for the treatment of cancer. Rat hepatomas were shown to demonstrate increased uptake and catabolism of [2-^{14}C]uracil when compared with normal liver tissue.[1] Furthermore, it was noted that fluorine could alter cellular metabolism when it was substituted for hydrogen in various biologic compounds. Based on these observations, Heidelberger et al[2] synthesized the fluoropyrimidine 5-fluorouracil (5-FU) and injected it into the peritoneal cavities of tumor-bearing mice and rats. The drug showed significant antitumor activity and appeared to be well tolerated.

Over the next 20 years, two central mechanisms of action for 5-FU were carefully established.[3,4] First, 5-FU is metabolized to 5-fluorouridine triphosphate (FUTP) and is incorporated into RNA. This interferes with RNA synthesis and function. Second, 5-FU is metabolized to 5-fluoro-2'-deoxyuridylate (FdUMP) and acts as a quasisubstrate for the enzyme thymidylate synthase in the conversion of deoxyuridylate (dUMP) and methylenetetrahydrofolate to thymidylate (dTMP) and dihydrofolate. This in turn reduces pools of available thymidylate synthase, leading to the depletion of dTMP and thymidine triphosphate (dTTP) and the accumulation of dUMP and deoxyuridine triphosphate (dUTP), thereby inhibiting DNA synthesis.

By 1978, 5-FU had been tested extensively in clinical trials of colorectal cancer, and had been combined with other agents such as semustine (methyl-CCNU) and vincristine. Although an improved response rate was documented with 5-FU in combination with these drugs, no improvement in survival could be demonstrated, and single-agent 5-FU remained the standard of care for colorectal cancer.[5] The optimal schedule for 5-FU, however, remained uncertain: two basic schedules, an intravenous loading schedule and a weekly intravenous schedule, emerged as the most popular regimens.[6]

PRECLINICAL STUDIES OF REDUCED FOLATES AND 5-FU

While oncologists were exploring the clinical uses of 5-FU, pharmacologists were seeking to optimize its antitumor activity. They found that the formation of the stable ternary complex between FdUMP, thymidylate synthase, and methylenetetrahydrofolate occurs rapidly, with the resultant inhibition of thymidylate synthase.[7] Dissolution of this complex occurs slowly and is independent of dUMP concentration. As the concentration of methylenetetrahydrofolate is increased from 0 to 3 mM, however, the half-life of this reaction can be increased from 36 to 840 minutes at 37°C.

In cell lines, this pharmacokinetic effect (i.e. the modulation of 5-FU) results in enhanced antitumor activity. Thus, the cytotoxicity of 5-fluoro-2'-deoxyuridine (FdUrd), an active metabolite of 5-FU, can be increased fourfold in the L1210 mouse leukemia cell line if the concentration of leucovorin (folinic acid, LV, D,L-5-formyltetrahydrofolate) is increased from 3 μM to 23 μM.[8] Similarly, leucovorin at a concentration of 10–20 μM enhances 5-FU inhibition threefold in the Friend murine erythroleukemia cell line and the human carcinoma Hep-2 cell line.[9,10] In 5-FU-resistant human colorectal adenocarcinoma cell lines, excess FdUMP in the absence of methylenetetrahydrofolate produces only a 50% reduction in thymidylate synthase activity; the addition of methylenetetrahydrofolate (54 μM) increases thymidylate synthase inhibition to 95%.[11]

EARLY CLINICAL STUDIES OF REDUCED FOLATES AND 5-FU

In a series of clinical trials, Bruckner et al[12] first explored the use of low-dose leucovorin (25–200 mg) in combination with high-dose 5-FU (25–35 mg/kg every 3 weeks). Initial studies suggested that leucovorin substantially increased the toxicity of 5-FU. Leukopenia and neurotoxicity were dose-limiting when this schedule was utilized. Once dose modifications were made, however, major responses were achieved in 19% of patients, including those patients whose tumor was refractory to the same schedule of 5-FU without leucovorin.

In France, Machover et al[13] initiated a trial of 5-FU and high-dose leucovorin in colorectal and gastric cancer. In this study, 35 patients with colorectal cancer received 5-FU (370–400 mg/m²/day) and high-dose leucovorin (200 mg/m²/day) simultaneously for 5 days every 3 weeks. Of 30 evaluable patients with measurable disease, 14 had been previously treated with unmodulated 5-FU. Major responses were documented in 56% of the chemotherapy-naive patients and in 21% of the pretreated patients. Toxicities included stomatitis, myelosuppression, and diarrhea. The authors concluded that patients with 5-FU-refractory colon cancer could still benefit from 5-FU if high-dose leucovorin was added. Cunningham et al[14] later reported similar results with high-dose leucovorin plus 5-FU administered either as a bolus or as a continuous infusion.

ROSWELL PARK REGIMEN: PHASE I–II TRIALS

In 1984, Rustum and colleagues[15] at the Roswell Park Cancer Institute completed a phase I–II study of 5-FU and high-dose leucovorin. Chemotherapy was given weekly for 6 weeks, followed by a 2-week rest period (see Figure 42.1). Leucovorin was given as a 2-hour infusion at 500 mg/m². The initial dose of 5-FU, given midway through the leucovorin infusion (after 1 hour), was 300 mg/m²/week, and, in the absence of dose-limiting toxicity, was escalated every second course to 600 mg/m²/week and then to 750 mg/m²/week. Major responses were observed in 9 of 23 patients (39%), including 6 of 12 patients who had previously received 5-FU alone. Grade 3/4 toxicity at a 5-FU dose of 600 mg/m² included diarrhea in

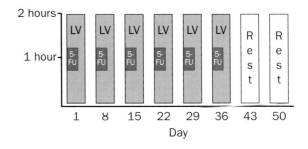

Figure 42.1 Schema for Roswell Park regimen (one cycle): 5-FU, 5-fluorouracil 600 mg/m² intravenous push (original) or 5-fluorouracil 500 mg/m² intravenous push (standard and adjuvant); LV, leucovorin 500 mg/m² intravenous bolus over 2 hours.

17% and leukopenia in 6% of patients. At a 5-FU dose of 750 mg/m², grade 3/4 toxicity increased significantly, with diarrhea occurring in 55% and leukopenia in 36% of patients. The recommended phase II dose was therefore 5-FU 600 mg/m²/week with leucovorin 500 mg/m²/week (see Figure 42.1).

With this 2-hour leucovorin infusion schedule, the peak plasma level for leucovorin ranged from 33 to 194 μM (mean 111 μM) and the peak plasma level for methylenetetrahydrofolate ranged from 2 to 23 μM (mean 11 μM). Both peak plasma levels were achieved within minutes after the start of the infusion. In a subsequent report, the authors added that the plasma level of L-leucovorin remained greater than 10 μM for 2 hours, with a mean elimination half-life ($t_{1/2}$) of 1.2 hours. Methyltetrahydrofolate plasma levels remained greater than 10 μM for more than 6 hours, with a mean $t_{1/2}$ of 7 hours. This increased the $t_{1/2}$ of 5-FU by 26%.[16]

Hines et al[17] achieved similar results with a weekly schedule of oral high-dose leucovorin and 5-FU that differed only slightly from that of the Roswell Park regimen. In this study, patients received oral leucovorin 500 mg/m² in divided doses over 3 hours and then 5-FU 600 mg/m² 2 hours later. Additionally, patients received a 3- to 4-week break rather than a 2-week rest between 6-week chemotherapy cycles. Of 31 patients with evaluable disease, 14 (45%; 95% confidence interval (CI) 28–63%) achieved a major response. Of these patients, 10 had received prior 5-FU-based chemotherapy. Among these previously treated patients, a 32% response rate was recorded. Responding patients had a median time to progression of 16 months and a median survival of 21 months. No grade 3 toxicities occurred. Grade 2 toxicities were notable for diarrhea (45%), emesis (19%), and myelosuppression (10%).

ROSWELL PARK REGIMEN IN ADVANCED DISEASE

Roswell Park regimen versus single-agent 5-FU

Early randomized studies attempted to validate the improved response rate that had been observed with high-dose leucovorin-modulated 5-FU at selected institutions. As part of a randomized phase II trial, Petrelli et al[18] compared the Roswell Park regimen with Ansfield's 'intravenous loading course schedule'.[6] The monthly loading schedule employed 5-FU 450 mg/m^2 daily for 5 days, followed by 5-FU 200 mg/m^2 every other day for 6 doses. Of 19 chemotherapy-naive patients who received this loading schedule, only 2 (11%) had a partial response. By contrast, 12 of 25 patients (48%) treated with the Roswell Park schedule had a major response. Toxicity requiring dose reduction on the Roswell Park regimen included diarrhea in 40%, stomatitis in 10%, and leukopenia in 10% of patients.

Similarly, the Gastrointestinal Tumor Study Group (GITSG) compared the Roswell Park regimen with maximally dose-intense monthly 5-FU (500–625 mg/m^2/day × 5 days) as well as with weekly low-dose leucovorin 25 mg/m^2 plus 5-FU 600 mg/m^2. In an initial 1987 report,[19] the authors were able to confirm the superior response rate of leucovorin-modulated 5-FU compared to prior GITSG studies of single-agent 5-FU. They cautioned, however, that the Roswell Park schedule caused a significant number of life-threatening toxicities and therefore recommended that 5-FU on this schedule be reduced from 600 mg/m^2 to 500 mg/m^2. While grade 3/4 leukopenia was greater for the dose-intensive single-agent 5-FU arm, other grade 3/4 toxicities such as diarrhea, mucositis, and nausea/vomiting increased with the leucovorin dose and were most prominent with the Roswell Park schedule (see Table 42.1). Response rates were 30% for the high-dose leucovorin arm, 19% for the low-dose leucovorin arm, and 12% for the single agent 5-FU arm. In their final report (see Table 42.1),[20] the authors concluded that high-dose weekly leucovorin plus 5-FU has a significantly higher response rate than either low-dose leucovorin plus 5-FU ($p = 0.046$) or single-agent 5-FU ($p < 0.01$). No statistical improvement in survival, however, was seen when the high-dose leucovorin arm was compared with either low-dose leucovorin plus 5-FU (p not given) or 5-FU alone ($p = 0.08$).

In Italy, two randomized trials compared weekly 5-FU with weekly 5-FU and leucovorin. The first of these studies, conducted by Nobile et al,[21] evaluated a modified Roswell Park schedule in 148 patients with advanced chemotherapy-naive colorectal cancer (see Table 42.1). The group treated with the modified Roswell Park regimen received 5-FU 600 mg/m^2 plus leucovorin 500 mg/m^2 weekly without the traditional 2-week break between cycles (see Table 42.1). The comparison cohort received weekly 5-FU 600 mg/m^2 alone, also without break. The likelihood of a major response was statistically more frequent ($p = 0.03$) in the patients given weekly 5-FU and leucovorin (23%) than in the single-agent 5-FU group (8%). The median time to progression also showed a trend ($p = 0.08$) in favor of the 5-FU/leucovorin-treated patients (5 months versus 3 months). The survival duration, however, was similar for both groups (median 11 months). Patients given the modified Roswell Park regimen experienced significantly more grade 3/4 diarrhea (20% versus 9%; $p = 0.045$) and conjunctivitis (27% versus 6%; $p = 0.003$), but other toxicities were relatively similar. Despite the apparent disparity in dose intensity between the two arms, patients allocated to receive 5-FU alone actually received a greater total dose of 5-FU per week. On this arm, 5-FU was ultimately given at a median of 600 mg/m^2/week versus 505 mg/m^2/week in the group that received leucovorin. Thus, it can be argued that maximal dose intensity was given in both arms. In contrast to the previous studies, 5-FU was administered by the same schedule in both arms. Potentiation of 5-FU by leucovorin was therefore independent of 5-FU schedule.

The second of these randomized Italian trials, conducted by Martoni et al,[22] compared a weekly regimen of 5-FU 600 mg/m^2 with a weekly regimen of 5-FU 600 mg/m^2 given halfway through a 1-hour infusion of intermediate-dose leucovorin 200 mg/m.^{2} Therapy was given for 6 weeks to both patient cohorts. Partial remissions were obtained in 1 of 30 patients (3%) who received 5-FU alone and in 9 of 34 patients (26%) allocated to the 5-FU/leucovorin arm ($p = 0.028$). A statistically insignificant trend in median time to progression (6 months versus 5 months) and median survival (10 months versus 7 months) was noted in favor of the 5-FU/leucovorin arm. A similar trend for increased diarrhea was observed in patients receiving the 5-FU/leucovorin arm, leading to a significant increase ($p = 0.011$) in the number of treatment interruptions.

These four trials and other studies comparing a monthly loading schedule of 5-FU with or without leucovorin were analyzed as part of the Advanced

Table 42.1 Weekly 5-FU and high-dose leucovorin versus weekly 5-FU with or without low-dose leucovorin (LV) in advanced colorectal cancer

Authors	Schedule	No. of patients	Response rate (%)	Grade 3/4 toxicity (%): diarrhea/mucositis/WBC	Survival (months)
GITSG[20] (1989)	LV 500 mg/m^2/2 h + 5-FU 600 mg/m^2 at 1 h weekly × 6 q2mos	109	30 ($p = 0.046$)	26/4/7	12.7 ($p = $ NS)
	LV 25 mg/m^2/2 h + 5-FU 600 mg/m^2 at 1 h weekly × 6 q2mos	112	19	14/0/4	10.4
Nobile et al[21] (1992)	LV 500 mg/m^2/2 h + 5-FU 600 mg/m^2 at 1 h weekly without break	70	23 ($p = 0.03$)	20/3/0 ($p = 0.045$ for diarrhea)	11
	5-FU 600 mg/m^2 weekly without break	72	8	9/1/0	11
Jaeger et al[26] (1996)	LV 500 mg/m^2/2 h + 5-FU 500 mg/m^2 at 1 h weekly × 6 (q8wks?)	148	22 ($p = $ NS)	27/0/1	12.7 ($p = $ NS)
	LV 20 mg/m^2/2 h + 5-FU 500 mg/m^2 at 1 h weekly × 6 (q8wks?)	143	18	16/0/1	12.5

Abbreviations: NS, not statistically significant; WBC, white blood cell count.

Colorectal Cancer Meta-Analysis Project.[23] In this meta-analysis of 1381 patients, major responses were noted in 181 of 803 patients (23%) receiving 5-FU and leucovorin versus 64 of 578 patients (11%) treated with 5-FU alone. These results were highly significant ($p < 10^{-7}$), with an odds ratio of 0.45. No survival advantage, however, was observed for the 5-FU/leucovorin group ($p = 0.57$; odds ratio 0.97), with a median survival of 11.5 months compared with 11 months in the 5-FU group. In a subgroup analysis of patients receiving weekly 5-FU with or without leucovorin, the response benefit for 5-FU/leucovorin was preserved with an odds ratio of 0.35 ($p < 10^{-5}$); again, no improvement in survival was noted (odds ratio 0.9; $p = 0.22$).

Roswell Park regimen versus weekly 5-FU and low-dose leucovorin

The therapeutic impact of high-dose leucovorin in the Roswell Park regimen is still debated among experts. Earlier, a randomized trial conducted by the Mayo Clinic/North Central Cancer Treatment Group (NCCTG) had demonstrated no improvement in survival when high-dose leucovorin (200 mg/m^2) was compared with low-dose leucovorin (20 mg/m^2), given daily for 5 days with 5-FU as part of a monthly loading regimen.[24,25] However, not until 1996 was the contribution of high-dose leucovorin addressed in the Roswell Park regimen. Jaeger et al[26] compared the Roswell Park regimen with weekly 5-FU and low-dose leucovorin in a randomized study of patients with advanced disease (see Table 42.1). In this experience, 148 patients received the Roswell Park regimen with 5-FU 500 mg/m^2 plus leucovorin 500 mg/m^2, while 143 patients received the same schedule except that the leucovorin dose was 20 mg/m^2. Although a greater number of major responses were recorded in patients receiving high-dose leucovorin (22% versus 18%), the difference was not statistically significant and median survival was essentially the same (12.7 versus 12.5 months for the low-dose leucovorin arm). The incidence of grade 3/4 diarrhea, however, was significantly greater on the high-dose leucovorin arm (27% versus 16%). The results of this study have convinced some oncologists to give weekly 5-FU and low-dose leucovorin to their patients with metastatic disease.

Roswell Park regimen versus Mayo Clinic regimen

By the late 1980s, the Mayo Clinic regimen and the Roswell Park regimen had emerged as the two most popular leucovorin-modulated 5-FU regimens for colorectal cancer in North America; both had been shown to lead to a higher likelihood of disease regression than 5-FU alone. Therefore, the Mayo Clinic/NCCTG decided to compare its schedule with the Roswell Park regimen in 372 patients with metastatic disease (see Table 42.2).[27] Patients assigned to the Mayo Clinic arm received leucovorin 20 mg/m² in an intravenous 'push', followed by 5-FU 425 mg/m² daily for 5 consecutive days on weeks 1, 4, and 8, and then every 5 weeks. Patients allocated to the Roswell Park arm received leucovorin 500 mg/m² as a 2-hour infusion and 5-FU 600 mg/m² 1 hour after the start of this infusion every week for 6 weeks, followed by a 2-week break, on an 8-week cycle. Major responses were recorded in 31% of patients on the Roswell Park arm versus 35% of patients on the Mayo Clinic arm ($p = 0.51$). There was no statistical difference in progression-free sur-

vival or overall survival. The Mayo Clinic regimen caused significantly more leukopenia and stomatitis than the Roswell Park regimen, whereas the latter caused significantly more diarrhea (see Table 42.2). Hospitalizations were more frequent (31% versus 21%; $p = 0.02$) and longer in patients given the Roswell Park arm, in large part because such hospitalizations were mandated by protocol design if four or more diarrheal stools occurred per day, reflecting concern over the toxic deaths that had occurred when the Roswell Park regimen had been utilized in the earlier GITSG trial.[19] In this NCCTG trial, however, the likelihood for toxic death was actually less in patients treated with the Roswell Park regimen (1.1% versus 2.7%; $p = 0.26$).

A modified Roswell Park regimen was also compared with the Mayo Clinic schedule as part of a large randomized phase II trial to examine various approaches to the modulation of 5-FU.[28] In this Southwest Oncology Group (SWOG) study, 85 patients were randomized to the Roswell Park arm. These patients received leucovorin 500 mg/m² as a 3-hour infusion, followed by 5-FU 600 mg/m² weekly for 6 weeks, followed by a 2-week break, on an 8-week cycle. A similar cohort of 85 patients received the standard Mayo Clinic schedule as in the NCCTG study.[27] With approximately 60 patients evaluable for response on each arm, the study was not powered to detect statistically significant differences in response

Table 42.2 Weekly 5-FU and high-dose leucovorin (LV) versus the Mayo Clinic regimen in advanced colorectal cancer

Authors	Schedule	No. of patients	Response rate (%)	Grade 3/4 toxicity (%): diarrhea/mucositis/ANC	Survival (months)
Buroker et al[27] (1994)	LV 500 mg/m²/2 h + 5-FU 600 mg/m² at 1 h weekly × 6 q8wks	179 (55*)	31 (p = NS)	32/2/5 (p < 0.01 for all)	10.7 (p = NS)
	LV 20 mg/m² bolus, then 5-FU 425 mg/m² daily × 5 q4–5wks	183 (56*)	35	18/24/29	9.3
Leichman et al[28] (1995)	LV 500 mg/m²/3 h, then 5-FU 600 mg/m² weekly × 8 weeks	60	21 (p = NS)	27/1/8	13 (p = NS)
	LV 20 mg/m² IVP, then 5-FU 425 mg/m² daily × 5 q4–5wks	61	27	12/14/47	14

Abbreviations: NS, not statistically significant; ANC, absolute neutrophil count; IVP, intravenous 'push'.
*Measurable disease.

Table 42.3 Grade 3/4 toxicities in SWOG trial of various 5-FU schedules in advanced colorectal cancer[a]

5-FU regimen	Schedule	Toxicity (%)				
		ANC	Platelets	Vomiting	Stomatitis	Diarrhea
Monthly 5-day bolus	5-FU 500 mg/m^2 IVP: d1–5 q5wks	47	5	2	5	10
Mayo Clinic regimen	LV 20 mg/m^2 IVP + 5-FU 425 mg/m^2 IVP: d1–5 q4–5wks	47	2	6	14	12
Roswell Park-type schedule	LV 500 mg/m^2/3 h, then 5-FU 600 mg/m^2 IVP: weekly × 6 q8wks	8	1	6	1	27
Continuous infusion	CI 5-FU 300 mg/m^2/d: d1–28 q5wks	1	0	4	6	6
Continuous infusion + LV	CI 5-FU 200 mg/m^2/d: d1–28 q5wks + LV 20 mg/m^2: d1,8,15,22 q5wks	1	0	5	11	11
24 h continuous infusion	24 h CI 5-FU 2600 mg/m^2 weekly	4	0	4	1	11
24 h continuous infusion + PALA	PALA 250 mg/m^2/15 min, then 24 h CI 5-FU 2600 mg/m^2: weekly	11	4	4	7	10

Abbreviations: LV, leucovorin; PALA, N-phosphonoacetyl-L-aspartate; IVP, intravenous 'push'; CI, continuous infusion; ANC, absolute neutrophil count.
[a] Modified from Leichman et al.[28]

or survival. Response rates were lower than had been reported in prior randomized trials, with a 27% response rate (95% CI 16–39%) for the Mayo Clinic regimen and 21% response rate (95% CI 11–32%) for the modified Roswell Park schedule. The median survival time was 14 months for patients given the Mayo Clinic arm and 13 months for those treated with the Roswell Park arm. Toxicities are listed in Table 42.3. Similar to the NCCTG study, grade 3/4 leukopenia and stomatitis were more frequent when the Mayo Clinic arm was utilized, and diarrhea was more severe when the Roswell Park arm was given (see Table 42.2). Additionally, two sepsis-related deaths (2.4%) occurred on the Mayo Clinic arm, whereas none were recorded on the Roswell Park arm.

Roswell Park regimen versus 5-FU infusional schedules

Most direct comparisons of bolus 5-FU/leucovorin with infusional 5-FU schedules have utilized the Mayo Clinic regimen. The only published trial that has directly compared a Roswell Park schedule with various infusional schedules is the aforementioned seven-arm study in advanced colon cancer by the SWOG.[28] As part of this study, a modified Roswell Park schedule (see Table 42.3) was compared with (1) continuous-infusion 5-FU 300 mg/m^2 for 4 weeks on a 5-week cycle, (2) continuous-infusion 5-FU 200 mg/m^2 plus weekly leucovorin 20 mg/m^2 for 4 weeks on a 5-week cycle, (3) 24-hour weekly continuous-infusion 5-FU 2600 mg/m^2, and (4) weekly N-phosphonoacetyl-L-aspartate (PALA) 250 mg/m^2 followed by 24-hour continuous-infusion 5-FU

2600 mg/m². Since only 58–63 patients were evaluable for response on each arm, the study was not powered to detect a statistically significant response or survival advantage. Response rates (and median survival) for the modified Roswell Park schedule and for the four other regimens were essentially equivalent at 21% (13 months), 29% (15 months), 26% (14 months), 15% (15 months), and 25% (11 months), respectively. Toxicities are listed in Table 42.3. The incidence of grade 3/4 diarrhea was less (6–11%) for the infusional schedules than the modified Roswell Park regimen (27%). Grade 3/4 granulocytopenia was also generally less on the infusional regimens; grade 3/4 stomatitis was higher for the prolonged infusion schedules, ranging from 6% to 11%.

The results of another randomized trial that compared a Roswell Park-like regimen with an infusional 5-FU schedule have been presented thus far only in abstract form.[29] In this cooperative group study of 1118 patients with previously untreated advanced colorectal cancer, patients were randomized to five treatment arms: (1) 5-FU 600 mg/m² plus leucovorin 600 mg/m² weekly, (2) 5-FU 2600 mg/m² given as a weekly 24-hour infusion, (3) 5-FU with oral leucovorin, (4) 5-FU with PALA, and (5) 5-FU with interferon-α-2a. Grade IV toxicity (primarily diarrhea) occurred in 23% of patients receiving the modified Roswell Park regimen and in 11% of patients receiving the weekly 24-hour infusion of 5-FU. Median survival for the Roswell Park-like schedule was 13.6 months and that for the 24-hour continuous-infusion arm was 14.8 months ($p = 0.8$). The authors concluded that the Roswell Park-like regimen was more toxic than the 24-hour infusional schedule but did not improve survival.

Roswell Park regimen in combination with other agents

In an early attempt to improve upon the Roswell Park regimen, a group led by the MD Anderson Cancer Center randomized patients with advanced colorectal cancer to the Roswell Park regimen with or without semustine.[30] Both groups received leucovorin 500 mg/m² and 5-FU 600 mg/m², utilizing the now 'standard' schedule. Additionally, one group received semustine 110 mg/m² on the first day of each 8-week cycle. The group with the added semustine experienced markedly increased toxicity, characterized primarily by increased myelosuppression but also by nausea and vomiting. Major responses were recorded in 28% of patients who received 5-FU/leucovorin and in 24% of patients who received 5-FU/leucovorin plus semustine. Median survival similarly favored patients who had received 5-FU/leucovorin without semustine (11.8 months versus 11.1 months). Although the study failed to show a benefit for semustine in combination with 5-FU and leucovorin, it provides a reliable standard for response and survival of the Roswell Park regimen in advanced disease.

More recently, with the development of irinotecan (CPT-11) and oxaliplatin, new approaches to the treatment of colorectal cancer are being examined. Both irinotecan and oxaliplatin have been shown to be active in 5-FU-refractory patients. After initial evaluation in the refractory disease setting, these agents are now being tested in previously untreated patients. The weekly Roswell Park schedule is particularly suited for the addition of irinotecan and oxaliplatin. Weekly irinotecan 125 mg/m² can be added to 5-FU 500 mg/m² and low-dose leucovorin 20 mg/m² when administered for 4 consecutive weeks followed by a 2-week break.[31] In a follow-up trial, this weekly triple combination was compared with the Mayo Clinic regimen and with weekly single-agent irinotecan in a three-arm study.[32] The response rate of the irinotecan/5-FU/leucovorin combination was superior to that of the Mayo Clinic regimen (50% versus 28%; $p < 0.0001$). Similarly, overall survival (14.8 months versus 12.6 months; $p = 0.042$) and progression-free survival (7.0 months versus 4.3 months; $p = 0.004$) were significantly better for the irinotecan combination. The irinotecan/5-FU/leucovorin arm was associated with more diarrhea (23% versus 13%) but less neutropenia (24% versus 43%) and less mucositis (2% versus 17%) than the Mayo Clinic regimen. Currently, this regimen is being compared by the GI Intergroup with other promising irinotecan and oxaliplatin combinations in patients with advanced colorectal cancer (NCCTG N9741).

Oxaliplatin has been successfully added to the Roswell Park regimen (5-FU 500 mg/m²) as part of a compassionate-use study currently underway in the USA. Through June of 1999, 1017 patients with 5-FU-refractory advanced colorectal cancer have been enrolled. Of these, 41% are being treated on the Roswell Park arm. Oxaliplatin 85 mg/m²/2 h is administered prior to 5-FU/leucovorin on weeks 1, 3, and 5, while 5-FU/leucovorin is given alone on weeks 2, 4, and 6. The safety profile appears to be similar to that of other studies incorporating the Roswell Park schedule (personal communication, Elizabeth Harvey, Sanofi Pharmaceuticals). Response and survival data compared with other oxaliplatin combinations are not yet available.

ROSWELL PARK REGIMEN AS ADJUVANT THERAPY

The Roswell Park regimen was first evaluated in the adjuvant setting by the National Surgical Adjuvant Breast and Bowel Project (NSABP) with the initiation of Protocol C-03 in 1987. In this trial, the NSABP compared the Roswell Park regimen with MOF (semustine, vincristine, and 5-FU) as postoperative therapy in 1081 patients with Dukes B and C colon cancer.[33] Patients randomized to the Roswell Park arm received 5-FU 500 mg/m^2 and leucovorin 500 mg/m^2 weekly for 6 weeks followed by a 2-week rest period (see Figure 42.1); a total of 6 cycles (i.e. about 1 year) of total treatment was given. After 3 years of follow-up, the disease-free survival (DFS) rate (73% versus 64%; $p = 0.0004$) and overall survival (OS) rate (84% versus 77%; $p = 0.003$) both favored the Roswell Park arm. Hematologic toxicity for the Roswell Park cohort was minimal, but 85% of these patients experienced diarrhea (28% grade 3/4), leading to 4 treatment-related deaths (0.77%).

In their next trial (Protocol C-04),[34] the NSABP compared the Roswell Park regimen with 5-FU/levamisole, which had been shown previously to be effective as postoperative therapy in stage III colon cancer. An additional treatment arm included 5-FU, leucovorin, and levamisole. Stage II and III patients were eligible to participate. Patients assigned to the Roswell Park arm received the standard schedule for a total of 6 cycles (46 weeks). Patients randomized to 5-FU/levamisole were 'loaded' with 5-FU 450 mg/m^2 for 5 days during the first month, and then continued this dose weekly for 48 weeks. Patients allocated to 5-FU/leucovorin/levamisole were given the Roswell Park regimen with the same dose of levamisole as in the 5-FU/levamisole arm. The 5-year DFS rate (65% versus 60%; $p = 0.04$) and OS rate (74% versus 70%; $p = 0.07$) favored the Roswell Park arm. Levamisole provided no added survival benefit to the Roswell Park regimen. Of the 2151 patients on this study, 41% had stage II colon cancer. In this group, the 5-year DFS rate (75% versus 71%) and OS rate (84% versus 81%) also favored the Roswell Park arm. Grade 3/4 toxicity occurred in 35% of patients on the Roswell Park regimen, and was primarily diarrhea (27%). Four treatment-related deaths (0.6%) were recorded on this arm.

In March 1999, the NSABP concluded accrual to their most recent adjuvant colorectal trial, Protocol C-06. In this phase III adjuvant study of patients with stage II/III colon cancer, patients were randomized to either the Roswell Park regimen or oral uracil/tegafur (UFT) with oral leucovorin. Data from this trial will take several years to mature. Thus, for the present time, the Roswell Park regimen remains the standard of care for the NSABP.

Following preliminary results suggesting that 5-FU/levamisole and the Mayo Clinic program of 5-FU/leucovorin were each effective in the adjuvant setting, the North American GI Intergroup decided to compare these schedules with the Roswell Park regimen in 3759 patients with high-risk stage II and stage III colon cancer.[35,36] In this study (INT-0089), patients were randomized to receive either the Roswell Park regimen for 32 weeks (4 cycles; 2 cycles less than NSABP Protocol C-04), the Mayo Clinic regimen for 28 weeks (6 cycles), or the 5-FU/levamisole regimen for 52 weeks. A fourth arm, in which levamisole was added to the Mayo Clinic schedule, was given over 32 weeks. No significant differences in 5-year DFS or 5-year OS were observed among these treatment arms. A 2-sided statistical comparison between the Mayo Clinic regimen and Roswell Park regimen yielded a p value of 0.57 for 5-year DFS and a p value of 0.70 for 5-year OS. The 5-year DFS/OS rates were 59%/66% for the Roswell Park regimen, 60%/67% for the Mayo Clinic regimen, and 56%/63% for the 12-month levamisole regimen. In contrast to the NSABP C-04 trial, stage II patients had to fulfill high-risk criteria for recurrence, and comprised only 20% of patients in this trial. In this group, the 5-year OS rate was 75% for the Roswell Park regimen and 77% for the Mayo Clinic regimen. In stage III patients, the 5-year OS rate was 63% for both groups. Overall grade 3–5 toxicity was lowest for the Roswell Park arm, occurring in 41% of patients. The 5-FU/levamisole and Mayo Clinic arms had higher overall toxicities, at 44% and 56% respectively. This was primarily due to the low incidence of grade 3–5 granulocytopenia (4%) and stomatitis (1%) in the Roswell Park group. By comparison, the incidences of severe granulocytopenia and stomatitis with the Mayo Clinic regimen were 24% and 18%, respectively. Diarrhea accounted for most of the grade 3–5 toxicity in the Roswell Park group, occurring in 30% of patients. This compared with 21% in the Mayo Clinic group and 11% in the 5-FU/levamisole group. The authors concluded that either the Roswell Park regimen or the Mayo Clinic regimen should represent the standard of care for resected high-risk colon cancer. However, it should be noted that these same authors (GI Intergroup) have chosen the Roswell Park regimen as the standard arm in their current postadjuvant chemotherapy trial for high-risk resected colon cancer (CALGB-89803).

CONCLUSIONS

After more than four decades of intensive studies, the optimal regimen for managing patients with colorectal cancer with 5-FU is still debated. 5-FU may be given as a weekly bolus, a monthly loading dose, a 24-hour infusion, a continuous infusion, or even as a daily pill. Although toxicities differ, none of these schedules has demonstrated a clear survival advantage, and therefore, cost, tolerance, convenience, and physician preference often dictate the regimen chosen (see Table 42.3).[79]

In colorectal cancer, most trials suggest that leucovorin enhances the response rate of bolus 5-FU.[12–23] In weekly regimens, the substitution of low-dose leucovorin (20–25 mg/m^2) for high-dose leucovorin (500 mg/m^2) appears to lessen the response rate of 5-FU by 4–11% (see Table 42.1).[18,26] The addition of weekly high-dose leucovorin, however, does not appear to have an impact upon survival in this disease.[18,21,26] Compared with low-dose leucovorin,

weekly high-dose leucovorin increases the incidence of grade 3/4 diarrhea by 11–12%.[18,26] Other toxicities, such as mucositis and leukopenia, appear relatively unaffected by leucovorin dose.

Originally, weekly 5-FU and high-dose leucovorin (i.e. the Roswell Park regimen: see Figure 42.1) was given with 5-FU 600 mg/m^2.[15,16] This dose, however, has proven to be too toxic,[19] and therefore all recent trials have used the lower dose of 500 mg/m^2/week. With this regimen, the medical oncologist can expect a major response in one quarter of patients, lasting a median of 6 months (see Table 42.4).[26,30] Additionally, 40% of patients will have stable disease. The median overall survival prior to the introduction of irinotecan as a second-line agent has been a little more than one year.

In advanced disease, the Mayo Clinic regimen and Roswell Park regimen show essentially the same response rate and overall survival (see Table 42.2).[27,28] The Roswell Park regimen induces more grade 3/4 diarrhea. The Mayo Clinic regimen, on the other

Table 42.4 Roswell Park regimen (5-FU 500 mg/m^2) in phase III trials

Stage IV patients	
Major response rate[24,27]	22–28%
Minor response/stable[24,27]	43%
Duration of response[24,27]	5–6 months
Time to progression[27]	7 months
Overall survival[a,24,27]	12–13 months
Postoperative chemotherapy	
5-year disease-free survival rate: stage II[39]	75%
5-year disease-free survival rate: stage III[39]	57%
5-year overall survival rate: stage II[39]	84%
5-year overall survival rate: stage H-R II[b,38]	75%
5-year overall survival rate: stage III[38,39]	63–67%
Grade III/IV toxicity	
Overall[38,39]	35–41%
Diarrhea[33,38,39]	27–30%
Nausea/vomiting[27,39]	5%
Granulocytopenia[33,38,39]	1–4%
Stomatitis[38,39]	1–2%
Treatment-related death[33,39]	0.6–0.8%

[a] Pre-irinotecan.
[b] Includes only high-risk stage II patients.

hand, causes more mucositis and leukopenia. Infusional 5-FU schedules also demonstrate similar response rates and survival.[28,29] Toxicities, however, are generally less with this type of treatment, but must be balanced by the cost and inconvenience of protracted intravenous pump therapy. New, active drugs in colorectal cancer may render these regimens obsolete. Already, the addition of irinotecan to weekly 5-FU and low-dose leucovorin has demonstrated a superior response rate and overall survival compared with the Mayo Clinic regimen.[32] Thus, the current GI Intergroup trial, coordinated by the NCCTG (N9741), uses the weekly irinotecan/5-FU/leucovorin combination as its standard arm.

As postoperative therapy, the 28-week Mayo Clinic regimen and the 32-week Roswell Park regimen have become the standard of care for high-risk colon cancer.[35,36] Survival statistics are essentially the same for the two schedules. A 5-year survival may be expected in three-quarters of high-risk stage II patients and in two-thirds of stage III patients (see Table 42.4). Grade 3/4 toxicities differ between the two regimens, but are less frequent overall (41% versus 56%) on the Roswell Park regimen.[36] For this reason, cooperative groups and community physicians have begun to favor the Roswell Park regimen. Thus, the current GI Intergroup trial, coordinated by the CALGB (C-89803), uses the Roswell Park regimen as its standard arm. Similarly, the NSABP has employed the Roswell Park regimen as its standard for its last two trials (Protocols C-04 and C-06), as well as its current study (Protocol C-07) in which patients are randomized to the Roswell Park regimen with or without oxaliplatin.

Thus, it is fair to say that the Roswell Park regimen, now almost 20 years since its inception, remains an excellent choice for both adjuvant and metastatic colorectal cancer. It is less toxic than the Mayo Clinic regimen and more convenient than the infusional schedules commonly employed in Europe. It represents the North American reference standard for adjuvant therapy in high-risk colon cancer.

REFERENCES

1. Rutman RJ, Cantarow A, Paschkis KE, Studies in 2-acetylaminofluorene carcinogenesis. III. The utilization of uracil-2-C[14] by pre-neoplastic rat liver and rat hepatoma. *Cancer Res* 1954; **14**: 119–23.

2. Heidelberger C, Chaudhuri NK, Danneberg P et al, Fluorinated pyrimidines, a new class of tumour-inhibitory compounds. *Nature* 1957; **179**: 663–6.

3. Evans RM, Laskin JD, Hakala MT, Assessment of growth-limiting events caused by 5-fluorouracil in mouse cells and in human cells. *Cancer Res* 1980; **40**: 4113–22.

4. Santi DV, McHenry CS, Sommer H, Mechanism of interaction of thymidylate synthase with fluorodeoxyuridylate. *Biochemistry* 1974; **13**: 471–80.

5. Moertel CG, Current concepts in cancer: chemotherapy of gastrointestinal cancer. *N Engl J Med* 1978; **299**: 1049–52.

6. Ansfield F, Klotz J, Nealon T, A phase III study comparing the clinical utility of four regimens of 5-fluorouracil. *Cancer* 1977; **39**: 34–40.

7. Danenberg PV, Danenberg KD, Effect of 5,10-methylenetetrahydrofolate on the dissociation of 5-fluoro-2'-deoxyuridylate from thymidylate synthetase: evidence for an ordered mechanism. *Biochemistry* 1978; **17**: 4018–24.

8. Ullman B, Lee M, Martin DW Jr, Santi DV, Cytotoxicity of 5-fluoro-2'-deoxyuridine: requirement for reduced folate cofactors and antagonism by methotrexate. *Proc Natl Acad Sci USA* 1978; **75**: 980–3.

9. Waxman S, Bruckner H, The enhancement of 5-fluorouracil antimetabolic activity by leucovorin, menadione and alpha-tocopherol. *Eur J Cancer Clin Oncol* 1982; **18**: 685–92.

10. Evans RM, Laskin JD, Hakala MT, Effect of excess folates and deoxyinosine on the activity and site of action of 5-fluorouracil. *Cancer Res* 1981; **41**: 3288–95.

11. Houghton JA, Maroda SJ Jr, Phillips JO, Houghton PJ, Biochemical determinants of responsiveness to 5-fluorouracil and its derivatives in xenografts of human colorectal adenocarcinomas in mice. *Cancer Res* 1981; **41**: 144–9.

12. Bruckner HW, Roboz J, Spigelman M et al, An efficient leucovorin–5-flurouracil sequence: dosage escalation and pharmacologic monitoring. In: *Advances in Cancer Chemotherapy. The Current Status of 5-Fluorouracil–Leucovorin Calcium Combination* (Bruckner HW, Rustum YM, eds). New York: Park Row, 1984: 49–53.

13. Machover D, Schwarzenberg L, Goldschmidt E, Treatment of advanced colorectal and gastric adenocarcinoma with 5-FU combined with high-dose folinic acid: a pilot study. *Cancer Treat Rep* 1982; **66**: 1803–7.

14. Cunningham J, Bukowski RM, Budd GT et al, 5-Fluorouracil and folinic acid: a phase I–II trial in gastrointestinal malignancy. *Invest New Drugs* 1984; **2**: 391–5.

15. Madajewicz S, Petrelli N, Rustum YM et al, Phase I–II trial of high-dose calcium leucovorin and 5-fluorouracil in advanced colorectal cancer. *Cancer Res* 1984; **44**: 4667–9.

16. Rustum YM, Trave F, Zakrzewski SF et al, Biochemical and pharmacologic basis for potentiation of 5-fluorouracil action by leucovorin. *J Natl Cancer Monogr* 1987; **5**: 165–70.

17. Hines JD, Zakem MH, Adelstein DJ, Rustum YM, Treatment of advanced-stage colorectal adenocarcinoma with fluorouracil and high-dose leucovorin calcium: pilot study. *J Clin Oncol* 1988; **6**: 142–6.

18. Petrelli N, Herrera L, Rustum Y et al, A prospective randomized trial of 5-fluorouracil versus 5-fluorouracil and high-dose leucovorin versus 5-fluorouracil and methotrexate in previously untreated patients with advanced colorectal carcinoma. *J Clin Oncol* 1987; **5**: 1559–65.

19. Bruckner HW, Petrelli NJ, Stablein D et al, Comparison of unique leucovorin and 5-fluorouracil 'escalating' and 'maximum' dosage strategies. *J Natl Cancer Monogr* 1987; **5**: 179–84.

20. Gastrointestinal Tumor Study Group, The modulation of fluorouracil with leucovorin in metastatic colorectal carcinoma: a prospective randomized phase III trial. *J Clin Oncol* 1989; **7**: 1419–26.

21. Nobile MT, Rosso R, Sertoli MR et al, Randomized comparison of weekly bolus 5-fluorouracil with or without leucovorin in metastatic colorectal carcinoma. *Eur J Cancer* 1992; **28A**: 1823–7.

22. Martoni A, Cricca A, Guaraldi M, Weekly regimen of 5-FU vs. 5-FU + intermediate dose folinic acid in the treatment of

advanced colorectal cancer. *Anticancer Res* 1992; **12:** 607–12.

23. Piedbois P, Buyse M, Rustum Y, Modulation of fluorouracil by leucovorin in patients with advanced colorectal cancer: evidence in terms of response rate. *J Clin Oncol* 1992; **10:** 896–903.

24. O'Connell MJ, A phase III trial of 5-fluorouracil and leucovorin in the treatment of advanced colorectal cancer. *Cancer* 1989; **63:** 1026–30.

25. Poon MA, O'Connell MJ, Moertel CG, Biochemical modulation of fluorouracil: evidence of significant improvement of survival and quality of life in patients with advanced colorectal carcinoma. *J Clin Oncol* 1989; **7:** 1407–18.

26. Jaeger E, Heike M, Bernhard H et al, Weekly high-dose leucovorin versus low-dose leucovorin combined with fluorouracil in advanced colorectal cancer: results of a randomized multicenter trial. *J Clin Oncol* 1996; **14:** 2274–9.

27. Buroker TR, O'Connell MJ, Wieand HS, Randomized comparison of two schedules of fluorouracil and leucovorin in the treatment of advanced colorectal cancer. *J Clin Oncol* 1994; **12:** 14–20.

28. Leichman CG, Fleming TR, Muggia FM et al, Phase II study of fluorouracil and its modulation in advanced colorectal cancer: a Southwest Oncology Group study. *J Clin Oncol* 1995; **13:** 1303–11.

29. O'Dwyer PJ, Ryan LM, Valone FH, Phase III trial of biochemical modulation of 5-fluorouracil by IV or oral leucovorin or by interferon in advanced colorectal cancer: an ECOG/CALGB phase III trial. *Proc Am Soc Clin Oncol* 1996; **15:** A469.

30. Jones, Jr. DV, Winn RJ, Brown BW, Randomized phase III study of 5-fluorouracil plus high dose folinic acid versus 5-fluorouracil plus folinic acid plus methyl-lomustine for patients with advanced colorectal cancer. *Cancer* 1995; **76:** 1709–14.

31. Saltz LB, Kanowitz J, Kemeny NE, Phase I clinical and pharmacokinetic study of irinotecan, fluorouracil, and leucovorin in patients with advanced solid tumors. *J Clin Oncol* 1996; **14:** 2959–67.

32. Saltz LB, Cox JV, Blanke C et al, Irinotecan plus fluorouracil and leucovorin for metastatic colorectal cancer. *N Engl J Med* 2000; **343:** 905–14.

33. Wolmark N, Rockette H, Fisher B et al, The benefit of leucovorin-modulated fluorouracil as postoperative therapy for primary colon cancer: results from National Surgical Adjuvant Breast and Bowel Protocol C-03. *J Clin Oncol* 1993; **11:** 1879–87.

34. Wolmark N, Rockette H, Mamounas E, Clinical trial to assess the relative efficacy of fluorouracil and leucovorin, fluorouracil and levamisole, and fluorouracil, leucovorin, and levamisole in patients with Dukes' B and C carcinoma of the colon: results from the National Surgical Adjuvant Breast and Bowel Project C-04. *J Clin Oncol* 1999; **17:** 3553–9.

35. Haller DG, Catalano PJ, Macdonald JS et al, Fluorouracil, leucovorin and levamisole adjuvant therapy for colon cancer: five-year final report of INT-0089. *Proc Am Soc Clin Oncol* 1998; **17:** A982.

36. Haller DG, Gastrointestinal Cancer Oral Session at the 34th Annual Meeting of the American Society of Clinical Oncology, Tuesday, May 19, 1998.

43

Infusional 5-FU: The 24-hour weekly approach

Claus-Henning Köhne

INTRODUCTION

Despite its limited activity as a single agent, especially when given as an intravenous bolus, 5-fluorouracil (5-FU) remains the chemotherapeutic agent of choice for advanced colorectal cancer. To enhance the efficacy of 5-FU, the optimal dose, schedule, method of administration, and biochemical modulation of 5-FU all continue to be investigated in clinical trials. 5-FU has a short plasma half-life of approximately 8–14 minutes.[1] The drug is cytotoxic mainly to cells in the S phase. Therefore, with bolus administration of 5-FU, only a small proportion of cells are susceptible, as compared with administration by continuous infusion of 5-FU. Plasma levels above a threshold of 1 μM are considered necessary for the cytotoxic effect, and are thus maintained for only a few hours. 5-FU clearance is faster for schedules with continuous infusion as compared with bolus administration.[2,3] The longer the infusion period of 5-FU, the lower is the tolerable dose of 5-FU. When 300 mg/m^2 5-FU are administered over several weeks, plasma steady-state concentrations of less than 1 μM are measured.[4] If infused over 4–5 days at a dose of 1 g/m^2, plasma steady-state concentrations are in the range of 1–3 μM.[5] With the use of weekly 24-hour continuous infusion with a dose of 2000–2600 mg/m^2, the plasma steady-state concentration is 6–8 μM.[5]

Preclinical data suggest that bolus 5-FU results mainly in disturbance of RNA function, while continuous-infusion 5-FU is DNA-directed via thymidylate synthase (TS) inhibition.[6] Sobrero and co-workers[2] observed that cell lines resistant to pulse 5-FU still retain sensitivity to prolonged exposure to the fluoropyrimidine, while cells resistant to continuous-infusion 5-FU are only partially sensitive to pulse 5-FU. Bolus and continuous-infusion 5-FU

have therefore been considered as two different drugs,[8] and the mode of administration of 5-FU may be critical for its antineoplastic activity. A Scandinavian group noted that 5-FU is less toxic but also less active when the same dose is given within 3 minutes or over a 20-minute period.[9] According to our own experience, twice the dose of 5-FU can be administered if given over a period of 2 hours as compared with bolus administration.[10] A dose–response relationship has been debated, with different slopes for the dose–response curves for bolus and continuous-infusion administration[11] (Figure 43.1). Infusion schedules differ in their intended 5-FU dose intensity, which is very high relative to conventional bolus regimens, especially in the first 4 weeks of administration (Table 43.1).

At least four infusional or high-dose 5-FU schedules are popular. Lokich and co-workers[12] used 5-FU in a dose of 300 mg/m^2 over a period of 28 days. Spanish investigators[13] developed a schedule of a weekly 48-hour continuous infusion of 5-FU in a dose of 3500 mg/m^2. A regimen of 5-FU bolus followed by a 24-hour continuous infusion in combination with folinic acid (FA, leucovorin) given on 2 consecutive days and repeated every 2 weeks is popular in France,[14] while a weekly 24-hour continuous infusion of 5-FU in a dose of 2600 mg/m^2 combined with folinic acid 500 mg/m^2 is widely used in Germany.[15] This schedule, originally designed by Ardalan and co-workers,[16] has been modified, and is now widely known in Europe as the AIO schedule.

Continuous-infusion 5-FU was pioneered by Seifert et al,[17] and, as reported by Lokich et al,[12] was superior to bolus 5-FU. The experience of six randomized trials investigating infusion 5-FU relative to bolus administration has been summarized in a meta-analysis using source data on 1219 patients.[18] The response rate was nearly doubled with

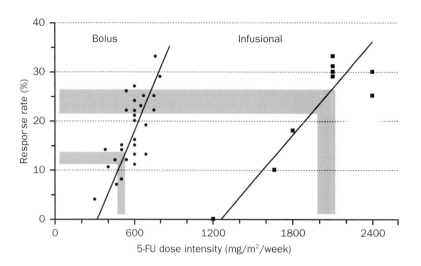

Figure 43.1 5-FU dose intensity and response. (Modified from Wils.[11])

Table 43.1 Different infusional 5-FU schedules and 5-FU dose intensity					
				Intended 5-FU dose intensity (mg/m²/week)	
Schedule				**4 weeks**	**8 weeks**
Spanish, TTD	5-FU weekly	3.5 mg/m²	48 h	3500	1800–3500
French, LV5FU2	FA	200 mg/m²	2 h	1000	1000
	5-FU	400 mg/m²	Bolus		
	5-FU	600 mg/m²	22 h		
	d1, 2	qw2			
German, AIO	FA	500 mg/m²	2 h	2600	1950
	5-FU	2.6 g/m²	24 h		
	weekly ×6, 2w rest				
US, Lokich	FU	300 mg/m²/d	CI	2100	1800
	d1–28				

FA, folinic acid (leucovorin); CI, continuous infusion.

infusional 5-FU (22% versus 14%; $p = 0.0002$), and also the median survival was prolonged (12.1 months versus 11.3 months; $p = 0.04$). The better antineoplastic activity was associated with lower gastrointestinal but higher haematological toxicity, while the hand–foot syndrome appears to be dose-limiting for infusional 5-FU.[19]

PHASE I/II STUDIES OF WEEKLY HIGH-DOSE INFUSIONAL 5-FU

Weekly high-dose 5-FU in a dose of 2.6 g/m[2] given over 24 hours was pioneered by Ardalan and co-workers. A total of 47 patients entered a randomized phase I study in which patients received 5-FU as a weekly 24-hour infusion with or without N-(phosphonoacetyl)-L-aspartic acid (PALA). For patients receiving 250 mg/m[2] PALA 24 hours prior to 5-FU, the 5-FU dose was escalated from 1000 mg/m[2] to 3400 mg/m[2], and for those without PALA, it was escalated from 1300 mg/m[2] to 3400 mg/m[2]. The maximum delivered 5-FU dose was 3400 mg/m[2] for both cohorts, when ataxia and myelosuppression appeared as limiting toxicity. The weekly administration of 2600 mg/m[2] 5-FU was recommended for further studies.[20] Haas and colleagues[21] confirmed the feasibility of this weekly high-dose infusional schedule, and failed in their attempt to further increase 5-FU to 2800, 3000, or 3250 mg/m[2] when given without the addition of PALA or any other modulator. As most patients required 5-FU dose reductions or treatment interruptions due to diarrhoea, 5-FU dose escalation beyond 2600 mg/m[2] was not feasible. This schedule was further combined with both PALA and folinic acid to take advantage of a potential double modulation.[16] The initial dose of 5-FU was incremented up to 2600 mg/m[2], when diarrhoea, mucositis, nausea, and vomiting prevented further escalation. Only 7 of the 14 patients treated with 2600 mg/m[2] were able to tolerate this treatment without interruption. The actual delivered 5-FU dose was 2100 mg/m[2] per week.[22] Interestingly, the maximum tolerable dose of 5-FU when given as a weekly 24-hour infusion did not differ if given alone or in combination with a biochemical modulator.

5-FU in combination with folinic acid alone was further investigated by Ardalan et al[22] in a phase II trial including 10 pretreated and 12 untreated patients. Grade 3 stomatitis and diarrhoea occurred in 3 patients. The overall objective response rate was 45%, and among previously untreated patients it was 58%. At the time it was published, this regimen appeared to be one of the most active and deserved

further evaluation in randomized trials. Also, Löffler and co-workers[23] reported on a high activity of a weekly 24-hour infusion of 5-FU 2000 mg/m[2] in combination with 500 mg/m[2] folinic acid as a 1-hour infusion and interferon (IFN)-α2b 3 MU subcutaneously, three times a week. Among 28 untreated patients, 75% responded to this regimen.

RANDOMIZED TRIALS OF WEEKLY HIGH-DOSE INFUSIONAL 5-FU AS A 24-HOUR INFUSION

Following the promising results of this regimen, investigators from the Eastern Cooperative Oncology Group (ECOG) and the Cancer and Leukemia Group B (CALGB)[24] studied 5-FU 2600 mg/m[2] given as a weekly 24-hour infusion (FU_{24h}), with or without PALA (250 mg/m[2]), compared with three 5-FU bolus schedules of weekly 5-FU 600 mg/m[2] with oral (125 mg/m[2]) or intravenous (600 mg/m[2]) folinic acid or 5-FU 750 mg/m[2]/day as an intravenous continuous infusion over 5 days followed by weekly bolus 5-FU 750 mg/m[2] and combined with IFN-α2a 9 MU subcutaneously 3 times a week. The results of the two 24-hour infusional schedules relative to the 5-FU/FA intravenous push regimen (the Roswell Park schedule), which was the internal reference arm, are listed in Table 43.2. The conclusion from this trial was that neither regimen was better than weekly bolus 5-FU/FA, but the weekly infusional regimens were less toxic and should be further investigated.

The Southwest Oncology Group (SWOG) conducted a seven-arm randomized trial with the following treatment arms:[25]

1. FU_{24h} (2600 mg/m[2]);
2. FU_{24h} plus PALA (250 mg/m[2]);
3. 5-FU continuous infusion (300 mg/m[2]);
4. 5-FU continuous infusion (200 mg/m[2]) plus intravenous low-dose folinic acid (20 mg/m[2] on days 1, 8, 15 and 22);
5. 5-FU bolus (500 mg/m[2] on days 1–5 every 5 weeks);
6. 5-FU 425 mg/m[2] plus folinic acid 20 mg/m[2] both given on days 1–5, repeated every 4–5 weeks);
7. folinic acid 500 mg/m[2] plus 5-FU 600 mg/m[2] weekly times six.

The internal reference treatment was 5-FU bolus alone. The response rate and median survival did not differ in any of these seven patient cohorts. It was concluded, however, that the infusional schedules warrant further investigation because of their lower

Table 43.2 Modulation of infusional 5-FU

	No. of patients	Response rate (%) (CR/PR)	p	Median survival (months)	p	Ref
5-FU bolus 500 mg/m² d1–5, qw5, versus	89	29		14		25
5-FU continuous infusion 200 mg/m²/d + FA 20 mg/m² i.v. weekly, versus	84	26	NS	14	NS	
FU$_{24h}$ 2600 mg/m² weekly, versus	85	15		15		
FU$_{24h}$ 2600 mg/m² weekly + PALA 250 mg/m² weekly	86	25	NS	11	NS	
(A) 5-FU 600 mg/m² i.v. push, FA 600 mg/m² 2 h infusion, weekly ×6, 2w rest, versus	224	16		12.9		24
(B) FU$_{24h}$ 2600 mg/m² weekly, versus	221	13		14.8		
(C) FU$_{24h}$ 2600 mg/m² weekly + PALA 250 mg/m² weekly	223	10	NS	12.9	NS	
FU$_{24h}$ 2600 mg/m² + FA 500 mg/m² 2 h, weekly ×6, versus	91	44		16.2		15
FU$_{24h}$ 2600 mg/m² + IFN-α 3 MU s.c. 3 ×/w, weekly ×6, versus	90	18	<0.05	12.7	<0.04	
FU$_{24h}$ 2600 mg/m² + FA + IFN-α, weekly ×6	49	27		19.6		
5-FU 425 mg/m² FA 20 mg/m²; d1–5, qw4–5	67	18		370 days		34
FU$_{24h}$ 2600 mg/m² + FA 500 mg/m² 2 h, weekly ×4, qw6	64	23[a]	NS	463 days	0.047	
5-FU 425 mg/m²; d1–5, qw4–5, versus FA 20 mg/m²	167 (104)[a]	11.5		12		35
FU$_{24h}$ 2600 mg/m² weekly ×6, qw8	166 (97)[a]	9.3		12.5		
FU$_{24h}$ 2600 mg/m² + FA 500 mg/m² 2 h, weekly ×6, qw8	164 (78)[a]	20.5	NS	13.2	NS	

[a]Patients evaluable for response, analysis preliminary.
FA, folinic acid (leucovorin); PALA, N-phosphonacetyl-L-aspartic acid; IFN-α, interferon-α; NS, not significant.

toxicity and slightly longer median survival. Nevertheless, PALA or low-dose weekly intravenous folinic acid are ineffective means to modulate infusional or high dose 5-FU.

The Arbeitsgemeinschaft für Internistische Onkologie (AIO) randomized 236 patients[15] to receive weekly high-dose infusional 5-FU (2600 mg/m^2: 5-FU$_{24h}$) in combination with a 2-hour infusion of folinic acid 500 mg/m^2 given prior to 5-FU (FU$_{24h}$/FA), or 5-FU$_{24h}$ combined with IFN-α 3 MU subcutaneously three times weekly (FU$_{24h}$/IFN) or both modulators in combination (FU$_{24h}$/FA/IFN). The three-drug regimen was associated with an excess of toxicity, and this arm was therefore closed early after the first planned interim analysis indicated equivalence in response rate relative to the use of FU$_{24h}$ plus folinic acid alone. The results of this trial were especially promising: the response rate of 44% observed in patients receiving FU$_{24h}$/FA was significantly superior to the administration of FU$_{24h}$/IFN (24%; $p < 0.05$). Those patients who achieved an objective response under the FU$_{24h}$/FA regimen maintained this response for a median of 11 months before tumour progression was observed. The time to tumour progression was also significantly longer for the folinic acid-modulated schedules: 6.8 or 6.3 months versus 3.8 months ($p < 0.004$). The median survival was longest for the folinic acid-containing schedules: 16.6 or 19.6 months versus 12.7 months for FU$_{24h}$/IFN. This difference was statistically significant ($p < 0.002$) (Figure 43.2). Of note, only very few patients received second-line treatment with irinotecan or oxaliplatin, which were not available at the time of the study.

The level of toxicity observed for FU$_{24h}$/FA was acceptable, and compared favourably with previous reports of two conventional 5-FU bolus regimens. When the survival data of the FU$_{24h}$/FA schedules were compared with previous experience of the group[10,26,27] with various modulated 5-FU/FA bolus schedules, the use of FU$_{24h}$/FA appeared to be particularly promising (Figure 43.3).

While the AIO trial was ongoing, several publications reported disappointing results regarding the ability of IFN-α to modulate 5-FU relative to 5-FU alone or 5-FU/FA.[28–31] With the exception of a single study that demonstrated increased response and time to progression but not survival,[32] IFN-α did not increase the response rate, time to progression, or survival in six other studies when combined with 5-FU and compared with different schedules of 5-FU with or without folinic acid. These reports contradict the preclinical findings of increased 5-FU cytotoxicity that provided a rationale for the clinical use of IFN-α. On the other hand, no preclinical investigations or clinical trials indicated the opposite, namely that IFN-α decreases the antineoplastic activity of 5-FU. Since FU$_{24h}$/FA was superior to FU$_{24h}$/IFN in our trial, one was tempted to speculate that FU$_{24h}$/FA would also be superior to 5-FU alone or to bolus 5-FU regimens. In a multivariate analysis, the treatment with FU$_{24h}$/FA remained as an independent prognostic parameter compared with other prognostic factors.[33] These data formed the hypothesis for randomized trials comparing 5-FU as a weekly 24-hour infusion versus the North Central Cancer Treatment Group (NCCTG)–Mayo Clinic regimen.

Weh and colleagues[34] reported on a small

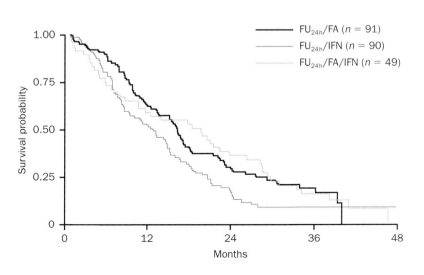

FU$_{24h}$/FA ($n = 91$)
FU$_{24h}$/IFN ($n = 90$)
FU$_{24h}$/FA/IFN ($n = 49$)

Figure 43.2 Survival in AIO Trial 2/93.[15]

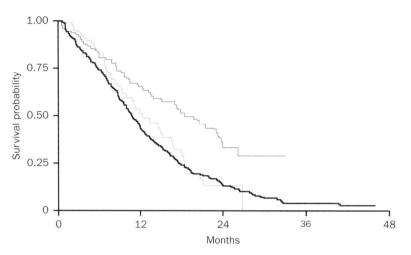

------------ Weekly high-dose 5-FU 24 h infusion + folinic acid (± IFN-α) (n = 121)[19]

------------ Weekly high-dose 5-FU 24 h infusion + IFN-α (n = 77)[19]

———— Bolus 5-FU + folinic acid (± dipyridamole, ± IFN-α) (n = 248)[20,21]

randomized phase III study comparing FU_{24h}/FA with the NCCTG–Mayo Clinic regimen. One course consisted of four weekly infusions (instead of the six infusions used in the AIO schedule) and was repeated after a therapy-free interval of two weeks. Seventy-six patients received the monthly regimen and 73 patients received FU_{24h}/FA. While the rate of objective responses did not differ significantly for the infusional or the bolus schedule (23.4% versus 17.9%, respectively), the rate of progressive disease was significantly higher for patients receiving the Mayo Clinic regimen (47.7% versus 18.8%; $p < 0.01$). Also, a significantly longer median survival for patients in the infusional arm of 463 days versus 370 days ($p = 0.047$) was observed (Table 43.2).

Recently, the EORTC Gastrointestinal Tract Cooperative Cancer Group (GITCCG) reported on preliminary results[35] of the randomized trial 40952 including 497 patients with metastatic colorectal cancer, from 59 centres. In this trial, 166 patients received weekly 2600 mg/m² 5-FU as a 24-hour infusion (FU_{24h}) alone and 164 patients folinic acid 500 mg/m² as a 2-hour infusion in addition to FU_{24h} (FU_{24h}/FA). All infusional regimens were repeated weekly times six followed by a rest period in week 7, and the regimen was reinitiated in week 8. The reference arm was the standard Mayo Clinic regimen, with 5-FU 425 mg/m² given as an intravenous push following low-dose folinic acid 20 mg/m² for 5 days and repeated on weeks 4 and 5 thereafter. This trial aimed to demonstrate superior survival for either of the high-dose infusional 5-FU schedules relative to

the Mayo Clinic regimen alone. The hypothesis was to increase the median survival from 12 to 18 months. Also, the contribution of folinic acid added to infusional 5-FU (FU_{24h}) could be investigated. All patients were untreated. However, adjuvant treatment was allowed if completed 6 months prior to study inclusion. Measurable disease was present in 56% of patients. Patients were encouraged to receive the treatment until progression or unacceptable toxicity. An average of 10% of patients had received prior adjuvant treatment, while the remainder were chemotherapy-naive. The response rate was preliminary at this time, with only 54–74% of patients having data available for response. Nevertheless, 11.5% and 9.3% of patients responded to the Mayo Clinic regimen or to FU_{24h}, respectively. Of patients receiving FU_{24h}/FA 20.5% achieved an objective response. This difference was not statistically significant (Table 43.2). The preliminary median progression-free survival was 4.1 months and 4.4 months for the Mayo Clinic regimen and FU_{24h}, respectively, and was statistically inferior to the 6.4 months of FU_{24h}/FA ($p = 0.02$) (Figure 43.4). The preliminary median survival was 12 months for patients receiving bolus 5-FU/FA, 12.5 months for patients on FU_{24h} alone, and 13.2 months for patients with FU_{24h}/FA treatment ($p = 0.2$). Thus, the study failed to show improved survival for either of the infusional 5-FU regimens. Available data on toxicity demonstrate 20% grade 3 or 4 diarrhoea in patients on the FU_{24h}/FA arm, versus 6% or 7% in patients treated with FU_{24h} alone or the Mayo Clinic regimen, respec-

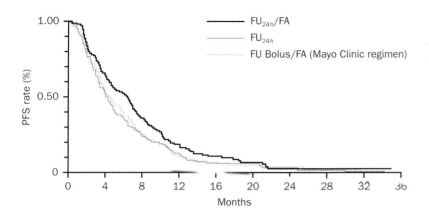

tively. Grade 3 or 4 stomatitis occurred in 3%, 7%, and 10% of patients on the FU_{24h}, FU_{24h}/FA, and Mayo Clinic regimens, respectively. Haematological toxicity was lowest in the FU_{24h}/FA arm (2.1% grade 3 or 4) and highest in the NCCTG–Mayo Clinic regimen (9%). While awaiting the final analysis, these data suggest that:

- weekly 24-hour infusional 5-FU plus folinic acid dose not increase survival compared with the standard bolus 5-FU/FA regimen;
- it increases the response rate from 9–12% to 21%, a difference that is not statistically significant at present;
- it prolongs progression-free survival by 50% compared with the standard bolus 5-FU/FA or FU_{24h} infusion without folinic acid;
- high-dose infusional 5-FU can be effectively modulated by folinic acid, resulting in a higher response rate and significantly longer progression-free survival compared with infusional FU_{24h} alone.

It is for these reasons that high-dose infusional FU_{24h}/FA is now the internal reference treatment for further EORTC trials, especially when progression-free survival is the major study endpoint.

PHASE I DATA WITH THE AIO SCHEDULE IN COMBINATION WITH IRINOTECAN

In a phase I trial, 26 patients with measurable metastatic colorectal cancer previously untreated were entered to receive FU_{24h}/FA in combination with irinotecan (CPT-11).[36] Fixed doses of irinotecan (80 mg/m²) and folinic acid (500 mg/m²) in combination with escalated doses of FU_{24h} ranging from 1800 to 2600 mg/m² were administered on a weekly times

four (dose level 1–4) or weekly times six (dose level 5–6) schedule. The dose of irinotecan was increased to 100 mg/m² on dose level 7. No dose-limiting toxicity was observed during the first cycles at dose levels 1–6. With the escalation of the irinotecan dose to 100 mg/m² at dose level 7, grade 3 or 4 diarrhoea occurred in 4 of 6 patients during the first cycle and the dose-limiting toxicity was achieved. The recommended doses for further studies were irinotecan 80 mg/m², folinic acid 500 mg/m² and FU_{24h} 2600 mg/m² given on a weekly times six schedule followed by a one-week rest period. Objective tumour responses were observed on every dose level and were achieved in 16 of 25 evaluable patients (64%; 95% confidence interval, CI, 45–83%). This experience was confirmed in 24 additional patients, who received the recommended dose, and 18 of these patients responded (response rate 75%; 95% CI 53–90%; unpublished data). The median survival has not been reached at 19 months. This regimen (with 5-FU 2300 mg/m²) has been studied together with the French LV5FU2 treatment plus irinotecan in a randomized trial,[37] and continues to be evaluated within the ongoing EORTC trial 40986 comparing FU_{24h}/FA with FU_{24h}/FA plus irinotecan.

24-HOUR INFUSIONAL 5-FU IN PATIENTS WITH LIVER METASTASES ONLY

Intra-arterial, regional treatment of patients with metastases confined to the liver appeared to be a promising means to improve response rate and probably survival.[38] Indeed, with intra-arterial administration, response rates of approximately 50% have been achieved, and the median survival has been in excess of 16 months. However, only in studies in which the intra-arterial administration of 5-FU was compared with best supportive care or suboptimal systemic chemotherapy was the median survival significantly prolonged.[39,40]

Patient selection is a potential reason for the good results of intra-arterial treatment. To support this hypothesis, we identified 169 patients with a Karnofsky performance index of 80 or better and metastatic disease affecting the liver only, determined by standard staging procedures including computer tomography evaluations.[41] All patients were chemotherapy-naive and were required to meet similar protocol entry criteria. Seventy-five patients were treated with modulated 5-FU bolus regimens within a randomized trial (51 patients)[26] and two phase II studies (24 patients).[10] Thirty-four individuals received weekly high-dose FU_{24h}/IFN and 60 patients were treated with FU_{24h}/FA with (21 patients) or without (39 patients) the addition of IFN-α. The latter 94 patients were treated with a randomized protocol of AIO.[15] The response rate (20–24%) and time to treatment failure (3.5–5.6 months) of the modulated bolus schedules or the FU_{24h}/IFN combination were inferior compared with published data with hepatic arterial infusion (HAI). However, patients receiving a combination including FU_{24h}/FA had a response rate of 48%, with 13% complete clinical responses, a median time to treatment failure of 9.3 months, and a 21-month median survival. Patients considered for HAI treatment are probably more rigorously examined to exclude extrahepatic tumour spread. Our patient group might therefore represent a more unfavourable population with a higher possibility of extrahepatic disease.

Nevertheless, the median survival time of 14.3 months observed in patients receiving modulated bolus schedules is very close to the median survival for HAI patients reported by the French and British trials.[39,40] Patients treated with a combination including FU_{24h}/FA had a median survival (21 months) exceeding that reported in studies with HAI (Figure 43.5). At least, these data support the favourable outcome of patients given effective systemic therapy such as high-dose 5-FU (Figure 43.4). The more that systemic chemotherapy is improved, the less may be the necessity for locoregional techniques to provide effective palliation in patients with metastases confined to the liver.

Patients with liver metastases should be considered for surgical resection.[42] In the case of a R0 resection with a margin of at least 1 cm, approximately one-third of patients will survive at least 5 years. If adverse factors such as age over 60 years, extension into the serosa or lymphatic spread of the primary cancer, time interval from primary tumour to metastasis of less than 2 years, size of largest metastasis greater than 5 cm, more than three hepatic metastases, surgical clearance of less than 1 cm, and elevated carcinoembryonic antigen (CEA) levels are present, then the prognosis is worse. If a patient has five or more of these adverse risk factors, the 2-year survival rate drops to 34%.[43]

We identified 50 inoperable patients with colorectal cancer hepatic metastases and at least five risk factors according to Nordlinger et al.[43] This group received high-dose infusional 5-FU modulated by IFN-α (FU_{24h}/IFN) or folinic acid (FU_{24h}/FA).[15] This

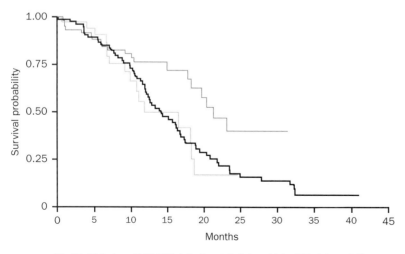

Figure 43.5 Survival of selected patients with Karnofsky performance index of 80 or better and metastases limited to the liver receiving different regimens of systemic intravenous 5-FU.[41]

——— Weekly high-dose 5-FU 24 h infusion + folinic acid (± IFN-α) (n = 60)

.... Weekly high-dose 5-FU 24 h infusion + IFN-α (n = 34)

——— Bolus 5-FU + folinic acid (± dipyridamole, ± IFN-α) (n = 75)

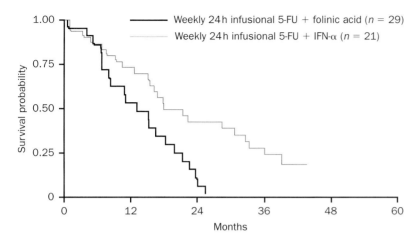

Figure 43.6 Survival of patients receiving high-dose infusional 5-FU with colorectal cancer metastases confined to the liver[44] and five or more risk factors according to Nordlinger et al.[43]

cohort had a 2-year survival rate of 40%, which compares favourably with the resected patients in Nordlinger's database (Figure 43.6). Obviously, such data have to be interpreted with caution. Nevertheless, they indicate the improvements achieved by infusional 5-FU plus folinic acid modulation, and also support the idea that patient selection contributes to the results obtained with locoregional treatment.

CONCLUSIONS

High-dose 5-FU given as a weekly 24-hour infusion appears to be one of the most effective ways to administer this agent. Biochemical modulation with $500 \, mg/m^2$ folinic acid is effective in this schedule: the response rate is doubled and the progression-free survival is significantly prolonged compared with weekly 24-hour infusion of high-dose 5-FU alone. However, the median survival of patients with metastatic colorectal cancer is not altered compared with conventional FU_{24h}/FA bolus regimens. The results with infusional FU_{24h}/FA observed in the subgroup of patients with liver metastasis only are speculative, but may indicate that good-risk patients benefit from FU_{24h}/FA. This regimen serves as an excellent basis for further developments involving the addition of one of the newer agents such as irinotecan or oxaliplatin.

ACKNOWLEDGEMENT

The author's work was supported by Deutsche Krebshilfe Grant 70-2292.

REFERENCES

1. Grem JL, McAtee N, Murphy RF et al, A pilot study of interferon alfa-2a in combination with fluorouracil plus high-dose leucovorin in metastatic gastrointestinal carcinoma. *J Clin Oncol* 1991; **9:** 1811–20.
2. Harris BE, Song R, Soong SJ, Diasio RB, Relationship between dihydropyrimidine dehydrogenase activity and plasma 5-fluorouracil levels with evidence for circadian variation of enzyme activity and plasma drug levels in cancer patients receiving 5-fluorouracil by protracted continuous infusion. *Cancer Res* 1990; **50:** 197–201.
3. Fraile RJ, Baker LH, Buroker TR et al, Pharmacokinetics of 5-fluorouracil administered orally, by rapid intravenous and by slow infusion. *Cancer Res* 1980; **40:** 2223–8.
4. Spicer DV, Ardalan B, Daniels JR et al, Reevaluation of the maximum tolerated dose of continuous venous infusion of 5-fluorouracil with pharmacokinetics. *Cancer Res* 1988; **48:** 459–61.
5. Grem JL, McAtee N, Steinberg M et al, A phase I trial of continuous infusion 5-fluorouracil plus calcium leucovorin in combination with N-(phosphonacetyl)-L-asparate in metastatic gastrointestinal adenocarcinoma. *Cancer Res* 1993; **53:** 4828–36.
6. Yonekura K, Basaki Y, Chikahisa L et al, UFT and its metabolites inhibit the angiogenesis induced by murine renal cell carcinoma, as determined by a dorsal air sac assay in mice. *Clin Cancer Res* 1999; **5:** 2185–91.
7. Sobrero AF, Aschele C, Guglielmi AP et al, Synergism and lack of cross-resistance between short-term and continuous exposure to fluorouracil in human colon adenocarcinoma cells. *J Natl Cancer Inst* 1993; **85:** 1937–44.
8. Sobrero AF, Aschele C, Bertino JR, Fluorouracil in colorectal cancer – a tale of two drugs: implications for biochemical modulation. *J Clin Oncol* 1997; **15:** 368–81.
9. Glimelius B, Jakobsen A, Graf W et al, Bolus injection (2–4 min) versus short-term (10–20 min) infusion of 5-fluorouracil in patients with advanced colorectal cancer: a prospective randomised trial. Nordic Gastrointestinal Tumour Adjuvant Therapy Group. *Eur J Cancer* 1998; **34:** 674–8.
10. Köhne CH, Wilke H, Hiddemann W et al, Phase II evaluation of 5-fluorouracil plus folinic acid and alpha 2b-interferon in metastatic colorectal cancer. *Oncology* 1997; **54:** 96–101.
11. Wils JA, High-dose fluoroouracil: a new perspective in the treatment of colorectal cancer? *Semin Oncol* 1992; **19:** 126–30.
12. Lokich JJ, Ahlgren JD, Gullo JJ et al, A prospective randomized

comparison of continuous infusion fluorouracil with a conventional bolus schedule in metastatic colorectal carcinoma: a Mid-Atlantic Oncology Program study. *J Clin Oncol* 1989; **7**: 425–32.

13. Aranda E, Cervantes A, Dorta J et al, A phase II trial of weekly high dose continuous infusion 5-fluorouracil plus oral leucovorin in patients with advanced colorectal cancer. The Spanish Cooperative Group for Gastrointestinal Tumor Therapy (TTD). *Cancer* 1995; **76**: 559–63.

14. de Gramont, Bosset JF, Milan C et al, A randomized trial comparing monthly low-dose leucovorin/fluorouracil bolus with bimonthly high-dose leucovorin/fluorouracil bolus plus continuous infusion for advanced colorectal cancer: a French intergroup study. *J Clin Oncol* 1997; **15**: 808–15.

15. Köhne CH, Schöffski P, Wilke H et al, Effective biomodulation by leucovorin of high dose infusional fluorouracil given as a weekly 24-hour infusion: results of a randomized trial in patients with advanced colorectal cancer. *J Clin Oncol* 1998; **16**: 418–26.

16. Ardalan B, Sridhar KS, Benedetto P et al, A phase I, II study of high-dose 5-fluorouracil and high-dose leucovorin with low-dose phosphonacetyl-L-aspartic acid in patients with advanced malignancies. *Cancer* 1991; **68**: 1242–6.

17. Seifert P, Baker LH, Reed ML, Vaitkevicius VK, Comparison of continuous infused 5-fluorouracil with bolus injection in treatment of patients with colorectal adenocarcinoma. *Cancer* 1975; **36**: 123–8.

18. Meta-analysis Group in Cancer, Efficacy of intravenous continuous infusion of fluorouracil compared with bolus administration in advanced colorectal cancer. *J Clin Oncol* 1998; **16**: 301–8.

19. Meta-analysis Group in Cancer, Toxicity of fluorouracil in patients with advanced colorectal cancer: effect of administration schedule and prognostic factors. *J Clin Oncol* 1998; **16**: 3537–41.

20. Ardalan B, Singh G, Silberman H, A randomized phase I and II study of short-term infusion of high-dose fluorouracil with or without N-(phosphonacetyl)-L-aspartic acid in patients with advanced pancreatic and colorectal cancers. *J Clin Oncol* 1988; **6**: 1053–8.

21. Haas NB, Hines JB, Hudes GR et al, Phase I trial of 5-fluorouracil by 24-hour infusion weekly. *Invest New Drugs* 1993; **11**: 181–5.

22. Ardalan B, Chua L, Tian EM et al, A phase II study of weekly 24-hour infusion with high-dose fluorouracil with leucovorin in colorectal carcinoma. *J Clin Oncol* 1991; **9**: 625–30.

23. Löffler TM, Weber FW, Hausamen TU, Double modulation of 5-fluorouracil (FU) with leucovorin (LV) and interferon-alpha-2b in metastatic colorectal cancer. Results of a pilot study. *Onkologie* 1991; **14**(Suppl): 25.

24. O'Dwyer PJ, Manola J, Valone FH et al, Fluorouracil modulation in colorectal cancer: lack of improvement with N-phosphonoacetyl-L-aspartic acid or oral leucovorin or interferon, but enhanced therapeutic index with weekly 24-hour infusion schedule – an Eastern Cooperative Oncology Group/Cancer and Leukemia Group B study. *J Clin Oncol* 2001; **19**: 2413–21.

25. Leichman CG, Fleming TR, Muggia FM et al, Phase II study of fluorouracil and its modulation in advanced colorectal cancer: a Southwest Oncology Group study. *J Clin Oncol* 1995; **13**: 1303–11.

26. Köhne CH, Hiddemann W, Schuller J et al, Failure of orally administered dipyridamole to enhance the antineoplastic activity of fluorouracil in combination with leucovorin in patients with advanced colorectal cancer: a prospective randomized trial. *J Clin Oncol* 1995; **13**: 1201–8.

27. Köhne CH, Daniel PT, Dörken B, The value of weekly high dose infusional 5-fluorouracil in the treatment of advanced colorectal cancer. *Tumori* 1997; **83**: S56–60.

28. Greco FA, Figlin R, York M et al, Phase III randomized study to

compare interferon alfa-2a in combination with fluorouracil versus fluorouracil alone in patients with advanced colorectal cancer. *J Clin Oncol* 1996; **14**: 2674–81.

29. Hill M, Norman A, Cunningham D et al, Royal Marsden phase III trial of fluorouracil with or without interferon alfa-2b in advanced colorectal cancer. *J Clin Oncol* 1995; **13**: 1297–302.

30. Seymour MT, Slevin ML, Kerr DJ et al, Randomized trial assessing the addition of interferon alpha-2a to fluorouracil and leucovorin in advanced colorectal cancer. Colorectal Cancer Working Party of the United Kingdom Medical Research Council. *J Clin Oncol* 1996; **14**: 2280–8.

31. Kosmidis PA, Tsavaris N, Skarlos D et al, Fluorouracil and leucovorin with or without interferon alfa-2b in advanced colorectal cancer: analysis of a prospective randomized phase III trial. Hellenic Cooperative Oncology Group. *J Clin Oncol* 1996; **14**: 2682–7.

32. Dufour P, Husseini F, Dreyfus B et al, 5-Fluorouracil versus 5-fluorouracil plus alpha-interferon as treatment of metastatic colorectal carcinoma. A randomized study. *Ann Oncol* 1996; **7**: 575–9.

33. Köhne CH, Hecker H, Schöffski P et al, Weekly high dose infusional (CI) 5-FU plus folinic acid (FA) has major impact on survival in patients with advanced colorectal cancer. Results of a multivariate analysis using RECPAM. *Proc Am Soc Clin Oncol* 1996; **15**: 201.

34. Weh HJ, Zschaber R, Braumann D et al, A randomized phase III study comparing weekly folinic acid (FA) and high dose 5-fluorouracil (5-FU) with monthly 5-FU/FA (days 1–5) in untreated patients with metastatic colorectal carcinoma. *Onkologie* 1998; **21**: 403–7.

35. Schmoll HJ, Köhne CH, Lorenz M et al, Weekly 24 h infusion of high dose (HD) 5-fluorouracil (FU24h) with or without folinic acid (FA) vs. bolus FU/FA (NCCTG/Mayo) in advanced colorectal cancer (CRC): a randomized Phase III study of the EORTC GITCCG and the AIO. *Proc Am Soc Clin Oncol* 2000; **19**: 241a.

36. Vanhoefer U, Harstrick A, Köhne CH et al, Phase I study of a weekly schedule of irinotecan, high-dose leucovorin, and infusional fluorouracil as first-line chemotherapy in patients with advanced colorectal cancer. *J Clin Oncol* 1999; **17**: 907–13.

37. Douillard JY, Cunningham D, Roth AD et al, Irinotecan combined with fluorouracil compared with fluorouracil alone as first-line treatment for metastatic colorectal cancer: a multicentre randomised trial. *Lancet* 2000; **355**: 1041–7.

38. Meta-Analysis Group in Cancer, Reappraisal of hepatic arterial infusion in the treatment of nonresectable liver metastases from colorectal cancer. *J Natl Cancer Inst* 1996; **88**: 252–8.

39. Allen Mersh TG, Earlam S, Fordy C et al, Quality of life and survival with continuous hepatic-artery floxuridine infusion for colorectal liver metastases. *Lancet* 1994; **344**: 1255–60.

40. Rougier P, Laplanche A, Huguier M et al, Hepatic arterial infusion of floxuridine in patients with liver metastases from colorectal carcinoma: long-term results of a prospective randomized trial. *J Clin Oncol* 1992; **10**: 1112–18.

41. Cohen AM, Kemeny NE, Köhne CH et al, Is intra-arterial chemotherapy worthwhile in the treatment of patients with unresectable hepatic colorectal cancer metastases? *Eur J Cancer* 1996; **32A**: 2195–205.

42. Fong Y, Cohen AM, Fortner JG et al, Liver resection for colorectal metastases. *J Clin Oncol* 1997; **15**: 938–46.

43. Nordlinger B, Guiguet M, Vaillant JC et al, Surgical resection of colorectal carcinoma metastases to the liver. A prognostic scoring system to improve case selection, based on 1568 patients. Association Francaise de Chirurgie. *Cancer* 1996; **77**: 1254–62.

44. Köhne CH, Lorenz M, Herrmann R, Colorectal cancer liver metastasis: local treatment for a systemic disease? *Ann Oncol* 1998; **9**: 967–71.

44

Infusional 5-fluorouracil: The bimonthly approach

Aimery de Gramont, Christophe Louvel, Thierry André, Christophe Tournigand, Frédérique Maindrault-Goebel, Pascal Artru, Marcel Krulik, for the GERCOR (Oncology Multidisciplinary Research Group)

INTRODUCTION

5-Fluorouracil (5-FU) is considered to be the standard treatment for patients with advanced colorectal cancer. This agent has been available for more than 40 years, and, to date, no other single agent has been shown to be more effective in the first-line treatment of advanced disease. However, when 5-FU is given alone, as an intravenous bolus, it is generally associated with tumour response rates of less than 20%. During the last two decades, several studies have indicated that the cytotoxicity of 5-FU can be enhanced either with continuous infusion[1–6] or with modulation by leucovorin (LV; folinic acid).[7–11] The first LV/5-FU protocols used 5-FU as a bolus.[10,11] A meta-analysis of clinical trials comparing 5-FU by bolus or continuous-infusion administration showed that infusion improved tumour response rates from 14% to 22%, and this translated to significantly enhanced patient survival.[12] Another meta-analysis of nine clinical trials comparing 5-FU regimens with or without LV found that the addition of LV improved tumour response rates from 11% to 23%.[13] However, increases in tumour response rates were not reflected in significantly enhanced patient survival (11.5 versus 11.0 months).

EVOLUTION OF THE BIMONTHLY REGIMEN

The bimonthly regimen was designed to combine both 5-FU continuous infusion and leucovorin modulation. In addition, a synergism between the administration of 5-FU by bolus and continuous infusion has been demonstrated in vitro.[14]

A series of trials were subsequently performed to evaluate the efficacy and safety of bimonthly LV/5-FU-based regimens in the management of patients with advanced colorectal cancer. The first bimonthly regimen to be investigated involved 2-day administration of high-dose LV plus 5-FU bolus and infusion of low-dose 5-FU (LV5FU2).[15,16] The initial LV5FU2 regimen was administered to 37 chemotherapy-naive patients with advanced colorectal cancer, and consisted of a 2-hour intravenous infusion of LV (200 mg/m^2), followed by an intravenous bolus of 5-FU (300 mg/m^2), then a 22-hour infusion of 5-FU (300 mg/m^2) (Figure 44.1). This procedure was repeated on the second treatment day, with the whole 2-day cycle being repeated 2 weeks later. The dose of 5-FU was increased in subsequent treatment cycles if unacceptable toxicity had not occurred. Treatment cycles were repeated until disease progression, or for 9 months in non-responders. In responders, treatment was readministered if there was progression of the disease after cessation of therapy. This regimen produced tumour responses in 54% of patients, with a median survival of 18 months. Moderate toxicity, including nausea and diarrhoea controllable by dose reduction, was observed. Although toxicity usually limits the dose of 5-FU that can be given by intravenous bolus to 350–400 mg/m^2 over 4–5 days, the use of continuous infusion allowed the monthly dose to reach 4000 mg/m^2 in the majority of patients.

The LV5FU2 approach permitted a doubling of the total administered dose of 5-FU compared with the monthly NCCTG–Mayo Clinic regimen (4000 mg/m^2 versus 2100 mg/m^2 per month – see Chapter 41), and this has been shown to be superior,

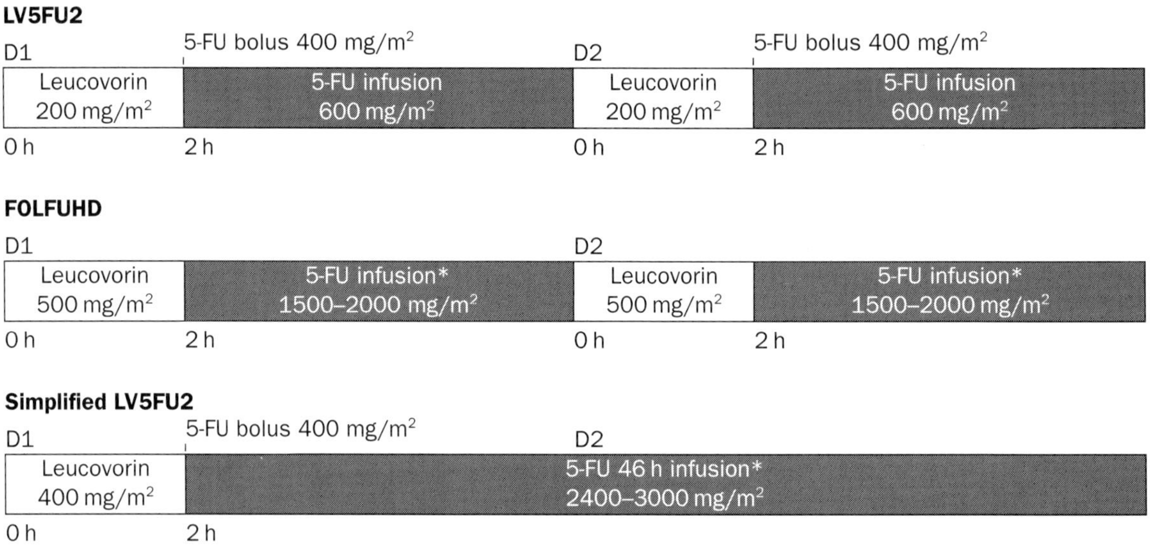

LV5FU2

FOLFUHD

Simplified LV5FU2

Figure 44.1 Outline of the three main LV/5-FU bimonthly regimens that have been investigated in patients with advanced colorectal cancer. Treatment cycles were repeated every 2 weeks. *The dose was administered at the lower level for two cycles, then at the higher level for subsequent cycles, if toxicity < WHO grade 2.

in terms of both tumour response rates and incidence of toxicity. The bimonthly LV5FU2 schedule has been extensively investigated in a French Intergroup study, and has been shown to produce a more favourable toxicity profile than the monthly 5-FU/LV regimen.[17] In a randomized trial of 433 previously untreated patients, the bimonthly LV5FU2 regimen (a 2-hour infusion of LV, 200 mg/m², followed by an intravenous bolus of 5-FU, 400 mg/m², and a 22-hour infusion of 5-FU, 600 mg/m² for 2 consecutive days) (Figure 44.1) was compared with the monthly NCCTG–Mayo Clinic regimen (an intravenous bolus of 5-FU, 425 mg/m²/day for 5 consecutive days). Significant improvements in tumour response rates were observed among patients receiving LV5FU2 (32.6%) compared with the NCCTG–Mayo Clinic regimen (14.4%). In addition, the median progression-free survival was significantly improved by the bimonthly regimen (27.6 weeks versus 22 weeks, $p = 0.0012$), although there was no significant difference in median survival between the two regimens (62.0 weeks versus 56.8 weeks, $p = 0.067$).[17] The bimonthly regimen was associated with more acceptable toxicity than the monthly regimen, with World Health Organization (WHO) grade 3–4 toxicities occurring in 11.1% of patients who received LV5FU2, compared with 23.9% for the NCCTG–Mayo Clinic regimen

($p = 0.0004$). Furthermore, the bimonthly regimen was associated with a reduced incidence of grade 3–4 granulocytopenia (1.9% versus 7.3%), diarrhoea (2.9% versus 7.3%), or mucositis (1.9% versus 12.7%).

Following on from these promising findings, a modified bimonthly regimen was investigated in 101 patients with advanced colorectal cancer (the FOLFUHD study: **fol**inic acid, 5-**FU h**igh **d**ose).[18] The regimen consisted of high-dose LV (500 mg/m²) plus a 22-hour infusion of high-dose 5-FU (1500–2000 mg/m²/day) on 2 consecutive days, repeated every 2 weeks (Figure 44.1). An overall response rate of 33.7% was reported, with 5 complete responses (5%) and 29 partial responses (28.7%). Survival outcomes were encouraging, with median progression-free and overall survival rates of 8 and 18 months respectively. The regimen was associated with low toxicity. WHO toxicity grades 3–4 were reported in 15% of patients, and included nausea (2%), diarrhoea (5.1%), mucositis (4%), neutropenia (4%), hand–foot syndrome (2%), and alopecia (4%). Furthermore, 15.2% of patients experienced no toxic effects with the bimonthly regimen, and a further 28.3% had only grade 1 toxicity. Overall, a total of 73% of the patients studied were able to receive the full planned dose of 5-FU (8 g/m²/month).

The results of FOLFUHD indicated that the bimonthly regimen could be modified by replacing the 5-FU bolus by a higher dose of 5-FU in the form of a continuous infusion without loss of efficacy or an increase in toxicity. Furthermore, the efficacy and low toxicity of FOLFUHD provided the opportunity to add other antitumour agents to the regimen with the aim of improving patient survival, as is discussed in Chapter 54.

THE SIMPLIFIED BIMONTHLY REGIMEN

The LV5FU2 regimen has recently been simplified so that, instead of requiring patients to come into hospital on 2 consecutive days every 2 weeks, the procedure requires only 2 hours at the hospital. A feasibility study has demonstrated that the new simplified regimen has antitumour efficacy combined with low toxicity.[19]

The simplified regimen, administered as outpatient therapy with disposable pumps, included a 2-hour infusion of the LV *l*-isomer 200 mg/m² on day 1, followed by a 5-FU bolus 400 mg/m² and a 46-hour infusion of 2400–3600 mg/m², every 2 weeks. 5-FU doses were increased according to toxicity. Forty-six patients aged 35–77 years, performance status 0–2, with measurable advanced colorectal cancer, were treated. The response rate was 41.3% (95% confidence interval 27.5–55.9%); stable disease was observed in 41.3% of patients and progression in 17.4%. The median progression-free survival was 8.7 months. At progression, 86% of the patients (38/44) received oxaliplatin and 66% (25/38) subsequently received irinotecan. The median overall survival was 25.8 months. Fourteen patients (30%) experienced grade 3-4 toxicity: five hand–foot syndrome (11%), five diarrhoea (11%), and four neutropenia (9%). This simplified, bimonthly regimen has a good toxicity profile, and appears to be even more active than the other LV/5-FU regimens.

CONCLUSIONS

The good therapeutic ratio of LV5FU2 explains why this regimen is now widely used in the treatment of advanced colorectal cancer. It has now been used in a number of randomized studies.[20–23] The low toxicity of the bimonthly regimens allows combination with other drugs – oxaliplatin in the FOLFOX regimens (the intermediate FOLFUHD regimen in the FOLFOX 1–3 regimens, LV5FU2 in the FOLFOX 4 regimen, and the simplified bimonthly regimen in the FOLFOX 6 and 7 regimens) or irinotecan with the simplified bimonthly regimen in the FOLFIRI regimen (see Chapter 54).

ACKNOWLEDGEMENT

The authors are grateful to Adis International for editorial development.

REFERENCES

1. Lokich JJ, Ahlgren JD, Gullo JJ et al, A prospective randomized comparison of continuous infusion fluorouracil with a conventional bolus schedule in metastatic colorectal carcinoma: a Mid-Atlantic Oncology Program study. *J Clin Oncol* 1989; **7**: 425–32.

2. Meta-analysis Group in Cancer, Efficacy of intravenous continuous infusion of fluorouracil compared with bolus administration in advanced colorectal cancer. *J Clin Oncol* 1998; **16**: 301–8.

3. Hansen RM, Quebbeman E, Anderson T, 5-Fluorouracil by protracted venous infusion. A review of current progress. *Oncology* 1989; **46**: 245–50.

4. Hansen RM, Ryan L, Anderson T et al, Phase III study of bolus versus infusion fluorouracil with or without cisplatin in advanced colorectal cancer. *J Natl Cancer Inst* 1996; **88**: 668–74.

5. Leichman CG, Fleming TR, Muggia FM et al, Phase II study of fluorouracil and its modulation in advanced colorectal cancer: a Southwest Oncology Group study. *J Clin Oncol* 1995; **13**: 1303–11.

6. Rougier PH, Paillot B, Laplanche A et al, End results of a multicenter randomized trial comparing 5-FU in continuous systemic infusion (CI) to bolus administration (B) in measurable metastatic colorectal cancer. *Proc Am Soc Clin Oncol* 1992; **11**: 163.

7. Evans RM, Laskin JD, Hakala MT, Effects of excess folates and deoxyinosine on activity and site of action of 5-fluorouracil. *Cancer Res* 1981; **41**: 3288–95.

8. Houghton JA, Maroda SJ, Philips JO et al, Biochemical determinants of responsiveness to 5-fluorouracil and its derivatives in xenografts of human colorectal adenocarcinoma in mice. *Cancer Res* 1981; **41**: 144–9.

9. Rustum YM, Trave F, Zakrzewski SF et al, Biochemical and pharmacologic basis for potentiation of 5-fluorouracil action by leucovorin. *NCI Monogr* 1987; **5**: 165–70.

10. Petrelli N, Douglass HO Jr, Herrera L et al, for the Gastrointestinal Tumor Study Group, The modulation of fluorouracil with leucovorin in metastatic colorectal carcinoma: a prospective randomized phase III trial. *J Clin Oncol* 1989; **7**: 1419–26.

11. Poon MA, O'Connell MJ, Moertel CG et al, Biochemical modulation of fluorouracil: evidence of significant improvement of survival and quality of life in patients with advanced colorectal carcinoma. *J Clin Oncol* 1989; **7**: 1407–18.

12. Meta-Analysis Group in Cancer, Efficacy of intravenous continuous infusion of fluorouracil compared with bolus administration in advanced colorectal cancer. *J Clin Oncol* 1998; **16**: 301–8.

13. Advanced Colorectal Cancer Meta-Analysis Project, Modulation of fluorouracil by leucovorin in patients with advanced colorectal cancer: evidence in terms of response rate. *J Clin Oncol* 1992; **10**: 896–903.

14. Sobrero AF, Aschele C, Guglielmi AP et al, Synergism and lack of cross-resistance between short-term and continuous exposure to fluorouracil in human colon adenocarcinoma cells. *J Natl Cancer Inst* 1993; **85**: 1937–44.

15. de Gramont A, Krulik M, Cady J et al, High-dose folinic acid and 5-fluorouracil bolus and continuous infusion in advanced colorectal cancer. *Eur J Cancer Clin Oncol* 1988; **24**: 1499–503.

16. de Gramont A, Vignoud J, Tournigand C et al, Oxaliplatin with high-dose leucovorin and 5-fluorouracil 48-hour continuous

infusion in pretreated metastatic colorectal cancer. *Eur J Cancer* 1997; **33:** 214–19.

17. de Gramont A, Bosset JF, Milan C et al, Randomized trial comparing monthly low-dose leucovorin and fluorouracil bolus with bimonthly high-dose leucovorin and fluorouracil bolus plus continuous infusion for advanced colorectal cancer: a French Intergroup Study. *J Clin Oncol* 1997; **15:** 808–15.

18. Beerblock K, Rinaldi Y, André T et al, Bimonthly high dose leucovorin and 5-fluorouracil 48-hour continuous infusion in patients with advanced colorectal carcinoma. Groupe d'Etude et de Recherche sur les Cancers de l'Ovaire et Digestifs (GERCOD). *Cancer* 1997; **79:** 1100–15.

19. Tournigand C, de Gramont A, Louvet C et al, A simplified bimonthly regimen with leucovorin and 5FU for metastatic colorectal cancer. *Proc Am Soc Clin Oncol* 1998; **17:** 274.

20. Seymour MT, Slevin M, Kerr DJ et al, Randomized trial assessing the addition of interferon-2α to fluorouracil and leucovorin in advanced colorectal cancer. *J Clin Oncol* 1996; **14:** 2280–8.

21. de Gramont A, Figer A, Seymour M et al, Leucovorin and 5-fluorouracil with or without oxaliplatin in advanced colorectal cancer. *J Clin Oncol* 2000; **18:** 2938–47.

22. Douillard JY, Cunningham D, Roth AD et al, Irinotecan combined with fluorouracil compared with flurouracil alone as first-line treatment for metastatic colorectal cancer: a multicentre randomised trial. *Lancet* 2000; **355:** 1041–7.

23. Maughan TS, James RD, Kerr D et al, Preliminary results of a multicentre randomised trial comparing 3 chemotherapy regimens (de Gramont, Lokich and raltitrexed) in metastatic colorectal cancer. *Proc Am Soc Clin Oncol* 1999; **18:** 262a.

45

Infusional 5-FU in the treatment of metastatic colorectal cancer: The 48-hour weekly approach

Andrés Cervantes, Eduardo Díaz-Rubio, Enrique Aranda, on behalf of the Spanish Group for Gastrointestinal Tumor Therapy (TTD)

INTRODUCTION

Since its introduction in clinical oncology more than 40 years ago, 5-fluorouracil (5-FU) remains the most useful drug in the treatment of patients with advanced colorectal cancer. Many schedules, dosages and routes of administration have been used for 5-FU, not only as a single agent, but also in combination with modulating compounds such as leucovorin (folinic acid), methotrexate, N-(phosphonoacetyl)-L-aspartic acid (PALA), interferon, dipyridamole and hydroxyurea, among others. Randomized trials using strict response criteria showed that the objective response rate that may be achieved with 5-FU, given as an intravenous push, lies in the range 10–15%. Despite some advances in the understanding of the metabolic pathways by which 5-FU may eventually produce tumour cell death, the impact of biomodulation on the natural history of the disease is limited, with some improvement in response rate, but without any significant effect on survival.[1] However, improvements in tumour-related symptoms are frequently seen, and, for this reason, palliative chemotherapy of metastatic colorectal cancer has a major role to play.

Although intravenous administration of 5-FU is the most widely accepted way to give the drug, the optimal schedule is still not settled. There are tumour cell kinetics as well as pharmacological considerations that may explain the low response rates observed in colorectal cancer when 5-FU is administered as a rapid bolus injection.

As with other antimetabolites, 5-FU is most effec-tive against tumour cells that are in active cell division. Colorectal cancer is a slowly growing tumour, with most tumour cells in G_0 or resting phase and only a small proportion in the susceptible S phase. This may be one of the reasons why 5-FU, when given by rapid push injection, will only kill a small proportion of malignant cells. On the other hand, owing to its rapid catabolism, the serum half-life of 5-FU is very short, not exceeding 11 minutes; therefore tumour cells are exposed to the drug for only a short period of time.

Prolonged intravenous infusion may circumvent these disadvantages. However, low serum concentrations of a drug may induce drug-resistant cell clones. The result of a meta-analysis of six randomized trials comparing bolus 5-FU versus infusional therapy in metastatic colorectal cancer confirms this hypothesis.[2] Infusional 5-FU produces a significantly higher response rate (22% versus 14%) and also a slightly better median survival than bolus treatment.

WEEKLY HIGH-DOSE 48-HOUR INFUSION OF 5-FU: HIGHER DOSE INTENSITY WITH BETTER THERAPEUTIC INDEX

To develop a theoretically optimal approach to the use of 5-FU in metastatic colorectal cancer, several factors have to be taken into account: high dose and appropriate dose intensity, prolonged exposure, limiting toxicity, ways of effective biomodulation, and feasibility of combination with new active agents such as oxaliplatin and irinotecan. A dose–response relationship has been suggested for 5-FU in colorectal cancer,[3] and it is clear that, by employing a continuous-infusion schedule, much higher dose intensity can be obtained. However, data supporting the concept of a dose–response relationship are mainly derived from retrospective analysis by a comparison of different trials. This means of analysis may be misleading, because a supposed dose–response relationship can simply reflect the fact that patients with better prognostic factors can tolerate higher doses of chemotherapy. Comparisons of different trials have many flaws because of widely varying selection criteria and means of assessing the response. Despite these problems, the collected data suggest that there is a dose–response relationship, and they underline the impact of the dose intensity of 5-FU. This applies not only for bolus injection of 5-FU, but also for continuous-infusion schedules.[4]

Investigators in Vancouver pioneered a number of ways to administer 5-FU by continuous infusions of short duration but at frequent intervals.[5] The best results, with an overall response rate of 30%, were achieved with a 48-hour 5-FU infusion of 60 mg/kg given weekly. The dose intensity of this schedule reached approximately 2500 mg/m^2/week, which was at that time considerably higher than with any other schedule. In a phase I–II trial design, it was shown that, when administered weekly in such a 48-hour infusional schedule, the maximum tolerated dose of 5-FU was 3500 mg/m^2/week, with a good toxicity profile and a response rate of 43% in non-pretreated patients.[6] When different ways of giving 5-FU are compared in order to define dose intensity (Table 45.1), it is found that bolus injection of 5-FU may give a maximum dose intensity of 500–750 mg/m^2/week, with myelosuppression as the limiting toxicity.[7,8] When the duration of the infu-

sion is prolonged to 5 days, the dose intensity achieved is almost doubled, but mucositis appears as the limiting toxic effect, and 3–4 weeks are needed for recovery before the next dose may be administered.[9,10] When 5-FU is given as a protracted infusion of at least 5 weeks, the daily dose goes down to 300 mg/m^2, but the dose intensity increases to 2100 mg/m^2/week. This indicates a threefold increase in dose intensity over bolus injection, with a significant improvement in response rate (30% versus 7%) in a randomized study.[7] The therapeutic index is also better, with fewer episodes of grade 3 or 4 toxicity, and evidence of the hand–foot syndrome as a prominent feature. However, no survival benefit could be found in this trial.

Prolonged continuous infusion of 5-FU produces relatively low plasma levels of 5-FU over a long time. Theoretically, this may facilitate the development of resistance, although there is no clinical evidence of this phenomenon. Some other schedules with weekly short-term infusions of 24- or 48-hour duration have been studied, in order to allow the delivery of higher dose intensity.[11,12] With those schedules, the tumour is exposed every week to higher plasma concentrations than with the protracted infusion, leading to higher dose intensity. This is particularly clear with the weekly 48-hour schedule, which achieves the highest dose intensity ever achieved with 5-FU, allowing the administration of 3500 mg/m^2/week.[6] A summary of several published studies of weekly 5-FU by 48-hour infusion is presented in Table 45.2.

Data on the 48-hour schedule have been developed by the Spanish Group for Gastrointestinal Tumour Therapy (TTD) and by the Gastrointestinal Tract Cooperative Group of the European Organization for Research and Treatment of Cancer (EORTC).[12–14] The European study tried to confirm

---

Table 45.1 A dose-intensity comparison of different routes of 5-FU administration

Dose (mg/m^2)	Infusion duration	Schedule	Dose intensity (mg/m^2/week)	Limiting toxicity	Ref.
500 × 5	i.v. push	5 weeks	500	Myelosuppression	7
750	i.v. push	Weekly	750	Myelosuppression	8
5000	120 h	Monthly	1250	Mucositis	9, 10
300	Protracted	Daily	2100	Hand–foot	7
2600	24 h	Weekly	2600	Diarrhoea	11
3500	48 h	Weekly	3500	Diarrhoea	12

Table 45.2 Data from phase II and III trials of weekly 48-hour continuous infusion of 5-FU as a single agent in advanced colorectal cancer patients

Phase	Dose	Dose intensity (mg/m²/week)	No. of patients	Response rate (%)	Toxicity WHO grade 3 + 4 (%)	Ref.
II	60 mg/kg	2500	30	30	14	5
II	3500 mg/m²	3500	83	39	21	12
III	60 mg/kg	1600	110	10	5	14
III	3500 mg/m²	3500	155	30	18	13

the activity observed by Shah et al[5] in a randomized trial comparing weekly high-dose infusional 5-FU (60 mg/kg) over a 48-hour period with or without methotrexate.[14] The addition of low-dose methotrexate led to a doubling of the response rate from 10% to 21% without any significant effect on survival. It may be important to consider that in this schedule the dose intensity of 5-FU was approximately 1600 mg/m²/week, which is below the maximum of 3500 mg/m²/week intended by the Spanish TTD trials. The suboptimal dose intensity administered may explain the low response rate obtained with infusional 5-FU alone.

However, in an extended multicentre phase II trial[12] and in a subsequent phase III randomized study,[13] the Spanish TTD group confirmed the results previously achieved in the early phase I–II trial.[6] The response rate was 38.5% in 83 patients registered in the phase II trial. The median administered dose intensity was 3000 mg/m²/week, ranging from 1800 to 3500 mg/m²/week. Grade 3 and 4 diarrhoea and mucositis were only reported in 11% and 12% of cases respectively. In the phase III trial, a total of 306 patients with advanced colorectal cancer and bidimensionally measurable disease were randomized to receive either 5-FU 425 mg/m² given by bolus injection on days 1–5 plus intravenous leucovorin 20 mg/m² every 4–5 weeks, or 5-FU 3500 mg/m²/week in a 48-hour continuous infusion. The main endpoint of the trial was assessment of response. Therapy was continued until disease progression. Second-line therapy and crossover were also allowed after progression. The response rate was 30.3% in 155 patients allocated to the continuous-infusion arm, with a 95% confidence interval (CI) ranging from 24% to 39%. This was significantly superior to the 19.2% response rate observed in the modulated 5-FU bolus arm. The trial was not pow-

ered to detect differences in survival or time to progression. A summary of the results of this trial is presented in Table 45.3. Another point of interest is the confirmation of a different toxicity profile and the excellent tolerance of the treatment. More hand–foot syndrome was observed in the infusional arm, though the proportion of severe mucositis or diarrhoea was 18% in both arms. Weekly 48-hour continuous infusion of 5-FU permits high dose intensity and a maximum tolerated dose superior to all other schedules, with an activity that is superior to single-agent bolus 5-FU with or without modulated leucovorin.

When the response rates obtained by different schedules of continuous infusion of 5-FU in several randomized trials[7,9,10,13–15] are plotted against the planned dose intensity, there seems to be a linear relationship. However, the analysis of dose intensity and response is mainly based on retrospective studies. Data from randomized studies to support the hypothesis of a relationship between dose intensity and response are lacking.

When protracted-infusional studies of 5-FU were analysed in terms of toxicity, myelosuppression was virtually absent. The hand–foot syndrome was the most prominent toxic effect.[7] A seven-arm trial with a screening design, including 620 patients with advanced colorectal cancer, compared several bolus, infusional, and modulated 5-FU schedules.[15] The single-agent protracted-infusion 5-FU was the better tolerated arm. Only 11% of patients presented grade 4 toxicity, particularly diarrhoea. Despite the high dose intensity achieved, the toxicity profile of weekly high doses of 5-FU in a 48-hour infusional schedule indicates excellent tolerance. In the EORTC trial, only 5% of the patients receiving 5-FU alone showed a grade 3–4 toxicity,[14] none of them having the hand–foot syndrome. As previously stated, the weekly 48-hour

Table 45.3 Summary of the results of the phase III trial comparing weekly 48-hour continuous infusion of 5-FU versus modulated bolus 5-FU in advanced colorectal cancer patients (median follow-up 38 weeks)[13]

Arm	No. of patients	Response rate (%)	95% CI	Time to progression (weeks)	Overall survival (weeks)
Modulated 5-FU bolus	151	19.2	12–29	23.5	42.5
Weekly high-dose 5-FU continuous infusion	155	30.3	24–39	25	48
p		<0.05		NS	NS

Abbreviations: 95% CI, 95% confidence interval; NS, not significant.

infusional treatment achieved the highest dose intensity of 5-FU ever reached. However, grade 4 toxicity was seen in only 10% of patients. In the previously cited multicenter phase III trial, the most frequent grade 3–4 toxicities observed among patients allocated to the infusional arm were diarrhoea (9%) and mucositis (9%). Severe hand–foot syndrome was detected in only 4% of patients, but 35% had this effect at grade 1–2. It is important to stress that almost half of the patients treated did not require a dose reduction due to toxicity, and the median dose intensity that could be given was $3000 \, mg/m^2/week$. Overall, weekly 48-hour infusions offer the possibility of achieving a high dose intensity of 5-FU, with a better response rate than the modulation of bolus 5-FU plus leucovorin and with an improved toxicity profile.

BIOMODULATION OF WEEKLY HIGH-DOSE 48-HOUR INFUSION OF 5-FU

It is sensible to try to improve the therapeutic activity of weekly high-dose continuous-infusion schedules of 5-FU by the addition of modulating agents, and several phase II and III studies have addressed this particular issue. Some European investigators have developed several forms of modulation for the 48-hour schedule (Table 45.4). The EORTC trial is the only randomized study showing that methotrexate was able to increase the antitumour activity of infusional 5-FU over 48 hours versus 5-FU alone.[14] The

response rate was 21% in the modulated arm, compared with 11% in the 5-FU-alone arm. Severe toxicity was also double in the modulated arm, rising to a 24% incidence of grade 3 and 4 episodes, mainly stomatitis, compared with a 5% incidence in the control arm. A point to underline in this study is the low dose intensity of 5-FU administered. At the beginning of therapy, four courses were given on a weekly basis. Thereafter, four more courses were given biweekly, meaning a total of 8 courses of therapy in 12 weeks. This implies a dose intensity of $1600 \, mg/m^2/week$. As can be seen from other studies of short-term infusional therapy, when 5-FU is modulated, the dose intensity of the drug goes down. In other words, 5-FU can be modulated only if a lower dose intensity of the drug is given.

In two consecutive phase II trials, the Spanish group showed that when very high-dose infusional 5-FU over 48 hours is modulated by oral leucovorin, there is a higher incidence of severe toxicity, while activity does not seem to increase.[16,17] In the first TTD study with $3000 \, mg/m^2$ of 5-FU plus oral leucovorin, 78% of patients suffered from severe toxicity. In many of them, dose reductions had to be made, and the actual dose intensity went down to $2000 \, mg/m^2/week$. When, in a second trial, also with oral leucovorin, the dose of 5-FU was reduced to $2000 \, mg/m^2/week$, a lower incidence of severe toxicity without loss of antitumour activity was observed, despite a reduction in the real dose intensity to $1600 \, mg/m^2/week$.

Table 45.4 Phase II–III trials of weekly 48-hour continuous infusions of biomodulated 5-FU in advanced colorectal cancer patients

Phase	Dose of 5-FU	Biomodulating agent	Dose intensity (mg/m^2/week)		No. of patients	Response rate (%)	Toxicity WHO grade 3 + 4 (%)	Ref.
			Planned	Achieved				
III	60 mg/kg	Methotrexate	1600	Not stated	106	21	14	14
II	3000 mg/m^2	Oral leucovorin	3000	2200	43	29	78	16
II	2000 mg/m^2	Oral leucovorin	2000	1600	110	37	40	17

In summary, oral modulation with leucovorin is not useful when weekly 5-FU is given over 48 hours at 5-FU doses higher than 3000 mg/m^2, owing to the appearance of intolerable toxicity without any evidence of increasing activity. A similar observation was also made from the meta-analysis of nine studies of leucovorin modulation. If high doses of 5-FU were used in the control arm, leucovorin was not able to improve the results.[1]

This finding reinforces the concept that when short-term 5-FU is given alone without any modulating drug, it is critical to give an adequate dose intensity. This approach will yield a response rate of 30%, with a tolerable toxicity. However, if the concept of modulation is applied, dose intensity is not of such critical importance. When effective modulation of infusional 5-FU schedules with leucovorin, PALA, or methotrexate is used, a similar antitumour activity is usually observed, despite a clear dose-intensity reduction and slightly worse toxicity profile.

COMBINATION OF OXALIPLATIN OR IRINOTECAN WITH WEEKLY HIGH-DOSE 48-HOUR INFUSION OF 5-FU

Considering the data on the activity of irinotecan and oxaliplatin combined with other infusional 5-FU regimens, the TTD group has developed two trials to study the feasibility of combining the 48-hour continuous infusion of 5-FU with either drug.

In a phase I–II design, our group has studied the combination of 5-FU with irinotecan. To determine the maximum tolerated dose (MTD) of a combination of irinotecan administered weekly in 30 minutes, just before a fixed dose of 5-FU (3000 mg/m^2) given over 48 hours, a classical phase I trial was performed.

Irinotecan was started at a dose of 60 mg/m^2 per week. A period of 6 weeks on therapy plus 2 more rest weeks were taken for the observation of toxicity. Table 45.5 shows data related to the toxicity observed at all dose levels studied. At the fourth step, when 90 mg/m^2 were added to the weekly high-dose 5-FU infusion, a total of four episodes of dose-limiting toxicity were observed in six patients. The main dose-limiting toxicity was diarrhoea in three cases and myelosuppression in only one patient. Thus this step represents the maximal tolerated dose, and the recommended dose for the subsequent phase II trial was 80 mg/m^2.

In a further phase II trial, 41 patients with measurable advanced colorectal cancer were treated with the recommended dose as first-line chemotherapy. Treatment was given continuously every week without any rest between courses. Response was assessed every 8 weeks. At the moment, only 21 patients have been assessed for response. Preliminary information suggests an active schedule, with 48% overall response rate (95% CI 26–70).[18]

To assess the feasibility of a combination of oxaliplatin and weekly high-dose continuous-infusion 5-FU in first-line chemotherapy, another phase II trial was performed by the TTD group. Oxaliplatin (85 mg/m^2) was given every 2 weeks as a 2-hour infusion just before the 48-hour infusion of 5-FU (3000 mg/m^2). For this trial, 90 patients with advanced colorectal cancer and measurable disease were accrued. When a first cohort of 59 patients were on therapy, a high proportion of cases of severe diarrhoea were reported. Of these, 27 (45%) presented NCI-CTC grade 3 or 4 diarrhoea, and the steering committee decided to lower the dose of 5-FU to 2250 mg/m^2 in this first cohort. A second cohort of 31 patients was further accrued, and started therapy

Table 45.5 Summary of the results of the phase I trial of a fixed dose of weekly 48-hour continuous infusion of 5-FU (3000 mg/m^2) combined with irinotecan

Irinotecan dose (mg/m^2)	No. of patients	Limiting toxicity	
		Haematological	Delayed diarrhoea
60	6	0	2 (1 G3, 1 G4)
70	3	0	0
80	3	0	2 G3
90	6	1 G4 neutropenia	3 G3

G3 and G4 indicate grades 3 and 4 toxicity according to the CTC-NCI criteria. The maximum tolerated dose was 90 mg/m^2 and the recommended dose for further phase II trial was 80 mg/m^2.

with the same schedule but with an initial dose of 5-FU of 2250 mg/m^2. In this second cohort, the proportion of patients presenting grade 3–4 diarrhoea went down to 20%. Grade 2 neurosensorial toxicity was observed also in 18 out of 90 patients. This combination of oxaliplatin and weekly high-dose continuous-infusion 5-FU has also proved to be active, with a 54% response rate in 72 assessed patients (95% CI 33–65%).[19]

REFERENCES

1. Advanced Colorectal Cancer Meta-Analysis Project, Modulation of fluorouracil by leucovorin in patients with advanced colorectal cancer: evidence in terms of response rate. *J Clin Oncol* 1992; **10**: 896–903.
2. The Meta-Analysis Group in Cancer, Efficacy of intravenous infusion of fluorouracil compared with bolus administration in advanced colorectal cancer. *J Clin Oncol* 1998; **16**: 301–8.
3. Hryniuk WM, Figueredo A, Goodyear M, Applications of dose intensity to problems of chemotherapy of breast and colorectal cancer. *Semin Oncol* 1987; **14**(Suppl 4): 3–11.
4. Wils J, High dose fluorouracil: a new perspective in the treatment of colorectal cancer. *Semin Oncol* 1992; **19**(Suppl 3): 126–30.
5. Shah A, MacDonald W, Goldie J et al, 5-FU infusion in advanced colorectal cancer: a comparison of three dose schedules. *Cancer Treat Rep* 1985; **69**: 739–42.
6. Díaz-Rubio E, Aranda E, Martín M et al, Weekly high-dose infusion of 5-fluorouracil in advanced colorectal cancer. *Eur J Cancer* 1990; **26**: 727–9.
7. Lokich JJ, Ahlgren JD, Gullo JJ et al, A prospective comparison of continuous infusion fluorouracil with a conventional bolus schedule in metastatic colorectal carcinoma. A Mid-Atlantic Oncology Program study. *J Clin Oncol* 1989; **7**: 425–33.
8. Ansfield F, Klots J, Nealon T et al, A phase III study comparing the clinical utility of four regimens of 5-fluorouracil. *Cancer* 1977; **39**: 34–40.
9. Kemeny N, Israel K, Niedzwiecki D et al, Randomized study of continuous infusion fluorouracil versus fluorouracil plus cis-

platin in patients with metastatic colorectal cancer. *J Clin Oncol* 1990; **8**: 313–18.
10. Díaz-Rubio E, Jimeno J, Antón A et al, A prospective randomized trial of continuous infusion 5-fluorouracil (5-FU) versus 5-FU plus cisplatin in patients with advanced colorectal cancer. *Am J Clin Oncol* 1992; **15**: 56–60.
11. Köhne CH, Wilke H, Schöffski P et al, High dose infusional 5-FU (HDFU) is superior compared to HDFU plus interferon. Final results of a multicenter randomized trial of the AIO. *Ann Oncol* 1996; **7**(Suppl 5): 2110.
12. Díaz-Rubio E, Aranda E, Camps C et al, A phase II study of weekly 48-hour infusion with high dose 5-fluorouracil in advanced colorectal carcinoma: an alternative to biochemical modulation. *J Infus Chemother* 1994; **4**: 58–61.
13. Aranda E, Díaz-Rubio E, Cervantes A et al, A phase III multicenter randomized study in advanced colorectal cancer: weekly high dose continuous infusion 5-fluorouracil versus fluorouracil plus leucovorin. *Ann Oncol* 1988; **9**: 727–31.
14. Blijham G, Wagener T, Wils J et al, Modulation of high-dose infusional fluorouracil by low-dose methotrexate in patients with advanced colorectal cancer: final results of a randomized European Organization for Research and Treatment of Cancer study. *J Clin Oncol* 1996; **14**: 2266–73.
15. Leichman CG, Fleming TR, Muggia FM et al, Phase II study of fluorouracil and its modulation in advanced colorectal cancer: a Southwest Oncology Group study. *J Clin Oncol* 1995; **13**: 1303–11.
16. Aranda E, Cervantes A, Dorta J et al, A phase II trial of weekly high dose continuous infusion 5-fluorouracil plus oral leucovorin in patients with advanced colorectal cancer. *Cancer* 1995; **76**: 559–63.
17. Aranda E, Cervantes A, Carrato A et al, Outpatient weekly high dose continuous infusion 5-fluorouracil plus oral leucovorin in patients with advanced colorectal cancer. A phase II trial. *Ann Oncol* 1996; **7**: 851–5.
18. Aranda E, Carrato A, Cervantes A et al, Irinotecan (CPT-11) in combination with high dose infusional 5-FU (TTD schedule) in advanced colorectal cancer. Preliminary results of a phase I/II study. *Proc Am Soc Clin Oncol* 2000; **19**: 1177.
19. Abad A, Navarro M, Sastre J, Cervantes A et al, Biweekly oxaliplatin plus weekly 48 hours continuous infusion in first line treatment in of advanced colorectal cancer. Preliminary results. *Proc Am Soc Clin Oncol* 1999; **18**: 1056.

46

Infusional 5-fluorouracil: Protracted infusion

Norwood R Anderson, Jacob J Lokich

INTRODUCTION

Initially synthesized in 1957 as a pyrimidine antagonist,[1] the fluorinated pyrimidine 5-fluorouracil (5-FU) remains the single most important chemotherapeutic agent in the treatment of colorectal cancer. Despite over four decades of extensive clinical use, significant controversy still exists regarding the optimal dose and schedule of administration for this foundational agent, however.

Recent technological advances in drug delivery systems and venous access devices have permitted investigation of a delivery system characterized by prolonged venous exposure in ambulatory settings. Such prolonged venous infusions (PVI) of 5-FU present an alternative mode of administration to the commonly employed bolus delivery schedules, routinely administered as a five times per week dose repeated every 28–35 days or as weekly doses for 6 weeks cycled every 8 weeks, both now co-administered with the modulating agent leucovorin (folinic acid).

Widespread acceptance of the PVI administration schedule has been hampered by concerns regarding the necessity for venous access systems and the cumbersome nature of most infusion pumps. Nonetheless, this mode of administration of 5-FU in colorectal cancer has added significantly to the general medical knowledge about the mechanisms of action of 5-FU, has been associated with antitumor activity equivalent to that of the more commonly utilized bolus administration schedules in advanced colorectal cancer, and, perhaps most significantly, has spurred the development of 5-FU derivatives and prodrugs that can be delivered on the ultimate prolonged 'infusion schedule' – namely, daily oral administration.

PHARMACOLOGIC RATIONALE FOR THE USE OF 5-FU ON A PVI SCHEDULE

As an antimetabolite, 5-FU is in many respects the prototypical agent to be considered for use on a PVI administration schedule. The major cytotoxic effects of 5-FU occur during S phase of the cell cycle, thus defining 5-FU as a classical cell-cycle-specific agent. In addition, its pharmacokinetic profile, with a mean plasma half-life of 11 minutes after bolus administration, makes it the ideal agent for use in a delivery system that assures prolonged drug exposure over time.[2] Similarly, its prolonged stability in aqueous solution permits its use for protracted periods of time without requiring frequent drug reservoir changes. Additionally, the inhibition of thymidylate synthase following a rapid bolus dose is short, with a dissociation half-life of approximately 6 hours, thereby favoring more prolonged exposure to the cytotoxic agent to induce greater tumor cell kill via enzymatic inhibition.[3] Lastly, at any one time, only approximately 3% of tumor cells are in S phase and susceptible to the cytotoxic effects of 5-FU, irrespective of the mode of administration, arguing forcefully for prolonged exposure to permit greater drug effect as cells cycle through S phase, where they are susceptible to the effects of the administered 5-FU.[4]

In addition to its well-documented cell-cycle specificity and pharmacokinetic profile, 5-FU exhibits considerable schedule dependence, which favors its utilization on a PVI administration schedule (Table 46.1). Early studies conducted on human epithelial cancer lines in vitro by Calabro-Jones et al[5] as well as by Drewinko and Yang[6] revealed that both increased dose and increased duration of exposure of the cell lines to 5-FU resulted in augmented tumor cell kill. At each concentration of 5-FU administered, there was an incremental increase in cell kill with

---

Table 46.1 5-Fluorouracil: rationale for infusional administration

- Prolonged stability in aqueous solution
- Cell-cycle specificity (S phase)
- Plasma half-life of 11 minutes
- Schedule dependence for cell kill
- Low percentage of tumor cells 'in cycle' at any one time
- Short thymidylate synthase inhibition

---

increased duration of exposure to the drug, indicating that a complex relationship between dose and duration of exposure exists for the optimal antitumor effect of administered drug.

PHASE I CLINICAL TRIALS OF PVI 5-FU

Building on the initial experience of Seifert et al[7] detailing a doubling of response rates from 22% to 44% for a 120-hour infusion of 5-FU as compared with the then-standard bolus administration of single-agent 5-FU, Lokich et al[8] performed the first formal phase I trial of PVI 5-FU. Reported in 1981, their report detailed a trial in which 17 patients with various advanced-stage cancers received 19 courses of PVI 5-FU at doses ranging from 200 to 600 mg/m²/day, with interruption of the infusion being dictated only by the development of dose-limiting toxicity. At doses of 300 mg/m²/day or less, the treatment did not require interruption for upwards of 60 days, whereas for doses in excess of 300 mg/m² day, the

duration of the PVI was reduced to less than 10 days (Table 46.2).

Stomatitis was the dose-limiting toxicity for the PVI administration. In addition, a new toxicity was also described with the prolonged administration schedule: palmar–plantar erythrodysesthesia (more commonly known by the less cumbersome title 'hand–foot syndrome'), characterized by painful, erythematous swelling of the hands and feet, which was completely reversible with discontinuation of the infusion but which progressed to severe disability if PVI 5-FU was continued.[9] This appearance of a newly described toxicity coincided with the finding that when given on a prolonged administration, 5-FU was associated with an almost complete absence of grade 3 and 4 myelosuppression (also described by Seifert et al), the usual dose-limiting toxicity of the bolus delivery systems. Thus, it appeared that when given as a PVI, 5-FU was a 'different drug' than when given by bolus administration. It now appears likely that these differences in toxicity relate to the fact that, with prolonged exposure, 5-FU metabolites are preferentially incorporated into tumor DNA, whereas, with short high-dose bolus schedules, tumor RNA is the target for cytotoxicity, thus indicating that, indeed, bolus and prolonged-exposure 5-FU may actually be different drugs.[10,11]

PHASE II CLINICAL TRIALS OF PVI 5-FU

Following the documentation of the maximally tolerated dose of PVI 5-FU (300 mg/m²/day), numerous single-institution phase II trials were conducted to assess the clinical efficacy of this delivery method in the treatment of advanced colorectal cancer (Table

---

Table 46.2 Phase I study of prolonged venous infusion of 5-fluorouracil: total cumulative dose and duration relative to daily dose rate of delivery[a]

No. of patients	Dose (mg/m²/day)	Mean duration[b] (days)	Mean total dose (g)
5	200	35 (30–47)	11.5
4	300	38 (30–60)	22.6
4	350	20 (19–23)	10.9
4	400	9 (7–12)	7.9
2	600	14 (9–18)	15.3

[a]From Lokich J, Bothe A, Fine N, Phase I study of protracted venous infusion of 5-fluorouracil. *Cancer* 1981; **48:** 2565–8.
[b]Range in parentheses.

Table 46.3 Single-arm phase II trials of prolonged venous infusion 5-fluorouracil in metastatic colorectal cancer: a compendium of results

Authors	No. of patients treated	No. of patients responding	Toxicity
Lelchman et al[12]	16	5 (31%)	Mucocutaneous
Belt et al[13]	20	10 (39%)	Stomatitis
			Hand–foot syndrome
Molina et al[14]	25	11 (44%)	Hand–foot syndrome
Wade et al[15]	100	53 (53%)	Mucocutaneous
			Hand–foot syndrome
Hansen et al[16]	91	30 (33%)	Hand–foot syndrome
			Mucocutaneous
Kuo et al[17]	26	11 (42%)	Mucocutaneous
			Hand–foot syndrome
Totals	284	120 (42%)	

46.3). In addition to being single-institution trials, all of these studies were single-armed and not randomized.[12–17] While many criticisms of these studies may be raised, collectively they documented that delivery of 5-FU on a PVI schedule was at least not inferior to the more commonly employed bolus system modulated by leucovorin. While response rates varying between 31% and 53% were universally considered to be non-reproducible in multi-institutional randomized trials, the verification of the total absence of myelosuppression indicated that there was a possible striking toxicity advantage for the PVI schedule of delivery as compared with the leucovorin-modulated bolus method of administration. Despite the increased response rates of these trials, no improvement in survival was noted when the PVI delivery was compared with the historic controls of bolus 5-FU.

In a complicated randomized phase II trial reported in 1995, the Southwest Oncology Group (SWOG) evaluated the toxicity and efficacy of seven 5-FU-containing chemotherapy regimens in 599 evaluable patients with measurable colorectal cancer.[18] Three schedules of leucovorin-modulated 5-FU were randomly compared with PVI 5-FU given for 28 days (with and without leucovorin) and with high-dose 24-hour 5-FU (with or without biochemical modulation with N-phosphonoacetyl-L-aspartate, PALA). All arms of the study enrolled between 84 and 88 patients. At a median follow-up of 37 months, there was a slight survival advantage for the single-

agent PVI 5-FU and the 24-hour high-dose single agent 5-FU infusion versus the other treatment arms (15 months median survival versus 11–14 months). This difference, however, did not reach statistical significance. Toxicity patterns were different in the bolus and infusional treatment arms, with considerably more grade 3 and 4 neutropenia occurring in the bolus arms and more diarrhea in the high-dose leucovorin-modulated 5-FU arms. Diarrhea and neutropenia were uncommon in the PVI 5-FU group.

RANDOMIZED PHASE III TRIALS OF PVI 5-FU WITH BOLUS SCHEDULES

In 1989, the Mid-Atlantic Oncology Program (MAOP) completed the first prospective phase III multi-institutional randomized trial comparing the efficacy of 5-FU bolus administration with PVI 5-FU in chemotherapy-naive patients with advanced measurable colorectal cancer.[19] In this study, 174 patients were randomly assigned to receive either a bolus loading schedule of 5-FU at 500 mg/m^2/day $\times$ 5 every 5 weeks versus a PVI dose of 300 mg/m^2/day for 70 consecutive days. Utilizing stringent response criteria requiring independent confirmation of documented responses, the tumor response rates were 7% (6/87 patients) for the bolus group and 30% (26/87 patients) for the PVI group – a statistically significant difference (Table 46.4).

Table 46.4 A prospective randomized comparison of prolonged venous infusional 5-fluorouracil with a conventional bolus schedule in metastatic colorectal cancer[a]

	Treatment arm	
	Infusional 5-FU	Bolus 5-FU
Total no. of patients	87	87
Median age (years)	64.6	61.1
Performance status 0–1	78 (90%)	81 (93%)
Response:		
Partial response	22 (25%)	6 (7%)
Complete response	4 (5%)	0
Total response	26 (30%)	6 (7%)
Median survival (months)	10.3	11.2
Toxicity:		
Grade 3–4 neutropenia	1 (1%)	17 (22%)
Grade 3–4 stomatitis	3 (4%)	10 (13%)
Hand–foot syndrome	20 (24%)	0
Drug-related death	0	4 (5%)

[a]From Lokich J, Ahlgren J, Gulb J et al, A prospective randomized comparison of continuous infusion fluorouracil with a conventional bolus schedule in metastatic colorectal carcinoma: a Mid-Atlantic Oncology Program study. *J Clin Oncol* 1989; **7:** 425–32.

In addition to showing marked difference in response rates for the two groups, the study further demonstrated differing patterns of toxicity in the two groups. Twenty-two percent of the bolus-treated patients developed grade 3–4 neutropenia, compared with only 1/87 patients in the PVI arm ($p < 0.001$). Additionally, four patients (5%) in the bolus arm died from sepsis associated with neutropenia, while there were no deaths in the PVI arm. Stomatitis occurred in both groups, with a trend to increased incidence in the bolus group, while 'hand–foot syndrome' was the most common toxicity with the PVI group, occurring in 24% (29/87) patients – but this toxicity was never life-threatening, although it did require dose attenuation or periods of withdrawal of therapy to allow spontaneous resolution of symptoms. Despite the impressive differences in toxicity and response highly favoring the PVI administration schedule, survival was similar for both groups, with median survivals of 10 months for the PVI 5-FU arm and 11 months for the bolus arm.

Subsequent to this initial MAOP report, three additional randomized phase III trials have been reported that compare PVI 5-FU with bolus single-agent 5-FU (Table 46.5). Each of these well-conducted trials enrolling a total of 789 additional patients[20–22] confirmed the response advantage for the PVI 5-FU compared with bolus administration. Despite total response rate improvement with the PVI 5-FU seen in all three trials, there was no statistically significant difference in overall survival between the bolus and infusional 5-FU schedules. Only the French cooperative trial, which utilized a schedule of 7 consecutive days of infusional 5-FU repeated every 21 days,[21] showed a small advantage in 'survival until progression' for the infusional schedule, which reached statistical significance (7 months versus 5 months for bolus). Toxicity analysis of these three additional trials confirmed the MAOP data that PVI 5-FU resulted in markedly decreased myelotoxicity compared with bolus delivery. The dose-limiting toxicity for infusional 5-FU was either

Table 46.5 5-Fluorouracil infusion: randomized phase III trials of infusion versus bolus in advanced colorectal cancer							
Group[a]	No. of patients	5-FU bolus (mg/m²)	5-FU infusion (mg/m²)	Response rate (%)		Survival (months)	
				Bolus	Infusion	Bolus	Infusion
MAOP[19]	174	500/d × 5 d q5wks	300/d × 70 d	7 (p = 0.001)	30	11.2	10.3
NCI-C[20]	184	450/d × 5 d q4wks	350/d × 14 d q4wks	6 (p = 0.34)	12	9.5	9.5
ECOG[22]	450	500/d × 5 d then weekly	300/d	19 (p = 0.12)	27	10.6	13
French[21]	155	500/d × 5 d q4wks	750/d × 7 d q3wks	8 (p = 0.02)	19	9	10

[a]MAOP, Mid-Atlantic Oncology Program; NCI-C, National Cancer Institute of Canada; ECOG, Eastern Cooperative Oncology Group.

'hand–foot syndrome' or mucocutaneous toxicity, with the PVI schedule being generally associated with an improved therapeutic index compared with bolus administration. Median survival was identical for bolus and PVI schedules in all studies, despite the toxicity and response advantage favoring the prolonged administration schedule.

SINGLE-AGENT PVI 5-FU VERSUS LEUCOVORIN-MODULATED 5-FU BOLUS

There is a paucity of direct randomized phase III trials comparing PVI 5-FU with the more commonly utilized combination of leucovorin-modulated 5-FU bolus. In 1992, however, Ahlgren[23] analyzed existing leucovorin–5-FU reports and the existing PVI 5-FU reports, looking for advantages and disadvantages of both administration schedules (Table 46.6). The results of the comparison of the data for a commonly employed leucovorin plus 5-FU bolus schedule (low-dose leucovorin modulation in the manner popularized by the North Central Cancer Treatment Group (NCCTG) and Mayo Clinic affiliates) contrasted with single-agent PVI 5-FU revealed overall median survivals of 11.5 months for the bolus group (173 patients) and 11.1 months for the PVI groups (255 patients). Toxicity for the PVI group was demonstra-

bly less than for the bolus group, particularly in the absence of myelotoxicity.

When taken together with the SWOG randomized phase II trial detailed above, these trials indicate that survival is not decreased with an infusional administration schedule as compared with a modulated bolus schedule, and that there is an improvement in therapeutic index with the infusional delivery, most noticeably with the marked decrease in neutropenia associated with the infusional system.

META-ANALYSIS OF PVI 5-FU COMPARED WITH BOLUS ADMINISTRATION

In 1998 the Meta-Analysis Group in Cancer reported two analyses comparing PVI 5-FU with bolus single-agent 5-FU in advanced colorectal cancer. One report detailed clinical response and median survival,[24] while the second analyzed the toxicity patterns of each schedule of administration.[25]

Clinical efficacy analysis

Utilizing results from six randomized clinical trials comparing various bolus 5-FU regimens with PVI 5-FU given for periods ranging from 7 days to

Table 46.6 5-Fluorouracil infusion: comparison of phase III trials of prolonged infusion versus low-dose leucovorin modulation from a literature review[a]

Institution and year[b]	Response	Median survival (months)	Toxicity[c] (%)		Treatment mortality
			Grade 3	Grade 4	
Protracted infusional 5-FU					
MAOP 1989	26/87 (30%)	10.3	27	0	0/87
MAOP 1991	29/83 (35%)	11.2	30	3	0/83
MAOP 1991	28/85 (33%)	11.8	42	4	0/85
Total	83/255 (32%)	11.1	33	3	0/255
5-FU/low-dose leucovorin (Mayo/NCCTG schedule)					
NCCTG 1989	16/37 (43%)	12.0	56	NR	0/37
NCCTG 1990	16/49 (33%)	13.7	NR	NR	1/89 (1%)
NCCTG 1991	29/87 (33%)	10	NR	NR	2/87 (2%)

[a]Adapted from Ahlgren J, Protracted infusion schedules of fluorouracil in colorectal cancer versus fluorouracil with modulators: differences and similarities. *J Infus Chemother* 1992; **2**: 128–37.
[b]MAOP, Mid-Atlantic Oncology Program; NCCTG, North Central Cancer Treatment Program.
[c]NR, not recorded.

continuation until toxicity,[18–22,26] data from 1219 patients were analyzed for clinical response to treatment and median survival. After removal of patients with non-measurable disease, 1103 patients were included for response analysis (Table 46.7). Seventy-six patients had received leucovorin-modulated bolus 5-FU, while 475 were treated with single-agent bolus and 552 with PVI administration. The tumor response rate was 22% in the PVI 5-FU arms (124/552), compared with 14% in the bolus-treated patients (76/551). The median duration of tumor response was 6.7 months for the bolus groups and 7.1 months for the PVI groups. The duration of 5-FU infusion did not apparently have an impact on the overall response benefit of the infusional delivery system.

Survival analysis was conducted on all 1219 patients, and showed a median survival of 11.3 months in the bolus groups, as compared with 12.1 months in the infusional groups. Prolonged survivals were seen in both groups, but there was a trend toward increased benefit for the infusional groups, with 39 infusional patients versus 23 bolus-treated patients, alive at 3 years and 16 infusional patients versus 4 bolus-treated patients alive at 4 years.

Concluding their analysis with the statement that PVI 5-FU is superior to bolus 5-FU in terms of tumor response and survival, even though the magnitude of benefit is small, the group confirmed the findings of previous phase II and III trials indicating that infusional delivery of 5-FU is a reasonable alternative to bolus delivery in the treatment of advanced colorectal cancer.

Toxicity analysis

In a second independent report analyzing toxicity patterns for bolus 5-FU and PVI 5-FU the Meta-Analysis Group analyzed the toxicity data from the

Table 46.7 Meta-analysis of prolonged venous infusion 5-FU compared with bolus 5-FU: clinical efficacy evaluation[a]

Study	Response	
	PVI 5-FU	Bolus 5-FU
5-FU alone	113/483	66/475
	(23.4%)	(13.9%)
5-FU + leucovorin	11/69	10/76
	(15.9%)	(13.1%)
Total	124/552	76/551
	(22.4%)	(13.8%)
	PVI 5-FU	Bolus 5-FU (all inclusive)
Median duration of tumor response (months)	7.1	6.7
Median survival	12.1	11.3

[a]Adapted from meta-analysis Group in Cancer, Efficacy of intravenous continuous infusion of fluorouracil compared with bolus administration in advanced colorectal cancer. *J Clin Oncol* 1998; **16**: 301–8.

1219 patients included in their earlier response analysis detailed above. Validating earlier phase II trials, they found that hematologic toxicity was uncommon among PVI-treated patients (4%), while grade 3 or 4 neutropenia occurred in 31% of bolus-treated patients. This difference was highly statistically significant ($p < 0.0001$). Predictably, hand–foot syndrome was significantly more common among the PVI-treated patients than in the bolus groups (34% versus 13%, respectively; $p < 0.0001$). Non-hematologic toxicities were equivalent in each of the treatment arms.

Taken together, these two meta-analyses confirm earlier studies indicating that the toxicity of PVI-administered 5-FU is principally cutaneous, while neutropenia dominates for the bolus delivery. Survival and tumor responses are nearly equivalent within the two schedules. The decreased incidence of neutropenia, combined with similar survival patterns, however, indicates that PVI 5-FU improves the therapeutic index of 5-FU in the setting of advanced colorectal cancer. Given these facts, it is reasonable to consider such prolonged schedules as first-line therapies in the treatment of patients with chemotherapy-naive advanced colorectal cancer.[27]

SPECIAL CONSIDERATIONS

Logistics of PVI delivery systems

Spurred by the development of hyperalimentation technology, prolonged ambulatory infusion of chemotherapeutic agents became logistically feasible in the latter half of the 1980s. The two major advances allowing this clinical utilization of the PVI schedule were the development and production of reliable venous access options and ambulatory infusion pumps. Both of these technical advances have been considerably improved in the past decade, with venous access devices now routinely utilized for bolus administration schedules as well as for infusional delivery. Virtually any style of ambulatory infusion pump (i.e. high-flow-rate, low-flow-rate, high-volume-reserve, low-volume-reserve, multi-variate programmable, or chronoprogrammable) is commercially available to be utilized with an effective venous access device, thus removing much of the concern about the logistical possibility of prolonged infusion that surrounded this method of 5-FU administration when it was first introduced into clinical practice.

Associated risks of infusional delivery systems

With advances in the technology of venous access devices along with increased surgical experience with their implantation, concerns regarding the risks of infection and venous thrombosis of the surgically implanted devices have gradually diminished. In an early report reviewing the complications of implanted venous catheters, Lokich et al[28] reported a 9% incidence of catheter-related infection (8/92 catheters), with only two of the eight patients developing bacteremia from the implanted devices. A review of the Cancer Center of Boston experience likewise showed that in a series of 600 patients with implanted venous access devices, there were 17 cases of access-related infection (2.8%), with 7 cases of documented bacteremia (1.2%) (C Moore, personal communication).

Venous thrombosis incited by the presence of the venous device remains the major potential morbidity of the surgically implanted delivery system, occurring variably in 16–30% of patients. With the use of prophylactic very low-dose warfarin (1 mg/day), Bern et al[29] reported a statistically significant decrease in the incidence of local thrombosis, which resulted in improved clinical efficacy and decreased requirement for device explantation.

In an analysis of the Royal Marsden Hospital experience with surgically implanted access ports, Ross and Cunningham[30] reported that 18% of implanted catheters were removed for various complications, including thrombosis in 4.7%, infection in 5.7%, catheter migration in 3.6%, local pain in 2.5%, and local port damage in 2.0%. They likewise indicated that 15% of 832 patients treated with infusional delivery systems developed access device complications that did not require catheter explantation and that quality-of-life issues were affected in 10–23% of their patients.

Cost analysis of infusional delivery of 5-FU

Direct cost comparisons for bolus and infusional 5-FU are fraught with complexity and great difficulty. Confounding issues of differences in toxicity patterns, quality-of-life issues, and ancillary cost issues such as time from work and time spent commuting to and from physicians' offices, as well as differences in treatment charges in differing geographic locales, make cost comparison of bolus and infusional systems extraordinarily difficult. Attempting to take these variables into consideration, however,

Anderson and Lokich[31] reported their analysis of the costs incurred for leucovorin-modulated 5-FU compared with that of PVI 5-FU. They concluded that costs associated with the two treatment schedules were comparable, but that confounding factors such as time out of work clouded the analysis.

In a later series of two reports analyzing infusional therapy in general and not specific for 5-FU, Lokich et al[32,33] also reported their analyses, concluding that the reimbursement differential for bolus versus infusional treatment for cancers of the colon and breast and lymphomas was not significant and that infusional schedules are no more costly than bolus schedules when costs for venous access device implantation were amortized over the entire life of the infusion. Similarly, a recent analysis of infusional 5-FU versus other treatment possibilities in women with metastatic breast cancer[34] indicated that infusional 5-FU was the most cost-effective treatment for women who already had a pre-existing venous access device in position when compared with three alternative therapies – capecitabine given orally, gemcitabine, and vinorelbine.

CONCLUSIONS

Prolonged venous infusion of 5-FU in the treatment of advanced colorectal cancer is currently both logistically and technologically feasible in an ambulatory setting. Significant numbers of clinical trials – both single-institution phase II and multi-institutional phase III – have detailed improved tumor responsiveness to infusional delivery, combined with significant amelioration of drug-associated toxicity and the virtual elimination of iatrogenic, drug-related deaths due to bacteremia complicating neutropenia.

While such advances in the treatment of patients with advanced colorectal cancer should be applauded, the fact remains that infusional therapy has not been translated into a significant survival advantage for most patients with these common cancers, and overall survival remains unsatisfactorily low at a median of 12–15 months irrespective of what delivery system or modulation of 5-FU is employed. Despite this fact, however, infusional 5-FU has proven to be equivalent to bolus-administered 5-FU. Because of the improved therapeutic index associated with the infusional system, protracted infusion should be considered as an alternative treatment to the commonly employed bolus delivery system in most patients presenting with advanced colorectal cancer, even as newer agents such as irinotecan and oxaliplatin are incorporated into infusional and bolus systems with the goal of improving tumor responsiveness and median survival while maintaining minimal clinical toxicity.

REFERENCES

1. Duschinsky R, Pleven B, Heidelberger C, The synthesis of 5-fluoropyrimidines. *J Am Chem Soc* 1957; **79:** 4559–60.

2. MacMillan W, Wolberg W, Welling P, Pharmacokinetics of 5-fluorouracil in humans. *Cancer Res* 1978; **38:** 3479–82.

3. Washtein W, Santi D, Assay of intracellular free and macro-molecular-bound metabolites of 5-fluorodeoxyuridine and 5-fluorouracil. *Cancer Res* 1979; **39:** 3397–404.

4. Shackney S, Cell kinetics and cancer chemotherapy. In: *Medical Oncology* (Calabresi P, Schein P, Rosenberg S, eds). New York: MacMillan, 1985: 41–60.

5. Calabro-Jones P, Byfield J, Ward J, Sharp T, Time–dose relationships for 5-fluorouracil cytotoxicity against human epithelial cancer cells in vitro. *Cancer Res* 1982; **42:** 4413–20.

6. Drewinko B, Yang L, Cellular basis for the inefficacy of 5-fluorouracil in human colon carcinoma. *Cancer Treat Rep* 1985; **69:** 1391–8.

7. Seifert P, Baker L, Reed M, Vaitkevicius V, Comparison of continuously infused 5-fluorouracil with bolus injection in treatment of patients with colorectal adenocarcinoma. *Cancer* 1975; **36:** 123–8.

8. Lokich J, Bothe A, Fine N, Phase I study of protracted venous infusion of 5-fluorouracil. *Cancer* 1981; **48:** 2565–8.

9. Lokich J, Moore C, Chemotherapy-associated palmar-plantar erythrodysesthesia syndrome. *Ann Intern Med* 1984; **101:** 798–800.

10. Sobrero A, Aschele C, Bertino J, Fluorouracil in colorectal cancer – a tale of two drugs: implications for biochemical modulation. *J Clin Oncol* 1997; **15:** 368–81.

11. Iyer L, Ratain M, 5-Fluorouracil pharmacokinetics: causes for variability and strategies for modulation in cancer chemotherapy. *Cancer Invest* 1999; **17:** 494–506.

12. Leichman L, Leichman C, Kinzie J et al, Long term low dose 5-fluorouracil in advanced measurable colon cancer: no correlation between toxicity and efficacy. *Proc Am Soc Clin Oncol* 1985; **4:** 86.

13. Belt R, Davidner M, Lyron M et al, Continuous low dose 5-fluorouracil for adenocarcinoma: confirmation of activity. *Proc Am Soc Clin Oncol* 1985; **4:** 90.

14. Molina R, Fabian C, Slavik M et al, Reversal of palmar–plantar erythrodysesthesia by B6 without loss of response in colon cancer patients receiving 200 mg/m sq/day continuous 5-FU. *Proc Am Soc Clin Oncol* 1987; **6:** 74.

15. Wade J, Herbst S, Greenberg A, Prolonged venous infusion of 5-fluorouracil for metastatic colon cancer: a follow-up report. *Proc Am Soc Clin Oncol* 1988; **7:** 94.

16. Hansen R, Quebbeman E, Ausman R et al, Continuous systemic 5-fluorouracil chemotherapy in advanced colorectal cancer: results in 91 patients. *J Surg Oncol* 1989; **40:** 177–81.

17. Kuo S, Finck S, Cho J et al, Continuous ambulatory infusional 5-fluorouracil chemotherapy in advanced colorectal cancer: a single institution retrospective study. *Proc Am Soc Clin Oncol* 1989; **8:** 126.

18. Leichman C, Fleming T, Muggia F et al, Phase II study of fluorouracil and its modulation in advanced colorectal cancer: a Southwest Oncology Group study. *J Clin Oncol* 1995; **13:** 1303–11.

19. Lokich J, Ahlgren J, Gullo J et al, A prospective randomized comparison of continuous infusion fluorouracil with a conventional bolus schedule in metastatic colorectal carcinoma: a Mid-Atlantic Oncology Program study. *J Clin Oncol* 1989; **7:** 425–32.

20. Weinerman B, Shah A, Fields A et al, Systemic infusion versus bolus chemotherapy in measurable colorectal cancer. *Am J Clin Oncol* 1992; **15:** 518–23.

21. Rougier P, Paillot B, Laplanche A et al, End results of a multicenter randomized trial comparing 5-FU in continuous systemic infusion to bolus administration in measurable metastatic colorectal cancer. *Proc Am Soc Clin Oncol* 1992; **11:** 465.

22. Hansen R, Ryan L, Anderson T et al, Phase III study of bolus versus infusion fluorouracil with or without cisplatin in advanced colorectal cancer. *J Natl Cancer Inst* 1996; **88:** 668–74.

23. Ahlgren J, Protracted infusion schedules of fluorouracil in colorectal cancer versus fluorouracil with modulators: differences and similarities. *J Infus Chemother* 1992; **2:** 128–37.

24. Meta-Analysis Group in Cancer, Efficacy of intravenous continuous infusion of fluorouracil compared with bolus administration in advanced colorectal cancer. *J Clin Oncol* 1998; **16:** 301–8.

25. Meta-Analysis Group in Cancer, Toxicity of fluorouracil in patients with advanced colorectal cancer: effect of administration schedule and prognostic factors. *J Clin Oncol* 1998; **16:** 3537–41.

26. Isacson S, 5-Fluorouracil and folinic acid in the treatment of colorectal carcinoma: a randomized trial of two different schedules of administration. Second International Conference on Gastro-Intestinal Cancer, Jerusalem, Israel, 1989 (oral presentation).

27. Koehne C, Midgley R, Seymour M et al, Advanced colorectal cancer: Which regimes should we recommend? *Ann Oncol* 1999; **10:** 877–82.

28. Lokich A, Bothe A, Benotti P et al, Complications and management of implanted venous access catheters. *J Clin Oncol* 1985; **3:** 710–17.

29. Bern M, Lokich J, Wallach S et al, Very low doses of warfarin can prevent thrombosis in central venous catheters. *Ann Intern Med* 1990; **112:** 423–8.

30. Ross P, Cunningham D, Protracted infusion of 5-FU for colorectal cancer. In: *Management of Colorectal Cancer* (Bleiberg H, Rougier P, Wilke H-J, eds). London: Martin Dunitz, 1998: 249–57.

31. Anderson N, Lokich J, Controversial issues in 5-fluorouracil infusion use. *Cancer* 1992; **70**(Suppl): 998–1002.

32. Lokich J, Moore C, Anderson N, Comparison of costs for infusion versus bolus chemotherapy administration: analysis of five standard chemotherapy regimens in three common tumors – Part one. *Cancer* 1996; **78:** 294–9.

33. Lokich J, Moore C, Anderson N, Comparison of costs for infusion versus bolus chemotherapy administration – Part two. *Cancer* 1996; **78:** 300–3.

34. Berkowitz N, Gupta S, Silberman G et al, Comparing the cost-effectiveness in the treatment of metastatic breast cancer. *Manag Care Cancer* 1999; **Sept/Oct:** 18–26.

47

Oral fluoropyrimidines in colorectal neoplasia

Melanie B Thomas, Paulo M Hoff

INTRODUCTION

Since its initial synthesis more than 40 years ago, 5-fluorouracil (5-FU) has become one of the most widely used chemotherapy agents, and is now included in nearly all adjuvant and palliative regimens used for colorectal cancer. 5-FU has been investigated as a single agent, in combination with biomodulators such as leucovorin (folinic acid), as part of complex bolus and continuous-infusion schedules, and for administration via intrahepatic arterial infusion. Each of the numerous routes of administration and dosing schedules for 5-FU has a distinct toxicity profile, and several studies and meta-analyses have shown that prolonged exposure to 5-FU and a high dose intensity may be important in maximizing the antitumor activity of this drug.[1–4]

Infusional regimens of 5-FU, which result in prolonged exposure of tumor cells to this agent, are widely used. Compared with bolus administration, continuous infusions of 5-FU are also associated with considerably lower toxicity (principally less mucositis and diarrhea), improved response rates, and possibly prolonged overall patient survival.[3,4] However, continuous infusion requires central access devices, with their attendant costs, inconvenience to patients, and potential for costly and morbid complications. These factors, along with patient preference for an oral regimen, have contributed to the development of oral 5-FU preparations.

The intent of this chapter is to review the development of oral fluoropyrimidine agents for colorectal cancer and to summarize their efficacy and future role in the treatment of this important disease.

PHARMACOLOGY OF FLUOROPYRIMIDINES

5-FU was one of the first rationally developed chemotherapy agents. The drug acts as a 'false' pyrimidine, differing from the naturally occurring base uracil by the addition of a fluoride at position 5. Researchers believe that the drug enters cells by cell-mediated processes and, once within the cell, undergoes conversion to 5-fluorouridine 5′-monophosphate (FUMP), 5-fluorouridine 5′-triphosphate (FUTP), and 5-fluoro-2′-deoxyuridine 5′-monophosphate (FdUMP). The cytotoxicity of fluorouracil is believed to be related to the following actions: (1) inhibition of thymidylate synthase by FdUMP, (2) incorporation of FUTP into cellular RNA, and (3) incorporation of fluorodeoxyuridine triphosphate (FdUTP) into cellular DNA (Figure 47.1).[5] The drug exerts several cytotoxic effects, including inhibition of DNA synthesis, induction of DNA strand breaks, and misincorporation of nucleotides into DNA and RNA.[6–8] 5-FU is an antimetabolite, and is most actively incorporated into cells during the S phase of the cell cycle.[5,8] Oral absorption is poor, and the drug was developed for parenteral administration. 5-FU pharmacokinetics are influenced by the dosing and administration schedule. Less than 10% of the parent drug is cleared in the urine; the balance is cleared by catabolism. Whether given by bolus or by continuous infusion, 5-FU readily penetrates the extracellular space as well as 'third spaces', such as cerebrospinal fluid, ascites, and pleural effusions. Most intravenously administered 5-FU is rapidly catabolized and is therefore unavailable for inhibition of cell growth. The clearance of 5-FU is governed by the activity of the cytosolic enzyme dihydropyrimidine dehydrogenase (DPD). The activity of DPD is inversely proportional to the amount of 5-FU available for conversion

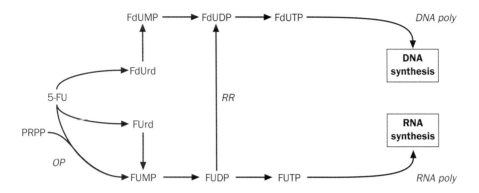

Figure 47.1 Intracellular pathways for 5-fluorouracil (5-FU). *Abbreviations:* FdUrd, 5-fluoro-2'-deoxyuridine (floxuridine); FdUMP/FdUDP/FdUTP, 5-fluoro-2'-deoxyuridine 5'-mono-/di-/triphosphate; FUrd, 5-fluorouridine; FUMP/FUDP/FUTP, 5-fluorouridine 5'-mono-/di-/triphosphate; PRPP, phosphoribosyl pyrophosphate; *OP*, orotate phosphoribosyltransferase; *RR*, ribonucleotide reductase; *DNA poly*, DNA polymerase; *RNA poly*, RNA polymerase.

to active nucleotide metabolites. Because the DPD levels in the gastrointestinal (GI) tract and plasma vary widely among patients, the bioavailability of 5-FU is also highly variable. The inter- and intra-individual variability of levels of DPD, and thus 5-FU, results from several factors, including genetic deficiencies, and variability of intestinal concentrations of DPD throughout the day.[8–11] 5-FU is commonly coadministered with biomodulating compounds such as leucovorin. The combination of 5-FU with leucovorin is based on the ability of leucovorin to raise cellular concentrations of reduced folates and thus to increase the stability of a ternary complex formed from the combination of FdUMP, thymidylate synthase, and reduced folate (methylated tetrahydrofolate).[12] The resulting increased stability of the ternary complex leads to prolonged inhibition of thymidylate synthase and thus to increased cytotoxicity.

RATIONALE FOR DEVELOPMENT OF ORAL FLUOROPYRIMIDINES

Continuous-infusion regimens have acceptable toxicity profiles and are possibly more cytotoxic than bolus schedules.[3,4] Researchers have shown great interest in developing oral regimens that would provide serum levels approximating those achieved by continuous infusion while reducing costs, increasing patient convenience, and avoiding morbidity. Owing to variable absorption from the GI tract and rapid clearance by DPD, 5-FU is not suitable for oral administration. However, researchers have developed several alternative formulations to circumvent

this problem while providing drug serum levels that approximate those achieved by continuous infusion. These include a variety of pharmacologic manipulations designed to overcome 5-FU degradation by enzymes in the GI tract. The sections that follow review current information regarding the most widely used oral formulations of 5-FU. Table 47.1 summarizes the activities and current status of these formulations.

Capecitabine

Capecitabine (Figure 47.2), an oral formulation of 5-FU, was developed as an alternative to intravenous 5-FU. Compared with the parenteral compound, capecitabine provides greater tumor selectivity while minimizing systemic exposure. The drug is well absorbed via the GI tract and is catabolized to the active drug by a series of three enzymes. Capecitabine is absorbed as an intact molecule

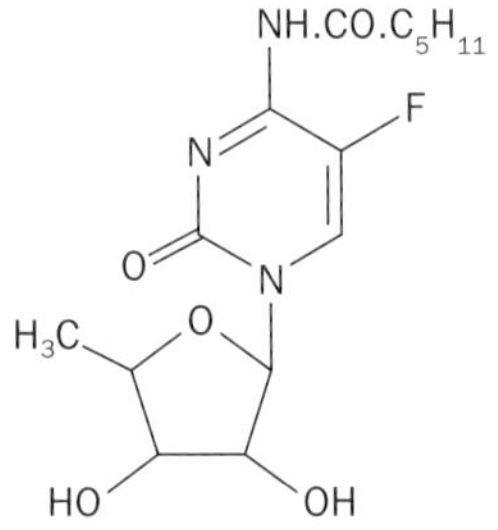

Figure 47.2 Chemical structure of capecitabine.

Table 47.1 Oral fluorinated pyrimidines

Agent	Preclinical advantages of intravenous 5-FU	Current status in the USA
UFT	Combines tegafur with uracil, a DPD inhibitor	Phase III (in combination)
UFT + leucovorin	Double modulation of 5-FU by uracil and leucovorin	Phase III trials in advanced colorectal cancer completed; NSABP (C-06); adjuvant trial in stage II and III colon cancer
Capecitabine	Higher 5-FU tumor concentrations compared with plasma and normal tissue; 'tumor selectivity'	FDA approved for breast cancer
S-1	DPD inhibition by CDHP (200 times that of uracil); reduction in diarrhea by potassium oxonate	Phase I
Eniluracil + oral 5-FU	Reproducible oral bioavailability of 5-FU; inactivation of tumoral DPD (a potential tumor-resistance mechanism); elimination of 5-FU catabolites, which may interfere with 5-FU activity	Phase III trial in advanced colorectal cancer ongoing
TAS-102	Combines a fluoropyrimidine (FTD) with a thymidine phosphorylase inhibitor	Phase I

through the intestinal mucosa,[13] is metabolized in the liver by carboxylesterase to 5'-deoxy-5-fluorocytidine (5'-DFCR), which is converted by cytidine deaminase to 5'-deoxy-5-fluorouridine (5'-DFUR, doxifluridine), mainly in the liver and in tumor tissues. Finally, 5'-DFUR is metabolized by thymidine phosphorylase, also known as platelet-derived endothelial cell growth factor (PD-ECGF), to 5-FU at the tumor site. Colorectal cancers, like many other solid tumors, tend to have high levels of PD-ECGF.[14,15] Levels of 5-FU in human cancer animal xenograft models were higher in those treated with orally administered capecitabine than in those treated with parenteral 5-FU.[14]

Capecitabine has been studied in phase I trials as a single agent on three schedules: (1) continuous oral twice-daily dosing; (2) twice-daily oral dosing for 14 days with a 7-day rest before resumption of the cycle; and (3) a fixed dose of leucovorin (60 mg/day) with either the continuous schedule or the intermittent schedule.[16–18] The dose-limiting toxicities in phase I trials were diarrhea, vomiting, and hand–foot syndrome (palmar–plantar erythrodysesthesia).

A large, randomized, open-label phase II trial conducted in Europe, North America, and Australia evaluated three schedules of capecitabine (continuous, intermittent, and intermittent with oral leucovorin) in metastatic colon cancer.[19] The addition of leucovorin seemed to increase the incidence of side-effects without a benefit on response rates or survival times. The response rates for the three schedules ranged from 21% to 24%; the median time to disease progression ranged from 127 days to 230 days, with the longest time to progression being seen in the capecitabine intermittent arm (without leucovorin). This schedule, which consists of twice-daily dosing for 14 days followed by 7 days' rest, was further evaluated in two phase III trials.

Results have been presented for two trials comparing capecitabine with 5-FU on the Mayo regimen ($425 \, \text{mg/m}^2$ per day 5-FU delivered as a bolus injection plus $20 \, \text{mg/m}^2$ per day for 5 days every 4 weeks) in patients with metastatic colon cancer.[20,21] Each of these large trials included more than 600 patients. In the trial conducted in 61 centers in the USA, Brazil, Canada, and Mexico, a total of 605 patients were randomized to receive either 2500 mg/m^2 per day capecitabine in divided daily doses for 14 days followed by 7 days' rest or the Mayo regimen described above.[20] Capecitabine was more active than 5-FU in the induction of tumor response, and the two groups showed similar times to tumor response and response durations. Times to disease progression and overall survival times were comparable for the two regimens, but the toxicity of capecitabine was less than that of 5-FU, with a substantially lower incidence of diarrhea, stomatitis, nausea, and alopecia. However, capecitabine was associated with a higher incidence of palmar–plantar erythrodysesthesia.

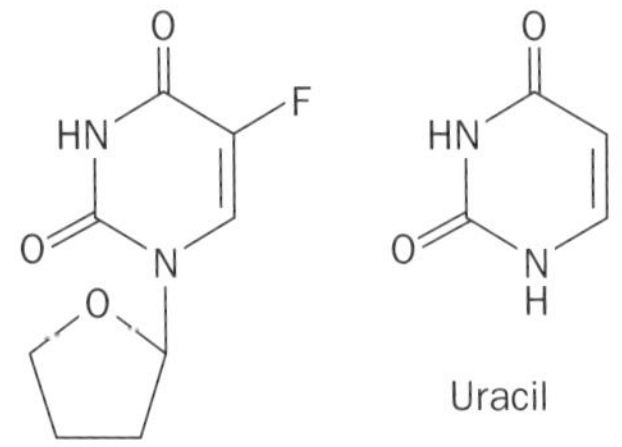

Figure 47.3 Chemical composition of UFT (uracil plus tegafur in a 4 : 1 molar ratio).

UFT plus leucovorin

UFT (Figure 47.3) is an oral antineoplastic drug that combines the DPD inhibitor uracil with the 5-FU prodrug tegafur in a 4 : 1 molar ratio. UFT was initially synthesized in Japan approximately 20 years ago, and has been widely used in a variety of solid tumors, including gastric, breast, colorectal, bladder, and head and neck cancers. Since the early 1990s, researchers have investigated UFT in numerous clinical trials in the USA and Europe.[22] UFT was rationally developed to exploit the fact that uracil competes with 5-FU for DPD and inhibits the degradation of the 5-FU generated by tegafur.[23,24] Tegafur (ftorafur), a 5-FU prodrug that was originally developed in the Soviet Union, is slowly metabolized by hepatic microsomal cytochrome P450.[25–27] After the conversion, the metabolism and cytotoxic activity of the 5-FU generated by tegafur are identical to those of parenteral 5-FU. Compared with 5-FU alone, administration of UFT results in higher concentrations of 5-FU in tumors.[22,28]

Owing to extensive prior experience with leucovorin in combination with 5-FU, UFT was combined with oral leucovorin in the USA. The addition of leucovorin to 5-FU regimens increases the intracellular concentrations of reduced folates, and stabilizes the FdUMP/thymidylate synthase enzyme complex, responsible for the drug's cytotoxic activity.[12] In phase I trials of UFT and leucovorin as a single agent in the USA, the total daily dose was divided into three doses given every 8 hours on a 5- or 28-day schedule. The dose-limiting toxicities of the 5- and 28-day schedules were neutropenia and diarrhea, respectively. The recommended phase II dose for the 28-day schedule was UFT 300–350 mg/m^2 per day and leucovorin 150 mg/day.[29] The rationale for the

28-day schedule with daily oral dosing of UFT plus leucovorin was to mimic the effects of a continuous infusion of 5-FU.

One trial in the USA studied 45 patients with previously untreated metastatic colorectal cancer using doses of 350 mg/m^2 per day of UFT plus 150 mg/day of leucovorin. The overall response rate was 42.2%. Diarrhea was the major dose-limiting toxicity, and the UFT dose was reduced to 300 mg/m^2 per day after the first 7 patients treated experienced this side-effect. No grade 3 or 4 neutropenia, mucositis, or hand–foot syndrome was observed.[30]

Because of the efficacy and favorable toxicity profile of this drug combination in phase II trials, two large, multinational phase III trials compared UFT plus leucovorin versus the Mayo regimen of 5-FU and leucovorin in patients with previously untreated advanced colon cancer. A regimen of UFT 300 mg/m^2 per day plus oral leucovorin 75 or 90 mg/day for 28 days every 5 weeks was compared with 5-FU 425 mg/m^2 per day plus leucovorin 20 mg/m^2 per day intravenously for 5 days every 4 weeks[31] or 5 weeks.[32] The larger study with 816 patients[31] reported similar overall response rates (12% for UFT plus leucovorin versus 15% for 5-FU plus leucovorin) and no statistically significant difference in survival times. In the second study, which included 380 patients,[32] the two regimens demonstrated similar times to disease progression, median survival times, and response rates. However, in both studies, the UFT plus leucovorin regimen showed significantly lower toxicity, with a lower incidence of grade 3 mucositis, myelosuppression, febrile neutropenia, and infections, and no notable hand–foot syndrome.[24]

The combination of UFT plus leucovorin has generated much interest owing to its potential in the adjuvant setting. Several groups have explored the oral agent as an alternative to conventional 5-FU given intravenously. The National Surgical Adjuvant Breast and Bowel Project (NSABP) has enrolled more than 1500 patients in the NSABP C-06 trial, which compared the conventional 5-FU plus leucovorin regimen with the UFT plus leucovorin regimen in patients with stages II and III colon cancer. The results of this trial are eagerly anticipated. The combination of UFT and leucovorin has also been explored as a radiation sensitizer in the treatment of pancreatic and rectal cancers.[33]

Eniluracil plus oral 5-FU

Because 5-FU is rapidly catabolized by endogenous DPD, the systemic levels of 5-FU produced from a given dose may vary greatly and render efficacy and toxicity unpredictable. The variable levels of intestinal DPD cause erratic oral absorption and preclude oral administration of 5-FU. In addition, some tumors contain high levels of DPD and are believed to be less likely to respond to 5-FU treatment. The metabolic byproducts of 5-FU may be largely responsible for the toxic side-effects, which are cardiac toxicity, neurotoxicity, hand–foot syndrome, and GI toxicity.[11,34]

Eniluracil (5-ethynyluracil, 776C85) is a potent irreversible inhibitor of DPD that completely prevents the catabolism of 5-FU.[11] The route of elimination of 5-FU changes from rapid catabolism to renal clearance. Eniluracil enables oral dosing of conventional 5-FU to replace intravenous bolus and continuous infusion of this agent.

A phase I trial conducted in the USA compared the maximum tolerated dose, toxicity, and pharmacokinetics of twice-daily oral 5-FU with eniluracil. Maximum inactivation of DPD was achieved using eniluracil doses ranging from 10 to 40 mg/day. The pharmacokinetic parameters of oral 5-FU were independent of the eniluracil dose. Concentrations of 5-FU in this oral regimen were comparable to steady-state levels obtained by continuous infusions of 5-FU. Toxicities included nausea, vomiting, mucositis, pain, dehydration, and constipation. Grade 3 or 4 side-effects included fatigue in 6% and diarrhea in 1% of patients.[11]

A subsequent multicenter phase II trial used a regimen of 1.0 mg/m^2 5-FU plus 10 mg/m^2 eniluracil, orally twice daily for 28 days followed by a 7-day rest. Owing to the low toxicity levels initially encountered, the doses of both agents were increased to 1.15 mg/m^2 and 11.5 mg/m^2, respectively. The overall response rate was 25%.[35] Currently, two phase III trials in patients with metastatic colorectal cancer are being conducted to compare this oral combination regimen with bolus 5-FU plus leucovorin. Other trials are comparing oral eniluracil plus oral 5-FU versus continuous-infusion 5-FU, oral eniluracil plus 5-FU in patients with colorectal cancer refractory to intravenous 5-FU, and a variety of schedule modifications using these two drugs.

S-1

S-1 is a novel oral fluoropyrimidine combination developed in Japan. The drug consists of tegafur and two 5-FU-modulating agents: 5-chloro-2,4-dihydroxypyrimidine (CDHP) and potassium oxonate (1,3,5-triazine 2,4(1H,3H)-dione-6-carboxylate) at fixed molar concentrations of 1 : 0.4 : 1. CDHP, a competitive inhibitor of 5-FU catabolism, is about 200 times more potent than uracil in inhibiting DPD.[36] When tegafur is combined with CDHP, the resulting 5-FU levels are maintained in both plasma and tumor. Potassium oxonate inhibits orotate phosphoribosyltransferase, the enzyme that phosphorylates 5-FU in the GI tract. Thus, potassium oxonate is expected to decrease the GI toxicity of 5-FU without interfering with its antitumor activity. The cytotoxic activity of S-1 is ultimately exerted by 5-FU through antimetabolite effects on DNA and RNA levels, as described above.

Phase I trials of S-1 have been conducted in Japan, Europe, and the USA. Japanese investigators administered S-1 to patients with advanced solid tumors for 28 consecutive days followed by a 14-day rest. In one Japanese study that compared once- versus twice-daily dosing schedules, the maximum tolerated doses of S-1 were 75–100 mg for the twice-daily regimen and 150–200 mg for the once-daily regimen. Toxicity was primarily hematologic, and GI side-effects were mild. Another phase I study treated 12 patients with fixed doses of S-1 according to ranges of body surface area (BSA). Patients with BSA < 1.25 m^2 received 40 mg twice daily, and patients with BSA > 1.5 m^2 were given 60 mg twice daily. This fixed-dose system, based on ranges of BSA, was used in all subsequent Japanese phase II trials.

Phase I studies in the USA and Europe used a dosing system based on actual BSA values. A European Organization for the Research and Treatment of Cancer (EORTC) study of 15 patients who received S-1 for 28 days followed by a 7-day rest used a starting dose of 25 mg/m^2 twice daily. At 45 mg/m^2 and 40 mg/m^2 twice daily, the dose-limiting toxicity of grade 3 or 4 diarrhea was reached.[37] A phase I study conducted at the University of Texas MD Anderson Cancer Center also evaluated a 28-day course of S-1 followed by 7 days of rest. The dose-limiting toxicity was diarrhea, as in the European study, and was reached at the dose of 35 mg/m² twice daily.[38]

Phase II studies in patients with gastric cancer were conducted in Japan, where S-1 was subsequently approved for use in this disease on the basis of a response rate of around 50%. The EORTC Early Clinical Studies Group has launched an early phase II study of S-1 for patients with advanced or metastatic gastric and colorectal cancer.

TAS-102

TAS-102 is a novel functional antitumor nucleoside. It is a 1 : 0.5 molar combination of 2′-deoxy-5-(trifluoromethyl)uridine (α,α,α-trifluorothymidine, FTD) and an inhibitor of thymidine phosphorylase (TPI). As discussed above, in human tumors, 5-FU is metabolized to FUMP and is then converted to the active nucleotide forms FUTP and FdUMP. The primary mechanism of cytotoxicity appears to be FdUMP inhibition of thymidylate synthase (TS) and thus inhibition of DNA synthesis. It has been postulated that resistance and/or ineffectiveness of 5-FU in cancer patients may be due to overexpression of intratumoral TS.[39] The antineoplastic antimetabolite FTD is a TS inhibitor similar to 5-FU.[40,41] However, when FTD is incubated with cancer cells at a high concentration for short periods, it is passively incorporated into DNA. This activity differs from the cytotoxic mechanism of 5-FU and 5-fluoro-2′-deoxyuridine (FdUrd, floxuridine), which inhibits TS.[42] After FTD is orally administered, it is rapidly degraded to an inactive form by thymidine phosphorylase (TP). Coadministration of TPI with FTD should increase the concentration of available FTD in the body, leading to augmentation of the cytotoxicity of FTD. Thymidine phosphorylase has been shown to be the same protein as PD-ECGF,[43] and a TPI may have antiangiogenic activity on its own. In preclinical studies, TAS-102 was effective against human tumors – both those that were highly sensitive to 5-FU and those characterized by innate and acquired resistance to 5-FU. Furthermore, TAS-102 has shown potent activity against primary carcinomas and against the processes of tumor-derived angiogenesis and metastasis. Phase I studies of TAS-102 are currently underway in the USA.

FUTURE DIRECTIONS

The fluoropyrimidines are an important part of the therapeutic arsenal against cancer. Gastrointestinal cancers are particularly sensitive to these agents, and 5-FU remains the cornerstone of treatment regimens for colorectal cancer. Compared with traditional, intravenous agents, the use of oral fluoropyrimidines brings important advantages, since they allow for a protracted dosing without the cost and risks associated with central venous catheters and portable pumps, while maintaining the lower toxicity associated with those regimens. Both oral capecitabine and oral UFT-plus-leucovorin regimens can be used instead of intravenous 5-FU in the treatment of colon cancer, and each of these regimens offers a more favorable safety profile. This type of therapy may be particularly attractive for treating frail or elderly patients who are unwilling to use the traditional intravenous agents.

The possibility of using the oral fluoropyrimidines as radiosensitizing agents has recently been explored, and has been shown to be feasible. This new use of oral agents opens a new field of research that could have important implications in the future treatment of common tumors such as rectal and head and neck cancers. The favorable safety profile of the oral fluoropyrimidines studied to date also makes them potential targets for use in combination with other drugs that have demonstrated activity when combined with intravenous 5-FU. Several trials are underway to explore combinations of oral fluoropyrimidines with agents such as irinotecan and oxaliplatin. Although the benefits seen in patient safety, comfort, and convenience would seem sufficient to justify the widespread use of oral fluoropyrimidines, research continues in an attempt to develop newer agents with improved therapeutic efficacy and safety profiles.

REFERENCES

1. International Multicentre Pooled Analysis of Colon Cancer Trials (IMPACT) investigators, Efficacy of adjuvant fluorouracil and folinic acid in colon cancer. *Lancet* 1995; **345:** 939–44.

2. Caudry M, Bonnel C, Floquet A et al, A randomized study of bolus fluorouracil plus folinic acid versus 21-day fluorouracil infusion alone or in association with cyclophosphamide and mitomycin C in advanced colorectal carcinoma. *Am J Clin Oncol* 1995; **18:** 118–25.

3. Lokich J, Infusional 5-FU: historical evolution, rationale, and clinical experience. *Oncology (Huntingt)* 1998; **12**(10 Suppl 7): 19–22.

4. Meta-analysis Group in Cancer, Efficacy of intravenous continuous infusion of fluorouracil compared with bolus administra-

tion in advanced colorectal cancer. *J Clin Oncol* 1998; **16**: 301–8.

5. Perry MC, *The Chemotherapy Source Book*, 2nd edn. Columbia, Missouri: Williams & Wilkins, 1997.

6. Almersjo OE, Gustavsson BG, Regardh CG et al, Pharmacokinetic studies of 5-fluorouracil after oral and intravenous administration in man. *Acta Pharmacol Toxicol* 1980; **46**: 329–36.

7. Diasio RB, Harris BE, Clinical pharmacology of 5-fluorouracil. *Clin Pharmacokinet* 1989; **16**: 215–37.

8. Grem JL, 5-Fluorouracil: forty-plus and still ticking. A review of its preclinical development. *Invest New Drugs* 2000; **18**: 299–313.

9. Diasio RB, Beavers TL, Carpenter JT, Familial deficiency of dihydropyrimidine dehydrogenase. Biochemical basis for familial pyrimidinemia and severe 5-fluorouracil-induced toxicity. *J Clin Invest* 1988; **81**: 47–51.

10. Diasio RB, Van Kuilenburg AB, Lu Z et al, Determination of dihydropyrimidine dehydrogenase (DPD) in fibroblasts of a DPD deficient pediatric patient and family members using a polyclonal antibody to human DPD. *Adv Exp Med Biol* 1994; **370**: 7–10.

11. Paff M, Baccanari D, Davis ST et al, Preclinical development of eniluracil: enhancing the therapeutic index and dosing convenience of 5-fluorouracil. *Invest New Drugs* 2000; **18**: 365–71.

12. Mini E, Trave F, Rustum YM et al, Enhancement of the antitumor effects of 5-fluorouracil by folinic acid. *Pharmacol Ther* 1990; **47**: 1–19.

13. Hoff PM, Royce M, Medgyesy D et al, Oral fluoropyrimidines. *Semin Oncol* 1999; **26**: 640–6.

14. Ishikawa T, Utoh M, Sawada N et al, Tumor selective delivery of 5-fluorouracil by capecitabine, a new oral fluoropyrimidine carbamate, in human cancer xenografts. *Biochem Pharmacol* 1998; **55**: 1091–7.

15. Miwa M, Ura M, Nishida M et al, Design of a novel oral fluoropyrimidine carbamate, capecitabine, which generates 5-fluorouracil selectively in tumours by enzymes concentrated in human liver and cancer tissue. *Eur J Cancer* 1998; **34**: 1274–81.

16. Budman DR, Capecitabine. *Invest New Drugs* 2000; **18**: 355–63.

17. Budman DR, Meropol NJ, Reigner B et al, Preliminary studies of a novel oral fluoropyrimidine carbamate: capecitabine. *J Clin Oncol* 1998; **16**: 1795–802.

18. Cassidy J, Dirix L, Bissett D et al, A phase I study of capecitabine in combination with oral leucovorin in patients with intractable solid tumors. *Clin Cancer Res* 1998; **4**: 2755–61.

19. Van Cutsem E, Findlay M, Osterwalder B et al, Capecitabine, an oral fluoropyrimidine carbamate with substantial activity in advanced colorectal cancer: results of a randomized phase II study. *J Clin Oncol* 2000; **18**: 1337–45.

20. Hoff PM, Ansari R, Batist G et al, Comparison of oral capecitabine (Xeloda) versus intravenous 5-fluorouracil plus leucovorin (Mayo Clinic regimen) as first-line treatment in 605 patients with metastatic colorectal cancer: results of a randomized phase III study. *J Clin Oncol* 2001; **19**: 2282–92.

21. Twelves C, Harper P, Van Cutsem E et al, A phase III trial (SO14796) of Xeloda™ (capecitabine) in previously untreated advanced/metastatic colorectal cancer. *Proc Am Soc Clin Oncol* 1999; **18**: 263a.

22. Hoff PM, Pazdur R, Benner SE et al, UFT and leucovorin: a review of its clinical development and therapeutic potential in the oral treatment of cancer. *Anticancer Drugs* 1998; **9**: 479–490.

23. Rustum YM, Mechanism-based improvement in the therapeutic selectivity of 5-FU prodrug alone and under conditions of metabolic modulation. *Oncology* 1997; **54**(Suppl 11): 7–11.

24. Hoff PM, The tegafur-based dihydropyrimidine dehydrogenase inhibitory fluoropyrimidines, UFT/leucovorin (ORZEL™) and S-1; a review of their clinical development and therapeutic potential. *Invest Drugs* 2000; **18**: 331–42.

25. Au JL, Sadee W, Activation of ftorafur [*R,S*-1-(tetrahydro-2-furanyl)-5-fluorouracil] to 5-fluorouracil and gamma-butyrolactone. *Cancer Res* 1980; **40**(8 Pt 1): 2814–19.

26. El Sayed YM, Sadee W, Metabolic activation of ftorafur [*R,S*-1-(tetrahydro-2-furanyl)-5-fluorouracil]: the microsomal oxidative pathway. *Biochem Pharmacol* 1982; **31**: 3006–8.

27. El Sayed YM, Sadee W, Metabolic activation of *R,S*-1-(tetrahydro-2-furanyl)-5-fluorouracil (ftorafur) to 5-fluorouracil by soluble enzymes. *Cancer Res* 1983; **43**: 4039–44.

28. Heggie GD, Sommadossi JP, Cross DS et al, Clinical pharmacokinetics of 5-fluorouracil and its metabolites in plasma, urine, and bile. *Cancer Res* 1987; **47**: 2203–6.

29. Pazdur R, Lassere Y, Diaz-Canton E et al, Phase I trial of uracil–tegafur (UFT) plus oral leucovorin: 28-day schedule. *Cancer Invest* 1998; **16**: 145–51.

30. Pazdur R, Lassere Y, Rhodes JA et al, Phase II trial of uracil and tegafur plus oral leucovorin: an effective oral regimen in the treatment of metastatic colorectal carcinoma. *J Clin Oncol* 1994; **12**: 2296–300.

31. Pazdur R, Douillard J-Y, Skillings JR et al, Multicenter phase III study of 5-fluorouracil (5-FU) or UFT in combination with leucovorin (LV) in patients with metastatic colorectal cancer. *Proc Am Soc Clin Oncol* 1999; **18**: 263a.

32. Carmichael J, Popieta T, Radstone D et al, Randomized comparative study of Orzel (oral uracil/tegafur (UFT) plus leucovorin (LV)) versus parenteral 5-fluorouracil (5-FU) plus LV in patients with metastatic colorectal cancer. *Proc Am Soc Clin Oncol* 1999; **18**: 264a.

33. Hoff PM, Brito R, Slaughter C et al, Preoperative UFT, oral leucovorin (LV) and radiotherapy (RT) for patients (PTS) with resectable rectal carcinoma: an oral regimen with complete pathological responses. *Proc Am Soc Clin Oncol* 1998; **17**: 223a.

34. Diasio RB, The role of dihydropyrimidine dehydrogenase (DPD) modulation in 5-FU pharmacology. *Oncology* 1998; **12**: 23–7.

35. Mani S, Hochster H, Beck T et al, Multicenter phase II study to evaluate a 28-day regimen of oral fluorouracil plus eniluracil in the treatment of patients with previously untreated metastatic colorectal cancer. *J Clin Oncol* 2000; **18**: 2894–901.

36. Tatsumi K, Fukushima M, Shirasaka T et al, Inhibitory effects of pyrimidine, barbituric acid and pyridine derivatives on 5-fluorouracil degradation in rat liver extracts. *Jpn J Cancer Res* 1987; **78**: 748–55.

37. van Groeningen CJ, Godefridus JP, Schornagel JH et al, Phase I clinical and pharmacokinetic study of oral S-1 in patients with advanced solid tumors. *J Clin Oncol* 2000; **18**: 2772–9.

38. Hoff PM, Wenske C, Medgyesy D et al, Phase I and pharmacokinetic (PK) study of the novel oral fluoropyrimidine, S-1. *Proc Am Soc Clin Oncol* 1999; **18**: 173a.

39. Leichman CG, Lenz HJ, Leichman L et al, Quantitation of intratumoral thymidylate synthase expression predicts for disseminated colorectal cancer response and resistance to protracted-infusion fluorouracil and weekly leucovorin. *J Clin Oncol* 1997; **15**: 3223–9.

40. Reyes P, Heidelberger C, Fluorinated pyrimidines. Mammalian thymidylate synthetase; its mechanism of action and inhibition by fluorinated nucleotides. *Mol Pharmacol* 1965; **1**: 14–30.

41. Heidelberger C, Anderson SW, Fluorinated pyrimidines. The tumor-inhibitory activity of 5-trifluoromethyl-2'-deoxyuridine. *Cancer Res* 1964; **24**: 1979–85.

42. Santi D, Sakai TT, Thymidylate synthetase. Model studies of inhibition by 5-trifluoromethyl-2'-deoxyuridylic acid. *Biochemistry* 1971; **10**: 3598–607.

43. Emura T, Suzuki N, Murukami Y et al, Invention of a novel antitumor agent, TAS-102. (1) Effect of 5-trifluorothymidine on 5-FU and FdUrd-resistant tumor cells. *Proc Am Assoc Cancer Res* 1997; **38**: 475.

48

5-FU in combination with DPD inhibitors

Robert B Diasio

INTRODUCTION

It has now been more than 40 years since the cancer chemotherapeutic agent 5-fluorouracil (5-FU) was first synthesized and introduced as a drug for treating colorectal cancer.[1] 5-FU is classified as an antimetabolite type of antineoplastic drug, being an analog of the naturally occurring pyrimidine uracil. It was synthesized to take advantage not only of this structural similarity to uracil but also the fact that uracil is a necessary growth factor for many tumors. 5-FU differs from uracil in having a fluorine atom substituted for a hydrogen atom in position 5 of the pyrimidine ring.

Although 5-FU has been used extensively since being introduced clinically in the late 1950s, there have been numerous attempts over the past four decades to develop 5-FU-like drugs with more desirable pharmacologic properties, in particular formulations that can be orally administered.[2] While numerous compounds have been synthesized, few have ultimately been approved for clinical use.

METABOLISM OF FLUOROPYRIMIDINE DRUGS

Similar to uracil and thymine, 5-FU can pass through the cell membrane and then be metabolized by the pyrimidine anabolic and catabolic pathways (see Figure 48.1).[1]

Anabolism results in the formation of the 5-FU

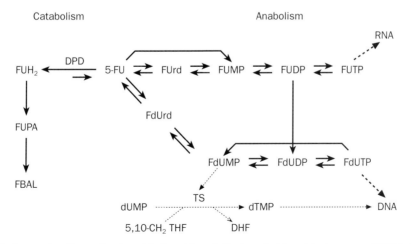

Figure 48.1 Metabolic overview illustrating the critical position of dihydropyrimidine dehydrogenase (DPD) in the metabolism of 5-fluorouracil (5-FU). FUH$_2$, 5-fluoro-5,6-dihydrouracil; FUPA, α-fluoro-β-ureidopropionate; FBAL, α-fluoro-β-alanine; FUrd, 5-fluorouridine; FUMP/FUDP/FUTP, 5-fluorouridine mono-/di-/triphosphate; FdUrd, 5-fluoro-2'-deoxyuridine (floxuridine); FdUMP/FdUDP/FdUTP, 5-fluoro-2'-deoxyuridine mono-/di-/triphosphate; TS, thymidylate synthase; dUMP, deoxyuridine monophosphate; dTMP, deoxythymidine monophosphate; 5,10-CH$_2$THF, N^5,N^{10}-methylenetetrahydrofolate; DHF, dihydrofolate.

nucleotide metabolites 5-fluorodeoxyuridine 5'-monophosphate (FdUMP), 5-fluorouridine 5'-triphosphate (FUTP), and 5-fluoro-2'-deoxyuridine 5'-triphosphate (FdUTP), which, through affecting indirectly or directly nucleic acid synthesis and/or function, can in turn block cell replication. This occurs through inhibition of thymidylate synthase or via incorporation of the 5-FU nucleotides FUTP and FdUTP into RNA and DNA, respectively.

While anabolism is clearly important to the cytotoxicity of 5-FU, over the past several years, there has been an increasing recognition of the important role of catabolism in 5-FU pharmacology, which regulates the amount of 5-FU that can be anabolized.[3] The first enzyme in catabolism, dihydropyrimidine dehydrogenase (DPD, also known as dihydrouracil dehydrogenase, dihydrothymine dehydrogenase, uracil reductase, and EC 1.3.1.2), is the critical rate-limiting step in the regulation of 5-FU metabolism.[4] DPD is responsible for converting more than 85% of clinically administered 5-FU to FUH_2 (5-fluoro-5,6-dihydrouracil: an inactive metabolite) in an essentially irreversible enzymatic step.[5]

IMPORTANCE OF DPD IN FLUOROPYRIMIDINE PHARMACOLOGY

DPD activity is known to vary, both within individual patients and from patient to patient, and has been shown to be responsible for much of the variability in the clinical pharmacology of 5-FU. The effects of variable DPD activity on the clinical pharmacology of 5-FU are summarized in Table 48.1.

Within a single patient, DPD activity can be shown to vary over a 24-hour period.[6] This intrapatient variation in DPD activity has been shown to be associated with a concomitant variation in 5-FU levels of patients receiving a constant intravenous (pro-tracted) infusion of 5-FU. The DPD activity has been shown to follow a circadian pattern with a peak and trough that can be plotted on a cosine wave.[6,7] The 5-FU levels in these patients also have a circadian pattern that is the inverse of the circadian pattern observed with the DPD levels. This finding has prompted some chemotherapists to propose the use of time-modified 5-FU infusions to optimize drug delivery during a 24-hour period as a potential benefit in the treatment of certain human cancers.[8]

DPD activity has also been shown to vary from patient to patient among patients who otherwise have similar liver function. This interpatient variation in DPD is now thought to be responsible for the large variation in 5-FU pharmacokinetics ($t_{1/2\beta}$ and clearance) observed from patient to patient. Following administration of an intravenous bolus of 5-FU, $t_{1/2\beta}$ was shown to vary almost fivefold among patients studied.[5] DPD enzyme activity in normal tissues (peripheral blood mononuclear cells and liver) was also shown to vary from individual to individual with a Gaussian (normal, or bell-shaped) distribution pattern, with as much as a sixfold variation from the lowest to the highest values.[9,10] It is now accepted that the wide variation in DPD activity observed from patient to patient is responsible for the wide variation in the $t_{1/2\beta}$ observed in population studies.

Although most individuals have DPD activity that varies within a Gaussian distribution, a small percentage (<5%) of the population has DPD activity that can be shown to be statistically significantly lower.[11–13] Such individuals are at a significant risk if subsequently treated with 5-FU. Normal catabolism of 5-FU does not occur, resulting in much more 5-FU being available for anabolism. Patients having decreased DPD activity (i.e. DPD deficiency) have a clinical presentation that is typical of a drug overdose after being treated with 5-FU. This is an

---

Table 48.1 Importance of variability in DPD activity in 5-FU pharmacology

- Variability in DPD activity over 24 hours (circadian variation) explains the variability in 5-FU blood levels observed in patients receiving continuous (protracted) continuous infusion of 5-FU; implication for time-modified therapy.
- Variability of 5-FU clinical pharmacokinetics ($t_{1/2\beta}$ and clearance) related to variability in DPD.
- Variability of 5-FU catabolism due to variability in gene expression of DPD in turn secondary to sequence changes in the DPD gene; genetic deficiency of DPD (pharmacogenetic syndrome).
- Variability in 5-FU bioavailability related to variability in DPD.
- Variability in 5-FU antitumor activity (i.e. resistance) may be related to variability in DPD expression in the tumor.
- Variability in toxicity due to 5-FU catabolites would be expected to vary with DPD levels.

example of a pharmacogenetic syndrome, with symptoms not being recognized until affected individuals are exposed to the drug.[14]

It is now recognized that variation in DPD activity from individual to individual is responsible for the apparent variation in bioavailability of 5-FU that has been described in patients who have been given oral 5-FU in the past.[15] As a result, until recently, there has been a recommendation that 5-FU not be administered orally. The erratic bioavailability has not been well understood, particularly since 5-FU has a relatively low molecular weight and a pK_a that should predict excellent absorption and hence oral bioavailability.[1] As noted below, the role of DPD in 5-FU bioavailability was not appreciated until pharmacokinetic studies with DPD inhibitors demonstrated that the plasma pharmacokinetics (AUC, i.e. the area under the plasma concentration × time curve) of oral 5-FU were essentially the same as those produced by intravenous 5-FU, suggesting almost 100% bioavailability.[16]

DPD activity expressed by tumors has also been shown to vary from individual to individual.[17] This is thought to explain the observed varied tumor response to 5-FU that has been noted in clinical studies.[18] Recent studies utilizing quantitative polymerase chain reaction (PCR) methods have demonstrated increased DPD expression in tumors from patients who were resistant to 5-FU, even when other factors (e.g. low thymidylate synthase expression) would have suggested sensitivity to 5-FU.[19]

Variation in DPD activity from individual to individual may also explain the variation in certain 5-FU toxicities observed in the cancer patient population. While many 5-FU toxicities (e.g. cytopenias, mucositis, and diarrhea) are thought to result from anabolism of 5-FU to nucleotides, which can interfere with nucleic acid synthesis and function, other toxicities (e.g. some neurotoxicities, cardiotoxicity, and possibly hand–foot syndrome) have been thought to result from 5-FU catabolites (see Figure 48.2).[15] This has led to the suggestion that if one decreases DPD activity it may be possible to lessen these toxicities due to 5-FU catabolites.

MODULATION OF DPD ACTIVITY FOR PHARMACOLOGIC BENEFIT

Over the past few decades, there have been many attempts to inhibit DPD in order to minimize the variability in 5-FU pharmacology produced by the variability in DPD in both healthy and tumor tissues. Inhibition of DPD activity in 5-FU-susceptible host tissue, such as gastrointestinal mucosa and bone marrow, theoretically should decrease the variability in clinical response to 5-FU from patient to patient, lessening the need for dosing adjustments. This would be a potential improvement over current therapeutic practice, in which dosing decisions are typically based on previous toxicity with the drug. Inhibition of DPD activity in tumor specimens is also attractive, particularly since many tumors appear to be resistant to 5-FU owing to increased DPD activity within the tumor, resulting in increased degradation and in turn less anabolism of 5-FU.

Table 48.2 lists several of the new 5-FU drugs that have recently entered clinical studies. Since the newer drugs were developed from earlier intermediate drugs, which in turn had been developed from 5-FU, one can subdivide these drugs into essentially three generations.[20] The first generation includes the parent drug 5-FU (which continues to be widely used, administered as an intravenous bolus or as a continuous or protracted infusion) and the nucleoside 5-fluoro-2'deoxyuridine (FdUrd, floxuridine)

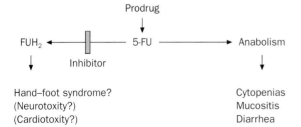

Figure 48.2 Toxicities associated with 5-FU secondary to anabolism and possibly secondary to catabolism. FUH_2, 5-fluoro-5,6-dihydrouracil.

Table 48.2 Generations of fluoropyrimidine drugs
I.   5-Fluorouracil (5-FU, FUra)
5-Fluoro-2'-deoxyuridine (FdUrd, FUDR, floxuridine)
II.   Tegafur (ftorafur)
5'Deoxy-5-fluorouridine (5'dFUrd, doxifluridine)
III.   (A)   Capecitabine
(B)   • Uracil + tegafur (UFT)
• S-1 (tegafur + 5-chloro-2,4-dihydroxypyridine + potassium oxonate)
• Eniluracil (ethynyluracil; 776C85)

which has for many years been used for hepatic arterial infusion. The second generation includes two drugs introduced in the 1970s: tegafur (ftorafur, 1-(2-tetrahydrofuranyl)-5-fluorouracil, whose structure is shown as part of Figure 48.5) and 5'-deoxy-5-fluorouridine (5'-dFUrd, doxifluridine). Both were synthesized as 5-FU prodrugs that can be administered orally. They have been extensively used in Japan, but not as much in other parts of the world. The third generation includes two subclasses. The first consists of the prodrug capecitabine, which represents a further modification of the second-generation drug 5'-dFUrd to gain pharmacologic benefit. As noted in Chapter 47, capecitabine must be activated to 5-FU via three enzymatic steps, 5'-dFUrd being formed as an intermediate. In this sense, capecitabine is actually a prodrug of a prodrug. The second subclass within the third generation of drugs comprises what are known as DPD-inhibiting fluoropyrimidine (DIF) drugs.

DPD-INHIBITORY FLUOROPYRIMIDINES (DIF)

Three DIF drugs have undergone relatively complete clinical evaluation. These are UFT, eniluracil, and S-1.[2,20] The three drugs differ both in the type of DPD 'inhibition' and in the degree and duration of inhibition produced. The rationale for using DIF drugs is shown in Figure 48.3. One first needs a source of 5-FU. This can be from 5-FU itself or from a prodrug that is converted to 5-FU. Secondly, one needs another drug that will interfere with (or inhibit) the catabolism of 5-FU. The resultant effect is that there is an increased exposure to 5-FU over time.

- Source of 5-FU
  - From 5-FU directly (e.g. with eniluracil), or from prodrugs (e.g tegafur) that are not active until converted to 5-FU
- DPD inhibition
  - Used to prevent 5-FU degradation and 'push' more 5-FU towards anabolism
- Effect
  - Increased exposure to 5-FU

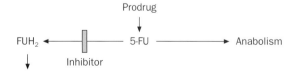

Figure 48.3 Rationale for using DPD-inhibitory fluoropyrimidine (DIF) drugs.

DPD inhibition also enables oral delivery of 5-FU (bioavailability >70%) and results in less variability in the pharmacokinetics of the fluoropyrimidines. In addition, by inhibiting the catabolic pathway, more 5-FU can enter the anabolic pathway and potentially increase the antitumor effect, which is theoretically important for tumors that have become resistant secondary to an increase of intratumoral DPD. Finally, inhibiting DPD may also decrease the incidence of some 5-FU toxicities (hand–foot syndrome, some forms of neurotoxicity, and possibly cardiotoxicity) that may be secondary to 5-FU catabolites.

UFT

UFT is the DIF drug that has been most widely used clinically.[21] It is a formulation consisting of the naturally occurring pyrimidine uracil mixed together with the fluoropyrimidine tegafur (ftorafur) in a 4:1 molar ratio. Figure 48.4 illustrates the mechanism by which UFT functions as a DIF drug. Initially tegafur is slowly metabolized to the pyrimidine 5-FU. The pyrimidine uracil in UFT is present in excess compared to 5-FU. Since uracil and 5-FU have similar substrate affinities for DPD,[4] they 'compete' at the level of DPD such that the 5-FU formed from tegafur is not degraded as rapidly and therefore is hypothesized to be present over a longer period of time. While not true 'inhibition' of DPD, the competition between 5-FU and uracil for DPD produces an effect similar to what is achieved with a true DPD inhibitor. In contrast to the true DPD inhibitors and inactivators described below, the effect of UFT on DPD is rapidly reversible. This rapidly reversible inhibition potentially avoids some of the problems observed with the earlier DPD inhibitors, and may account for a more favorable toxicity profile compared with some of these[22] as well as some of the

Modulation at level of DPD

Uracil (U) and tegafur are present in a 4 : 1 molar ratio. Excess uracil competes with 5-FU for DPD (effectively 'inhibiting' 5-FU catabolism)

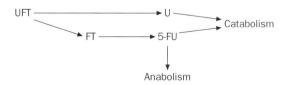

Figure 48.4 Mechanism of action of UFT.

newer DIF drugs (e.g. eniluracil). Extensive data from Japan, as well as from Europe, South America, and the USA, demonstrate that orally administered UFT has antitumor activity in several tumor types (particularly breast and colon cancer), either as a single agent or combined with leucovorin.[23–25] Large phase III studies conducted thus far have shown that it is at least as effective as intravenously infused 5-FU. Furthermore, the toxicity profile has proven quite tolerable, with mainly the same characteristic fluoropyrimidine toxicities (e.g diarrhea and nausea) seen at the maximal tolerated dose, but without the neutropenia or febrile neutropenia typically seen with intravenous bolus regimens of 5-FU. Other toxicities, in particular hand–foot syndrome and neurologic and cardiologic toxicities, are less frequent.[26] As noted above (see Figure 48.2), it has been suggested that these toxicities may be secondary to 5-FU catabolites. Such catabolites are less likely to form from UFT, possibly accounting for the decreased incidence of these toxicities. While currently approved in numerous countries throughout the world, including Asia, South America, and Europe, UFT failed to win approval from the FDA in the USA owing to several concerns, including doubt about whether equivalence to the Mayo Clinic regimen of 5-FU and leucovorin had been demonstrated, as well as concern about failure to demonstrate convincingly the role of uracil in the formulation mix.

S-1

In Japan, there have been several attempts to improve on fluoropyrimidine therapy by designing a drug containing a component to decrease the occurrence of diarrhea, which has remained a bothersome toxicity with many of the fluoropyrimidine regimens. S-1 is a triple-drug combination (see Figure 48.5), consisting of the prodrug tegafur, together with a DPD inhibitor 5-chloro-2,4-dihydroxypyridine (CDHP), and potassium oxonate in a molar ratio of 1:0.4:1, respectively.[27] This combination not only provides the sustained 5-FU release from the prodrug (tegafur) and DPD inhibitor, but also utilizes potassium oxonate to theoretically lessen the risk of gastrointestinal toxicity, particularly diarrhea. Potassium oxonate has been shown in preclinical studies to selectively inhibit 5-FU phosphorylation by the enzyme orotate phosphoribosyltransferase; this inhibition has been suggested to occur in the gastrointestinal tract more than in the tumor.[28] Preclinical studies have been encouraging, demonstrating excellent antitumor activity.[29] Clinical studies, thus far, have demonstrated S-1 to be quite tolerable.[30–32] Based on its clinical efficacy in gastric cancer and the decreased incidence of diarrhea, S-1 has been approved in Japan.[33] Unfortunately, early clinical studies in Western Europe and the USA have been notable because diarrhea continues to be the dose-limiting toxicity.[34] The basis for this is unclear, but may be secondary to genetic differences in drug metabolism in the different populations.

ENILURACIL

Eniluracil (ethynyluracil or GW776C85) is a newer, more potent type of DPD inhibitor that was synthesized as a specific inactivator of DPD.[35] This compound is a pyrimidine possessing a structure similar to both uracil and 5-FU.[36] The mechanism by which this drug works is shown in Figure 48.6. It forms a covalent bond with a cysteine amino acid within the DPD enzyme, resulting in permanent inactivation of DPD activity until new enzyme is synthesized. Initial

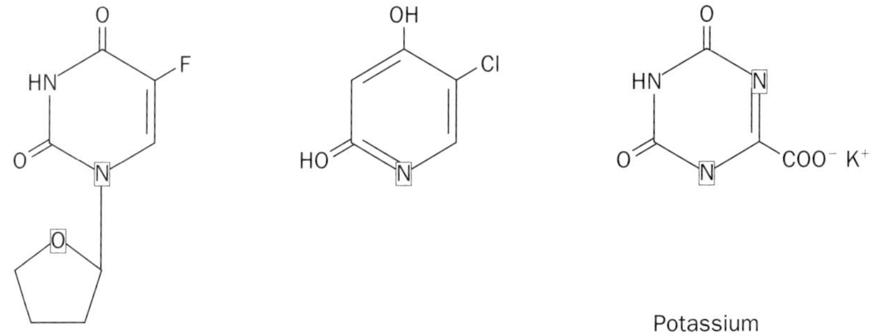

Figure 48.5 Composition of S-1.

Tegafur		5-Chloro-2,4-dihydroxypridine		Potassium oxonate
1	:	0.4	:	1

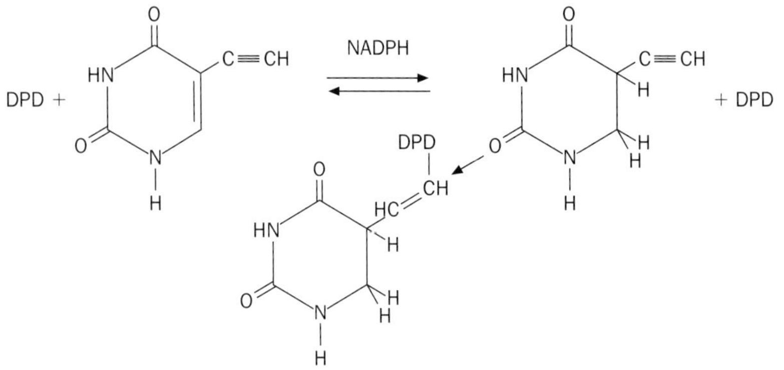

Figure 48.6 Mechanism of action of eniluracil (ethynyluracil).

phase I and II clinical studies with eniluracil demonstrated that DPD was rapidly and completely inactivated, with inhibition maintained for more than 1 day at clinically used doses.[37,38] Unfortunately, recently completed phase III studies[39,40] have demonstrated inferiority compared to a Mayo Clinic regimen of 5-FU and leucovorin in colorectal cancer, leading to suspension of clinical development in late 2000. This drug theoretically remains interesting as a potential pharmacologic method for reversing 5-FU resistance due to DPD overexpression within tumors.

SUMMARY AND FUTURE DIRECTIONS

DPD-inhibiting fluoropyrimidines (DIF drugs) provide a new strategy by which 5-FU may be administered orally at reduced doses. While not a substitute for protracted intravenous infusion, DIF drugs produce an effect somewhat similar to continuous infusion of 5-FU. Inhibition of DPD also results in potentially less intrapatient or interpatient variability in 5-FU pharmacokinetics, and (at least theoretically) is a means by which 5-FU resistance may be reversed and certain 5-FU toxicities may be decreased. Thus far, clinical studies with several of these drugs demonstrate tolerable toxicities. Worldwide clinical use of at least one of these drugs, single-agent UFT (or the combination of UFT and leucovorin) has demonstrated that this oral fluoropyrimidine can achieve similar therapeutic efficacy as that obtained with the more standardized intravenous regimen of 5-FU. Future experimental uses of DPD inhibitors might include consideration for use together with prodrugs such as capecitabine to lessen some of the toxicities that may be associated with continuous exposure to 5-FU (from capecitabine) and, in turn, continuous exposure to 5-FU catabolites. Lastly, it

remains of theoretical interest to use strong DPD inhibitors such as eniluracil not as a means of oral delivery of 5-FU, but rather to specifically overcome 5-FU resistance due to DPD overexpression in tumors.

REFERENCES

1. Daher GC, Harris BE, Diasio RB, Metabolism of pyrimidine analogues and their nucleosides. In: *Metabolism and Reactions of Anticancer Drugs*, Vol 1 (*International Encyclopedia of Pharmacology and Therapeutics*) (Powis G, ed). Oxford: Pergamon Press, 1994: 55–94.
2. Diasio RB, Oral administration of fluorouracil: a new approach utilizing modulators of dihydropyrimidine dehydrogenase activity. *Cancer Ther* 1999; **2**: 97–106.
3. Diasio RB, Lu Z, Zhang R, Shahinian HS, Fluoropyrimidine catabolism. In: *Concepts and Mechanisms, and New Targets for Chemotherapy* (Muggia FM, ed). Norwell, MA: Kluwer Academic, 1995: 71–93.
4. Lu Z-H, Zhang R, Diasio RB, Purification and characterization of dihydropyrimidine dehydrogenase from human liver. *J Biol Chem* 1992; **267**: 17102–9.
5. Heggie GD, Sommadossi JP, Cross DS et al, Clinical pharmacokinetics of 5-fluorouracil and its metabolites in plasma, urine, and bile. *Cancer Res* 1987; **47**: 2203–6.
6. Harris BE, Song R, Soong SJ, Diasio RB, Relationship of dihydropyrimidine dehydrogenase activity and plasma 5-fluorouracil levels: evidence for circadian variation of 5-fluorouracil levels in cancer patients receiving protracted continuous infusion. *Cancer Res* 1990; **50**: 197–201.
7. Zhang R, Diasio RB, Pharmacologic basis for circadian pharmacodynamics. In: *The Scientific Basis for Optimized Cancer Therapy* (Hrushesky WJM, ed). Boca Raton, FL: CRC Press, 1994: 60–103.
8. Giacchetti S, Perpoint B, Zidani R et al, Phase III multicenter randomized trial of oxaliplatin added to chronomodulated fluorouracil–leucovorin as first-line treatment of metastatic colorectal cancer. *J Clin Oncol* 2000; **18**: 136–47.
9. Lu Z, Zhang R, Diasio RB, Dihydropyrimidine dehydrogenase activity in human peripheral blood mononuclear cells and liver: population characteristics, newly identified patients, and clinical implication in 5-fluorouracil chemotherapy. *Cancer Res* 1993; **53**: 5433–8.
10. Lu Z, Zhang R, Diasio RB, Dihydropyrimidine dehydrogenase

activity in human liver: population characteristics and clinical implication in 5-FU chemotherapy. *Clin Pharmacol Ther* 1995; **58**: 512–22.

11. Diasio RB, Beavers TL, Carpenter JT, Familial deficiency of dihydropyrimidine dehydrogenase: biochemical basis for familial pyrimidinemia and severe 5-fluorouracil-induced toxicity. *J Clin Invest* 1988; **81**: 47–51.

12. Harris BE, Carpenter JT, Diasio RB, Severe 5-fluorouracil toxicity secondary to dihydropyrimidine dehydrogenase deficiency: a potentially more common pharmacogenetic syndrome. *Cancer* 1991; **68**: 499–501.

13. Johnson MJ, Hageboutros A, Wang K et al, Life-threatening toxicity in a dihydropyrimidine dehydrogenase deficient patient following treatment with topical 5-fluorouracil. *Clin Cancer Res* 1999; **5**: 2006–11.

14. Diasio RB, Pharmacogenetics. In: *Cancer Chemotherapy and Biotherapy*, 3rd edn (Chabner BA, Longo DL, eds). Philadelphia: Lippincott Williams & Wilkins, 2001.

15. Diasio RB, Clinical implications of dihydropyrimidine dehydrogenase (DPD) inhibition. *Oncology (Huntington)* 1999; **13**(Suppl 3): 17–21.

16. Baker SD, Diasio RB, O'Reilly S et al, Phase I and pharmacologic study of oral 5-fluorouracil on a chronic daily schedule in combination with the dihydropyrimidine dehydrogenase inactivator eniluracil. *J Clin Oncol* 2000; **18**: 915–26.

17. Jiang W, Lu Z, He Y, Diasio RB, Dihydropyrimidine dehydrogenase activity in hepatocellular carcinoma; implication for 5-fluorouracil-based chemotherapy. *Clin Cancer Res* 1997; **3**: 395–9.

18. Diasio RB, Dihydropyrimidine dehydrogenase and resistance to 5-fluorouracil. *Prog Exp Tumor Res* 1999; **36**: 115–23.

19. Salonga D, Danenberg KD, Johnson M et al, Gene expression levels of dihydropyrimidine dehydrogenase and thymidylate synthase together identify a high percentage of colorectal tumors responding to 5-fluorouracil. *Clin Cancer Res* 2000; **6**: 1322–7.

20. Diasio RB, Improving 5-fluorouracil chemotherapy with novel orally administered fluoropyrimidines. *Drugs* 1999; **58**(Suppl 3): 119–26.

21. Majima H, Phase I and preliminary phase II study of co-administration of uracil and FT-207 (UFT therapy). *Gan To Kagaku Ryoho* 1980; **7**: 1383–7.

22. Naguib FN, el Kouni MH, Cha S, Structure–activity relationship of ligands of dihydrouracil dehydrogenase from mouse liver. *Biochem Pharmacol* 1989; **38**: 1471–80.

23. Takino T, Clinical studies on the chemotherapy of advanced cancer with UFT (uracil plus futraful preparation). *Gan To Kagaku Ryoho* 1980; **7**: 1804–12.

24. Pazdur R, Lassere Y, Diaz-Canton E et al, Phase I trial of uracil–tegafur (UFT) plus oral leucovorin: 14-day schedule. *Invest New Drugs* 1997; **15**: 123–8.

25. Vanhoefer U, Wilke H, Oral fluoropyrimidine-based combination therapy in gastrointestinal cancer. *Oncology (Huntington)* 2001; **15**(Suppl 2): 79–84.

26. Sun W, Haller D, UFT in the treatment of colorectal and breast cancer. *Oncology (Huntington)* 2001; **15**(Suppl 2): 49–56.

27. Shirasaka T, Shimamato Y, Ohsimo H et al, Development of a novel form of oral 5-fluorouracil derivative (S-1) directed to the potentiation of the tumor selective cytotoxicity of 5-fluorouracil by two biochemical modulators. *Anticancer Drugs* 1996; **7**: 548–57.

28. Shirasaka T, Shimamato Y, Fukushima M, Inhibition by oxonic acid of gastrointestinal toxicity of 5-fluorouracil without loss of its antitumor activity in rats. *Cancer Res* 1993; **53**: 4004–9.

29. Fukushima M, Satake H, Uchida J et al, Preclinical antitumor efficacy of S-1: a new oral formulation of 5-fluorouracil on human tumor xenografts. *Int J Oncol* 1998; **13**: 693–8.

30. Hoff PM, The tegafur-based dihydropyrimidine dehydrogenase inhibitory fluoropyrimidines, UFT/leucovorin (ORZEL) and S-1: a review of their clinical development and therapeutic potential. *Invest New Drugs* 2000; **18**: 331–42.

31. Shirasaka T, Yamamitsu S, Tsuji A, Taguchi T, Conceptual changes in cancer chemotherapy: from an oral fluoropyrimidine prodrug, UFT, to a novel oral fluoropyrimidine prodrug, S-1, and low-dose FP therapy in Japan. *Invest New Drugs* 2000; **18**: 315–29.

32. Ohtsu A, Baba H, Sakata Y et al, Phase II study of S-1, a novel oral fluoropyrimidine derivative, in patients with metastatic colorectal carcinoma. S-1 Cooperative Colorectal Carcinoma Study Group. *Br J Cancer* 2000; **83**: 141–5.

33. Koizumi W, Kurihara M, Nakano S, Hasegawa K, Phase II study of S-1, a novel oral derivative of 5-fluorouracil, in advanced gastric cancer. For the S-1 Cooperative Gastric Cancer Study Group. *Oncology* 2000; **58**: 191–7.

34. van Groeningen CJ, Peters GJ, Schornagel JH et al, Phase I clinical and pharmacokinetic study of oral S-1 in patients with advanced solid tumors. *J Clin Oncol* 2000; **18**: 2772–9.

35. Baccanari DP, Davis ST, Knick VC, Spector T, 5-Ethynyluracil: effects on the pharmacokinetics and antitumor activity of 5-fluorouracil. *Proc Natl Acad Sci USA* 1993; **90**: 11064–8.

36. Spector T, Porter DJT, Nelson DJ et al, 5-Ethynyluracil (776C85), a modulator of the therapeutic activity of 5-fluorouracil. *Drugs Future* 1994; **19**: 566–71.

37. Baker SD, Khor SP, Adjei AA et al, Pharmacokinetics, oral bioavailability, and safety study of fluorouracil in patients treated with 776C85, an inactivator of dihydropyrimidine dehydrogenase. *J Clin Oncol* 1996; **14**: 3085–96.

38. Schilsky RL, Burris H, Ratain M et al, Phase I clinical and pharmacologic study of 776C85 plus 5-fluorouracil in patients with advanced cancer. *J Clin Oncol* 1998; **16**: 1450–7.

39. Van Cutsem, E, Sorensen J, Cassidy J et al, International phase III study of oral eniluracil (EU) plus 5-fluorouracil (5-FU) versus intravenous (IV) 5-FU plus leucovorin (LV) in the treatment of advanced colorectal cancer (ACC). *Proc Am Soc Clin Oncol* 2001; **20**: 522.

40. Levin J, Schilsky R, Burris H et al, North American phase III study of oral eniluracil (EU) plus oral 5-fluorouracil (5-FU) versus intravenous (IV) 5-FU plus leucovorin (LV) in the treatment of advanced colorectal cancer (ACC). *Proc Am Soc Clin Oncol* 2001; **20**: 523.

49

Irinotecan: Mechanism of action

Udo Vanhoefer, Youcef M Rustum

INTRODUCTION

DNA topoisomerase I (TOP-I) plays a key role in DNA replication and transcription, and possibly in DNA recombination and repair.[1–4] Human TOP-I mRNA and protein expression increases during cell proliferation, and is regulated by a complex system of negative and positive transcription factors, including NF-κB, NF-IL-6 (C/EBP family), factor Sp1, octamer transcription factor, cAMP-responsive element-binding protein (CREB/ATF), and members of the Myc-related family of basic helix–loop–helix/leucine-zipper proteins.[5–12] Recent data suggest that the phosphorylation state of TOP-I is one of the key mechanisms of post-translational regulation, involving protein kinase C and casein II-associated tyrosine kinase.[13–15] Phosphorylation of the serine residues increases TOP-I relaxation activity, while dephosphorylation inhibits TOP-I function.[13,14] There is evidence that TOP-I function may additionally be altered by other nuclear proteins (e.g. nucleolin, p53, and hsp).[16–18]

For the cytotoxic mechanism of irinotecan, the following TOP-I-mediated steps of functional DNA alterations are of importance:[2,4,19–21]

1. TOP-I relaxes torsionally strained supercoiled duplex DNA by becoming covalently linked by its tyrosine hydroxyl group (position 723) to the 3′-phosphate at the DNA break site, resulting in an enzyme-linked single-strand nick in the phosphodiester backbone of DNA.
2. This enyzme-bridged single-strand DNA break allows the intact DNA strand to pass through.
3. After rotation of the intact DNA strand, DNA religation is initiated – the exposed 5′-hydroxyl group of the cleaved DNA strand attacks the tyrosyl phosphate bond, the tyrosine residue is released from the phosphate, and the DNA-strand break is resealed.

MOLECULAR MECHANISM OF CYTOTOXICITY

Irinotecan is a semisynthetic derivative of the plant alkaloid camptothecin (Figure 49.1). In contrast to other camptothecin derivatives (e.g. topotecan and 9-aminocamptothecin) irinotecan is in vivo enzymatically converted by carboxylesterase to its most active cytotoxic metabolite 7-ethyl-10-hydroxycamptothecin (SN-38), which has at least a more than 200-fold higher cytotoxic activity in vitro.[22,23] Reversible pH-dependent hydrolysis establishes an equilibrium between the pharmacologically active closed lactone ring form of SN-38 and the inactive open-ring hydroxy acid form (Figure 49.2).[24] SN-38 is referred to as a topoisomerase I interactive agent, and exerts its cytotoxic mechanism by generating intermediate forms of drug-stabilized covalent DNA/TOP-I complexes. The collision of these drug-stabilized enzyme-bridged DNA breaks (referred to as cleavable complexes) with moving replication forks may lead to cell death due to replication arrest and replication fork disassembly, as well as chromosomal fragmentation (Figure 49.3).[1,25–31] An important feature in terms of mechanism of cytotoxic action is that SN-38 exerts its cytotoxicity by trapping cleavable complexes rather than by inhibition of TOP-I enzyme function. There is evidence that camptothecin derivatives trap TOP-I predominantly in actively transcribed genes.[32,33] In addition, cytogenetic data indicate two distinct interactions of SN-38 with DNA: immediate induction of chromatin breaks independent of DNA synthesis, and induction of chromatid breaks associated with radical chromosome configuration dependent on DNA synthesis.[34] The role of cellular ubiquitin (UB) in processing cleavage complex formation of TOP-I, which has been observed independently of DNA replication

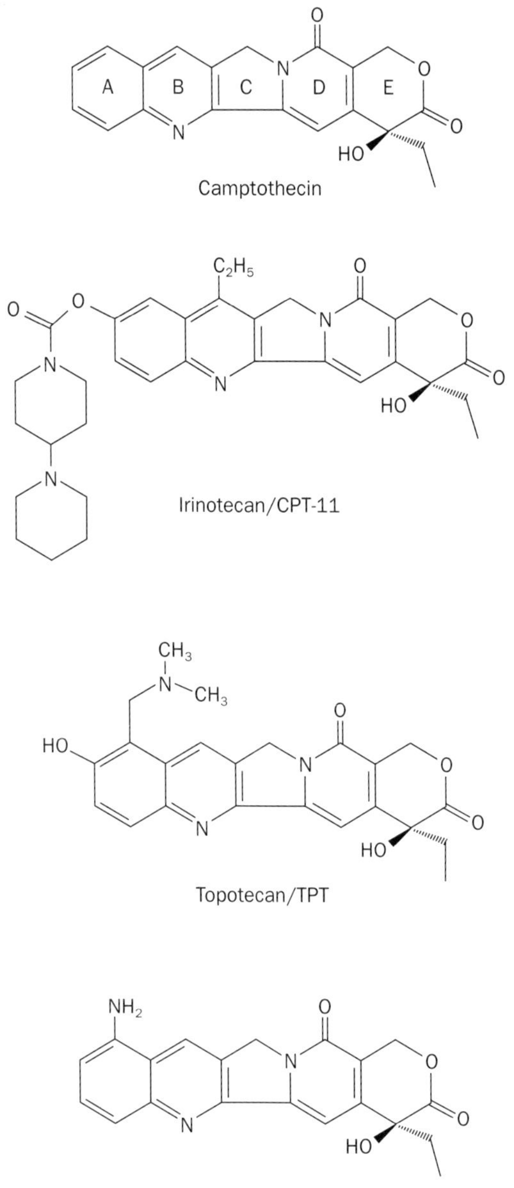

Figure 49.1 Chemical structures of camptothecin and its derivatives.

after exposure to camptothecin derivatives and the destruction of these multi-UB–TOP-I conjugates by 26S proteasome, needs to be further evaluated.[35] There is also evidence that multi-UB–TOP-I complexes may play an important role in resistance to TOP-I-interactive agents. In addition, in vitro and in vivo studies indicate that prolonged exposure time to irinotecan (or SN-38 in cell culture) may enhance antitumor efficacy.[36]

CELLULAR DETERMINANTS OF CYTOTOXICITY

Studies on cell cultures may indicate that high levels of TOP-I mRNA and protein expression predict for tumor response to camptothecin derivatives.[37–40] Furthermore, increased TOP-I expression and activity in human tumor samples were found, when compared to normal colon mucosa, using RT-PCR, immunoblotting, or measurements of enzyme activity.[41,42] However, evaluation of human cancer cell lines and tumor samples revealed that TOP-I expression varies widely between individuals.[43] Furthermore, no correlation was found between the level of TOP-I expression in human biopsy samples and clinical resistance to irinotecan or topotecan.[44–46]

Since epidermal growth factor receptor (EGFR) alters cell cycle regulation by promoting cells in S phase, it may be hypothesized that EGFR expression may be related to higher sensitivity to S-phase-specific cytotoxic drugs (e.g. camptothecin derivatives).[47] However, in these preclinical studies, only EGFR expression has been determined, but not EGFR autophosphorylation. Furthermore, data from our study indicate that the addition of non-cytotoxic concentrations of specific EGFR-tyrosine kinase inhibitors enhances sensitivity to SN-38 in vitro (Vanhoefer et al, manuscript in preparation).

Exposure to SN-38 induced in vitro mitochondrial Bax dimerization, while the cytosolic Bax was retained in the monomeric state (Rustum et al, manuscript in preparation). Since dimerization of mitochondrial Bax and downstream events (e.g. cytochrome *c* release and activation of caspases) have been associated with increased drug-induced apoptotic cell death, changes in Bcl-2/Bax expression may predict for response to SN-38.[48] Recently, A253 cells with low endogenous Bcl-2/Bax protein and negative for p53 were transfected with *bax* cDNA resulting in about a 50-fold increase in Bax protein expression.[49] In vitro, A253/Bax turned out to be about 14-fold more responsive to SN-38, which translated to curative treatment options in vivo (80% versus 20% cure rate for A253/Bax versus A253/Vec, respectively).[50] Furthermore, it has been shown that *bcl-2* gene expression prevents induction of SN-38-related apoptosis in L1210 murine leukemia cells.[51] The data suggest an important role of Bcl-2/Bax in drug sensitivity to irinotecan.

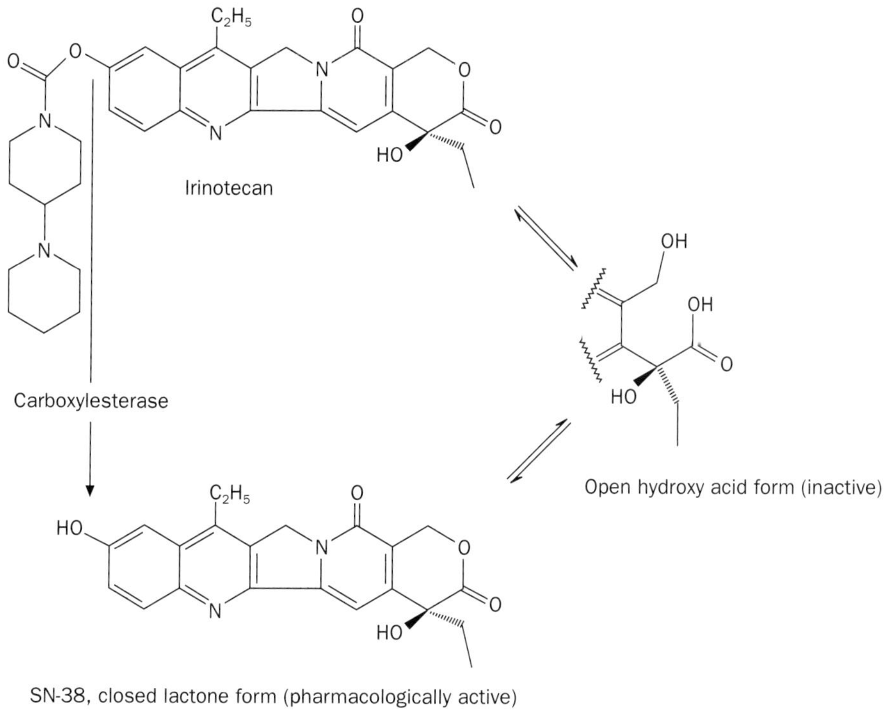

C₂H₅

Irinotecan

Open hydroxy acid form (inactive)

Carboxylesterase

C₂H₅

SN-38, closed lactone form (pharmacologically active)

Figure 49.2 Conversion of irinotecan to its active metabolite SN-38, and the equilibrium between the active lactone and inactive hydroxy acid forms.

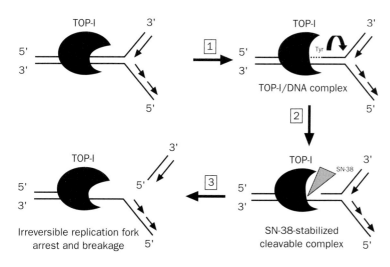

Figure 49.3 Cytotoxic mechanism of SN-38. (1) Topoisomerase I (TOP-I) binds to supercoiled DNA by becoming covalently linked with its tyrosine hydroxyl group (position 723) to the 3'-phosphate at the DNA break site, resulting in an enzyme-linked single-strand nick in the phosphodiester backbone of DNA; the intact DNA strand may then pass through. (2) SN-38 binds to the TOP-I/DNA complex, resulting in stabilization of the cleavable complex. (3) Moving DNA replication forks collide with SN-38-stabilized enzyme-bridged DNA breaks, and lead to cell death due to replication arrest and replication fork disassembly.

In addition, human tumor carboxylesterase activity has been correlated with cytotoxicity of irinotecan.[52]

Taken together, it is unlikely that TOP-I expression alone is sufficient to predict for response to irinotecan (SN-38). Other factors, such as drug uptake, drug activation (e.g. tumor carboxylesterase activity) and metabolism, distraction DNA repair capacity, and TOP-I phosphorylation, may also be important cellular determinants of response to irinotecan.

MECHANISMS OF RESISTANCE TO IRINOTECAN

Acquired resistance to TOP-I-interactive drugs in preclinical models has been related to downregulation of TOP-I gene and protein expression as well as to alterations in TOP-I gene structure and function (e.g. point mutations, deletions, and rearrangements of the TOP-I gene).[53–61] In vitro data suggest that decreased activity of carboxylesterase may also alter the antitumor activity of irinotecan, owing to decreased enzymatic conversion of irinotecan to its cytotoxic metabolite SN-38.[62] Furthermore, UDP-glucuronosyltransferase (UGT) conjugates SN-38 into its almost inactive glucuronide. Therefore, increased UGT activity may confer resistance to SN-38.[63] Increased topoisomerase II (TOP-II) expression has also been related to resistance to TOP-I-interactive agents – this is of importance because DNA TOP-I and -II perform related functions, and TOP-II has been shown to compensate for TOP-I function.[64–66] While positively charged camptothecin derivatives (e.g. topotecan) may be transported by the multidrug-resistance gene (*MDR1*) product P_{170}-glycoprotein and by the multidrug-resistance protein (MRP), both drug transporters appear not to confer resistance to irinotecan or SN-38.[67–72] It is of interest that significant mRNA and protein expression of P_{170}-glycoprotein and MRP have been demonstrated in colorectal cancer by immunohistochemistry and RT-PCR methods.[73,74] Thus, the low clinical efficacy of topotecan in colorectal cancer might be at least partially related to altered drug accumulation.[75–78] Resistance to SN-38 has been related to altered drug accumulation in two topotecan- or mitoxantrone-selected cell lines (T8 and MX3, respectively) with expression of BCRP/MXR/ABCP, an ATP-binding cassette (ABC) membrane transporter protein, but lacking MRP and P_{170}-glycoprotein expression.[79,80] There is evidence that overexpression of the mitoxantrone-resistance half-transporter (MXR) alone is sufficient to confer resistance to SN-38, independent of the cellular UGT activity.[81]

Ehrlichman and co-workers[82] demonstrated that the HER family tyrosine kinase inhibitor CI1033 induces antiproliferative effects in colorectal HCT-8 and glioblastoma T98G cells. The increased sensitivity was associated with higher induction of SN-38-stabilized covalent DNA/TOP-I complexes, but not with alterations in EGFR autophosphorylation and TOP-I enzymatic function. Further studies revealed that the quinazoline-based HER family tyrosine kinase inhibitor is a competitive substrate for BCRP function, resulting in increased cellular drug uptake and retention of SN-38.

RATIONALE FOR COMBINATION THERAPY

In preclinical studies, schedule-dependent cytotoxic interactions have been reported for the combination of thymidylate synthase (TS) inhibitors with either irinotecan itself or its active metabolite SN-38.[83–89]

In vitro data showed a cytotoxic synergism for the sequence SN-38 followed by 5-fluorouracil (5-FU), while the opposite schedule resulted in additive or antagonistic cytotoxic interactions.[84,86–88] Using irinotecan itself in cell culture, synergistic cytotoxic interactions were seen if irinotecan (IC_{20}) preceded 5-FU (IC_{50}) in SW620, HT-29, and SNU-C4 colon cancer cells, associated with increased DNA damage.[86]

The antitumor activity of 5-FU in combination with irinotecan was evaluated in several in vivo tumor models.[89,90] Using nude mice bearing human 5-FU-sensitive HCT-8 colon tumor xenografts and rats with advanced ward tumors, different schedules of irinotecan in combination with 5-FU showed significant antitumor activity. The sequential administration of irinotecan followed 24 hours later by 5-FU was the most active in both in vivo tumor models. Similar results were observed in 5-FU (bolus)-resistant HT29-R1 tumor xenografts in nude mice, demonstrating increased therapeutic efficacy for the schedule of irinotecan followed by 5-FU bolus.[89]

The combination of SN-38 and 5-FU induced a prolonged inhibition of TS and increased the incorporation of 5-FU derivatives (e.g. FdUTP) into DNA – results that may explain the cytotoxic synergism between both drugs.[85,88] Recent data suggest that the lack of dTTP consumption due to SN-38-mediated inhibition of DNA synthesis increases cellular dTTP pools, resulting in an inhibition of dCMP deaminase activity. Inhibition of dCMP deaminase itself will produce cellular depletion of dUMP, an endogenous nucleotide that competes with FdUMP – the main cytotoxic metabolite of 5-FU – for TS. Thus, SN-38-mediated inhibition of dUMP synthesis would be expected to potentiate the cytotoxicity of 5-FU by enhanced inhibition of TS activity.[88] In addition, in vivo data indicate that the mechanisms of cytotoxic synergism between irinotecan and 5-FU may also implicate (a) recruitment of cells by irinotecan into S phase, and (b) increased expression of Bax, associated with apoptosis.[49]

Short term exposure to SN-38 followed by raltitrexed, a specific and potent direct inhibitor of TS, also resulted in cytotoxic synergism at broad dose–effect ranges in vitro – data that are similar to those obtained for 5-FU.[83] This synergism was completely lost under conditions of more prolonged drug exposure. The opposite sequence of raltitrexed followed by SN-38 or a simultaneous exposure resulted in almost additive cytotoxic interactions.

The cellular pharmacology of the combination of SN-38 with the diaminocyclohexane (DACH) platinum derivative oxaliplatin has been described recently.[91,92] The combination of SN-38 and oxaliplatin showed in vitro cytotoxic synergism in the colon cancer cell line HT29, with a maximum effect when oxaliplatin was administered first.[92] The molecular mechanism of this synergism was explained by altered oxaliplatin interstrand crosslink repair machinery. These data suggest that oxaliplatin DNA adduct formation leads to increased SN-38-induced DNA elongation inhibition, and thereby alters TOP-I function. In contrast, results obtained in HCT-8 colon tumor cells showed that the sequence of SN-38 followed by oxaliplatin was associated with synergistic cytotoxic interactions, while the opposite sequence resulted in antagonism.[91] The synergism in HCT-8 cells was associated with G_2/M checkpoint arrest in the cell cycle, but was not attributed to alterations in oxaliplatin–DNA adduct formation or TOP-I expression.

The use of irinotecan in combination therapy is discussed further in Chapters 52–56.

PREVENTION OF IRINOTECAN-INDUCED DIARRHEA

Diarrhea induced by irinotecan represents one of the most common dose-limiting toxicities independent of the schedule of drug administration. SN-38 glucuronide – a detoxified SN-38 metabolite – is hydrolyzed by intestinal β-glucuronidase to active SN-38, which may damage intestinal epithelium cells and lead clinically to diarrhea.[93–95] A rat model with a profile of dose-limiting toxicities similar to those observed clinically was developed and used to evaluate the role of interleukin-15 (IL-15) in the modulation of the therapeutic selectivity of irinotecan.[96] IL-15 offered complete and sustained selective protection against irinotecan-induced delayed diarrhea, and reduced lethality in rats. It also moderately potentiated the antitumor activity of irinotecan in rats bearing advanced colorectal cancer. Morphologic examination of rat intestinal tissues after treatment with a lethal dose of irinotecan revealed dramatic protection of duodenal and colon tissue architecture by IL-15, while irinotecan alone caused serious damage to duodenal villi and colon crypts.[96] Furthermore, oral administration of a new synthetic lipopeptide (JBT-3002) protected mice from irinotecan-induced intestinal injury by enhanced expression of IL-15 in lamina propria cells.[97]

These results suggest that IL-15 can provide significant protection from irinotecan-induced intestinal toxicity, with maintenance of antitumor activity, resulting in an increased irinotecan therapeutic index.

ACKNOWLEDGEMENTS

This work was supported in part by a grant of the Deutsche Forschungsgemeinschaft (DFG RA119/17-2) (UV) and by CA66761-07 from the National Cancer Institute, Bethesda, MD(YR).

REFERENCES

1. Chen AY, Liu LF, DNA topoisomerases: essential enzymes and lethal targets. *Annu Rev Pharmacol Toxicol* 1994; **34**: 191–218.
2. Pommier Y, Pourquier P, Fan Y et al, Mechanisms of action of eukaryotic DNA topoisomerase I and drugs targeted to the enzyme. *Biochim Biophys Acta* 1998; **1400**: 83–106.
3. Pommier Y, Eukaryotic DNA topoisomerase I: Genome gatekeeper and its intruders, camptothecins. *Semin Oncol* 1996; **23**: 3–10.
4. Wang JC, DNA topoisomerase. *Annu Rev Biochem* 1996; **65**: 635–92.
5. Duguet M, Lavenot C, Harper F et al, DNA topoisomerases from rat liver: physiological variations. *Nucleic Acids Res* 1983; **11**: 1059–75.
6. Heiland S, Knippers R, Kunze N, The promoter region of the human type-I-DNA-topoisomerase gene protein binding sites and sequences involved in transcriptional regulation. *Eur J Biochem* 1993; **217**: 813–22.
7. Kunze N, Klein M, Richter A et al, Structural characterization of the human DNA topoisomerase I gene promoter. *Eur J Biochem* 1990; **194**: 323–30.
8. Kunze N, Yang G, Dölberg M et al, Structure of the human type I DNA topoisomerase gene. *J Biol Chem* 1991; **266**: 9610–16.
9. Romig H, Richter A, Expression of the type I DNA topoisomerase gene in adenovirus-5 infected human cells. *Nucleic Acids Res* 1990; **18**: 801–8.

10. Heiland S, Knippers R, The human topoisomerase I gene promoter is regulated by NF-IL6. *Mol Cell Biol* 1995; **12:** 6623–31.

11. Leteurtre F, Kohlhagen G, Fesen MR et al, Effects of DNA methylation on topoisomerase I and II cleavage activities. *J Biol Chem* 1994; **11:** 7893–990.

12. Piret B, Schoonbroodt S, Piette J, The ATM protein is required for sustained activation of NF-κB following DNA damage. *Oncogene* 1999; **13:** 2261–71.

13. Pommier Y, Kerrigan D, Hartmann KD et al, Phosphorylation of mammalian DNA topoisomerase I and activation by protein kinase C. *J Biol Chem* 1990; **16:** 9418–22.

14. Samuels DS, Shimizu Y, Shimizu N, Protein kinase C phosphorylates DNA topoisomerase I. *FEBS Lett* 1989; **259:** 57–60.

15. Tse-Dinh YC, Wong TW, Goldberg AR, Virus- and cell-encoded tyrosine protein kinases inactivate DNA topoisomerases in vitro. *Nature* 1984; **312:** 785–6.

16. Ciavarra RP, Goldman C, Wen KK et al, Heat stress induces hsp70/nuclear topoisomerase I complex formation in vivo: evidence for hsp70-mediated, ATP-independent reactivation in vitro. *Proc Natl Acad Sci USA* 1994; **91:** 1751–5.

17. Gobert C, Bracco L, Rossi F et al, Modulation of DNA topoisomerase I activity by p53. *Biochemistry* 1996; **35:** 5778–86.

18. Haluska P Jr, Rubin EH, A role for the amino terminus of human topoisomerase I. *Adv Enzyme Regul* 1998; **38:** 253–62.

19. Stewart L, Redinbo MR, Qiu X et al, A model for the mechanism of human topoisomerase I. *Science* 1998; **279:** 1534–41.

20. Redinbo MR, Stewart L, Kuhn P et al, Crystal structure of human topoisomerase I in covalent and noncovalent complexes with DNA. *Science* 1998; **279:** 1504–13.

21. Takahashi M, Matsuda M, Kojima A et al, Human immunodeficiency virus type 1 reverse transcriptase: enhancement of activity by interaction with cellular topoisomerase I. *Proc Natl Acad Sci USA* 1995; **92:** 5694–8.

22. Lavelle F, Bissery MC, André S et al, Preclinical evaluation of CPT-11 and its active metabolite SN-38. *Semin Oncol* 1996; **23** (Suppl 3): 11–20.

23. Rivory LP, Bowles MR, Robert J et al, Conversion of irinotecan (CPT-11) to its active metabolite, 7-ethyl-10-hydroxy-camptothecin (SN-38) by human liver carboxylesterase. *Biochem Pharmacol* 1996; **52:** 1103–11.

24. Satoh R, Hosokawa M, Atsumi R et al, Metabolic activation of CPT-11, 7-ethyl-10-[4-(1-piperidino)-1-piperidino]carbonyloxy camptothecin, a novel antitumor agent, by carboxylesterase. *Biol Pharm Bull* 1994; **17:** 662–4.

25. Covel JM, Jaxel C, Kohn KW et al, Protein-linked DNA strand breaks induced in mammalian cells by camptothecin, an inhibitor of topoisomerase I. *Cancer Res* 1989; **49:** 5016–22.

26. Fan Y, Kohn KW, Shi LM et al, Molecular modelling studies of the DNA topoisomerase I ternary complex with camptothecin. *J Med Chem* 1998; **41:** 2216–26.

27. Hsiang YH, Lihou MG, Liu LF, Arrest of replication forks by drug-stabilized topoisomerase I-DNA cleavable complexes as a mechanism of cell killing by camptothecin. *Cancer Res* 1989; **49:** 5077–82.

28. Hsiang YH, Liu LF, Identification of mammalian DNA topoisomerase I as an intracellular target of the anticancer drug camptothecin. *Cancer Res* 1988; **48:** 1722–6.

29. Ryan AJ, Squires S, Strutt HL et al, Camptothecin cytotoxicity in mammalian cells is associated with the induction of persistent double strand breaks in replicating DNA. *Nucleic Acids Res* 1991; **19:** 3295–300.

30. Ryan AJ, Squires S, Strutt HL et al, Different fates of camptothecin-induced replication fork-associated double-strand DNA breaks in mammalian cells. *Carcinogenesis* 1994; **15:** 823–8.

31. Tsao YP, Russo A, Nyamuswa G et al, Interaction between replication forks and topoisomerase I-DNA cleavable complexes: studies in a cell-free SV40 DNA replication system. *Cancer Res* 1993; **53:** 5908–14.

32. Egyhazi E, Durban E, Microinjection of anti-topoisomerase I immunoglobulin G into nuclei of chironomus tentans salivary gland cells leads to blockage of transcription elongation. *Mol Cell Biol* 1987; **7:** 4308–18.

33. Zhang H, Wang JC, Liu LF, Involvement of DNA topoisomerase I in transcription of human ribosomal RNA genes. *Proc Natl Acad Sci USA* 1988; **85:** 1060–4.

34. Voigt W, Matsui S, Yin MB et al, Topoisomerase I inhibitor SN38 can induce DNA damage and chromosomal aberrations independent from DNA synthesis. *Anticancer Res* 1998; **18:** 3499–506.

35. Desai SD, Liu LF, Vazquez-Abad D et al, Ubiquitin-dependent destruction of topoisomerase I is stimulated by the antitumor drug camptothecin. *J Biol Chem* 1997; **272:** 24159–64.

36. Houghton PJ, Cheshire PJ, Hallman JD et al, Efficacy of topoisomerase I inhibitors, topotecan and irinotecan, administered at low dose levels in protracted schedules to mice bearing xenografts of human tumors. *Cancer Chemother Pharmacol* 1995; **36:** 393–403.

37. Goldwasser F, Bae I, Valenti M et al, Topoisomerase I-related parameters and camptothecin activity in the colon carcinoma cell lines from the national cancer institute anticancer screen. *Cancer Res* 1995; **55:** 2116–21.

38. Ishikawa H, Kawano MM, Okada K et al, Expressions of DNA topoisomerase I and II gene and the genes possibly related to drug resistance in human myeloma cells. *Br J Haematol* 1993; **83:** 68–74.

39. McLeod HL, Keith WN, Variation in topoisomerase I gene copy number as a mechanism for intrinsic drug sensitivity. *Br J Cancer* 1996; **74:** 508–12.

40. Pommier Y, Leteurtre F, Fesen MR et al, Cellular determinants of sensitivity and resistance to DNA topoisomerase inhibitors. *Cancer Invest* 1994; **12:** 530–42.

41. Husian I, Mohler JL, Seigler HF et al, Elevation of topoisomerase I messenger RNA, protein, and catalytic activity in human tumors: demonstration of tumor-type specificity and implications for cancer chemotherapy. *Cancer Res* 1994; **54:** 539–46.

42. Staley BE, Samowith WS, Bronstein IB et al, Expression of DNA topoisomerase I and DNA topoisomerase II-alpha in carcinoma of the colon. *Mod Pathol* 1999; **12:** 356–61.

43. McLeod HL, Douglas F, Oates M et al, Topoisomerase I and II activity in human breast, cervix, lung and colon cancer. *Int J Cancer* 1994; **59:** 607–11.

44. Ohashi N, Fujiwara Y, Yamaoka N et al, No alteration in DNA topoisomerase I gene related to CPT-11 resistance in human lung cancer. *Jpn J Cancer Res* 1996; **87:** 1280–7.

45. Takatani H, Oka M, Fukuda M et al, Gene mutation analysis and quantitation of DNA topoisomerase I in previously untreated non-small cell lung carcinomas. *Jpn J Cancer Res* 1997; **88:** 160–5.

46. van der Zee AGJ, Hollema H, de Jong S et al, P-glycoprotein expression and DNA topoisomerase I and II activity in benign tumors of the ovary and in malignant tumors of the ovary, before and after platinum/cyclophosphamide chemotherapy. *Cancer Res* 1991; **51:** 5915–20.

47. Ling YH, Donato NJ, Perez-Soler R, Sensitivity to topoisomerase I inhibitors and cisplatin is associated with epidermal growth factor receptor expression in human cervical squamous carcinoma ME180 sublines. *Cancer Chemother Pharmacol* 2001; **47:** 473–80.

48. Yin MB, Toth K, Cao S et al, Involvement of cyclin D1–CDK-5 overexpression and MCM3 cleavage in bax-associated spontaneous apoptosis and differentiation in an A253 human head

and neck carcinoma xenograft model. *Int J Cancer* 1999; **83**: 341–8.

49. Guo B, Yin MB, Toth K et al, Dimerization of mitochondrial bax is associated with increased drug response in bax-transferred A253 cells. *Oncol Res* 1999; **11**: 97–9.

50. Guo B, Cao S, Toth K et al, Overexpression of Bax enhances antitumor activity of chemotherapeutic agents in human head and neck squamous cell carcinoma. *Clin Cancer Res* 2000; **6**: 718–24.

51. Kondo S, Yin D, Morimura T, Takeuchi J, bcl-2 gene prevents induction of apoptosis in L1210 murine leukemia cells by SN-38, a metabolite of the camptothecin derivative CPT-11. *Int J Oncol* 1994; **4**: 649–54.

52. Chen SF, Rothenberg LM, Clark G et al, Human tumor carboxylesterase activity correlates with CPT-11 cytotoxicity in vitro. *Proc Am Assoc Cancer Res* 1994; **35**: 365 (abst).

53. Andoh T, Ishii K, Suzuki Y et al, Characterization of a mammalian mutant with a camptothecin-resistant DNA topoisomerase I. *Proc Natl Acad Sci* 1987; **84**: 5565–9.

54. Benedetti P, Fiorani P, Capuani L et al, Camptothecin resistance from a single mutation changing glycine 363 of human DNA topoisomerase I to cysteine. *Cancer Res* 1993; **53**: 4343–8.

55. Fujimori A, Harker WG, Kohlhagen G et al, Mutation at the catalytic site of topoisomerase I in CEM/C2, a human leukemia cell line resistant to camptothecin. *Cancer Res* 1995; **55**: 1339–46.

56. Gromova I, Kjeldsen E, Svejstrup IQ et al, Characterization of an altered DNA catalysis of a camptothecin-resistant eukaryotic topoisomerase I. *Nucleic Acids Res* 1993; **21**: 593–600.

57. Kanzawa F, Sugimoto Y, Minato K et al, Establishment of a camptothecin analogue (CPT-11)-resistant cell line of human non-small cell lung cancer: characterization and mechanism of resistance. *Cancer Res* 1990; **50**: 5919–24.

58. Kapoor R, Slade DL, Fujimori A et al, Altered topoisomerase I expression in two subclones of human CEM leukemia selected for resistance to camptothecin. *Oncol Res* 1995; **7**: 83–95.

59. Eng WK, McCabe FL, Tan KB et al, Development of a stable camptothecin-resistant subline of P388 leukemia with reduced topoisomerase I content. *Mol Pharmacol* 1990; **38**: 471–80.

60. Sugimoto Y, Tsukahara S, Oh-Hara T et al, Decreased expression of DNA topoisomerase I in camptothecin-resistant tumor cell lines as determined by a monoclonal antibody. *Cancer Res* 1990; **50**: 6925–30.

61. Tan KB, Mattern MR, Eng WK et al, Nonproductive rearrangement of DNA topoisomerase I and II genes: correlation with resistance to topoisomerase inhibitors. *J Natl Cancer Inst* 1989; **81**: 1732–5.

62. Kojima A, Hackett N, Crystal RG, Reversal of CPT-11 resistance of lung cancer cells by adenovirus-mediated gene transfer of the human carboxylesterase cDNA. *Cancer Res* 1998; **58**: 4368–74.

63. Takahashi T, Fujiwara Y, Yamakido M et al, The role of glucuronidation in 7-ethyl-10-hydroxycamptothecin resistance in vitro. *Jpn J Cancer Res* 1997; **88**: 1211–17.

64. Sugimoto Y, Tsukahara S, Oh-Hara T et al, Elevated expression of DNA topoisomerase II in camptothecin-resistant human tumor cell lines. *Cancer Res* 1990; **50**: 7962–5.

65. Friedman HS, Dolan ME, Kaufmann SH et al, Elevated DNA polymerase alpha, DNA polymerase beta, and DNA topoisomerase II in a melphalan-resistant rhabdomyosarcoma xenograft that is cross-resistant to nitrosoureas and topotecan. *Cancer Res* 1994; **54**: 3487–93.

66. Holm C, Covey JM, Kerrigan D et al, Differential requirement of DNA replication for the cytotoxicity of DNA topoisomerase I and II inhibitors in Chinese hamster DC3F cells. *Cancer Res* 1989; **49**: 6365–8.

67. Hendrick CB, Rowinsky EK, Grochow LB et al, Effect of P-gly-

68. Jansen WJM, Hulscher TM, van Ark-Otte J et al, CPT-11 sensitivity in relation to the expression of P170-glycoprotein and multidrug resistance-associated protein. *Br J Cancer* 1998; **77**: 359–65.

69. Ma J, Maliepaard M, Nooter K et al, Reduced cellular accumulation of topotecan: a novel mechanism of resistance in a human ovarian cancer cell line. *Br J Cancer* 1998; **77**: 1645–52.

70. Mattern MR, Hofman GA, Polsky RM et al, In vitro and in vivo effects of clinically important camptothecin analogues on multidrug-resistant cells. *Oncol Res* 1993; **5**: 467–74.

71. Hapke G, Vanhoefer U, Harstrick A et al, Antitumor efficacy of irinotecan (CPT-11) and topotecan in nude mice bearing tumor xenografts that express the multidrug resistance protein (MRP). *Onkologie* 1999; **22**: 844 (abst).

72. Vanhoefer U, Müller MR, Hilger RA et al, Reversal of MDR1-associated resistance to topotecan by PAK-200S, a new dihydropyridine analogue, in human cancer cell lines. *Br J Cancer* 1999; **81**: 1304–10.

73. Filipits M, Suchomel RW, Dekan G et al, Expression of the multidrug resistance-associated protein (MRP) gene in colorectal carcinomas. *Br J Cancer* 1997; **75**: 208–12.

74. Tomonaga M, Oka M, Narasaki F et al, The multidrug resistance-associated protein gene confers drug resistance in human gastric and colon cancers. *Jpn J Cancer Res* 1996; **87**: 1263–70.

75. Creemers GJ, Ferrits CHJ, Plating ASTh et al, Phase II study with topotecan (T) administered as a 21-day continuous infusion to patients with colorectal cancer. *Eur J Cancer* 1995; **31A**(Suppl 5): 700 (abst).

76. Creemers GJ, Wanders J, Gamucci T et al, Topotecan in colorectal cancer: a phase II study of the EORTC early clinical trials group. *Ann Oncol* 1995; **8**: 844–6.

77. Rowinsky EK, Baker SD, Burks K et al, High-dose topotecan with granulocyte-colony stimulating factor in fluoropyrimidine-refractory colorectal cancer: a phase II and pharmacodynamic study. *Ann Oncol* 1998; **9**: 173–80.

78. Macdonald JS, Benedetti JK, Modiano M et al, Phase II evaluation of topotecan in patients with advanced colorectal cancer. *Invest New Drugs* 1997; **15**: 357–9.

79. Maliepaard M, van Gastelen MA, de Jong LA et al, Overexpression of the BCRP/MXR/ABCP gene in a topotecan-selected ovarian tumor cell line. *Cancer Res* 1999; **59**: 4559–63.

80. Yang CHJ, Horton JK, Cowan KH et al, Cross-resistance to camptothecin analogues in a mitoxantrone-resistant human breast carcinoma cell line is not due to DNA topoisomerase I alterations. *Cancer Res* 1995; **55**: 4004–9.

81. Brangi M, Litman T, Ciotti M et al, Camptothecin resistance: role of the ATP-binding cassette (ABC), mitoxantrone-resistance half-transporter (MXR), and potential for glucuronidation in MXR-expressing cells. *Cancer Res* 1999; **59**: 5938–46.

82. Erlichman C, Boerner SA, Hallgren CG et al, The HER tyrosine kinase inhibitor CI1033 enhances cytotoxicity of 7-ethyl-10-hydroxycamptothecin and topotecan by inhibiting breast cancer resistance protein-mediated drug efflux. *Cancer Res* 2001; **61**: 739–48.

83. Aschele C, Baldo C, Sobrero AF et al, Schedule-dependent synergism between raltitrexed and irinotecan in human colon cancer cells in vitro. *Clin Cancer Res* 1998; **4**: 1323–30.

84. Guichard S, Cussac D, Hennebelle I et al, Sequence-dependent activity of the irinotecan-5FU combination in human colon-cancer model HT-29 in vitro and in vivo. *Int J Cancer* 1997; **73**: 729–34.

85. Guichard S, Hennebelle I, Bugat R, Canal P, Cellular interac-

tions of 5-fluorouracil and the camptothecin analogue CPT-11 (irinotecan) in a human colorectal carcinoma cell line. *Biochem Pharmacol* 1998; **55:** 667–76.

86. Mans DRA, Grivicich I, Peters GJ et al, Sequence-dependent growth inhibition and DNA damages formation by the irinotecan–5–fluorouracil combination in human colon carcinoma cell lines. *Eur J Cancer* 1999; **35:** 1851–61.

87. Mullany S, Svingen PA, Kaufmann SH et al, Effect of adding the topoisomerase I poison 7-ethyl-10-hydroxycamptothecin (SN38) to 5-fluorouracil and folinic acid in HCT-8 cells: elevated dTTP pools and enhanced cytotoxicity. *Cancer Chemother Pharmacol* 1999; **42:** 391–9.

88. Pavillard V, Formento P, Rostagno P et al, Combination of irinotecan (CPT-11) and 5-fluorouracil with an analysis of cellular determinants of drug activity. *Biochem Pharmacol* 1998; **56:** 1315–22.

89. Vanhoefer U, Hapke G, Harstrick A et al, Schedule-dependent antitumor efficacy of irinotecan (CPT-11) in 5-FU resistant human colon tumor xenograft HT29R1. *Proc Am Soc Cancer Res* 1999; **40:** 728.

90. Rustum YM, Cao S, New drugs in therapy of colorectal cancer: preclinical studies. *Semin Oncol* 1999; **26:** 612–29.

91. Erlichman C, Scott B, Kaufmann SC, Mechanism of synergy between oxaliplatin and the topoisomerase I inhibitor SN-38. *Clin Cancer Res* 1999; **5**(Suppl): 615 (abst).

92. Zeghari-Squalli N, Raymond E, Cvitkovic E et al, Cellular pharmacology of the combination of the DNA topoisomerase I inhibitor SN-38 and the diaminocyclohexane platinum derivative oxaliplatin. *Clin Cancer Res* 1999; **5:** 1189–96.

93. Takasuna K, Hagiwara T, Hirohashi M et al, Inhibition of intestinal microflora β-glucuronidase modifies the distribution of the active metabolite of the antitumor agent, irinotecan hydrochloride (CPT-11) in rats. *Cancer Chemother Pharmacol* 1998; **42:** 280–6.

94. Takasuna K, Hagiwara T, Hirohashi M et al, Involvement of β-glucuronidase in intestinal microflora in the intestinal toxicity of the antitumor camptothecin derivative irinotecan hydrochloride (CPT-11) in rats. *Cancer Res* 1996; **56:** 3752–7.

95. Gupta E, Lestingi TM, Mick R et al, Metabolic fate of irinotecan in humans: correlation of glucuronidation with diarrhea. *Cancer Res* 1994; **54:** 3723–5.

96. Cao S, Black JD, Troutt AB et al, Interleukin 15 offers selective protection from irinotecan-induced intestinal toxicity in a preclinical animal model. *Cancer Res* 1998; **58:** 3270–4.

97. Shinohara H, Killion JJ, Bucana CD et al, Oral administration of the immunomodulator JBT-3002 induces endogenous interleukin 15 in intestinal macrophages for protection against irinotecan-mediated destruction of intestinal epithelium. *Clin Cancer Res* 1999; **5:** 2148–56.

50

Oxaliplatin: Mechanism of action and preclinical activity

Eric Raymond, Stephen Chaney, Esteban Cvitkovic

INTRODUCTION

Drugs that contain platinum, such as cisplatin and carboplatin, have been considered for many years to be among the most active anticancer agents in a variety of human tumours.[1] However, the occurrence or development of intrinsic or acquired resistance has been a major clinical problem associated with platinum-based therapy, with cisplatin and carboplatin sharing the same spectrum of antitumour activity and cross-resistance in most tumour types. During the last 30 years, thousands of analogues have been synthesized to overcome cellular resistance, enlarge the spectrum of activity, and reduce toxicity. Among the platinum derivatives, compounds bearing the 1,2-diaminocyclohexane (DACH) carrier ligand have demonstrated antitumour activity in cell lines with acquired cisplatin resistance, and appear to be active in several tumour types that are intrinsically resistant to cisplatin and carboplatin.[1-4] While several analogues have been tested in laboratory and clinical studies, only oxaliplatin has met the clinical criteria for safety and efficacy for a complete clinical development and registration.[5-7]

For many years, several new agents have been investigated for use in the treatment of advanced colorectal cancer.[8] Most of the successful drugs are thymidylate synthase (TS) inhibitors, including 5-fluorouracil (5-FU),[9,10] raltitrexed, UFT (uracil plus tegafur), and capecitabine. More recently, irinotecan (CPT-11), a topoisomerase I inhibitor deriving from captothecin, has also joined the armamentarium of drugs with clinical activity in patients with advanced colorectal cancer.[11,12] However, drugs such as cisplatin and carboplatin have consistently been shown to be inactive in clinical trials in colorectal cancer, either as single agents or in combination with other drugs, despite a perceived synergism with thymidylate synthase inhibitors and topoisomerase I inhibitors in preclinical and clinical studies in several other tumour types. The relative resistance of colon cancer cells to cisplatin (and carboplatin) remains poorly understood, but is thought to be related to an intrinsically high level of expression of several resistance mechanisms, including non-specific inactivation and efflux at the cytoplasmic level and specific DNA-adduct repair mechanisms at the nuclear level. The activity of oxaliplatin against colorectal cancer has been recognized both from the compilation of results from a number of clinical trials and from laboratory studies showing activity in colon cancer cells expressing intrinsic and acquired resistance to cisplatin and carboplatin. While the mechanisms of action of cisplatin and oxaliplatin appear similar in many ways, including DNA binding, adduct formation, strand breaks, and subsequent apoptosis, the reasons why oxaliplatin has more potent cytotoxic activity than cisplatin in colon cancer cells remain poorly understood. From a chemical standpoint, this differential in the resistance to cisplatin and oxaliplatin appears to be linked to the presence of the DACH carrier ligand (Figure 50.1). This DACH carrier ligand is retained in the DNA adducts formed by oxaliplatin, and could affect the mechanisms of DNA-damage recognition and repair classically involved in resistance to cisplatin.[13-18] Thus the DACH moiety might explain at least in part the greater cytotoxicity of oxaliplatin compared with cisplatin in colon cancer cells.

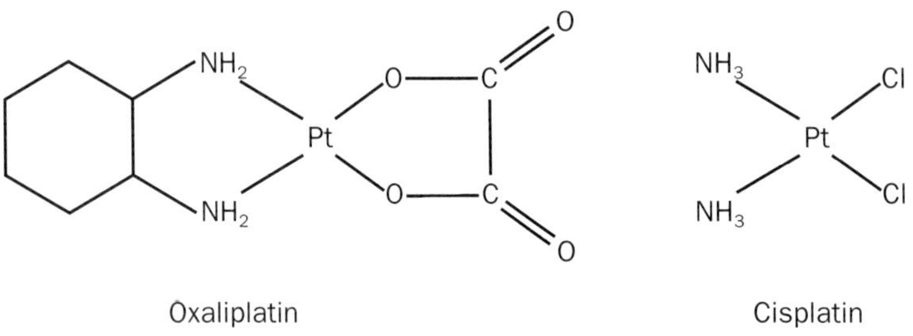

Figure 50.1 Chemical structures of oxaliplatin and cisplatin.

MECHANISMS OF ACTION AND CELLULAR PHARMACOLOGY

Oxaliplatin interacts principally at the DNA level, inducing several types of primary lesions that block DNA replication and RNA transcription. By far the most frequent type is represented by intrastrand adducts, in which the platinum is bound covalently to guanine (G) and adenine (A) residues; for example in A2780 ovarian cells, most adducts are Pt–GG and Pt–AG intrastrand crosslinks,[19] accounting for almost all detectable lesions. The other types of primary lesions are interstrand crosslinks and DNA–protein crosslinks. Investigations performed with naked DNA in vitro showed that oxaliplatin and cisplatin bind to similar G-rich regions of DNA, inducing intra- and interstrand crosslinks and strand breaks.[19,20] At equimolar concentrations, the levels of interstrand crosslinks and strand breaks were significantly less for oxaliplatin than for cisplatin.[19,20] In cells, the difference in adduct level between these two compounds appears smaller, suggesting enhancement of adduct formation by intracellular biotransformation of oxaliplatin to more reactive species.[19]

In A2780 cells, both oxaliplatin and cisplatin induce early and persistent strand breaks, inhibiting DNA synthesis and the induction of apoptosis.[21] However, the amount of platinum bound to cellular DNA is significantly less for oxaliplatin compared with cisplatin at equimolar concentrations. Thus oxaliplatin adducts appear to be more potent than cisplatin adducts at inducing apoptotic fragmentation.[21]

Ex vivo and in vivo pharmacokinetics in A2780 cells show that the rate of protein binding is high and similar for oxaliplatin and cisplatin, ranging from 85% to 88% within the first five hours. In whole blood, about one-third of oxaliplatin binds to erythrocytes within two hours.[22] This raised the question of whether the red blood cell could serve as a reservoir for cytotoxic DACH–Pt complexes. However, 83% of the platinum in red blood cells is irreversibly bound to membrane and cytosolic proteins.[15,22] In addition, biotransformation studies have shown that the majority of the ultrafilterable platinum in the red blood cells is complexed with sulphur-containing amino acids and glutathione.[15] These complexes are non-toxic to rat dorsal root ganglia in vitro,[23] and display no cytotoxicity towards human colon carcinoma cells in culture.[13] Thus it appears unlikely that the red blood cell serves as a reservoir for reactive platinum complexes.

IN VITRO STUDIES OF OXALIPLATIN AS A SINGLE AGENT

The cytotoxic activity of oxaliplatin against a variety of cell lines of human origin has been investigated (Table 50.1). These include ovarian, colon, breast, bladder, melanoma, and glioma cell lines, as well as embryonic tumours and leukaemia. Several methods have been used, including cell count, microtetrazoline (MTT) assay, and a clonogenic assay. Oxaliplatin was given either as a short 2-hour exposure, or by continuous exposure ranging from 24 hours to 96 hours. From the data summarized in Table 50.1, it appears that oxaliplatin has a broad cytotoxic effect in a number of cell lines, including colon, ovarian, and lung cancer lines, with IC_{50} (the concentration at which there is growth inhibition in 50% of the cells treated) values ranging from 0.5 to 240 μM in colon cells,[22,24] 0.12 to 19.8 μM in ovarian cells,[24,25] and 2.6 to 6.1 μM in lung cells.[26] Using a human cloning assay that tests the drug on tumour specimens taken directly from patients, oxaliplatin is active against breast, colon, and gastric cancer, renal cell carcinomas, and sarcomas.[27]

Using cisplatin tests on human cell lines as a benchmark, a comparison with oxaliplatin shows that the cytotoxicity of oxaliplatin is dissimilar to that of cisplatin. For example, a 24-hour exposure to oxaliplatin and cisplatin in the HT29 cell line led to IC_{50} values of 0.97 and 20.4 μM respectively.[25] In contrast, a 72-hour exposure to oxaliplatin and cisplatin

Table 50.1 Cytotoxicity of oxaliplatin as a single agent in vitro in a panel of colon cancer cell lines

Cell line	Origin	Assay	Duration of exposure (h)	IC$_{50}$ (μM)		Ref
				Oxaliplatin	Cisplatin	
HT29	Human	MTT	72	0.5		25
		MTT	24	0.97 ± 0.09	20.4 ± 1.68	25
		Cell count	48	2.11 ± 1.1		30
Colo 205	Human	MTT	2	10		43
SW620	Human	MTT	2	35		43
CAL14	Human	MTT	2	130		43
WIDR	Human	MTT	2	240		43
CACO2	Human	Cell count	48	5.9 ± 1.7		30
HCT116	Human	Clonogenic	60 min/d × 4 d	approx. 6 μM	approx. 6 μM	36
		Cell count	24	10.2 ± 4.9	2.7 ± 1.5	47
		Cell count	72	6.9 ± 0.2	19.7 ± 0.4	17
Colo 320 DM	Human	Cell count	24	4.6 ± 1.7	8.6 ± 1.0	47

MTT, microtetrazoline.

in the DLD-1 cell line led to IC$_{50}$ values of 21.5 and 6.6 μM respectively.

Interestingly, in vitro, the cytotoxicity of oxaliplatin depends on the duration of exposure, the drug being more effective with longer exposure duration. For example, in the A2780 ovarian cell line, the cytotoxicities of oxaliplatin in an MTT assay were 0.25 μM and 19.8 μM when the drug was given as 72-hour and 24-hour exposures respectively.[22,25] This was also observed in a cloning assay with cancer cells taken directly from patients, with a two-fold increase in the response rate after increasing the duration of exposure to oxaliplatin from 1 hour to 14 days.[27]

POTENCY OF OXALIPLATIN IN RESISTANT MODELS

Using the Drug Discovery Program from the National Cancer Institute (COMPARE), the DACH compounds, including oxaliplatin, were shown to have a different spectrum of activity than cisplatin and carboplatin.[24] Therefore oxaliplatin has been tested in vitro and in vivo against cell lines and tumour models selected for resistance to cisplatin. These include human ovarian, lung, cervix, and colon cancer and leukaemia cell lines. Resistance to cisplatin ranged from 8- to 80-fold compared with

the parental lines. The methods used included both cell counts and the MTT assay. The duration of treatment ranged from 2 to 72 hours for single exposure and 60 min/day × 4 for intermittent exposure. In cisplatin-resistant cell lines, the cross-resistance with oxaliplatin was mild, IC$_{50}$ values ranging from 0.19 to 14.3 μM. When a direct comparison was made with cisplatin, oxaliplatin generally had lower IC$_{50}$ values, as shown in Table 50.2. The data indicate that the activity of oxaliplatin is maintained in several mouse leukaemia (L1210/DDP, L1210 PtR4, L1210DDP5), human non-small cell lung cancer PC14/CDDP, cervical squamous cell carcinoma KB CP(20), and ovarian A2780-E(80) cells resistant to cisplatin.[24,28,29] In addition, oxaliplatin activity was not affected by resistance to 5-FU and doxorubicin in HT29 and MCF-7 cancer cell lines respectively.[30] Using the human cloning assay in resistant tumours, 1-hour exposures in 5.0 and 10.0 μg/ml of oxaliplatin led to 7.4% and 23.4% response rates respectively. This study showed that concentrations of oxaliplatin above 5 μg/ml have activity in some tumours that are unresponsive to cisplatin.

Resistance to platinum anticancer agents can result from decreased accumulation, increased inactivation by glutathione, or an increased ability of the cells to tolerate Pt–DNA adducts. However, cisplatin-resistant cell lines with decreased

Table 50.2 Cytotoxicity of oxaliplatin as a single agent in vitro in cell lines resistant to cisplatin

Cell line Parental	Resistant	Type of resistance (×fold)	Origin	Assay	Duration of exposure (h)	IC$_{50}$ (μM) Oxaliplatin	Cisplatin	Ref
Cervix KB3-1	KBCP	Cisplatin (×20)	Human	MTT	96	2.27 ± 1.2	78 ± 15	24
Ovarian A2780	A2780E	Cisplatin (×80)	Human	MTT	96	4.7 ± 0.9	92 ± 11	24
	A2780/CP	Cisplatin (×18)	Human	MTT	72	0.33		22
	A2780/CP	Cisplatin (×20)	Human	Cell count	72	25.4 ± 5.2	79 ± 4	17
	A2780C13	Cisplatin (×13)	Human	Cell count	48	13.5 ± 4.6		30
	A2780C10	Cisplatin (×8)	Human	MTT	72	0.19 ± 0.09		32
	A2780C25	Cisplatin (×12)	Human	MTT	72	2.2 ± 0.14		32
	A2780C70	Cisplatin (×32)	Human	Cell count	72	6.7 ± 0.2	124 ± 10	17
Lung PC-9	PC9/CDDP	Cisplatin (×11)	Human	Cell count	72	13.3 ± 0.7	11.0 ± 1.6	29
PC-14	PC14/CDDP	Cisplatin (×10)	Human	Cell count	72	14.3 ± 2	20.8 ± 3.3	29
Ovarian A2780	A2780/LOHP	Oxaliplatin (×4)	Human	MTT	72	0.9		22
Leukaemia L1210	L1210/CP	Cisplatin (×11)	Murine	MTT	72	0.1		22
Colon HT29	HT29-5-FU	5-FU (×6)	Human	Cell count	48	1.7 ± 0.8		30
Breast MCF-7	MCF-7/mdr	Doxorubicin (×2)	Human	Cell count	48	12.2 ± 9.1		30

accumulation of cisplatin also show decreased accumulation of carboplatin, ormaplatin, and oxaliplatin.[28] In addition, increased intracellular levels of glutathione have been shown to be associated with resistance to both cisplatin and oxaliplatin.[31,32] However, most cisplatin-resistant cell lines display an increased ability to tolerate cisplatin–DNA adducts, but retain a high degree of sensitivity to the presence of oxaliplatin–DNA adducts.[17] Thus a great deal of research has been focused on the nature of the DNA adducts formed by cisplatin and oxaliplatin and the mechanisms by which cells tolerate Pt–DNA adducts. Previous studies have shown that oxaliplatin can form the same major adducts (primarily GG and AG intrastrand diadducts) in the same proportions as cisplatin.[19,20] A recent molecular modelling study also suggests that the conformation of oxaliplatin–GG adducts is very similar to that of cisplatin–GG adducts, except for the presence of the bulky DACH ligand in the major groove of DNA.[33] However, it is possible that the DACH ligand may affect the flexibility of DNA containing the adducts.

The major mechanisms that affect the ability of cells to tolerate Pt–DNA adducts are nucleotide excision repair, post-replication repair, and mismatch repair. In addition, these processes may be affected by the presence in the cell of damage-recognition proteins that bind to Pt–DNA adducts. Because the genome is exposed to a wide variety of DNA-damaging agents, nucleotide excision repair has an extremely broad specificity. Thus it is not surprising that nucleotide excision repair does not appear to discriminate between oxaliplatin and cisplatin adducts.[16] In contrast, the mismatch-repair protein hMutSα binds to cisplatin adducts, but not to oxaliplatin adducts.[34] Furthermore, defects in mismatch repair are associated with a modest resistance to cisplatin, but not to oxaliplatin.[34–36] The mechanism of this effect is not known with any certainty. However, it has been proposed that the binding of the mismatch-repair complex to the Pt–DNA adducts may directly initiate a signal transduction pathway leading to cell-cycle arrest and/or apoptosis.[34,36] Alternatively, the mismatch-repair complex may prevent net replicative bypass of the adducts, thus leading to the presence of persistent gaps in the DNA, which serve as signals for apoptosis.

Post-replication repair (which is often referred to as replicative bypass) also discriminates between cisplatin and oxaliplatin adducts. Most cisplatin-resistant cell lines appear to show increased replicative bypass of cisplatin adducts, but not of oxaliplatin adducts.[17] The mechanism by which replicative bypass discriminates between cisplatin and oxali-

platin adducts is likely to be complex. Human pol β,[19] yeast pol ζ,[19] human pol γ,[19] and human pol η[37] have all been shown to replicate past oxaliplatin–GG adducts more efficiently than cisplatin–GG adducts. Of these polymerases, pol β, pol ζ, and/or pol η could, in theory, participate in the replicative bypass of Pt–DNA adducts in vivo. However, the specificity of these translesion polymerases for bypass of cisplatin and oxaliplatin adducts is different from the specificity of replicative bypass that is seen in cisplatin-resistant cell lines. Thus, while the level of expression of translesion polymerases such as pol β, pol ζ, and pol η may determine the extent of replicative bypass, the specificity of replicative bypass is likely to be influenced by other factors. For example, cell lines with defects in mismatch repair show increased replicative bypass of cisplatin adducts, but not of oxaliplatin adducts.[17] This is thought to be due to 'futile cycles' of translesion synthesis, followed by mismatch-repair removal of the newly synthesized strand. This would result in the presence of persistent gaps in the DNA, which would directly or indirectly lead to cell death. Thus loss of mismatch-repair activity leads to increased net replicative bypass of those adducts that are recognized by the mismatch-repair complex. Since cisplatin adducts are preferentially recognized by the mismatch-repair complex, loss of mismatch repair leads to preferential bypass of cisplatin adducts. Finally, Pt–DNA damage-recognition proteins have also been shown to block translesion synthesis past Pt–DNA adducts.[18] Thus those Pt–DNA damage-recognition proteins that bind to cisplatin and oxaliplatin DNA adducts with different efficiencies could also impart specificity to the process of replicative bypass.[18]

Over 25 cellular proteins have been discovered that bind to Pt–DNA adducts. All of these Pt–DNA damage-recognition proteins are proteins that bind to bent or bendable DNA, and normally play important roles in chromatin structure, transcription, repair, recombination, and/or damage recognition. The role of these proteins in determining the response to platinum anticancer agents has not been determined, but they have been proposed to block nucleotide excision repair and replicative bypass of the adducts,[18] hijack essential transcription factors, and/or act as 'damage sensors' that initiate signal transduction pathways leading to cell-cycle arrest or apoptosis. Two of the three Pt–DNA damage-recognition proteins that have been evaluated in detail bind with significantly different affinities to cisplatin and oxaliplatin adducts.[18] The extent to which different resistance mechanisms are thought to affect the cytotoxicity of cisplatin and oxaliplatin is summarized in Table 50.3.

Table 50.3 Mechanisms of resistance to cisplatin and oxaliplatin

Mechanisms of resistance	Cisplatin	Oxaliplatin
Cytoplasmic level[13]		
Decreased diffusion through the cell membrane	+ +	+ +
Increased efflux from cancer cells	+ +	+ +
Increased inactivation by glutathione in the cytoplasm	+ + +	+ + +
Nuclear level[16–18]		
Increased quenching	+	+
Increased excision repair	+ + +	+ + +
Increased post-replication repair	+ + +	+
Decreased mismatch repair	+ + +	±
Recognition of adducts by damage-recognition proteins	+ +	+

Resistance to platinum compounds in colon cancer might be, at least in part, due to mutations of genes involved in DNA mismatch repair. Mutations of mismatch-repair genes are found in about 15% of sporadic tumours at the time of diagnosis, and are characterized by a microsatellite instability, replication-error-positive (RER⁺) phenotype. Mutations of the mismatch-repair mechanism are also frequently found in patients with hereditary non-polyposis colorectal cancers (HNPCC). To date, six genes encoding proteins involved in the mismatch repair have been identified. Mutations of *hMSH2* and *hMLH1* are the most frequent, representing 45–49% of all mutations in cancer cells with an RER⁺ phenotype. Interestingly, the RER⁺ phenotype seems to be more frequently observed in advanced stages of colorectal cancer. Furthermore, and most importantly, the acquisition of mismatch-repair deficiency during tumour progression and/or as a consequence of previous chemotherapy treatment is a highly prevalent phenomenon in solid tumours[38] and notably in cancers of the colon.[39,40] This is usually through a lack of transcription of the *hMLH1* gene promoter as a result of hypermethylation.[39,40]

In summary, mismatch repair, replicative bypass (post-replication repair), and Pt–DNA damage-recognition proteins all discriminate between cisplatin and oxaliplatin DNA adducts. In addition, the extent and specificity of replicative bypass is likely to be determined by translesion DNA polymerase(s), mismatch-repair activity, and Pt–DNA damage-recognition proteins. Research over the next few years will be focused on evaluating the relative importance of these proteins in determining the overall cellular response to cisplatin and oxaliplatin. Ideally, it may be possible to utilize this information to identify molecular markers that would predict the relative efficacy of cisplatin and oxaliplatin chemotherapy. In cases where the mechanism(s) of resistance are unknown, it may be possible to predict responsiveness to oxaliplatin using a cloning assay with tumour specimens taken from the patient,[27] or by immunohistochemistry of tumoral biopsies.[41]

PRECLINICAL NEUROTOXICITY

The neurotoxicity of oxaliplatin has been compared with that of cisplatin and ormaplatin in Wistar rats by morphometric analysis of the dorsal root ganglia by Holmes et al.[26] Oxaliplatin caused non-significant changes in all three morphometric parameters measured (neuronal cell area, nuclear area, and cells with multiple nucleoli), and was considered to be less neurotoxic than either cisplatin or ormaplatin in that model system.[23]

Similar results were obtained with an in vitro assay using embryonic rat dorsal root ganglia explant cultures.[23] The plasma biotransformations of oxaliplatin appear to offer an explanation for its reduced neurotoxicity compared with ormaplatin. Following oxaliplatin infusion in both rats and humans, oxaliplatin is the major platinum complex in plasma at all times tested. In contrast,

Pt(DACH)Cl$_2$ is the major platinum complex in plasma following ormaplatin infusion in both rats and humans. The plasma Pt(DACH)Cl$_2$ concentration is 30- to 50-fold lower following oxaliplatin infusion than following ormaplatin infusion. All other plasma biotransformation products are identical and are present at the same concentrations following ormaplatin and oxaliplatin infusion. The striking difference in Pt(DACH)Cl$_2$ levels is likely to be significant, since experiments with rat dorsal root ganglia explant cultures have shown that Pt(DACH)Cl$_2$ is fourfold more neurotoxic than oxaliplatin.[23] Thus, differences in the severity of the neurotoxicity associated with ormaplatin and oxaliplatin treatment appear to be directly related to differences in the biotransformations of these two compounds.

Screnci et al[42] correlated the peripheral sensory neurotoxicity of the DACH–platinum complexes oxaliplatin and ormaplatin with their stereochemistry. The R,R enantiomers of ormaplatin, oxaliplatin, and their dichloro metabolites produced peripheral sensory neurotoxicity at lower cumulative doses and at earlier times than the S,S enantiomers. There was no difference in the platinum concentration in blood or tissues for the different platinum enantiomers. Thus the mechanism of stereoselective neurotoxicity of oxaliplatin is not completely known.

IN VITRO AND IN VIVO STUDIES OF OXALIPLATIN-BASED COMBINATIONS
(see Tables 50.4–50.6)

Oxaliplatin has been combined with TS inhibitors, topoisomerase I inhibitors, other platinum compounds such as cisplatin and carboplatin, taxanes, mitomycin C, cyclophosphamide, and more recently a recombinant adenovirus replicating selectively in p53-deficient cells.

Antimetabolites

Combination with a variety of TS inhibitors, including 5-FU, AG337, and UFT in vitro and/or in vivo showed additive or synergistic effects. In vitro, oxaliplatin given simultaneously with 5-FU had a synergistic effect in HT29 colon cancer cells, MDA-MB-231 breast cancer cells and A2008 ovarian cancer cells.[30] In vivo, 5-FU potentiated oxaliplatin antitumour activity against HT29 xenografts.[10,30] A number of investigations of oxaliplatin with 5-FU in colon cancer cells showed synergy with no sequence dependence. However, cytotoxicity was significantly

different according to the 5-FU exposure type (short > mixed > continuous exposure). Moreover, leucovorin (folinic acid) increased significantly the cytotoxicity of the FUFOL regimen in vitro.[43,44]

The combination of oxaliplatin with the TS inhibitor AG337 displayed synergistic effects both in vitro in the A2008 ovarian cell line and in vivo against GR murine mammary tumours.[8,30] In vivo, the combination of oral UFT plus leucovorin plus oxaliplatin treatment had an increased antitumour activity compared to oxaliplatin or UFT plus leucovorin alone.[45] In a model of peritoneal colon carcinomatosis in rats, oxaliplatin had synergistic activities with 5-FU, mitomycin C, and cyclophosphamide.[46]

Other antimetabolites, such as gemcitabine, displayed synergistic effects with oxaliplatin in two different colon cancer cell lines (HCT116 and Colo 320 DM). The cytotoxic effect was sequence-dependent, gemcitabine followed by oxaliplatin being more cytotoxic than the opposite sequence. When a comparison was made with cisplatin, the effects of the oxaliplatin–gemcitabine combinations were superior to those of cisplatin–gemcitabine combinations.[47]

Platinum compounds

Based on the NCI COMPARE program results, classical platinum compounds were combined with DACH–platinum compounds, and synergy was observed both in vitro and in vivo. In vitro, the combination of oxaliplatin and cisplatin showed at least additive and possibly synergistic effects.[24] In vivo, simultaneous injection of oxaliplatin and cisplatin or carboplatin resulted in synergistic antitumour activity against murine leukaemia L1210, 70% of animals being cured with the latter combination.[48,49]

Topoisomerase I inhibitors

Oxaliplatin was combined with irinotecan in vivo and with its active metabolite SN38 in vitro. In vitro, SN38 showed synergistic effects when combined with oxaliplatin in the HT29 colon cancer cell line. The cytotoxicity of this combination was sequence-dependent, oxaliplatin followed by SN38 being more cytotoxic than the opposite sequence or simultaneous administration. The supra-additive toxicity observed with oxaliplatin and SN38 was associated with evidence of reciprocal interactions: prior exposure to oxaliplatin enhanced the toxic effects of SN38, with a more pronounced S-phase block. A high rate of DNA fragmentation was detectable in cells at 48 hours, con-

Table 50.4 Cytotoxicity of oxaliplatin (OXA) in combination in vitro[a]

Combination	Tumour types		Results	Schedule dependence	Comments	Ref
SN38/OXA/FUFOL	Colon:	WIDR SW620	Synergy	Yes: SN38 484 prior to OXA/FUFOL	—	43
SN38/OXA	Colon:	HT29	Synergy	Oxaliplatin prior to SN38	SN38 slows down oxaliplatin-induced interstrand crosslink repair	51
OXA/cisplatin	Cervix:	KB3-1 KBCP	At least additive	Not evaluated	—	24
	Ovarian:	A2780 A2780/E80				
OXA/gemcitabine	Colon:	HCT116 Colo 320 DM	Synergy	Gemcitabine prior to oxaliplatin	Oxaliplatin was superior to cisplatin in the same combinations	47
	Leukaemia:	CEM				
OXA/5-FU ± FA[b]	Colon:	Colo 205 SW620 CAL14 WIDR	Synergy	FA significantly enhances the effect of OXA/5-FU	Short exposure to 5-FU has later cytotoxicity in combination with oxaliplatin	43
OXA/5-FU	Colon:	HT29 HT29-5-FU	Synergy in colon and ovarian and additive effect in breast cancer	Not performed	—	30
	Breast:	MCF-7 MCF-7/mdr				
	Ovarian:	A2008 A2008C13				
OXA/AG337	Ovarian:	A2008 A2008C13	Synergy	Not performed	—	30

[a] The statistical method used throughout was that of Chou and Talalay.
[b] FA, folinic acid (leucovorin).

Table 50.5 Activity of oxaliplatin as a single agent in vivo

Tumour type	Resistance to cisplatin	Dose range (mg/kg)[a]	Route[b]	Antitumour activity	Ref
L1210 murine leukaemia	No	3–10	i.p.	++ (> cisplatin)	54
		6–8	i.v.	± (= cisplatin)	54
		NS	s.c.	++ (> cisplatin)	54
L1210 murine leukaemia	No	NS	i.p.	++ (> cisplatin)	55
L1210/DDP murine leukaemia	Yes	3.1–6.2	i.p.	++ (> cisplatin)	56
AKR murine leukaemia	Yes	5–7.5	i.p.	++ (= cisplatin)	54
LGC murine leukaemia	Yes	5	i.p.	++ (> cisplatin)	54
Glasgow osteogenic carcinoma	No	10.2	i.v.	++	52
HT29 human colon xenograft	No	10	i.p.	++	30
HCT116 + 3 human colon xenograft	No	12	i.p.	++ (= cisplatin)	36
HCT116 human colon xenograft	Yes (low-level)	12	i.p.	++ (> cisplatin)	36
GR1 murine mammary tumour	No	10	i.p.	++	30
GR1 1 murine mammary tumour	No	10	i.p.	++	51

[a] NS, not specified.
[b] i.p., intraperitoneal; i.v., intravenous; s.c., subcutaneous.

Table 50.6 Activity of oxaliplatin (OXA) in combination in vivo[a]

Combinations	Mice	Tumour type	Results	Comments	Ref
OXA/cyclophosphamide	BDFI	L1210 leukaemia	Modest additivity	—	46
OXA/cyclophosphamide/5-FU	BDFI	L1210 leukaemia	Supra additivity effects	—	46
OXA/5-FU	Nude	HT29 colon	Additive	—	30
	GR-1	Mammary tumours	Additive		
OXA/carboplatin	B6D2 F1	L1210 leukaemia	Synergy	—	48
OXA/UFT	Nude	HT29 colon	Additive	Better effects with leucovorin	45
OXA/FUFOL	BDIX	DHD/K2-TRb colon	Synergy	Synergy mentioned with mitomycin C and cyclophosphamide	57
OXA/irinotecan	GR-1	Mammary tumours	Additive	—	51
OXA/irinotecan	B6D2	GOS sarcoma	Additive at best	—	52
OXA/paclitaxel	Nude	MU-522 lung	Additive effects	—	58
OXA/paclitaxel/tirapazamine	Nude	MU-522 lung	Additive effects	—	59

[a] Schedule dependence was not evaluated in any of these studies.

firming that S-phase-arrested cells were undergoing apoptosis. DNA- and RNA-synthesis inhibition following topoisomerase-I-mediated DNA damage may also slow the reversion of oxaliplatin-induced interstrand crosslinks.[50,51] The oxaliplatin/irinotecan combination was also active in vivo against GR1 mouse mammary tumour.[51] However, the activity of the same combination was not superior to the activity of oxaliplatin alone in an osteogenic sarcoma model.[52,53]

CONCLUSIONS

Convergent laboratory data indicate that oxaliplatin is at least as efficient as cisplatin in cancer cells sensitive to platinum agents. Moreover, a number of cancer cells either primarily or secondarily resistant to cisplatin remain sensitive to oxaliplatin. This preclinical aspect of the mechanism of action of oxaliplatin is best exemplified by several clinical trials showing that colon cancers primarily resistant to cisplatin are sensitive to oxaliplatin either alone or in combination with 5-FU or irinotecan. Specific molecular events at the origin of human carcinogenesis of colon cancer, such as mismatch-repair deficiency, indicate that oxaliplatin may be the DNA-interacting agent of choice in this indication. Similarly, ovarian cancers sensitive to cisplatin remain sensitive to oxaliplatin, with a better clinical tolerance, allowing the treatment of patients with a bad performance status and patients with an impaired renal function. In addition, preclinical studies showed a marked in vitro synergy with most of the TS and topoisomerase I inhibitors available for prescription. These preclinical observations translated into a supra-additive activity in vivo, and were often associated with good results in clinical trials based on the preclinical studies described above, clinical trials investigating the effects of oxaliplatin with 5-FU, raltitrexed, irinotecan, and topotecan have been performed or are ongoing, and are reported elsewhere in this book.

REFERENCES

1. Cvitkovic E, A historical perspective on oxaliplatin: rethinking the role of platinum compounds and learning from near misses. *Semin Oncol* 1998; **25**: 1–3.

2. Cvitkovic E, Ongoing and unsaid on oxaliplatin: the hope. *Br J Cancer* 1998; **77**(Suppl 4): 8–11.

3. Llory JF, Soulie P, Cvitkovic E, Misset JL, Feasibility of high-dose platinum delivery with combined carboplatin and oxaliplatin. *J Natl Cancer Inst* 1994; **86**: 1098–9.

4. Soulie P, Bensmaine A, Garrino C et al, Oxaliplatin/cisplatin (L-OHP/CDDP) combination in heavily pretreated ovarian cancer. *Eur J Cancer* 1997: **33**: 1400–6.

5. Raymond E, Chaney SG, Taamma A, Cvitkovic E, Oxaliplatin: a review of preclinical and clinical studies. *Ann Oncol* 1998; **9**: 1053–71.

6. Raymond E, Faivre S, Woynarowski JM, Chaney SG, Oxaliplatin: mechanism of action and antineoplastic activity. *Semin Oncol* 1998; **25**: 4–12.

7. Soulie P, Raymond E, Brienza S, Cvitkovic E, Oxaliplatin: the first DACH platinum in clinical practice. *Bull Cancer* 1997; **84**: 665–73.

8. Ducreux M, Louvet C, Bekradda M, Cvitkovic E, Oxaliplatin for the treatment of advanced colorectal cancer: future directions. *Semin Oncol* 1998; **25**: 47–53.

9. Andre T, Louvet C, Raymond E et al, Bimonthly high-dose leucovorin, 5-fluorouracil infusion and oxaliplatin (FOLFOX3) for metastatic colorectal cancer resistant to the same leucovorin and 5-fluorouracil regimen. *Ann Oncol* 1998; **9**: 1251–3.

10. de Gramont A, Vignoud J, Tournigand C et al, Oxaliplatin with high-dose leucovorin and 5-fluorouracil 48-hour continuous infusion in pretreated metastatic colorectal cancer. *Eur J Cancer* 1997; **33**: 214–19.

11. Boige V, Raymond E, Armand JP, Irinotecan: various administration schedules, study of drug combinations, phase I experience. *Bull Cancer* 1998 (Dec): 26–32.

12. Monnet I, Brienza S, Hugret F et al, Phase II study of oxaliplatin in poor-prognosis non-small cell lung cancer (NSCLC), ATTIT. Association pour le Traitement des Tumeurs Intra Thoraciques. *Eur J Cancer* 1998; **34**: 1124–7.

13. Luo FR, Wyrick SD, Chaney SG, Cytotoxicity, cellular uptake, and cellular biotransformations of oxaliplatin in human colon carcinoma cells. *Oncol Res* 1998; **10**: 595–603.

14. Luo FR, Yen TY, Wyrick SD, Chaney SG, High-performance liquid chromatographic separation of the biotransformation products of oxaliplatin. *J Chromatogr B Biomed Sci Appl* 1999; **724**: 345–56.

15. Luo FR, Wyrick SD, Chaney SG, Biotransformations of oxaliplatin in rat blood in vitro. *J Biochem Mol Toxicol* 1999; **13**: 159–69.

16. Reardon JT, Vaisman A, Chaney SG, Sancar A, Efficient nucleotide excision repair of cisplatin, oxaliplatin, and bis-aceto-ammine-dichloro-cyclohexylamine-platinum(iv) (JM216) platinum intrastrand DNA diadducts. *Cancer Res* 1999; **59**: 3968–71.

17. Vaisman A, Varchenko M, Umar A et al, The role of hMLH1, hMSH3, and hMSH6 defects in cisplatin and oxaliplatin resistance: correlation with replicative bypass of platinum–DNA adducts. *Cancer Res* 1998; **58**: 3579–85.

18. Vaisman A, Lim SE, Patrick SM et al, Effect of DNA polymerases and high mobility group protein 1 on the carrier ligand specificity for translesion synthesis past platinum–DNA adducts. *Biochemistry* 1999; **38**: 11026–39.

19. Saris CP, van de Vaart PJM, Rietbroek RC, Blommaert FA, In vitro formation of DNA adducts by cisplatin, lobaplatin and oxaliplatin in calf thymus DNA in solution and in cultured human cells. *Carcinogenesis* 1996; **17**: 2763–9.

20. Woynarowski JM, Chapman WG, Napier C et al, Sequence- and region-specificity of oxaliplatin adducts in naked and cellular DNA. *Mol Pharmacol* 1998; **54**: 770–7.

21. Faivre S, Woynarowski JM, Oxaliplatin effects on DNA integrity and apoptosis induction in human tumor cells. *Proc Am Assoc Cancer Res* 1998; **39**: 158.

22. Pendyala L, Kidani Y, Perez R et al, Cytotoxicity, cellular accumulation and DNA binding of oxaliplatin isomers. *Cancer Lett* 1995; **97**: 177–84.

23. Luo FR, Wyrick SD, Chaney SG, Comparative neurotoxicity of oxaliplatin, ormaplatin, and their biotransformation products utilizing a rat dorsal root ganglia in vitro explant culture model. *Cancer Chemother Pharmacol* 1999; **44**: 29–38.

24. Rixe O, Ortuzar W, Alvarez M et al, Oxaliplatin, tetraplatin, cisplatin, and carboplatin: spectrum of activity in drug-resistant cell lines and in the cell lines of the National Cancer Institute's Anticancer Drug Screen Panel. *Biochem Pharmacol* 1996; **52:** 1855–65.

25. Pendyala L, Creaven PJ, In vitro cytotoxicity, protein binding, red blood cell partitioning, and biotransformation of oxaliplatin. *Cancer Res* 1993; **53:** 5970–6.

26. Holmes J, Stanko J, Varchenko M et al, Comparative neurotoxicity of oxaliplatin, cisplatin, and ormaplatin in a Wistar rat model. *Toxicol Sci* 1998; **46:** 342–51.

27. Raymond A, Lawrence R, Izbicka E et al, Activity of oxaliplatin against human tumor colony-forming units. *Clin Cancer Res* 1998; **4:** 1021–9.

28. Kraker A, Steinkampf RW, Moore CW, Transport of Cis-Pt and Cis-Pt analogs in sensitive and resistant murine leukemia cell lines. *Proc Am Assoc Cancer Res* 1986; **27:** 286.

29. Fukuda M, Ohe Y, Kanzawa F et al, Evaluation of novel platinum complexes, inhibitors of topoisomerase I and II in non-small cell lung cancer (NSCLC) sublines resistant to cisplatin. *Anticancer Res* 1995; **15:** 393–8.

30. Raymond E, Buquet-Fagot C, Djelloul S et al, Antitumor activity of oxaliplatin in combination with 5-fluorouracil and the thymidylate synthase inhibitor AG337 in human colon, breast and ovarian cancers. *Anticancer Drugs* 1997; **8:** 876–85.

31. Pendyala L, Creaven PJ, Perez R et al, Intracellular glutathione and cytotoxicity of platinum complexes. *Cancer Chemother Pharmacol* 1995; **36:** 271–8.

32. el-akawi Z, Abu-hadid M, Perez R et al, Altered glutathione metabolism in oxaliplatin resistant ovarian carcinoma cells. *Cancer Lett* 1996; **105:** 5–14.

33. Scheeff ED, Briggs JM, Howell SB, Molecular modeling of the intrastrand guanine–guanine DNA adducts produced by cisplatin and oxaliplatin. *Mol Pharmacol* 1999; **56:** 633–43.

34. Fink D, Nebel S, Aebi S et al, The role of DNA mismatch repair in platinum drug resistance. *Cancer Res* 1996; **56:** 4881–6.

35. Nebel S, Fink D, Nehme A et al, Role of the DNA mismatch repair proteins in the recognition of platinum DNA adducts. *Proc Am Assoc Cancer Res* 1997; **38:** 359.

36. Fink D, Zheng H, Nebel S et al, In vitro and in vivo resistance to cisplatin in cells that have lost DNA mismatch repair. *Cancer Res* 1997; **57:** 1841–5.

37. Vaisman A, Masutani C, Hanaoka F, Chaney SG, Efficient translesion replication past oxaliplatin and cisplatin GpG adducts by human DNA polymerase eta. *Biochemistry* 2000; **39:** 4575–80.

38. Mackay HJ, Cameron D, Rahilly M et al, Reduced MLH1 expression in breast tumors after primary chemotherapy predicts disease-free survival. *J Clin Oncol* 2000; **18:** 87–93.

39. Strathdee G, MacKean M, Illand M et al, A role for methylation of the hMLH1 promoter in loss of hMLH1 expression and drug resistance. *Oncogene* 1999; **18:** 2335–41.

40. Herman JG, Umar A, Polyak K et al, Incidence and functional consequences of hMLH1 promoter hypermethylation in colorectal carcinoma. *Proc Natl Acad Sci USA* 1998; **95:** 6870–5.

41. Fink D, Nebel S, Norris PS et al, The effect of different chemotherapeutic agents on the enrichment of DNA MMR-deficient tumour cells. *Br J Cancer* 1998; **77:** 703–8.

42. Screnci D, Er HM, Hambley TW et al, Stereoselective peripheral sensory neurotoxicity of diaminocyclohexane platinum enantiomers related to ormaplatin and oxaliplatin. *Br J Cancer* 1997; **76:** 502–10.

43. Fischel JL, Etienne MC, Formento P, Milano G, Search for the optimal schedule for the oxaliplatin/5-fluorouracil association

44. Metzger G, Massari C, Etienne MC et al, Spontaneous or imposed circadian changes in plasma concentrations of 5-fluorouracil coadministered with folinic acid and oxaliplatin: relationship with mucosal toxicity in patients with cancer. *Clin Pharmacol Ther* 1994; **56:** 190–201.

45. Louvet C, Coudray AM, Tournigand C et al, Synergistic antitumoral activity of combined UFT, folinic acid and oxaliplatin against human colorectal HT29 cell xenografts in athymic nude mice. *Anticancer Drugs* 2000; **11:** 579–82.

46. Gale GR, Loretta M, Atkins LM et al, Potentiating action of 5-fluorouracil when used in combination with platinum compounds and cyclophosphamide in treatment of advanced L1210 leukemia. *Bioinorg Chem* 1987; **8:** 445–51.

47. Faivre S, Raymond E, Woynarowski JM, Cvitkovic E, Supraadditive effect of 2′,2′-difluorodeoxycytidine (gemcitabine) in combination with oxaliplatin in human cancer cell lines. *Cancer Chemother Pharmacol* 1999; **44:** 117–23.

48. Mathe G, Chenu E, Bourut C, Florentin I, Experimental study of three platinum complexes: CDDP, CBDCA and L-OHP on L1210 leukemia. *Proc Am Assoc Cancer Res* 1989; **30:** 471.

49. Mathe G, Kidani Y, Segiguchi M et al, Oxalato-platinum or *l*-OHP, a third-generation platinum complex: an experimental and clinical appraisal and preliminary comparison with cis-platinum and carboplatinum. *Biomed Pharmacother* 1989; **43:** 237–50.

50. Goldwasser F, Bozec L, Zeghari-Squalli N, Misset JL, Cellular pharmacology of the combination of oxaliplatin with topotecan in the IGROV-1 human ovarian cancer cell line. *Anticancer Drugs* 1999; **10:** 195–201.

51. Zeghari-Squalli N, Raymond E, Cvitkovic E, Goldwasser F, Cellular pharmacology of the combination of the DNA topoisomerase I inhibitor SN-38 and the diaminocyclohexane platinum derivative oxaliplatin. *Clin Cancer Res* 1999; **5:** 1189–96.

52. Bissery MC, Vrignaud P, Lavelle F, In vivo evaluation of the irinotecan–oxaliplatin combination. *Proc Am Assoc Cancer Res* 1998; **39:** 526–7.

53. Mailliet P, Segal-Bendirdjian E, Kozelka J et al, Asymmetrically substituted ethylenediamine platinum(II) complexes as antitumor agents: synthesis and structure–activity relationships. *Anticancer Drug Des* 1995; **10:** 51–73.

54. Mathe G, Kidani Y, Noji M et al, Antitumour activity of L-OHP in mice. *Cancer Lett* 1985; **27:** 135–43.

55. Machida S, Ito Y, Kojima T et al, Comparative studies of antitumor activities of oxalate-(trans-1-1,2-cyclohexane diamine)platinum(II) and cis-dichlorodiaminoplatinum(II). In: *Proceedings of International Congress of Chemotherapy 1985*, Vol. 14: 461.

56. Tashiro T, Kawada Y, Sakurai Y, Kidani Y, Antitumor activity of a new platinum complex, oxalato (trans-1-1,2-diaminocyclohexane)platinum(II): new experimental data. *Biomed Pharmacother* 1989; **43:** 251–60.

57. Genne P, Duchamp O, Brienza S et al, Oxaliplatin (L-OHP) in combination with 5-fluorouracil (5FU), mitomycin C (MTC) or cyclophosphamide (CPM) in a model of peritoneal carcinomatosis induced by colon cancer cells in BD IX rats. *Proc Am Assoc Cancer Res* 1997; **38:** 319.

58. Skou G, Mangold G, Dexter D, Von Hoff DD, Comparison of an oxaliplatin–Taxol versus carboplatin–Taxol regimen in the treatment of the MV-522 human lung tumor xenograft. *Proc Am Assoc Cancer Res* 1996; **37:** 375.

59. Debner J, Dexter D, Mangold G et al, Evaluation of oxaliplatin–tirapazamine–Taxol combinations in the MV-522 human lung carcinoma xenograft model. *Proc Am Assoc Cancer Res* 1997; **38:** 312.

51

Raltitrexed and the new thymidylate synthase inhibitors

Hugo ER Ford, David Cunningham

INTRODUCTION

Thymidylate synthase

Thymidylate synthase (TS) is a critical enzyme in the de novo synthesis of thymidylate (dTMP), which is the only nucleotide specifically required for DNA synthesis. The enzyme acts by reductive methylation of 2′-deoxyuridylate (dUMP), requiring the donation of a methyl group. This is provided by the folate cofactor 5,10-methylenetetrahydrofolate. In this respect, it is one of a number of folate-dependent enzymes involved in purine and thymidine nucleotide synthesis and metabolism (Figure 51.1).

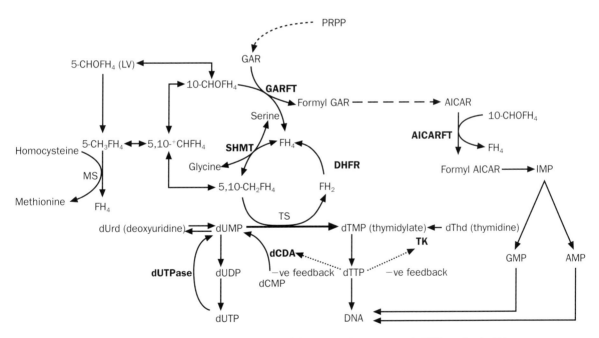

Figure 51.1 The role of thymidylate synthase (TS) and other folate-dependent enzymes in DNA synthesis. FH$_4$, tetrahydrofolate; TK, thymidine kinase; DHFR, dihydrofolate reductase; MS, methionine synthetase; SHMT, serine hydroxymethyltransferase; dCDA, deoxycytidylate deaminase; GARFT, glycinamide ribonucleotide formyltransferase; AICARFT, aminoimidazolecarboxamide ribonucleotide formyltransferase; PRPP, phosphoribosyl pyrophosphate; IMP, inositol monophosphate; AMP, adenosine monophosphate; GMP, guanidine monophosphate; LV, leucovorin.

5-Fluorouracil (5-FU), via one of its active metabolites 5-fluoro-2'-deoxyuridine monophosphate (FdUMP), inhibits TS by binding to the pyrimidine-binding site of the enzyme and the subsequent formation of a stable ternary complex with the enzyme and the folate cofactor.[1] There is evidence that other 5-FU metabolites (principally FUTP) are incorporated into RNA, which may also account for some of the cytotoxicity seen with this drug.[2] Preclinical observations have suggested that TS inhibition may be more prominent with prolonged exposures to 5-FU, whereas the RNA effects may be more prominent when shorter exposures are employed.[3] In addition, clinical studies have shown that there is no reduction in response rate or survival when infused 5-FU regimens are compared with bolus schedules, although toxicity is reduced.[4] Drug development programmes have therefore focused on the development of newer specific inhibitors of TS based on the structure of the folate cofactor.

Uptake and polyglutamation of antifolate TS inhibitors

In assessing this class of drugs, it is relevant to examine the properties and metabolism of natural folates, and how these relate to potential resistance mechanisms and the properties of individual compounds (Figure 51.2). In nature, reduced folates are largely transported into the cell by the reduced folate carrier (RFC), and subsequently metabolized by the enzyme folylpolyglutamate synthetase (FPGS) to polyglutamated forms. The higher-chain-length polyglu-

tamates are retained intracellularly, since they are not readily effluxed by the RFC. These polyglutamates are, however, thought to be substrates for folylpolyglutamate hydrolase (FPGH, γ-GH), which cleaves the glutamate residues by hydrolysis.[5] The total intracellular folate pool thus may exist in a state of equilibrium between higher- and lower-chain-length polyglutamates. Polyglutamation of antifolates has potential advantages in chemotherapy, since it may allow for prolonged intracellular retention, and hence less frequent dosing. In addition, for a number of antifolates, the polyglutamated species show increased potency compared with the parent compounds.[6,7] The requirement for polyglutamation does, however, provide a potential resistance mechanism, since cells expressing low amounts of FPGS may be relatively resistant to compounds that are a substrate for this enzyme, particularly where the polyglutamated forms possess greater activity, as above.[8]

RALTITREXED

Preclinical development

The first folate-based TS inhibitor to receive a product licence was raltitrexed (Tomudex, ZD1694).[9] This compound has a quinazoline structure (Figure 51.3), and the parent drug has a k_i for isolated TS of 60–90 nM.[9,10] The drug undergoes rapid intracellular polyglutamation by FPGS, however, and the higher-length polyglutamates are up to 70-fold more potent inhibitors of the isolated enzyme. In addition, in

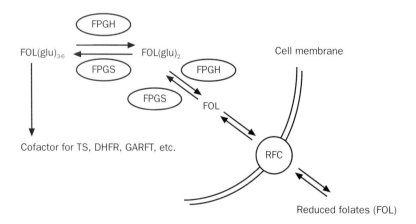

Figure 51.2 Cellular handling of natural folates. FPGS, folylpolyglutamate synthetase; FPGH, folylpolyglutamate hydrolase; RFC, reduced folate carrier.

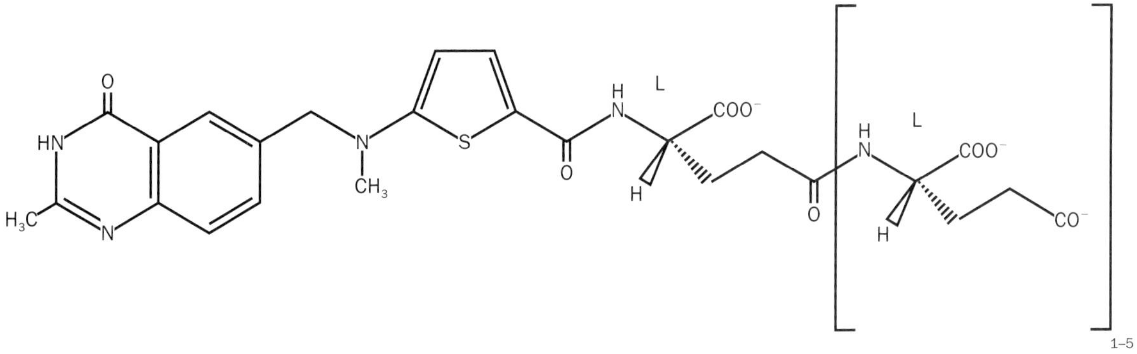

Figure 51.3 Structure of raltitrexed and its polyglutamates.

vitro studies found that polyglutamation leads to a high degree of potency even after short exposures, owing to prolonged TS inhibition after extracellular drug removal.[11] The property of prolonged tissue retention was subsequently confirmed by in vivo studies, and supported the use of an infrequent dosing schedule.[12] Preclinical data also suggested that raltitrexed could act as a radiosensitizing agent, and supported investigation of raltitrexed combined with fractionated radiotherapy.[13]

Phase I studies

One phase I study showed the dose-limiting toxicities (DLT) of raltitrexed to be lethargy, diarrhoea and neutropenia, with a maximum tolerated dose (MTD) of 3.5 mg/m², and these investigators recommended that the dose for phase II evaluation should be 3.0 mg/m² 3-weekly.[14] In another study, carried out in the USA, DLT (which were identical) were not seen until 4.5 mg/m², and the recommended dose from this trial was 4.0 mg/m² 3-weekly.[15] The current recommended dose of raltitrexed is 3.0 mg/m² 3-weekly. Studies of raltitrexed in patients with renal impairment showed that the area under the plasma concentration–time curve (AUC) was approximately doubled in patients with creatinine clearance less than 65 ml/min, and that the terminal half-life was also prolonged. This study also showed an increase in adverse events in the group of patients with renal impairment.[16] For this reason, it is recommended that patients with creatinine clearance less than 25 ml/min should not receive raltitrexed. Patients

with creatinine clearance less than 65 ml/min should receive only 50% of the standard dose, and the dosing interval in these patients should be extended to 4 weeks.

Phase II studies

Raltitrexed went into phase II study at a dose of 3.0 mg/m² every 3 weeks. Phase II trials[17–19] yielded significant response rates in advanced colorectal (26%) and breast (23%) cancer. In addition, there was some evidence of activity in pancreatic, ovarian and non-small cell lung cancer. On the basis of these results, phase III studies were initiated in advanced colorectal cancer, randomizing raltitrexed against 5-FU-based regimens.

Phase III studies

There have now been four large randomized studies comparing raltitrexed with a variety of different 5-FU regimens;[20–23] the available results from these studies are summarized in Table 51.1. In three of the studies, the dose chosen was 3.0 mg/m² every 3 weeks. Based on the results of the second phase I study, one of the trials included a regimen of raltitrexed 4.0 mg/m² 3-weekly as a third arm. Toxicity was unacceptable in this group of patients, however, and this arm of the study was closed early. Data analysis was performed only on the other two study arms of 5-FU and raltitrexed 3.0 mg/m² 3-weekly. Over all the trials, response rates were

Table 51.1 Randomized clinical studies with raltitrexed and 5-FU/LV[a]

Trial and regimen[a]	No. of patients	Response rate (%)	OS[b] (months)	PFS[c] (months)	Leukopenia (%)	Stomatitis (%)	Diarrhoea (%)
European study	439						
5-FU 425 mg/m² + LV 20 mg/m² daily × 5 q 28 d	216	16.7	10.2	3.6	30[d]	22[d]	14
Raltitrexed 3.0 mg/m² q 21 d	223	19.3	10.1	4.8	14[d]	2[d]	14
US study	427						
5-FU 425 mg/m² + LV 20 mg/m² daily × 5 q 28 d	210	15.2	12.7[d]	5.3[d]	41[d]	10	12
Raltitrexed 4.0 mg/m² or 3.0 mg/m² q 21 d	217	14.3	9.7[d]	3.1[d]	16[d]	3	9
International study	495						
5-FU 400 mg/m² + LV 200 mg/m² daily × 5 q 28 d	248	18.0	12.3	5.1[c]	11.9	15.6[d]	18.1
Raltitrexed 3.0 mg/m² q 21 d	247	19.0	10.9	3.9[c]	5.3	1.2[d]	9.7
MRC-CR06	905						
de Gramont schedule[e] q 14 d	303	24	10	6[d,f]	nya[g]	nya	nya
5-FU 300 mg/m²/d continuous infusion	301	26	10	6[d,f]	nya	nya	nya
Raltitrexed 3.0 mg/m² q 21 d	301	20	10	5[d,f]	nya	nya	nya

[a]LV, leucovorin. [b]Overall survival. [c]Progression-free survival. [d]Statistically significant. [e]LV 200 mg/m² + 5-FU 400 mg/m² bolus + 5-FU 600 mg/m² 22 h continuous infusion d1 and 2 repeated q 14 d. [f]PFS was not an endpoint in this study, so data must be interpreted with caution. [g]Not yet available.

similar for raltitrexed and all the 5-FU regimens studied. All of the studies for which complete data are currently available showed significant reduction in proliferating-tissue toxicity for raltitrexed compared with bolus 5-FU regimens. In particular, there was less stomatitis and leukopenia. Survival data from three of the four studies showed no difference in overall survival between the raltitrexed and 5-FU groups; however, in the US trial, survival was significantly inferior in the raltitrexed arm. This was the study that had initially had a 4.0 mg/m^2 arm, and although the data analysed were from the cohort of patients treated at the lower dose only, there is evidence that the initial poor results from the high-dose arm may have influenced clinicians' judgement and impaired the validity of the study data. However, in two of the three studies where progression-free survival (PFS) was a trial endpoint, there was a small but statistically significant reduction in PFS for those patients treated with raltitrexed, and this should also be considered when evaluating the data from these trials.

Toxicity

As will be seen from the above data, raltitrexed is in general well tolerated. The incidence of significant grade 3 or 4 toxicity has been less with raltitrexed than with 5-FU in all published data series, and the large body of data now available has confirmed that the most common toxicities experienced are leukopenia, diarrhoea and asthenia. Many patients experience elevations in hepatic transaminases (aminotransferases) following treatment with raltitrexed (so-called 'transaminitis'); however, these elevations are asymptomatic, tend to improve with subsequent treatments, and are not dose-limiting. This effect is also seen with other antifolates, and is not specific to raltitrexed. In addition, a small proportion of patients will experience cutaneous toxicity, most often manifested as a bilateral lower limb cellulitis. This condition may respond to steroids; however, it can be so severe as to necessitate the discontinuation of therapy. The combination of severe diarrhoea and neutropenia occurs in a small percentage of patients treated with raltitrexed (approximately 3% in the Royal Marsden series of 127 consecutive patients[24]). Unless promptly treated with intensive supportive therapy, this condition has a very high morbidity and mortality. It is therefore

imperative that, despite the generally excellent toxicity profile of this drug, patients treated with raltitrexed should be closely observed for signs of toxicity and there should be a low threshold for admission to hospital should these symptoms occur. There is also evidence (see above) that impaired renal function significantly affects the excretion of raltitrexed, and failure to adhere to the recommended dose modifications in patients with reduced creatinine clearance or with previous toxic events is likely to result in increased morbidity and mortality.[16,25] Preclinical models show that administration of leucovorin can ameliorate the effects of raltitrexed-induced toxicity in mice.[26] The mechanism for this is presumed to be competition for transport and alteration of polyglutamate homeostasis. Although there has been no clinical evidence in support of this, it is therefore suggested that in the event of grade 3/4 diarrhoea coupled with neutropenia, consideration should be given to the administration of leucovorin 25 mg/m^2 every 6 hours in addition to standard supportive-care measures.[27]

Cross-resistance between raltitrexed and 5-FU

As both raltitrexed and 5-FU share TS as a target, alteration in TS levels or expression clearly have the potential to affect sensitivity to both drugs. High TS gene expression has been shown to confer resistance to 5-FU and leucovorin (5-FU/LV),[28] and similar results are emerging for raltitrexed. Because of the different biochemical properties and metabolism of these two drugs, however, it is likely that there will be some mechanisms that are not shared and hence some potential for non-cross-resistance between the agents. Further support for this hypothesis is provided by early data from a clinical study of patients treated with raltitrexed, suggesting that overexpression of dihydropyrimidine dehydrogenase (DPD) and thymidine phosphorylase (TP), which are both independent predictors of 5-FU resistance, may not affect response to raltitrexed.[29] One published retrospective study of 50 patients treated with infused 5-FU or 5-FU plus mitomycin C after failure to respond to raltitrexed showed only one response, and this in a patient who received mitomycin C.[30] However, preliminary data from a prospective study of raltitrexed after 5-FU failure showed objective responses in 7 of 45 patients.[31] These figures are comparable to those for other agents used as second-line therapy in colorectal cancer, and, if confirmed in larger studies, would suggest that raltitrexed might have a role in this setting.

Combination with other cytotoxic agents

Because of its manageable side-effect profile and convenient outpatient dosing regimen, raltitrexed is an ideal candidate for combination with other cytotoxic agents. Preliminary results have been published from the following combinations:

Raltitrexed and irinotecan

In vitro studies show sequence- and schedule-dependent synergy for the combination of raltitrexed and SN38, the active metabolite of irinotecan. In particular, synergy seems to depend on the SN38 being administered prior to raltitrexed.[32,33] A phase I study carried out at the Royal Marsden Hospital in patients with gastrointestinal-tract cancers combined 3-weekly short infusions of irinotecan followed by raltitrexed.[34] Toxicity was less than expected, and the dose-limiting toxicity was asthenia. In particular, diarrhoea and neutropenia were uncommon. A response rate of 20% across all dose levels in heavily pretreated patients was seen, and the recommended phase II dose was set at irinotecan 350 mg/m^2 and raltitrexed 3.0 mg/m^2 every 21 days, which are the full recommended single-agent doses of these drugs. Phase II evaluation at these doses is underway.

Raltitrexed and oxaliplatin

A phase II study has been carried out using a 3-weekly schedule of oxaliplatin 130 mg/m^2 and raltitrexed 3.0 mg/m^2. Early reports of the data from this study are impressive, with an overall response rate of over 50%, and stable disease in a further 23% of the 40 patients treated. Again toxicity was low, with grade 3/4 diarrhoea in 3 cases (7.5%) and grade 3/4 neutropenia in 6 cases (15%). In contrast to trials of 5-FU and oxaliplatin, where grade 3 neurotoxicity occurs in up to 18% of patients, grade 3 neurotoxicity was not seen.[35]

Raltitrexed and 5-FU

Preclinical work has suggested that the ternary complex formed by 5-FdUMP, TS and raltitrexed may be at least as stable as that formed with 5,10-methylenetetrahydrofolate.[36] In addition, the potential for

non-cross-resistance provides a rationale for the evaluation of this combination. Preclinical studies suggest sequence-specific effects, with optimum cytotoxicity achieved when 5-FU is preceded by raltitrexed.[37] Early results are available from two phase I studies of the combination of raltitrexed with 5-FU. In the first study, patients were treated with a weekly 24-hour infusion of 5-FU, with raltitrexed given on days 8, 29 and 3-weekly thereafter. Raltitrexed was dose-escalated from 2.6 to 3.0 mg/m^2, and 5-FU was subsequently escalated to 2800 mg/m^2 without significant DLT in males, although the MTD in females was reached at a dose of 5-FU 2400 mg/m^2 weekly and raltitrexed 3.0 mg/m^2 3-weekly. Significant antitumour activity was seen, with 9 of 16 patients treated at the four highest dose levels responding.[38] In the second study, raltitrexed was given immediately prior to a bolus injection of 5-FU every 3 weeks. In the latter part of this trial, the 5-FU dose was fixed at 1200 mg/m^2, and raltitrexed was dose-escalated. The reported data show that no DLT had been seen with the doses of raltitrexed 5.5 mg/m^2 and 5-FU 1200 mg/m^2 3-weekly, and that this schedule was also active provided that attention is paid to pretreatment assessment of renal function and adequate monitoring of toxicity while patients are receiving treatment, raltitrexed provides a useful alternative treatment option.[39] Interestingly, both these studies have shown that raltitrexed appears to modify the pharmacokinetics of 5-FU, with an increase in maximum plasma concentration (C_{max}) and AUC.

Alternative schedules

Initial in vivo and pharmacokinetic studies suggested that because of the prolonged intracellular retention seen with raltitrexed, a 3-weekly dosing schedule would be appropriate for patients with normal renal function (see above). Recent studies of the duration of the biological effect of raltitrexed by measuring the elevation of plasma 2'-deoxyuridine (dUrd), a surrogate marker of TS inhibition, have suggested that, at least in normal proliferating tissues, the duration of TS inhibition may be less than 7 days.[29] In view of this, a phase I study of a 2-weekly regimen has been carried out.[40] This study has found the MTD at this schedule to be 2.0 mg/m^2 every 14 days, and studies are planned to combine the drug at this schedule with the commonly used 2-weekly 'de

Gramont' 5-FU/LV regimen, and to compare efficacy in combination with other agents. Weekly schedules are also under evaluation, and it is thus possible that alternative regimens may become available, particularly for use in combination.

Current place in therapy

A recent large study of raltitrexed compared with 5-FU in the adjuvant setting (PETACC-1) closed early owing to excessive toxicity in the raltitrexed arm, and no efficacy data for adjuvant raltitrexed are therefore available. Figure 51.4 shows survival figures for raltitrexed in advanced colorectal cancer compared with pooled data from 43 studies of different 5-FU regimens. It appears from current information that overall survival is similar for raltitrexed and 5-FU. In view of concerns over toxicity and the suggestion of inferior PFS with single-agent raltitrexed, 5-FU-based therapy remains the preferred treatment for most clinicians. Raltitrexed is, however, clearly indicated in those patients for whom 5-FU is contraindicated or impractical for geographical or administrative reasons. With its manageable toxicity profile and convenient schedule, it will be an important drug for use in combination chemotherapy of colorectal cancer, and the results of ongoing studies will further clarify this.

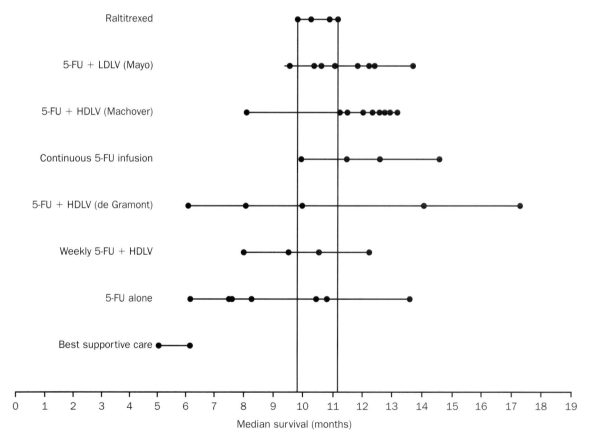

Figure 51.4 Pooled survival data from 43 clinical studies in patients with advanced colorectal cancer. HDLV, high-dose leucovorin; LDLV, low-dose leucovorin. From Cunningham D, *Br J Cancer* 1998; **77**(Suppl 2): 15–21.

LY231514 (MULTITARGETED ANTIFOLATE, MTA)

MTA was developed from the structure of the glycinamide ribonucleotide formyltransferase (GARFT) inhibitor lometrexol, but was found to be a potent inhibitor of TS that, like raltitrexed, is extensively and rapidly polyglutamated to more active species. The structure of MTA, a pyrrolo[2,3-d]pyrimidine-based molecule, is shown in Figure 51.5. It was observed that cells were only partly protected against the cytotoxic effects of MTA by thymidine, and, moreover, in early clinical trials, responses to the drug were seen in patients with disease resistant to both raltitrexed and 5-FU.[41] Further isolated enzyme studies have shown that this drug is active against a number of folate-dependent enzymes, particularly GARFT and dihydrofolate reductase (DHFR), as well as to a lesser extent aminoimidazole-carboxamide ribonucleotide formyltransferase (AICARFT) and C-1 synthetase.[42] The drug is active in colorectal cancer, and two phase II studies in this disease at a dose of 500–600 mg/m^2 3-weekly gave objective response rates of 17% and 15%.[43,44] The pattern of toxicity with MTA is similar to that seen with raltitrexed, with DLT of myelosuppression, particularly neutropenia, and fatigue. Rash and mucositis were also seen. It is hoped that the multiple loci of action of this drug may help to overcome the emergence of resistance to pure TS inhibition, although TS remains the principal target.

NON-POLYGLUTAMABLE TS INHIBITORS: ZD9331

While polyglutamation has potential advantages in antitumour therapy, it also provides a potential mechanism for resistance by tumours expressing low levels of FPGS or overexpressing FPGH. In vitro studies against a variety of cell lines appeared to confirm that raltitrexed activity was reduced in cell lines expressing low levels of FPGS.[45,46] Research effort was therefore directed at the development drugs that would retain the potency of raltitrexed against TS, but would not be substrates for FPGS. ZD9331 is the most advanced in development of these compounds;[47] its structure is shown in Figure 51.6. Preclinical studies confirmed that ZD9331 was active in low-FPGS-expressing cell lines, and in phase I tri-

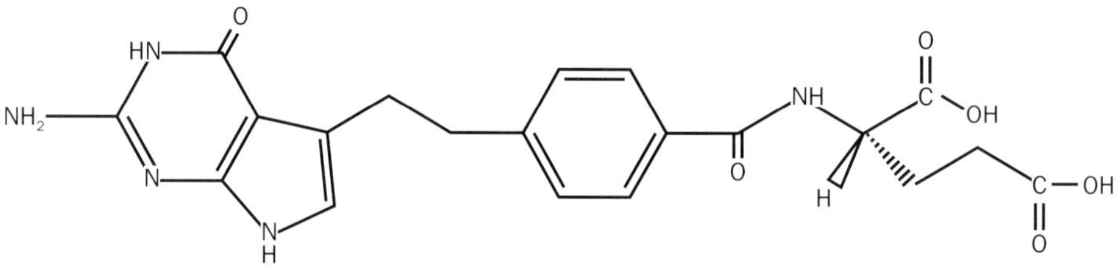

Figure 51.5 Structure of LY231514 (multitargeted antifolate, MTA).

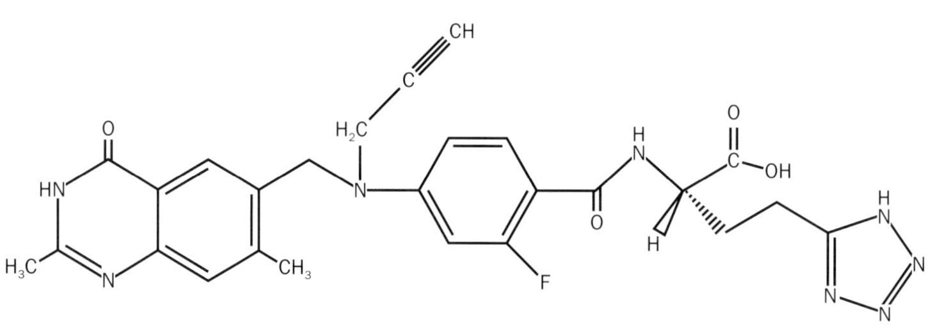

Figure 51.6 Structure of ZD9331.

als, evidence of activity was seen in ovarian, breast and colorectal cancer.[48,49] As with raltitrexed, DLT are myelosuppression and gastrointestinal toxicity. In contrast with raltitrexed, however, preclinical data showed rapid elimination from tissues after plasma levels fell to non-cytotoxic levels. Pharmacokinetic data from the phase I trials demonstrated a long elimination half-life of up to 75 hours in humans. It may be that this property will allow a similarly convenient dosing schedule to raltitrexed, while overcoming at least one possible resistance mechanism. This may imply both a different spectrum of activity and a different toxicity profile. The drug has recently entered phase II study, and results will be eagerly awaited.

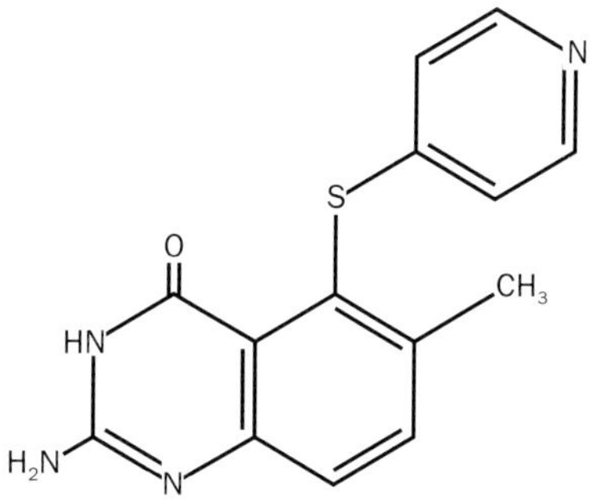

Figure 51.7 Structure of nolatrexed (Thymitaq, AG337)

NON-CLASSICAL (LIPOPHILIC) TS INHIBITORS

As outlined above, the cellular uptake of the so-called classical antifolates such as raltitrexed, MTA, ZD9331 and methotrexate is largely by a saturable carrier-mediated mechanism: the reduced folate carrier or RFC. These drugs may also be internalized by the folate receptor, and this area is under investigation. It is possible that downregulation or mutation of these proteins might provide a mechanism of resistance to these drugs. Agouron Pharmaceuticals therefore developed a series of compounds, based on the crystal structure of *E. coli* TS, that bind to the enzyme at the folate-binding site but lack a glutamate moiety.[50] These compounds are lipophilic, entering the cell by a process of passive diffusion, and they lack substrate activity for FPGS. The culmination of this programme was nolatrexed (Thymitaq, AG337), whose structure is shown in Figure 51.7. This potent TS inhibitor, with a k_i for isolated human TS of approximately 11 nM, was shown in phase I studies to require prolonged intravenous administration,[51,52] and the schedule finally chosen was a 5-day infusion repeated 3-weekly. Oral administration was also effective. In a phase II study, nolatrexed in a 5-day infusion of 800 mg/m²/day repeated 3-weekly showed evidence of activity in colorectal cancer, with 1 partial remission and 3 biological responses (50% fall in carcinoembryonic antigen) in the 17 patients studied.[53] Despite this, and activity in other tumour types (principally head and neck cancer and pancreatic cancer), there are currently no plans for this drug to be developed further.

CONCLUSIONS

TS inhibition remains the mainstay of chemotherapy for colorectal cancer. Although 5-FU remains the benchmark against which other treatments must be assessed, recent developments indicate that the future standard of care is likely to be combination chemotherapy. The task confronting the clinician, and future clinical trials, is to choose the best available treatment from a range of effective drugs. Each of the new TS inhibitors has distinctive properties and the potential to overcome various resistance mechanisms (Figure 51.8). Currently, it is not practicable to establish cohorts of patients likely to benefit from specific compounds on a mass scale, and therefore development prospects are limited. In the future, however, we must hope that diagnostic technology is sufficiently widely available to ensure that we reap the full benefits of the extensive research and development programmes that have resulted in this rationally designed range of compounds directed against the same important target. For the present, in addition to providing a valuable treatment alternative to 5-FU, raltitrexed and the other new TS inhibitors provide the opportunity for maximizing the convenience and minimizing the toxicity of combination regimens while maintaining a high level of efficacy. The development of TS inhibitors sets a standard for rational drug design in cancer chemotherapy that will have applications far beyond the field of colorectal cancer, and provides considerable optimism with regard to future programmes of development of drugs directed at other novel targets.

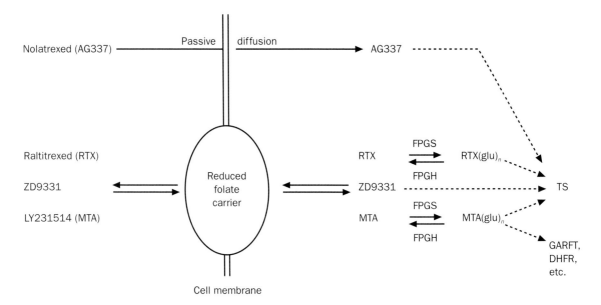

Figure 51.8 Folate-based TS inhibitors: different pathways for uptake and retention. For abbreviations, see Figures 51.1 and 51.2.

REFERENCES

1. Sommer A, Santi DV, Purification and amino acid analysis of an active site peptide from thymidylate synthase containing covalently bound 5′-fluoro-2′-deoxyuridylate and methylene tetrachloride. *Biochem Biophys Res Commun* 1974; **57**: 689–96.

2. Mandel HG, Incorporation of 5-fluorouracil into RNA and its molecular consequences. *Prog Mol Subcell Biol* 1969; **1**: 82–135.

3. Aschele C, Sobrero A, Faderan MA, Bertino JR, Novel mechanism(s) of resistance to 5-fluorouracil in human colon cancer (HCT-8) sublines following exposure to two different clinically relevant dose schedules. *Cancer Res* 1992; **52**: 1855–64.

4. Meta-analysis Group in Cancer, Efficacy of continuous infusion of fluorouracil compared with bolus administration in advanced colorectal cancer. *J Clin Oncol* 1998; **16**: 301–8.

5. McGuire JJ, Coward JK, Pteroylpolyglutamates: biosynthesis, degradation, and function. *Folates Pterins* 1984; **1**: 135–90.

6. Chabner BA, Allegra CJ, Curt GA et al, Polyglutamation of methotrexate. Is methotrexate a prodrug? *J Clin Invest* 1985; **76**: 907–12.

7. Harrap KR, Jackman AL, Newell DR et al, Thymidylate synthase: a target for anticancer drug design. *Adv Enzyme Regul* 1989; **29**: 161–79.

8. McGuire JJ, Heitzman KJ, Haile WH et al, Cross-resistance studies of folylpolyglutamate synthetase-deficient, methotrexate-resistant CCRF- CEM human leukemia sublines. *Leukemia* 1993; **7**: 1996–2003.

9. Jackman AL, Taylor GA, Gibson W et al, ICI D1694, a quinazoline antifolate thymidylate synthase inhibitor that is a potent inhibitor of L1210 tumor cell growth in vitro and in vivo: a new agent for clinical study. *Cancer Res* 1991; **51**: 5579–86.

10. Ward WHJ, Kimbell R, Jackman AL, Kinetic characteristics of ICI D1694: a quinazoline antifolate which inhibits thymidylate synthase. *Biochem Pharmacol* 1992; **43**: 2029–31.

11. Jackman AL, Kimbell R, Brown M et al, Quinazoline thymidylate synthase inhibitors: methods for assessing the contribution of polyglutamation to their in vitro activity. *Anti-Cancer Drug Design* 1995; **10**: 555–72.

12. Aherne GW, Ward E, Lawrence N et al, Comparison of plasma and tissue levels of ZD1694 ('Tomudex'), a highly polyglutamable quinazoline thymidylate synthase inhibitor, in preclinical models. *Br J Cancer* 1998; **77**: 221–6.

13. Teicher BA, Ara G, Chen YN et al, Interaction of tomudex with radiation in vitro and in vivo. *Int J Oncol* 1998; **13**: 437–42.

14. Clarke SJ, Hanwell J, De Boer M et al, Phase I trial of ZD1694, a new folate-based thymidylate synthase inhibitor, in patients with solid tumors. *J Clin Oncol* 1996; **14**: 1495–503.

15. Grem JL, Sorensen JM, Cullen E et al, A phase I study of raltitrexed, an antifolate thymidylate synthase inhibitor, in adult patients with advanced solid tumors. *Clin Cancer Res* 1999; **5**: 2381–91.

16. Judson I, Maughan TS, Beale P et al, Effects of impaired renal function on the pharmacokinetics of raltitrexed (Tomudex, ZD1694). *Br J Cancer* 1998; **78**: 1188–93.

17. Cunningham D, Zalcberg J, Smith I et al, 'Tomudex' (ZD1694): a novel thymidylate synthase inhibitor with clinical antitumour activity in a range of solid tumours. *Ann Oncol* 1996; **7**: 179–82.

18. Zalcberg JR, Cunningham D, Van Cutsem E et al, ZD1694: a novel thymidylate synthase inhibitor with substantial activity in the treatment of patients with advanced colorectal cancer. Tomudex Colorectal Study Group. *J Clin Oncol* 1996; **14**: 716–21.

19. Smith I, Jones A, Spielmann M et al, A phase II study in advanced

breast cancer: ZD1694 (Tomudex) a novel direct and specific thymidylate synthase inhibitor. *Br J Cancer* 1996; **74:** 479–81.

20. Cunningham D, Zalcberg JR, Rath U et al, Final results of a randomised trial comparing 'Tomudex' (raltitrexed) with 5-fluorouracil plus leucovorin in advanced colorectal cancer. 'Tomudex' Colorectal Cancer Study Group. *Ann Oncol* 1996; **7:** 961–5.

21. Cocconi G, Cunningham D, van Cutsem E et al, Open, randomized, multicenter trial of raltitrexed versus fluorouracil plus high-dose leucovorin in patients with advanced colorectal cancer. Tomudex Colorectal Cancer Study Group. *J Clin Oncol* 1998; **16:** 2943–52.

22. Cunningham D, Mature results from three large controlled studies with raltitrexed ('Tomudex'). *Br J Cancer* 1998; **77**(Suppl 2): 15–21.

23. Maughan TS, James RD, Kerr D et al, Preliminary results of a multicentre randomised trial comparing 3 chemotherapy regimens (de Gramont, Lokich and raltitrexed) in metastatic colorectal cancer. *Proc Am Soc Clin Oncol* 1999; **18:** 262a (Abst 1007).

24. Ford HER, Cunningham D, Safety of raltitrexed. *Lancet* 1999; **354:** 1824–5.

25. Garcia-Vargas JE, Sahmoud T, Smith MP, Green S, Qualitative and chronological assessment of toxicities during treatment with raltitrexed (Tomudex) in 861 patients: implications for patient management. *Eur J Cancer* 1999; **35**(Suppl 4): S72 (Abst 222).

26. Farrugia DC, Aherne GW, Brunton L et al, Leucovorin rescue from raltitrexed (Tomudex)–induced antiproliferative effects: in vitro cell line and in vivo mouse studies. *Clin Cancer Res* 2000; **6:** 3646–56.

27. Jackman AL, Farrugia DC, Gibson W et al, ZD1694 (Tomudex): a new thymidylate synthase inhibitor with activity in colorectal cancer. *Eur J Cancer* 1995; **31A:** 1277–82.

28. Leichman CG, Lenz HJ, Leichman L et al, Quantitation of intratumoral thymidylate synthase expression predicts for disseminated colorectal cancer response and resistance to protracted-infusion fluorouracil and weekly leucovorin. *J Clin Oncol* 1997; **15:** 3223–9.

29. Farrugia D, Ford HER, Cunningham D et al, Genomic study of patients with advanced colorectal cancer treated with raltitrexed ('Tomudex'). *Proc Am Soc Clin Oncol* 1999; **18:** 268a (Abst 1029).

30. Farrugia DC, Norman AR, Cunningham D, Single agent infusional 5-fluorouracil is not effective second-line chemotherapy after raltitrexed (Tomudex™) in advanced colorectal cancer. *Eur J Cancer* 1998; **34:** 987–91.

31. Horikoshi N, Aiba K, Kurihaba M et al, Phase II study of 'Tomudex' in chemotherapy pretreated patients with advanced colorectal cancer. *Proc Am Soc Clin Oncol* 1999; **18:** 257a (Abst 988).

32. Aschele C, Baldo C, Sobrero AF et al, Schedule dependent synergism between raltitrexed and irinotecan in human colon cancer cells in vitro. *Clin Cancer Res* 1998; **4:** 1323–30.

33. Kimbell R, Jackman AL, In vitro studies with ZD1694 (Tomudex™) and SN38 in human colon tumour cell lines. In: *Chemistry and Biology of Pteridines and Folates* (Pfleiderer W, Rokos H, eds). Blackwell Science, Oxford 1997: 249–52.

34. Ford HER, Cunningham D, Ross PJ et al, Phase I study of irinotecan and raltitrexed in patients with advanced gastrointestinal tract adenocarcinoma. *Br J Cancer* 2000; **83:** 146–52.

35. Bennouna J, Seitz JF, Paillot B et al, Tomudex (raltitrexed) plus oxaliplatin (Eloxatin) in previously untreated metastatic colorectal cancer (MCRC) patients: an active combination. *Eur J Cancer* 1999; **35**(Suppl 4): S75 (Abst 237).

36. Van der Wilt CL, Pinedo HM, Kuiper CM et al, Biochemical basis for the combined antiproliferative effect of AG337 or ZD1694 and 5-fluorouracil. *Proc Am Assoc Cancer Res* 1995; **36:** 379 (Abst 2260).

37. Jackman AL, Kimbell R, Ford HER, Combination of raltitrexed with other cytotoxic agents: rationale and preclinical observations. *Eur J Cancer* 1999; **35**(Suppl 1): S3–8.

38. Mayer S, Harstrick A, Muller C et al, Phase I study of Tomudex combined with protracted infusion of 5-FU in patients with metastatic colorectal cancer. *Ann Oncol* 1999; **98**(9 Suppl 2): 110 (Abst 633).

39. Bertino JM, Schwartz GK, Kemeny N et al, Raltitrexed ('Tomudex') plus 5-fluorouracil (5-FU): improved palliation as second line therapy in patients with metastatic colorectal cancer. *Proc Am Soc Clin Oncol* 1999; **18:** (Abst 949) 247a.

40. Farrugia D, Ford HE, Tischkowitz M et al, Initial results of a phase I study of raltitrexed (Tomudex) given every 14 days (q14). *Proc Am Soc Clin Oncol* 2000; **19:** 194 (Abst 756).

41. Rinaldi DA, Burris HA, Dorr FA et al, Initial phase I evaluation of the novel thymidylate synthase inhibitor, LY231514, using the modified continual reassessment method for dose escalation. *J Clin Oncol* 1995; **13:** 2842–50.

42. Shih C, Chen VJ, Gossett LS et al, LY231514, a pyrrolo[2,3-d]pyrimidine-based antifolate that inhibits multiple folate-requiring enzymes. *Cancer Res* 1997; **57:** 1116–23.

43. Cripps MC, Burnell M, Jolivet J et al, Phase II study of first-line LY231514 (multi-targeted antifolate) in patients with locally advanced or metatstatic colorectal cancer: an NCIC Clinical Trials Group Study. *Ann Oncol* 1999; **10:** 1175–9.

44. John W, Picus J, Blanke CD et al, Activity of multi-targeted antifolate (pemetrexed disodium, LY231514) in patients with advanced colorectal carcinoma: results from a phase II study. *Cancer* 2000; **88:** 1807–13.

45. Jackman AL, Kelland LR, Kimbell R et al, Mechanisms of acquired resistance to the quinazoline thymidylate synthase inhibitor ZD1694 (Tomudex) in one mouse and three human cell lines. *Br J Cancer* 1995; **71:** 914–24.

46. Takemura Y, Kobayashi H, Gibson W et al, The influence of drug-exposure conditions on the development of resistance to methotrexate or ZD1694 in cultured human leukaemia cells. *Int J Cancer* 1996; **66:** 29–36.

47. Jackman AL, Kimbell R, Aherne GW et al, Cellular pharmacology and in vitro activity of a new anticancer agent ZD9331: a water soluble non-polyglutamatable quinazoline-based inhibitor of thymidylate synthase. *Clin Cancer Res* 1997; **3:** 911–21.

48. Goh BC, Ratain M, Bertucci D et al, Phase I study of ZD9331 on a 5-day short infusion schedule given every 3 weeks. *Proc Am Soc Clin Oncol* 1999; **18:** 170a (Abst 653).

49. Rees C, Beale P, Trigo J et al, Phase I trial of ZD9331, a non-polyglutamable thymidylate synthase inhibitor given as a five day continuous infusion every 3 weeks. *Proc Am Soc Clin Oncol* 1999; **18:** 171a (Abst 657).

50. Webber SE, Bleckman TM, Attard J et al, Design of thymidylate synthase inhibitors using protein crystal structures: the synthesis and biological evaluation of a novel class of 5-substituted quinazolinones. *J Med Chem* 1993; **36:** 733–46.

51. Rafi I, Taylor GA, Calvete JA et al, Clinical pharmacokinetic and pharmacodynamic studies with the nonclassical antifolate thymidylate synthase inhibitor 3,4-dihydro-2-amino-6-methyl-4-oxo-5-(4-pyridylthio)-quinazolone dihydrochloride (AG337) given by 24-hour continuous intravenous infusion. *Clin Cancer Res* 1995; **1:** 1275–84.

52. Rafi I, Boddy AV, Calvete JA et al, Preclinical and phase I clinical studies with the nonclassical antifolate thymidylate synthase inhibitor nolatrexed dihydrochloride given by prolonged administration in patients with solid tumors. *J Clin Oncol* 1998; **16:** 1131–41.

53. Belani CP, Lembersky B, Ramanathan R et al, A phase II trial of Thymitaq in patients with adenocarcinoma of the colon. *Proc Am Soc Clin Oncol* 1997; **16:** 272a (Abst 965).

52

New combinations in colorectal cancer

François Goldwasser, Esteban Cvitkovic, Patrice Hérait

INTRODUCTION

For nearly 40 years, 5-fluorouracil (5-FU) was the sole cytotoxic agent with significant activity in advanced colorectal cancer.[1,2] During the 1970s and 1980s, elucidation of the complex biochemical pathways that 5-FU follows in cells and its mechanisms of action (thymidylate synthase inhibition, and DNA and RNA incorporation) has led to the development of several biochemical modulation strategies designed to enhance the cytotoxic effects of the drug. Amongst many, the prevalent standard is the addition of folinic acid (FA, leucovorin), which results in an increased response rate, but results of meta-analyses have failed to show increased survival when it is added to bolus 5-FU.[3] Modulation with methotrexate, N-phosphonoacetyl-L-aspartate (PALA) or levamisole has led to very modest gains compared with 5-FU/FA.[4,5] The development of hybrid regimens, combining bolus and infusional administration and biochemical modulators, has led to increased response rates and 2–3 months' increase in time to progression.[6–8] Besides 5-FU modulation, most attempts to improve systemic treatment have consisted of empirically adding drugs to 5-FU.[1,2] Nitrosoureas were extensively studied as an addition to 5-FU schedules. Response rates of 10–15% have been reported for carmustine (BCNU), lomustine (CCNU), chlorozotocin, and semustine (methyl-CCNU). The addition of semustine to 5-FU (MOF- or MF-type regimens) resulted in response rates ranging from 4% to 40%. Most of these responses were partial and lasted less than 6 months.[2,8] Nitrosoureas were definitively abandoned because of the lack of difference in time-related parameters and the risk of secondary leukaemia.[9] Attempts to substitute or add other agents did not result in clinically meaningful differences.[2,10] The addition of cisplatin to 5-FU has been evaluated based on preclinical studies demonstrating synergy between these two agents. Although initial phase II studies produced response rates of 30–40%, several randomized trials have subsequently failed to demonstrate any advantage of the combination over 5-FU alone in terms of time to progression or survival.[11,12]

During the last 10 years, we have seen the emergence of two new active antitumour agents with mechanisms of action independent of thymidylate synthase inhibition (TSI); irinotecan (CPT-11) and oxaliplatin.

Irinotecan is a DNA topoisomerase I (topo I) inhibitor.[13] Its antitumour activity is mainly effected by its metabolite SN38, through the stabilization of covalent topo I–DNA complexes.[14] These stabilized complexes are thought to collide with replication forks during DNA synthesis, leading to DNA double-strand breakages.[13,15] Interference by these covalent cleavable complexes in RNA transcription probably explains the persistence of a cytotoxic effect outside S phase.[14] The mechanism of action of irinotecam is discussed in detail elsewhere in this volume (see Chapter 49). Irinotecan has proven to be an effective drug for colorectal cancer patients whose tumors no longer respond to 5-FU treatment.[16–18] Furthermore, two large phase III clinical trials demonstrated that the combination of irinotecan and 5-FU/FA is superior to 5-FU/FA alone as a first-line treatment of metastatic colorectal cancer patients,[19,20] based on response rate, progression-free survival,[19,20] and survival (in one trial[19]).

Oxaliplatin, a third-generation platinum compound, is a diaminocyclohexane platinum, which is responsible for the formation of mainly intrastrand DNA adducts.[21,22] These DNA adducts differ from those of cisplatin or carboplatin by their repair capability: oxaliplatin-induced DNA damage has a higher cytotoxic potency, which is unchallenged in mismatch-repair deficient cells, accounting for the activity of oxaliplatin in cisplatin-resistant cell lines and cancer patients.[23] This non-recognition by the mismatch-repair complex is of major importance, since the mismatch-repair deficiency, linked specifically to hereditary non-polyposis colon cancer (HNPCC) carcinogenesis, is also prevalent in approximately half of advanced colorectal cancers because of epigenetic tumoral phenomena (e.g. hypermethylation of the *hMLH1* gene promoter[24–27]). Oxaliplatin cytotoxicity is synergistic both in vitro and in vivo with 5-FU and other TSIs,[28,29] and is addressed in detail elsewhere in this volume (see Chapter 50). The response rate of single-agent oxaliplatin in 139 5-FU-resistant patients was 10%,[30] while response rates consistently superior to 20% have been reported in patients progressing on 5-FU/FA alone and subsequently treated with oxaliplatin plus 5-FU/FA, even when the same 5-FU regimen was pursued.[31,32] The addition of oxaliplatin to 5-FU/FA as first-line treatment of metastatic colorectal cancer patients resulted in more than a twofold increase in response rate and a significant increase in time-related disease progression parameters[33,34] in two phase III randomized trials.

Since both irinotecan and oxaliplatin are cytotoxic through a TSI-independent mechanism, the combination of oxaliplatin with irinotecan appeared to be an attractive therapeutic option as salvage therapy in patients who had failed 5-FU. Both irinotecan and oxaliplatin have been used in combination with several schedules of either 5-FU/FA or raltitrexed, and have been combined together. The almost simultaneous availability of both agents as first prescription choices in 5-FU-pretreated patients – and very recently in first-line regimens for advanced disease – has rapidly changed the therapeutic results in advanced colorectal cancer. This has led to a renewed interest in individual patient management, including systematic attempts at surgical resections of metastases, and long-term disease control management beyond the simple palliation offered by 5-FU treatment that has been prevalent over the past three decades.

In this chapter, we summarize combination regimens that include either or both of these new antitumour agents, investigated and reported as recently as the year 2000.

PRECLINICAL RATIONALE FOR OXALIPLATIN- AND IRINOTECAN-BASED COMBINATIONS

Oxaliplatin plus thymidylate synthase inhibitors

Synergy is well documented between cisplatin and S-phase-acting antimetabolites, such as cytarabine,[35] 5-FU,[36] and gemcitabine.[37] The synergy is mostly attributed to DNA and RNA synthesis inhibition by the S-phase-dependent agent, which hampers reversal of platinum-induced DNA damage. The in vitro synergy reported between 5-FU or other TSIs and oxaliplatin[29] might be related to the same mechanism. The synergy between oxaliplatin and 5-FU has also been observed in vivo in transplantable tumour models.[28,29] A detailed analysis of these results is presented in Chapter 50.

Irinotecan plus thymidylate synthase inhibitors

The preclinical evidence of the benefit of combining a DNA topo I inhibitor with 5-FU is not well established: the 5-FU-induced DNA synthesis inhibition may protect the tumour cells from lethal collisions between covalent topo I–DNA complexes and advancing replication forks.[15] Hence this transient protective effect might explain in part the schedule dependence found in vitro,[38,39] where antagonism is mostly seen when 5-FU is given prior to irinotecan and synergy is seen when the DNA topo I inhibitor is given first. Furthermore, these results are supported by an in vivo study.[40] Recent in vitro studies have reported the same schedule dependence for the combination of irinotecan with raltitrexed.[41]

Oxaliplatin plus irinotecan

In agreement with other in vitro studies combining alkylating agents,[42] including cisplatin,[43,44] with a camptothecin derivative, a synergy was found between oxaliplatin and topotecan[45] or SN38, the active metabolite of irinotecan.[46,47] The mechanism of the synergy is attributed to a reciprocal intracellular interaction: (1) the inhibition of topo I and the inhibition of both RNA and DNA synthesis following topo I-mediated DNA damage tend to slow down the reversion of oxaliplatin-induced DNA damage;[46] (2) oxaliplatin-induced DNA damage and DNA distortion might stimulate topo I cleavage activity and thus enhance the effect of agents acting through the stabilization of covalent topo I–DNA complexes.[45,48]

RESULTS OF COMBINATION TRIALS

Combinations of oxaliplatin with thymidylate synthase inhibitors

The initial clinical development of oxaliplatin was based exclusively in France for over five years. It focused on advanced colorectal cancer patients on combination therapy with 5-FU/FA because of preliminary in vivo evidence of synergy between oxaliplatin and 5-FU.[28] From 1989 to 1996, the studies with oxaliplatin by Lévi et al were done using a chronomodulated continuous infusion of 5-FU/FA and oxaliplatin[49–51] (see also Chapter 55). The same group compared this mode of administration with constant-rate infusion,[49,52,53] and later intensified the treatment using a '4–10' regimen (4 days on/10 days off, every 2 weeks) instead of a '5–16' (5 days on/16 days off, every 3 weeks).[54,55] After the groundbreaking work of Lévi et al, the group led by de Gramont also developed this combination with their 48 hour/every 2 weeks hybrid bolus/infusion 5-FU/FA regimens (FOLFOX) and evaluated the feasibility of several schedules to intensify the therapy.[31–33,56–61] The experiences of both groups with several hundred patients favour the every 2 weeks use of oxaliplatin in combination with 5-FU/FA, with an increase in both dose density and dose intensity of the combination regimen delivery (Tables 52.1 and 52.2). See also the discussion of the FOLFOX regimens in Chapter 54.

Table 52.1 Antitumour activity of oxaliplatin plus 5-fluorouracil (5-FU) and folinic acid (FA) in previously treated patients with metastatic colorectal cancer

Study design[a]	Ref	No. of patients	Response rate (%)	Median PFS[b] (months)	Median survival (months)
FOLFOX 1 every 2 weeks Oxaliplatin: 130 mg/m² days 1 and 28 FA: 500 mg/m² days 1 and 2 5-FU CI: 1500–2000 mg/m² days 1 and 2	57	13	31	—	—
FOLFOX 2 every 2 weeks Oxaliplatin: 100 mg/m² day 1 FA: 500 mg/m² days 1 and 2 5-FU CI: 1500–2000 mg/m²/24 h days 1 and 2	31	46	46	7	17
FOLFOX 3 every 2 weeks Oxaliplatin: 85 mg/m² day 1 FA: 500 mg/m² days 1 and 2 5-FU CI: 1500 mg/m² days 1 and 2	32	30	20	6	10
FOLFOX 4 every 2 weeks Oxaliplatin: 85 mg/m² day 1 FA: 200 mg/m² days 1 and 2 5-FU bolus: 400 mg/m² days 1 and 2 5-FU CI: 600 mg/m² days 1 and 2	58	57	23.5	5.1	11.1
Chronotherapy 5 days every 3 weeks Oxaliplatin: 25 mg/m²/d FA: 300 mg/m²/d 5-FU: 700 mg/m²/d	50	42	55	10	13
Chronotherapy 4 days every 2 weeks Oxaliplatin: 20–25 mg/m²/d FA: 300 mg/m²/d 5-FU: 700 mg/m²/d	54	37	40	10.3	16.9

[a]CI, continuous infusion.
[b]Progression-free survival.

Table 52.2 Antitumour activity of oxaliplatin plus 5-fluorouracil (5-FU) and folinic acid (FA) in previously untreated patients with metastatic colorectal cancer

Study design	Ref	No. of patients	Response rate (%)	Median PFS[a] (months)	Median survival (months)
Chronotherapy 5 days every 3 weeks Oxaliplatin: 25 mg/m²/d FA: 300 mg/m²/d 5-FU: 700 mg/m²/d		46	59	11	15
versus	50				
Chronotherapy 4 days every 2 weeks Oxaliplatin: 25 mg/m²/d FA: 300 mg/m²/d 5-FU: 700–1000 mg/m²/d		90	67	—	19
Flat infusion 5 days every 3 weeks Oxaliplatin: 20 mg/m²/d FA: 300 mg/m²/d 5-FU: 600 mg/m²/d		47	32	8	14.9
versus	52				
Chronotherapy 5 days every 3 weeks Oxaliplatin: 20 mg/m²/d FA: 300 mg/m²/d 5-FU: 600 mg/m²/d		45	53	11	19
Flat infusion 5 days every 3 weeks Oxaliplatin: 25 mg/m²/d FA: 300 mg/m²/d 5-FU: 600 mg/m²/d	53	93	29	7.9	16.9

[a]Progression-free survival.

Antitumour activity in 5-FU-pretreated patients (Table 52.1)

When oxaliplatin was added to the same 5-FU/FA regimen on which the tumour progressed, several clinical studies reproducibly found response rates superior to those expected with oxaliplatin alone.[31,32,51–55] The results of prospective phase II clinical trials are summarized in Table 52.1. A retrospective analysis reported 721 patients treated with many different regimens of 5-FU with or without FA in the extended-access, compassionate-use programmes.[62] Hence the antitumour activity of the combination has been evaluated in more than 1000 previously pretreated patients with 5-FU/FA-resistant metastatic colorectal cancer. The 5-FU resistance was defined restrictively as having imaging (or, in a smaller proportion, clinical) evidence of disease progression while on 5-FU-based treatment. The response rate of the combination was consistently found to be higher than 20% (20–55%), with minor responses and prolonged stabilizations leading to tumour control in over 60% of patients. The median progression-free survival in all of these experiences is greater than 9 months. The first feasibility trial was the FOLFOX 1 regimen. A new regimen (FOLFOX 2) aimed to increase the dose intensity of oxaliplatin, which was given at a dose of 100 mg/m² every 2 weeks (instead of every other cycle).[31] The same bimonthly regimen of high-dose FA and continuous-infusion 5-FU with a dose of 85 mg/m² of oxaliplatin was later developed to decrease the incidence of neurosensory toxicity, and was called FOLFOX 3.[32] To obtain the same dose intensity as that recommended based on single-agent phase II studies (namely 130 mg/m² every 3 weeks), a multicentre phase II trial assessed the efficacy of adding 85 mg/m² of oxaliplatin every 2 weeks to the same specific hybrid 48 hours every 2 weeks 5-FU/FA regimen (either FOLFOX 3 or FOLFOX 4) on which they had progressed.[58] The regimens allowing the highest dose intensity of 5-FU and oxaliplatin seemed to be those associated with the best tumour response rate and the longest median survival[61] (see also Chapter 55). The FOLFOX 6 regimen is addressing the issues of the immediate haematological toxicity related to the mode of administration of 5-FU and of the cumulative neurosensory toxicity of oxaliplatin. A dose of 100 mg/m² of oxaliplatin is combined with a shorter infusion of 5-FU given at a higher dose (400 mg/m² leucovorin followed by 2400–3000 mg/m² of 5-FU).[59] A FOLFOX 7 regimen with a dose of oxaliplatin of 130 mg/m² is currently being investigated to address the issues of the dose response of oxaliplatin and of the management of its cumulative neurotoxicity.[60] The work of Lévi et al in 5-FU-pretreated and -resistant patients is also extensive, but is less systematic in its approach to data analysis since it does not always specify clinical 5-FU resistance and the relationship with response.[50,54]

Antitumour activity in first-line therapy (Tables 52.2 and 52.3)

At least four phase II and two controlled phase III studies have evaluated the antitumour activity of oxaliplatin combined with 5-FU/FA in chemotherapy-naive patients.[33,34,52–55] Two of these phase II studies included both previously pretreated and chemotherapy-naive patients. Since surgical resection is considered to be the most potentially curative treatment for colorectal cancer with hepatic metastases, investigators have sought to increase the fraction of patients eligible for surgical metastasis removal after tumour shrinkage on aggressive chemotherapy.[63] In one study,[63] the addition of oxaliplatin to 5-FU/FA given as a chronomodulated infusion allowed up to 50% of patients with initially inoperable liver metastases to undergo surgical resection.

The first European phase III study randomly assigned 200 patients to receive a 5-day chronomodulated infusion of 700 mg/m²/day of 5-FU and 300 mg/m²/day of FA with or without 125 mg/m² of oxaliplatin given as a 6-hour infusion on the first day of each cycle. Each course was repeated every 21 days. A second multicentre European trial included 420 patients and randomized a 2-hour infusion of 200 mg/m²/day of FA followed by a 5-FU bolus of 400 mg/m² and a 22-hour infusion of 600 mg/m²/day of 5-FU for 2 consecutive days every 2 weeks, either alone or combined with 85 mg/m² of oxaliplatin given on day 1.

The addition of oxaliplatin did not compromise the delivered dose intensity of 5-FU/FA, and significantly improved the antitumour efficacy of the regimen in the two studies. Markedly improved response rates (more than twofold over the control arm) were observed in the oxaliplatin-containing arms (see Table 52.3). Most important in both studies was the fact that median progression-free survival increased from 6 months with 5-FU/FA to 9 months in patients receiving the oxaliplatin-containing chemotherapy. It is of note that the median survival was superior to 16 months in both studies (see Table 52.3), which is the highest median survival observed in a large multicentre trial setting. The higher rate of crossover may have had a major influence on the lack of survival difference significance.

The combination of oxaliplatin or irinotecan with the same LV5FU2 regimen in a randomized phase II study has been reported and is discussed below.

Safety

The addition of oxaliplatin to 5-FU/FA resulted in an increased frequency of diarrhoea, mucositis, and neutropenia. Grade 4 neutropenia was reported in 15% and 36.9% patients following the FOLFOX 3 and FOLFOX 4 regimens respectively,[58] in 8% of patients following 5-day infusion with constant rate, and in 3% of patients using a 5-day chronomodulated infusion.[61] Grade 4 diarrhoea was experienced by 5% of the patients treated by either FOLFOX 3 or FOLFOX 4.[58] Grade 3–4 diarrhoea occurred in 43% of the patients who received oxaliplatin in the first trial, and in 12% in the second one. Less than 2% of the patients had severe haematotoxicity in the first study, and 12% in the second. Cumulative neurosensory toxicity with moderate functional impairment was reported in 13% and 18% of patients treated with oxaliplatin in the first and second studies respectively. Hence the first oxaliplatin-based regimen was more diarrhoeaogenic but induced less neutropenia than the second regimen. The neurosensory toxicity, seen with a 10% prevalence after

Table 52.3 Phase III randomized trials of combinations of either irinotecan or oxaliplatin with 5-fluorouracil/folinic acid (5-FU/FA) as first-line treatment of metastatic colorectal cancer

Study design	Ref	Treatment modalities[a]	Response rate (%)	Median PFS[b] (months)	Median[b] survival (months)
(A) FA/5-FU, 169 patients (B) Irinotecan + FA/5-FU, 169 patients	19	(A) LV5FU2 or AIO (B) • Irinotecan 180 mg/m² followed by LV5FU2 q2wks, or • Irinotecan 80 mg/m² followed by AIO, weekly × 6, q7wks	23 41	4.4* 6.7 ($p < 0.001$)	14 16.8 ($p = 0.03$)
(A) Irinotecan + FA/5-FU, 231 patients (B) FA/5-FU, 226 patients (C) Irinotecan, 226 patients	20	(A) Irinotecan 125 mg/m² followed by 20 mg/m² FA, 5-FU 500 mg/m² bolus, weekly × 4, q6wks (B) FA 20 mg/m², 5-FU 425 mg/m² daily × 5 q28d (C) Irinotecan 125 mg/m² weekly × 4, q6wks	39 21 ($p < 0.001$) 18	7.0 4.3 ($p = 0.004$) 4.2	14.8 12.6 ($p = 0.004$) 12.0
420 patients LV5FU2 vs LV5FU2 + oxaliplatin	33	LV5FU2 ± oxaliplatin 85 mg/m² q2wks	LV5FU2: 22.3 LV5FU2 + oxaliplatin: 50.7 ($p = 0.0001$)	6.2 9.0 ($p = 0.0003$)	14.7 16.2 (Wilcoxon $p = 0.05$)
Chronomodulated 5-FU/FA vs 5-FU/FA + oxaliplatin, 200 patients	34	5-FU 700 mg/m²/d FA 300 mg/m²/d over 5 days q21d ± oxaliplatin 125 mg/m² d1 over 6 h	5-FU/FA: 16 5-FU/FA oxaliplatin: 53 ($p < 0.001$)	6.1 8.7 ($p = 0.048$)	19.9 19.4

[a] The LV5FU2 regimen is FA 200 mg/m² over 2 h before 5-FU 400 mg/m² over 2 h, followed by 5-FU 600 mg/m² over 22 h, every other week. The AIO regimen is FA 500 mg/m² over 2 h followed by 5-FU 2600 mg/m² as a 24 h continuous intravenous infusion every other week.

[b] PFS, progression-free survival; NA, not available.

700 mg/m[2] of oxaliplatin, and consistently present in all patients receiving doses greater than 1000 mg/m[2], was the cumulative treatment-limiting toxicity.[64] Grade 3 neurosensory toxicity was found when a cumulative dose of more than 700 mg/m[2] of oxaliplatin was reached. Since the neuropathy, which is consistently reversible within a few months of oxaliplatin discontinuation, was a late toxic event closely correlated with cumulative dosing,[64] its occurrence reflected the effectiveness of the therapeutic combination, which could be maintained for months without disease progression. To reduce this toxicity, new regimens of 5-FU/FA and oxaliplatin (FOLFOX 3 and 4) have been successively introduced with a dose reduction of oxaliplatin from 130 mg/m[2] to 85 mg/m[2], which appears to be the optimal dose using the every 2 weeks schedule. The percentage of patients experiencing cumulative grade 3 sensory neuropathy was 27.5% using the FOLFOX 3 regimen and 15.8% with FOLFOX 4.[58]

In a randomized trial comparing a 5-day treatment with 5-FU, FA, and oxaliplatin given by either constant-rate or chronomodulated infusion, the chronomodulated arm was associated with a significant reduction of severe grade 4 toxicity requiring hospital admission, as well as of the incidence of severe mucosal toxicity (14% versus 76%).[53] The chronotherapy halved the incidence of functional impairment from peripheral sensitive neuropathy (16% versus 31%).[53]

The combination was well tolerated even in performance status 2–3, heavily pretreated patients (including those with more than three previous chemotherapy regimens), with a wide variety of 5-FU-containing regimens, as shown in the retrospective analysis of the European compassionate-use programme.[62]

A large randomized multicentre phase III clinical trial is presently underway to compare the antitumour efficacy and the toxicity of the combination of 5-FU/FA and oxaliplatin given every 2 weeks, using either a FOLFOX regimen[33] or the '4–10' chronomodulated infusion.[54,55] This study will compare head to head the results of these two combination regimens using an every 2 weeks schedule. Moreover, this study will also specify whether the increase in dose intensity and tolerability reported with chronomodulation may have a clinical impact on the percentage of patients who may have surgical resections of initially unresectable metastases. Of major interest, phase III clinical trials are ongoing to evaluate the benefit of the addition of oxaliplatin to 5-FU/FA in the adjuvant setting, with results expected to be available in 2002.

The combination of oxaliplatin with raltitrexed is active and feasible, and can be given easily in an outpatient setting, without the need for infusional devices.[65,66] The antitumor activity of this combination has recently been evaluated in a multicentre phase II study in advanced colorectal cancer patients.[66] Raltitrexed was given at 3 mg/m[2] as a 15-minute infusion, followed 45 minutes later by oxaliplatin 130 mg/m[2], as a 2-hour infusion, every 3 weeks. The objective response rate was 62% in 63 evaluable patients. The median time to progression was 6.3 months. The median survival was at least 13 months and the 1-year survival rate was 56.4%. A surgical resection of the metastases could be performed after chemotherapy in eight (12%) patients. The most frequent Common Toxicity Criteria grade 3–4 toxic effects were neutropenia (16.5% of patients), nausea (10.5% of patients), and diarrhoea (9.0% of patients).

COMBINATIONS OF IRINOTECAN WITH THYMIDYLATE SYNTHASE INHIBITORS

A variety of 5-FU and irinotecan schedules have been tested in combination (Tables 52.4 and 52.5), and see also Chapter 53. The patients included in these studies either had solid tumours of some sort[73,74] or were restricted to those with gastrointestinal neoplasias – predominantly[71] or exclusively[72,75,76,79–85] colorectal cancers. 5-FU was administered weekly[71,73,76] or daily × 5;[68,80] hybrid 5-FU/FA (LV5FU2) was given for 48 hours biweekly,[77,79,82] for 24 hours biweekly,[83,84] as a 5-, 7-, or 14-day infusion,[69,70,73] or in a chronomodulated schedule;[73] irinotecan was given weekly,[71,74,76] every other week,[72,77,79,82] or every 3[73,75] or 4[68,69] weeks. Alternated schedules, with irinotecan or 5-FU/FA every other cycle, were also tested.[80,85]

Diarrhoea is a common toxic side-effect of irinotecan and 5-FU, and was expected to be the main dose-limiting toxicity. In fact, less than half of the patients in the phase I studies had diarrhoea as the dose-limiting toxicity.[69,70,76,77] As for single-agent therapy, diarrhoea did not appear to be related to the irinotecan schedule, but rather to the 5-FU regimen. Diarrhoea was the dose-limiting toxicity when most diarrhoeogenic schedules of 5-FU were used – either infusional 5-FU[69,70,77] or a weekly bolus.[20,71,73,76] Using infusional 5-FU, it was consistently possible to maintain a high dose intensity of both 5-FU and irinotecan, and promising antitumour activity was reported. In contrast, concomitant bolus administration of 5-FU seemed to be associated with severe haematotoxicity (with neutropenia as the dose-

Table 52.4 Combinations of irinotecan with 5-fluorouracil/folinic acid (5-FU/FA) or raltitrexed: phase I clinical trials

Patients (pts) and schedules[a]	Ref	Dose range[a]	Dose-limiting toxicities	Recommended doses[b]
33 gastrointestinal cancer pts (31 ACRC) irinotecan + raltitrexed q3wks	67	Irinotecan: 175–400 mg/m^2 Raltitrexed: 2.6–3.0 mg/m^2	Asthenia	irinotecan: 350 mg/m^2 raltitrexed: 3.0 mg/m^2
41 pts, including 38 ACRC irinotecan d1 or 6, 5-FU bolus d1–5, q3wks	68	Irinotecan: 200–350 mg/m^2 5-FU bolus: 375 mg/m^2	Neutropenia	irinotecan: 300 mg/m^2 5-FU: 375 mg/m^2/d
38 ACRC pts irinotecan + 7-day CI 5-FU q4wks	69	Irinotecan: 50–250 mg/m^2 5-FU 7-day CI: 400 mg/m^2/d	Neutropenia, diarrhoea	irinotecan: 250 mg/m^2 5-FU: 400 mg/m^2/d RR: 11%
20 ACRC pts irinotecan q2wks + 5-day CI 5-FU, d3–7	70	Irinotecan: 100–175 mg/m^2 5-FU: 5-day CI 600 mg/m^2/d	Neutropenia, diarrhoea	MTD not reached RR: 26%
42 pts, including 38 CRC weekly irinotecan + 5-FU/FA 4 wks repeated q6wks	71	Irinotecan: 100–150 mg/m^2 FA: 20 mg/m^2 5-FU: bolus 210–500 mg/m^2	Neutropenia	irinotecan: 125 mg/m^2 FA: 20 mg/m^2 5-FU: 500 mg/m^2 RR: 17%
1st-line ACRC irinotecan + 5-FU/FA q2wks	72	Irinotecan: 150–200 mg/m^2 FA: 250 mg/m^2 5-FU: bolus 600–950 mg/m^2	Neutropenia	irinotecan: 200 mg/m^2 FA: 250 mg/m^2 5-FU: 850 mg/m^2 RR: 45%
31 pts with advanced solid tumours (14 ACRC) irinotecan q3wks + CI 5-FU over 14 days	73	Irinotecan: 150–350 mg/m^2 5-FU: 250–300 mg/m^2 CI over 14 days	Febrile neutropenia	irinotecan:350 mg/m^2 5-FU: 250 mg/m^2

74	15 pts, all tumours irinotecan + 5-FU weekly for 6 weeks	Irinotecan:60–80 mg/m² 5-FU 3000 mg/m² 48 h CI	Not yet available	MTD not reached
75	14 ACRC pts irinotecan d1 + Chronomodulated 5-FU/FA over 5 days every 3 weeks	Irinotecan: 175–275 mg/m² FA: 150 mg/m²/d 5-FU: 700–900 mg/m²/d	Not yet available	MTD not reached
76	26 ACRC pts weekly irinotecan + weekly FA/5-FU over 24 h × 6 wks, 1 wk rest (AIO)	Irinotecan: 80 mg/m² FA: 500 mg/m² 5-FU: 1800–2600 mg/m² over 24 h	Diarrhoea	irinotecan: 80 mg/m² + FA 500 mg/m² + 5-FU 2600 mg/m² RR: 64%
77	55 ACRC pts irinotecan + LV5FU2*	Irinotecan: 100–300 mg/m² + LV5FU2	Diarrhoea and fatigue	irinotecan: 80–200 mg/m² + full doses of LV5FU2

[a](A)CRC, (advanced) colorectal cancer; CI, continuous infusion; LV5FU2, see footnote *a* to Table 52.3.
[b] RR, response rate; MTD, maximum tolerated dose.

Table 52.5 Combinations of irinotecan with 5-fluorouracil/folinic acid (5-FU/FA) or raltitrexed: phase II clinical trials

Study design[a]	Ref	Treatment modalities[b]	Response rate (%)
ACRC, irinotecan + raltitrexed (10 patients)	78	Irinotecan: 300 or 350 mg/m² d1 + 3 mg/m² raltitrexed d2, q3wks	30
3rd-line ACRC, irinotecan + 5-FU/FA (33 patients)	79	Irinotecan: 180 mg/m² d1 FA: 400 mg/m² followed by 5-FU bolus 400 mg/m² and 46 h CI of 2400–3000 mg/m² q2wks	6 (+6% stabilizations)
ACRC, alternated schedule, weekly irinotecan + Mayo Clinic (70 patients)	80	• Weekly irinotecan: 100 mg/m² d1, 8, 15, 22, alternated with: • FA 20 mg/m²/d, 5-FU bolus 425 mg/m²/d, days 43–47 q10wks	26
ACRC, alternated schedule, irinotecan + Mayo Clinic (33 patients)	81	• Irinotecan: 350 mg/m², alternated with: • FA 20 mg/m²/d, 5-FU bolus 425 mg/m²/d, days 22–26 q10wks	31
Randomized phase II, 1st-line CRC: (A) LV5FU2 (29 patients) versus (B) irinotecan + LV5FU2 (59 patients) 1st-line CRC, irinotecan + LV5FU2 (34 patients)	82 83	(A) LV5FU2: FA 100 mg/m² 2 h, 5-FU bolus 400 mg/m², 5-FU 600 mg/m² over 22 h, q2wks (B) Irinotecan: 180 mg/m² followed by LV5FU2 irinotecan: 180 mg/m² followed by FA 200 mg/m² 2 h, 5-FU 400 mg/m² bolus, 5-FU 600 mg/m² over 22 h, q2wks	21 40 27
ACRC irinotecan + LV5FU2 (44 patients)	84	Irinotecan: 180 mg/m² followed (d1–2) by FA 200 mg/m² 2 h, 5-FU 400 mg/m² bolus, 5-FU 600 mg/m² over 22 h, q2wks	22

[a](A)CRC, (advanced) colorectal cancer.
[b]CI, continuous infusion.

limiting toxicity),[68,71,72] requiring dose reduction, which led to reduced dose intensity of both agents. Albeit conceptually interesting, the alternating-administration combinations now appear less attractive, given the good tolerability, the higher dose-intensity and the antitumour activity of schedules in which the two drugs are administered simultaneously.

Two phase III studies, one in Europe and one in the USA, evaluated the effect of the addition of irinotecan to 5-FU/FA for first-line treatment of advanced colorectal cancer patients.[19,20] In the European study, 387 patients were randomized to receive 5-FU/FA given with or without irinotecan. Two of the most common European modalities of administration of 5-FU/FA were used: based either on the LV5FU2 regimen (FA 200 mg/m² over 2 hours before 5-FU 400 mg/m² over 2 hours, followed by 5-FU 600 mg/m² over 22 hours every other week) or on the AIO regimen (FA 500 mg/m² over 2 hours, followed by 2600 mg/m^2 5-FU as a 24-hour continuous intravenous infusion every week). This arm was compared with irinotecan combined with the same modalities of administration of 5-FU. The irinotecan dose was 80 mg/m^2 weekly in combination with the AIO 5-FU/FA regimen, and 180 mg/m^2 every other week with LV5FU2.

All the criteria for efficacy were significantly better in the irinotecan arm (see Table 52.3): increased overall response rate, including 4% versus 0% of complete remissions ($p < 0.001$), as well as time-related parameters. The median duration of responses and disease stabilizations was 8.6 versus 6.2 months ($p < 0.001$); the median time to progression and the median survival were also significantly improved (see Table 52.3) with a 1-year survival rate of 69% versus 59% ($p = 0.03$). Forty-two percent of the patients in the irinotecan-containing arm experienced grade 3–4 neutropenia, versus 11% in the 5-FU/FA arm. The frequency of febrile neutropenia was also higher in the irinotecan arm (5% versus 1%), and one patient in this arm died from sepsis. Grade 3–4 diarrhoea was observed in 22% of the patients receiving irinotecan versus 10% of the patients treated with 5-FU/FA. Quality-of-life assessment showed similar results in the two treatment groups.

In the three-arm study reported by Saltz et al,[20] irinotecan 125 mg/m^2 followed by FA 20 mg/m^2 and 5-FU 500 mg/m^2 bolus, weekly for 4 consecutive weeks, in a 6-week cycle, was compared with single-agent irinotecan and with the Mayo Clinic 5-FU/FA-alone regimen. The addition of irinotecan to 5-FU/FA also resulted in an almost twofold higher response rate than 5-FU/FA alone or irinotecan alone (see Table 52.3). The combination arm was complicated with more diarrhoea but less mucositis, less grade 4 neutropenia, and less febrile neutropenia than the 5-FU/FA arm. This decreased myelotoxicity in the combination might be partly due to the weekly bolus regimen of 5-FU/FA, which yields less neutropenia than the Mayo Clinic regimen used in the control arm. However, a reduction in dose intensity due to omission of the last infusions of the cycle using this weekly schedule may also have contributed to this phenomenon, and it will be interesting to compare the respective dose intensities of irinotecan and 5-FU in the final publication. Alternatively, the decreased myelotoxicity might be due to the aforementioned interaction between 5-FU and irinotecan at the cellular level leading to antagonism when the antimetabolite was given in vitro prior to topo I-mediated DNA damage.[45–48] The combination of irinotecan and 5-FU/FA has been evaluated in a study comparing the effect of the sequence of a FOLFOX regimen until treatment failure followed by FOLFIRI (see Chapter 54) versus the reverse sequential treatment (FOLFIRI followed by FOLFOX).[86] In this study, the same hybrid 48-hour 5-FU/FA regimen was used in combination with either 180 mg/m^2 of irinotecan (FOLFIRI) or 100 mg/m^2 of oxaliplatin every two weeks (FOLFOX). The primary endpoint of this interesting study is the time to disease progression after both therapeutic regimens, and is still not reached at this time. Only results for the first-line treatments are currently available. The response rates to the first-line regimen were similar; 60% versus 63% with FOLFOX and FOLFIRI respectively. Toxicity was similar in both regimens, except for alopecia with FOLFIRI and neurosensory toxicity with FOLFOX.[86]

The combination of irinotecan with raltitrexed has also been tested.[67,78] The recommended doses using an every 3 weeks schedule were the full doses of each agent given alone: 350 mg/m^2 of irinotecan with 3.0 mg/m^2 of raltitrexed. The main toxicity was asthenia, while an ongoing phase II trial suggests response rates similar to those seen with 5-FU/FA.[78]

Combinations of oxaliplatin with irinotecan

The combination of the two new agents oxaliplatin and irinotecam appeared very attractive, since their mechanism of action is completely independent of thymidylate synthase inhibition, and led to supra-additive activity in preclinical models.[46] This combination therapy is the most recent, and (in contrast to the combination of 5-FU/FA and oxaliplatin or 5-FU/FA and irinotecan) only preliminary reports from small numbers of patients, all of them 5-FU-pretreated and most of them resistant, are available. The antitumour activity of this new combination is already very promising. The results of the phase I and II clinical trials are worth noting because most of the patients were resistant and frequently truly refractory to optimal therapy with 5-FU with or without FA. In this population of colorectal cancer patients with particularly bad prognosis, tumour responses were rapidly and commonly observed, and outright progression was very rare. One study also included patients after failure of single-agent irinotecan, with responses also reported in this patient subset.[87]

To date, six studies have evaluated four schedules, and are presented in Table 52.6:

• two phase I studies in gastrointestinal tumour patients and one phase II trial in advanced

Table 52.6 Combinations of irinotecan with oxaliplatin

Schedule[a]	Ref	Dose-limiting toxicities	Recommended doses (mg/m²)		Dose intensity at recommended doses (mg/m²/week)[b]
Phase I every 3 weeks	88	Diarrhoea, febrile neutropenia	Irinotecan: Oxaliplatin:	200 85	66.6
Randomized phase II every 3 weeks versus alternated schedule LV5FU2–irinotecan/LV5FU2–oxaliplatin	89	Neutropenia	Irinotecan: Oxaliplatin:	200 85	28.3
Phase I every 2 weeks	87 90	Neutropenia	Irinotecan: Irinotecan: Oxaliplatin:	175 (PS 0–1)[c] 150 (PS 2) 85	87.5 75 42.5
Phase I/II weekly irinotecan (d1, 8, 15) and oxaliplatin every 2 weeks repeated every 4 weeks, + G-CSF	91	Neutropenia (without G-CSF), diarrhoea (with G-CSF)	Irinotecan: Oxaliplatin:	80 85	60 42.5
Phase I weekly irinotecan + weekly oxaliplatin, 4 weeks, every 6 weeks	92	Diarrhoea, febrile neutropenia	Irinotecan: Oxaliplatin:	65 60	43.3 40

[a]LV5FU2, see footnote *a* to Table 52.3; G-CSF, granulocyte colony-stimulating factor.
[b]Calculated over a 6-week period.
[c]PS, performance status.

colorectal cancer using a once every 3 weeks schedule;[88,89]

- irinotecan given weekly, plus oxaliplatin every other week;[91]
- both irinotecan and oxaliplatin given every 2 weeks;[87,90]
- both given weekly for 4 consecutive weeks, repeated every 6 weeks.[92]

The once every 3 weeks schedule was the first to be investigated. Two parallel phase I studies were carried out and published in the same paper.[88] Oxaliplatin, given as a 2-hour intravenous infusion, was followed by a 30-minute irinotecan infusion. Dose levels in the trials ranged from 85 to 110 mg/m² for oxaliplatin and 150 to 250 mg/m² for irinotecan. Thirty-nine patients with gastrointestinal tumours, including 24 with colorectal cancer, received 216 treatment cycles, with all but 6 having failed 5-FU chemotherapy. The maximum tolerated dose was oxaliplatin 110 mg/m² plus irinotecan 200 mg/m² in one study and oxaliplatin 110 mg/m² plus irinotecan 250 mg/m² in the other. The dose-limiting toxicities were those of irinotecan, namely febrile neutropenia and delayed diarrhoea. The recommended doses for phase II studies were oxaliplatin 85 mg/m² and irinotecan 200 mg/m². At these doses, grade 3 and 4 toxicities were emesis in 42% of patients, neutropenia in 33% (febrile episodes in 17%), peripheral neuropathy in 25%, delayed diarrhoea in 17%, and thrombocytopenia in 8%. An increased toxicity of irinotecan in patients with Gilbert's syndrome was noted.[93] No pharmacokinetic interaction was detected between oxaliplatin and irinotecan or SN38. The results of the first randomized phase II study using irinotecan/oxaliplatin every 3 weeks confirmed these results, with a response rate of 28% (plus 45% additional disease stabilizations) and a median time to progression of 10 months.[88] This result compares favourably with the results of either irinotecan alone[16–18] or oxaliplatin alone.[20]

In the once every 2 weeks schedule, a fixed dose of 85 mg/m[2] of oxaliplatin was combined with a dose of irinotecan ranging from 100 to 200 mg/m[2]. One hundred and eighty-six cycles were administered to 23 gastrointestinal cancer patients, including 11 colorectal cancer patients. Incomplete recovery at day 15 was more limiting than febrile neutropenia or diarrhoea with this schedule. The maximal tolerated dose of irinotecan was 200 mg/m[2], with incomplete neutrophil recovery at day 15. Grade 3 oxaliplatin-induced neurotoxicity was cumulative and limiting in 39% of patients. The recommended dose was 175 mg/m[2] of irinotecan plus 85 mg/m[2] of oxaliplatin, without need for granulocyte colony-stimulating factor (G-CSF) support. The treatment was feasible in an outpatient setting. A dose of 150 mg/m[2] of irinotecan was recommended in patients with a performance status of 2. It is worth noting that this schedule allowed the highest dose intensity for both agents to be reached. The doses of oxaliplatin and irinotecan are those recommended every 2 weeks in combination with 5-FU/FA. In combination with 85 mg/m[2] of oxaliplatin, the dose of irinotecan recommended every 2 weeks is close to the dose recommended every 3 weeks (175 mg/m[2] compared with 200 mg/m[2]). In turn, the once every 3 weeks schedule resulted in the lowest dose intensity of oxaliplatin and thus the lowest incidence of neurosensory cumulative toxicity. Weekly administration of irinotecan led to the lowest dose intensity of this agent. Reproducible evidence of clinical activity was observed in 5-FU-resistant colorectal cancer patients using any of the schedules tested. This was also the case in some irinotecan-resistant patients.[87] More recently, we have seen clinical activity of irinotecan in patients having disease progression while on 5-FU/FA and oxaliplatin. The objective response rate in advanced colorectal cancer patients was high in all studies.[87–91] Moreover, the very low (<10%) rate of outright disease progression seen, with a time to progression of over 7 months in mostly 5-FU-resistant patients, is the major point of interest.

TOWARDS TRITHERAPY?

The recent availability of two new agents in addition to thymidylate synthase inhibitors has led naturally to the assessment of three-drug combination regimens for colorectal cancer therapy, as has been the case for other tumour types. Although tritherapy preclinical models have not been assessed, the different mechanisms of action and resistance, the additivity (or synergism) observed with the three possible double combinations, and the different safety profiles provide enough rationale for their clinical investigation. Most trials are ongoing or only recently completed, and have been reported only in abstract form.[89,94,95] Here again, two main strategies have been tested: either the three drugs are given on the same day or they are given as alternating bitherapy regimens. The paradigm of the latter option is to avoid the possible overlap of toxic events (which is more of a concern than with bitherapy) at the expense of decreased dose-intensity delivery of the individual agents.

The first published approach was an alternating regimen using the LV5FU2 regimen every 2 weeks combined alternately with irinotecan 180 mg/m[2] or oxaliplatin 85 mg/m[2].[89] This regimen was randomly assigned versus the two-drug combination of irinotecan, 200 mg/m[2] and oxaliplatin 85 mg/m[2] given together every 3 weeks to patients with 5-FU-resistant metastatic colorectal cancer. The rationale for this study was to assess the benefit of adding 5-FU to irinotecan plus oxaliplatin in the clinical setting of 5-FU failure. Although it was a randomized phase II trial without planned comparison, all efficacy parameters appeared better with the irinotecan/oxaliplatin bitherapy than with alternating tritherapy (response rate 23% versus 6%; median time to progression 9 months versus 8 months and median survival 12 months versus 10 months). Nonetheless, the time to progression was remarkably long in both arms, taking into account the documented clinical 5-FU resistance required for accrual. Febrile neutropenia occurred more frequently with tritherapy (13% of patients) than with bitherapy (3%), as did severe diarrhoea (19% versus 10%). Severe vomiting and cumulative oxaliplatin neuropathy, in turn, occurred more frequently with bitherapy. It may be worth speculating that the lower-efficacy results of tritherapy could be due to the lower dose intensities of irinotecan and oxaliplatin (the two drugs thought to be more active in this situation of 5-FU failure) obtained with this alternating approach, which cannot be compensated by the introduction of a third less active drug. Likewise, the well-documented clinical synergism of 5-FU with oxaliplatin, even in situations of 5-FU resistance, is probably compromised by the low dose intensity of oxaliplatin (21.25 mg/m^2/week planned dose intensity with this schedule). It appears from such data that the true benefit of tritherapy approaches should be further tested in 5-FU-naive patients.

A study with another alternating schedule is ongoing (L Cals, personal communication). 5-FU is given according to the AIO weekly regimen at a dose of 2600 mg/m^2 over a 24-hour continuous infusion, without FA, for 4 consecutive weeks every 6 weeks. Every other week, either irinotecan or oxaliplatin is added to 5-FU at increasing doses (60/40, 60/60, and 80/60 mg/m^2 respectively). So far, 14 patients have been enrolled. The maximum tolerated dose is not reached at dose level III (80/60 mg/m^2, which are the individual recommended doses of irinotecan and oxaliplatin respectively with this 5-FU regimen),[76] while antitumour activity has been observed. An increased 5-FU dose (3000 mg/m^2) is now being considered. Once the recommended dose has been determined, chemotherapy-naive patients will be treated to assess the efficacy of this combination.

Another study, reported by Lerebours et al,[94] has evaluated the three drugs given together in a phase I, dose-escalating design. Fixed doses of CPT-11 (200 mg/m^2) and oxaliplatin (85 mg/m^2), corresponding to the recommended doses of the two-drug regimen, were given every 3 weeks in addition to increasing doses of 5-FU, given as a continuous intravenous infusion over 96 hours. Fourteen patients were entered at two dose levels. The dose of 3000 mg/m^2 of 5-FU was considered to be the maximum tolerated dose, with febrile neutropenia and diarrhoea being the dose-limiting toxicities. The dose of 2000 mg/m^2/cycle of 5-FU is recommended for phase II studies. To date, no responses have been observed among the 7 heavily pretreated colorectal cancer patients.

An ongoing study, reported by Conroy et al,[95] tests the concomitant administration of irinotecan and oxaliplatin at escalating doses and the full-dose LV5FU2 regimen every 2 weeks. The dose of irinotecan was escalated from 90 to 220 mg/m^2 and that of oxaliplatin from 60 to 85 mg/m^2. Thirty-five patients with miscellaneous tumours were enrolled. The limiting toxicities were febrile neutropenia, diarrhoea, and peripheral neuropathy. The maximum tolerated dose of this combination was deemed to be oxaliplatin 85 mg/m^2 and irinotecan 220 mg/m^2. The recommended doses for further phase II studies were oxaliplatin 85 mg/m^2 and irinotecan 180 mg/m^2. At these doses, only 2 of 9 patients experienced a dose-limiting toxicity in the first cycle. It is of note that the recommended doses of both oxaliplatin and irinotecan in the three-drug regimen are the same as those recommended in two-drug combinations – either with each drug combined with LV5FU2 or with the two combined together every 2 weeks – suggesting that the triple addition does not lead to additional unmanageable toxicity. Furthermore, two complete and three partial responses were observed in the nine pretreated colorectal cancer patients entered in this study.

Although the results are very preliminary, the first experiments with tritherapy suggest that the combination of the three drugs on the same day is feasible and well tolerated and results in high dose intensity, at least when combined with the LV5FU2 regimen.[95]

Although to the best of our knowledge, no such study is planned, the combination of irinotecan, oxaliplatin, and raltitrexed, all given over short infusions on the same day every 3 weeks, should be considered, because of its very easy and convenient schedule, the good tolerance and high dose intensity reached when 5-FU, irinotecan, and oxaliplatin are given together, and the promising results of both oxaliplatin/raltitrexed[65,66] and irinotecan/raltitrexed[67,78] combinations.

DISCUSSION

Whilst it is very encouraging that more treatment options are available for patients with advanced colorectal cancer, this leads unavoidably to new unanswered questions. What is the best combination for first-line chemotherapy? Will a three-drug regimen be a better option than any two-drug regimen? What are the optimal schedules of 5-FU/oxaliplatin and irinotecan in combination? Which regimen provides the best balance between clinical activity and toxicity? Is it possible to prospectively identify patients who are most likely to respond, become resectable, or be resistant to each specific regimen?

Is combination therapy better than single-agent chemotherapy?

In second-line treatment, several studies have evaluated the effect of the addition of oxaliplatin to 5-FU/FA. This combination was reproducibly found to show an increased response rate and a longer time to progression.[31,32,51–55] Furthermore, the availability of experienced surgical teams led to a high rate of metastasis removal after cytoreductive chemotherapy.[63] In 5-FU-pretreated patients, the combination of irinotecan with oxaliplatin appeared more efficient than monotherapy with either agent alone.[16,18,30,89,91] Little information is available concerning the potential benefit of the addition of irinotecan to 5-FU/FA in second-line treatment as compared with irinotecan alone. Although it has not been assessed specifically, a randomized comparison of irinotecan versus infusional 5-FU showed evidence of activity of infusional 5-FU in second-line treatment, suggesting a potential additive effect.[18]

In the first-line treatment of advanced disease, several randomized studies have demonstrated an increased antitumour effect in treatment with 5-FU/FA plus either irinotecan[18,19] or oxaliplatin[33,34] in comparison with the same 5-FU/FA regimen alone. Reproducible differences in response rate and time to progression were observed in favour of the addition of oxaliplatin to 5-FU/FA.[33,34] The same results and, moreover, a survival advantage were observed when irinotecan was combined with 5-FU/FA.[19]

What is the best initial bitherapy for advanced colorectal cancer patients? We do not have sufficient information yet to answer this question. The ongoing randomized controlled clinical trial comparing the two sequences, FOLFOX followed by FOLFIRI or FOLFIRI followed by FOLFOX, may provide interesting information in this regard.[86] Of major interest is the very large trial currently being conducted in the USA by the North Central Cancer Treatment Group (NCCTG) (R

Goldberg, personal communication). Scheduled to include 1800 patients in six different arms, it compares, in a random allocation design, the possibly outdated Mayo Clinic reference regimen with a variety of irinotecan/5-FU and oxaliplatin/5-FU regimens, and even goes so far as to introduce as a front-line regimen a non-5-FU-containing arm – the oxaliplatin/irinotecan combination given every 3 weeks, as reported by Wasserman et al.[88] Table 52.7 shows a summary of its design. The main efficacy endpoint is progression-free survival, which seems appropriate given the second- and third-line regimens currently available.

Is increased-dose-intensity delivery of the available two-drug combinations a worthwhile goal in advanced colorectal cancer?

The incrementalist approach to dosing delivery is one of the inspiring tenets of anticancer chemotherapy,[96] but its clinical application in combination regimens for solid tumours, another paradigm of chemotherapy, has seen its potential limited by additive toxicities compromising dose-intensity delivery, and has not always resulted in major survival differences, especially since second- and third-line regimens have become available and are effective.

There is a relationship between 5-FU dose intensity and the objective tumour response rate in solid

Table 52.7 Summary of treatment arms in the NCCTG trial[a]

Arm	Treatment[b]	Patients (total 1800)
1	Weekly irinotecan/weekly bolus 5-FU/FA	300
2	Every 3 weeks irinotecan/bolus 5-FU/FA, Mayo regimen	300
3	Weekly irinotecan, weekly 24-hour CI 5-FU/FA	300
4	Oxaliplatin every 3 weeks, Mayo regimen 5-FU/FA	300
5	FOLFOX 2, oxaliplatin every 2 weeks + LV5FU2	300
6	Oxaliplatin every 3 weeks	300

[a]The primary efficacy endpoint is progression-free survival.
[b]CI, continuous infusion.

tumours[97] and in advanced colorectal cancer patients (see Chapter 55). In 381 patients with previously untreated metastatic colorectal cancer who were treated with 5-FU, FA, and oxaliplatin (using either flat or chronomodulated infusion), a retrospective analysis of two randomized phase III trials and two phase II studies indicated an increase in the objective response rate from 30% with $900 \, mg/m^2/week$ of 5-FU, to 50 with $1050 \, mg/m^2/week$, and over 60% with more than $1300 \, mg/m^2/week$ $(r = 0.96; p = 0.002)$ (see Chapter 55). A trend towards a dose–response relationship was suggested during the initial phase I studies with irinotecan.[98] In combination, no study has been prospectively designed to specify the role of oxaliplatin dose intensity within the therapeutic dose range, although investigators noticed a correlation when results were retrospectively analysed in the phase II setting (see Chapter 55). The every 3 weeks schedule of 5-FU/FA and oxaliplatin has tended to be replaced by the more intensified every 2 weeks schedules.[54,55,58–60] Similarly, even if the results are more preliminary, it also seems that the combination of irinotecan with oxaliplatin is more active using the every 2 weeks schedule, which is also the regimen providing the highest dose intensity of both irinotecan and oxaliplatin.[87–92]

Among each type of combination, many regimens and schedules have been proposed: Can we already determine the optimal schedule?

Many administration schedules have been proposed for 5-FU, as well as for irinotecan and oxaliplatin, without evidence of a clear advantage. Hence it is not realistic to determine which, among the multiple possible combinations (not all of which have yet been tested), is optimal. Nevertheless, some trends appear, although as yet there are no randomized trials supporting them:

- Infusional regimens of 5-FU with or without FA, active mainly on thymidylate synthase, seem better tolerated in combination regimens than bolus 5-FU/FA. This may be due to the relatively low myelotoxicity of these infusional regimens. The combination of infusional 5-FU-containing regimens was used in all phase III trials but one.[19,20,33,34]
- The every-other-week schedules may be the best regimens in terms of dose intensity of all compounds for the combinations of oxaliplatin with irinotecan[87,90] or of each of them with 5-FU/FA.[19,54,55,58–60]

- Since the combination of irinotecan with 5-FU/FA was initially feared to be too toxic owing to the possible addition of the same dose-limiting toxicities (i.e. neutropenia and diarrhoea), sequential treatments were developed. Alternation of irinotecan alone with bolus 5-FU daily × 5 plus low-dose FA was assessed in two studies.[80,81] The results are acceptable in terms of both tolerance and antitumour activity (with a response rate of about 30%). One of these studies has shown that, with each patient being his or her own control, severe neutropenia and diarrhoea were experienced by different patients on irinotecan or 5-FU. This may explain why the concomitant administration of the drugs does not lead to increased toxicity. Thus the dose intensity and response rates observed with non-alternated regimens appear more attractive. Moreover, further and very preliminary results with tritherapy[95] seem to confirm the higher dose intensity and the absence of increased toxicity when all drugs are given together.

For the time being, the only schedules that can be recommended are those verified as being superior in adequate phase III trials, i.e. the LV5FU2 regimen with either oxaliplatin or irinotecan every 2 weeks,[19,33] the 4-day chronomodulated infusion of 5-FU/FA and oxaliplatin,[34] or the AIO regimen with irinotecan weekly.[19] The above-mentioned large ongoing North American trial may further clarify the best amongst the many options available (see Table 52.7).

Is 5-FU essential in second-line combinations with new agents after failure of a 5-FU-based regimen?

For oxaliplatin and 5-FU, the answer is clearly yes. However, the preliminary data on the feasibility and activity of thymidylate-synthase-independent combinations (irinotecan/oxaliplatin) make this a very valid question. The only trial aimed at addressing this question was that of Becouarn et al,[89] which showed that there is no advantage in adding 5-FU in this situation. Reports of several ongoing and recently completed studies will address the potential of the oxaliplatin/irinotecan regimen, such as in the ambitious large North American trial mentioned above. However, the alternating design of the tritherapy-regimen arm considerably decreased the dose intensity of both irinotecan and oxaliplatin. Nevertheless, this question cannot be answered satisfactorily in the absence of optimal, dose-intensive tritherapy regimens.

Is tritherapy superior to bitherapy? Which endpoints?

While bitherapy may allow a better dose intensity of both agents, tritherapy might be beneficial despite dose reduction, because of the enlarged spectrum of antitumour activity covering three different targets instead of two, without cross-resistance. If, in addition, there is no loss in dose intensity, as suggested by one study,[95] it is reasonable to expect that tritherapy could show better therapeutic outcome. Future randomized trials comparing optimal tritherapy with bitherapy regimens are warranted to answer this question. If, in turn, the three-drug regimens are not superior to the two-drug regimens, the next question would be to determine what is the most effective sequence of drug administration for the three available bitherapy regimens. The ongoing randomized clinical trial comparing FOLFIRI followed by FOL-FOX and FOLFOX followed by FOLFIRI will partially answer this question, with regard to the preferable sequence of introduction of oxaliplatin and irinotecan. Furthermore, prospective tumour molecular target assessment may help to define the best initial option in a given patient. So far, the level of thymidylate synthase appears to be a determinant for the response to 5-FU-based chemotherapy.[99,100] The predictive values for chemosensitivity of other molecular markers, such as tumour dihydropyrimidine dehydrogenase levels,[101,102] p53,[103–105] microsatellite instability and mismatch-repair protein expression,[24–27] and topoisomerase I,[13,14] are undergoing evaluation. Even the consecrated role of 5-FU as a necessary and essential component of first-line treatment deserves to be challenged and compared with irinotecan plus oxaliplatin.

Which goal for which patient?

A decade ago, palliation was the common reasonable therapeutic goal proposed to advanced colorectal cancer patients. The presence of new active agents has transformed this situation. Long-term disease control or even curability in a small fraction of patients has become a realistic therapeutic proposal. The efficacy of second-line therapies is already a welcome reality, and third-line treatments are possible in many patients with advanced disease.

Finally, the choice of the combination therapy will depend on the therapy goal in a given advanced colorectal cancer patient:

- Aggressive front-line therapy with a curative intent to turn initially unresectable metastases into resectable metastases is presently conceivable. In this case, the patient is expected to have a few months' presurgical chemotherapy combining two or three agents as often as possible (i.e. weekly or every 2 weeks), to provide the maximal dose intensity of each agent and a fast objective response.
- Conversely, in the adjuvant setting and for palliative treatment of non-operable patients, in the elderly, or in patients with altered performance status, to avoid life-threatening toxicity, treatment tolerability becomes an important criterion by which to choose the most appropriate initial combination chemotherapy. A study evaluating the survival and quality of life of patients treated with palliative chemotherapy, comparing simultaneous and sequential approaches, would also be interesting in this regard.

CONCLUSIONS

This survey of therapeutic options in the treatment of colorectal cancer, either recently reported or currently under investigation, reveals a very exciting array of possibilities for the near future. Ongoing clinical trials will better determine the benefit of an initial aggressive approach with different regimens combining 5-FU/LV or other thymidylate synthase inhibitors with oxaliplatin and irinotecan, but will also optimize and further the clinical benefit of a palliative therapeutic outlook. In less than a decade, colorectal cancer has switched from having the status of a chemotherapy-refractory disease to that of being chemotherapy-sensitive, partially as a result of a more rational use of 5-FU/FA but mostly owing to the introduction of irinotecan and oxaliplatin in clinical practice. Median survivals in the latest generation of multicentre phase III trials range from 14 to 19 months, representing a gain of at least 40% over the decades-old standard 5-FU/FA. The possibility of cure or long-term disease control should concern an increasing proportion of patients – either those with metastatic disease who are capable of undergoing surgical resection of their metastases after intensive chemotherapeutic cytoreduction, or those with locally advanced disease, with the introduction of more efficient adjuvant combination regimens.

REFERENCES

1. Carter SK, Large bowel cancer: the current status of treatment. *J Natl Cancer Inst* 1976; **56**: 3–12.

2. Moertel CG, Chemotherapy of gastrointestinal cancer. *N Engl J Med* 1978; **299**: 1049–52.

3. Advanced Colorectal Cancer Meta-Analysis Project, Modulation of fluorouracil by leucovorin in patients with advanced colorectal cancer: evidence in terms of response rate. *J Clin Oncol* 1989; **10**: 896 903.

4. Poon MA, O'Connell MJ, Moertel CG et al, Biochemical modulation of fluorouracil: Evidence of significant improvement of survival and quality of life in patients with advanced colorectal carcinoma. *J Clin Oncol* 1989; **7**: 1407–12.

5. Nordic Gastrointestinal Tumor Adjuvant Therapy Group, Superiority of sequential methotrexate, fluorouracil and leucovorin to fluorouracil alone in advanced symptomatic colorectal carcinoma: a randomized trial. *J Clin Oncol* 1989; **7**: 1437–42.

6. Sobrero AF, Aschele C, Bertino JR et al, Fluorouracil in colorectal cancer – a tale of two drugs: implications for biochemical modulation. *J Clin Oncol* 1997; **15**: 368–81.

7. De Gramont A, Bosset JF, Milan C et al, Radomized trial comparing monthly low-dose leucovorin and fluorouracil bolus with bimonthly high-dose leucovorin and fluorouracil bolus plus continuous infusion for advanced colorectal cancer: a French Intergroup study. *J Clin Oncol* 1997; **15**: 808–15.

8. Moertel CG, Schutt AJ, Hahn RG et al, Therapy of advanced colorectal cancer with a combination of 5-fluorouracil, methyl-1,3-cis(2-chloroethyl)-1-nitrosourea, and vincristine. *J Natl Cancer Inst* 1975; **54**: 69–71.

9. Boice JD Jr, Greene MH, Killen JY Jr et al, Leukemia after adjuvant chemotherapy with semustine (methyl-CCNU). *N Engl J Med* 1986; **314**: 119–24.

10. Buroker T, Kim PN, Groppe C et al, 5-FU infusion with mitomycin C versus 5-FU infusion with methyl CCNU in the treatment of advanced colon cancer. *Cancer* 1978; **42**: 1228–33.

11. Loehrer PJ, Turner S, Kubilis P et al, A prospective randomized trial of fluorouracil versus fluorouracil plus cis-platin in the treatment of metastatic colorectal cancer: a Hoosier Oncology Group Trial. *J Clin Oncol* 1988; **6**: 642–8.

12. Kemeny N, Israel K, Niedzwiecki D et al, Randomized study of continuous infusion fluorouracil versus fluorouracil plus cis-platin in patients with metastatic colorectal cancer. *J Clin Oncol* 1990; **8**: 313–18.

13. Pommier Y, Pourquier P, Fan Y et al, Mechanism of eukaryotic DNA topoisomerase I and drugs targeted to the enzyme. *Biochim Biophys Acta* 1998; **1400**: 83–106.

14. Goldwasser F, Bae I, Valenti M et al, Topoisomerase I-related parameters and camptothecin activity in the colon carcinoma cell lines from the National Cancer Institute Anticancer Screen. *Cancer Res* 1995; **55**: 2116–21.

15. Hsiang YH, Lihou MG, Liu LF, Arrest of DNA replication by drug-stabilized topoisomerase I–DNA cleavable complexes as a mechanism of cell killing by camptothecin. *Cancer Res* 1989; **49**: 5077–82.

16. Rougier P, Bugat R, Douillard JY et al, Phase II study of irinotecan in the treatment of advanced colorectal cancer in chemotherapy-naive patients and patients pretreated with fluorouracil-based chemotherapy. *J Clin Oncol* 1997; **15**: 251–60.

17. Cunningham D, Pyrhonen S, James RD et al, Randomized trial of irinotecan plus supportive care versus supportive care alone after fluorouracil failure for patients with metastatic colorectal cancer. *Lancet* 1998; **352**: 1413–18.

18. Rougier P, Van Cutsem E, Bajetta E et al, Randomized comparison of irinotecan versus fluorouracil by continuous infusion after fluorouracil failure in patients with metastatic colorectal cancer. *Lancet* 1998; **352**: 1407–12.

19. Douillard JY, Cunningham D, Roth AD et al, Irinotecan combined with fluorouracil compared with fluorouracil alone as first-line treatment for metastatic colorectal cancer: a multicentre randomised trial *Lancet* 2000; **355**: 1041–7.

20. Saltz LB, Cox JV, Blanke C et al, Irinotecan plus fluorouracil and leucovorin for metastatic colorectal cancer. Irinotecan study group. *N Engl J Med* 2000; **343**: 905–14.

21. Raymond E, Faivre S, Woynarowski JM et al, Oxaliplatin: mechanism of action and antineoplastic activity. *Semin Oncol* 1998; **25**(2 Suppl 5): 4–12.

22. Raymond E, Chaney S, Taamma A et al, Preclinical and clinical studies of oxaliplatin. *Ann Oncol* 1998; **9**: 1053–71.

23. Rixe O, Ortuzar W, Alvarez M et al, Oxaliplatin, tetraplatin, cisplatin and carboplatin: spectrum of activity in drug-resistant cell lines and in the cell lines of the national cancer institute's anticancer drug screen panel. *Biochem Pharmacol* 1996; **52**: 1855–65.

24. Cunningham JM, Christensen ER, Tester DG et al, Hypermethylation of the hMLH1 promoter in colon cancer with microsatellite instability. *Cancer Res* 1998; **58**: 3455–60.

25. Thibodeau SN, French AJ, Cunningham JM et al, Microsatellite instability in colorectal cancer: Different mutator phenotypes and the principal involvement of hMLH1. *Cancer Res* 1998; **58**: 1713–18.

26. Thibodeau SN, French AJ, Roche PC et al, Altered expression of hMSH2 and hMSH1 in tumors with microsatellite instability and genetic alterations in mismatch repair genes. *Cancer Res* 1996; **56**: 4836–40.

27. Herman JG, Umar A, Polyak K et al, Incidence and functional consequences of hMLH1 promoter hypermethylation in colorectal carcinoma. *Proc Natl Acad Sci USA* 1998; **95**: 6870–5.

28. Mathé G, Kidani Y, Segiguchi M et al, Oxalato-platinum or L-OHP, a third generation platinum complex: an experimental and clinical appraisal and preliminary comparison with cis-platinum and carboplatinum. *Biomed Pharmacother* 1989; **43**: 237–50.

29. Raymond E, Buquet-Fagot C, Djelloul S et al, Antitumor activity of oxaliplatin in combination with 5-fluorouracil and the thymidylate synthase inhibitor AG337 in human colon, breast and ovarian cancers. *Anticancer Drugs* 1997; **8**: 876–85.

30. Machover D, Diaz-Rubio E, De Gramont A et al, Two consecutive phase II studies of oxaliplatin (L-OHP) for treatment of patients with advanced colorectal carcinoma who were resistant to previous treatment with fluoropyrimidines. *Ann Oncol* 1996; **7**: 95–8.

31. de Gramont A, Vignoud J, Tournigand C et al, Oxaliplatin with high-dose leucovorin and 5-fluorouracil 48-hour continuous infusion in pretreated metastatic colorectal cancer. *Eur J Cancer* 1997; **33**: 214–19.

32. André T, Louvet C, Raymond E et al, Bimonthly high-dose leucovorin and 5-fluorouracil infusion and oxaliplatin (FOLFOX 3) for metastatic colorectal cancer resistant to the same leucovorin and 5-fluorouracil regimen. *Ann Oncol* 1998; **9**: 1251–3.

33. De Gramont A, Figer A, Seymour M et al, A randomized trial of leucovorin (LV) and 5-fluorouracil (5FU) with or without oxaliplatin in advanced colorectal cancer (CRC). *Proc Am Soc Clin Oncol* 1998; **17**: 257a (Abst 985).

34. Giacchetti S, Perpoint B, Zidani R et al, Phase III multicenter randomized trial of oxaliplatin added to chronomodulated fluorouracil–leucovorin as first-line treatment of metastatic colorectal cancer. *J Clin Oncol* 2000; **18**: 136–47.

35. Fram RJ, Rochibaud N, Bishov SD et al, Interactions of *cis-*

diaminedichloroplatinum(II) with 1-b-D-arabinofuranosylcytosine in Lovo colon carcinoma cells. *Cancer Res* 1987; **47:** 3360–5.

36. Esaki T, Nakano S, Tatsumoto T et al, Inhibition by 5-fluorouracil of *cis*-diaminedichloroplatinum(II)-induced DNA interstrand cross-link removal in HST-1 human squamous carcinoma cell line. *Cancer Res* 1992; **52:** 6501–6.

37. Bergman AM, Ruiz van Haperen VWT, Veerman G et al, Synergistic interaction between cisplatin and gemcitabine in vitro. *Clin Cancer Res* 1996; **2:** 521–30.

38. Akutsu M, Suzuki K, Tsunoda S et al, Effect of SN-38 in combination with other anticancer agents against Dauji cells. *Jpn J Cancer Chemother* 1994; **21:** 1607–11.

39. Zeghari-Squalli N, Micret JL, Goldwasser F, Mechanism of the in vitro interaction between SN38 and 5-FU. *Proc Am Assoc Cancer Res* 1997; **38:** 3 (Abst 19).

40. Houghton JA, Cheshire PJ, Hallman II JD et al, Evaluation of irinotecan in combination with 5-fluorouracil or etoposide in xenograft models of colon adenocarcinoma and rhabdomyosarcoma. *Clin Cancer Res* 1996; **2:** 107–18.

41. Aschele C, Baldo C, Sobrero AF et al, Schedule-dependent synergism between raltitrexed and irinotecan in human colon cancer cells in vitro. *Clin Cancer Res* 1998; **4:** 1323–30.

42. Schwartz GN, Teicher BA, Eder JP et al, Modulation of antitumor alkylating agents by novobiocin, topotecan, and lonidamine. *Cancer Chemother Pharmacol* 1993; **32:** 455–62.

43. Chou TC, Motzer RJ, Tong V et al, Computerized quantitation of synergism and antagonism of Taxol, topotecan, and cisplatin against human teratocarcinoma cell growth: a rational approach to clinical protocol design. *J Natl Cancer Inst* 1994; **86:** 1517–24.

44. Goldwasser F, Valenti M, Torres R et al, Potentiation of cisplatin cytotoxicity by 9-aminocamptothecin. *Clin Cancer Res* 1996; **2:** 687–93.

45. Goldwasser F, Bozec L, Zeghari-Squalli N et al, Cellular pharmacology of the combination of oxaliplatin with topotecan in the IGROV-1 human ovarian cancer cell line. *Anticancer Drugs* 1999; **10:** 195–201.

46. Zeghari-Squalli N, Raymond E, Cvitkovic E, Goldwasser F, Cellular pharmacology of the combination of the DNA topoisomerase I inhibitor SN-38 and the diaminocyclohexane platinum derivative oxaliplatin. *Clin Cancer Res* 1999; **5:** 1189–96.

47. Fischel JL, Rostagno P, Formento P et al, Ternary combination of irinotecan, fluorouracil-folinic acid and oxaliplatin: results on human colon cancer cell lines. *Br J Cancer* 2001; **84:** 579–85.

48. Pommier Y, Pourquier P, Strumberg D et al, Multiple mechanisms for activation of topoisomerase-mediated DNA damage. *Proc Am Assoc Cancer Res* 1999; **40:** 773–4.

49. Caussanel JP, Lévi F, Brienza S et al, Phase I trial of 5-day continuous venous infusion of oxaliplatin at circadian rhythm modulated rate compared with constant rate. *J Natl Cancer Inst* 1990; **82:** 1046–50.

50. Lévi F, Misset JL, Brienza S et al, A chronopharmacologic phase II clinical trial with 5-fluorouracil, folinic acid, and oxaliplatin using an ambulatory multichannel programmable pump: high antitumor effectiveness against metastatic colorectal cancer. *Cancer* 1992; **69:** 893–900.

51. Lévi F, Soussan A, Adam R et al, A phase I–II trial of five-day continuous intravenous infusion of 5-fluorouracil delivered at circadian rhythm modulated rate in patients with metastatic colorectal cancer. *J Infus Chemother* 1995; **5:** 153–7.

52. Lévi F, Zidani R, Vannetzel JM et al, Chronomodulated versus fixed-infusion-rate delivery of ambulatory chemotherapy with oxaliplatin, fluorouracil, and folinic acid (leucovorin) in patients with colorectal cancer metastases: a randomized multi-institutional trial. *J Natl Cancer Inst* 1994; **86:** 1608–17.

53. Lévi F, Zidani R, Misset J-L et al, Randomised multicentre trial of chronotherapy with oxaliplatin, fluorouracil, and folinic acid in metastatic colorectal cancer. *Lancet* 1997; **350:** 681–6.

54. Bertheault-Cvitkovic F, Jami A, Ithzaki M et al, Biweekly intensified ambulatory chronomodulated chemotherapy with oxaliplatin, fluorouracil, and leucovorin in patients with metastatic colorectal cancer. *J Clin Oncol* 1996; **14:** 2950–8.

55. Lévi F, Zidani R, Brienza S et al, A multicenter evaluation of intensified ambulatory chronomodulated chemotherapy with oxaliplatin (L-OHP), 5-fluorouracil (5-FU), and leucovorin (LV) as initial treatment of patients with colorectal cancer. *Cancer* 1999; **85:** 2532–40.

56. Gérard B, Bleiberg H, Vandaele D et al, Oxaliplatin combined to 5-fluorouracil and folinic acid: an effective salvage therapy in patients with advanced colorectal cancer. *Anticancer Drugs* 1998; **9:** 301 5

57. de Gramont A, Gastiaburu J, Tournigand C et al, Oxaliplatin with high-dose folinic acid and 5-fluorouracil 48 h infusion in pretreated metastatic colorectal cancer. *Proc Am Soc Clin Oncol* 1994; **13:** 220.

58. André T, Bensmaine MA, Louvet C et al, Multicenter phase II study of bimonthly high-dose leucovorin, fluorouracil infusion, and oxaliplatin for metastatic colorectal cancer resistant to the same leucovorin and fluorouracil regimen. *J Clin Oncol* 1999; **17:** 3560–8.

59. Gilles-Amar V, Garcia ML, Sebille A et al, Evolution of severe sensory neuropathy with oxaliplatin combined to the bimonthly 48 h leucovorin and 5-fluorouracil regimens in metastatic colorectal cancer. *Proc Am Soc Clin Oncol* 1999; **18:** 246a (Abst 944).

60. Maindrault-Goebel F, De Gramont A, Louvet C et al, High-dose oxaliplatin with the simplified 48 h bimonthly leucovorin and 5-fluorouracil regimen in pretreated metastatic colorectal cancer. *Proc Am Soc Clin Oncol* 1999; **18:** 265a (Abstr 1017).

61. Bleiberg H, de Gramont A, Oxaliplatin plus 5-fluouracil: clinical experience in patients with advanced colorectal cancer. *Semin Oncol* 1998; **25**(2 Suppl 5): 32–49.

62. Brienza S, Bensmaine MA, Soulie P et al, Oxaliplatin added to 5-fluorouracil-based therapy (5-FU ± FA) in the treatment of 5-FU-pretreated patients with advanced colorectal carcinoma (ACRC): results from the European compassionate-use program. *Ann Oncol* 1999; **10:** 1311–16.

63. Giacchetti S, Itzhaki M, Gruia G et al, Long-term survival of patients with unresectable colorectal cancer liver metastases following infusional chemotherapy with 5-fluorouracil, leucovorin, oxaliplatin, and surgery. *Ann Oncol* 1999; **10:** 663–9.

64. Extra J-M, Marty M, Brienza S, Misset J-L, Pharmacokinetics and safety profiles of oxaliplatin. *Semin Oncol* 1998; **25**(2 Suppl 5): 13–22.

65. Fizazi K, Ducreux M, Ruffié P et al, Phase I, dose-finding and pharmacokinetic study of raltitrexed combined with oxaliplatin in patients with advanced cancer. *J Clin Oncol* 2000; **18:** 2293–300.

66. Douillard JY, Michel P, Gamelin E et al, Raltitrexed (Tomudex) plus oxaliplatin: an active combination for first-line chemotherapy in patients with metastatic colorectal cancer. *Proc Am Soc Clin Oncol* 2000; **19:** 250a (Abst 971).

67. Ford HER, Cunningham D, Ross PJ et al, Open label dose finding phase I study of irinotecan hydrochloride and raltitrexed in patients with advanced gastrointestinal tract adenocarcinoma. *Proc Am Soc Clin Oncol* 1999; **18:** 176a (Abst 678).

68. Benhammouda A, Bastian G, Rixe O, A phase I and pharmacokinetic study of CPT-11 and 5-FU in combination. *Proc Am Soc Clin Oncol* 1997; **16:** 202 (Abst 710).

69. Shimada Y, Topoisomerase I inhibitors: combination chemotherapy with CPT-11 in gastrointestinal cancers. In: *Proceedings of 2nd International Conference on Gastrointestinal Malignancies*, 1995: 18 (Abst 32).

70. Yamao T, Shimada Y, Shirao K, Phase I study of CPT-11 combined with sequential 5-FU in metastatic colorectal cancer. *Proc Am Soc Clin Oncol* 1996; **15**: 481 (Abst 1527).

71. Saltz L, Kanowitz J, Kemeny NE et al, Phase I clinical and pharmacokinetic study of irinotecan, fluorouracil, and leucovorin in patients with advanced solid tumors. *J Clin Oncol* 1996; **14**: 2959–67.

72. Comella P, Casaretti R, De Vita F et al, Concurrent irinotecan and 5-fluorouracil plus levo-folinic acid given every other week in the first-line management of advanced colorectal carcinoma: a phase I study of the Southern Italy Cooperative Oncology Group. *Ann Oncol* 1999; **10**: 915–21.

73. Sastre J, Paz-Ares L, Diaz-Rubio E et al, Phase I dose finding study of irinotecan (CPT-11) over a short iv infusion combined with a fixed dose of 5-fluorouracil (5-FU) over a protracted iv infusion in patients (pts) with advanced solid tumors. *Proc Am Soc Clin Oncol* 1998; **18**: 201a (Abst 775).

74. Aranda E, Carrato A, Cervantes A et al, Phase I/II study of escalating doses of weekly irinotecan (CPT-11) in combination with 5-fluorouracil (5-FU) (48 h continuous i.v. infusion) in patients with advanced solid tumors. *Proc Am Soc Clin Oncol* 1999; **18**: 277a (Abst 1064).

75. Garufi C, Dogliotti L, Pace R et al, A phase I study of CPT-11 plus chronomodulated (chrono) 5-fluorouracil (5-FU) and L-folinic acid (FA) in advanced colorectal cancer (ACC). *Proc Am Soc Clin Oncol* 1998; **17**: 291a (Abst 1120).

76. Vanhoefer U, Harstrick A, Kohne CH et al, Phase I study of a weekly schedule of irinotecan, high-dose leucovorin, and infusional fluorouracil as first-line chemotherapy in patients with advanced colorectal cancer. *J Clin Oncol* 1999; **17**: 907–13.

77. Ducreux M, Ychou M, Seitz JF et al, Irinotecan combined with bolus fluorouracil, continuous infusion fluorouracil, and high-dose leucovorin every two weeks (LV5FU2 regimen): a clinical dose-finding and pharmacokinetic study in patients with pretreated metastatic colorectal cancer. *J Clin Oncol* 1999; **17**: 2901–8.

78. Nobile MT, Gozza A, Simoni C et al, Combination phase II study of irinotecan (CPT-11) and raltitrexed (Tomudex) in advanced colorectal cancer. *Proc Am Soc Clin Oncol* 1999; **18**: 294a (Abst 1129).

79. André T, Louvet C, Maindrault-Goebel F et al, CPT-11 (irinotecan) addition to bimonthly, high-dose leucovorin and bolus and continuous-infusion 5-fluorouracil (FOLFIRI) for pretreated metastatic colorectal cancer. *Eur J Cancer* 1999; **35**: 1343–7.

80. Rothenberg ML, Pazdur R, Rowinsky EK et al, A phase II multicenter trial of alternating cycles of irinotecan and 5FU/LV in patients with previously untreated metastatic colorectal cancer. *Proc Am Soc Clin Oncol* 1997; **16**: 266a (Abst 944).

81. Barone C, Pozzo C, Starkhammar H et al, CPT-11 alternating with 5-FU/folinic acid: a multicentre phase II study in first line chemotherapy of metastatic colorectal cancer. *Proc Am Soc Clin Oncol* 1997; **16**: 270a (Abst 957).

82. Maiello E, Giuliani F, Gebbia V et al, Bi-monthly folinic acid and 5-fluorouracil bolus and continuous infusion alone or with irinotecan for advanced colorectal cancer: preliminary results of a phase II randomized trial of the Southern Italy Oncology Group. *Proc Am Soc Clin Oncol* 1999; **18**: 242a (Abst 929).

83. Kalbakis K, Kandylis N, Stavrakakis J et al, First line chemotherapy with 5-fluorouracil, leucovorin and irinotecan in advanced colorectal cancer: a multicenter phase II study. *Proc Am Soc Clin Oncol* 1999; **18**: 257a (Abst 989).

84. Durrani ASK, Benhammouda A, Gil-Delgado MA et al, Combination of irinotecan with leucovorin and 5-FU in advanced colorectal carcinoma. *Proc Am Soc Clin Oncol* 1999;

18: 282a (Abst 1083).

85. Van Cutsem E, Pozzo C, Stakhammar H et al, A phase II study of irinotecan alternated with five days bolus of 5-fluorouracil and leucovorin in first-line chemotherapy of metastatic colorectal cancer. *Ann Oncol* 1998; **9**: 1199–204.

86. Tournigand C, Louvet C, André T et al, FOLFIRI followed by FOLFOX or FOLFOX followed by FOLFIRI in metastatic colorectal cancer: Which is the best sequence? Safety and preliminary efficacy results of a randomized phase III study. *Proc Am Soc Clin Oncol* 2000; **19**: 245a (Abst 949).

87. Rothenberg ML, McKinney J, Hande KR et al, A phase I clinical and pharmacokinetic trial of oxaliplatin and irinotecan (CPT-11) given every two weeks to patients with refractory solid tumors. *Proc NCI-Am Assoc Cancer Res* 1999; **12** (Abst 948).

88. Wasserman E, Cuvier C, Lokiec F et al, Combination of oxaliplatin plus irinotecan in patients with gastrointestinal tumors: results of two independent phase I studies with pharmacokinetics. *J Clin Oncol* 1999; **17**: 1751–9.

89. Becouarn Y, Mousseau M, Gamelin E et al, Final results of CPT-11 and L-OHP combination as alternated combination of LV5FU2 + CPT-11/LV5FU2 + L-OHP in 5-FU resistant advanced colorectal cancer. *Proc Am Soc Clin Oncol* 2000; **19**: 245a (Abst 948).

90. Goldwasser F, Gross-Goupil M, Tigaud J-M et al, Dose escalation of CPT-11 in combination with oxaliplatin using an every two weeks schedule: A phase I study in advanced gastrointestinal cancer patients. *Ann Oncol* 2000; **11**: 1463–70.

91. Scheithauer W, Kornek GV, Raderer M et al, Combined irinotecan and oxaliplatin plus granulocyte colony-stimulating factor in patients with advanced fluoropyrimidine/leucovorin-pretreated colorectal cancer. *J Clin Oncol* 1999; **17**: 902–6.

92. Kemeny N, Tong W, Stockman J et al, Phase I trial of weekly oxaliplatin and irinotecan in previously treated patients with metastatic colorectal cancer. *Proc Am Soc Clin Oncol* 2000; **19**: 245a (Abst 948).

93. Wasserman E, Myara A, Lokiec F et al, Severe CPT-11 toxicity in patients with Gilbert's syndrome: two case reports. *Ann Oncol* 1997; **8**: 1049–51.

94. Lerebours F, Cottu P, Hocini H et al, Oxaliplatin, irinotecan, and 4-day continuous infusion 5-fluorouracil every three weeks: a phase I study in advanced gastrointestinal tumors. *Proc Am Soc Clin Oncol* 2000; **19**: 313a (Abst 1237).

95. Conroy T, Seitz JF, Capodano G et al, Phase I study of the triple combination of oxaliplatin + irinotecan + LV5FU2. *Proc Am Soc Clin Oncol* 2000; **19**: 236a (Abst 921G).

96. Schabel FM Jr, The use of tumor growth kinetics in planning 'curative' chemotherapy of advanced solid tumors. *Cancer Res* 1969; **29**: 2384–90.

97. Hryniuk WM, The importance of dose intensity in the outcome of chemotherapy. In: *Important Advances in Oncology* (De Vita VT, Holman S, Rosenberg SA, eds). JB Lippincott: Philadelphia, 1988: 121–42.

98. Abigerges D, Chabot GG, Armond JP et al, Phase I and pharmacologic studies of the camptothecin analog irinotecan administered every 3 weeks in cancer patients. *J Clin Oncol* 1995; **13**: 210–21.

99. Aschele C, Debernardis D, Casazza S et al, Immunohistochemical quantitation of thymidylate synthase expression in colorectal cancer metastases predicts for clinical outcome to fluorouracil-based chemotherapy. *J Clin Oncol* 1999; **17**: 1760–70.

100. Cascinu S, Aschele C, Barni S et al, Thymidylate synthase protein expression in advanced colon cancer: correlation with the site of metastasis and the clinical response to leucovorin-modulated bolus 5-fluorouracil. *Clin Cancer Res* 1999; **5**: 1996–9.

101. Ishikawa T, Sekiguchi F, Fukase Y et al, Positive correlation between the efficacy of capecitabine and doxifluridine and the ratio of thymidine phosphorylase to dihydropyrimidine dehydrogenase activities in tumors in human cancer xenografts. *Cancer Res* 1998; **58**: 685–90.

102. Ishikawa Y, Kubota T, Otani Y et al, Dihydropyrimidine dehydrogenase activity and messenger RNA level may be related to the antitumor effect of 5-fluorouracil on human tumor xenografts in nude mice. *Clin Cancer Res* 1999; **5**: 883–9.

103. Goh H-S, Yao J, Smith DR, p53 point mutation and survival in colorectal cancer patients. *Cancer Res* 1995; **55**: 5217–21.

104. Lenz H-J, Hayashi K, Salonga D et al, p53 point mutations and thymidylate synthase messenger RNA levels in disseminated colorectal cancer; an analysis of response and survival. *Clin Cancer Res* 1998; **4**: 1243–50.

105. Ahnen DJ, Feigl P, Quan G et al, Ki-ras mutation and p53 overexpression predict the clinical behavior of colorectal cancer: a Southwest Oncology Group Study. *Cancer Res* 1998; **58**: 1149–58.

53

Irinotecan: Combination chemotherapy

Hansjochen Wilke, Udo Vanhoefer, Wolf Achterrath

INTRODUCTION

During the past few decades, the overall prognosis of colorectal cancer has not essentially changed. It remains one of the major causes of cancer death in developed countries, and about 40–50% of patients will die of their disease, predominantly due to metastatic spread. Until the late 1980s, therapeutic options for patients with advanced colorectal cancer were almost exclusively based on fluoropyrimidines. Single-agent 5-fluorouracil (5-FU) predominantly administered as intravenous bolus injection was the standard of care for more than 30 years until it was replaced in the early 1990s by the combination of 5-FU plus folinic acid (FA, leucovorin), which demonstrated a greater antineoplastic activity than 5-FU alone.[1] With bolus 5-FU/FA administered either five times daily every 4 weeks (the Mayo regimen; see Chapter 41) or once-weekly × 6 (the Roswell Park regimen; see Chapter 42), an overall response rate of about 20% and median survival times of 12 months were achieved.[1] Further improvements in the systemic treatment of colorectal cancer occurred with the introduction of infusional 5-FU/FA regimens administered once-weekly as a 24- or 48-hour infusion or on a biweekly 48-hour infusional schedule. Compared with bolus 5-FU/FA, infusional 5-FU/FA induced higher response rates (30–40%), longer progression-free intervals/times to progression (6–7 months), and median survival times of up to 17 months.[2,3] In the past decade, a number of new compounds have been developed and introduced into the clinic that demonstrated activity in colorectal cancer; these include oxaliplatin, raltitrexed, oral 5-FU-prodrugs (capecitabine, UFT, and S1), and irinotecan.

IRINOTECAN: CLINICAL ACTIVITY

Irinotecan (CPT-11) is a semisynthetic derivative of the natural alkaloid camptothecin, and belongs to a new class of antineoplastic agents, called topoisomerase I interactive compounds.[4–7] Since its introduction into the clinic, irinotecan has undergone a comprehensive evaluation as a single agent and in combination chemotherapy in first-line as well as in second-line therapy of colorectal cancer.

Irinotecan was evaluated as first-line chemotherapy in Europe and in the USA in five non-randomized phase II studies with a total of 224 response-evaluable patients.[8–12] Mean overall response rates of 24% and 2% respectively have been achieved with the 'European' once-every-three-weeks schedule and the US weekly × 4 schedule. The median response duration ranged from 8 to 9 months and the median survival time was 12 months. Randomized trials comparing irinotecan with bolus 5-FU/FA showed that irinotecan was at least as effective as the generally accepted standard bolus 5-FU/FA.[13,14]

Clinically relevant activity was also shown in patients who had failed prior 5-FU/FA therapy. With the above-mentioned irinotecan schedules, an overall response rate of 13% (95% confidence interval (CI) 11.5–14.5%) and a tumour growth control rate (complete or partial response or no change) of 50% (95% CI 48–52%) were achieved in more than 1800 patients treated in 20 studies.[9,10,15–32] The median response duration ranged from 6 to 8 months and the median survival time from 7 to 13 months. The clinical benefit of second-line irinotecan as assumed from these data was confirmed by two randomized trials that compared irinotecan either with best supportive care or with the best estimated infusional 5-FU regimen in patients with resistance to conventional 5-FU regimens.[33,34] The encouraging single-agent activity of irinotecan led to broad investigation of irinotecan-containing combinations in colorectal cancer.

IRINOTECAN IN COMBINATION WITH OTHER CYTOTOXIC DRUGS

Phase I trials

Irinotecan in combination with fluoropyrimidines with or without FA[35–50]

In association with bolus 5-FU with or without FA, irinotecan was investigated in five different dose and time schedules.[36–38,40,44,45] The recommended doses being determined in the various phase I trials are listed in Table 53.1. The dose-limiting toxicities of these bolus 5-FU/FA plus irinotecan regimens were either neutropenia or a combination of neutropenia and diarrhoea.

These phase I studies suggested that irinotecan can be combined with various 5-FU regimens, and prompted the initiation of further phase I studies using irinotecan in combination with higher doses of 5-FU with or without FA, given by intravenous infusion over 24 or 48 hours[35,48,49] (Table 53.1). When all drugs were administered in a weekly × 6 schedule, the dose-limiting toxicity was diarrhoea for the 24-hour[49] and 48-hour[35] schedules of 5-FU/FA. With a biweekly schedule of irinotecan plus 5-FU/FA (the de Gramont schedule; see Chapter 44), the dose-limiting toxicities were neutropenia and diarrhoea.[39] With a once-every-3-weeks schedule of irinotecan in combination with FA-modulated 5-FU over 48 hours, the dose-limiting toxicity again consisted of a combination of neutropenia and diarrhoea.[40] In these trials with irinotecan and infusional 5-FU/FA, significant response rates were observed. Overall response rates of 69% and 48% respectively have been achieved in the first-line treatment of colorectal cancer with the combination of irinotecan and infusional 5-FU/FA given as the weekly × 6 24-hour schedule[39] and with the weekly combination of irinotecan and 5-FU as a 48-hour infusion.[35] In patients with 5-FU-pretreated colon cancer, response rates of 23% and 33% respectively have been reported for irinotecan in combination with 5-FU/FA (de Gramont schedule) and for irinotecan plus chronomodulated 5-FU/FA.[39,42]

Table 53.1 summarizes phase I trial results combining irinotecan with 5-FU given as continuous infusion over several days, with or without FA.[42,43,47]

Irinotecan plus raltitrexed

Irinotecan was combined with raltitrexed in three phase I studies in patients with solid tumours.[51–53] Asthenia was found as the dose-limiting toxicity in two studies with recommended doses of irinotecan 350 mg/m^2 and raltitrexed 3 mg/m^2 given once every 3 weeks and diarrhoea as dose-limiting toxicity in one study (recommended doses of irinotecan 210 mg/m^2 and raltitrexed 2.5 mg/m^2, given every 2 weeks).

Irinotecan plus oxaliplatin with or without 5-FU/FA

Six phase I studies were performed with the combination of irinotecan and oxaliplatin in patients with advanced gastrointestinal tumours.[54–59] A once-every-2-weeks schedule and a once-every-3-weeks schedule were investigated in three separate studies each. The dose-limiting toxicities were neutropenia for the 3-weekly schedules (recommended doses irinotecan 200 mg/m^2 and oxaliplatin 85 mg/m^2 or irinotecan 175 mg/m^2 and oxaliplatin 130 mg/m^2) and neutropenia and diarrhoea for the biweekly schedule (recommended doses irinotecan 85 mg/m^2 and oxaliplatin 175 mg/m^2). These combinations induced overall response rates of 29%, 38%, and 55% in patients with colorectal cancer and prior exposure to 5-FU.[54,56,59] The recommended doses for a weekly × 4 schedule of irinotecan and oxaliplatin on day 1 were 50 mg/m^2 and 60 mg/m^2 respectively (the dose-limiting toxicities were diarrhoea and neutropenia), with an overall response rate of 24% in 49 previously treated patients.[57] When irinotecan was combined with oxaliplatin and infusional 5-FU/FA, the recommended doses for the combination were 175 mg/m^2 of irinotecan and 100 mg/m^2 of oxaliplatin on day 1, followed by FA (200 mg/m^2) and 5-FU (3800 mg/m^2) as a 48-hour infusion every 2 weeks.[58]

Irinotecan plus UFT

Eighteen patients with pretreated colorectal cancer were accrued into a dose-finding trial with fixed doses of UFT (uracil plus ftorafur; 250 mg/m^2, days 1–21) and escalating doses of irinotecan (80–120 mg/m^2, day 1; recommended dose for phase II trials 120 mg/m^2).[60] Cycles were repeated every 4 weeks. There was a 66% rate of tumour stabilization, but no responses were observed. A Spanish trial conducted in 25 patients recommended irinotecan in a dose of 250 mg/m^2 on day 1 and UFT/FA orally on days 1–14 in doses of 300 mg/m^2 and 45 mg/m^2 respectively.[62]

Irinotecan plus capecitabine

One trial combined irinotecan weekly × 6

Table 53.1 Phase I studies of irinotecan with 5-fluorouracil (5-FU) with or without folinic acid (FA)

Refs	No. of evaluable patients	Schedule and recommended doses		Dose-limiting toxicity
Irinotecan and 5-FU short-time infusion				
44	27	Irinotecan:	125 mg/m^2 i.v. weekly for 4 weeks	Neutropenia
		FA:	20 mg/m^2 i.v. weekly for 4 weeks	
		5-FU:	500 mg/m^2 i.v. bolus for 4 weeks, q6wks	
38	31	Irinotecan:	200 mg/m^2 i.v. d1	Neutropenia
		FA:	250 mg/m^2 i.v. d2	Diarrhoea
		5-FU:	850 mg/m^2 i.v. bolus d2; q2wks	
36	36	Irinotecan:	300 mg/m^2 i.v. d1	Neutropenia
		5-FU:	375 mg/m^2 i.v. bolus d1–5; q4wks	
41	47	Irinotecan:	275 mg/m^2 i.v. d1	Neutropenia
		FA:	20 mg/m^2 i.v. d2–5	Diarrhoea
		5-FU:	400 mg/m^2 i.v. 90 min, d2–5; q4wks	
45	23	Irinotecan:	250 mg/m^2	Diarrhoea
		FA:	20 mg/m^2 i.v. d1–5; q4wks	Neutropenia
		5-FU:	425 mg/m^2 i.v. d1–5	
46	18	Irinotecan:	210 mg/m^2 i.v. d1; q2wks	Diarrhoea
		FA:	60 mg/m^2 i.v. d1 + 2	Neutropenia
		5-FU:	500 mg/m^2 i.v. d1 + 2	
Irinotecan with 5-FU 24 h or 48 h infusion				
48,49	47	Irinotecan:	80 mg/m^2 i.v. weekly for 6 weeks	Diarrhoea
		FA:	500 mg/m^2 i.v. weekly for 6 weeks	
		5-FU:	2600 mg/m^2 i.v. 24 h weekly for 6 weeks; q8wks	
39	55	Irinotecan:	180–200 mg/m^2 i.v. d1	Not reached
		FA:	200 mg/m^2 i.v. d1 + 2	
		5-FU:	400 mg/m^2 i.v. bolus, d1 + 2	
		5-FU:	600 mg/m^2 i.v. 22 h d1 + 2; q2wks	
50	83	Irinotecan:	400 mg/m^2 i.v. d1	Neutropenia
		FA:	250 mg/m^2 i.v. d1	Diarrhoea
		5-FU:	3500 mg/m^2 i.v. 48 h d1; q3wks	
35	41	Irinotecan:	80 mg/m^2 i.v., d1, weekly	Diarrhoea
		5-FU	3000 mg/m^2 48 h, d1; weekly	
Irinotecan and 5-FU protracted infusion				
43	42	Irinotecan:	350 mg/m^2 i.v. d1	Diarrhoea
		5-FU:	600 mg/m^2/d, d2–5 as protracted infusion	Neutropenia
42	26	Irinotecan:	350 mg/m^2 i.v. d1	Neutropenia
		FA:	150 mg/m^2/d as protracted infusion for 5 days	Diarrhoea
		5-FU:	700 mg/m^2/d as protracted infusion for 5 days	
47	31	Irinotecan:	300 mg/m^2 i.v. d1	Neutropenia
		5-FU:	250 mg/m^2/d as protracted infusion for 14 days	

(70–80 mg/m²) with capecitabine (1000–1250 mg/m², on days 1–14 and 22–35, twice daily). An overall response rate of 42% was achieved in 19 response-evaluable patients.

Irinotecan plus mitomycin

Irinotecan (150–200 mg/m², on days 1 and 8) and mitomycin 8–10 mg/m², on day 1) were administered every 4 weeks in 52 pretreated patients.[61] The recommended doses for irinotecan and mitomycin were 175 mg/m² and 10 mg/m² respectively. Five objective responses were observed.

Phase II trials

Irinotecan plus 5-FU/FA

Three phase II trials with irinotecan either 350 mg/m² on day 1 every 3 weeks or 100 mg/m² weekly for 4 weeks alternated with the Mayo regimen of 5-FU/FA were conducted as first-line chemotherapy in patients with advanced colorectal cancer.[64–66] In all trials, the overall response rate was about 30% and the median survival times were 16–18 months.

A response rate of 31% was reported with a weekly × 6 schedule of irinotecan (70 mg/m²) and bolus 5-FU (450 mg/m²) and FA (200 mg/m²),[67] and a weekly × 4 schedule of irinotecan plus bolus 5-FU/FA (the Saltz regimen) resulted in an overall response rate of 35% in 34 response-evaluable patients.[68]

Eight trials investigated irinotecan in association with infusional 5-FU/FA. Overall response rates of 26% and 75% were achieved with irinotecan plus 5-FU/FA according to the de Gramont schedule[69,70] and of 50% with a simplified de Gramont schedule.[71] A confirmed response rate of 72% was reported with a weekly × 6 schedule of irinotecan (80 mg/m²) and a 24-hour infusion of 5-FU (2000 mg/m²) plus FA (200 mg/m²)[72] and a rate of 48% with the Spanish schedule.[35] In three other small trials with infusional 5-FU/FA plus irinotecan, overall response rates of 24%, 45%, and 57% were achieved.[73–75]

Four randomized trials compared irinotecan/5-FU/FA-based regimens with 5-FU/FA administered according to the de Gramont, Mayo Clinic, or Saltz regimen as first-line chemotherapy for advanced disease.[76–79] In one trial, 102 patients received either the de Gramont regimen alone or the same 5-FU/FA schedule in combination with irinotecan. Responses were observed in 18% and 40% of evaluable patients respectively.[76] A three-arm trial used in addition to these regimens an alternating treatment with irinotecan and infusional 5-FU/FA, and confirmed the efficacy of the regimens stated above in terms of response rates.[77] One study enrolled 117 patients, and compared a weekly × 4 schedule of irinotecan at a dose of 125 mg/m² in combination with FA (20 mg/m²)/5-FU (500 mg/m²) (the Saltz regimen) with either 350 mg/m² of irinotecan alternating with 5-FU/FA (the Mayo regimen), or the Mayo regimen alone. The overall response rates were 47%, 39%, and 24% respectively.[78] In another randomized phase II trial, irinotecan/5-FU/FA (Saltz regimen) was compared with irinotecan/infusional 5-FU/FA (de Gramont regimen) and with irinotecan/5-FU/FA (Mayo regimen). The response rates were 44%, 39%, and 41% respectively.[79]

As salvage chemotherapy, the combination of irinotecan plus infusional 5-FU/FA (the modified or original de Gramont schedule) was investigated in two non-randomized phase II trials in patients with prior exposure to 5-FU/FA-based chemotherapies.[80,81] Depending on the previous chemotherapy regimens, a response rate of 6% was achieved in patients who had failed 5-FU/FA and 5-FU/FA/oxaliplatin (third-line chemotherapy) and a rate of 22% in less extensively pretreated patients. With the Saltz schedule of irinotecan and bolus 5-FU/FA, 6 out of 14 previously 5-FU-treated patients (43%) responded.[82]

Irinotecan plus oxaliplatin with or without 5-FU/FA

The combination of irinotecan plus oxaliplatin administered with granulocyte colony-stimulating factor (G-CSF) support induced encouraging objective response rates of 42% and 37% in 5-FU/FA-pretreated colorectal cancer patients in phase II trials.[83,84] A randomized trial comparing an alternating schedule of irinotecan/5-FU/FA and oxaliplatin/5-FU/FA (both of the de Gramont type) (arm A) with irinotecan/oxaliplatin (arm B) resulted in 16% and 28% objective response rates and median times to progression of 8 and 10 months in pretreated patients.[85] In a randomized phase II trial, 92 patients were allocated either to oxaliplatin/irinotecan or to raltitrexed alone, with response rates of 42% and 20% respectively.[86]

The combination of irinotecan/oxaliplatin plus two different schedules of infusional 5-FU/FA induced 57% objective responses in 30 response-evaluable patients who had progressed on other previous chemotherapies. However, three treatment-related deaths were observed.[87] Updated results of this trial using the doses recommended for phase II

Table 53.2 Randomized phase III trials with irinotecan, 5-fluorouracil (5-FU), and folinic acid (FA)

Refs	Regimen	No. of patients	Confirmed response rate (%)	p-value	Median time to progression (months)	p-value	Median survival (months)	p-value
77	Irinotecan/5-FU/FA	198	35	0.005	6.7	0.001	17.4	0.032
	5-FU/FA	187	21		4.4		14.1	
14, 78	Irinotecan/5-FU/FA	225	39	0.0001	7.0	0.004	14.8	0.042
	5-FU/FA	219	21		4.3		12.6	

trials reported a response rate of 69% and no treatment-related death.[88] In three other trials with this three-drug combination, response rates of 40%, 58%, and 67% were observed.[89–91] In 101 5-FU-refractory patients, three different combinations (irinotecan plus LV5FU2, oxaliplatin plus LV5FU2, and oxaliplatin/irinotecan) were compared.[92] The response rates were 12%, 23%, and 17%, and the median survival times 12 months, 11.5 months, and 11 months. No treatment-related death occurred.

Irinotecan plus raltitrexed

Three trials investigated irinotecan/raltitrexed in patients without prior chemotherapy for metastatic disease.[93–95] Irinotecan ($300–350 \, mg/m^2$) was combined with raltitrexed in doses of $2.6 \, mg/m^2$ or $3.0 \, mg/m^2$ once every 3 weeks. Overall response rates of 53% (16/30), 30% (7/23), and 40.6% (13/32) were observed in both trials – but so were significant toxicities requiring substantial dose reductions in two trials.[93,94]

Irinotecan plus mitomycin

In a randomized phase II trial, mitomycin was combined either with irinotecan or with oxaliplatin in a total of 64 response-evaluable patients failing 5-FU-based therapy.[96] The observed response rates were similar with both regimens (21% and 16%). The median time to disease progression appeared to be longer with irinotecan/mitomycin (7.0 months versus 5.2 months).

Irinotecan plus capecitabine

In a small phase II trial, 21 response-evaluable patients were treated with two different schedules of irinotecan plus capecitabine. An encouraging 71% of objective responses was achieved.[97]

Phase III trials

The promising results being achieved with 5-FU/FA/irinotecan combinations in the phase I and II evaluation programmes prompted the initiation of two large randomized international trials comparing the efficacy, toxicity, and quality of life for this combination with more frequently used 5-FU/FA-alone regimens as first-line chemotherapy in patients with metastatic colorectal cancer[14,98] (Table 53.2).

In the first trial, which was conducted in the USA, Canada, Australia and New Zealand, a weekly combination of irinotecan, FA, and 5-FU was chosen, based on the phase I trial reported by Saltz and co-workers.[14] The control arm with which this combination was compared was a conventional 5-FU/low-dose FA schedule (the Mayo Clinic regimen). A third arm consisted of single-agent irinotecan. Owing to the statistical design of this study, a statistical comparison with the other two study arms was not foreseen for the irinotecan-alone arm. The stratification criteria were performance status, age, time from diagnosis and prior adjuvant therapy (more than 12 months since completion of adjuvant 5-FU). The statistical analysis involved time to progression (TTP) as the main endpoint of the trial, as well as time to treatment failure (TTF), response rate, overall survival, safety, and quality of life as secondary study endpoints. The number of patients necessary for the statistical evaluation (220 patients per treatment arm) was based on the assumption that the 5-FU/FA/irinotecan treatment arm would be associated with a 40% improvement in TTP relative to the 5-FU/FA control arm. While the schedules of 5-FU administration differed, the trial was designed with the knowledge that the 5-FU dose intensity in the combination arm ($333 \, mg/m^2/week$) would be lower than the planned 531 mg/m^2/week in the control arm. This design helped to ensure that any incremental beneficial effects of the irinotecan/5-FU/FA regimen could be attributed definitively to irinotecan. From May 1996 until May 1998, a total of 683 patients were enrolled, with similar numbers of patients in each treatment group. These patients constituted the intent-to-treat population on which all efficacy analyses were performed. Accounting for patients who were never treated, or were treated on another treatment arm, the remaining 667 patients were analysed for drug administration, safety, and quality of life. The treatment arms were well balanced for gender, median age, median performance status, and prior adjuvant therapy, as well as for disease-related risk factors. Of note, only about 10% of patients had received prior adjuvant 5-FU treatment. Concerning the main endpoint of this study, the median TTP was statistically significantly longer with the combination than with 5-FU/FA alone (7.0 months versus 4.3 months; unstratified log-rank test, $p = 0.004$). This difference remained significant ($p = 0.002$) when a stratified log-rank test was applied. When adjusted for significant prognostic factors in a multivariate analysis, treatment with irinotecan/5-FU/FA remained a significant factor for survival, with a hazard ratio of 0.64 (95% CI 0.51–0.79). The median TTP with irinotecan alone was 4.2 months. The treatment with the irinotecan-containing combination was also associated with a statistically higher confirmed objective response rate (39% versus 21%; $p = 0.0001$) compared with 5-FU/FA alone, and with a statistically longer TTF. The objective response rate with irinotecan alone was 18%. Of note also, the median survival time with irinotecan/5-FU/FA was significantly longer than with 5-FU/FA alone (14.8 months versus 12.6 months; $p = 0.042$). When accounting for the impact of significant prognostic factors of baseline lactate dehydrogenase (LDH), performance status, white blood cell count, extent of organ involvement, and total bilirubin in a multiple regression analysis, irinotecan/5-FU/FA treatment was again significantly associated with improved survival, with a p-value of 0.037. The median survival with irinotecan alone was 12.0 months. Summarizing the efficacy data, irinotecan/5-FU/FA was statistically significantly superior to 5-FU/FA with respect to TTP, TTF, response rate, and survival. Single-agent irinotecan and the conventional 5-FU/FA regimen were similar in terms of response rates, median TTP, median TTF, and median overall survival. Grade 3 and 4 diarrhoea was seen in 23% of patients in the irinotecan/5-FU/FA arm and in 13% in the 5-FU/FA arm.

The highest incidence of severe diarrhoea (grade 3 and 4) was seen with irinotecan alone (31%). On the other hand, 5-FU/FA alone showed a significantly higher incidence of grade 4 neutropenia (42%) compared with either irinotecan/5-FU/FA (24%) or irinotecan alone (12%). Furthermore, neutropenic fever and mucositis were also seen more frequently in the 5-FU/FA arm. Quality of life was assessed during treatment using the EORTC QLQ C30. It could be demonstrated that treatment with irinotecan/5-FU/FA had no detrimental effect on overall quality of life and global health status compared with 5-FU/FA or irinotecan alone.

In the second multinational, multicentre randomized trial (Study V 303), conducted in Europe and South Africa, an infusional schedule of 5-FU was used.[98] This 5-FU/FA schedule was either the weekly 24-hour infusion of 5-FU in combination with high-dose FA (500 mg/m^2) (the modified AIO regimen) or the biweekly de Gramont bolus and infusional regimen. Participating centres had to choose one of the two schedules. Depending on the 5-FU/FA schedule, irinotecan was given in the experimental treatment arm either in a dose of 80 mg/m^2 weekly $\times$ 6 in association with the AIO schedule (5-FU 2300 mg/m^2 and FA 500 mg/m^2) or in a dose of 180 mg/m^2 every 2 weeks together with the de Gramont schedule. Except for the time since completion of adjuvant 5-FU treatment (over 6 months) and the fact that prior pelvic irradiation was permitted, the study entry criteria were the same as in the Saltz trial. The main endpoint of Study V 303 was response rate, with the assumption that the irinotecan/5-FU/FA combination would be associated with a 40% improvement in response rate, and it was estimated that at least 169 patients per study arm were required to meet the study objectives. Secondary endpoints were TTP, TTF, overall survival, safety, and quality of life. Altogether, 387 patients previously untreated with chemotherapy (other than adjuvant) for advanced colorectal cancer were accrued into this trial (188 in the 5-FU/FA-alone group and 199 in the irinotecan/5-FU/FA group) from May 1997 to February 1998. Two patients (one in each arm) received no study treatment because consent was withdrawn, and they were not included in the efficacy analysis. Approximately one-quarter of the patients were randomized to the AIO regimens and approximately three-quarters to the de Gramont regimens. There was a good balance for known risk factors, with the exception of a slight excess of rectal primaries in the combination arm. A higher proportion of patients than in the American trial had received prior adjuvant chemotherapy (25% versus 10% respectively). For the intention-to-treat population, the confirmed response rates were 35% for the combination and 21% for the 5-FU/FA-alone arm. This difference was statistically significant, with a *p*-value of less than 0.005. In the response-evaluable population, the response rate was 49% for the combination and 31% for 5-FU/FA ($p < 0.001$). The TTP results also showed a statistically highly significant difference in favour of the combination treatment (6.7 months versus 4.4 months; $p < 0.001$). When TTP was compared with a stratified log-rank test including the four stratification factors, the results were also statistically significant ($p = 0.002$). This remained so when adjusted by the Cox regression process for prognostic factors such as involved organ sites and baseline serum LDH. The hazard ratio indicates a 41% reduction in the risk of progression. A survival advantage for early combination therapy with irinotecan/5-FU/FA was confirmed in Study V 303. The median survival time with combination treatment was 17.4 months, versus 14.1 months among those patients randomized to only 5-FU/FA. When comparing this difference using the unstratified log-rank test, the result was statistically significant, with a *p*-value of 0.032. Again, when considering prognostic factors, irinotecan/5-FU/FA treatment was significantly associated with improved survival ($p = 0.045$). The response analysis by regimen showed overall response rates of 51% and 38% for the weekly × 6 and for the biweekly regimen using the combination of irinotecan and 5-FU/FA. The weekly and biweekly 5-FU/FA-alone regimens produced 29% and 21% overall response rates respectively. Concerning toxicities, a higher incidence of neutropenia grade 3 and 4 occurred with the combination (42% versus 11%, $p < 0.01$); however, this did not result in a significantly higher rate of neutropenic fever or infection. Severe diarrhoea (grade 3 and 4) was less frequent with 5-FU/FA alone (10%) compared with the combination treatment (22%). As in the US study, the addition of irinotecan to 5-FU/FA had no negative impact on overall health status and quality of life.

Based on the results of these two studies, it can be concluded that the addition of irinotecan to 5-FU/FA resulted in a significantly longer time to progression, progression-free survival, and – what is especially noteworthy – also in a significantly longer survival time and a significantly higher objective response rate without impairing quality of life. The combined analysis of these phase III trials confirmed that the combination of irinotecan with 5-FU/FA as first-line therapy is superior to 5-FU/FA alone (with improvements in time to progression ($p < 0.001$) and overall survival ($p < 0.009$)).[99] Therefore the combination of irinotecan with 5-FU/FA has to be considered as a new reference first-line treatment for patients with metastatic colorectal cancer.

CONCLUSIONS

The developments that have been made in the past few years clearly show that chemotherapy of advanced, metastatic colorectal cancer is a clinically meaningful approach as first-line therapy as well as salvage therapy. In that context, irinotecan in combination chemotherapy is an important step ahead in the management of colorectal cancer, and contributes to an improved prognosis for this disease.

REFERENCES

1. The Advanced Colorectal Cancer Meta-Analysis Project, Modulation of fluorouracil by leucovorin in patients with advanced colorectal cancer: evidence in terms of response. *J Clin Oncol* 1992; **10**: 896–903.
2. Köhne CH, Schöffski P, Wilke H et al, Effective biomodulation by leucovorin of high-dose infusion fluorouracil given as a weekly 24-hour infusion: results of a randomized trial in patients with advanced colorectal cancer. *J Clin Oncol* 1998, **16**: 418–26.
3. de Gramont A, Bosset JF, Milan C et al, Randomized trial comparing monthly low-dose leucovorin and fluorouracil bolus with bimonthly high-dose leucovorin and fluorouracil bolus plus continuous infusion for advanced colorectal cancer: a French intergroup study. *J Clin Oncol* 1997; **15**: 808–15.
4. Chen AY, Liu LF, DNA topoisomerases: essential enzymes and lethal targets. *Annu Rev Pharmacol Toxicol* 1994; **34**: 191–218.
5. Lavelle F, Bissery MC, André S et al, Preclinical evaluation of CPT-11 and its active metabolite SN-38. *Semin Oncol* 1996; **23**(Suppl 3): 11–20.
6. Pommier Y, Eukaryotic DNA topoisomerase I: genome gatekeeper and its intruders, camptothecins. *Semin Oncol* 1996; **23**(Suppl 3): 3–10.
7. Wisemann LR, Markham A, Irinotecan: a review of its pharmacological properties and clinical efficacy in the management of advanced colorectal cancer. *Drugs* 1996; **52**: 606–23.
8. Conti JA, Kemeny NE, Saltz LB et al, Irinotecan is an active agent in untreated patients with metastatic colorectal cancer. *J Clin Oncol* 1996; **14**: 709–15.
9. Pitot HC, Wender DB, O'Connell MJ et al, Phase II trial of irinotecan in patients with metastatic colorectal carcinoma. *J Clin Oncol* 1997; **8**: 2910–19.
10. Rougier P, Bugat R, Douillard JY et al, Phase II study of irinotecan in the treatment of advanced colorectal cancer in chemotherapy-naive patients and patients pretreated with fluorouracil-based chemotherapy. *J Clin Oncol* 1997; **15**: 251–60.
11. Irigoyen AL, Firvida JL, Vazquez S et al, Phase II trial of irinotecan (CPT-11) in patients with not pretreated advanced colorectal cancer. *Proc Am Soc Clin Oncol* 1998; **17**: 279a.
12. Ychou M, Kramar A, Raoul JL et al, Final results of a phase II study using CPT-11 high dose (500 mg/m²) as first line chemotherapy in patients with metastatic colorectal cancer (MCRC). *Proc Am Soc Clin Oncol* 2000; **19**: 966.
13. Pozzo C, Pyrhönen S, Bodrogi I et al, A randomized phase II

trial assessing irinotecan (IRI) and 5FU/folinic acid (LV), 'Mayo regimen', in first line palliative chemotherapy patients with metastatic colorectal cancer. *Eur J Cancer* 1999; **35**(suppl 4): S70.

14. Saltz LB, Cox JV, Blanke C et al, Irinotecan plus fluorouracil and leucovorin for metastatic colorectal cancer. *N Engl J Med* 2000; **343**: 905–14.

15. Van Cutsem E, Rougier P, Droz JP et al, Clinical benefit of irinotecan (CPT-11) in metastatic colorectal cancer resistant to 5-FU. *Proc Am Soc Clin Oncol* 1997; **16**: 268a.

16. Rothenberg ML, Hainsworth JD, Rosen L et al, Phase II study of irinotecan (CPT-11) 250 mg/m² given every-other-week in previously treated colorectal cancer patients. *Proc Am Soc Clin Oncol* 1998; **17**: 284a.

17. Van Cutsem E, Cunningham D, Ten Bokkel Huinink WW et al, Clinical activity and benefit of irinotecan (CPT-11) in patients with colorectal cancer truly resistant to 5-fluorouracil (5-FU). *Eur J Cancer* 1999; **35**: 54–9.

18. Tsavaris N, Polyzos A, Georgoulias V et al, Irinotecan (CPT-11) in patients with advanced colon carcinoma (ACC) relapsing after 5-fluorouracil (5-FU)–leucovorin (LV) combination. *Proc Am Soc Clin Oncol* 1998; **17**: 304a.

19. Anton A, Aranda E, Carrato A et al, Phase II study of irinotecan (CPT-11) in the treatment of patients with advanced colorectal cancer resistant to 5-fluorouracil (5-FU) based chemotherapy. The experience of TTD Spanish Cooperative Group. *Proc Am Soc Clin Oncol* 1998; **17**: 278a.

20. Frontini L, Labianca R, Sobrero A et al, Irinotecan (CPT-11) is effective as second-line chemotherapy in advanced colorectal cancer: a phase II trial of GISCAD (Italian Group for the Study of Gastrointestinal Cancer). *Proc Am Soc Clin Oncol* 1999; **18**: 260a.

21. Hoeffken K, Ridwelsky C, Wein A et al, Phase II study of irinotecan as second line chemotherapy in metastatic colorectal cancer. *Proc Am Soc Clin Oncol* 1999; **18**: 244a.

22. Santoro A, Santoro M, Maiorino L et al, Irinotecan (CPT-11) in patients with 5-FU refractory metastatic colorectal carcinoma. *Proc Am Soc Clin Oncol* 1999; **18**: 251a.

23. Vicent JM, Aparicio J, Lizon J et al, 5-FU-highly resistant advanced colorectal cancer patients treated with CPT-11. A phase II trial. *Proc Am Soc Clin Oncol* 1999; **18**: 303a.

24. Rothenberg ML, Eckardt JR, Kuhn JG et al, Phase II trial of irinotecan in patients with progressive or rapidly recurrent colorectal cancer. *J Clin Oncol* 1996; **14**: 1128–35.

25. Rothenberg ML, Cox JV, Russell F et al, A multicenter, phase II trial of weekly irinotecan (CPT-11) in patients with previously treated colorectal carcinoma. *Cancer* 1999; **85**: 786–95.

26. Van Cutsem E, Dirix L, Van Laethem J et al, A randomized phase II trial of three different regimens of irinotecan (CPT-11): a fixed dose of 350 mg/m², or an individual dose optimisation (B) or a risk factor optimisation in patients with metastatic colorectal cancer (MCRC) previously treated with 5-FU. *Proc Am Soc Clin Oncol* 2000; **19**: 946.

27. Huinink WT, Moiseyenko V, Glimelius B et al, A randomised phase II multicenter trial of irinotecan (CPT 11) using different schedules in patients (pts) with metastatic colorectal cancer (MCRC). *Proc Am Soc Clin Oncol* 2000; **19**: 951.

28. Navarro M, Losa F, Carcia-Alfonso P et al, Phase II trial of irinotecan (CPT-11) in patients with advanced colorectal cancer refractory to one previous adjuvant 5-FU schedule. *Proc Am Soc Clin Oncol* 2000; **19**: 1135.

29. Schöffski P, Vanhöfer U, Kirchner G et al, Phase II study of irinotecan as second line chemotherapy in metastatic colorectal cancer after prior exposure to infusional 5-FU-based chemotherapy. *Proc Am Soc Clin Oncol* 1151; **19**: 1151.

30. Sasaki K, Takasaka H, Hirata K et al, Weekly low dose irinotecan for advanced colorectal cancer on an outpatient treatment basis. *Proc Am Soc Clin Oncol* 2000; **19**: 1245.

31. Adenis A, Douillard J, Lacroix H et al, Randomized phase II–III trial of oxaliplatin (OXA) with 5-fluorouracil (5FU) continuous infusion (CI) versus a control arm with either 5FU or irinotecan (CPT 11) in previously treated metastatic colorectal cancer (MCRC) patients (pts). *Proc Am Soc Clin Oncol* 2000; **19**: 1088.

32. Michael M, Moore MJ, Hedley D et al, A phase II study of irinotecan (CPT-11) as palliative therapy in refractory advanced colorectal cancer. *Proc Am Soc Clin Oncol* 1999; **18**: 243a.

33. Cunningham D, Pyrhönen S, James RD et al, Randomised trial of irinotecan plus supportive care versus supportive care alone after fluorouracil failure for patients with metastatic colorectal cancer. *Lancet* 1998; **352**: 1413–18.

34. Rougier P, Van Cutsem E, Bajetta E et al, Randomised trial of irinotecan versus fluorouracil by continuous infusion after fluorouracil failure in patients with metastatic colorectal cancer. *Lancet* 1998; **352**: 1407–12.

35. Aranda E, Carrato A, Cervantes A et al, Irinotecan (CPT-11) in combination with high-dose infusional 5-FU (Ttd schedule) in advanced colorectal cancer (Crc): preliminary results of a phase I/II. *Proc Am Soc Clin Oncol* 2000; **19**: 1280A.

36. Benhammouda A, Bastian G, Rixe O et al, A phase I and pharmacokinetic study of CPT-11 and 5-FU in combination. *Proc Am Soc Clin Oncol* 1997; **16**: 202a.

37. VanEcho DA, Levy S, Phase II study of a weekly schedule of irinotecan (C), high dose leucovorin (LV), and infusional fluorouracil (FU) in patients with advanced colorectal cancer (CRC): preliminary report. *Proc Am Soc Clin Oncol* 2000; **19**: 1199.

38. Comella P, Casaretti R, De Vita F et al, Concurrent irinotecan and 5-fluorouracil plus levo-folinic acid given every other week in the first-line management of advanced colorectal carcinoma: a phase I study of the Southern Italy Cooperative Oncology Group. *Ann Oncol* 1999; **10**: 915–21.

39. Ducreux M, Ychou M, Seitz JF et al, Irinotecan combined with bolus fluorouracil, continuous infusion fluorouracil, and high-dose leucovorin every two weeks (LV5FU2 regimen): a clinical dose-finding and pharmacokinetic study in patients with pretreated metastatic colorectal cancer. *J Clin Oncol* 1999; **17**: 2901–8.

40. Falcone A, Danesi R, Allegrini G et al, Escalating dose irinotecan (CPT-11) immediately prior or after 5-fluorouracil (5-FU) 48 hours infusion + leucovorin (LV): pharmacokinetic and pharmacodynamic interactions in chemotherapy-naïve metastatic colorectal cancer patients. *Proc Am Soc Clin Oncol* 1999; **18**: 241a.

41. Fonseca R, Goldberg RM, Erlichman C et al, Phase I study of the combination of CPT-11/5-FU and leucovorin (LV). *Proc Am Soc Clin Oncol* 1998; **17**: 203a.

42. Garufi C, Dogliotti L, D'Attino RM et al, Irinotecan and chronomodulated infusion of 5-fluorouracil folinic acid in the treatment of patients with advanced colorectal cancer: A phase 1 study. *Cancer* 2001; **91**: 712–20.

43. Kakolyris S, Souglakos J, Kouroussis C et al, A dose finding study of irinotecan (CPT-II) plus a four-day continuous 5-fluorouracil infusion in advanced colon cancer. *Oncology* 2001; **60**: 201–13.

44. Saltz LB, Kanowitz J, Kemeny NE et al, Phase I clinical and pharmacokinetic study of irinotecan, fluorouracil, and leucovorin in patients with advanced solid tumors. *J Clin Oncol* 1996; **14**: 2959–67.

45. Kuehr T, Ruff P, Boussard B et al, CPT-11 and 5-fluorouracil (5-FU/FA) Mayo Clinic regimen in advanced colorectal cancer (ACRC) as front line therapy – a phase I/II study. *Proc Am Soc Clin Oncol* 2001; **20**: 2221.

46. Ristamaki R, Glimelius B, Linne T et al, A phase I/II study of CPT-11 combined with 5-fluorouracil (5FU)/folinic acid (FA) as Nordic schedule as first line therapy in patients with metastatic colorectal cancer (MRCR). *Ann Oncol* 2000; **11**(Suppl 4): 47 (Abst 201).

47. Sastre H, Paz-Ares L, Diaz-Rubio E et al, Phase I dose finding study of irinotecan (CPT-11) over a short IV infusion combined with a fixed dose of 5-fluorouracil (5-FU) over a protracted IV infusion in patients with advanced solid tumors. *Proc Am Soc Clin Oncol* 1998; **17**: 201a.

48. Vanhoefer U, Harstrick A, Köhne CH et al, Phase I study of a weekly schedule of irinotecan, high-dose leucovorin, and infusional fluorouracil as first-line chemotherapy in patients with advanced colorectal cancer. *J Clin Oncol* 1999; **17**: 907–13.

49. Vanhoefer U, Harstrick A, Achterrath W et al, Extended phase I study of a weekly schedule of irinotecan (CPT-11), leucovorin and infusional 5-FU as first-line chemotherapy in metastatic colorectal cancer. *Clin Cancer Res* 1999; **5**(Suppl): 3799s.

50. Falcone A, Allegrini G, Masi G et al, Irinotecan in combination with leucovorin and 5-fluorouracil 48 hours continuous infusion: a phase I study with pharmacokinetic, DNA damage and topoisomerase I/DNA complexes evaluation in chemotherapy naïve metastatic colorectal cancer patients. *Proc Am Soc Clin Oncol* 1998; **17**: 290a.

51. Ford HER, Cunningham D, Ross PJ et al, Open label dose finding phase I study of irinotecan hydrochloride and raltitrexed in patients with advanced gastrointestinal tract adenocarcinoma. *Proc Am Soc Clin Oncol* 1999; **18**: 176a.

52. Sun W, Stevenson JP, Gallagher M et al, Phase I and pharmacokinetic trial of irinotecan (CPT-11) and Tomudex administered as sequential IV infusions, D1 and D2, repeated every 21 days. *Clin Cancer Res* 1999; **5**(Suppl): 3799s.

53. Colucci G, Giuliani F, Giotta F et al, Irinotecan (CPT-11) and raltitrexed (Tomudex) combination therapy in the treatment of advanced colorectal cancer (ACC): a phase I/II study. *Proc Am Soc Clin Oncol* 2001; **20**: 146a (Abst 580).

54. Goldwasser F, Gross-Goupil M, Tigaud JM et al, Dose escalation of CPT-11 in combination with oxaliplatin using an every two weeks' schedule: a phase 1 study in advanced gastrointestinal cancer patients. *Ann Oncol* 2000; **11**: 1463–70.

55. Rothenberg ML, McKinney J, Hande KR et al, A phase I clinical and pharmacokinetic trial of oxaliplatin and irinotecan (CPT-11) given every two weeks to patients with refractory solid tumors. *Clin Cancer Res* 1999; **5**(Suppl): 3853s.

56. Wasserman E, Cuvier E, Lokiec F et al, Combination of oxaliplatin plus irinotecan in patients with gastrointestinal tumors: results of two independent phase I studies with pharmacokinetics. *J Clin Oncol* 1999; **17**: 1751–9.

57. Kemeny N, Tong W, Dilauro J et al, Phase I/II trial of weekly oxaliplatin (Oxa) and irinotecan (CPT-11) in previously treated patients with metastatic colorectal cancer. *Proc Am Soc Clin Oncol* 2001; **20**: 133a (Abst 529).

58. Falcone A, Masi G, Pfanner E et al, Phase I–II study of irinotecan (CPT-11), oxaliplatin (LOHP), leucovorin (LV) and 5-fluorouracil (5-FU) 46 hours continuous infusion (C.I.) in metastatic colorectal cancer patients. *Proc Am Soc Clin Oncol* 2000; **19**: 1161.

59. Hoff PM, Aguayo-Gonzales A, Boggard K et al, Phase I trial of oxaliplatin and CPT-11 administered once every three weeks to patients with metastatic colorectal cancer (MCC). *Proc Am Soc Clin Oncol* 2001; **20**: 137a (Abst 543).

60. Escudero P, Vicente A, Herrero A et al, Phase I–II trial of irinotecan (CPT-11) over a short IV weekly infusion combined with a fixed dose of UFT in second line advanced colorectal carcinoma (ACRC). *Proc Am Soc Clin Oncol* 2000; **19**: 1136.

61. Comella P, Biglietto M, Casaretti R et al, Irinotecan and mitomycin C in 5-fluorouracil-refractory colorectal cancer patients. A phase I/II study of the Southern Italy Cooperative Oncology Group. *Oncology* 2001; **60**: 127–33.

62. Castellano D, Gravalos P, Garcia-Alfonso B et al, Phase I/II study of escalating doses of irinotecan (CPT-11) in combination with UFT/folinic acid (FA) in patients (pts) with advanced col-

63. Schleucher N, Tewes M, Achterrath W et al, Extended phase I study of capecitabine in combination with a weekly schedule of irinotecan as first-line chemotherapy in metastatic colorectal cancer. *Proc Am Soc Clin Oncol* 2001; **20**: 141a (Abst 561).

64. Rothenberg ML, Pazdur R, Rowinsky EK et al, A phase II multicenter trial of alternating cycles of irinotecan (CPT-11) and 5-FU/LV in patients with previously untreated metastatic colorectal cancer. *Proc Am Soc Clin Oncol* 1997; **18**: 266a.

65. Van Cutsem E, Pozzo C, Starkhammar H et al, A phase II study of irinotecan alternated with five days bolus of 5-fluorouracil and leucovorin in first-line chemotherapy of metastatic colorectal cancer. *Ann Oncol* 1998; **9**: 1199–204.

66. Salvador J, Moreno-Nogueira JA, Reina J et al, Irinotecan (CPT-11) alternated with Mayo Clinic regimen as treatment of first-line metastatic colorectal cancer (CRC). *Proc Am Soc Clin Oncol* 2000; **19**: 1247.

67. Kalofonos HP, Papakostas P, Christodoulou C et al, A phase II trial with CPT-11, folinic acid (LV) and 5-fluorouracil (FU) in patients with metastatic colorectal carcinoma. *Proc Am Soc Clin Oncol* 2000; **19**: 1091.

68. Munoz A, Rivera F, Giron CG et al, Multi-institutional confirmatory study of weekly irinotecan (CPT-11), leucovorin (LV) and 5-fluorouracil (5-FU in previously untreated advanced colorectal cancer (CRC) patients (Pts) in clinical setting. *Proc Am Soc Clin Oncol* 2001; **20**: 111b (Abst 2196).

69. Kalbakis K, Kandylis N, Stavrakakis J et al, First line chemotherapy with 5-fluorouracil (5-FU), leucovorin (LV) and irinotecan (CPT-11) in advanced colorectal cancer: a multicenter phase II study. *Proc Am Soc Clin Oncol* 1991; **18**: 257a.

70. Ramos M, Romero C, Amenedo M et al, A phase II study of irinotecan (CPT-11) and 5-fluorouracil/folinic acid (5-FU/FA) ('de Gramont') in advanced colorectal cancer (CRC). *Proc Am Soc Clin Oncol* 2001; **10**: 108b (Abst 2183).

71. Ducreux M, Marti P, Raoul J et al, Phase II study of high-dose irinotecan (CPT-11) combined with 5-fluorouracil/folinic acid (LV5FU2) in 1st line metastatic colorectal cancer (MCRC). *Proc Am Soc Clin Oncol* 2001; **20**: 115b (Abst 2210).

72. Lipp R, Hegewichs-Becker S, Göthert J et al, Decrease of severe toxicities by reducing the 5-FU-dosage in the combination therapy with CPT-11/5-FU/FA weekly in patients with advanced colorectal cancer. *Onkologie* 1999; **22**(Suppl 1): 84.

73. Yoshioka T, Ohtsu A, Hyodo I et al, Phase II study of a combination of irinotecan and 5-day infusional 5-fluorouracil in patients with metastatic colorectal cancer. A Japanese Clinical Oncology Group (JCOG) Study 9703. *Proc Am Soc Clin Oncol* 2000; **19**: 1142.

74. Vazquez S, Mel J, Sabin P et al, Irinotecan (CPT-11) in combination with 5-fluorouracil/folinic acid (5-FU/FA) as a weekly schedule in previously untreated patients with metastatic colorectal cancer (MCRC). *Proc Am Soc Clin Oncol* 2000; **19**: 1249.

75. Bernabe Caro R, Salvador J, Reina J et al, Biweekly schedule of irinotecan (CPT-11) and 5-fluorouracil (5-FU) as first line treatment in advanced colorectal cancer (CRC). *Proc Am Soc Clin Oncol* 2001; **20**: 109b (Abst 2187).

76. Graeven U, Ridwelski K, Manns M et al, Irinotecan (CPT-11) with bolus 5-fluorouracil (5-FU) and folinic acid (FA) in patients with previously untreated metastatic colorectal cancer: an active and safe regimen. *Proc Am Soc Clin Oncol* 2000; **19**: 952.

77. Labianca R, Martoni A, Galligioni E et al, CPT-11 alternated with leucovorin + 5-fluorouracil (LV5FU2) regimen in advanced colorectal cancer (ACC): a multicenter randomized phase II trial. *Proc Am Soc Clin Oncol* 2001; **20**: 135a (Abst 535).

78. Maiello E, Gebbia V, Giuliani F et al, 5-Fluorouracil and folinic acid with or without CPT-11 in advanced colorectal cancer patients: a multicenter randomized phase II study of the

Southern Italy Oncology Group. *Ann Oncol* 2000; **11:** 1045–51.

79. Ben Ayed F, Khalfallah S, Tujakowski J et al, CPT-11 combined or alternated with 5-fluorouracil/folinic acid (5-FU/FA) in advanced colorectal cancer (CRC). *Proc Am Soc Clin Oncol* 2001; **20:** 135a (Abst 536).

80. André T, Léuvet C, Maindrault-Goebel F et al, CPT-11 (irinotecan) addition to bimonthly, high-dose leucovorin and bolus and continuous-infusion 5-fluorouracil (FOLFIRI) for pretreated metastatic colorectal cancer. *Eur J Cancer* 1999; **35:** 1343–7.

81. Gil Delgado MA, Guinet F, Castaing D et al, Prospective phase II trial of irinotecan, 5-fluorouracil, and leucovorin in combination as salvage therapy for advanced colorectal cancer. *Am J Clin Oncol* 2001; **24:** 101–5.

82. Salgado M, Firvida J, Mata J et al, A phase II study of weekly irinotecan (CPT-11) combined with folinic acid and 5-FU in pretreated advanced colorectal cancer (CRC) patients. *Proc Am Soc Clin Oncol* 2000; **19:** 1157.

83. Scheithauer W, Kornek GV, Raderer M et al, Combined irinotecan and oxaliplatin plus granulocyte colony-stimulating factor in patients with advanced fluoropyrimidine/leucovorin-pretreated colorectal cancer. *J Clin Oncol* 1999; **17:** 902–6.

84. Kretzschmar A, Thuss-Patience PC, Grothey A et al, Weekly combination of oxaliplatin (Ox) and irinotecan (Iri) in 5-FU resistant metastatic colorectal cancer (CRC). *Proc Am Soc Clin Oncol* 2001; **20:** 136a (Abst 540).

85. Yves B, Mousseau M, Gamelin E et al, Final results of CPT-11 and L-OHP combination versus alternated combination of LV5FU2 + CPT/11/LV5FU2 + LOHP in 5FU resistant advanced colorectal cancer (ACRC). *Proc Am Soc Clin Oncol* 2000; **19:** 978.

86. Scheithauer W, Kornek GV, Ulrich-Pur H et al, Irinotecan (CPT-11) plus oxaliplatin (L-OHP) in advanced colorectal cancer (ACC): a randomized phase II study. *Proc Am Soc Clin Oncol* 2001; **20:** 135a (Abst 538).

87. Calvo E, Gonzales-Cao M, Cortes J et al, Combined irinotecan, oxaliplatin, 5-FU in patients with metastatic colorectal cancer (MCC). *Proc Am Soc Clin Oncol* 2000; **19:** 1008.

88. Calvo E, Cortes J, Rodriguez J et al, Irinotecan, oxaliplatin plus 5-FU/leucovorin in advanced colorectal cancer. *Proc Am Soc Clin Oncol* 2001; **20:** 136a (Abst 542).

89. Souglakos J, Kakolyris S, Athanasiadis C et al, Irinotecan (CPT-11) plus oxaliplatin (LOHP) plus infusional 5-fluorouracil (5-FU) and leucovorin (LV) as first line treatment for metastic colorectal cancer (MCC): a phase II trial. *Proc Am Soc Clin Oncol* 2001; **20:** 118b (Abst 2223).

90. Gil-Delgado M, Bastian G, Guinet F et al, Final results of oxaliplatin (LOHP) + irinotecan (CPT-11) and FU-FOL (LV5FU2) combination and pharmacokinetic (PK) analysis in advanced colorectal cancer (ACRC) patients (pts). *Proc Am Soc Clin Oncol* 2001; **20:** 140a (Abst 558).

91. Masi G, Allegrini G, Lencioni M et al, Irinotecan (CPT-11), oxaliplatin (LOHP), leucovorin (LV) and 5-fluorouracil (5-FU) 48 hrs continuous infusion every two weeks in metastatic colorectal cancer patients (pts). *Proc Am Soc Clin Oncol* 2001; **20:** 136a (Abst 539).

92. Rougier P, Lepille D, Doullard J et al, Final results of a randomized phase II study of three combinations CPT-11 + LV5FU2, L-OHP + LV5FU2, and CPT-11 + L-OHP in 5-FU resistant advanced colorectal cancer (ACRC). *Proc Am Soc Clin Oncol* 2001; **20:** 142a (Abst 566).

93. Carnaghi C, Zucali P, Rimassa L et al, Promising activity of irinotecan (CPT 11) and raltitrexed (ZD 1694) as first line chemotherapy in metastatic colorectal cancer (MCC). *Proc Am Soc Clin Oncol* 2000; **19:** 1211.

94. Nobile M, Gozza A, Heouaine A et al, Irinotecan (CPT 11) and raltitrexed (Tomudex) in advanced colorectal cancer: a phase II study. *Proc Am Soc Clin Oncol* 2000; **19:** 1220.

95. Escudero P, Espinosa J, Milla A et al, An ongoing phase II study of raltitrexed (Tomudex) plus irinotecan in advanced colorectal cancer. *Proc Am Soc Clin Oncol* 2001; **20:** 120b (Abst 2230).

96. Scheithauer W, Kornek GV, Brugger S et al, Randomized phase II study of irinotecan plus mitomycin (MMC) versus oxaliplatin plus MMC in patients with advanced fluoropyrimidine/leucovorin-pretreated colorectal cancer (ACC). *Onkologie* 1999; **22**(Suppl 1): 78.

97. Cassata A, Stani SC, Alu M et al, Ongoing phase II trial with two schedules of irinotecan (CPT-11) in combination with capecitabine as first line chemotherapy in patients with advanced colorectal cancer. *Proc Am Soc Clin Oncol* 2001; **20:** 144a (Abst 573).

98. Douillard JY, Cunningham D, Roth AD et al, Irinotecan combined with fluorouracil compared with fluorouracil alone as first-line treatment for metastatic colorectal cancer: a multicentre randomised trial. *Lancet* 2000; **355:** 1041–7.

99. Saltz LB, Douillard J, Pirotta N et al, Combined analysis of two randomized trials comparing irinotecan (C), fluorouracil (F), leucovorin (L) vs F alone as first-line therapy of previously untreated metastatic colorectal cancer (MCRC). *Proc Am Soc Clin Oncol* 2000; **19:** 938.

54

Bimonthly leucovorin–5-fluorouracil with oxaliplatin or irinotecan: The FOLFOX and FOLFIRI regimens

Aimery de Gramont, Christophe Louvet, Thierry André, Christophe Tournigand, Frédérique Maindrault-Goebel, Pascal Artru, Marcel Krulik, for the GERCOR (Oncology Multidisciplinary Research Group)

INTRODUCTION

Oxaliplatin is a novel platinum derivative and the first platinum compound to demonstrate significant efficacy in the treatment of advanced colorectal cancer (see also Chapter 50). In vitro and in vivo preclinical studies on colorectal cancer have shown that oxaliplatin is active against colorectal cell lines and is synergistic with 5-fluorouracil (5-FU).[1] Furthermore, phase II trials of oxaliplatin monotherapy in previously treated or untreated patients with colorectal cancer have shown response rates of between 10% and 24%, with acceptable toxicity.[2–4] Oxaliplatin has also been used in combination with leucovorin (LV; folinic acid) and 5-FU continuous infusion. The first studies concerned a 5-day chronomodulated regimen.[5] Irinotecan (CPT-11) is a semisynthetic camptothecin analogue that has activity against advanced colorectal cancer cells[6] – see also Chapter 49. Phase II trials have demonstrated that this agent is effective in patients whose disease has progressed on 5-FU-based therapy.[7–9] The efficacy and low toxicity of the bimonthly LV/5-FU regimens[10–13] allowed combination with the other active antitumour drugs in colorectal cancer therapy. FOLFOX (**fol**inic acid, 5-**FU**, **oxa**liplatin) and FOLFIRI (**fol**inic acid, 5-**FU**, **iri**notecan) refer to a series of trials combining bimonthly 48-hour LV/5-FU regimens with oxaliplatin or irinotecan at different doses.[14]

OXALIPLATIN

First-line therapy

The first studies of combined therapy with oxaliplatin and LV/5-FU involved a chronomodulated regimen administered to 93 patients with metastatic colorectal cancer, of whom 49% had received previous treatment with radiotherapy or chemotherapy[5] – see also Chapter 55. High-dose 5-FU ($700 \, \mathrm{mg/m^2/day}$) plus LV ($300 \, \mathrm{mg/m^2/day}$) and oxaliplatin ($25 \, \mathrm{mg/m^2/day}$) were administered by continuous infusion for 5 days, and the cycle was repeated every 3 weeks. Objective responses were observed in 58% of patients, and the median and progression-free survival times were 10 months and 15 months respectively and were independent of treatment history. These encouraging results led to further investigation of the role of oxaliplatin in 5-FU-based regimens. A randomized phase III study of the same chronomodulated regimen for first-line treatment produced a significantly higher response rate compared with flat administration of the drugs (49.5% versus 30% respectively).[15] However, the interaction between 5-FU and oxaliplatin has subsequently been shown to be independent of any chronomodulated schedule.[16]

The benefit of adding oxaliplatin to LV/5-FU in the first-line therapy of patients with metastatic colorectal cancer has been demonstrated in two large international, multicentre, randomized phase III trials.[17,18] The first study involved 200 patients who received a chronomodulated LV/5-FU regimen, with or without oxaliplatin, 125 mg/m^2, as a 6-hour infusion.[17] Objective tumour responses were observed in 53% of patients in the combination arm, compared with only 16% of patients receiving LV/5-FU alone ($p < 0.0001$). After a median follow-up period of 47 months, the median progression-free survival was significantly greater in the oxaliplatin group compared with the controls (8.7 months versus 6.1 months respectively, $p = 0.048$). However, overall survival rates were similar in both groups (19.9 months and 19.4 months respectively). Nonetheless, combination therapy allowed more patients to undergo potentially curative surgery of metastases than in those receiving LV/F-FU alone (32% versus 21% respectively).

In the second randomized study, the role of oxaliplatin in combination with 2-day administration of high-dose LV plus 5-FU bolus and low-dose infusional 5-FU (LV5FU2; see Chapter 44) in the first-line therapy of advanced colorectal cancer was evaluated in 420 patients.[18] Subjects received LV5FU2 with or without oxaliplatin (85 mg/m^2, administered as a 2-hour infusion), and were followed up for a median period of 28 months. Objective tumour responses were achieved in 51% of patients receiving the combination, compared with 22% of those allocated to LV5FU2 alone ($p = 0.0001$). Progression-free survival was significantly improved in the oxaliplatin group compared with the control group (9.0 months versus 6.2 months respectively, $p = 0.0001$). The 1-year survival rates were 69% in the oxaliplatin group and 59% for the controls, although this difference was not significant. However, metastectomy was possible in twice as many subjects receiving oxaliplatin as among those receiving LV5FU2 alone (6.7% versus 3.3% respectively).

In both of these large studies, the addition of oxaliplatin to LV/5-FU regimens was associated with significant differences in tumour response rates and progression-free survival. Although a survival benefit was not demonstrated in these studies, this cannot be ruled out on the basis of these results alone. It is possible that a survival benefit was obscured owing to the crossover from the control group to the oxaliplatin arm that occurred in both trials. In the first of these studies, 57% of patients allocated to the LV/5-FU control arm received oxaliplatin as second-line therapy, and therefore comparison of the overall survival rates in the two treatment arms may be misleading. Importantly, multivariate analysis of the second randomized study showed that oxaliplatin was a strong independent predictor of overall survival.[18]

Second-line therapy

The efficacy of various doses of oxaliplatin in combination with 48-hour bimonthly regimens of LV/5-FU has also been evaluated as second-line therapy among patients whose tumours were resistant to LV/5-FU. Various doses and schedules of administration have been evaluated, with the aim of defining the regimen that provides optimal efficacy with minimal toxicity.

A feasibility study (FOLFOX 1) used the bimonthly intermediate LV/5-FU regimen, FOLFUHD (**fol**inic acid, 5-**FU h**igh **d**ose; see Chapter 44), with oxaliplatin (130 mg/m^2) added at every other treatment cycle (Figure 54.1).[19] A response rate of 31% was observed in 13 patients who received the FOLFOX 1 regimen, with median and progression-free survival times of 6 and 11 months, respectively (Table 54.1). The low level of toxicity associated with the FOLFOX 1 regimen led to the design of FOLFOX 2, in which the total dose of oxaliplatin was increased to 100 mg/m^2, administered at every treatment cycle to 46 patients.[20] The dose of 5-FU was 1500 mg/m^2/day for the first two treatment cycles, and this was increased to 2000 mg/m^2/day in subsequent cycles if the maximal toxicity remained below WHO grade 2. Major limiting toxicities were neutropenia and peripheral neuropathy. Grade 3–4 neutropenia occurred in 18 patients (39%), although in all but 4 patients (9%) a reduction in the dose of 5-FU produced reversal of this adverse effect. In addition, grade 2–3 peripheral neuropathy was observed in 15 patients (33%), of whom 3 were able to resume oxaliplatin therapy after recovery.

In terms of efficacy, the FOLFOX 2 regimen produced a high response rate of 46%, with median and progression-free survival times of 7 months and 17 months respectively. The high response rate observed in this study among patients whose disease was already refractory to LV/5-FU was attributed to an effective synergy between the FOLFUHD regimen and oxaliplatin. The positive outcome of FOLFOX 2 prompted further trials in which the dose of the 5-FU infusion was reduced to 1500 mg/m^2/day, and that of oxaliplatin to 85 mg/m^2 (FOLFOX 3, Figure 54.1).[21,22] The FOLFOX 4 regimen used the modified bimonthly LV5FU2 regimen (see Chapter 44) in combination with oxaliplatin (85 mg/m^2) (Figure 54.1). Both regimens were administered to patients whose disease had progressed while receiving the LV/5-FU regimen alone, and the studies confirmed the synergistic effects of oxaliplatin when administered with LV/5-FU. However, the response rates were much lower than those observed with the FOLFOX 2

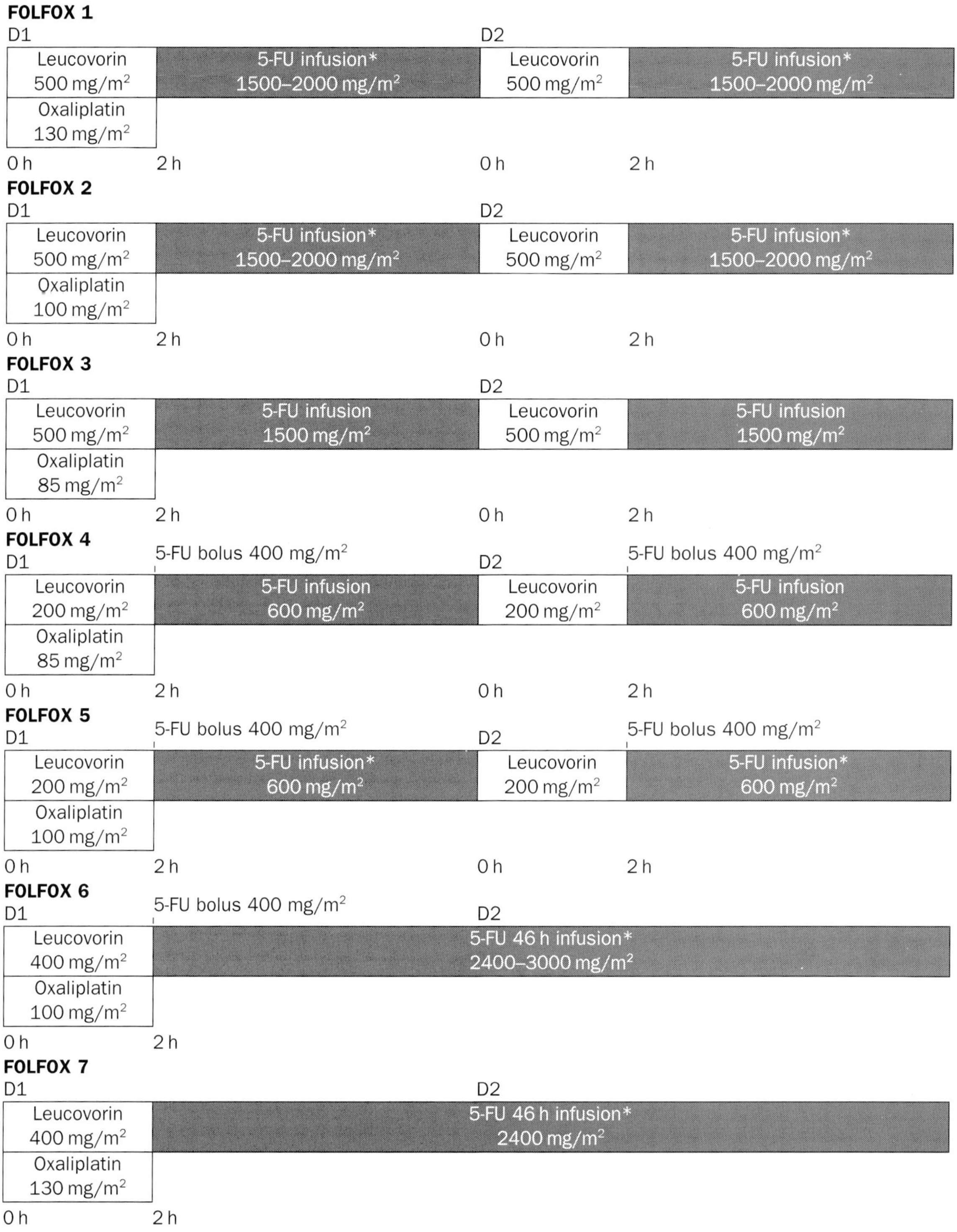

FOLFOX 1

D1		D2	

| Leucovorin 500 mg/m² | 5-FU infusion* 1500–2000 mg/m² | Leucovorin 500 mg/m² | 5-FU infusion* 1500–2000 mg/m² |
| Oxaliplatin 130 mg/m² | | | |

0 h   2 h   0 h   2 h

FOLFOX 2

D1		D2	

| Leucovorin 500 mg/m² | 5-FU infusion* 1500–2000 mg/m² | Leucovorin 500 mg/m² | 5-FU infusion* 1500–2000 mg/m² |
| Oxaliplatin 100 mg/m² | | | |

0 h   2 h   0 h   2 h

FOLFOX 3

D1		D2	

| Leucovorin 500 mg/m² | 5-FU infusion 1500 mg/m² | Leucovorin 500 mg/m² | 5-FU infusion 1500 mg/m² |
| Oxaliplatin 85 mg/m² | | | |

0 h   2 h   0 h   2 h

FOLFOX 4

D1   5-FU bolus 400 mg/m²   D2   5-FU bolus 400 mg/m²

| Leucovorin 200 mg/m² | 5-FU infusion 600 mg/m² | Leucovorin 200 mg/m² | 5-FU infusion 600 mg/m² |
| Oxaliplatin 85 mg/m² | | | |

0 h   2 h   0 h   2 h

FOLFOX 5

D1   5-FU bolus 400 mg/m²   D2   5-FU bolus 400 mg/m²

| Leucovorin 200 mg/m² | 5-FU infusion* 600 mg/m² | Leucovorin 200 mg/m² | 5-FU infusion* 600 mg/m² |
| Oxaliplatin 100 mg/m² | | | |

0 h   2 h   0 h   2 h

FOLFOX 6

D1   5-FU bolus 400 mg/m²   D2

| Leucovorin 400 mg/m² | 5-FU 46 h infusion* 2400–3000 mg/m² |
| Oxaliplatin 100 mg/m² | |

0 h   2 h

FOLFOX 7

D1	D2

| Leucovorin 400 mg/m² | 5-FU 46 h infusion* 2400 mg/m² |
| Oxaliplatin 130 mg/m² | |

0 h   2 h

Figure 54.1 Regimens used in the FOLFOX 1–7 studies. Treatment cycles were repeated every 2 weeks. Oxaliplatin was administered at every other cycle in FOLFOX 1, and at every cycle in FOLFOX 2–6. *The dose was administered at the lower level for two cycles, then at the higher level for subsequent cycles, if toxicity < WHO grade 2.

Table 54.1 Summary of the findings of the FOLFOX studies, in which LV/5-FU was administered with oxaliplatin in the second-line therapy of advanced colorectal cancer

Regimen[a]	No. of patients	Response rate (%)	Median PFS[b] (months)	Median survival (months)
FOLFOX 1	13	31	6	11
FOLFOX 2	46	46	7	17
FOLFOX 3	30	20	6	10
FOLFOX 3	40	18	4.6	10.6
FOLFOX 4	57	23	5.1	11.1
FOLFOX 6	60	27	5.3	10.8
FOLFOX 7	34	44	6.2	12.6

[a]Note that there were two FOLFOX 3 studies and FOLFOX 5 was not conducted.
[b]Progression-free survival.

regimen (18–23% versus 46%). Similarly, survival times were shorter, with median progression-free survivals of 4.6–6.0 months and median survivals of 10.0–11.1 months being reported. As expected, toxicity rates were lower in FOLFOX 3 and 4 compared with FOLFOX 2: grade 2–3 peripheral neuropathy was observed in 13–27% of patients, while grade 3–4 neutropenia occurred in 15–20%.

The FOLFOX 5 regimen involved the addition of oxaliplatin 100 mg/m^2 to LV5FU2, although this was not evaluated in a clinical trial. Instead, subsequent trials have used the new simplified regimen (see Chapter 44) because this has been found to be more convenient for patients, with the same low toxicity as LV5FU2 while being at least as effective.[13] FOLFOX 6 used the new simplified regimen in combination with oxaliplatin at 100 mg/m^2 (Figure 54.1). Among the 60 patients treated, the overall tumour response rate was 27%.[23] The median progression-free survival was 5.3 months, and the median survival was 10.8 months. However, retrospective analysis of the oxaliplatin dose intensity administered in the FOLFOX 6 study indicated that the scheduled dose was not administered to most patients in the FOLFOX 6 trial. This may account for the poorer outcome of patients receiving the FOLFOX 6 regimen compared with FOLFOX 2. In addition, limiting toxicities were comparable in FOLFOX 6 compared with FOLFOX 2: grade 3–4 neutropenia was observed in 24% of patients and grade 2–3 peripheral neuropathy in 41%.

The findings of the previous FOLFOX trials indicate that the dose intensity of oxaliplatin may be important in determining the efficacy of the triple-agent regimen.[24] No other factor, such as age, number of metastatic sites, carcinoembryonic antigen (CEA) level, or response to first-line therapy, appeared to influence the response to second-line therapy. In the most recent trial (FOLFOX 7), a higher dose intensity of oxaliplatin (130 mg/m^2) was added to the simplified LV/5-FU regimen in an attempt to improve tumour response rates in patients with advanced colorectal cancer resistant to previous therapy with LV/5-FU.[25] Among the first 34 patients treated, a high tumour response rate of 44% was observed. In order to limit the incidence of toxicity, the FOLFOX 7 regimen was stopped after eight treatment cycles. Patients were then evaluated every 2 months, and the FOLFOX 7 regimen was resumed if there was progression of the disease. The results of the trial indicate that the FOLFOX 7 regimen was well tolerated. In particular, the limiting toxicities of grade 3 sensory neuropathy (6.1% of patients) and grade 3–4 neutropenia (8.1%) occurred less frequently than with all of the other FOLFOX regimens. Importantly, median progression-free survival (6.2 months) and median survival (12.6 months) were not adversely affected by the break in therapy. These encouraging results have led to the investigation of the FOLFOX 7 regimen in the first-line treatment of advanced colorectal cancer. A trial (the OPTIMOX study, aimed at identifying the optimal FOLFOX regimen), is currently underway to compare the efficacy of FOLFOX 7 with FOLFOX 4 in previously untreated patients.

IRINOTECAN

The first large randomized phase III trial compared best supportive care alone or in combination with irinotecan as second-line therapy in 279 patients.[26] A significant survival advantage was demonstrated in the irinotecan group compared with patients receiving supportive care only (1-year overall survival rate 36.2% versus 13.8%, $p = 0.001$). Furthermore, irinotecan had no adverse effect on performance status or overall quality of life. In another phase III trial, irinotecan was associated with significantly improved survival ($p = 0.035$) compared with 5-FU infusion in patients with metastatic colorectal cancer who had failed to respond to first-line 5-FU regimens.[27] The median survival duration was 10.8 months for the irinotecan group, compared with 8.5 months for patients receiving 5-FU, and the 1-year survival rates were 45% and 32% respectively. Importantly, the increased survival was not gained at the expense of quality of life, and both treatment regimens were well tolerated.

Preclinical and phase I–II studies have demonstrated a potential synergy when irinotecan is combined with 5-FU and LV[28,29] – see also Chapter 53. In view of the potential clinical benefit of this combination, the addition of irinotecan to the simplified bimonthly LV/5-FU regimen has been investigated recently in a phase II study of patients with advanced colorectal cancer resistant to LV/5-FU plus oxaliplatin (FOLFOX regimens). The FOLFIRI trial evaluated LV/5-FU in combination with irinotecan as third-line therapy in 33 patients, and showed that this combination has clinical activity in these heavily pretreated patients.[30] Diarrhoea and neutropenia were the main limiting toxicities, and were observed at grade 3–4 severity in 12% and 15% of patients respectively. Overall, 30% of patients experienced grade 3–4 toxicities, which were amenable to treatment or dose reduction, and the tolerability of the regimen was regarded as good. Objective tumour responses were observed in 6% of patients, with median and progression-free survival times of 9.9 months and 4.1 months respectively. The FOLFIRI trial thus indicates that third-line therapy is beneficial for some patients with metastatic colorectal cancer. In view of these findings, the FOLFIRI regimen is currently being evaluated in the first- and second-line treatment of advanced colorectal cancer. Further development of the FOLFIRI regimen – the FOLFIRI 2 study with irinotecan administered after 5-FU,[31] and the FOLFIRI 3 study with two doses of irinotecan – are ongoing (Figure 54.2).

Other regimens of LV/5-FU plus irinotecan have been investigated in the first-line treatment of advanced colorectal cancer. A large randomized

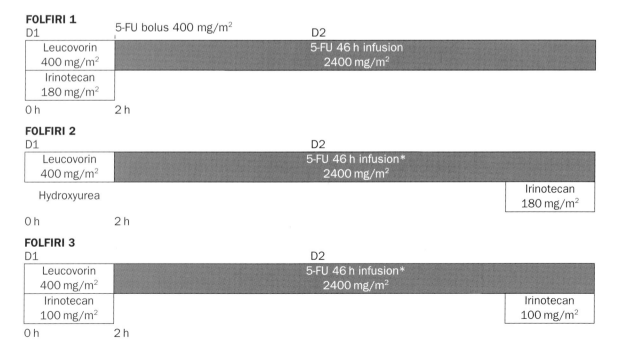

Figure 54.2 Regimens used in the FOLFIRI studies. Treatment cycles were repeated every 2 weeks.

clinical trial has demonstrated that the administration of irinotecan plus the weekly LV/5-FU regimen is associated with significantly higher tumour response rates than either regimen alone in previously untreated patients with advanced colorectal cancer.[32] Objective responses were recorded in 40% of patients receiving the three-drug combination, compared with 18% receiving irinotecan and 22% in the LV/5-FU group. Furthermore, progression-free and median survivals were significantly increased by the three-drug regimen.

A further phase III trial has evaluated the outcome of two commonly used LV/5-FU regimens, including bimonthly LV5FU2 in a majority of patients, with or without irinotecan in the first-line therapy of advanced colorectal cancer.[33] The results indicate that tumour response rates, progression-free survival, and overall survival were all improved among patients receiving irinotecan plus LV/5-FU. Furthermore, the combination had acceptable tolerability. In view of the antitumour activity that has been demonstrated with the three-drug combination, the role of irinotecan plus LV/5-FU is currently being investigated in a range of settings, including the postoperative treatment of colorectal cancer and first- and second-line treatment of metastatic disease.

CONCLUSIONS

During the last decade, considerable progress has been made in the development of LV/5-FU regimens that optimize antitumour efficacy while minimizing toxicity in the management of advanced colorectal cancer. The use of continuous infusions has permitted the administration of high doses of LV and 5-FU, leading to enhanced efficacy with acceptable toxicity. Furthermore, the relatively low toxicity of bimonthly LV/5-FU regimens has provided the opportunity to add other antitumour agents, such as oxaliplatin and irinotecan, with the possibility of improving tumour response rates and patient survival. The availability of these novel agents provides additional therapeutic options for tumours that are resistant to LV/5-FU regimens. Several studies of LV/5-FU regimens are currently in progress, and these aim to identify chemotherapeutic regimens that can produce both improved tumour response rates and prolonged survival in patients with advanced colorectal cancer. An ongoing study by the GERCOR (Oncology Multidisciplinary Research Group) is comparing FOLFOX 6 followed by FOLFIRI with FOLFIRI followed by FOLFOX 6 in order to define the best therapeutic sequence.[34]

ACKNOWLEDGEMENT

The authors are grateful to Adis International for editorial development.

REFERENCES

1. Raymond E, Faivre S, Woynarowski JM, Chaney SG, Oxaliplatin: mechanism of action and antineoplastic activity. *Semin Oncol* 1998; **25**(Suppl 5): 4–12.
2. Becouarn Y, Ychoul M, Ducreux M et al, A phase II trial of oxaliplatin as first-line chemotherapy in metastatic colorectal cancer patients. *J Clin Oncol* 1998; **8**: 2739–44.
3. Diaz-Rubio E, Sastre J, Zaniboni A et al, Oxaliplatin as single agent in previously untreated colorectal carcinoma patients: a phase II multicentric study. *Ann Oncol* 1998; **9**: 105–8.
4. Machover D, Diaz-Rubio E, de Gramont A et al, Two consecutive phase II studies of oxaliplatin (L-OHP) for treatment of patients with advanced colorectal carcinoma who were resistant to previous treatment with fluoropyrimidines. *Ann Oncol* 1996; **7**: 95–8.
5. Lévi F, Misset JL, Brienza S et al, A chronopharmacologic phase II clinical trial with 5-fluorouracil, folinic acid, and oxaliplatin using an ambulatory multichannel programmable pump: high antitumor effectiveness against metastatic colorectal cancer. *Cancer* 1992; **69**: 893–900.
6. Shimada Y, Rothenberg M, Hilsenbeck SG et al, Activity of CPT-11 (irinotecan hydrochloride), a topoisomerase inhibitor, against human tumour colony-forming units. *Anticancer Drugs* 1994; **5**: 20–6.
7. Ducreux M, Ychoul M, Seitz JF et al, Irinotecan combined with bolus fluorouracil, continuous infusion fluorouracil, and high-dose leucovorin every two weeks (LV5FU2 regimen): a clinical dose-finding and pharmacokinetic study in patients with pre-treated metastatic colorectal cancer. *J Clin Oncol* 1999; **17**: 2901–8.
8. Pitot HC, Wender DB, O'Connell MJ et al, Phase II trial of irinotecan in patients with metastatic colorectal carcinoma. *J Clin Oncol* 1997; **15**: 2910–19.
9. Rougier P, Bugat R, Douillard Y et al, Phase II study of irinotecan in the treatment of advanced colorectal cancer in chemotherapy-naïve patients and patients pretreated with fluorouracil-based chemotherapy. *J Clin Oncol* 1997; **15**: 251–60.
10. de Gramont A, Krulik M, Cady J et al, High-dose folinic acid and 5-fluorouracil bolus and continuous infusion in advanced colorectal cancer. *Eur J Cancer Clin Oncol* 1988; **24**: 1499–503.
11. de Gramont A, Bosset JF, Milan C et al, Randomized trial comparing monthly low-dose leucovorin and fluorouracil bolus with bimonthly high-dose leucovorin and fluorouracil bolus plus continuous infusion for advanced colorectal cancer: a French Intergroup study. *J Clin Oncol* 1997; **15**: 808–15.
12. Beerblock K, Rinaldi Y, André T et al, Bimonthly high dose leucovorin and 5-fluorouracil 48-hour continuous infusion in patients with advanced colorectal carcinoma. Groupe d'Etude et de Recherche sur les Cancers de l'Ovaire et Digestifs (GERCOD). *Cancer* 1997; **79**: 1100–15.
13. Tournigand C, de Gramont A, Louvet C et al, A simplified bimonthly regimen with leucovorin and 5FU for metastatic colorectal cancer. *Proc Am Soc Clin Oncol* 1998; **17**: 274.
14. de Gramont A, Louvet C, André T et al, A review of GERCOD trials of bimonthly leucovorin plus 5 fluorouracil 48-h continuous infusion in advanced colorectal cancer: evolution of a regimen. *Eur J Cancer* 1998; **34**: 619–26.
15. Lévi F, Zidani R, Misset JL, Randomised multicentre trial of

chronotherapy with oxaliplatin, fluorouracil, and folinic acid in metastatic colorectal cancer. International Organization for Cancer Chronotherapy. *Lancet* 1997; **350:** 681–6.

16. Raymond E, Buquet-Fagot C, Djelloul S et al, Antitumour activity of oxaliplatin in combination with 5-fluorouracil and the thymidylate synthase inhibitor AG337 in human colon, breast and ovarian cancers. *Anticancer Drugs* 1997; **8:** 876–85.

17. Giacchetti S, Perpoint B, Zidani R et al, Phase III multicenter randomized trial of oxaliplatin added to chronomodulated fluorouracil–leucovorin as first-line treatment of metastatic colorectal cancer. *J Clin Oncol* 2000; **18:** 136–47.

18. de Gramont A, Figer A, Seymour M et al, Leucovorin and 5-fluorouracil with or without oxaliplatin in advanced colorectal cancer. *J Clin Oncol* 2000; **18:** 2938–47.

19. de Gramont A, Gastiaburu J, Tournigand C et al, Oxaliplatin with high-dose folinic acid and 5-fluorouracil 48 hour infusion in pretreated metastatic colorectal cancer. *Proc Am Soc Clin Oncol* 1994; **13:** 220.

20. de Gramont A, Vignoud J, Tournigand C et al, Oxaliplatin with high-dose leucovorin and 5-fluorouracil 48-hour continuous infusion in pretreated metastatic colorectal cancer. *Eur J Cancer* 1997; **33:** 214–19.

21. André T, Louvet C, Raymond E et al, Bimonthly high-dose leucovorin, 5-fluorouracil infusion and oxaliplatin (FOLFOX 3) for metastatic colorectal cancer resistant to the same leucovorin and 5-fluorouracil regimen. *Ann Oncol* 1998; **9:** 1–3.

22. André T, Bensmaine MA, Louvet C et al, Multicenter phase II study of bimonthly high-dose leucovorin, fluorouracil infusion, and oxaliplatin for metastatic colorectal cancer resistant to the same leucovorin and fluorouracil regimen. *J Clin Oncol* 1999; **17:** 3560–8.

23. Maindrault-Goebel F, Louvet C, André T et al, for the GERCOR, Oxaliplatin added to the simplified bimonthly leucovorin and 5-fluorouracil regimen as second-line therapy for metastatic colorectal cancer (FOLFOX 6). *Eur J Cancer* 1999; **35:** 1338–42.

24. Maindrault-Goebel F, de Gramont A, Louvet C et al, Evaluation of oxaliplatin dose-intensity in bimonthly leucovorin and 48-hour 5-fluorouracil continuous infusion regimens (FOLFOX) in pretreated metastatic colorectal cancer. *Ann Oncol* 2000; **11:** 1477–83.

25. Maindrault-Goebel F, de Gramont A, Louvet C et al, for the GERCOR, High-dose intensity oxaliplatin added to the simpli-

fied bimonthly leucovorin and 5-fluorouracil regimen as second-line therapy for metastatic colorectal cancer (FOLFOX 7). *Proc Am Soc Clin Oncol* 1999; **18:** 265.

26. Cunningham D, Pyrhonen S, James RD et al, Randomized trial of irinotecan plus supportive care versus supportive care alone after fluorouracil failure for patients with metastatic colorectal cancer. *Lancet* 1998; **352:** 1413–18.

27. Rougier P, Van Cutsem E, Bajetta E et al, Randomised trial of irinotecan versus fluorouracil by continuous infusion after fluorouracil failure for patients with metastatic colorectal cancer. *Lancet* 1998; **352:** 1407–12.

28. Mullany S, Svingen PA, Kaufmano SH et al, Effect of adding the topoisomerase 1 poison 7-ethyl 10-hydroxycamptothecin (SN 38) to 5-fluorouracil and folinic acid in HCT8 cells: elevated dTTP pools and enhanced cytotoxicity. *Cancer Chemother Pharm* 1998; **42:** 391–9.

29. Ducreux M, Ychou M, Seitz JF et al, Irinotecan combined with bolus fluorouracil, continuous infusion fluorouracil, and high-dose leucovorin every two weeks (LV5FU2 regimen): a clinical dose-finding and pharmacokinetic study in patients with pretreated metastatic colorectal cancer. *J Clin Oncol* 1999; **17:** 2901–8.

30. André T, Louvet C, Maindrault-Goebel F et al, CPT-11 (irinotecan) addition to bimonthly, high-dose leucovorin and bolus and continuous-infusion 5-fluorouracil (FOLFIRI) for pretreated metastatic colorectal cancer. *Eur J Cancer* 1999; **35:** 1343–7.

31. Mabro M, André T, Louvet C et al, Bimonthly leucovorin, 5-fluorouracil infusion and hydroxyurea followed by CPT-11 (irinotecan) in pretreated patients with metastatic colorectal cancer. *Proc Am Soc Clin Oncol* 2000; **19:** 294a.

32. Saltz LB, Cox JV, Blanke C et al, Irinotecan plus fluorouracil and leucovorin for metastatic colorectal cancer. Irinotecan Study Group. *N Engl J Med* 2000; **343:** 905–14.

33. Douillard JY, Cunningham D, Roth AD et al, Irinotecan combined with fluorouracil compared with flurouracil alone as first-line treatment for metastatic colorectal cancer: a multicentre randomised trial. *Lancet* 2000; **355:** 1041–7.

34. Tournigand C, Louvet C, André T et al, FOLFIRI followed by FOLFOX or FOLFOX followed by FOLFIRI in metastatic colorectal cancer: Which is the best sequence? Safety and preliminary efficacy results of a randomized phase III study. *Proc Am Soc Clin Oncol* 2000; **19:** 245a.

55

Chronomodulation of chemotherapy against metastatic colorectal cancer

Francis Lévi, Sylvie Giacchetti

INTRODUCTION

The adaptation of drug delivery to circadian rhythms (chronotherapy) has been implemented in patients with metastatic colorectal cancer in order to improve chemotherapy tolerability and efficacy. The application of this concept in this disease has been based upon the following:

- the experimental chronopharmacology of the active drugs: 5-fluorouracil (5-FU), floxuridine, methotrexate, mitomycin C, oxaliplatin, and irinotecan;
- the occurrence of near-normal circadian rhythms in groups of colorectal cancer patients;
- the availability of multichannel programmable-in-time pumps allowing chronotherapy to be administered without hospitalization.

Chronomodulated delivery schedules with sinusoidally varying flow rates along a 24-hour time scale have been designed in order to minimize drug exposure of normal cells at the circadian times when they are most susceptible to damage. This strategy has been applied to single-agent 5-FU, oxaliplatin, and irinotecan, and mostly to combination therapy with 5-FU–leucovorin (LV) or 5-FU–LV–oxaliplatin. Phase I, II, and III clinical trials have shown that chronotherapy significantly increases the tolerable doses of these drugs and improves antitumour activity in patients with metastatic colorectal cancer. These safe conditions of drug delivery led to the first demonstration of the high activity of 5-FU–LV–oxaliplatin. Chronotherapy with these three drugs also allowed surgical removal of previously unresectable liver or lung metastases. This novel medicosurgical management of metastases now provides some hope for curability of metastatic disease in patients with unresectable colorectal cancer metastases. This chapter will review the experimental and clinical rationales of cancer chronotherapy, summarize our knowledge of the drug-delivery systems needed for its implementation, and review the relevant clinical data available.

RATIONALE FOR CHRONOMODULATION OF CHEMOTHERAPY

Circadian system physiology

Biological functions of living beings are organized on a 24-hour time scale. These circadian rhythms are generated by a clock mechanism involving at least nine specific circadian genes. This circadian oscillator controls the rhythmic expression of cell functions at both transcriptional and translational levels (Figure 55.1).[1–4] These cellular rhythms are coordinated by the suprachiasmatic nuclei (SCN), which are located in the hypothalamus.[5,6] The SCN help adjust the rhythms to the environmental cycles, in particular to the alternation of light and darkness over 24 hours.[4]

Under such synchronization, mammals with normal circadian function display circadian rhythms in rest–activity as well as in cellular metabolism and proliferation. These latter rhythms influence anticancer drug pharmacology and ultimately tolerability and/or antitumour efficacy of cancer treatments.[7,8]

The easy recording of the rest–activity cycle has further supported its use as a reference rhythm for

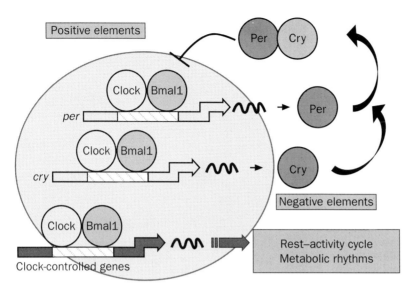

Figure 55.1 Molecular mechanisms of cellular circadian clocks in mammals. Positive elements include Clock and Bmal1 proteins. These proteins form heterodimers in the cell nucleus, which activate the transcription of *per* and *cry* genes. The protein outputs of these genes, Per and Cry, also heterodimerize in the cytoplasm, enter the nucleus, and suppress the gene-activation processes that are triggered by Clock–Bmal1. This feedback loop also regulates the transcription of several other genes, such as those responsible for vasopressin and transcription factors, including *dbp* and *tef*.

circadian timing of medications, and more recently for assessing circadian system function in cancer patients.

Chronopharmacology of relevant anticancer drugs

Toxicity rhythms
Circadian dosing time influences the extent of toxicity of about 30 anticancer drugs in mice or rats.[7,8] This effect is characteristic of the agents that are active against colorectal cancer, both longstanding ones such as 5-FU, floxuridine, methotrexate, and mitomycin C as well as recent drugs such as oxaliplatin and irinotecan[9–17] (Figure 55.2).

For all of these drugs, the difference in survival rate varied by two- to eightfold according to the dosing time of a potentially lethal dose in mice. Thus, the same dose could either kill 80% of the mice or spare the life of 90% of them. The least toxic time was located near the middle of the rest span of mice (day) for 5-FU[9] and for irinotecan,[15,16] and in the second half of the activity span (night) for methotrexate, floxuridine, mitomycin C, and oxaliplatin.[11–14,17] The lethal toxicity of these drugs mainly involved cellular

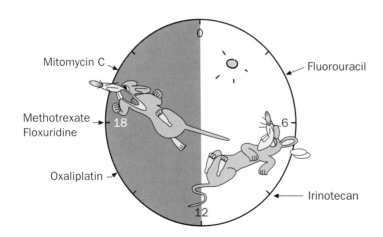

Figure 55.2 Circadian rhythms in tolerability of anticancer drugs in mice or rats. Only those agents that are known to be active against colorectal cancer are shown. The survival rate was two- to eightfold higher if a potentially lethal dose of a drug was injected at the circadian time indicated with an arrow, as compared with an administration 12 hours earlier or later. These drug tolerability rhythms are coupled to the rest–activity cycle of these animals, synchronized with a regular alternation of 12 hours of light and 12 hours of darkness.

damage to both bone marrow and intestinal mucosa. These tissues usually displayed synchronous rhythms in their susceptibility to the same agent.

Chronopharmacological mechanisms involve circadian changes in drug pharmacokinetics and/or susceptibility rhythms of target tissues.

Drug disposition

Times of high toxicity corresponded to the longest plasma elimination half-life for methotrexate.[12] This was not the case for 5-FU or oxaliplatin.[18,19] Conversely, platinum concentration in spleen and gut mucosa was least following oxaliplatin dosing, at its least toxic time.[17] These and other results suggest that toxicity rhythms may more closely match cellular changes in drug uptake or efflux than circadian plasma pharmacokinetics (reviewed in references 7 and 8).

Cellular mechanisms

Circadian changes in cellular enzymatic activities by two- to eightfold appear to contribute to the chronopharmacology of antimetabolites (Table 55.1). Thus, dihydrofolate reductase (DHFR), a target enzyme for methotrexate cytotoxity, peaks at 18 hours after light onset (HALO, middle of the activity span) in the liver of mice. The activity of dehydropyrimidine dehydrogenase (DPD), the rate-limiting catabolic enzyme of fluoropyrimidines, peaks in the early light span (early rest) in mouse or rat tissues. Conversely, the activities of uridine phosphorylase (URDP), orotate phosphoribosyltransferase (OPRT), and deoxythymidine kinase (TK) – all three of which are involved in the anabolism of the cytotoxic forms of the fluoropyrimidines (5-fluoro-2'-deoxyuridine 5'-monophosphate and 5-fluorouridine 5'-monophosphate) – peak

Table 55.1 Rhythms in enzymatic activities involved in fluoropyrimidine chronopharmacology in rodents synchronized with an alternation of 12 hours of light and 12 hours of darkness.[10,20–24] Mice or rats rest during the light span and are active during the dark span

Synchronizer phase		Peak		Trough	
		Enzyme	Organ	Enzyme	Organ
Light	Early to mid	DPD	Liver, Bone marrow	OPRT URDP TK DHFR	Liver
				TK	Spleen
	Late	TS	Tongue, Bone marrow	TS	Small intestine
Darkness	Early to mid	OPRT URDP TK DHFR	Liver	DPD	Liver, Bone marrow
		TK	Spleen	TS	Tongue, Bone marrow
		TS	Small intestine		
	Late	TS	Tongue, Bone marrow		

DPD, dehydropyrimidine dehydrogenase; OPRT, orotate phosphoribosyltransferase; URDP, uridine phosphorylase; TK, deoxythymidine kinase; DHFR, dihydrofolate reductase; TS, thymidylate synthase.

near the middle of darkness (mid activity) in mice or rats.[10,20–22] More recently, thymidylate synthase (TS) activity was found to peak in the late activity span in mouse small intestine, tongue, and bone marrow. A second peak was also found in the late rest span in both of the latter organs.[23] This enzyme is one of the main targets of 5-FU cytotoxicity. The cellular rhythm in TS activity as well as that in DPD activity seem to be controlled by the circadian oscillator at both transcriptional and translational levels.[23,24] All of the data concur to support a better tolerability of 5-FU in the first half of the light span in mice or rats.

Cellular resistance to many cytostatics involves reduced glutathione. Its concentration in liver cells doubles along the 24-hour time scale: lowest and highest values respectively occur near dark onset and near light onset. Synchronous rhythms were found for thiol groups in kidney and in intestine. The results support the better tolerability of platinum complexes and several alkylating drugs in the second half of darkness.[25–27]

Finally, O^6-alkylguanine-DNA alkyltransferase (AGTase), a DNA repair enzyme of alkylated DNA, was about sixfold higher at 19 HALO (second half of activity span) as compared with 7 HALO (second half of rest span) in mouse liver. This rhythm contributes to the better murine tolerability of cystemustine, a nitrosourea, in the second half of darkness.[28]

These data point towards an essential role for rhythmic enzymatic mechanisms in the cellular detoxification of chemotherapy damage to healthy cells.

Antitumour efficacy

Dosing time not only affects drug tolerability, but may also modify anticancer efficacy, as was first shown with cytosine arabinoside against mouse L1210 leukaemia.[29] Similarly, 5-FU displayed increased efficacy against murine colon tumours (CO36 and CO38) following dosing in the early rest span, when it was less toxic.[30] Recently, oxaliplatin has been found to display increased efficacy against murine Glasgow osteosarcoma following dosing near the middle of the activity span, when this drug is also best tolerated. Furthermore, dosing irinotecan near the middle of the light span (rest) and oxaliplatin near the middle of the dark span (activity) was found to be mandatory for this combination to display synergistic activity in this model.[31] Thus, most experimental data support a link between the rhythm in drug tolerability and anticancer efficacy (reviewed in references 7 and 8). These observations led to incremental approaches in chronopharmacological combination of drugs, which documented

that the rate of tumour cures could be brought up from 25% to 80% or more with adequately circadian-scheduled chemotherapy involving up to five cytostatics.[32]

In summary, the experimental model tells us that the circadian rhythm in drug tolerability can be used for two purposes. An improvement in quality of life can result from the dosing-time-related reduction of chemotherapy toxicity, while dose and efficacy remain similar to standard schedules of delivery. An improvement in survival can result from the administration of a higher maximum tolerated dose at the least toxic circadian time as compared with other dosing times.

Rhythms in relevant human tissues

Proliferative activity (DNA synthesis) in haematopoietic or oral mucosa progenitor cells vary by 50% or more along the 24-hour time scale in healthy subjects. This is also the case for ex vivo DNA synthetic activity in human rectal mucosa or skin. For these four tissues, lower mean values in DNA synthesis occurred between midnight and 04 : 00 h at night, while higher mean values occurred between 08 : 00 h and 20 : 00 h.[33–40] Reduced glutathione also varied rhythmically in human bone marrow, yet intersubject variability appeared to be larger than that of proliferative indices.[38,41] The activity of DPD in human mononuclear cells increased by about 50% between 10 : 00 h and midnight both in healthy subjects and in cancer patients[42–44] (Figure 55.3). The circadian time structure of oral mucosa has recently been well documented with regard to both the expression of circadian genes (per, clock, tim, bmal1, cry) and of cell-cycle-related proteins (cyclins, p53) as well as activity of TS, a target enzyme for 5-FU cytotoxicity.[45–47]

Mitotic index and/or DNA synthesis have been used to evaluate the proliferative activity of many experimental and human breast, ovarian, or lymphomatous tumours. Data suggest that well-differentiated slowly growing tumours retain a circadian time structure, whereas poorly differentiated rapidly growing tumours tend to lose it[48,49] (reviewed in reference 50).

Drug chronopharmacokinetics

A short intravenous infusion of 5-FU or methotrexate was associated with modifications of plasma and/or urinary pharmacokinetics according to dosing

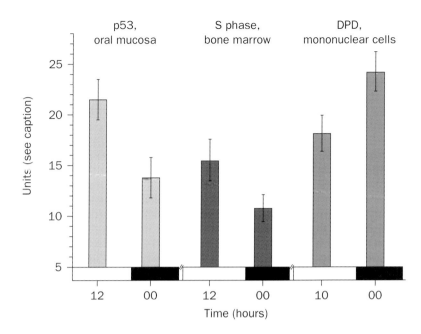

Figure 55.3 Twenty-four hour changes in human normal tissues. Mean ± SEM near peak and trough ($p < 0.05$, for each variable). p53 expression (% positive cells) was measured in the oral mucosa of healthy subjects.[45] The proportion of bone marrow cells in S phase (%) was assessed in cancer patients.[38] DPD activity in mononuclear cells was determined in 12 patients with metastatic colorectal cancer (nmol/min/mg protein).[44] A 4-hour span, located between midnight and 04 : 00 h, corresponds to a low point in the DNA synthetic activity of bone marrow and oral mucosa (as well as skin and rectal mucosa – data not shown). Circulating mononuclear cells also display higher DPD activity at these times.

time.[51,52] Physiological rhythms in urinary excretion or plasma proteins contributed to methotrexate chronopharmacokinetics.[51]

The most striking results, however, came from flat intravenous infusion of chemotherapeutic agents. To the best of our knowledge, seven such clinical investigations have been reported for 5-FU. In six of them, 5-FU was infused at a flat rate for 1–5 days.[53–58] The mean plasma 5-FU level nearly doubled from a trough near midday to a maximum near 01 : 00 h to 04 : 00 h at night. However, after a 14-day venous infusion of 5-FU, the plasma 5-FU rhythm peaked near noon in nine patients with gastrointestinal malignancy.[43] In this study, DPD activity in circulating mononuclear cells displayed a circadian rhythm, with a peak occurring near 01 : 00 h at night, i.e. 12 hours of phase with the 5-FU rhythm.[43] The DPD rhythm was similar to that found in healthy subjects or in untreated cancer patients.[42,44] Thus, 5-FU clearance was least near 01 : 00 h at night when this drug was injected as a bolus or continuously infused at a dose of more than 500 mg/m²/day for 1–5 days.[52–58] Conversely, this parameter was highest near 13 : 00 h when 5-FU was infused for 14 days at a dose of less than 300 mg/m², with a 24-hour mean plasma level about one-twentieth of that observed during 4- or 5-day infusion (16 ng/ml versus 340 ng/ml).[43] Most

likely, high-dose flat infusion or bolus injection of 5-FU saturates DPD activity, which no longer represents a relevant mechanism of the 5-FU plasma concentration rhythm, but rather protects normal cells against 5-FU cytotoxicity in a circadian-dependent manner.[54]

Well-known interindividual differences in 5-FU clearance warrant analysis of rhythmicity relative to each patient's 24-hour mean level, especially in studies involving small groups of patients.[53] The use of a Bayesian method was an interesting approach to the further demonstration of a circadian rhythm in 5-FU plasma concentration in a rather large patient population.[57] Indeed, the average circadian pattern was similar on all infusional days in patients with bladder or gastrointestinal metastatic cancer and in those receiving prior cisplatin, or concurrent flat infusion of leucovorin alone or associated with oxaliplatin. Nevertheless, interindividual changes in circadian rhythmicity have been observed in all these studies, and have sometimes been judged as prominent.[58] Recent data in patients with lung cancer indicate that morning hydrocortisone can help synchronize the 5-FU plasma concentration rhythm.[59]

Similarly, circadian changes also characterized flat infusion of leucovorin, although with a lower amplitude (10%) than 5-FU.[54]

DRUG-DELIVERY DEVICES FOR CHRONOMODULATING CHEMOTHERAPY

Technology: first- and second-generation injectors

The availability of multichannel programmable-in-time ambulatory pumps has been indispensable for the administration of chronomodulated infusions. The first device of its kind was a four-channel programmable pump equipped with four 30 ml reservoirs (IntelliJect, Aguettant, Lyon, France).

Two devices from a second generation of multichannel programmable-in-time pumps are now available. The Z-pump (Zambon-Inphardial, Antibes, France) is a two-channel injector that can be equipped with one or two 100 ml reservoirs, and thus appears appropriate for chronomodulated delivery of two drugs, such as 5-FU and leucovorin. The Mélodie pump (Aguettant-Santé, Lyon, France) is a four-channel device that can be programmed with user-friendly software under Windows on a PC, and can accommodate any reservoir volume and delivery profile (Table 55.2). The use of both of these devices has been approved by the European Community. The Mélodie pump is also approved by the US Food and Drug Administration. This latter device has been extensively used for ongoing chronotherapy protocols.

The use of these pumps has necessitated the documentation of the compatibility of 5-FU, leucovorin oxaliplatin, and irinotecan with the reservoirs and the stability of these drugs under these conditions during the protocol duration: 5 days for 5-FU, leucovorin, and oxaliplatin (Figure 55.4) and 6 hours for irinotecan (Figure 55.5).

Drug pharmacokinetics during chronomodulated infusions

Plasma concentrations of 5-FU, active folates, and oxaliplatin have been studied along the course of chronomodulated infusions.

Circadian changes in 5-FU plasma levels matched the sinusoidal delivery waveform over the four or five infusional days rather well (Figure 55.6).[54,58,60,61] Chronomodulated delivery of 5-FU and l-leucovorin with peak flow rates at 4:00 h was associated with markedly reduced interpatient variability in the plasma levels of both 5-FU and l-leucovorin as compared with constant-rate infusions or with chronomodulated administrations with peak flow rates at 13:00 h or at 19:00 h.[60] These three latter schedules displayed increased toxicity as compared with the former one. Although the average time course of plasma 5-FU and l-leucovorin concentrations closely matched chronomodulated delivery of 5-FU–LV with a peak at 04:00 h, this was not the case for plasma methyltetrahydrofolate, a metabolite that reflects the intracellular active form of l-leucovorin. The circadian maximum of methyltetrahydrofolate was found at about 2 hours after l-leucovorin peak delivery.[61]

The 'free' platinum plasma concentration reflected the chronomodulated flow rate of oxaliplatin, but accumulation was patent from the first to the fourth infusional day. The estimated area under the curve

---

Table 55.2 Approved drug-delivery devices used for multiple-drug chronotherapy in gastrointestinal malignancies

Model	Manufacturer	Main characteristics	Main drugs
Z-pump	Zambon-Inphardial (Antibes, France)	Two 100 ml reservoirs; programmable on a PC or pump or via a code-bar (laser printer)	5-FU, leucovorin
Mélodié	Aguettant-Santé (Lyon, France)	Four reservoirs of any capacity; programmable on a PC; one or two independent line(s); actual drug-delivery report	5-FU, leucovorin, with or without oxaliplatin or irinotecan

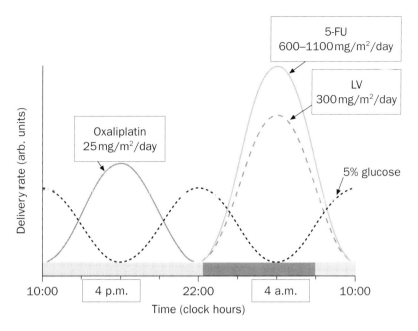

Figure 55.4 Schedule for intravenous chronomodulated infusion of 5-FU, leucovorin (LV), and oxaliplatin. This 24-hour cycle was repeated automatically for 5 consecutive days followed by a 16-day interval, or for 4 days followed by a 10-day interval. This complex drug-delivery pattern has been administered to fully ambulatory patients using a programmable multichannel pump.[74,79–82]

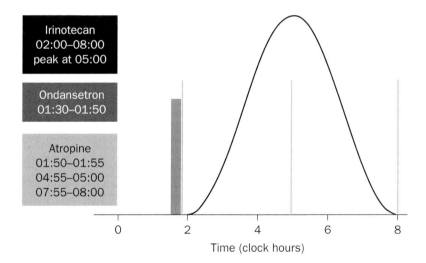

Figure 55.5 Schedule for intravenous chronomodulated infusion of irinotecan. This 6-hour chronomodulated delivery was combined with the automatic administration of supportive medications including ondansetron and atropine sulfate. This complex drug-delivery pattern has been administered to fully ambulatory patients using a programmable multichannel pump.[73]

(AUC) of both total and 'free' platinum was significantly higher in patients receiving chronomodulated oxaliplatin, with a peak at 07 : 00 h or at 16 : 00 h as compared with 01 : 00 h. The results suggested that extraplasmatic diffusion of oxaliplatin was greatest in the late evening or early night hours, possibly as a result of the circadian rhythms that modulate cell membrane fluidity, plasma proteins, blood flow, capillary resistance, and renal functions.[62]

These pharmacokinetic studies ensured that an appropriate target rhythm in tissue exposure was produced by the chosen chronomodulated schedule for 5-FU. They suggest that the delivery patterns of leucovorin and oxaliplatin could be amenable to further optimization in some patients.[61–63]

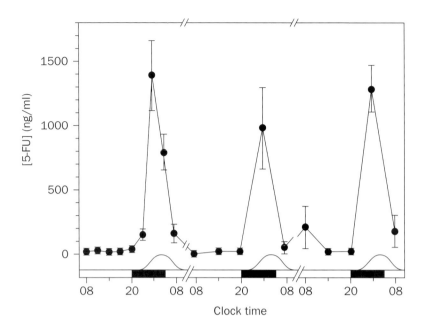

Figure 55.6 Twenty-four-hour changes in 5-FU plasma levels, during a 5-day chronomodulated infusion of 5-FU (600 mg/m²/day), *dl*-leucovorin (300 mg/m²/day) and oxaliplatin (20 mg/m²/day) in 6 patients with metastatic colorectal cancer.[54] The drug-delivery scheme is shown in Figure 55.4.

TOLERABILITY AND EFFICACY OF CHRONOTHERAPY

Overall strategy and hypothesis

To achieve a high dose intensity, we aimed at reducing treatment toxicity as much as possible so that doses could be increased compared with standard chemotherapeutic schedules. For this purpose, we adapted the drug-infusion rate to circadian rhythms. The hypothesis was that high doses of all drugs and proper circadian scheduling of drug delivery were needed to achieve clinical synergy.[8]

The main results of phase I, II and III clinical trials will be briefly reviewed here in order to define the role of chronotherapy in the medicosurgical management of patients with metastatic colorectal cancer.

Drug delivery in the chronomodulated schedules varied sinusoidally along the 24-hour time scale (see above). Times of maximum flow rate were extrapolated from murine experiments. For these reasons, peak delivery was scheduled at 4 : 00 h for 5-FU and leucovorin, at 16 : 00 h for oxaliplatin, and at 05 : 00 h for irinotecan.

Maximum tolerated dose and antitumour activity (phase I–II)

5-FU with or without leucovorin
5-FU has remained the main active drug against col-

orectal cancer. A dose–response relationship characterizes the antitumour efficacy of 5-FU against colorectal cancer.[64]

The infusion rate of 5-FU alone was chronomodulated along the 24-hour time scale for 5 consecutive days (every 3 weeks), with peak delivery at 04 : 00 h and no infusion from 16 : 00 h to 22 : 00 h. Thirty-five patients with metastatic colorectal cancer participated in this phase I–II trial, with intrapatient dose escalation according to defined toxicity criteria. As a result of good tolerability (<8% courses with severe, WHO grade 3, toxic symptoms), the recommended dose could be escalated up to 1400 mg/m²/day or more for 5 days in 80% of assessable patients. This represents a 40–100% increase in dose or dose intensity as compared with 5-day flat infusion, for which the recommended dose is 800–1000 mg/m²/day for 5 days every 3–4 weeks.[65]

Phase I trials have evaluated the tolerability and recommended dose of chronomodulated infusions of various 5-FU–LV combination schedules. In a Canadian study, 5-FU was infused for 14 days, with low-dose leucovorin. Both drugs were infused according to a quasisinusoidal 24-hour rhythmic chronomodulated pattern with peak flow rate near 04 : 00 h at night. The maximum tolerated dose (MTD) was 250 mg/m²/day of 5-FU (3500 mg/m²/course) with 20 mg/m²/day of leucovorin. The authors suggested that peak delivery early at night (22 : 00 h) could further improve tolerance in some patients.[66]

A phase I study established the MTD of the combination of 5-FU and *l*-leucovorin given as a 5-day chronomodulated infusion every 3 weeks to ambulatory patients with metastatic colorectal cancer. Thirty-four patients were included. The dose-limiting toxicities were stomatitis and diarrhoea. The recommended doses are 900 mg/m^2/day for 5-FU combined with 150 mg/m^2 for *l*-leucovorin. Objective responses were achieved in 8 of 20 untreated patients and in 1 of 13 previously treated ones.[67]

The low toxicity profile and the apparently dose-related antitumour activity led to further intensification of this regimen. Both drugs were delivered near MTD as chronomodulated infusions for 4 days instead of 5 and every 2 weeks rather than every 3. The antitumour efficacy and tolerability of this intensified 5-FU–LV schedule (FF4–10) was investigated in a European multicentre phase II trial that registered 100 patients with previously untreated metastatic colorectal cancer. While the leucovorin dose remained fixed (150 mg/m^2/day of *l*-leucovorin or 300 mg/m^2/day of *dl*-leucovorin), the 5-FU dose was escalated in the absence of grade 2 or greater toxicity from 900 mg/m^2/day in the first course to 1000 mg/m^2/day in the second and 1100 mg/m^2/day in the third. The dose-limiting toxicity of this regimen was grade 3 hand–foot syndrome, which was encountered in 38% of patients (8% of courses). The median 5-FU dose intensity was 1800 mg/m^2/week and the objective response rate, as assessed from computed tomography (CT) scans reviewed by an independent panel, was 41% (95% CI 31.5–50.5%). The median survival was 17 months, with 18.6% of the patients alive at 3 years.[68] A 45% objective response rate was obtained by another team.[69]

Oxaliplatin

The International Organization for Cancer Chronotherapy (IOCC), which later became the Chronotherapy Group of the European Organization for Research and Treatment of Cancer (EORTC), was the first to report oxaliplatin activity in metastatic colorectal cancers in monotherapy and in combination with 5-FU–LV. The time of least toxicity as extrapolated from murine data was 16 : 00 h. The phase I trial compared a 5-day flat infusion of oxaliplatin with a chronomodulated one in 25 patients. The recommended dose per course was 125 mg/m^2 for flat infusion. This dose level is close to that subsequently established for a standard 2-hour or 6-hour infusion of this drug once every 3 weeks. The recommended oxaliplatin dose for single-agent chronother-apy was 175 mg/m^2/course.[70] In a multicentre phase II trial, 29 patients with metastatic colorectal cancer received a 5-day chronomodulated infusion of oxaliplatin. This study confirmed the recommended dose of 175 mg/m^2 and documented a 10% objective response rate in heavily pretreated patients.[71]

Irinotecan

Delayed diarrhoea and haematological toxicity usually prevent increases in the irinotecan dose to 500 mg/m^2 or more. However, these dose levels seem to enhance the antitumour activity of this drug.[72] Since irinotecan toxicity varied according to the time of its administration in mice,[15,16] a proper circadian scheduling of irinotecan delivery could well decrease its toxicity and allow a safe increase in tolerable dose. A feasibility study of chronomodulated infusion of irinotecan was performed in 27 patients with heavily pretreated metastatic colorectal cancer. Irinotecan chronotherapy was given at an initial dose of 350 mg/m^2/course, with intrapatient escalation in subsequent courses according to tolerability. Each course consisted of a 6-hour chronomodulated infusion of irinotecan, with a peak at 05 : 00 h, as extrapolated from studies in mice. Ondansetron and atropine sulfate (0.75 mg) were automatically delivered with irinotecan using a multichannel programmable pump. A median of 6 courses was given (range 1–19). The irinotecan dose could be escalated to more than 350 mg/m^2 in 66% of the patients and for 59% of the courses. An objective response was achieved in 3 patients (11%) and disease remained stable in 13 patients. Surgery of metastases was performed in 3 patients receiving irinotecan chronotherapy as third-line treatment. This schedule allowed the irinotecan dose intensity to be maintained for up to six courses, with acceptable tolerability and efficacy.[73] A randomized multicentre trial is now comparing single-agent irinotecan chronotherapy with standard infusion of this drug.

5-FU, leucovorin, and oxaliplatin combination

Since single-drug solutions of 5-FU, leucovorin, or oxaliplatin remain stable at ambient temperature and under normal lighting conditions for 5 days or more, this three-drug combination chemotherapy was further amenable to continuous ambulatory infusion.

A phase II study of a 5-day schedule of chronomodulated chemotherapy with 5-FU, leucovorin, and oxaliplatin (chrono FFL) was performed in 93 patients with unresectable colorectal metastases. Forty-six of these patients had received previous chemotherapy. Courses were repeated every 21 days. A 58% objective response rate was achieved.

Moreover, all treatments were administered on an outpatient basis, and less than 10% of the 784 courses given were associated with severe toxicity. The median overall survival was 16 months irrespective of prior chemotherapy, with a 17% survival rate at 3 years in chemotherapy-naive patients. We related the high antitumour efficacy of chrono FFL both to the presence of oxaliplatin and to chronomodulation, which allowed us to safely deliver high drug doses.[74]

5-FU, leucovorin, and carboplatin combination

A single-institution phase II study of chronomodulated 5-FU, leucovorin, and carboplatin was performed in 60 patients with metastatic colorectal cancer, 50% of whom had failed up to three chemotherapy regimens. The chronomodulated delivery pattern of carboplatin (40 mg/m²/day) was similar to that of oxaliplatin. The daily doses of 5-FU and leucovorin were 700 and 300 mg /m²/day respectively. Courses lasted 4 days and were repeated every 2 weeks. Grade 3–4 granulocytopenia was encountered in 29% of the patients, and was the main dose-limiting toxicity. An objective response was achieved in 47% of the patients, and in 69% of 13 chemotherapy-naive patients. The median survival of the 60 patients was 14.6 months.[75] The good therapeutic index of this regimen now warrants further evaluation.

Chronomodulated 5-FU with concurrent radiation therapy

The MTD of a chronomodulated infusion of 5-FU combined with concurrent radiation therapy for 5 weeks was investigated in 18 patients with primary locally advanced or unoperable rectal cancer.[76] All the patients completed the whole treatment course and were subsequently resectable, so that the activity of the regimen was fully assessable. The MTD of 5-FU was 275 mg/m²/day. Seven patients had a sphincter-sparing procedure and 10 had an abdominoperineal resection. Five complete pathological resections were obtained (28%). The authors recommended a further evaluation of combined chronomodulated infusion of 5-FU and radiation therapy as neoadjuvant treatment of rectal cancer. The feasibility of combining chronotherapy and radiotherapy has been independently confirmed.[77] An international trial testing the clinical relevance of this approach is starting within the EORTC in biliary cancer (EORTC 5991), and is being discussed for rectal cancer.

Table 55.3 summarizes the recommended doses for chronomodulated infusion regimens.

Efficacy of chronotherapy in randomized phase III trials

Contribution of oxaliplatin

The role of addition of oxaliplatin to chronomodulated 5-FU–LV was investigated in a multicentre, open randomized phase II–III study. Two hundred patients from 15 centres, with previously untreated measurable metastases from colorectal cancer, were randomly assigned to receive chronomodulated 5-FU and leucovorin (700 and 300 mg/m²/day respectively; peak delivery rate at 04 : 00) with or without oxaliplatin. The latter (125 mg/m²) was given as a 6-hour flat infusion from 10 : 00 h to 16 : 00 h on the first day of each course every 3 weeks. This infusion schedule was devised to remain close to the time of least toxicity of oxaliplatin. Response, the main judgement criterion, was assessed with an extramural review of CT scans. Severe toxicity (grade 3–4) was minimal in patients receiving chronomodulated 5-FU–LV ($\leqslant$5% per patient; $\leqslant$1% per course). Grade 3–4 diarrhoea occurred in 43% of the patients given oxaliplatin (10% of courses), and less than 2% of the patients displayed grade 3 or 4 leukoneutropenia or thrombocytopenia. Thirteen percent of patients had moderate functional impairment from peripheral sensory neuropathy (WHO modified grade 2). An objective response was obtained in 16% of the patients of 5-FU–LV (95% CI 9–24%) as compared with 53% of those receiving additional oxaliplatin (95% CI 42–63%) ($p < 0.001$). The median progression-free survival times were 6.1 months with 5-FU–LV (95% CI 4.1–7.4 months) and 8.7 months (95% CI 7.4–9.2 months) with oxaliplatin and 5-FU–LV ($p = 0.048$). Following treatment failure, 57% of the patients in the 5-FU–LV group received the three-drug combination. With a minimum follow up of 3 years, median survival times and 3-year survival rates were similar in both treatment groups (19.9 months versus 19.4 months and 30% versus 23.5% respectively) (Table 55.4). Thus the addition of oxaliplatin to chronomodulated 5-FU–LV displayed acceptable toxicity and an improved response rate, but did not improve survival in patients with metastatic colorectal cancer.[78] The discrepancy between a large effect upon tumour response and an apparent lack of effect upon survival may result from (1) prolonged treatment administration, which was possible because of the good tolerability of chronomodulated infusion; (2) other therapeutic measures, including administration of oxaliplatin to 57% of the patients from the chronomodulated 5-FU–LV-only arm, after failure of this modality, as well as surgical resection of metastases; (3) insufficient power to detect a survival difference.

Table 55.3 Recommended doses of chronomodulated chemotherapy

Drugs	Dose range and schedule tested	Time of peak delivery	Tumour type (no. of patients)	Recommended dose	Refs
5-FU	800—1900 mg/m^2/d × 5 d q21d	4 : 00 h	Colorectal (35)	1400 mg/m^2/d × 5 d q21d	65
5-FU *l*-leucovorin (LV)	600–1100 mg/m^2/d 150 mg/m^2/d × 5 d q21d	4 : 00 h	Colorectal (34)	900 mg/m^2/d × 5 d q21d	67
5-FU *l*-LV	200–300 mg/m^2/d 5–20 mg/m^2/d × 14 d q28d	4 : 00 h	Solid tumour (14)	MTD: 250 mg/m^2/d of 5-FU and 20 mg/m^2/d of *l*-LV	66
5-FU *l*-LV or *dl*-LV	900–1100 mg/m^2/d 150–300 mg/m^2/d × 4 d q14d	4 : 00 h	Colorectal (100)	5-FU: 900 mg/m^2/d *l*-LV: 150 mg/m^2/d	68
Oxaliplatin	25–40 mg/m^2/d, × 5 d q21d flat vs chrono	16 : 00 h	Breast or liver (23)	Chronomodulated: 35 mg/m^2/d × 5 d (flat: 25 mg/m^2/d × 5 d)	70
Oxaliplatin	30–40 mg/m^2/d, × 5 d q21d	16 : 00 h	Colorectal (29)	Median dose: 35 mg/m^2/d × 5 d	71
5-FU LV Oxaliplatin	600–800 mg/m^2/d 300 mg/m^2/d 20 mg/m^2/d, × 5 d q21d	4 : 00 h 16 : 00 h	Colorectal (93)	700 mg/m^2/d 300 mg/m^2/d 20 mg/m^2/d	74
5-FU LV Oxaliplatin	700–1100 mg/m^2/d 300 mg/m^2/d 25 mg/m^2/d, × 4 d q14d	4 : 00 h 16 : 00 h	Colorectal (103)	850 mg/m^2/d 300 mg/m^2/d 25 mg/m^2/d	81, 82
5-FU LV Carboplatin	700 mg/m^2/d 300 mg/m^2/d 40 mg/m^2/d, × 4 d q14d	4 : 00 h 16 : 00 h	Colorectal (60)	700 mg/m^2/d 300 mg/m^2/d 40 mg/m^2/d	75

Contribution of chronomodulation

The role of chronomodulated delivery of all three drugs was investigated in two consecutive European multicentre, phase III studies that compared flat versus chronomodulated infusion of the same three-drug combination in patients with previously untreated metastatic colorectal cancer.

A first randomized trial was then undertaken in 92 patients. Grade 3 or 4 main toxicity (which was stomatitis) was fivefold higher with constant-rate infusion than with chronotherapy (89% versus 18%). Chronotherapy achieved a 22% increase in 5-FU dose intensity as compared with flat infusion. The response rate, the main judgement criterion, was significantly increased from 32% with flat infusion to 53% with chronotherapy. The median progression-

Table 55.4 Contribution of oxaliplatin: phase III randomized trial[78]

	Chronomodulated 5-FU–LV[a]		
	Alone	With oxaliplatin	*p*
Patients	100	100	
Hospitalization	3	13	0.01
Mucositis (grade 3–4)	4	10	0.10
Diarrhoea (grade 3–4)	5	43	0.001
Peripheral neuropathy			
(grade 2, functional impairment)	0	13	0.001
Objective responses	16	53	0.001
Progression-free survival			
(months)	6.1	8.7	0.048
Survival (months)	19.9	19.4	NS

[a]5 days on/16 days off.

free survival and survival of all patients were 8 months and 14.9 months respectively in the flat arm, and 11 months and 19 months in the chronotherapy schedule.[79]

A second multicentre trial registered 186 patients. Severe stomatitis was incurred by 76% on the flat-infusion regimen as compared with 14% of those on chronotherapy. Cumulative peripheral sensory neuropathy with functional impairment was reported in 31% of patients on constant delivery and in 16% of patients on chronotherapy. This latter schedule allowed administration of a higher dose of 5-FU (700 mg/m²/day) than flat infusion (500 mg/m²/day) and a 22% greater dose intensity. The objective response rate was 51% on chronotherapy and 29% on constant-rate delivery. The median survival was 16 months in both modalities, possibly because 24% of the patients crossed over from the flat schedule to chronotherapy (Table 55.5). In this European multicentre randomized setting, the most active chronomodulated schedule was also the least toxic.[80]

Dose intensity, response rate, and survival

The results from both of these latter studies led us to further increase the density and intensity of the chronotherapy schedule. This involved its administration for 4 days every 2 weeks (10 days' interval, chrono FFL 4–10) rather than for 5 days every 3 weeks (16 days' interval, chrono FFL 5–16).

An intrapatient 5-FU dose-escalation scheme was performed in 50 patients with metastatic colorectal cancer (37 previously treated and 13 chemotherapy-naive). Courses were repeated every 14 days, 5-FU being escalated by 100 mg/m²/day in each patient when toxicity was less than grade 2. Median 5-FU and oxaliplatin dose intensities were increased by 32% and 18% respectively, as compared with our previous 5 days on/16 days off phase II protocol. The objective response rate was 40% (95% CI 24–57%) in previously treated patients and 69% (95% CI 48–90%) in chemotherapy-naive patients. The median progression-free survival was 9.3 months (95% CI 6.6–11.2 months). The median survival was 16.9 months in previously treated patients and 20.7 months in chemotherapy-naive patients.[81] This highly effective fully ambulatory outpatient regimen was subsequently confirmed in a European multicentre phase II trial involving 90 patients. The main acute toxicities were WHO grade 3 or 4 diarrhoea (41% of patients, 8.2% of courses), stomatitis (30% of patients, 5.1% of courses). The overall objective response rate was 66% (95% CI 56–76%). The median progression-free survival and overall survival were 8.4 months (95% CI 5.9–10 months) and 18.5 months (95% CI 13.2–23.8 months) respectively.[82]

Figure 55.7 summarizes the relationship between the 5-FU dose intensity and the objective response rate in those multicentre trials that involved chemotherapy-naive patients.

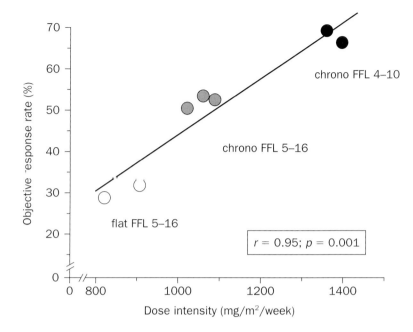

Figure 55.7 Relationship between 5-FU dose intensity and objective response rate in patients with previously untreated metastatic colorectal cancer. All these patients received 5-FU, leucovorin, and oxaliplatin as a 5 days on/16 days off regimen, either at a constant rate (flat FFL 5–16) or chronomodulated over 24 hours (chrono FFL 5–16), or as a 4 days on/10 days off regimen chronomodulated over 24 hours (chrono FFL 4–10). Results are from three randomized phase III trials[78–80] and from phase II trials.[81,82]

SURGERY OF METASTASES AFTER CHRONOTHERAPY: A NEW STRATEGY WITH CURATIVE INTENT

The achievement of a 50% or greater objective response rate with the three-drug chronomodulated regimen allowed surgical resection of metastases in a substantial proportion of patients.[83] In a retrospective study, we examined the outcome of patients with initially unresectable colorectal metastases who underwent infusional chemotherapy with 5-FU, leucovorin, and oxaliplatin, followed by surgery at the Hôpital Paul Brousse, Villejuif, France.[84] The cohort involves 389 patients, with a median follow-up of 5.5 years and a minimum follow-up of 3.5 years. Out of these 389 patients, 151 had unresectable liver-only metastases and have been analysed. Seventy-seven patients (51%) underwent liver surgery with curative intent; 58 patients had a complete resection. A complete histological response was documented in 4 patients. The median overall survival of the 151 patients with liver-only disease was 24 months (95% CI 19–28 months), with 28% surviving at 5 years (95% CI 20–35%) (Figure 55.8). The 77 operated patients had a median overall survival of 48 months (95% CI 25–71 months). The estimated 5-year survival rate of the operated patients was 50% (95% CI 38–61%). The median overall survival of the 58 patients in complete resection has not been reached. For comparison, the median overall survival of the 74 non-operated patients was 15.5 months (95% CI 13.5–17.5 months).[84] The surgery-related morbidity rate was less than 10%, and was comparable to that observed in patients with primary resection.[83]

Thus, combining effective and safe chemotherapy and surgery altered the natural history of primary unresectable colorectal cancer metastases. This study further emphasized the need for an active collaboration between surgeons and oncologists.

Figure 55.9 summarizes the relationship between the objective response rate produced by infusional 5-FU–LV–oxaliplatin and the rate of patients who could subsequently undergo a complete surgical resection of metastases within the multicentre setting of our group.

CONCLUSIONS AND PERSPECTIVES

The method of chronomodulation, consisting in the extrapolation of the times of least toxicity of chemotherapy from mice to human beings, has been validated in patients with metastatic colorectal cancer using clinical phase III trial methodology. It has led to the recognition of the activity of a new drug, oxaliplatin, against colorectal cancer, and has given rise to a new curative-intent management of patients with metastatic disease.

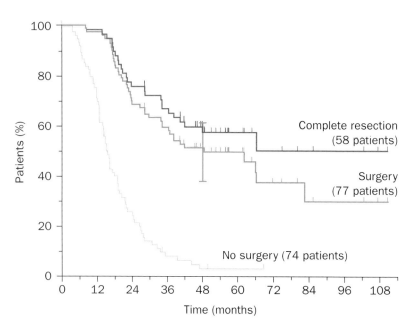

Figure 55.8 Survival of 151 patients with previously unresectable liver metastases from colorectal cancer treated with chronomodulated 5-FU–LV–oxaliplatin prior to reconsideration of surgery of metastases. Survival curves are drawn according to surgery outcome. The median survival was 15.5 months in the 74 non-operated patients and 48 months in the 77 operated patients. In those 58 patients with macroscopically complete resection, the median survival has not been reached at 5 years.[84]

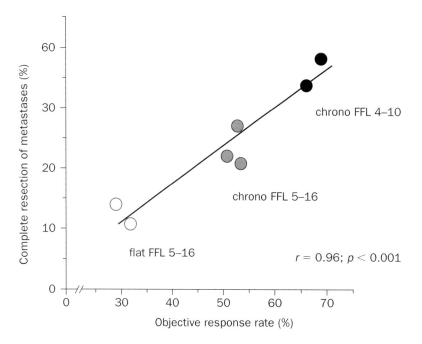

Figure 55.9 Relationship between objective response rate and rate of postsurgical complete responses in chemotherapy-naive patients with previously unresectable metastases from colorectal cancer (same dataset as in Figure 55.7).

Survival or quality of life as endpoints

Chronomodulated delivery of 5-FU–LV and oxaliplatin decreased toxicity, increased dose intensity, and improved antitumour activity in terms of response rate. The data are supportive of a survival improvement. Thus, intensified chronotherapy regimens seem to produce even better patient outcome.[82] The Chronotherapy Group of the EORTC is currently investigating the role of chronomodulation of the three-drug combination in patients with metastatic colorectal cancer with respect to survival and quality

Table 55.5 Contribution of chronomodulation: phase III randomized trial[80]

	5-FU–LV–oxaliplatin		
	Constant-rate infusion	Chronomodulated delivery[a]	*p*
Patients	93	93	
Hospitalization	31	10	0.01
Mucositis (grade 3–4)	74	14	0.001
Diarrhoea (grade 3–4)	26	29	NS
Peripheral neuropathy			
(grade 2, functional impairment)	31	16	0.01
Objective responses	29	50	0.003
Progression-free survival			
(months)	7.9	9.8	0.2
Survival (months)	16.9	15.9	NS

[a]5 days on/16 days off.

of life in a multicentre randomized trial (EORTC 05963).

New drugs and combinations

Over the last few years, two new drugs, irinotecan and oxaliplatin, have demonstrated modest yet definitive activity against colorectal cancer, similar to that of 5-FU. Our experience makes it clear that combinations of these agents should benefit considerably from chronopharmacological optimization. Because chronomodulated infusions are usually better tolerated than standard administration modalities, early phase II combination trials should allow us to safely and fully explore the antitumour efficacy potential of a new regimen. Clinical studies of chronomodulated combinations of irinotecan and 5-FU–LV, with or without oxaliplatin, are currently ongoing[85] (C Garufi, personal communication; H Curé and J Chipponi, personal communication; F Lévi and S Giacchetti, ongoing pilot study).

Neoadjuvant and adjuvant chronotherapy

The combination of chronotherapy with surgery has achieved long-term survival in patients with previously unresectable metastases from colorectal cancer.

The role of this effective and well-tolerated chemotherapy regimen needs to be further assessed as a neoadjuvant treatment in these patients within randomized trials. The relevance of chronotherapy to improve disease-free survival or survival also deserves to be evaluated in adjuvant situations, i.e. in patients with poor-prognosis Dukes B2 or C colon cancer. The combination of chronomodulated infusions with radiation therapy also represents an area of ongoing development of neoadjuvant chronotherapy in gastrointestinal malignancies, at both experimental and clinical levels[77,86] (Protocol EORTC 5991).

Circadian rhythmicity as a prognostic factor

Prognostic factors have a strong influence on the natural history of colorectal cancer liver metastases. Combinations of several of these factors led to median survival times varying from 3.8 to 21.3 months in the absence of specific therapy.[87–89] Cancer-associated alterations of the circadian system may constitute an additional prognostic factor for outcome, especially in patients receiving chronotherapy.

Thus, the 'group chronotherapy' approach, where all patients receive the same chronomodulated chemotherapy regimen, relies on the fact that groups of cancer patients who enter clinical trials exhibit significant circadian rhythms in almost every variable investigated.[7,8,90,91] Nevertheless, investigations of rhythms in individual patients and/or in subgroups of cancer patients with very advanced disease and/or with a poor performance status have shown marked alterations in circadian rhythms (reviewed in reference 50). The relevance of the rest–activity circadian cycle for quality of life and survival was prospectively investigated in 200 patients with metastatic colorectal cancer receiving chronotherapy. Patients with a marked rest–activity cycle had a better quality of life and a longer survival than those with poor rhythmicity. Survival at 2 years was fivefold higher in patients with a marked rhythm. Multivariate analysis indicated that the prognostic value of circadian rhythmicity in rest–activity was independent of that of well-known prognostic factors such as performance status or tumour burden.[92] An ongoing multicentre study is further investigating the relevance of circadian rhythms for outcome in patients receiving conventional versus chronomodulated chemotherapy (an additional study to EORTC 5963). The administration of specific supportive care for treating circadian-system dysfunctions may become indicated in patients with disturbed circadian function, prior to delivery of chronotherapy.

ACKNOWLEDGEMENTS

We are indebted to all our colleagues and friends from Hôpital Paul Brousse and from the Chronotherapy Group of the European Organization for Research and Treatment of Cancer. This chapter could not have been written without their active scientific contribution and exciting discussions throughout the past several years.

We thank M Lévi for fine editorial assistance and the Association pour la Recherche sur le Temps Biologique et la Chronothérapie, Hôpital Paul Brousse, Villejuif, for supporting these research activities.

REFERENCES

1. Touitou Y, Haus E (eds), *Biologic Rhythms in Clinical and Laboratory Medicine.* Berlin: Springer-Verlag, 1992.
2. Redfern PH, Lemmer B (eds), *Handbook of Experimental Pharmacology.* Berlin: Springer-Verlag, 1996.
3. Dunlap JC, Molecular bases for circadian clocks. *Cell* 1999; **96:** 271–90.
4. Brown SA, Schibler U, The ins and outs of circadian timekeeping. *Curr Opin Genet Develop* 1999; **9:** 588–94.
5. Klein DC, Moore RY, Reppert SM, *Suprachiasmatic Nucleus. The Mind's Clock.* Oxford: Oxford University Press, 1991.
6. Moore RY, Entrainment pathways and the functional organization of the circadian system. *Prog Brain Res* 1996; **111:** 103–19.
7. Lévi F, Chronotherapy for gastrointestinal cancers. *Curr Opin Oncol* 1996; **8:** 334–41.
8. Lévi F, Chronopharmacology of anticancer agents. In: *Handbook of Experimental Pharmacology.* Vol. 125: *Physiology and Pharmacology of Biological Rhythms.* Chap 11: *Cancer Chemotherapy* (Redfern PH, Lemmer B, eds). Berlin: Springer-Verlag, 1996: 299–331.
9. Burns ER, Beland SS, Effect of biological time on the determination of the LD50 of 5-fluorouracil in mice. *Pharmacology* 1984; **28:** 296–300.
10. Zhang R, Lu Z, Liu T et al, Relationship between circadian-dependent toxicity of 5-fluorodeoxyuridine and circadian rhythms of pyrimidine enzymes: possible relevance to fluoropyrimidine chemotherapy. *Cancer Res* 1993; **53:** 2816–22.
11. Von Roemeling R, Hrusheksy WJM, Determination of the therapeutic index of floxuridine by its circadian infusion pattern. *J Natl Cancer Inst* 1990; **82:** 386–93.
12. English J, Aherne GW, Marks V, The effect of timing of a single injection on the toxicity of methotrexate in the rat. *Cancer Chemother Pharmacol* 1982; **9:** 114–17.
13. Klein F, Danober L, Roulon A et al, Circadian rhythms in murine tolerance for the anticancer agent mitomycin-C (Mit-C). *Annu Rev Chronopharmacol* 1989; **5:** 367–70.
14. Sothern RB, Haus R, Langevin TR et al, Profound circadian stage dependence of mitomycin-C toxicity. *Annu Rev Chronopharmacol* 1989; **5:** 389–92.
15. Ohdo S, Makinosumi T, Ishizaki T et al, Cell cycle-dependent chronotoxicity of irinotecan hydrochloride in mice. *J Pharmacol Exp Ther* 1997; **283:** 1383–8.
16. Filipski E, Lévi F, Vadrot N et al, Circadian changes in irinotecan toxicity in mice. *Proc Am Assoc Cancer Res* 1997; **38:** 305(Abst 2048).
17. Boughattas N, Lévi F, Fournier C et al, Circadian rhythm in toxicities and tissue uptake of 1,2-diamminocyclohexane(trans-1)oxalatoplatinum(ii) in mice. *Cancer Res* 1989; **49:** 3362–8.
18. Codacci-Pisanelli G, Van Der Wilt C, Pinedo H et al, Antitumor activity, toxicity and inhibition of thymidilate synthase of prolonged administration of 5-fluorouracil in mice. *Eur J Cancer* 1995; **31A:** 1517–25.
19. Boughattas NA, Hecquet H, Fournier C et al, Comparative pharmacokinetics of oxaliplatin (l-OHP) and carboplatin (CBDCA) in mice with reference to circadian dosing time. *Biopharm Drug Disp* 1994; **15:** 1–13.
20. Malmary-Nebot M, Labat C, Casanovas A et al, Aspect chronobiologique de l'action du methotréxate sur la dihydrofolate réductase. *Ann Pharm Fr* 1985; **43:** 337–43.
21. El Kouni MH, Naguib FNM, Park KS et al, Circadian rhythm of hepatic uridine phosphorylase activity and plasma concentration of uridine in mice. *Biochem Pharmacol* 1990; **40:** 2479–85.
22. Naguib FNM, Soong SJ, El Kouni MH, Circadian rhythm of orotate phosphoribosyltransferase, pyrimidine nucleoside phosphorylases and dihydrouracil dehydrogenase in mouse liver. *Biochem Pharmacol* 1993; **45:** 667–73.
23. Lincoln DW, Hrushesky WJM, Wood PA, Circadian organization of thymidylate synthase (TS) activity in normal tissues: a possible basis for 5-fluorouracil chronotherapeutic advantage. *Int J Cancer* 2000; **88:** 479–85.
24. Porsin B, Formento JL, Filipski E et al, Dihydropyrimidine dehydrogenase circadian rhythm in both enzyme activity and gene expression from mouse liver. Submitted.
25. Belanger PM, Labrecque G, Biological rhythms in hepatic drug metabolism and biliary systems. In: *Biologic Rhythms in Clinical and Laboratory Medicine* (Touitou Y, Haus E, eds). Berlin: Springer-Verlag, 1992: 403–9.
26. Li XM, Metzger G, Filipski E et al, Pharmacologic modulation of reduced glutathione (GSH) circadian rhythms by buthionine sul-

foximine (BSO): relationship with cisplatin (CDDP) toxicity in mice. *Toxicol Appl Pharmacol* 1997; **143:** 281–90.

27. Li XM, Metzger G, Filipski E et al, Modulation of nonprotein sulfhydryl compounds rhythm with buthionine sulfoximine: relationship with oxaliplatin toxicity in mice. *Arch Toxicol* 1998; **72:** 574–9.

28. Martineau-Pivoteau N, Cussac-Buchdahl C, Chollet P et al, Circadian variation in O^6-methylguanine-DNA methyltransferase activity in mouse liver. *Anticancer Drugs* 1996; **7:** 1–7.

29. Haus E, Halberg F, Scheving L et al, Increased tolerance of leukemic mice to arabinosylcytosine with schedule-adjusted to circadian system. *Science* 1972; **177:** 80–2.

30. Peters GJ, Van Dijk J, Nadal JC et al, Diurnal variation in the therapeutic efficacy of 5-fluorouracil against murine colon cancer. *In Vivo* 1987; **1:** 113–18.

31. D'Attino RM, Filipski E, Granda TG et al, Irinotecan (CPT-11) and oxaliplatin (*l*-OHP) synergistic activity at specific circadian times in tumor-bearing mice. *Proc Am Assoc Cancer Res* 2000; **41:** Abst 1268.

32. Scheving LE, Burns ER, Halberg F et al, Combined chronochemotherapy of L1210 leukemic mice using β-D-arabino-furanosylcytosine, cyclophosphamide, vincristine, methylprednisolone and *cis*-diamminedichloroplatinum. *Chronobiologia* 1980; **17:** 33–40.

33. Buchi KN, Moore JG, Hrushesky WJM et al, Circadian rhythm of cellular proliferation in the human rectal mucosa. *Gastroenterology* 1991; **101:** 410–15.

34. Killman SA, Cronkite ZEP, Fliedner TM et al, Mitotic indices of human bone marrow cells. 1. Number and cytologic distribution of mitoses. *Blood* 1962; **19:** 743–50.

35. Mauer AM, Diurnal variation of proliferative activity in the human bone marrow. *Blood* 1965; **26:** 1–7.

36. Smaaland R, Laerum OD, Lote K et al, DNA synthesis in human bone marrow is circadian stage dependent. *Blood* 1991; **77:** 2603–11.

37. Smaaland R, Laerum OD, Sothern RB et al, Colony-forming unit–granulocyte–macrophage and DNA synthesis of human bone marrow are circadian stage-dependent and show covariation. *Blood* 1992; **79:** 2281–7.

38. Smaaland R, Abrahamsen JF, Svardal AM, DNA cell cycle distribution and glutathione (GSH) content according to circadian stage in bone marrow of cancer patients. *Br J Cancer* 1992; **66:** 39–45.

39. Brown WR, A review and mathematical analysis of circadian rhythms in cell proliferation in mouse, rat and human epidermis. *J Invest Dermatol* 1991; **97:** 273–80.

40. Warnakulasuriya KAAS, MacDonald DG, Diurnal variation in labelling index in human buccal epithelium. *Arch Oral Biol* 1993; **38:** 1107–11.

41. Smaaland R, Svardal AM, Lote K et al, Glutathione content in human bone marrow and circadian stage relation to DNA synthesis. *J Natl Cancer Inst* 1991; **83:** 1092–8.

42. Tuchman M, Roemeling RV, Lanning RM et al, Sources of variability of dihydropyrimidine dehydrogenase activity in human blood mononuclear cells. *Annu Rev Chronopharmacol* 1989; **5:** 399–402.

43. Harris B, Song R, Soong S et al, Relationship between dihydropyrimidine dehydrogenase activity and plasma 5-fluorouracil levels: evidence for circadian variation of plasma drug levels in cancer patients receiving 5-fluorouracil by protracted continuous infusion. *Cancer Res* 1990; **50:** 197–201.

44. Langouët AM, Metzger G, Comisso M, Plasma concentration of 5-fluorouracil and mononuclear cell dihydropyrimidine dehydrogenase activity in patients treated with different chronomodulated schedules. *Biol Rhythm Res* 1995; **26:** 409 (Abst 135).

45. Bjarnason GA, Jordan RCK, Sothern RB, Circadian variation in the expression of cell-cycle proteins in human oral epithelium. *Am J Pathol* 199; **154:** 613–22.

46. Bjarnason GA, Jordan RCK, Wood PA et al, Circadian expression of clock genes in human oral epithelium and skin: association with cell cycle progression. *Am J Pathol* 2001; **158:** 1793–801.

47. Lévi F, Zidani R, Llory JF et al, for the International Organization for Cancer Chronotherapy, Final efficacy update at 7 years of flat vs chronomodulated infusion (chrono) of oxaliplatin, 5-fluorouracil and leucovorin as first line treatment of metastatic colorectal cancer. *Proc Am Soc Clin Oncol* 2000; **19:** 242a (Abst 936).

48. Klevecz R, Shymko R, Braly P, Circadian gating of S phase in human ovarian cancer. *Cancer Res* 1987; **47:** 6267–71.

49. Smaaland R, Lote K, Sothern RB et al, DNA synthesis and ploidy in non-Hodgkin's lymphomas demonstrate variation depending on circadian stage of cell sampling. *Cancer Res* 1993; **53:** 3129–38.

50. Mormont MC, Lévi F, Circadian system alterations during cancer processes: a review. *Int J Cancer* 1997; **70:** 1–10.

51. Koren G, Ferrazini G, Sohl H et al, Chronopharmacology of methotrexate pharmacokinetics in childhood leukemia. *Chronobiol Intern* 1992; **9:** 434–8.

52. Nowakowska-Dulawa E, Circadian rhythm in 5-fluorouracil (FU) pharmacokinetics and tolerance. *Chronobiologia* 1990; **17:** 27–35.

53. Petit E, Milano G, Lévi F et al, Circadian varying plasma concentration of 5-FU during 5-day continuous venous infusion at constant rate in cancer patients. *Cancer Res* 1988; **48:** 1676–9.

54. Metzger G, Massari C, Etienne MC et al, Spontaneous or imposed circadian changes in plasma concentrations of 5-fluorouracil coadministered with folinic acid and oxaliplatin: relationship with mucosal toxicity in cancer patients. *Clin Pharmacol Ther* 1994; **56:** 190–201.

55. Fleming GF, Schilsky RL, Mick R et al, Circadian variation of 5-fluorouracil (5-FU) and cortisol plasma levels during continuous-infusion 5-FU and leucovorin (LV) in patients with hepatic or renal dysfunction. *Proc Am Soc Clin Oncol* 1994; **13:** 139 (Abst 352).

56. Thiberville L, Compagnon C, Moore N et al, Plasma 5-fluorouracil and alpha-fluoro-beta-alanin accumulation in lung cancer patients treated with continuous infusion of cisplatin and 5-fluorouracil. *Cancer Chemother Pharmacol* 1994; **35:** 64–70.

57. Bressolle F, Joulia JM, Pinguet F et al, Circadian rhythm of 5-fluorouracil population pharmacokinetics in patients with metastatic colorectal cancer. *Cancer Chemother Pharmacol* 1999; **44:** 295–302.

58. Takimoto CH, Yee LK, Venzon DJ et al, High inter- and intrapatient variation in 5-fluorouracil plasma concentrations during a prolonged drug infusion. *Clin Cancer Res* 1999; **5:** 1347–52.

59. Joly AC, Monnet I, Chouaid C et al, Continuous infusion of 5-fluorouracil and non-small cell lung cancer (NSCLC): circadian rhythms and influence of a corticotherapy. In: *Proceedings of the 28th European Symposium on Clinical Pharmacology Berlin*, 14–16 October 1999: Abst 195.

60. Langouët AM, Metzger G, Comisso M et al, Plasma drug concentration control through time-programmed administration. *Proc Am Assoc Cancer Res* 1996; **37:** 196 (Abst 1253).

61. Assier I, Leger-Enreille A, Bargnoux PJ et al, Relationship of dose-limiting toxicity (DLT) with plasma 5-fluorouracil (5-FU) accumulation during chronomodulated (CM) infusion of 5-FU and l-folinic acid (FA). *Proc Am Assoc Cancer Res* 1996; **37:** 180 (Abst 1232).

62. Lévi F, Metzger G, Massari C, Milano G, Oxaliplatin. Pharmacokinetics and chronopharmacological aspects. *Clin Pharmacokinet* 2000; **36:** 1–21.

63. Chevalier V, Kwiatkovsky F, Cure H et al, A new prognostic indicator in metastatic colo-rectal cancer treated by chronomodu-

lated infusion of high-dose 5-fluorouracil and l-folinic acid. *Proc Am Assoc Cancer Res* 2000; **41:** 281–2 (Abst 1792).

64. Hryniuk WM, The importance of dose intensity in the outcome of chemotherapy. In: *Important Advances in Oncology* (DeVita VT, Holman S, Rosenberg SA, eds). Philadelphia: JB Lippincott, 1988: 121–42.

65. Lévi F, Soussan A, Adam R et al, A phase I–II trial of five-day continuous intravenous infusion of 5-fluorouracil delivered at circadian rhythm modulated rate in patients with metastatic colorectal cancer. *J Infus Chemother* 1995; **5:** 153–8.

66. Bjarnason GA, Kerr IG, Doyle N et al, Phase I study of 5-fluorouracil and leucovorin by a 14-day circadian infusion in metastatic adenocarcinoma patients. *Cancer Chemother Pharmacol* 1993; **33:** 221–8.

67. Garufi C, Lévi F, Aschelter AM et al, A phase I trial of five day chronomodulated infusion of 5-fluorouracil and *l*-folinic acid in patients with metastatic colorectal cancer. *Eur J Cancer* 1997; **33:** 1566–71.

68. Curé H, Chevalier V, Adenis A et al, Phase II trial of chronomodulated infusion of high-dose 5-fluorouracil and *l*-folinic acid in previously untreated patients with metastatic colorectal cancer. Submitted.

69. Jolivet J, Létourneau Y, Colorectal cancer chronotherapy: implementation in general hospitals and clinical results. In: *Biological Clocks. Mechanisms and Applications* (Touitou Y, ed). Amsterdam: Elsevier, 1998: 483–90.

70. Caussanel JP, Lévi F, Brienza S et al, Phase I trial of 5-day continuous infusion of oxaliplatinum at circadian-modulated vs constant rate. *J Natl Cancer Inst* 1990; **82:** 1046–50.

71. Lévi F, Perpoint B, Garufi C et al, Oxaliplatin activity against metastatic colorectal cancer. A phase II study of 5-day continuous venous infusion at circadian rhythm modulated rate. *Eur J Cancer* 1993; **29:** 1280–4.

72. Abigerges D, Chabot GG, Armand JP et al, Phase I and pharmacologic studies of the camptothecin analog irinotecan administered every 3 weeks in cancer patients. *J Clin Oncol* 1995; **13:** 210–21.

73. Giacchetti S, Zidani R, Goldwasser F et al, Chronomodulated CPT-11. A pilot study. *Proc Am Soc Clin Oncol* 1999; **18:** 259a (Abst 996).

74. Lévi F, Misset JL, Brienza S et al, A chronopharmacologic phase II clinical trial with 5-fluorouracil, folinic acid and oxaliplatin using an ambulatory multichannel programmable pump. High antitumor effectiveness against metastatic colorectal cancer. *Cancer* 1992; **69:** 893–900.

75. Focan C, Kreutz F, Focan-Henrard D, Moeneclaey N, Chronotherapy with 5-fluorouracil, folinic acid and carboplatin for metastatic colorectal cancer; an interesting therapeutic index in a phase II trial. *Eur J Cancer* 2000; **36:** 341–7.

76. Marsh RD, Chu NM, Vauthey JN et al, Preoperative treatment of patients with locally advanced unresectable rectal adenocarcinoma utilizing continuous chronobiologically shaped 5-fluorouracil infusion and radiation therapy. *Cancer* 1996; **78:** 217–25.

77. Penberthy DR, Rich TA, Shelton III CH et al, A pilot study of chronomodulated infusional 5-fluorouracil chemoradiation for pancreatic cancer. *Ann Oncol* 2001; **12:** 681–4.

78. Giacchetti S, Perpoint B, Zidani R et al, for the International Organization of Cancer, Phase III multicenter randomized trial of oxaliplatin added to chronomodulated fluorouracil–leucovorin as first line treatment of metastatic colorectal cancer. *J Clin Oncol* 2000; **18:** 136–47.

79. Lévi F, Zidani R, Vannetzel JM et al, Chronomodulated versus fixed infusion rate delivery of ambulatory chemotherapy with oxaliplatin, 5-fluorouracil and folinic acid in patients with colorectal cancer metastases. A randomized multiinstitutional trial. *J Natl Cancer Inst* 1994; **86:** 1608–17.

80. Lévi F, Zidani R, Misset JL, for The International Organization for Cancer Chronotherapy, Randomized multicentre trial of chronotherapy with oxaliplatin, fluorouracil, and folinic acid in metastatic colorectal cancer. *Lancet* 1997; **350:** 681–6.

81. Bertheault-Cvitkovic F, Jami A, Ithzaki M et al, Biweekly dose intensification of circadian chronotherapy with 5-fluorouracil, folinic acid and oxaliplatin in patients with metastatic colorectal cancer. *J Clin Oncol* 1996; **14:** 2950–8.

82. Lévi F, Zidani R, Brienza S et al, for the International Organization for Cancer Chronotherapy, A multicenter evaluation of intensified ambulatory chronomodulated chemotherapy with oxaliplatin, fluorouracil and leucovorin as initial treatment of patients with metastatic colorectal cancer. *Cancer* 1999; **85:** 2532–40.

83. Bismuth H, Adam R, Lévi F et al, Resection of nonresectable liver metastases from colorectal cancer after neoadjuvant chemotherapy. *Ann Surg* 1996; **224:** 509–22.

84. Giacchetti S, Itzhaki M, Gruia G et al, Long term survival of patients with unresectable colorectal liver metastases following infusional chemotherapy with 5-fluorouracil, folinic acid, oxaliplatin and surgery. *Ann Oncol* 1999; **10:** 1–7.

85. Garufi C, Dogliotti L, D'Attino RM et al, Irinotecan (CPT-11) and chronomodulated infusion of 5-fluorouracil and folinic acid (CPT-11/FF$_{5-16}$) in patients with advanced colorectal cancer: a phase I study. *Cancer* 2001; **51:** 712–20.

86. Kirichenko AV, Rich TA, Radiation enhancement by 9-aminocamptothecin: the effect of fractionation and timing of administration. *Int J Radiat Oncol Biol Phys* 1999; **44:** 659–64.

87. Stangl R, Altendorf-Hofmann A, Charnley RM, Scheele J, Factors influencing the natural history of colorectal liver metastases. *Lancet* 1994; **343:** 1405–10.

88. Rougier Ph, Milan C, Lazorthes F et al, Prospective study of prognostic factors in patients with unresected hepatic metastases from colorectal cancer. *Br J Surg* 1995; **82:** 1397–400.

89. Lahr CJ, Soong SJ, Cloud G et al, A multifactorial analysis of prognostic factors in patients with liver metastases from colorectal carcinoma. *J Clin Oncol* 1983; **11:** 720–6.

90. Mormont MC, Hecquet B, Bogdan A et al, Non-invasive estimation of the circadian rhythm in serum cortisol in patients with ovarian or colorectal cancer. *Int J Cancer* 1998; **78:** 421–4.

91. Mormont MC, Lévi F, Cancer chronotherapy: principles, applications and perspectives. In: *Cancer Medicine*, 5th edn (Holland JF, Frei E III, Bast RC, Kufe DW et al, eds). Hamilton, Ontario: BC Decker, 2001.

92. Mormont MC, Waterhouse J, Bleuzen P et al, Marked 24-h rest–activity rhythms are associated with better quality of life, better response and longer survival in patients with metastatic colorectal cancer and good performance status. *Clin Cancer Res* 2000; **6:** 3038–45.

56

Which treatment in first line? The US approach

Michael J O'Connell

HISTORICAL BACKGROUND

The chemotherapeutic treatment of metastatic colorectal cancer in the USA began with the discovery of 5-fluorouracil (5-FU) in the late 1950s. Single-agent activity was demonstrated using a variety of dosage administration schedules. The most widely adopted 5-FU schedules in the USA were an 'intensive course' ('bolus daily × 5') regimen or a weekly schedule.[1–3] Although response rates predictably varied among the various uncontrolled trials, approximately 20% of patients experienced an objective tumor response that was almost always partial and lasted only a few months. There was no credible evidence from controlled clinical trials that single-agent 5-FU could improve patient survival.

Based upon the striking success of 'empiric' combination chemotherapy in certain childhood tumors and hematologic malignancies such as Hodgkin's disease in the 1970s, a wide variety of combination chemotherapy regimens were tested against metastatic colorectal cancer. The principle was to combine active agents with different mechanisms of action and non-overlapping toxicities. Many drugs were combined with 5-FU in this manner, including such agents as mitomycin C, semustine (methyl-CCNU), cisplatin, vincristine, and hydroxyurea. Unfortunately, this strategy did not result in any therapeutic gain against advanced colorectal cancer,[4] and exposed patients to a variety of unpleasant and sometimes dangerous side-effects.

BIOCHEMICAL MODULATION OF 5-FU BY LEUCOVORIN

5-FU acts primarily by blocking thymidylate synthase in tumor cells (see also Chapters 38 and 41–46), and thereby interferes with DNA synthesis. This inhibition is enhanced by the addition of leucovorin (folinic acid),[5] which increases the intracellular levels of reduced folates. In some preclinical systems, a high concentration of leucovorin was necessary to achieve the optimal cytotoxic effect;[6] however, in others,[7] low leucovorin concentrations were sufficient. These observations led to the development of two schedules of combining 5-FU and leucovorin for the treatment of colorectal cancer: a weekly regimen using high doses of leucovorin[8] and an intensive-course regimen using both high and low doses of leucovorin.[9,10]

Various combinations of 5-FU and leucovorin were shown to produce an improvement in objective tumor response rates,[8–12] and some demonstrated a small but statistically significant improvement in patient survival[9,10] compared with single-agent 5-FU. A meta-analysis confirmed the improvement in tumor response associated with leucovorin-modulated 5-FU, but failed to ascertain any significant improvement in survival[13] for patients with advanced disease.

Randomized clinical trials subsequently demonstrated no advantage to the use of high doses of leucovorin compared with low doses in conjunction with intensive-course 5-FU,[9,10] and no difference between weekly 5-FU plus high-dose leucovorin and intensive-course 5-FU plus low-dose leucovorin[14] in the treatment of advanced colorectal cancer.

IRINOTECAN

Irinotecan (CPT-11) is an inhibitor of the enzyme topoisomerase I (see also Chapters 49 and 52–54). It blocks DNA replication, resulting in multiple single-strand DNA breaks.[15] It has definite single-agent activity in patients with colorectal carcinoma, and can produce tumor response rates in 15–20% of patients previously treated with 5-FU.[16–18]

Irinotecan was shown to provide a significant sur-

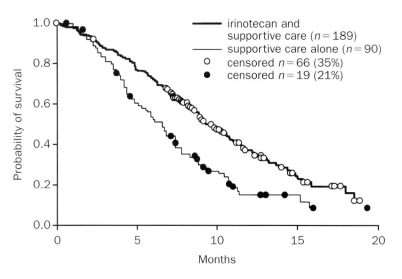

Figure 56.1 Survival of patients with advanced colorectal cancer who had failed a prior 5-FU regimen for metastatic disease. Reproduced with permission from Cunningham D, Pyrhonen S, James RD et al, Randomized trial of irinotecan plus supportive care versus supportive care alone after fluorouracil failure for patients with metastatic colorectal cancer. *Lancet* 1998; **352:** 1413–18.[19]

vival advantage over supportive care in a randomized clinical trial involving patients previously treated with 5-FU[19] (see Figure 56.1). These results were confirmed on comparing such 5-FU-refractory patients treated with irinotecan versus others treated with infusional regimens of 5-FU.[20] These data led to Food and Drug Administration (FDA) approval of irinotecan as second-line treatment for patients with advanced colorectal cancer in the USA. Since both weekly and every-three-week regimens of irinotecan had been shown to be active in phase II trials, each of these regimens was approved by the FDA.

IRINOTECAN PLUS 5-FU PLUS LEUCOVORIN

In consideration of the data previously discussed, it was logical to explore the addition of irinotecan to the combination of 5-FU and leucovorin for the first-line treatment of patients with metastatic colorectal cancer. A prospectively randomized clinical trial reported at the 1999 meeting of the American Society of Clinical Oncology indicated significant improvement in tumor response and time to progression in advanced colorectal cancer patients treated with irinotecan plus 5-FU plus leucovorin compared with 5-FU and leucovorin alone, and a third treatment arm of single-agent irinotecan.[21] The long-term follow-up of this trial[22] confirmed these findings, and also documented a significant improvement in patient survival (see Figure 56.2). Furthermore, a second controlled clinical trial also showed significant improvements in tumor response, time to progression, and survival when irinotecan was added to a

continuous-infusion schedule of 5-FU[23] for the first-line treatment of advanced colorectal cancer. These data (see Table 56.1) served as the basis for FDA approval (in April 2000) of the combination of irinotecan plus 5-FU plus leucovorin as first-line treatment for metastatic colorectal cancer. The dosage administration schedule of the irinotecan, 5-FU, leucovorin regimen from this trial is summarized in Table 56.2.

Irinotecan combined with 5-FU and leucovorin can reasonably be considered a 'standard' treatment based on the controlled clinical trials summarized above. However, there are several factors that must be taken into consideration to put these findings in clinical perspective.

1. The magnitude of the benefit of adding irinotecan to the combination of 5-FU and leucovorin is small. In the pivotal study,[22] the confirmed tumor response rate was 39%, the median progression-free survival was 7.0 months, and the median survival was 14.8 months. The median survival of patients who received irinotecan in combination with 5-FU and leucovorin was 2.2 months longer than that of the control group receiving 5-FU and leucovorin alone. There was no evidence of improved long-term patient survival. The limited impact of treatment on patient survival is highlighted in Figure 56.3, where the survival data from the trial reported by Saltz et al[22] are replotted on a time axis extending to 5 years.

2. Irinotecan has been associated with sometimes severe and life-threatening toxicity, predominately profuse diarrhea and leukopenia.[16–18] The

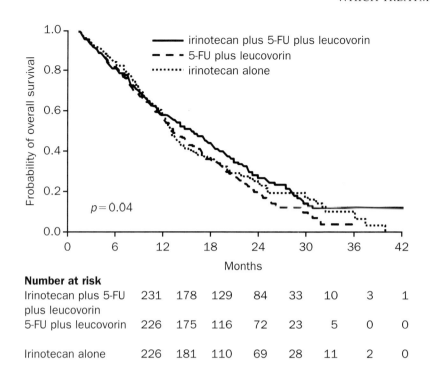

Number at risk

Irinotecan plus 5-FU plus leucovorin	231	178	129	84	33	10	3	1
5-FU plus leucovorin	226	175	116	72	23	5	0	0
Irinotecan alone	226	181	110	69	28	11	2	0

Kaplan–Meier estimates of overall survival; the *p* value was derived from a log-rank test comparing the triple-drug group with the two-drug group

Table 56.1 Comparative efficacy of 5-FU plus leucovorin versus (LV) 5-FU plus leucovorin plus irinotecan as first-line treatment in patients with metastatic colorectal cancer

Study and regimen	Tumor response rate (%)	Median progression-free survival (months)	Median survival (months)
Saltz et al[22]			
Irinotecan + 5-FU + LV	39[a]	7.0	14.8
	$p < 0.001$	$p = 0.004$	$p = 0.04$
5-FU + LV	21[a]	4.3	12.6
Douillard et al[23]			
Irinotecan + 5-FU + LV	49	6.7	17.4
	$p < 0.001$	$p < 0.001$	$p = 0.03$
5-FU + LV	31	4.4	14.1

[a]Tumor response confirmed radiographically.

Table 56.2 Dosage administration schedule of irinotecan, 5-FU, and leucovorin in the pivotal clinical trial[22]

Drug	Dose (mg/m^2)	Route	Frequency[a]
Irinotecan	125	Intravenous (90 min)	Weekly × 4
5-FU	500	Intravenous	Weekly × 4
Leucovorin	20	Intravenous	Weekly × 4

[a]Cycles repeated every 6 weeks.

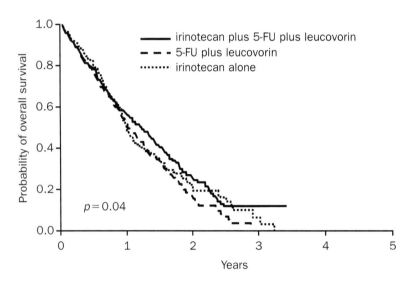

Figure 56.3 Replotted survival curves from Figure 58.2, with the time axis extending to 5 years.

diarrhea is usually manageable through the aggressive use of high-dose loperamide at the first sign of loose stools, and judicious dose reductions in patients who manifest toxicity. Leukopenia is a particular problem in patients with reduced bone marrow reserves, such as rectal cancer patients who have received pelvic irradiation, and the elderly. More experience in a larger patient population will be valuable in further assessing any incremental toxicity associated with the addition of irinotecan to the 5-FU/leucovorin combination.

3. Irinotecan adds substantially to the financial cost of palliative chemotherapy. Using the average wholesale prices (AWP) in the USA, the approximate cost of chemotherapy drugs per month of treatment with the 'Saltz' regimen in a patient with body surface area of 1.8 m^2 is $3770. This compares with $90 per month for intensive-course 5-FU and low-dose leucovorin without irinotecan, as used in the control arm of the Saltz trial. This increased cost must be weighed against improvement in treatment outcome as one factor in clinical decision making.

4. It is not clear whether the *sequential* use of less intensive chemotherapy regimens, such as 5-FU plus leucovorin followed by single-agent irinotecan at the time of tumor progression, could produce similar clinical results to those observed with the use of irinotecan as part of the initial regimen. This strategy might be of particular relevance in patients with slowly growing metastatic disease, the elderly, and those with comorbid conditions that might decrease their tolerance of intensive combination chemotherapy. On the other hand, the use of irinotecan combined with 5-FU and leucovorin might be of special value in medically fit patients with rapidly progressive

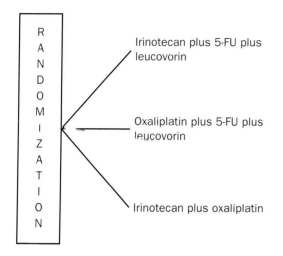

Irinotecan plus 5-FU plus leucovorin

Oxaliplatin plus 5-FU plus leucovorin

Irinotecan plus oxaliplatin

Figure 56.4 Schema of Intergroup Protocol N9741 for first-line treatment of patients with advanced colorectal cancer.

disease, or those with metastatic disease marginally resectable for cure because of the well-documented improvement in tumor response rates with irinotecan combination chemotherapy.

CONCLUSIONS

The currently preferred first-line treatment for many patients with metastatic colorectal cancer in the USA is irinotecan combined with 5-FU and leucovorin given on a weekly administration schedule, acknowledging the limitations discussed above. This recommendation is made in recognition of consistent data from several controlled clinical trials[19-23] indicating reproducible antitumor activity in this disease.

Further clinical research is sorely needed to make more substantive advances in the treatment of metastatic colorectal cancer. To this end, a national Intergroup clinical trial currently ongoing in the USA is comparing irinotecan combined with 5-FU and leucovorin with a regimen of infusional 5-FU and leucovorin combined with another promising drug – oxaliplatin[24-26] – and the combination of irinotecan and oxaliplatin without 5-FU (Figure 56.4 – see also Chapters 50 and 52–54). Perhaps the most beneficial role of these new drug regimens will be shown by controlled trials in the surgical adjuvant setting, where an incremental improvement in long-term survival or cure seems a realistic possibility.

REFERENCES

1. Ramirez G, Korbitz BC, Davis HL Jr, Ansfield FJ, Comparative study of monthly courses versus weekly doses of 5-fluorouracil (NSC-19893). *Cancer Chemother Rep Part 1* 1969; **53**: 243–7.
2. Ansfield F, Klotz J, Nealon T et al, A phase III study comparing the clinical utility of four regimens of 5-fluorouracil: a preliminary report. *Cancer* 1977; **39**: 34–40.
3. Hahn RG, Moertel CG, Schutt AJ, Bruckner HW, A double-blind comparison of intensive course 5-fluorouracil by oral vs. intravenous route in the treatment of colorectal carcinoma. *Cancer* 1975; **35**: 1031–5.
4. O'Connell MJ, Schutt AJ, Moertel CG et al, A randomized clinical trial of combination chemotherapy in advanced colorectal cancer. *Am J Clin Oncol* 1987; **10**: 320–4.
5. Park J, Collins JM, Gazdar AF et al, Enhancement of fluorinated pyrimidine-induced cytotoxicity by leucovorin in human colorectal carcinoma cell lines. *J Natl Cancer Inst* 1988; **80**: 1560–4.
6. Rustum YM, Trave F, Zakrzewski SF et al, Biochemical and pharmacologic basis for potentiation of 5-fluorouracil action by leucovorin. *NCI Monogr* 1987; **5**: 165–70.
7. Keyomarsi K, Moran RG, Folinic acid augmentation of the effects of fluoropyrimidines on murine and human leukemic cells. *Cancer Res* 1986; **46**: 5229–35.
8. Petrelli N, Douglass HO Jr, Herrara L et al, The modulation of fluorouracil with leucovorin in metastatic colorectal carcinoma: a prospective randomized phase III trial. Gastrointestinal Tumor Study Group. *J Clin Oncol* 1989; **7**: 1419–26.
9. Poon MA, O'Connell MJ, Moertel CG et al, Biochemical modulation of fluorouracil: evidence of significant improvement of survival and quality of life in patients with advanced colorectal carcinoma. *J Clin Oncol* 1989; **7**: 1407–17.
10. Poon MA, O'Connell MJ, Wieand HS et al, Biochemical modulation of fluorouracil with leucovorin: confirmatory evidence of improved therapeutic efficacy in advanced colorectal cancer. *J Clin Oncol* 1991; **9**: 1967–72.
11. Erlichman C, Fine S, Wong A et al, A randomized trial of fluorouracil and folinic acid in patients with metastatic colorectal carcinoma. *J Clin Oncol* 1988; **6**: 469–75.
12. Doroshow JH, Bertrand M, Multhauf P et al, Prospective randomized trial comparing 5-FU versus 5-FU and high dose folinic acid for treatment of advanced colorectal cancer. *Proc Am Soc Clin Oncol* 1987; **6**: 96.
13. Advanced Colorectal Cancer Meta-Analysis Project, Modulation of fluorouracil by leucovorin in patients with advanced colorectal cancer: evidence in terms of response rate. *J Clin Oncol* 1992; **10**: 896–903.
14. Buroker TR, O'Connell MJ, Wieand HS et al, Randomized comparison of two schedules of fluorouracil and leucovorin in the treatment of advanced colorectal cancer. *J Clin Oncol* 1994; **12**: 14–20.
15. Creemers GJ, Lund B, Verweij J, Topoisomerase I inhibitors: topotecan and irinotecan. *Cancer Treat Rev* 1994; **20**: 73–96.
16. Pitot HC, Wender DB, O'Connell MJ et al, Phase II trial of irinotecan in patients with metastatic colorectal carcinoma. *J Clin Oncol* 1997; **15**: 2910–19.
17. Rougier P, Bugat R, Douillard JY et al, Phase II study of irinotecan in the treatment of advanced colorectal cancer in chemotherapy-naive patients and patients pretreated with fluorouracil-based chemotherapy. *J Clin Oncol* 1997; **15**: 251–60.
18. Rothenberg ML, Eckardt JR, Kuhn JC et al, Phase II trial of irinotecan in patients with progressive or rapidly recurrent colorectal cancer. *J Clin Oncol* 1996; **14**: 1128–35.
19. Cunningham D, Pyrhonen S, James RD et al, Randomized trial of irinotecan plus supportive care versus supportive care alone

after fluorouracil failure for patients with metastatic colorectal cancer. *Lancet* 1998; **352:** 1413–18.

20. Rougier P, Van Cutsem E, Bajetta E et al, Randomised trial of irinotecan versus fluorouracil by continuous infusion after fluorouracil failure in patients with metastatic colorectal cancer. *Lancet* 1998; **352:** 1407–12.

21. Saltz LB, Locker PK, Pirotta N et al, Weekly irinotecan, leucovorin, and fluorouracil is superior to daily × 5 leucovorin/fluorouracil in patients with previously untreated metastatic colorectal cancer. *Proc Am Soc Clin Oncol* 1999; **18:** 233a (Abst 898).

22. Saltz LB, Cox JV, Blanke C et al, Irinotecan plus fluorouracil and leucovorin for metastatic colorectal cancer. *N Engl J Med* 2000; **343:** 905–14.

23. Douillard JY, Cunningham D, Roth AD et al, Irinotecan combined with fluorouracil compared with fluorouracil alone as first-line treatment for metastatic colorectal cancer: a multicentre randomised trial. *Lancet* 2000; **355:** 1041–7.

24. Cvitkovic E, Ongoing and unsaid on oxaliplatin: the hope. *Br J Cancer* 1998; **4:** 8–11.

25. Diaz-Rubio E, Sastre J, Zaniboni A et al, Oxaliplatin as single agent in previously untreated colorectal carcinoma patients: a phase II multicentric study. *Ann Oncol* 1998; **9:** 105–8.

26. de Gramont A, Figer A, Seymour M et al, Leucovorin and fluorouracil with or without oxaliplatin as first-line treatment in advanced colorectal cancer. *J Clin Oncol* 2000; **18:** 2938–47.

57

Which treatment in first line? The European approach

Philippe Rougier, Harry Bleiberg

INTRODUCTION

In industrialized countries, colorectal cancer is the second most common malignancy after lung cancer in men and breast cancer in women. In Europe in 1990, there were approximately 170 000 new cases and over 90 000 deaths due to the disease.[1] It is generally considered that half of the patients presenting with colorectal cancer have or will further develop metastatic disease. When surgery is not possible, the efficiency of chemotherapy has been clearly established in first-line as well as in second-line treatment.

WHAT TREATMENTS ARE CURRENTLY AVAILABLE?

The 5-fluorouracil story

5-Fluorouracil (5-FU) was synthesized in 1957.[2] Various schedules of bolus 5-FU have been designed. Current response rates were considered to be around 20%, based on an estimation of available clinical trials with response rates ranging from 0% to 87%.[3] This wide variability of response rates was probably due to patient heterogeneity and inadequate, non-standardized, response measurements. Further well-conducted studies showed that the true response rate of 5-FU did not exceed 10–15%. The first investigation with bolus 5-FU and folinic acid (FA, leucovorin) started in 1982.[4] Many studies were initiated, most of which demonstrated a superiority of 5-FU/FA as compared with 5-FU alone in terms of response rate. A meta-analysis of all available data revealed a response rate of 23% with the 5-FU/FA combination as compared with 11% for 5-FU alone. No difference of survival was disclosed, although one should keep in mind that most of these trials

were designed to identify a difference in response rate only[5] (Table 57.1).

The most commonly used bolus 5-FU/FA regimens include the Mayo Clinic schedule (given monthly for 5 days with low-dose FA: 5-FU 450 mg/m^2, FA 20 mg/m^2),[6] the Machover schedule (given monthly for 5 days with high-dose FA: 5-FU 400 mg/m^2, FA 200 mg/m^2 2-hour infusion),[4] and the Roswell Park schedule (given weekly: 5-FU 500 mg/m^2, FA 500 mg/m^2 2-hour infusion).[7] The most commonly used infusional 5-FU regimens include the Lokich regimen (given as a protracted infusion: 5-FU 300 mg/m^2),[8] or the optimized protocols such as the de Gramont schedule (given as a 48-hour both bolus and continuous infusion bimonthly: 5-FU 400 mg/m^2 bolus and 600 mg/m^2 continuous infusion, FA 200 mg/m^2 2-hour infusion on days 1 and 2),[9] the TTD regimen (given as a 48-hour infusion weekly: 5-FU 3000 mg/m^2),[10] the AIO regimen (given as a 24-hour infusion weekly: 5-FU 2600 mg/m^2, FA 500 mg/m^2),[11] and an infusional regimen with pharmacokinetic optimization[12] (Table 57.2).

Many controversies still remain regarding which of these regimens is the most active and should be seen as a reference. Although there are no direct comparisons of the various bolus regimens or the optimized infusional regimens, it can generally be assumed that all bolus 5-FU regimens are similar, as are all optimized infusional ones, and that their use is more dependent on local tradition and organization than on a scientific basis. Response rates derived from phase III studies of bolus 5-FU/FA and of the infusional 5-FU may vary from less than 10%[13] to more than 40%[6] for the bolus regimens and from 12%[14] to 41%[11] for the infusional regimens. Median survival times overlap even more and (besides the best supportive-care studies, which give a median

Table 57.1 Modulation and method of administration of 5-fluorouracil (5-FU) in colorectal cancer: synthesis of meta-analyses of randomized trials performed on individual data (Meta-analysis Group)

Ref	Treatment[a]	No. of patients	Reponse rate (%)	Survival (months)
5	5-FU	1381	11 $p < 10^{-7}$	11 NS
	5-FU/FA		23	11.5
15	5-FU bolus	1219	14 $p = 0.0002$	11.3 $p = 0.04$
	5-FU CI		22	12.1

[a]FA, folinic acid (leucovorin); CI, continuous infusion.
NS, not significant.

survival time of 5–7 months) range between 8.5 and 14 months for most bolus regimens and between 6.5 and 15 months for most infusional regimens. This great variability of response for a given schedule is probably due to patient selection criteria and prognostic factors.

Trials have compared the activity of infusional 5-FU with a bolus 5-FU[9,10,12,15,16] (Table 57.2). Although in the Lokich trial using protracted 5-FU, the response rates were 30% and 7%, respectively ($p < 0.001$), the corresponding median survivals did not differ greatly (10.3 and 11.2 months; $p = 0.379$).[8] In the FFCD–GERCOR trial, the response rate was twice as high for infusional as for bolus 5-FU (32.6% versus 14.4%; $p = 0.0004$) and the progression-free survival was improved, but there was no significant difference in overall survival (median 14.3 months versus 13.1 months; $p = 0.067$).[9] A recent comparison of the AIO regimen to the Mayo Clinic one designed to identify a difference in progression-free survival showed a two-month difference in favour of the AIO regimen.[16] Supporting these single-trial data, a meta-analysis of studies comparing infusional versus bolus 5-FU suggested an advantage in terms of response rate and survival in favour of the infusional treatment.[17]

The toxicity profile of infusional 5-FU appears more favourable, with less leukopenia (1% versus 20%[8]), granulocytopenia (1.9% versus 7.3%[9]), thrombocytopenia (1% versus 3%[8] and 1.9% versus 7.3%[9]), stomatitis (3% versus 11%[8] and 1.9% versus 7.3%[9]), and diarrhoea (2.9% versus 7.3%[9]). The hand–foot

syndrome was observed mainly with infusional 5-FU (23%).[8] Owing to the lack of undisputable scientific evidence of the superiority of one regimen over another in terms of overall survival, all of these regimens are utilized worldwide, with bolus 5-FU (Mayo and Roswell Park regimens) mainly being given in the USA, and infusional 5-FU (de Gramont, AIO, TTD) mainly being given in Europe.

During the last ten years or so, it has also become apparent that treating patients with chemotherapy should significantly improve survival as compared with treating them with best supportive care only (median survival 6 months versus 12 months),[18] and that the administration of systemic chemotherapy at an early stage, before symptoms are present, may also significantly improve survival as compared with giving it when patients are symptomatic (median survival 7 months versus 12 months).[19]

Oral 5-FU prodrugs have been developed for more than 20 years; however, it is only recently that the results of the phase III trials comparing UFT (uracil plus tegafur)[13,20] and capecitabine[21,22] with the Mayo Clinic regimen have suggested comparable levels of activity in terms of response rate and survival and a better tolerability (Table 57.3).

New drugs

The last five years or so have witnessed the development of three new agents active in colorectal cancer. Raltitrexed is an inhibitor of thymidylate synthase,

Table 57.2 Randomized trials testing optimized infusional 5-fluorourcil (5-FU), modulated or not by folinic acid (FA), compared with the 5-FU/FA Machover or Mayo Clinic regimens in patients with metastatic colorectal cancer

Ref	Treatment	No. of patients	Response rate (%)	Progression-free survival	Overall survival
9	5-FU/FA Machover	433	14 $p = 0.002$	22 weeks $p = 0.0012$	57 weeks $p = 0.067$
	LV5FU2 (do Gramont)		33	28 weeks	62 weeks
10	5-FU/FA Mayo Clinic	306	19 $p < 0.05$	23.5 weeks NS	12.5 weeks NS
	5-FU 48 h/week		30	25 weeks	48 weeks
12	5-FU/FA 8 h/week	208	18 $p < 0.0004$	?	13 months $p = NS$
	The same + pharmacokinetic monitoring		35		16 months
16	5-FU/FA Mayo Clinic 5-FU 2.6 g/m²/week	497	?	4 months 4.4 months $p = 0.03$	NS
	5-FU 2.6 g/m² + FA 500 mg/m²/week			6.4 months	

NS: not significant.

oxaliplatin is a diaminocyclohexane platinum complex acting as an alkylating agent and creating DNA adducts different from those of cisplatin, and irinotecan (CPT-11), which is a specific and potent topoisomerase 1 inhibitor acting through its active metabolite SN38. As single agents, their response rates are around 20% and their median survival times range from 10 to 15 months, which are in the range of what has been obtained with most of the 5-FU regimens.[23,24]

For more than 40 years, 5-FU alone or modulated by FA was the only possible treatment for advanced colorectal cancer. Today, many agents and many options are available. Preclinical studies have suggested that the combination of 5-FU, raltitrexed, oxaliplatin, and irinotecan could be synergistic.[25] This synergism is strongly suggested by non-randomized comparisons of the combinations of 5-FU/FA with irinotecan or oxaliplatin and of

raltitrexed with oxaliplatin. It has been further demonstrated in randomized studies of 5-FU/FA with oxaliplatin and irinotecan[26-28] (Table 57.4). The combination of 5-FU/FA with oxaliplatin or irinotecan turned out at the end of the 1990s to be the most active treatment available in advanced colorectal cancer.

Adding oxaliplatin to the 5-FU/FA de Gramont schedule led to a response rate of 51% and a progression-free survival of 8.8 months for the combination, as compared with 22% and 6.1 months for 5-FU/FA alone.[28] Based on the current concept that second and further treatment should equalize overall survival, and following the guidelines adopted by the American Society for Clinical Oncology,[29] progression-free survival could be considered as a valid endpoint to evaluate the activity of the treatment combination (Table 57.4).

In Europe, a combination of irinotecan 180 mg/m²

Table 57.3 Randomized trials testing the new oral 5-FU prodrugs UFT and capecitabine versus the 5-FU/FA Mayo Clinic regimen in patients with metastatic colorectal cancer

Ref	Protocol	No. of patients	Overall response rate (%)	Time to progression (months)	Survival (months)
20	5-FU/FA Mayo	816	15 NS	?	? NS
	UFT + FA		12	?	?
13	5-FU/FA Mayo	380	9 NS	3.3 NS	11.9 NS
	UFT + FA		11	3.4	12.2
21	5-FU/FA Mayo	605	15.5 $p = 0.02$	4.4 NS	?
	Capecitabine		26.2	5.1	
22	5-FU/FA Mayo	602	17.9 $p = 0.013$	4.8 NS	?
	Capecitabine		26.6	5.3	

NS, not significant.

with the biweekly 5-FU/FA de Gramont schedule every 2 weeks or 80 mg/m^2 with the AIO 5-FU/FA schedule weekly × 6 every 7 weeks showed a confirmed response rate of 35%, a progression-free survival of 6.7 months, and a median survival of 17.4 months, as compared with 22%, 4.4 months, and 14.1 months, respectively, for the corresponding 5-FU/FA-alone regimens ($p < 0.001$, $p < 0.001$, $p = 0.031$ respectively)[26] (Table 57.4). The number of patients included in the AIO arm was too small to allow any separate evaluation of this regimen, which is being further investigated in a trial of the EORTC (40986).

In the USA, a combination of irinotecan 125 mg/m^2 with 5-FU 500 mg/m^2 and FA 20 mg/m^2 bolus weekly, for 4 weeks every 6 weeks, showed a response rate of 39%, a progression-free survival of 5.0 months, and a median survival of 14.9 months, as compared with 21%, 3.8 months, and 12 months, respectively, for the 5-FU/FA-alone arm ($p = 0.04$)[27] (Table 57.4).

Based on our analysis, the most active treatments today include a combination of 5-FU, FA, and irinotecan or oxaliplatin, and lead to two important questions:

- Should this type of treatment be given to every patient?
- Is there no room left for one of the 5-FU/FA regimens or for the oral prodrugs?

Developing a strategy implies that parameters other than response rates and overall survival should also be taken into account. These should include patients' physical as well as psychological characteristics, tumour characteristics, the likelihood of secondary curative resection in the case of good tumour response, and finally the biological features of the tumour.

Table 57.4 Randomized trials testing the efficacy of irinotecan and oxaliplatin in combination with 5-FU/FA in patients with metastatic colorectal cancer

Ref	Protocol	No. of patients	Overall response rate (%)	Time to progression (months)	Survival (months)
14	5-FU/FA chronomodulated	100	16 $p < 0.001$	6.1 $p = 0.048$	19.4 NS
	The same + oxaliplatin	100	53	8.7	19.9
28	LV5FU2[a]	210	22 $p = 0.0001$	6.2 $p = 0.0003$	14.7 $p = 0.12$
	LV5FU2 + oxaliplatin	210	51	9	16.2
26	5-FU/FA[b]	187	22 $p < 0.005$	4.4 $p < 0.001$	14.1 $p = 0.031$
	The same + irinotecan	198	35	6.7	17.4
27	5-FU/FA Mayo[c]	226	21	4.3	12.6
	Weekly irinotecan alone	231	—	—	—
	Weekly 5-FU/FA + irinotecan	223	39	7 $p = 0.004$	14.8 $p = 0.04$

[a]LV5FU2 (de Gramont): 200 mg/m^2 FA i.v. for 2 h and 400 mg/m^2 5-FU bolus followed by 600 mg/m^2 5-FU i.v. over 22 h, days 1 and 2 every 2 weeks.

[b]Patients received either the LV5FU2 (de Gramont) regimen or the AIO infusional 5-FU regimen (500 mg/m^2 FA with 2.3 g/m^2 5-FU i.v. administered over 24 h every week).

[c]Mayo Clinic regimen: 20 mg/m^2 FA and 425 mg/m^2 5-FU, both administered as an i.v. bolus for 5 consecutive days every 4 weeks.

NS, not significant.

IMPORTANCE OF PROGNOSTIC FACTORS FOR RESPONSE AND SURVIVAL

For a decade or so, it has been clear that many factors influence response rates and survival, especially patient status, number of tumour sites, white blood cell (WBC) count, haemoglobin, and lactate dehydrogenase (LDH) level, all of which must be considered today when making a choice of chemotherapy regimen.[30] Tumour characteristics will also play a major role in the future, because some may predict resistance or sensitivity or toxicity to certain drugs. We shall briefly summarize how these prognostic factors may be integrated into a chemotherapeutic strategy.

Role of patient status

The benefit of combined chemotherapy in first-line treatment has been demonstrated in selected populations of patients who have volunteered to participate in clinical trials, who have good performance status, no serious concomitant disease and often age below 75 years. Nothing or very little is known on the harm/benefit of these treatments in patients with a poorer performance status and/or with extensive multiple metastases. In all of the reported trials, the most important prognostic factor was the performance status, and this was well illustrated in the largest meta-analysis ever done in metastatic colorectal patients receiving 5-FU-based chemotherapy.[30] The real gain in survival for patients in poor condition remains unknown, and should be explored by strategic trials focusing on this subgroup of patients. Age is also an important issue. In the palliative and adjuvant setting, there is undoubtedly an efficacy of chemotherapy for patients older than 70 years, although it is a little more toxic and less efficient than for younger patients.[31] The capacity of patients to face potentially severe toxicity should therefore be considered, and for each patient all of these factors should be taken into account. Therefore it may be reasonable in patients who are not fit for heavy chemotherapy to recommend one of the well-established 5-FU/FA regimens as first-line chemotherapy.

Role of tumour extension

It is known that in the case of multiple metastatic sites, bulky tumour, or biological abnormalities related to the presence of tumour dissemination (such as high LDH level and/or high WBC count), the prognosis is poor.[30] The benefit of combined chemotherapy in first-line treatment for such patients is not clearly established. However, data from the comparison of the de Gramont and Mayo Clinic schedules suggest that more effective chemotherapy could control the disease and improve survival. Indeed, the number of deaths occurring during the first two months following the first treatment administration, which correspond perhaps to very advanced cases, may be decreased by using combined chemotherapy as first-line treatment; there were 22 deaths in the 5-FU/FA-alone arm, compared with only 2 in the 5-FU/FA/oxaliplatin arm[28] (A de Gramont, personal communication).

Conversely, patients with metastases confined to the liver or the lung who are nevertheless not resectable for reasons of multiplicity, large volume, or bad location seem to be amenable to curative surgery if chemotherapy can induce a major shrinkage of the tumour.[32] This approach is undoubtedly useful for a small proportion of patients. However, the deleterious effect of inappropriate chemotherapy and surgery in unfit patients is a matter of concern,

so that criteria of resectability and patient selection need to be properly defined in specific trials before embarking patients on heavy combined treatments.

Even in cases of resectable liver or lung metastases, one may expect an improvement in disease-free and overall survival by adding neoadjuvant and/or adjuvant chemotherapy to surgery. An EORTC trial is testing this hypothesis and comparing immediate surgery versus surgery with a perioperative chemotherapy (preoperative and, if active, postoperative) using a 5-FU/FA/oxaliplatin combination (EORTC–GITCCG trial 40983).

Biological characteristics

The biological characteristics of the tumour will probably play an important role in chemotherapy strategy, and may influence the indications and choice of specific drugs according to these characteristics.

Biological factors predictive for tumour chemosensitivity

Gene expression and enzyme activity have been identified in vitro as predictors of response to certain chemotherapy products. For instance, a high thymidylate synthase (TS) expression is correlated with resistance to 5-FU and raltitrexed,[33] and *p53* mutation and apoptotic index seem to be predictive for response to 5-FU/FA combinations.[34] However, it is difficult to get tumour samples and characterize their gene expression for prediction of resistance to specific drugs, although this will probably become more and more feasible in the future with the development of biological techniques and their automation.[34]

The enzymes topoisomerase I and II,[35] dihydropyrimidine dehydrogenase (DPD),[36] UGT1A1,[37] and methylenetetrahydrofolate reductase (MTHFR)[38] have also been identified as possible predictors for response and toxicity to chemotherapy. However, it is difficult to obtain reliable results from these specific assays, and they are unlikely to be employed in the clinic in the short term.

Predictive factors for survival and recurrence rate

More molecular determinants of tumour progression in CRC will be defined in the future, but today some of these factors seem specific enough to be considered in ongoing trials. For instance, stage II (Dukes B) patients with mutations in codon 12 or 13 of the Ki-*ras* gene are at higher risk of developing lymph node metastases.[39] Wild-type p53 or Bcl-2 expression is a factor predicting better overall survival in patients with colorectal cancer,[40,41] and circulating p53 antibodies have been shown to be correlated with poorer survival.[42] Expression of β-catenin, which is a component of the E-cadherin adhesion complex, seems to predict a higher rate of liver and distant metastases and a poorer survival.[43,44] Angiogenesis is also important, and vascular endothelial growth factor (VEGF) expression seems to predict distant recurrence in stage II colon cancer patients.[45]

However, presently most of these factors have no impact on our strategy in the normal clinical setting. Only two of them will probably be routinely used in the short term: TS expression, which has a prognostic importance and predicts resistance to 5-FU, and the RER phenotype (presence or absence of a replication error: positive phenotype = RER$^+$; negative = RER$^-$). This RER phenotype has begun to change the treatment policy for colorectal cancer. In fact, it is now accepted that there are at least two different kinds of colorectal cancer, based on their molecular characteristics. The most frequent, accounting for approximately 85% of cases, has loss of heterozygosity (LOH) phenotype with chromosomal mutations in oncogenes or suppressor genes such as *FAP*, Ki-*ras*, and *p53*.[34] This type of colorectal cancer (MSS – for 'microsatellite stability') appears to be associated with a worse prognosis and less chemosensitivity. The second type (accounting for approximately 15% of cases) is characterized by chromosomal instability resulting from frequent mismatch repairs (MMR) of DNA and is frequently of RER$^+$ phenotype; it is usually termed MSI (for 'microsatellite instability'). This MSI colorectal cancer is predominantly observed in younger patients and in the proximal colon, and recent biological studies conducted on the tumours of patients who had participated in previous randomized trials have suggested that patients with MSI had a better prognosis[46,47] and a better chemosensitivity. In a recent study, MSI patients had an excellent survival rate after adjuvant 5-FU/levamisole (90% at 5 years) compared with MSI patients who had not received adjuvant chemotherapy (35% at 5 years) and with MSS patients.[48]

ROLE AND PLACE OF SECOND-LINE CHEMOTHERAPY

Today in Europe, patients with advanced colorectal cancer may receive further chemotherapy after failure of a first-line treatment. Treatment strategy following a first-line chemotherapy is extensively discussed in Chapter 58. There is some indirect evidence that patients receiving successive treatments may enjoy prolonged survival. Median survival time has moved from 5–6 months when only best supportive care is given,[18] to 12 months with 5-FU/FA bolus,[6] to 19 months when second-line treatments are systematically given.[14] Second-line therapy may induce major responses, and, in some cases, curative surgery may be performed successfully.[32]

CONCLUSIONS

The need for a strategy is related to the fact that chemotherapy still remains poorly active, with 1–3% complete responses, 30–50% partial responses, and another 30–40% stable disease. Duration of response or stabilization does not exceed 6 months. Although combination therapy increases the likelihood of response by 30–50% and the median survival by, at best, 3 months, no real breakthrough in complete response rate has been obtained. The use of a triple therapy combining all the available agents, including 5-FU/FA, irinotecan, and oxaliplatin, that is presently being investigated does not seem to induce a meaningful difference in response rate, and there is no increase in complete response rate compared with the combinations of 5-FU/FA with irinotecan or oxaliplatin. More information is required on the activity of new first-line combinations using the various agents together or sequentially. Today, the evidence at hand suggests that starting with a 5-FU/FA regimen combined with (in any order) oxaliplatin or irinotecan, and then moving, upon progression, to a second-line treatment with the combination not used as first-line chemotherapy gives the patient the greatest chance of having a prolonged survival of around 20 months (in a prospective randomized trial).[49] However, the use of a combination as front-line treatment is not completely established, and using a strategy starting with a 5-FU/FA regimen and moving to a combination chemotherapy as second- and third-line chemotherapy only in the case of progression has led to a median survival of about 24 months.[50] Clinical trials comparing the most appealing upfront triple combination with the sequential approach will be one of the priorities of the next few years.

REFERENCES

1. Parkin D, Whelan S, Ferlay J et al, *Cancer Incidence in Five Continents.* Lyon: IARC, Scientific Publication 143, 1997.

2. Heidelberg C, Chandhari NK, Danenberg P et al, Fluorinated pyrimidines: a new class of tumour inhibitory compounds. *Nature* 1957; **179:** 663–6.

3. Carter SK. Large bowel cancer: the current status of treatment. *J Natl Cancer Inst* 1976; **56:** 3–10.

4. Machover D, Schwarzenberg L, Goldsmith E et al, Treatment of advanced colorectal and gastric adenocarcinoma with 5-FU combined with high-dose folinic acid: a pilot study. *Cancer Treat Rep* 1982; **66:** 1803–7.

5. Advanced Colorectal Cancer Meta-Analysis Project, Modulation of fluorouracil by leucovorin in patients with advanced colorectal cancer: evidence in terms of response rate. *J Clin Oncol* 1992; **10:** 896–903.

6. Poon MA, O'Connel MJ, Wieand HS et al, Biochemical modulation of fluorouracil with leucovorin: confirmatory evidence of improved therapeutic efficacy advanced colorectal cancer. *J Clin Oncol* 1991; **9:** 1967–72.

7. Madajewicz S, Petrelli N, Rustum YM et al, Phase I–II trial of high-dose calcium leucovorin and 5-fluorouracil in advanced colorectal cancer. *Cancer Res* 1984; **44:** 4667–9.

8. Lokich JJ, Ahlgren JD, Gullo JJ et al, Prospective randomised comparison of continuous infusion fluorouracil with a conventional bolus schedule in metastatic colorectal carcinoma. A Mid Atlantic Oncology Programme study. *J Clin Oncol* 1989; **7:** 425–32.

9. De Gramont A, Bosset JF, Milan Ch et al, Randomised trial comparing monthly low-dose leucovorin and fluorouracil bolus with bimonthly high-dose leucovorin and fluorouracil bolus plus continuous infusion for advanced colorectal cancer. A French Intergroup study. *J Clin Oncol* 1997; **15:** 808–15.

10. Aranda E, Diaz-Rubio E, Cervantes A et al, Randomized trial comparing monthly low-dose leucovorin and fluorouracil for advanced colorectal cancer: a Spanish Cooperative Group for Gastro-Intestinal Tumor Therapy (TTD) study. *Ann Oncol* 1998; **9:** 727–31.

11. Köhne CH, Schöffski P, Käufer C et al, Effective biomodulation by leucovorin of high-dose infusion fluorouracil given as a weekly 24-hour infusion: results of a randomised trial in patients with advanced colorectal cancer. *J Clin Oncol* 1998; **16:** 418–26.

12. Gamelin E, Jacob J, Danquechin-Dorval EM et al, Multicentric randomized trial comparing in weekly treatment of advanced colorectal cancer (CRC) intensified 5-fluorouracil and folinic acid (FA) with 5-FU pharmacokinetic monitoring to a constant dose calculated with body surface area. *Proc Am Soc Clin Oncol* 1998; **17:** 270a.

13. Carmichael J, Popiela T, Radstone D et al, Randomised comparative study of ORZEL® (oral uracil/tegafur (UFT®) plus leucovorin (LV) versus parenteral 5-fluorouracil (5-FU) plus LV in patients with metastatic colorectal cancer. *Proc Am Soc Clin Oncol* 1999; **18:** 264a.

14. Giacchetti S, Perpoint MC, Zidani B et al, Phase III multicenter randomised trial of oxaliplatin added to chronomodulated fluorouracil-leucovorin as first-line treatment of metastatic colorectal cancer. *J Clin Oncol* 2000; **18:** 136–47.

15. Rougier Ph, Paillot B, Laplanche A et al, 5-Fluorouracil (5-FU) continuous intra-venous infusion (CVI) compared with bolus administration. Final results of a randomised trial in metastatic colorectal cancer. *Eur J Cancer* 1997; **33:** 1789–93.

16. Schmoll HJ, Köhne CH, Lorenz M et al, Weekly 24 h infusion of high-dose (HD) 5-fluorouracil (5-FU/FA NCCTG/Mayo) in advanced colorectal cancer (CRC): a randomised phase III study of the EORTC–GITCCG and the AIO. *Proc Am Soc Clin Oncol* 2000; **19:** 241a.

17. Meta-Analysis Group in Cancer, Efficacy of intravenous continuous infusion of 5-fluorouracil compared with bolus administration in advanced colorectal cancer. *J Clin Oncol* 1998; **16:** 301–8.

18. Scheithauer W, Rosen H, Kornek GV et al, Randomised comparison of combination chemotherapy plus supportive care with supportive care alone in patients with metastatic colorectal cancer. *BMJ* 1993; **306:** 752–5.

19. Nordic Gastrointestinal Tumor Adjuvant Therapy Group, Expectancy or primary chemotherapy in patients with advanced asymptomatic colorectal cancer: a randomised trial. *J Clin Oncol* 1992; **10:** 904–11.

20. Pazdur R, Douillard JY, Skilling JR et al, Multicentric phase III study of 5-fluorouracil (5FU) or UFT® in combination with leucovorin (LV) in patients with metastatic colorectal cancer. *Proc Am Soc Clin Oncol* 1999; **18:** 263a.

21. Cox JV, Pazdur R, Thibault A et al, A phase III trial of Xeloda™ (capecitabine) in previously untreated advanced/metastatic colorectal cancer. *Proc Am Soc Clin Oncol* 1999; **18:** 265a.

22. Twelves C, Harper P, Van Cutsem E et al, A phase III trial (SO14796) of Xeloda™ (capecitabine) in previously untreated advanced/metastatic colorectal cancer. *Proc Am Soc Clin Oncol* 1999; **18:** 263a.

23. Becouarn Y, Ychou M, Ducreux M et al, Phase II trial of oxaliplatin as first-line chemotherapy in metastatic colorectal cancer patients. *J Clin Oncol* 1998; **16:** 2739–44.

24. Rougier Ph, Bugat R, Douillard JY et al, Phase II study of irinotecan in the treatment of advanced colorectal cancer in chemotherapy-naïve patient and patients pretreated with fluorouracil-based chemotherapy. *J Clin Oncol* 1997; **15:** 251–60.

25. Raymond E, Chaney SG, Taama A et al, Oxaliplatin: a review of preclinical and clinical studies. *Ann Oncol* 1998; **9:** 1053–71.

26. Douillard JY, Cunningham D, Roth AD et al, Irinotecan combined with fluorouracil compared with fluorouracil alone as first-line treatment for metastatic colorectal cancer: a multicentre randomised trial. *Lancet* 2000; **355:** 1041–7.

27. Saltz LB, Cox JV, Blanke Ch et al, Irinotecan plus fluorouracil and leucovorin for metastatic colorectal cancer. *N Engl J Med* 2000; **343:** 905-14.

28. De Gramont A, Figer A, Seymour M, A randomised trial of leucovorin (LV) and 5-fluorouracil (5FU) with or without oxaliplatin in advanced colorectal cancer (CRC). *Proc Am Soc Clin Oncol* 1998; **17:** 257a.

29. Outcomes of Cancer Treatment for Technology Assessment and Cancer Treatment Guidelines. Adopted in July 1995 by the American Society of Clinical Oncology. *J Clin Oncol* 1996; **14:** 671–9.

30. Köhne C, Hecker H, Survival as a function of response to first and second line treatment: a mathematical model for patients with colorectal cancer. *Proc Am Soc Clin Oncol* 2001; **20:** 139.

31. Popescu RA, Norman A, Ross PJ et al, Adjuvant or palliative chemotherapy for colorectal cancer in patients 70 years or older. *J Clin Oncol* 1999; **17:** 2412–18.

32. Bismuth H, Adam R, Levi F et al, Resection of unresectable liver metastases from colorectal cancer after neoadjuvant chemotherapy. *Ann Surg* 1996; **224:** 509–22.

33. Paradiso A, Simone G, Petroni S et al, Thymidylate synthase and p53 primary tumour expression as predictive factors for advanced colorectal cancer patients. *Br J Cancer* 2000; **82:** 560–7.

34. Sobrero A, Kerr D, Glimelius B et al, New directions in the treatment of colorectal cancer: a look to the future. *Eur J Cancer* 2000; **36:** 559–66.

35. Kim R, Ohi Y, Inoue H, Toge T, Expression and relationship between topoisomerase 1 and 11 alpha genes in tumor and normal tissues in oesophageal, gastric and colon cancers. *Anticancer Res* 1999; **19:** 5393–8.

36. Danenberg K, Salonga J, Park J et al, Dihydropyrimidine dehydrogenase and thymidylate synthase gene expression identify a high percentage of colorectal tumours responding to FU. *Proc Am Soc Clin Oncol* 1998; **17:** 258a.

37. Iyer L, Janisch L, Das S et al, UGT1A1 promoter genotype correlates with pharmacokinetics of irinotecan (CPT-11). *Proc Am Soc Clin Oncol* 2000; **19:** 178a.

38. Stevensen J, Redlinger M, Kluijtmans LAJ et al, Polymorphisms in the methylene tetrahydrofolate reductase (MTHFR) gene and toxicity produced by the thymidylate synthase inhibitor tomudex in a phase I clinical trial. *Proc Am Soc Clin Oncol* 2000; **19:** 179a.

39. Thebo JS, Sonagore AJ, Reinhold DS, Stapleton SR, Molecular staging of colorectal cancer: K-ras mutation analysis of lymph nodes upstages Dukes B patients. *Dis Col Rectum* 2000; **43:** 155–9.

40. Sinicrope FA, Hart J, Hsu HA et al, Apoptotic and mitotic indices predict survival rates in lymph node-negative colon carcinoma. *Clin Cancer Res* 1999; **5:** 1793–804.

41. Elwell A, Xiong YP, Chang M et al, p53, p21 and thymidylate synthase (TS) protein expression: associations with recurrence in stage II and III rectal cancer. *Proc Am Soc Clin Oncol* 1997; **16:** 258a.

42. Shiota G, Ishida M, Noguchi N et al, Circulating p53 antibody in patients with colorectal cancer: relation to clinicopathologic features and survival. *Dig Dis Sci* 2000; **45:** 122–8.

43. Hugh TJ, Dillon SA, Taylor BA et al, Cadherin–catenin expression in primary colorectal cancer: a survival analysis. *Br J Cancer* 1999; **80:** 1046–51.

44. Hugh TJ, Dillon SA, O'Dowd G et al, Beta-catenin expression in primary and metastatic colorectal carcinoma. *Int J Cancer* 1999; **82:** 504–11.

45. Takahashi Y, Tucker SL, Kitadai Y et al, Vessel counts and expression of vascular endothelial growth factor as prognostic factors in node negative colon cancer. *Arch Surg* 1997; **132:** 541–6.

46. Halling KC, French AJ, McDonnell SK et al, Microsatellite instability and 8p allelic imbalance in stage B2 and C colorectal cancers. *J Natl Cancer Inst* 1999; **91:** 1295–303.

47. Gryfe R, Kim HK, Hsieh E et al, Tumor microsatellite instability and clinical outcome in young patients with colorectal cancer. *N Engl J Med* 2000; **342:** 69–77.

48. Elsaleh H, Joseph D, Grieu F et al, Association of tumor site and sex with survival benefit from adjuvant chemotherapy in colorectal cancer. *Lancet* 2000; **355:** 1745–50.

49. Tournigand C, Louvet C, Quinaux E et al, FOLFIRI followed by FOLFOX versus FOLFOX followed by FOLFIRI in metastatic colorectal cancer (MCRC): final results of a phase III study. *Proc Am Soc Clin Oncol* 2001; **20:** 124a.

50. Bleiberg H. Brienza S, Gerard B, Oxaliplatin combined with a high dose 24-hour continuous 5FU infusion and folinic acid based regimen in patients (pts) with advanced colorectal cancer (CRC). *Proc Am Soc Clin Oncol* 1999; **18:** 241a.

58

Treatment strategies after first-line therapy

Eric Van Cutsem, Chris Verslype

INTRODUCTION

In the last decade, the value of first-line treatment for patients with advanced colorectal cancer has been demonstrated and widely accepted. Response rates of 20–30%, a median survival of 12–14 months, and a quality-of-life benefit compared with best supportive care have been demonstrated with 5-fluorouracil (5-FU) and folinic acid (FA, leucovorin). The oral fluoropyrimidines capecitabine and UFT (uracil plus tegafur), and the specific thymidylate synthase inhibitor raltitrexed, are also active drugs in the treatment of advanced colorectal cancer.[1,2] Recently, it has been shown that combination treatment with 5-FU/FA/irinotecan and with 5-FU/FA/oxaliplatin induces significantly higher response rates (40–50%) and a longer time to tumour progression (TTP) or progression-free survival (PFS) compared with 5-FU/FA. The median survival is significantly prolonged for the combination 5-FU/FA/irinotecan compared with 5-FU/FA.[3–5] These new data influence the approach to patients with metastatic colorectal cancer.

The choice of first-line treatment also clearly influences the selection of a specific protocol for salvage treatment when the first-line treatment has failed. Until a few years ago, the second-line treatment of patients with advanced colorectal cancer after failure of first-line chemotherapy was very controversial. In the last few years, however, several phase II studies have shown that there are several effective second-line treatment options, and recently it has been shown in two large randomized phase III trials that effective second-line treatment can prolong survival and maintain quality of life over a longer period. These recent studies, as well as the development of new treatment options, have changed the therapeutic approach to patients with advanced colorectal cancer after failure of first-line treatment. From 50% to 70% of patients with metastatic colorectal cancer are still in good condition after failure of first-line treatment, and are therefore possible candidates for second-line treatment.

DIFFICULTIES IN THE INTERPRETATION OF PHASE II STUDIES IN SECOND-LINE TREATMENT

There are several major problems in the interpretation of the phase II studies regarding the value of second-line treatment for metastatic colorectal cancer.

- Most studies have included a relatively small number of patients.
- The definition of a second-line population of patients with advanced colorectal cancer is very heterogeneous. In some studies, patients have been pretreated with chemotherapy for advanced disease, without specifying the regimen or the response to first-line treatment. Patients have sometimes been treated with an inadequate or suboptimal first-line regimen, or have not always had progressive disease during or after first-line treatment. In contrast, in other studies, only carefully selected refractory patients have been treated. Resistance can – and probably should – be defined as the presence of clear progression on computed tomography scan (two successive imaging investigations within 6 months showing more than 25% growth in target lesions or the appearance of new lesions) while on first-line treatment or within 3–6 months after stopping first-line treatment. Most studies have also lacked an independent external review of the responses.
- It is also important to define the endpoints for palliative treatment in the second-line setting very accurately. Various parameters of activity have been reported in different clinical studies: the number of patients with an objective response

(response rate, RR), the number of patients without progression on second-line treatment after prior progression on first-line treatment (this is the number of responses plus tumour stabilizations, and in this setting is often indicated as the number of patients with tumour growth control), TTP, PFS, median survival, and quality of life.

Comparisons between different phase II studies using different patient populations, inclusion criteria, methods of assessment, and endpoints are therefore not always possible.

SECOND-LINE TREATMENT AFTER FAILURE WITH 5-FU/FA

Several treatment options have been studied most often in phase II studies, while the role of irinotecan in the second-line treatment of metastatic colorectal cancer has been evaluated in two prospective randomized phase III trials. The options include:

- intensified 5-FU with or without FA, and infusional 5-FU with or without FA;
- irinotecan in monotherapy and in combination with 5-FU/FA;
- oxaliplatin in monotherapy and in combination with 5-FU/FA;
- intrahepatic chemotherapy.

Intensified and infusional 5-FU/FA

It has been shown that 5-FU administered as a continuous infusion is superior to 5-FU bolus in terms of tumour response, and achieves a slight increase in overall survival ($p = 0.04$), although the survival times were close (12.1 months versus 11.3 months) in first-line treatment of advanced colorectal cancer.[6,7] It has also been shown that infusional 5-FU/FA is more active than a bolus regimen of 5-FU/FA.[8,9] The response rate and TTP are superior for infusional regimens compared with bolus regimens, but the median survivals were identical in first-line treatment of metastatic colorectal cancer.[8] Preclinical evidence is also strongly supportive of the concept that bolus 5-FU predominantly kills cells via an RNA-directed mechanism, whilst infusional 5-FU is cytotoxic via thymidylate synthase inhibition.[10] Experimental evidence that infusional 5-FU eradicates resistance to bolus 5-FU is also available.[11]

Therefore several trials have been performed to evaluate the role of an infusional regimen of 5-FU with or without FA after progression on a bolus regimen of 5-FU with or without FA. Published results concern small studies with a heterogeneous selection of regimens and methods of assessment, the great majority having no independent review of responses. The response rates for this second-line treatment range from 0% to 35%. From 10% to 70% of patients had tumour stabilization.[12–18] It is also noteworthy that most of the objective responses observed with 5-FU-based second-line regimens occurred either in patients who had previously responded to 5-FU or in patients who had previously received suboptimal doses of 5-FU. Combinations of 5-FU continuous infusion with cisplatin or cisplatin/epirubicin do not seem to offer any advantage over protocols with infusional 5-FU with or without FA, but add more toxicity.[19]

In a randomized phase III trial in 5-FU-resistant patients, it was shown that single-agent irinotecan prolonged median survival compared with an infusional regimen of 5-FU with or without FA (weekly 24-hour 5-FU/FA, biweekly 48-hour bolus plus infusional 5-FU/FA, or protracted continuous-infusion 5-FU)[20] (see below). On the basis of this study and results with oxaliplatin, an intensified or infusional 5-FU regimen is no longer considered a standard second-line option for patients with a truly 5-FU-resistant metastatic colorectal cancer.[21]

Irinotecan

The water-soluble camptothecin derivative irinotecan (CPT-11), a DNA topoisomerase I inhibitor, has a unique mechanism of action.

In preclinical studies, irinotecan demonstrated notable antitumour activity against several tumour types, including colorectal cancer. The initial clinical development of this drug was as a single agent in the second-line treatment of advanced colorectal cancer. In Europe, the drug was developed as a 3-weekly regimen (350 mg/m^2 every 3 weeks), while in the USA, a weekly regimen (100–125 mg/m^2/week for 4 consecutive weeks out of 6) was developed. The first European studies were conducted in a total of 455 patients presenting with histologically documented metastatic colorectal cancer. A response rate of 13% (95% confidence interval 9.7–16.8%) was reported in 363 progressive patients. Disease stabilization was achieved in 42% of patients.[22–25] The median duration of response was 7.5 months. The stabilization rate was 42%. The median duration of stabilization was 5 months and the TTP was 4 months. The median survival was 9.5 months (Table 58.1). In three US studies, a response rate of 13% and a stabilization rate of

49% were found in 304 patients. The TTP was 4 months and the median survival 9 months (Table 58.1).[26–28] Based on the high rate of tumour growth control observed, irinotecan was approved in many countries for the second-line treatment of 5-FU-resistant metastatic colorectal cancer. It has indeed been demonstrated that stabilization of progressive colorectal cancer is associated with both prolonged survival and subjective improvement. Analysis of the relationship between tumour response and survival in chemotherapy of advanced colorectal cancer has shown that any degree of objective tumour response of 4 months' duration is associated with definite survival advantage.[29] The survival advantage confirmed by a stable disease was almost as great as that associated with a partial response. In a prospective study of quality of life using interviews or questionnaires during chemotherapy for advanced colorectal cancer, benefit in terms of quality of life was associated with an antitumour effect that did not necessarily have to be sufficiently large to qualify as an objective response according to the World Health Organization (WHO) criteria.[30] In the phase II studies with irinotecan, it has been suggested that tumour growth control is reflected in clinical benefit, in terms of improvement and stabilization of weight and performance status and pain relief.[23] The major toxicities with irinotecan were grade 3 for diarrhoea, neutropenia, nausea and vomiting, and alopecia.[24]

Two randomized studies in 5-FU-resistant colorectal cancer have been performed simultaneously in Europe with primary endpoint the survival of patients. In one study, patients with 5-FU-refractory advanced colorectal cancer (second- or third-line treatment) were randomized between best supportive care or irinotecan 350 mg/m^2 every 3 weeks.[31] In a similar study, patients were treated in second line after 5-FU failure, with irinotecan 350 mg/m^2 every 3 weeks or infusional 5-FU with or without FA (biweekly 48-hour regimen, weekly 24-hour regimen, or protracted infusional regimen).[20] In both studies, a significantly longer survival was shown for patients

Table 58.1 Irinotecan in 5-FU-resistant advanced colorectal cancer: phase III studies[25,28]

Irinotecan dose and schedule	No. of patients evaluable for response	RR (%)	SD (%)	TTP (months)	Median survival (months)
350 mg/m^2 q3wks	363	13	42	4	9.5
100–125 mg/m^2/wk × 4; 2 wks rest	304	13	49	4	9.0

Abbreviations: RR, response rate; SD, stable disease; TTP, time to tumour progression.

Table 58.2 Randomized phase II studies of irinotecan versus best supportive care (BSC)[31] **and irinotecan versus infusional 5-FU**[20] **in refractory colorectal cancer**

	No. of patients	Median survival (months)	1-year survival rate (%)
Irinotecan	189	9.2[a]	36
BSC	90	6.5	14
Irinotecan	127	10.8[b]	45
Infusional 5-FU	129	8.5	32

[a]$p = 0.0001$; [b]$p = 0.035$.

treated with irinotecan (Table 58.2). The quality of life was also significantly better for patients treated with irinotecan compared with patients treated with best supportive care alone, and was similar for patients treated with irinotecan and with infusional 5-FU.[20,31]

These two pivotal trials have been the base for the worldwide acceptance that patients with advanced colorectal cancer can benefit from second-line treatment with an active agent and that irinotecan is a standard option for patients with 5-FU-refractory advanced colorectal cancer.

Several randomized phase II studies have studied the most optimal regimen for single-agent irinotecan. In the first study, irinotecan was administered weekly (125 mg/m^2), biweekly (250 mg/m^2), or three-weekly (350 mg/ml^2), or as a continuous infu-sion (10 mg/m^2/day 14-day continuous infusion every 3 weeks) (Table 58.3). It was concluded that the three-weekly and biweekly regimens showed better tolerance and induced higher response rates.[32] In another study, irinotecan as a three-weekly regimen was administered at a dose of 350 mg/m^2, at a dose adapted to toxicity, or at a dose adapted to prognostic factors (Table 58.4). Is was concluded that the best regimen was an individual dose optimization according to toxicity, starting with a dose of 250 mg/m^2, and increasing to 350 mg or 500 mg/m^2 if no major toxicity occurred.[33]

More recently, irinotecan has been developed in association with 5-FU and FA. As well as bolus regimens,[34] infusional regimens[35,36] have been developed. The role of the association of 5-FU/FA plus irinote-

---

Table 58.3 Randomized phase II study of different regimens of irinotecan in 5-FU/FA-resistant colorectal cancer (174 patients)[32]

Irinotecan dose and regimen	RR (%)	Diarrhoea grade 3–4 (%)	Neutropenia grade 3–4 (%)
350 mg/m^2/day q3wks	17	10	34
125 mg/m^2/day q1w	8	24	25
250 mg/m^2/day q2wks	17	13	28
10 mg/m^2/day 14-day CI q3wks	2	25	9

Abbreviations: RR, response rate; CI, continuous infusion.

Table 58.4 Randomized phase II trial of three different regimens of irinotecan at 3-week intervals in 5-FU-resistant colorectal cancer (164 patients)[33]

Irinotecan dose and regimen	RR (%)	Diarrhoea grade 3–4 (%)	Neutropenia grade 3–4 (%)
350 mg/m^2 q3wks	8	31	48
250 mg/m^2 q3wks, increased to 350–500 mg/m^2 according to toxicity	13	21	31
250 or 350 or 500 mg/m^2 q3wks, according to risk-factor analysis	9	27	44

can in 5-FU-resistant patients has been investigated in a few small phase II studies. No phase III data are available, and nor are there any data comparing the activity of irinotecan as single agent with a combination of 5-FU and irinotecan in second-line treatment of advanced colorectal cancer. The small phase II studies in second line with the combination of 5-FU/FA and irinotecan seem to indicate that this regimen is also active in second-line treatment. In a dose-finding study, a response rate of 22% was found in 55 patients with 5-FU-resistant colorectal cancer,[36] while another study showed a response rate of 7% in third-line treatment.[37] The toxicity of the combination of 5-FU/FA and irinotecan seems to be lower than that of single-agent irinotecan.

The question therefore remains open regarding the most optimal regimen of irinotecan in the treatment of 5-FU-refractory advanced colorectal cancer.

Oxaliplatin

Oxaliplatin is a new-generation platinum compound. In vitro activity has been shown in colon cancer cell lines sensitive and resistant to cisplatin, and in cell lines with primary or acquired resistance to 5-FU. In vitro and in vivo studies have also shown an additive or synergistic antitumour effect with 5-FU.[38]

Several studies with oxaliplatin as a single agent have been performed in advanced colorectal cancer. For previously untreated patients, response rates of 20% and 24% were shown in two small phase II stud-

ies.[39,40] For 5-FU-pretreated patients, two phase II studies have been reported with single-agent oxaliplatin at a dose of 130 mg/m^2 every 3 weeks. An overall response rate of 10% was observed. In a study with a chronomodulated regimen of oxaliplatin, the response rate was also 10%[41] (Table 58.5). Several small phase II studies have shown response rates of 21–46% with a combination of oxaliplatin and 5-FU/FA[40–47] (Table 58.5). These studies, however, contain a heterogeneous study population and heterogeneous criteria for 5-FU resistance. In a large, multicentre European trial, 234 strictly defined 5-FU-resistant patients with advanced colorectal cancer were evaluated.[21] The responses were reviewed by independent external experts. Oxaliplatin at a dose of 130 mg/m^2 every 3 weeks or 85 mg/m^2 every 2 weeks was added to the first-line regimen of 5-FU/FA during or after which there was tumour progression. Several groups of patients were treated: 5 days' bolus 5-FU/FA (Mayo Clinic regimen), weekly high-dose 24-hour infusional 5-FU/FA, short-infusional 5-FU/FA on days 1 and 2, every 2 weeks, and protracted continuous-infusion 5-FU. The overall response rate was 14% according to the investigators and 10% according to the independent experts. There was stable disease in 36% of patients. The tumour growth control rate was 50%. The median progression-free survival was 4.0 months and the median survival 11.0 months[21] (Table 58.6). Tolerance of oxaliplatin was acceptable. The results of this large, strictly performed trial seem to be more realistic than the results of the small phase II trials in

---

Table 58.5 Oxaliplatin in pretreated colorectal cancer: phase II studies

Ref	No. of patients	Regimen	RR (%)	SD (%)
42	53	Oxaliplatin	11	41
40	48	Oxaliplatin	10	42
41	29	Oxaliplatin (chrono)	10	24
43	46	Oxaliplatin + 5-FU/FA	46	46
44	24	Oxaliplatin + 5-FU/FA	21	37
45	60	Oxaliplatin + 5-FU/FA	27	45
46	25	Oxaliplatin + 5-FU/FA (chrono)	28	—
47	37	Oxaliplatin + 5-FU/FA (chrono)	40	51
21	234	Oxaliplatin + 5-FU/FA	14[a]	36

Abbreviations: RR, response rate; SD, stable disease; chrono, chronomodulated regimen.
[a]External review of responses (independent experts: RR = 10% in ref. 21).

Table 58.6 Oxaliplatin added to 5-FU/FA in advanced colorectal cancer refractory to the same 5-FU/FA regimen[21]

Regimen	No. of patients	Response rate (%)		Stable disease (%)	1-year survival rate (%)
		Investigators	Expert		
Oxaliplatin 130 mg/m^2 + daily × 5 5-FU/FA	115	18	13	36	43
Oxaliplatin 85 mg/m^2 + weekly 5-FU/FA 24 h	57	14	7	26	43
Oxaliplatin 85 mg/m^2 + biweekly 5-FU/FA d1–2	56	5	5	45	46
All regimens[a]	233	14	10	36	44

[a]Progression-free survival 4.0 months; median survival 11.0 months.

heterogeneous study populations. The results are also very similar to those obtained with irinotecan as a single agent in phase II studies.

Randomized phase III studies with oxaliplatin in second-line treatment of 5-FU-refractory colorectal cancer have not, however, been performed, and nor have randomized studies comparing oxaliplatin as a single agent with combinations of 5-FU/FA and oxaliplatin. The question of whether 5-FU/FA adds to the activity of oxaliplatin in second-line treatment is therefore not completely answered.

Irinotecan and oxaliplatin

Combining irinotecan with oxaliplatin for the treatment of 5-FU-refractory colorectal cancer is a logical approach in view of their different mechanisms of action. Experience is still limited, however.

The association of irinotecan and oxaliplatin with or without 5-FU has been investigated in several phase I studies. In a phase II study, a response rate of 42%, including 2 complete remissions (6%) in 36 patients with metastatic colorectal cancer, who had progressed while receiving or within 6 months after discontinuing palliative chemotherapy with 5-FU/FA, has been reported.[48] The median time to treatment failure was 7.5 months. Treatment consisted of oxaliplatin 85 mg/m^2 on days 1 and 15 and irinotecan 80 mg/m^2 on days 1, 8, and 15 every 4 weeks, with or without granulocyte colony-stimulating factor (G-CSF).[49] Further studies of this

interesting combination are needed in order to evaluate its activity and tolerability in 5-FU-refractory advanced colorectal cancer.

In a randomized phase II study, 101 patients with 5-FU-refractory advanced colorectal cancer were treated with 5-FU/FA/irinotecan (biweekly infusional regimen), with 5-FU/FA/oxaliplatin (biweekly infusional regimen), or with irinotecan (200 mg/m^2) plus oxaliplatin (85 mg/m^2) every 3 weeks. The respective response rates were 11%, 21%, and 15%; the stable disease rates were 52%, 50%, and 46%; the durations of response were 8.1, 6.7, and 6.5 months; and the median survivals were 12.2 months, 11.5 months, and 11.0 months for the combination 5-FU/FA oxaliplatin and irinotecan/oxaliplatin.[49]

SECOND-LINE TREATMENT AFTER COMBINATION CHEMOTHERAPY

No data from well-performed trials are available in the literature regarding the role of second-line chemotherapy after failure of a first-line regimen of 5-FU/FA/irinotecan or 5-FU/FA/oxaliplatin. In view of the different mechanisms of action, it seems logical to consider an oxaliplatin-containing regimen for patients who are candidates for second-line treatment after progression on an irinotecan-containing regimen, and vice versa. The impact on survival and the possible clinical benefit for patients of this approach are still unknown. The GERCOR (Oncology Multidisciplinary Research Group) is performing a randomized trial of sequential treatment with 5-FU/FA/irinotecan followed by 5-FU/FA/oxaliplatin versus 5-FU/FA/oxaliplatin followed by 5-FU/FA/irinotecan.[50] This type of sequential study is very important to determine the role of different treatment strategies.

SECOND-LINE TREATMENT AFTER FAILURE WITH OTHER DRUGS

Although no data are available in the literature from clinical trials on second-line treatment for patients with metastatic colorectal cancer after progression on the oral fluoropyrimidines and on raltitrexed, the same approach can be proposed as for patients who fail with 5-FU/FA. It can be expected that irinotecan- and oxaliplatin-containing regimens will be active in this setting.

RESEARCH TOPICS

Our knowledge of colorectal cancer has expanded over the last years. The range of treatment options for patients with metastatic disease has become larger. The number of unanswered questions in relation to treatment strategies after first-line failure is therefore increasing. These questions include the following:

- What is the best regimen of irinotecan and of oxaliplatin?
- What is the best sequence of treatment?
- Is there a role for third-line treatment?
- What is the role of intrahepatic chemotherapy?
- What are the clinical and molecular predictive factors for response for treatment of patients with advanced colorectal cancer?
- What is the role of new combinations, such as irinotecan plus oxaliplatin, raltitrexed combinations, and combinations with the oral fluoropyrimidines (capecitabine and UFT/FA) in 5-FU-refractory patients?
- What is the role of agents that act on new targets, such as angiogenesis inhibitors, vascular endothelial growth factor (VEGF) inhibitors, epidermal growth factor (EGF) inhibitors and farnesyltransferase inhibitors?

CONCLUSIONS

A large proportion of patients with metastatic colorectal cancer who fail first-line treatment are still good candidates for second-line treatment. The value of an active second-line treatment for patients with metastatic disease who fail with 5-FU/FA has been demonstrated in a randomized phase III trial in comparison with best supportive care. Both a survival benefit and a quality-of-life benefit have been shown for irinotecan compared with best supportive care. A survival benefit has also been shown for irinotecan compared with infusional 5-FU/FA regimens. Combination regimens of irinotecan and 5-FU/FA are less toxic than single-agent irinotecan, and are also active in the second-line treatment of 5-FU-resistant colorectal cancer. Randomized phase III trials with this combination have not, however, been performed in 5-FU-refractory disease.

Oxaliplatin as a single agent and in combination with 5-FU/FA is active in 5-FU/FA-resistant colorectal cancer. It is generally accepted that the combination of 5-FU/FA and oxaliplatin is additive or synergistic. However, in 5-FU-refractory advanced disease, no randomized trials of oxaliplatin or its combination with 5-FU/FA have been performed.

The search for prognostic factors and for predictive factors for response, and well-designed trials of new combinations and of sequential treatment regimens, can contribute to progress in the treatment of metastatic colorectal cancer.

REFERENCES

1. Punt C, New drugs in the treatment of colorectal carcinoma. *Cancer* 1998; **83:** 679–89.
2. Van Cutsem E, Peeters M, Developments in fluoropyrimidine therapy for gastrointestinal cancer. *Curr Opin Oncol* 1999; **11:** 312–17.
3. Saltz L, Cox J, Blanke C et al, Irinotecan plus fluorouracil and leucovorin for metastatic colorectal cancer. *N Engl J Med* 2000; **343:** 905–14.
4. Douillard JY, Cunningham D, Roth AD et al, Irinotecan combined with fluorouracil compared with fluorouracil alone as first-line treatment for metastatic colorectal cancer: a multicentre randomised trial. *Lancet* 2000; **355:** 1041–6.
5. de Gramont A, Figer A, Seymour M et al, Leucovorin and fluorouracil with or without oxaliplatin as first line treatment in advanced colorectal cancer. *J Clin Oncol* 2000; **18:** 2938–47.
6. The Meta-Analysis Group in Cancer, Efficacy of intravenous continuous infusion of fluorouracil compared with bolus administration in advanced colorectal cancer. *J Clin Oncol* 1998; **16:** 301–8.
7. The Meta-Analysis Group in Cancer, Toxicity of fluorouracil in patients with advanced colorectal cancer: effect of administration schedule and prognostic factors. *J Clin Oncol* 1998; **16:** 3537–41.
8. de Gramont A, Bosset J, Milan C et al, Randomized trial comparing monthly low-dose leucovorin-5-fluorouracil bolus with bimonthly high dose leucovorin–5-fluorouracil bolus plus continuous infusion for advanced colorectal cancer: a French Intergroup study. *J Clin Oncol* 1997; **15:** 808–15.

9. Aranda E, Diaz-Rubio E, Cervantes A et al, Randomized trial comparing monthly low-dose leucovorin and fluorouracil bolus with weekly high-dose 48-hour continuous-infusion fluorouracil for advanced colorectal cancer: a Spanish Cooperative Group for Gastrointestinal Tumor Therapy (TTD) study. *Ann Oncol* 1998; **9:** 727–31.

10. Sobrero A, Aschele C, Bertino J, Fluorouracil in colorectal cancer – a tale of two drugs: implications for biochemical modulation. *J Clin Oncol* 1997; **15:** 368–81.

11. Sobrero A, Kerr D, Glimelius B et al, New directions in the treatment of colorectal cancer: a look to the future. *Eur J Cancer* 2000; **36:** 559–66.

12. Weh HJ, Wilke HJ, Dierlamm J et al, Weekly therapy with folinic acid (FA) and high-dose 5-fluorouracil (5-FU), 24-hour infusion in pretreated patients with metastatic colorectal carcinoma. *Ann Oncol* 1994; **5:** 233–7.

13. Sobrero A, Nobile MT, Gugliemi A et al, Phase II study of 5-fluorouracil plus leucovorin and interferon 2β in advanced colorectal cancer. *Eur J Cancer* 1992; **28:** 850–2.

14. Findlay M, Hill A, Cunningham D et al, Protracted venous infusion of 5-fluorouracil in advanced and refractory colorectal cancer. *Ann Oncol* 1994; **5:** 239–43.

15. Conti JA, Kemeny NE, Saltz LB et al, Continuous infusion fluorouracil/leucovorin and bolus mitomycin C as a salvage regimen for patients with advanced colorectal cancer. *Cancer* 1995; **75:** 769–74.

16. Valone FH, Kohler M, Fisher K et al, A Northern California Oncology Group randomized trial of leucovorin plus 5-fluorouracil versus sequential methotrexate, 5-fluorouracil and leucovorin in patients with advanced colorectal cancer who failed treatment with 5-fluorouracil or 5-fluorodeoxyuridine alone. *NCI Monograph* 1987; **5:** 175–7.

17. Palmieri G, Gridelli C, Airoma G et al, Second-line chemotherapy of advanced colorectal cancer with sequential high-dose methotrexate and 5-fluorouracil. *J Chemother* 1991; **3:** 55–60.

18. Cascinu S, Fedeli A, Luzi Fedeli S, Catalano G, Salvage chemotherapy in colorectal cancer patients with good performance status and young age after failure of 5-fluorouracil/leucovorin combination. *J Chemother* 1992; **4:** 46–9.

19. Ahlgren JD, Trocki O, Gullo JJ et al, Protracted infusion of 5-FU with weekly low dose cisplatin as second line therapy in patients with metastatic colorectal cancer who have failed 5-FU monotherapy. *Cancer Invest* 1991; **9:** 27–33.

20. Rougier P, Van Cutsem E, Bajetta E et al, Randomised trial of irinotecan versus fluorouracil by continuous infusion after fluorouracil failure in patients with metastatic colorectal cancer. *Lancet* 1998; **352:** 1407–12.

21. Van Cutsem E, Szanto J, Roth A et al, Evaluation of the addition of oxaliplatin (oxa) to the same Mayo or German 5FU regimen in advanced refractory colorectal cancer (ARCRC). *Proc Am Soc Clin Oncol* 1999; **18:** 234a.

22. Rougier P, Bugat R, Douillard J et al, Phase II study of Irinotecan in the treatment of advanced colorectal cancer in chemotherapy-naive patients and patients pretreated with fluorouracil-based chemotherapy. *J Clin Oncol* 1997; **15:** 251–60.

23. Van Cutsem E, Cunningham D, Ten Bokkel Huinink WW et al, Clinical activity and benefit of irinotecan (CPT-11) in patients with colorectal cancer truly resistant to 5-fluorouracil (5-FU). *Eur J Cancer* 1999; **35:** 54–9.

24. Van Cutsem E, Peeters M, L'irinotecan en monothérapie dans le traitement des cancers colorectaux: résultats des études de phase II. *Bull Cancer* 1998; Numero spécial: 33–7.

25. Van Cutsem E, Rougier P, Droz J et al, Clinical benefit of irinotecan (CPT-11) in metastatic colorectal cancer. *Proc Am Soc Clin Oncol* 1997; **16:** 268a.

26. Rothenberg ML, Eckardt JR, Kuhn JG et al, Phase II trial of irinotecan in patients with progressive or rapidly recurrent colorectal cancer. *J Clin Oncol* 1996; **14:** 1128–35.

27. Conti JA, Kemeny NE, Saltz LB et al, Irinotecan is an active agent in untreated patients with metastatic colorectal cancer. *J Clin Oncol* 1996; **14:** 709–15.

28. Van Hoff D, Rothenberg M, Pitot H et al, Irinotecan (CPT-11) therapy for patients with previously treated metastatic colorectal cancer (CRC): overall results of FDA-reviewed pivotal US clinical trials. *Proc Am Soc Clin Oncol* 1997; **16:** 228a.

29. Graf W, Pahlman L, Bergström R, Glimelius B, The relationship between an objective response to chemotherapy and survival in advanced colorectal cancer. *Br J Cancer* 1994; **70:** 559–63.

30. Glimelius B, Hoffman K, Graf W et al, Quality of life during chemotherapy in patients with symptomatic advanced colorectal cancer. *Cancer* 1994; **73:** 556–62.

31. Cunningham D, Pyrhönen S, James R et al, Randomised trial of irinotecan plus supportive care versus supportive care alone after fluorouracil failure for patients with metastatic colorectal cancer. *Lancet* 1998; **352:** 1413–18.

32. Ten Bokkel Huinink W, Moiseyenko V, Glimelius B et al, A randomised phase II multicenter trial of irinotecan (CPT-11) using different schedules in patients (pts) with metastatic colorectal cancer (MCRC). *Proc Am Soc Clin Oncol* 2000; **19:** 245a.

33. Van Cutsem E, Dirix L, Van Laethem J et al, A randomized phase II trial of three different regimens of irinotecan (CPT-11): a fixed dose of 350 mg/m^2 (A), or an individual dose optimisation (B) or a risk factor optimisation (C) in patients with metastatic colorectal cancer (MCRC) previously treated with 5-FU. *Proc Am Soc Clin Oncol* 2000; **19:** 244a.

34. Saltz L, Kanowitz J, Kemeny N et al, Phase I clinical and pharmacokinetic study of irinotecan, fluorouracil and leucovorin in patients with advanced solid tumours. *J Clin Oncol* 1996; **14:** 2959–67.

35. Vanhoefer U, Harstrick A, Köhne C et al, Phase I study of a weekly schedule of irinotecan, high-dose leucovorin and infusional fluorouracil as first line chemotherapy in patients with advanced colorectal cancer. *J Clin Oncol* 1999; **17:** 907–13.

36. Ducreux M, Ychou M, Seitz J et al, Irinotecan combined with bolus fluorouracil, continuous infusion fluorouracil and high dose leucovorin every two weeks (LV5FU2 regimen): a clinical dose-finding and pharmacokinetic study in patients with pretreated metastatic colorectal cancer. *J Clin Oncol* 1999; **17:** 2901–8.

37. André T, Louvet C, Maindrault-Goebel F et al, CPT-11 (irinotecan) addition to bimonthly, high dose leucovorin and bolus and continuous-infusion 5-fluorouracil (FOLFIRI) for pretreated metastatic colorectal cancer. *Eur J Cancer* 1999; **35:** 1343–7.

38. Raymond E, Chaney SG, Taamma A, Cvitkovic E, Oxaliplatin: a review of preclinical and clinical studies. *Ann Oncol* 1998; **9:** 1053–71.

39. Becouarn Y, Ychou M, Ducreux M et al, Oxaliplatin (L-OHP) as first-line chemotherapy in metastatic colorectal cancer (MCRC) patients: preliminary activity/toxicity report. *Proc Am Soc Clin Oncol* 1997; **16:** 229a.

40. Diaz-Rubio E, Sastre J, Zaniboni A et al, Oxaliplatin as single agent in previously untreated colorectal carcinoma patients: a phase II multicentric study. *Ann Oncol* 1998; **9:** 105–8.

41. Lévi F, Perpoint B, Garufi C et al, Oxaliplatin activity against metastatic colorectal cancer. A phase II study of five-day continuous venous infusion at circadian rhythm modulated rate. *Eur J Cancer* 1993; **29A:** 1280–4.

42. Machover D, Diaz-Rubio E, de Gramont A et al, Two consecutive phase II studies of oxaliplatin (L-OHP) for treatment of patients with advanced colorectal carcinoma who were resistant to previous treatment with fluoropyrimidines. *Ann Oncol* 1996; **7:** 95–8.

43. de Gramont A, Vignoud J, Tournigand C et al, Oxaliplatin with

high-dose leucovorin and 5-fluorouracil 48-hour continuous infusion in pretreated metastatic colorectal cancer. *Eur J Cancer* 1997; **33**: 214–19.

44. Andre T, Bensmaine MA, Louvet C et al, Addition of oxaliplatin (Eloxatin) to the same leucovorin (LV) and 5-fluorouracil (5-FU) bimonthly regimen after progression in patients (pts) with metastatic colorectal cancer (MCRC): preliminary report. *Proc Am Soc Clin Oncol* 1997; **16**: 270a.

45. Maindrault-Goebel F, Louvet C, André T et al, Oxaliplatin added to simplified bimonthly leucovorin and 5-fluorouracil regimen as second-line therapy for metastatic colorectal cancer (FOLFOX6). *Eur J Cancer* 1999; **35**: 1338–42.

46. Garufi C, Brienza S, Bensmaine MA et al, Addition of oxaliplatin (l-OHP) to chronomodulated (CM) 5-fluorouracil (5-FU) and folinic acid (FA) for reversal of acquired chemoresistance in patients with advanced colorectal cancer. *Proc Am Soc Clin Oncol* 1995; **14**: 192.

47. Bertheault-Cvitkovic F, Jami A, Ithzaki M et al, Biweekly intensi-fied ambulatory chronomodulated chemotherapy with oxali-platin, fluorouracil, and leucovorin in patients with metastatic colorectal cancer. *J Clin Oncol* 1996; **14**: 2950–8.

48. Scheithauer W, Kornek G, Raderer M et al, Combined irinotecan and oxaliplatin plus granulocyte colony-stimulating factor in patients with advanced fluoropyrimidine/leucovorin pretreated colorectal cancer. *J Clin Oncol* 1999; **17**: 902–6.

49. Lepile D, Douillard JY, Marre A et al, Essai randomisé de phase II évaluant 3 associations en traitement de seconde ligne du can-cer colorectal métastatique (CCRM): LV5FU2 + CPT11 vs LV5FU2 + LOPH vs LOPH + CPT11. *Gastroenterol Clin Biol* 2000; **24**: A183.

50. Tournigand C, Louvet C, Andre T et al, FOLFIRI followed by FOLFOX or FOLFOX followed by FOLFIRI in metastatic colorec-tal cancer: Which is the best sequence? Safety and preliminary efficacy results of a randomized phase III study. *Proc Am Soc Clin Oncol* 2000; **19**: 245a.

59

Drug development in colorectal cancer: Viewpoint of the United States cooperative groups

David L Grinblatt, Richard L Schilsky

INTRODUCTION

The development of novel chemotherapy agents and regimens for the treatment of patients with colorectal cancer remains an important focus of cooperative group research in the USA. New drugs are initially evaluated in single- or limited-institutional phase I trials that are less suited for cooperative group efforts. Agents with promising levels of activity and acceptable toxicity are subsequently evaluated in phase II and phase III cooperative group trials in the USA. Often, new agents and combinations are initially evaluated in patients with metastatic disease for evidence of activity prior to testing in the adjuvant setting. The cooperative groups provide an excellent opportunity for the design and conduct of large multicenter phase III trials to compare new therapies with accepted standard treatment. The evaluation of new molecular markers for potential prognostic significance is also an important goal of adjuvant trials conducted by the cooperative groups. In addition, the cooperative groups are beginning to explore phenotypic differences in tumors for the role these differences play in variability in response to particular chemotherapy agents. Finally, biological agents, whose activity may be greatest in patients with minimal residual disease, may best be evaluated by novel protocol designs being developed by the US cooperative groups.

The results of recent phase III trials have established the combination of 5-fluorouracil (5-FU) and leucovorin (LV, folinic acid) with irinotecan as the standard treatment in patients with metastatic disease.[1] The various regimens using this combination are discussed in detail elsewhere in this volume (see Chapters 41–46). However, the recent identification of new active agents has fueled the development of new trials to test these agents as second-line therapy and in combination with 5-FU/LV and irinotecan as first-line therapy for metastatic disease, when appropriate. The combination of 5-FU and leucovorin remains the standard treatment in the adjuvant therapy of patients with stage III colorectal cancer and stages II–III rectal cancer.[2] Additional trials are testing new combinations as neoadjuvant and adjuvant therapies and as radiation sensitizers for stage III disease. The US cooperative groups have mounted a number of new trials in all of these settings to develop improved therapies for patients with colorectal cancer.

ORAL FLUOROPYRIMIDINES

Fluoropyrimidines have been a central component in the treatment of colorectal cancer since the introduction of 5-FU in 1957. The use of protracted infusion of 5-FU has been demonstrated to improve response and survival while diminishing toxicity in some settings when compared with intermittent bolus administration.[3] Biochemical modulation with agents such as N-(phosphonoacetyl)-L-aspartate (PALA), methotrexate, trimetrexate, leucovorin and interferon-α (IFN-α) has been studied in a number of clinical trials.[4] The recent development of oral fluoropyrimidines offers the benefit of improved patient convenience while delivering prolonged exposure with a potential for reduced toxicity.[5] These oral formulations are being tested with a variety of modulators as well as in combination with other new agents in cooperative group trials.

Tegafur (ftorafur), a 5-FU precursor, was the first such agent to be widely used. It is hydroxylated and converted to 5-FU by hepatic microsomal enzymes, resulting in enhanced and sustained 5-FU levels in hepatic tumors. When tegafur was studied as an intravenous bolus in the USA, it had increased toxicity compared with 5-FU – particularly neurologic toxicity. The oral form, studied in Japan, using prolonged administration of divided daily doses, resulted in antitumor activity with reduced toxicity.[6] Tegafur is not subject to degradation by the enzyme dihydropyrimidine dehydrogenase (DPD) in the gastrointestinal tract, since it is activated to 5-FU only after absorption and transport to the liver. Tegafur has been combined with uracil in an agent known as UFT. Uracil competitively inhibits DPD, resulting in increased and sustained levels of 5-FU in tissue. Phase I studies of UFT performed in the USA evaluated this agent in combination with oral leucovorin in three divided daily doses for 28 consecutive days followed by a 1-week break, repeated every 35 days. The dose-limiting toxicity was diarrhea.[7] Phase II trials have established the activity of UFT in previously untreated patients with metastatic colorectal cancer, with an overall response rate of approximately 25% and with higher response rates reported when it was used in combination with oral leucovorin.[8] Two randomized phase III trials of UFT with leucovorin versus parenteral 5-FU with leucovorin in patients with metastatic colorectal cancer have recently been reported, and show no differences in overall response rate, median time to progression, or overall survival, but significantly less myelosuppression and mucositis with the UFT/leucovorin regimen.[9,10]

A recently completed trial by the National Surgical Adjuvant Breast and Bowel Project (NSABP), known as the C-06 trial, randomized patients with stage III colon cancer to receive either weekly intravenous 5-FU and leucovorin for 6 weeks, repeated every 8 weeks, or UFT with leucovorin daily for 28 days, repeated every 35 days (Figure 59.1). Each treatment was continued for 6 months. No outcome data are available yet from this trial. Correlative studies will examine the prognostic significance of *p53* mutations, *DCC* ('deleted in colon cancer') gene deletion, proliferation status, and thymidylate synthase (TS) expression. This is the only adjuvant trial of an oral fluoropyrimidine conducted by the US cooperative groups, and will yield important data on the comparative activity of UFT and leucovorin versus the current standard as well as the relationship of biological prognostic markers to clinical outcomes.

Capecitabine, an oral fluoropyrimidine carbamate, is absorbed as an intact molecule through the intestinal mucosa before transport to the liver, where it is metabolized to deoxy-5-fluorouridine (doxifluridine). This molecule is then converted to 5-FU by the enzyme thymidine phosphorylase, which is more abundant in tumor tissue than in normal tissue. This selective activation to 5-FU by tumor tissue has the potential to provide greater efficacy with reduced toxicity to normal tissues.[11] In a study of 19 patients who underwent surgical resection of primary tumors and/or liver metastases, tumor selectivity was demonstrated by a ratio of 5-FU in tumor to that in healthy tissue of 3.21 in primary tumors and 1.41 in liver metastases. Plasma levels of 5-FU were 14-fold less than the levels in primary tumor and 8-fold less than the levels in liver metastases, suggesting intratumoral rather than systemic conversion of doxifluridine to 5-FU.[12] The activity of capecitabine has been demonstrated even in 5-FU-resistant cell lines.[13] Dose-limiting toxicities in phase I trials were diarrhea, vomiting, and hand–foot syndrome.[14] In a large randomized, phase II trial evaluating three schedules of capecitabine (continuous, intermittent, and intermittent with leucovorin) in patients with metastatic colorectal cancer, the response rates ranged from 21% to 24%. The longest time to disease progression

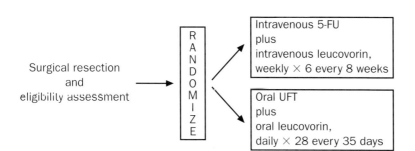

Figure 59.1 A clinical trial comparing oral uracil tegafur (UFT) plus leucovorin (LV) with 5-fluorouracil (5-FU) plus LV in the treatment of patients with stages II and III carcinoma of the colon (NSABP C-06).

was noted in the intermittent capecitabine arm without leucovorin. The addition of leucovorin resulted in increased toxicity and lower cumulative doses of capecitabine.[15] The intermittent schedule consists of 2500 mg/m^2 in two divided doses daily for 2 weeks followed by 1 week of rest, and was recently compared with bolus 5-FU and leucovorin in two phase III trials. Preliminary results revealed an improved response rate in the capecitabine arm compared with the standard arm for both studies, although there were no significant differences in progression-free or overall survival. The toxicity profile was more favorable in the capecitabine arms as well.[16,17]

The North Central Cancer Treatment Group (NCCTG) is currently evaluating capecitabine as a radiation sensitizer in a phase I study (NCCTG 984652) in patients with locally unresectable, residual, or recurrent colorectal cancer localized in the pelvis. This trial seeks to determine the maximally tolerated dose (MTD) of capecitabine in combination with pelvic radiotherapy and to obtain preliminary evidence of therapeutic activity. The capecitabine is administered on a twice-daily schedule continuously for 6 weeks, with radiation given on a Monday–Friday schedule. The use of continuous-infusion 5-FU as a radiation sensitizer has become standard in the adjuvant treatment of rectal cancer, and the eventual phase III testing of an oral agent in this setting could result in a new standard treatment.

Ethynyluracil (eniluracil) irreversibly inhibits DPD, resulting in enhanced absorption and bioavailability of oral 5-FU. Eniluracil is well tolerated, with only grade 1–2 toxicities, including anorexia, asthenia, nausea, and emesis.[18] It prolongs the half-life of 5-FU to 4.5–5.0 hours, with 28-day regimens of twice-daily administration resulting in steady-state plasma levels that are similar to those achieved with protracted 5-FU infusions.[19] Diarrhea and fatigue were the most common significant toxicities in phase II trials, and an overall response rate of 29% was observed in patients with metastatic colon carcinoma using the 28-day schedule. In addition, stable disease after two cycles was noted in 57% of patients.[20]

The Cancer and Leukemia Group B (CALGB) completed a phase II study of oral eniluracil, 5-FU, and leucovorin in previously untreated patients with advanced colorectal cancer (CALGB 9683). The overall response rate was 13%, with a median survival of 12.6 months. However, grade 3–5 toxicity (primarily neutropenia) was encountered in 85% of patients, with 37% of patients hospitalized for toxicity. The schedule used in this trial was 7 days of eniluracil in combination with oral 5-FU and leucovorin on days 2–6, repeated every 28 days.[21] The NCCTG performed a trial of eniluracil and oral 5-FU without leucovorin on a similar 7 out of 28 day schedule (NCCTG 954651), and preliminary data presented in abstract form suggest that less toxicity was encountered.[22]

A North American phase III study of oral eniluracil and oral 5-FU given for 28 out of 35 days versus intravenous 5-FU and leucovorin given daily for 5 days every 28 days in patients with advanced colorectal cancer was recently completed and analyzed. The results of this trial demonstrated a median survival of 58 weeks with the oral agents and 63 weeks with intravenous therapy ($p = 0.31$). The safety profiles of both regimens were acceptable, with a statistically significant increased rate of neutropenia with the intravenous regimen. However, these data, in combination with those from a European trial of similar design that demonstrated inferior survival with eniluracil/5-FU, has resulted in the halting of the development of this oral combination.[23]

For further discussion of oral fluoropyrimidines, see Chapter 47.

IRINOTECAN

Irinotecan (CPT-11) is a semisynthetic derivative of camptothecin, a plant alkaloid extracted from the *Camptotheca acuminata* tree. Its activity is derived from irreversibly binding the enzyme topoisomerase I, thereby producing DNA strand breaks that trigger the onset of apoptosis.[24] Phase I studies established the MTD as 125 mg/m^2 given weekly for 4 weeks in a 6-week cycle.[25] Two phase II studies of the agent in patients previously treated with at least one 5-FU-containing regimen demonstrated an overall response rate of 14.5%, with an additional 53.9% having stable disease after at least two cycles of therapy.[26]

The NCCTG completed a multicenter phase II study of irinotecan as a single agent in 31 previously untreated patients with metastatic colon cancer, and demonstrated a response rate of 29%, with all of the responses being partial responses. An additional 52% of patients had a minor response or stable disease. Diarrhea and myelosuppression were the most common serious toxicities.[27]

The CALGB recently completed a phase III randomized trial of 5-FU and leucovorin with or without irinotecan after curative resection for patients with stage III colon cancer (CALGB 89803) (Figure 59.2). This trial enrolled a total of 1260 patients. The NCCTG, Eastern Cooperative Oncology Group (ECOG), and Southwest Oncology Group (SWOG) participated in this intergroup trial. The regimen of irinotecan, 5-FU and leucovorin used in this trial is based on a phase I/II trial conducted at the Memorial Sloan-Kettering Cancer Center. A phase III randomized comparison of this weekly three-drug combination with 5-FU and leucovorin given for 5 days a month in previously untreated metastatic colon cancer was recently completed. The results demonstrated a statistically significant improvement in response rate, time to treatment failure, and survival in favor of the irinotecan-containing regimen.[28] The irinotecan is given at a dose of 125 mg/m^2 given weekly for 4 weeks along with 5-FU 500 mg/m^2 and leucovorin 20 mg/m^2, followed by a 2-week rest period. Objectives of the CALGB adjuvant trial include comparing the overall survival and disease-free survival of the two groups. The trial includes a comprehensive assessment of the prognostic or predictive value of several tissue-based and molecular markers (thymidylate synthase, p53, p21, p27, vascular endothelial growth factor (VEGF), microvascular density, 18q loss of heterozygosity, and microsatellite instability). In addition, the importance of thymidylate synthase and topoisomerase 1 expression and tumor sensitivity to 5-FU and irinotecan will be explored in this trial.

For further discussion of irinotecan as a single agent and in combination therapy, see Chapters 49 and 52–54.

OXALIPLATIN

Oxaliplatin (*trans*-1-diaminocyclohexane oxalatoplatinum(II)) is a novel platinum derivative with demonstrated activity in colorectal cancers. In vitro studies have shown synergistic or additive cytotoxicity with fluoropyrimidines and irinotecan.[29] A phase II trial of oxaliplatin in combination with bolus 5-FU and leucovorin in patients with advanced colorectal cancer who had failed previous therapy with bolus 5-FU and leucovorin yielded a response rate of 13%, with a median time to progression of 4.3 months. Improvement in the baseline performance status was noted in 47% of patients. Additional attempts at combining oxaliplatin with 5-FU and leucovorin have utilized infusional schedules of 5-FU, with the other agents being given as a bolus. Phase I trials of the combination of oxaliplatin and irinotecan yielded a recommended phase II dose of oxaliplatin 200 mg/m^2 and irinotecan 85 mg/m^2 given every three weeks. Diarrhea and neutropenia were the dose-limiting toxicities.[30] Other phase I trials of these two agents have defined a 28-day schedule, with irinotecan at a dose of 80 mg/m^2 on days 1, 8, and 15 and oxaliplatin at a dose of 85 mg/m^2 on days 1 and 15.[31]

A phase I study by the ECOG of preoperative radiation therapy with concurrent escalating doses of oxaliplatin and protracted continuous-infusion 5-FU followed by surgery and adjuvant oxaliplatin, 5-FU,

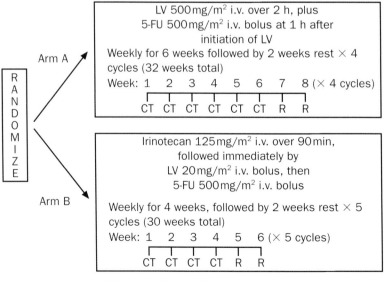

Figure 59.2 Phase III intergroup trial of irinotecan plus 5-fluorouracil/leucovorin (5-FU/LV) versus 5-FU/LV alone after curative resection for patients with stage III colon cancer (CALGB 89803).

CT, chemotherapy; R, rest

and leucovorin in patients with locally advanced rectal carcinoma (E 1297) is currently underway. This study seeks to determine the maximally tolerated dose of oxaliplatin biweekly when combined preoperatively with concurrent radiotherapy and continuous-infusion 5-FU in this population of patients. Additional objectives include the assessment of the resectability of T4 rectal cancers and pathologic complete response rates of T3 and T4 rectal cancers after this therapy. The CALGB has recently begun a similar phase I/II trial of preoperative radiation with weekly oxaliplatin and continuous-infusion 5-FU in patients with locally advanced rectal cancer (CALGB 89901).

The NCCTG has opened a phase II study of oxaliplatin and 5-FU with leucovorin in patients with unresectable hepatic metastases from colorectal carcinoma (NCCTG 974651). The objectives of this trial are to evaluate the efficacy of the combination in converting patients with unresectable hepatic metastases to candidates for hepatic resection, as well as to assess the response rate, toxicity, and overall survival of the treatment. The oxaliplatin will be given over 2 hours on day 1, followed by leucovorin over 2 hours along with bolus 5-FU, followed by a 22-hour infusion of 5-FU, repeated every 2 weeks.

A randomized phase III trial by the NCCTG (N9841) seeks to compare irinotecan with the combination of oxaliplatin, 5-FU, and leucovorin in patients with advanced colorectal carcinoma previously treated with 5-FU (Figure 59.3). If the combination is demonstrated to have equivalent efficacy with less toxicity compared with irinotecan, it could

become the established standard as second-line therapy in advanced colorectal cancer.

The largest study by the US cooperative groups for advanced colorectal cancer currently underway is a phase III trial of different combination regimens. This trial, led by the NCCTG (N9741), initially included six arms but currently includes three arms. The trial will compare time to progression after treatment with irinotecan/5-FU/LV versus oxaliplatin/5-FU/LV versus irinotecan/oxaliplatin (Figure 59.4). In addition, the trial will compare the toxicity, response rates, time to treatment failure, and survival in the three treatment groups. Quality-of-life parameters are being assessed as well in this landmark trial. The accrual is currently planned at 1125 patients.

The irinotecan/5-FU/LV treatment arm in this study was developed at the Memorial-Sloan Kettering Cancer Center. This regimen consists of irinotecan, 5-FU, and leucovorin given weekly for 4 weeks, followed by a 2-week rest, repeated every 6 weeks.[32] The second arm utilizes a 22-hour infusion of 5-FU after oxaliplatin and leucovorin given every 2 weeks. In the third arm, consisting of oxaliplatin and irinotecan, the two drugs are given every 2 weeks.

It is projected that this trial will complete accrual in 2 years. The CALGB and the National Cancer Institute of Canada (NCI-C) Clinical Trials Group are participating with the NCCTG in this important trial.

For further discussion of oxaliplatin as a single agent and in combination therapy, see Chapters 50 and 52–54.

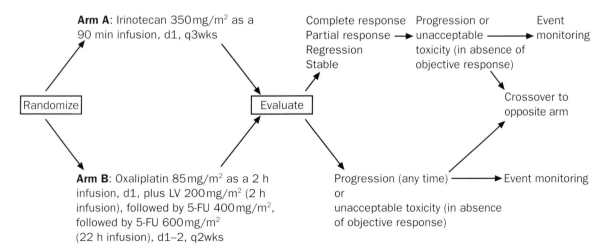

Figure 59.3 A randomized phase III equivalence trial of irinotecan versus oxaliplatin/5-fluorouracil (5-FU)/leucovorin (LV) in patients with advanced colorectal carcinoma previously treated with 5-FU (NCCTG N9841).

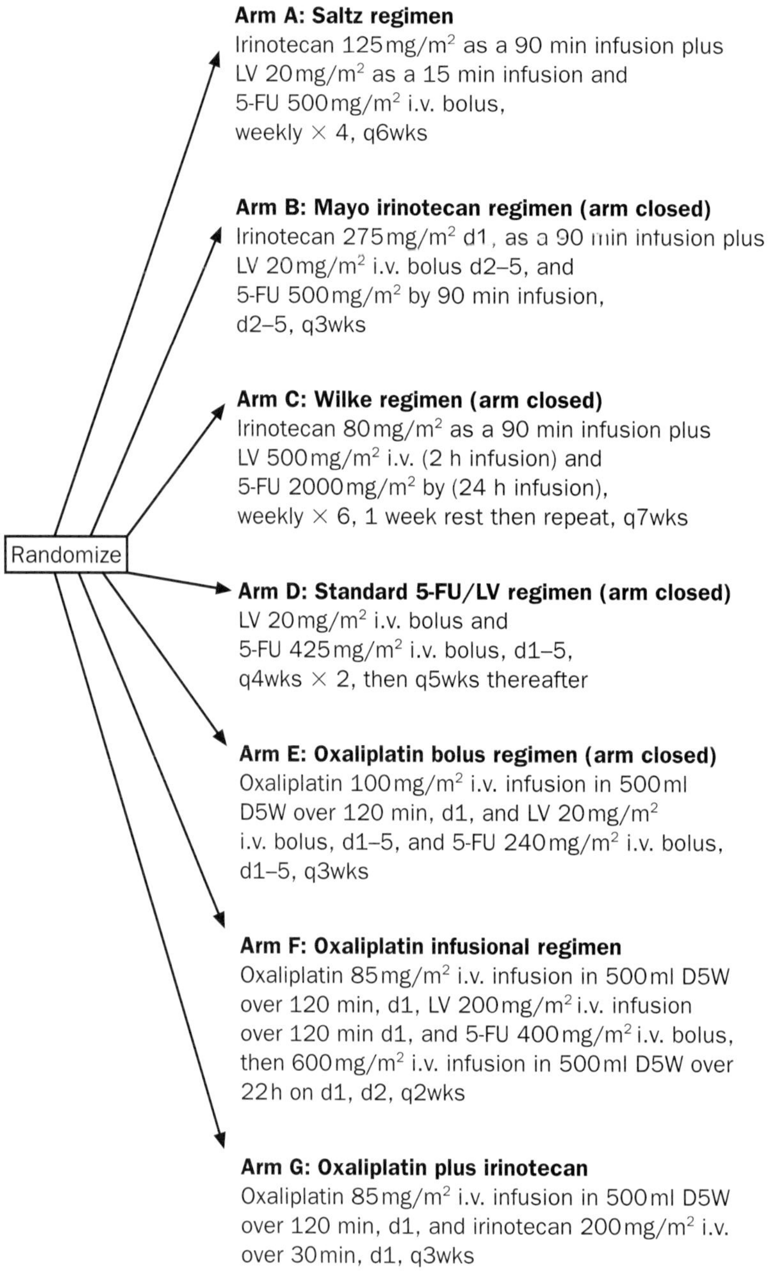

Arm A: Saltz regimen
Irinotecan 125 mg/m^2 as a 90 min infusion plus
LV 20 mg/m^2 as a 15 min infusion and
5-FU 500 mg/m^2 i.v. bolus,
weekly × 4, q6wks

Arm B: Mayo irinotecan regimen (arm closed)
Irinotecan 275 mg/m^2 d1, as a 90 min infusion plus
LV 20 mg/m^2 i.v. bolus d2–5, and
5-FU 500 mg/m^2 by 90 min infusion,
d2–5, q3wks

Arm C: Wilke regimen (arm closed)
Irinotecan 80 mg/m^2 as a 90 min infusion plus
LV 500 mg/m^2 i.v. (2 h infusion) and
5-FU 2000 mg/m^2 by (24 h infusion),
weekly × 6, 1 week rest then repeat, q7wks

Arm D: Standard 5-FU/LV regimen (arm closed)
LV 20 mg/m^2 i.v. bolus and
5-FU 425 mg/m^2 i.v. bolus, d1–5,
q4wks × 2, then q5wks thereafter

Arm E: Oxaliplatin bolus regimen (arm closed)
Oxaliplatin 100 mg/m^2 i.v. infusion in 500 ml
D5W over 120 min, d1, and LV 20 mg/m^2
i.v. bolus, d1–5, and 5-FU 240 mg/m^2 i.v. bolus,
d1–5, q3wks

Arm F: Oxaliplatin infusional regimen
Oxaliplatin 85 mg/m^2 i.v. infusion in 500 ml D5W
over 120 min, d1, LV 200 mg/m^2 i.v. infusion
over 120 min d1, and 5-FU 400 mg/m^2 i.v. bolus,
then 600 mg/m^2 i.v. infusion in 500 ml D5W over
22 h on d1, d2, q2wks

Arm G: Oxaliplatin plus irinotecan
Oxaliplatin 85 mg/m^2 i.v. infusion in 500 ml D5W
over 120 min, d1, and irinotecan 200 mg/m^2 i.v.
over 30 min, d1, q3wks

Randomize

Figure 59.4 A randomized phase III trial of two different regimens of irinotecan plus 5-fluorouracil (5-FU) and leucovorin (LV), two different regimens of oxaliplatin plus 5-FU and LV, and one regimen of oxaliplatin plus irinotecan compared with 5-FU and LV as initial treatment of patients with advanced adenocarcinoma of the colon and rectum (NCCTG N9741).

MONOCLONAL ANTIBODY 17-1A (MoAb 17-1A)

The monoclonal antibody (MoAb) 17-1A is a murine IgG2a directed against a transmembrane glycoprotein expressed on many adenocarcinomas. This antibody results in both antibody-dependent cellular cytotoxicity and complement-mediated cytolysis of tumor cells.[33] A multi-institutional phase II trial in patients with metastatic colorectal cancer produced a response rate of only 7%. However, the mechanisms through which this agent exerts its cytolytic effect are likely to be more significant in the adjuvant or minimal residual disease setting.[34]

A large phase III intergroup trial coordinated by the CALGB is currently testing the activity of MoAb 17-1A as adjuvant therapy following resection for patients with stage II adenocarcinoma of the colon (CALGB 9581). Eligible patients are randomized to either five doses of the antibody given every 28 days following surgical resection or observation alone (Figure 59.5). This international trial has been joined by SWOG, ECOG, and the NCI-C Clinical Trials Group, as well as the Cancer Research Campaign Clinical Trials Unit (CRCTU) and the European Organization for Research and Treatment of Cancer (EORTC), with an overall planned accrual of 2100 patients. Objectives of the trial include comparing survival and disease-free survival between the treatment and observation groups. In addition, alterations in cell-cycle-related genes, markers of metastatic potential (*DCC* gene), cellular differentiation, DNA ploidy, cell proliferation, and tumor angiogenesis will be assessed to determine their role in predicting recurrence and overall survival. This trial should yield important results regarding not only the activity of this novel antibody but also the predictive value of phenotypic and genotypic changes for relapse in early-stage colorectal tumors.

NOVEL TRIAL DESIGNS FOR CYTOSTATIC AGENTS

As new agents are being developed, with novel mechanisms of biological activity, new paradigms for evaluating efficacy are becoming necessary. This is important both for the agents whose activity is best demonstrated in the setting of minimal residual disease (e.g. immunomodulatory therapies) and for agents with cytostatic rather than cytotoxic activity (e.g. angiogenesis inhibitors).

Hepatic resection is a proven effective modality for the treatment of select patients with metastatic colorectal cancer confined to the liver. Numerous studies have demonstrated that as many as 40% of carefully selected patients with hepatic metastases remain disease-free at 2 years.[35] The majority of patients will progress, however, within this time frame. Although data exploring the utility of regional and systemic chemotherapy in this setting are emerging, this remains an excellent setting in which to evaluate the efficacy of agents that may delay or interfere with disease progression. The CALGB has recently embarked on a program to test novel agents in this setting of minimal residual disease in which cytostatic activity can be assessed by evaluating relapse-free survival following hepatic metastatectomy.

The burgeoning development of new agents with activity in colorectal cancer has fueled important new trials by the US cooperative groups to define the role of these agents in a variety of settings. The next decade promises to be an important one, with an opportunity to define active regimens to replace 5-FU and leucovorin as standard treatment in this disease. In addition, novel agents, developed through enhanced understanding of the molecular basis of carcinogenesis and cell proliferation, will no doubt result in continued progress in these diseases.

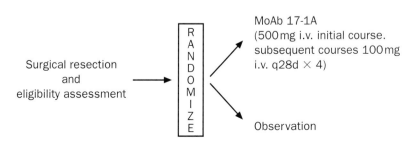

Figure 59.5 Phase III randomized study of adjuvant immunotherapy with monoclonal antibody (MoAb) 17-1A versus no adjuvant therapy following resection for stage II (modified Astler–Coller B2) adenocarcinoma of the colon (CALGB 9581).

REFERENCES

1. Saltz LB, Cox JV, Blanke C et al, Irinotecan plus fluorouracil and leucovorin for metastatic colorectal cancer. Irinotecan Study Group. *N Engl J Med* 2000; **343:** 905–14.

2. Moertel CG, Chemotherapy of colorectal cancer. *N Engl J Med* 1994; **330:** 1136–42.

3. The Meta-Analysis Group in Cancer, Efficacy of intravenous continuous infusion of fluorouracil compared with bolus administration in advanced colorectal cancer. *J Clin Oncol* 1998; **16:** 301–9.

4. Allegra CJ, Green JL, Antimetabolites. In: *Cancer: Principles and Practice of Oncology*, 5th edn (DeVita VT, Hellman S, Rosenberg SA, eds). Philadelphia: Lippincott, 1997: 432–52.

5. Brito RA, Medgyesy D, Zukowski TM et al, Fluoropyrimidines: a critical evaluation. *Oncol* 1999; **57**(Suppl 1): 2–8.

6. Taguchi T, Experience with UFT in Japan. *Oncology (Huntingt)* 1997; **11:** 30–4.

7. Hoff PM, Pazdur R, Benner SE, Canetta R, UFT and leucovorin: a review of its clinical development and therapeutic potential in the oral treatment of cancer. *Anti Cancer Drugs* 1998; **9:** 479–90.

8. Sulkes A, Benner SE, Canetta RM, Uracil – ftorafur, an oral fluoropyrimidine active in colorectal cancer. *J Clin Oncol* 1998; **16:** 3461–75.

9. Carmichael J, Popiela T, Radstone D et al, Randomized comparative study of Orzel (oral uroacil/tegafur (UFT) plus leucovorin) versus parenteral 5-fluorouracil plus leucovorin in patients with metastatic colorectal cancer. *Proc Am Soc Clin Oncol* 1999; **18:** 264a (Abst 1015).

10. Pazdur R, Douillard JY, Skillings JR et al, Multicenter phase III study of 5-fluorouracil or UFT in combination with leucovorin in patients with metastatic colorectal cancer. *Proc Am Soc Clin Oncol* 1999; **18:** 2263a (Abst 1009).

11. Miwa M, Ura M, Nishida N et al, Design of a novel fluoropyrimidine carbamate, capecitabine, which generates 5-fluorouracil selectively in tumors by enzymes concentrated in human liver and cancer tissues. *Eur J Cancer* 1998; **34:** 1274–81.

12. Schuller J, Cassidy J, Reigner B et al, Tumor selective activation of capecitabine in colorectal cancer patients. *Oncologie* 1997; **70**(Suppl 1): Abstract A 732.

13. Cao S, Luk M, Ishitsuka H, Rustunm YM, Antitumor activity of capecitabine against fluorouracil sensitive and resistant tumors. *Proc Am Soc Clin Oncol* 1997; **16:** 226a (Abst 795).

14. Budman DR, Meropol NJ, Reigner B et al, Preliminary studies of a novel fluoropyrimidine carbamate: capecitabine. *J Clin Oncol* 1998; **16:** 1795–802.

15. Findlay M, Van Cutsen E, Kocha W et al, A randomized phase II study of Xeloda (capecitabine) in patients with advanced colorectal cancers. *Proc Am Soc Clin Oncol* 1997; **16:** 227a (Abst 798).

16. Cox JV, Pazdur R, Thibault A et al, A phase III trial of Xeloda (capecitabine) in previously untreated advanced/metastatic colorectal cancer. *Proc Am Soc Clin Oncol* 1999; **18:** 265a (Abst 1016).

17. Twelves C, Harper P, Van Catsem E et al, A phase III trial of Xeloda (capecitabine) in previously untreated advanced/metastatic colorectal cancer. *Proc Am Soc Clin Oncol* 1999; **18:** 263a (Abst 1010).

18. Schilsky RL, Hohneker J, Ratain MJ et al, Phase I clinical and pharmacologic study of 5FU plus eniluracil in patients with advanced cancer. *J Clin Oncol* 1998; **16:** 1450–7.

19. Baker S, Khor S, Adjej A et al, Pharmacokinetics, oral bioavailability and safety study of fluorouracil in patients treated with 776C85, an inactivator of dihydropyrimidine dehydrogenase. *J Clin Oncol* 1996; **14:** 3085–96.

20. Mani S, Beck T, Chevlen E et al, A phase II open-label study to evaluate a 28-day regimen of oral 5-FU plus 776C85 for the treatment of patients with previously untreated metastatic colorectal cancer. *Proc Am Soc Clin Oncol* 1998; **17:** 281A.

21. Meropol NJ, Niedzwicki D, Hollis D et al, Phase II study of oral eniluracil, 5-fluorouracil, and leucovorin in patients with advanced colorectal carcinoma. *Cancer* 2001; **91:** 1256–63.

22. Goldberg RM, Kugler J, Sargent DJ et al, A phase II trial of oral 776C85 plus a five day regimen of oral 5-FU in untreated patients with metastatic colorectal cancer. NCCTG study. *Proc Am Soc Clin Oncol* 1998; **17:** 282a (Abst 1084).

23. Levin J, Schilsky RL, North American phase III study of oral eniluracil plus oral 5-fluorouracil (5-FU) versus intravenous 5-FU plus leucovorin in the treatment of advanced colorectal cancer. *Proc Am Soc Clin Oncol* 2001; **20:** Abst 523.

24. Kunimoto T, Nitta K, Tanaka T et al, Antitumor activity of 7-ethyl-10-[4-(piperidino)-1-piperidino]carbonyloxy-camptothecin, a novel, water-soluble derivative of camptothecin, against murine tumors. *Cancer Res* 1987; **47:** 5944–7.

25. Rothenberg ML, Kuha JG, Burris HA III et al, Phase I and pharmacokinetic trial of weekly CPT-11. *J Clin Oncol* 1993; **11:** 2194–204.

26. Rothenberg ML, Cox JV, DeVore RF et al, A multicenter phase II trial of weekly irinotecan (CPT-11) in patients with previously treated colorectal carcinoma. *Cancer* 1999; **85:** 786–95.

27. Pilot HC, Wender R, O'Connell MJ et al, A phase I trial of CPT-11 (irinotecan) in patients with metastatic colorectal cancer: a NCCTG study. *Proc Am Soc Clin Oncol* 1994; **13:** a573.

28. Saltz LB, Douillard J-Y, Pirotta N et al, Combined analysis of two phase III randomized trials comparing irinotecan (C), fluorouracil (F), leucovorin (L) vs F alone as first-line therapy of previously untreated metastatic colorectal cancer (MCRC). *Proc Am Soc Clin Oncol* 2000; **19:** Abst 938.

29. Raymond E, Faivre S, Woynarowski JM et al, Oxaliplatin: mechanism of action and antineoplastic activity. *Semin Oncol* 1998; **25**(2 Suppl 5): 4–12.

30. Wasserman E, Goldwasser F, Ouldacki M et al, CPT-11/oxaliplatin every 3 weeks: An active combination in colorectal cancer. *Proc Am Assoc Cancer Res* 1998; **39:** A2190.

31. Scheithauer W, Kornek GV, Rubere M et al, Combined irinotecan and oxaliplatin plus granulocyte-colony stimulating factor in patients with advanced fluoropyrimidine/leucovorin pretreated colorectal cancer. *J Clin Oncol* 1999; **17:** 902–6.

32. Saltz LB, Kanowitz J, Kemeny N, Phase I clinical and pharmacokinetic study of irinotecan, fluorouracil and leucovorin in patients with advanced solid tumors. *J Clin Oncol* 1996; **14:** 2959–67.

33. Adams DO, Hall T, Steplewski Z et al, Tumors undergoing rejection induced by monoclonal antibodies of the IgG2a isotype contain increased numbers of macrophages activated for a distinctive form of antibody-dependent cytolysis. *Proc Natl Acad Sci USA* 1984; **81:** 3506–10.

34. Wadler S, The role of immunotherapy in colorectal cancer. *Semin Oncol* 1991; **18**(Suppl): 27–38.

35. Fong Y, Cohen AM, Fortner JG et al, Liver resection for colorectal metastases. *J Clin Oncol* 1997; **15:** 938–46.

60

Drug development in colorectal cancer: Viewpoint of the European cooperative groups

Jacques Wils

INTRODUCTION

Drug development in advanced colorectal cancer in Europe has focused on the incorporation of the two most promising 'new' drugs in this disease, irinotecan (CPT-11) and oxaliplatin, in treatment protocols. These studies have been conducted and analysed by the pharmaceutical companies manufacturing these drugs, in cooperation with individual investigators. Both cytotoxic agents were first investigated in second-line therapy (see Chapters 49 and 50, and also Chapters 54–56) and then recently in first-line therapy.[1-3]

The next step will obviously be the assessment of these drugs in the adjuvant setting, and for this purpose large-scale cooperative trials are needed.

TREATMENT OF ADVANCED DISEASE

Studies investigating best supportive care in patients with metastatic colorectal cancer reported a median survival of approximately 6 months and 7–11 months for good-risk patients with tumour confined to the liver only. Data from chemotherapy trials with bolus 5-fluorouracil (5-FU) plus leucovorin (LV, folinic acid) in the 1980s and early 1990s reported a median survival of usually not more than 12 months. The new generation of trials using infusional 5-FU programmes consistently observed a median survival exceeding 15–16 months. These data may reflect a stepwise progress that has been achieved over time, through the development of chemotherapy mainly from bolus to infusional 5-FU. The first experience with irinotecan or oxaliplatin in first-line treatment in combination with infusional 5-FU appears to indicate a further improvement in treatment outcome. In the studies assessing the addition of oxaliplatin to infusional 5-FU/LV, no significant survival differences were detected,[1,2] which could be explained partly by crossover treatment upon relapse. In the trial conducted by the Aventis company that compared infusional 5-FU/LV with infusional 5-FU/LV plus irinotecan, a significant survival difference was detected, the relative improvement in median survival being 23% (14.1 versus 17.4 months).[3]

Other important trials in first-line treatment are still ongoing and include a European Organization for Research and Treatment of Cancer (EORTC) study comparing weekly 24-hour infusional high-dose 5-FU plus leucovorin (HD-FU/LV) with HD-FU/LV plus irinotecan. In this trial, patients who relapse after 5-FU/LV and are suited for further treatment will be offered irinotecan added to the infusional regimen (Table 60.1). Another trial, with five arms, has been initiated in the UK by the Colorectal Cancer Group of the Medical Research Council. This study assesses upfront irinotecan or oxaliplatin plus infusional 5-FU/LV (biweekly 48-hour infusion) versus the sequential treatment after infusional 5-FU/LV (Trial C-08). The drugs will be added to the infusional regimen upon relapse. The control or 'standard' arm consists of infusional 5-FU/LV; single agent irinotecan will be offered to patients upon relapse (Table 60.2). The UK trial especially aims to answer the question whether the upfront use of these new drugs in combination with infusional 5-FU is to be preferred over their sequential use in second-line therapy.

Table 60.1 Design of EORTC trial 40986

Arm A (reference arm): First-line HD-FU/LV; upon relapse, irinotecan will be added

Arm B: First-line HD-FU/LV plus irinotecan

HD-FU/LV, weekly 24-hour infusional high-dose 5-fluorouracil plus leucovorin.

Table 60.2 Design of MRC/CRC trial C-08

Arm A (reference arm): First-line 5-FU/LV; upon relapse, 5-FU/LV will be discontinued and patients will receive single-agent irinotecan (if appropriate)

Arm B: First-line 5-FU/LV; upon relapse add irinotecan

Arm C: First-line 5-FU/LV plus irinotecan

Arm D: First-line 5-FU/LV; upon relapse add oxaliplatin

Arm E: First-line 5-FU/LV plus oxaliplatin

5-FU/LV, biweekly 48-hour infusional 5-fluorouracil plus leucovorin ('De Gramont'). Randomization is one-third in Arm A and one-sixth in each of the other four arms.

Some clinicians follow the idea of a stepwise administration from less active regimens (modulated 5-FU bolus schedules) as first-line treatment to more potent schedules (such as infusional 5-FU programmes) as second-line treatment, followed by salvage therapy with oxaliplatin/5-FU or irinotecan/5-FU in selected patients. This view is supported by the lack of a clear survival advantage for the infusional regimens relative to modulated bolus 5-FU schedules. And indeed, to offer an effective salvage treatment after failure of a standard regimen might have contributed to the survival of over 15–16 months reported in the newer trials. On the other hand, a median time to tumour progression of 3–5 months associated with 5-FU bolus regimens necessitates the start of second-line therapy in every second patient already at this time. In addition, the condi-

tion of some patients might have deteriorated during bolus 5-FU, precluding second-line treatment. With the infusional programmes, patients have a greater chance to respond, which is then associated with a longer time to treatment failure (about 7 months) and probably a lower percentage of patients unsuitable for second-line therapy.

Therefore infusional 5-FU is considered a more appropriate first-line treatment by many European groups. To increase the efficacy of the first-line treatment with combinations of infusional 5-FU/LV plus oxaliplatin or irinotecan upfront might a be a step forward, but it seems to be too early at present to advocate this strategy for all patients.

Thus the question of combined versus sequential treatment with infusional 5-FU and the new drugs is of importance for most European investigators.

ADJUVANT THERAPY

Introduction

After many years, during which the assumption prevailed that adjuvant chemotherapy was of no benefit in patients with resected adenocarcinoma of the colon, data from several large US studies published from the late 1980s have caused a marked shift in surgical and medical opinion. Although results in patients with Dukes stage B disease have not shown a clear benefit, the efficacy of adjuvant chemotherapy has definitely been shown in those with stage C colon cancer. As a result, the Mayo regimen of bolus 5-FU with low-dose leucovorin (see Chapter 41) and the weekly Roswell Park regimen (see Chapter 42) have become widely accepted as standard adjuvant therapy in these patients.

To investigate alternatives to the bolus regimens in the adjuvant treatment of resected stage C adenocarcinoma of the colon, two large European trials, PETACC-1 (first Pan-European Trial for Adjuvant Treatment of Colon Cancer) and PETACC-2 (second Pan-European Trial) have been set up. These trials will provide valuable European data to add to those from the USA. They aim to assess the place of raltitrexed in the adjuvant treatment of resected stage C colon cancer, and compare infusional and bolus 5-FU regimens. A third study, comparing infusional 5-FU/LV with infusional 5-FU/LV plus irinotecan (PETACC-3), has more recently been initiated.

The current position

Results available today strongly support the use of postoperative adjuvant chemotherapy, particularly in patients with Dukes stage C colon cancer. Available data indicate bolus 5-FU with leucovorin, given for 6–8 months, to be at least as effective as bolus 5-FU plus levamisole for 12 months. Thus the Mayo regimen of 5-FU 425 mg/m^2 (370 mg/m^2 in some centres) plus leucovorin 20 mg/m^2 for 5 days every 4–5 weeks[4,5] and the Roswell Park regimen of 5-FU 500 mg/m^2 plus leucovorin 500 mg/m^2, weekly × 6, every 8 weeks are currently considered by most European investigators to be the standard adjuvant treatment in patients with resected stage C colon cancer. However, regimens based on bolus 5-FU need frequent administration, and may be associated with considerable toxicity, particularly mucositis and leukopenia,[6] which necessitates dose reduction and/or delay in treatment.[7] Indeed, in one study from the USA,[8] toxicity of WHO grade 3 severity or greater was reported in 35% of patients who received 5-FU plus leucovorin, 36% of those who received 5-FU, leucovorin, and levamisole, and 28% of those who received 5-FU plus levamisole. Although these data are derived from a mixture of bolus 5-FU/LV schedules and from patients treated in the adjuvant setting, as well as from patients with advanced disease, there is interest in the use of agents in adjuvant therapy that are at least as effective as modulated bolus 5-FU but that have more favourable tolerability profiles or less complex administration schedules.

European clinical studies of adjuvant treatment in Dukes C colon cancer

Large studies of the efficacy of adjuvant chemotherapy in resectable colon cancer have to date been carried out mainly by investigators in the USA. European trials in this area of study mainly aimed to confirm data from the USA or focused on intraportal treatment (see Chapter 15). Examples of trials assessing systemic therapy are 5-FU/LV versus control (France and Italy),[9] 5-FU/levamisole versus control (Netherlands and Denmark), and a study from the UK comparing different 5-FU/LV/levamisole combinations (QUASAR-1).[10] None of these trials resulted in outcomes different from what had already been achieved in the USA.

Intraportal chemotherapy alone or in combination with systemic treatment was studied by the EORTC,[11] the SAKK (Swiss Group for Clinical Cancer Research),[12] and groups from Italy[13] and the UK.[14] Lastly, a small but interesting study from the Netherlands with active specific immunotherapy has been published.[15] All studies took a long time to complete accrual.

Clinical research in oncology is a very demanding field and constantly full of challenges. It was felt that the way forward for the rapid development of new active anticancer agents in this setting was through collaboration among the existing national and international groups in Europe with the support of the pharmaceutical industry. Therefore European collaborative groups created PETACC (Pan-European Trials in Adjuvant Colon Cancer), a consortium for jointly running large-scale clinical trials in the field of adjuvant colorectal cancer research. The PETACC model has been presented at major oncology meetings, and has received much attention worldwide.[16]

Two European studies have been initiated to determine the efficacy of raltitrexed and various infusional 5-FU regimens relative to currently accepted adjuvant treatment. In order to recruit the large numbers of patients needed, these studies involved the collaboration of the cooperative groups gathered in PETACC, with the addition of individual centres and groups worldwide with interest in these trials.

Raltitrexed (Tomudex), a direct and specific inhibitor of thymidylate synthase (TS), appeared to be an interesting new candidate for the adjuvant therapy of surgically managed cancer of the colon (see Chapter 51). Over 1000 patients had been studied in one multi-institutional phase II and three multinational phase III trials. These studies demonstrated equivalence of raltitrexed compared with the Mayo regimen and the Machover schedule (5-FU plus high-dose LV) with respect to response rates not exceeding 20%.[17–19] The median time to progression was significantly less for patients treated with raltitrexed in two studies,[18,19] and the median survival was inferior in one study.[19] The clinical relevance of these minor differences, however, was felt to be debatable, because the median time to progression and survival were not different from what had been reported before in a number of clinical trials with bolus 5-FU/LV in advanced colorectal cancer. Raltitrexed was associated with a transient increase in aminotransferases (transaminases), which appears to be specific to this new compound. The quality-of-life dimensions measured in these studies demonstrated no differences except for a greater impact of nausea and vomiting in the cohort treated with raltitrexed. The convenient administration schedule for this drug is also of interest, since it reduces the frequency of hospital attendance by patients, with attendant beneficial effects on quality of life and on healthcare resource consumption.

The first study (PETACC-1) compared raltitrexed with the Mayo regimen as postsurgical adjuvant treatment in patients with Dukes stage C colon cancer who had undergone curative radical resection within the 42 days preceding enrolment. Primary objectives were to determine recurrence-free and overall survival rates; the secondary objective was to compare the toxicities of the two regimens. The study was supported by the AstraZeneca company.

After randomization of 1835 patients within 15 months, unfortunately PETACC-1 was closed by the sponsor to further randomization before the target accrual of 2800 patients. The reason for this action was that the independent data monitoring committee (IDMC) had recommended a temporary suspension of recruitment due to an excess of drug-related fatalities in the raltitrexed arm. The IDMC also recommended that a further safety and efficacy evaluation should be carried out. The PETACC Steering Committee agreed to follow these recommendations, and also felt that the observed excess mortality in the presence of a milder toxicity profile in terms of gastrointestinal and bone marrow toxicity was puzzling and needed further investigation. The sponsor, however, after having undertaken an unscheduled review of 'interim' efficacy data, which were not seen either by the IDMC or the Steering Committee, decided to close the trial. As a result, the planned statistical methods section of the protocol had to be amended, and the true benefit or lack of benefit of raltitrexed will become difficult, if not impossible, to assess.

A second study (PETACC-2) continues to be carried out to compare the Mayo regimen (5-FU 370 or 425 mg/m^2 plus leucovorin 20 mg/m^2 for 5 days every 4 weeks for 6 cycles) with three high-dose infusional 5-FU regimens. Interest in such a comparison stems from observations indicating that 5-FU acts in different ways depending on whether it is administered over a short period as an intravenous bolus injection or rapid infusion (e.g. up to 15 minutes), or as a prolonged infusion.[20] Furthermore, most studies comparing infusional 5-FU with or without leucovorin with modulated bolus regimens have shown a higher response rate, a safe toxicity profile, and a trend for superior survival. Three infusional regimens (24-hour weekly HD-FU/LV, 48-hour weekly HD-FU, and 48-hour biweekly infusional 5-FU/LV) are being assessed in the infusional arm of the trial; these regimens have not been compared directly but the assumption is that no major differences exist.

A third study, comparing infusional 5-FU/LV with infusional 5-FU/LV plus irinotecan has recently been initiated in cooperation with Aventis (PETACC-3).

Other studies are being conducted by the pharmaceutical companies, and include infusional 5-FU with or without oxaliplatin (MOZAIC trial) and capecitabine versus the Mayo regimen (X-ACT trial). Both of these trials have completed accrual. A large trial conducted in Europe by GlaxoSmithKline was recently reported which compared the antibody 17-1A (edrocolomab) with 5-FU/LV or with 5-FU/LV plus edrocolomab. Edrocolomab alone was significantly inferior to 5-FU/LV, and the addition of the antibody to 5-FU/LV did not improve results.[21]

CONCLUSIONS

This is an exciting and interesting time for all those involved in the treatment of patients with adenocarcinoma of the colon. Now that the benefit of adjuvant chemotherapy for patients with Dukes stage C disease has been clarified, mainly in US centres, it is time to move to the next stage of research to assess the benefit of alternatives to the Mayo and Roswell Park regimens. These alternatives include raltitrexed and various infusional 5-FU regimens with or without irinotecan or oxaliplatin. Furthermore, the oral 5-FU prodrugs are of potential interest because they may mimic infusional 5-FU and because of their easy route of administration (see Chapter 47).

Controversial as the decision for premature closure of PETACC-1 may be,[22] and regardless of the issues encountered in the process that has led to an early termination of this trial, in many other respects this study has been successful. Recruitment has exceeded expectations, and confidence remains that the PETACC intergroup structure is an appropriate way forward for conducting clinical trials in the field of adjuvant treatment of colorectal cancer within reasonable time periods.

To match the power of the US studies in European centres, it is necessary to organize collaborative efforts, with the global involvement of experienced teams.

Now that many other different options for studies in the adjuvant treatment have become available, such as irinotecan, oxaliplatin, oral 5-FU prodrugs, active immunotherapy, 'mechanism-based' new agents and combinations of these, there will be strong competition among different companies to launch trials and to recruit patients. In fact, some trials are coordinated completely by the pharmaceutical companies. It is important that we reflect carefully on how to improve the way of interacting with the pharmaceutical industry for future trials, particularly on how to preserve independent research and enforce strict clinical trial methodology and procedures.

Lastly, the challenge is how, on the basis of biological markers and new molecular targets (thymidylate synthase, topoisomerase I, epidermal growth factor, vascular endothelial growth factor, etc.), we should select the armentarium of new agents that have become available, alone or in combination regimens, as best treatment for individual patients.

REFERENCES

1. de Gramont A, Figer A, Seymour M et al, Leucovorin (LV) and fluorouracil with or without oxaliplatin as first-line treatment in advanced colorectal cancer (CRC). *J Clin Oncol* 2000; **18:** 2938–47.
2. Giacchetti S, Perpoint B, Zidani R et al, Phase III multicenter randomized trial of oxaliplatin addition to chronomodulated fluorouracil-leucovorin as first-line treatment of metastatic colorectal cancer. *J Clin Oncol* 2000; **18:** 136–47.
3. Douillard JY, Cunningham D, Roth AD et al, Irinotecan combined with fluorouracil compared with fluorouracil alone as first-line treatment for metastatic colorectal cancer: a randomized trial. *Lancet* 2000; **355:** 1041–7.
4. Poon MA, O'Connell MJ, Wieand HS et al, Biochemical modulation of fluorouracil: evidence of significant improvements in survival and quality of life in patients with advanced colorectal carcinoma. *J Clin Oncol* 1989; **7:** 1407–18.
5. O'Connell MJ, Maillard JA, Kahn MJ et al, Controlled trial of fluorouracil and low dose leucovorin given for six months as postoperative adjuvant therapy for colon cancer. *J Clin Oncol* 1997; **15:** 246–50.
6. Petrelli N, Douglas Jr HO, Herrera L et al, The modulation of fluorouracil with leucovorin in metastatic colorectal carcinoma: a prospective randomized phase III trial. *J Clin Oncol* 1989; **7:** 1419–26.
7. Advanced Colorectal Cancer Meta-Analysis Project, Modulation of fluorouracil by leucovorin in patients with advanced colorectal cancer: evidence in terms of response rate. *J Clin Oncol* 1992; **10:** 896–903.
8. Wolmark N, Rockette H, Mamounas EP et al, Clinical trial to assess the relative efficacy of fluorouracil and leucovorin, fluorouracil and levamisole, and fluorouracil, and leucovorin, and levamisole in patients with Dukes' B and C carcinoma of the colon: results from National Surgical Adjuvant Breast and Bowel Project C-04. *J Clin Oncol* 1999; **17:** 3553–9.
9. International Multicentre Pooled Analysis of Colon Cancer Trials Investigators, Efficacy of adjuvant fluorouracil and folinic acid in colon cancer. *Lancet* 1995; **345:** 939–44.
10. QUASAR Collaborative Group, Comparison of fluorouracil with additional levamisole, higher-dose folonic acid, or both, as adjuvant chemotherapy for colorectal cancer: a randomised trial. *Lancet* 2000; **355:** 1588–96.
11. Rougier Ph, Sahmoud T, Nitti D et al, Adjuvant portal vein infusion of fluorouracil and heparin in colorectal cancer: a randomised trial. *Lancet* 1998; **351:** 1677–81.
12. Laffer U, Maibach R, Metzger U et al, Randomized trial of adjuvant perioperative chemotherapy in radically resected colorectal cancer (SAKK 40/87). *Proc Am Soc Clin Oncol* 1998; **17:** 256a.
13. Labianca R, Boffi L, Marsoni S et al, A randomized trial of intraportal (IP) versus systemic (SY) versus IP + SY adjuvant chemotherapy in patients (pts) with resected Dukes B–C colon carcinoma (CC). *Proc Am Soc Clin Oncol* 1999; **18:** 264a.
14. James RD, Intraportal 5FU and perioperative radiotherapy (RT) in the adjuvant treatment of colorectal cancer (CRCa) – 3681 patients randomised in the UK Coordinating Committee on Cancer Research (UKCCCR) AXIS trial. *Proc Am Soc Clin Oncol* 1999; **18:** 264a.
15. Vermorken J, Claessen AM, van Tinteren H et al, Active specific immunotherapy for stage II and III human colon cancer: a randomized trial. *Lancet* 1999; **353:** 345–50.
16. Wils J, The establishment of a large collaborative trial programme in the adjuvant treatment of colon cancer. *Br J Cancer* 1998; **77**(Suppl): 23–8.
17. Cunningham D, Zalcberg JR, Rath U et al, 'Tomudex' (ZD 1694): results of a randomized trial in advanced colorectal cancer demonstrate efficacy and reduced mucositis and leucopenia. *Eur J Cancer* 1995; **31A:** 1945–54.
18. Harper P, Advanced colorectal cancer (ACC): results from the latest raltitrexed Tomudex[R] (raltitrexed) comparative study. *Proc Am Soc Clin Oncol* 1997; **16:** 228a.
19. Pazdur R, Vincent M, Raltitrexed (Tomudex) versus 5-fluorouracil and leucovorin (5-FU + LV) in patients with advanced colorectal cancer (ACC): results of a randomized, multicenter, North American trial. *Proc Am Soc Clin Oncol* 1997; **16:** 228a.
20. Sobrero AF, Aschele C, Bertino JR, Fluorouracil in colorectal cancer – a tale of two drugs: implications for biochemical modulation. *J Clin Oncol* 1997; **15:** 368–81.
21. Punt CJ, Nagy A, Douillard JY et al, Edrocolomab (17-1A antibody) alone or in combination with 5-fluorouracil based chemotherapy in the adjuvant treatment of stage III colon cancer: results of a phase III study. *Proc Am Soc Clin Oncol* 2001; **20:** 123a.
22. Editorial: Drug-company decision to end cancer trial. *Lancet* 1999; **354:** 1045.

61

New chemotherapy approaches in colorectal cancer

Richard M Goldberg, Charles Erlichman

INTRODUCTION

In this chapter, we shall discuss selectively some novel therapeutic targets identified through a better understanding of tumor biology (specifically, matrix metalloproteinases, farnesyltransferase, mitogen-activated kinase, and angiogenesis). The roles of fluoropyrimidines, specific thymidylate synthase inhibitors, irinotecan, and oxaliplatin are described elsewhere in the book. This discussion of novel targets and agents that are being developed to affect these agents is not intended to be all-inclusive. As these agents progress through clinical trials, their role in the management of colorectal cancer will be defined.

MATRIX-METALLOPROTEINASE INHIBITORS

Matrix metalloproteinases (MMPs) are enzymes that degrade proteins and the tissue extracellular matrix to permit remodeling in physiologic processes such as wound healing and pregnancy and in pathologic processes such as cancer and rheumatoid arthritis.[1–3] These proteins are classified into a family of enzymes consisting of more than 20 members and exhibit specific well-defined functional properties. They are all proteinases that degrade at least one component of the extracellular matrix, contain a zinc ion, are inhibited by chelating agents and tissue inhibitors of matrix metalloproteinases (TIMPs), require proteolytic activation, and share common amino acid sequences.[4] Historically, the enzymes have been subcategorized into collagenases, gelatinases, stromelysins, and membrane-type MMPs. The individual enzymes have been assigned a number (e.g. MMP-1).[5,6] Table 61.1 lists some of these MMPs.

The MMPs are secreted as proenzymes. Most are produced by normal stromal cells, but some originate in tumor cells. As noted above, all known MMPs must undergo proteolytic cleavage to form the active moiety.[7–10] At least three regulatory mechanisms have been identified, including the need for proteolytic activation and its regulation, the regulation of the genes encoding the proenzymes by cytokines, and the presence and concentrations of endogenous TIMPs. There is also a series of membrane-type matrix metalloproteinases (MT-MMPs) that are overexpressed in malignant tissue.[11] On binding to extracellular MMPs, these MT-MMPs promote proteolytic cleavage of the MMPs. This observation suggests the possibility that an activation cascade exists.[12] The gene expression of different MMPs may be positively or negatively affected by cytokines such as transforming growth factor β (TGF-β), interleukin-1 (IL-1), tumor necrosis factor α (TNF-α), interferon-γ (IFN-γ), epidermal growth factor (EGF), platelet-derived growth factor (PDGF), and basic fibroblast growth factor (bFGF).[13] Additionally, TIMPs can bind to these MT-MMPs, such that they inhibit the activation of the MMPs. MMPs and TIMPs appear to be regulated independently in some circumstances, as well as in concert, sometimes in a reciprocal manner.[14,15] The full spectrum of enzymes, proteins, cytokines, and other potential components of this system, as well as the regulatory mechanisms of their complex array of interactions (both in normal physiology and in pathologic processes such as invasive malignancy), have not been fully elucidated.

Both tumor cells and normal cells, including monocytes/macrophages, connective-tissue cells, and endothelial cells, may produce MMPs. These enzymes are apparently integral to the processes by which malignant cells pass through normal epithelium, penetrate the basement membrane, invade blood vessels or lymphatics, enter the circulation, and extravasate from the vascular system to establish distant metastases.[16]

Table 61.1 Matrix metalloproteinases

MMP	Name	Substrate	Tissue localization
1	Interstitial collagenase	Collagens (I, II, III, V, VII, X)	Connective-tissue cells, monocytes/macrophages, endothelial cells
2	Gelatinase A	Gelatin, elastin, collagens (IV, V, VII, X, XI), fibronectin	Most cell types, tumor cells
3	Stromelysin-1	Proteoglycans, gelatins, fibronectin, laminins, collagens (III, IV, V, IX)	Connective-tissue cells, monocytes/macrophages, endothelial cells, tumor cells
7	Matrilysin	Gelatins, fibronectin, elastin, proteoglycans	Monocytes, tumor cells, connective-tissue cells
8	Neutrophil collagenase	Collagens (I, II, III), gelatin	Neutrophils
9	Gelatinase B	Gelatin, elastin, collagens (IV, V, VII, X, XI), fibronectin	Connective-tissue cells, monocytes/macrophages, tumor cells
10	Stromelysin-2	Proteoglycans, gelatins, fibronectin, laminins, collagens (III, IV, V, IX)	Macrophages, tumor cells

Tumor angiogenesis is dependent on both proliferation of endothelial cells (see below) and the invasion of these cells into stroma to form blood vessels. MMPs appear to play a role in this latter step. Hence, this complex system may contribute to tumor invasion, metastasis, and neovascularization. These physiologic roles make the pharmacologic regulation of MMPs a very attractive potential target for antitumor therapy, despite the somewhat daunting complexity of the processes as they are currently understood.

Studies have been performed in clinical material demonstrating high levels of several specific MMPs (MMP-1, MMP-2, MMP-7, and MMP-9) in colorectal cancer,[17–19] and there appears to be a correlation between tumor growth and MMP activity. These results support the rationale for design of MMP inhibitors (MMPIs) to complement classic cytotoxic agents and their testing in colorectal cancer. Clinical development of a number of MMPIs is currently underway.[20,21] Batimastat, marimastat, AG3319, AG3340, CGS 27023A, Ro-32-3555, and BAY 12-9566 are seven compounds that have undergone preclinical evaluation. Batimastat and marimastat are peptides designed to be homologous with the peptide sequence surrounding the cleavage point in collagen that is targeted by interstitial collagenases.[22] Activity was noted in a number of preclinical models.[23–27] The

clinical utility of these peptides was limited by their poor oral bioavailability. Initial clinical trials of batimastat were abandoned because of difficulties with solubility, formulation, and administration. Ongoing studies of marimastat have demonstrated that this is a tolerable oral treatment. A trial in 70 patients with refractory colorectal cancer required patients to have an elevated and rising carcinoembryonic antigen (CEA) level before treatment began with varying doses of marimastat for at least 28 days.[28] Twice-daily dosing with 20–25 mg was associated with reasonable tolerance, limited by musculoskeletal toxicity, and more often associated with stable CEA levels than single daily doses. Further work is in progress to determine whether any clinical activity can be observed in other tumor types, including breast, gastric, glioblastoma, pancreatic, and lung cancer patients.[29]

Based upon the X-ray crystallographic profile of the three-dimensional structure of the active sites of MMPs, medicinal chemists have designed non-peptidic compounds that bind to the active site of MMPs.[30] AG3340 is such a compound, which functions as a selective inhibitor of the gelatinases MMP-2 and MMP-9, as well as MMP-3, MMP-13, and MMP-14.[31] AG3340 has been shown to delay tumor growth when mice, implanted with

COLO-320DM colon tumors and treated with 100 mg/kg twice daily, were compared with untreated controls.[32] Tumor angiogenesis, as assessed by CD31 staining, was also inhibited. The results in xenograft models are encouraging, with tumor regression when combined with chemotherapy, inhibition of tumor growth when started shortly after tumor inoculation in vivo, and growth inhibition of tumor when started after human tumor engraftment in nude mice. AG3340 has been tested in healthy male volunteers.[33] Human trials in patients with non small cell lung cancer and prostate cancer are underway.

BAY 12-9566 is a non-peptide fenbufen derivative with inhibitory activity for MMP-1, and with lesser inhibition noted for MMP-2 and -3. Activity has been noted in Lewis lung carcinoma and B16 melanoma xenograft models.[34] Phase I trials in patients with refractory advanced cancer have established a safe oral dose of 800 mg twice daily.[35] Trials in ovarian, pancreatic, small cell lung, and colon cancer patients have been initiated. Recently, further development of BAY 12-9566 as an antitumor agent has been put on hold because an early analysis of a randomized trial in small cell lung cancer indicated a shortened time to cancer progression and a shorter time of survival (JM Sorensen, Bayer Corporation, September 1999, personal communication).

Several other MMPIs are in earlier stages of development.[22] These include CGS 27023 (an inhibitor of MMP-1, -2, -3, -9), D2163, and D1927. Pharmaceutical company and academic scientists will continue to synthesize and test additional drugs as the potential for MMPIs undergoes further refinement.

FARNESYLTRANSFERASE INHIBITORS

Ras is a small guanine triphosphate-binding protein, which is an important component of a signal-transduction pathway used by a variety of growth factors to initiate cell proliferation.[36–40] Mutation of the ras oncogene, which occurs in approximately 50% of all colorectal cancers, leads to a constitutive expression of this oncogene and stimulates tumor proliferation. In most colon cancers in which ras is not mutated and constitutively expressed, stimulation by insulin-like growth factor (IGF) and EGF may contribute significantly to the proliferative component of colon carcinogenesis. Ras can be activated[41] by IGF or EGF binding to their respective receptors. Ras normally exists in an inactive guanine diphosphate membrane-bound state (Ras-GDP) and, when activated by a growth factor binding to its respective receptor or as a consequence of mutation, becomes a

guanine triphosphate membrane-bound form (Ras-GTP).[42] The addition of a farnesyl group to a cysteine residue on the Ras protein is catalyzed by the enzyme farnesyltransferase (FT). This step is required for the Ras protein to become activated. Insertion of mutated ras has been associated with transformation to the malignant phenotype, both in vitro and in vivo. An understanding of this biochemical process has led to identification of the FT enzyme as a potential target for antitumor effects. Investigations have focused on developing inhibitors of the tetrapeptide-binding site of FT. Inhibitors of FT (FTIs) have been developed as peptidomimetics, or bisubstrate inhibitors, or identified from compound libraries. These agents are potent inhibitors of FT in the nanomolar range.[43–58] Inhibition of FT has resulted in growth inhibition in ras-transformed cells, both in vitro and in vivo.[54,59–68] The treatment in vivo requires long-term administration of the FTI. Cessation of inhibitor administration leads to regrowth of the tumors in vivo. A report has suggested that resistance to FT inhibition may develop.[69] Currently four agents are undergoing clinical evaluation: R115777, SCH66336, L-778,123, and GMS214662.[70–76] Questions remain to be addressed regarding these compounds before clinical utility can be defined. Among these, is whether inhibition of this pathway, which is important in the farnesylation of other intracellular proteins, will result in novel toxicities or side-effects.[77] Another question is whether farnesylation of Ras is necessary for Ras processing.[78] Can the downstream proliferative effects of Ras be mediated by other pathways when the Ras pathway is inhibited? Since preclinical data indicate that long-term administration of the FTI is necessary to suppress tumor growth, the mechanism of action appears to be cytostatic rather than cytotoxic. This suggests that combinations of FTIs with cytotoxic agents or radiation[79] might result in a more potent therapeutic effect than either alone. Combination studies of FTIs and chemotherapy are underway. The clinical toxicities of these agents tend to be nausea, vomiting, diarrhea, and myelosuppression.[80] How this will affect the ability to combine these agents with fluoropyrimidines, irinotecan, and oxaliplatin remains to be determined.

ANGIOGENESIS INHIBITORS

Angiogenesis is a fundamental step in the growth and metastasis of tumors.[6,81–84] Without neurovascularization, tumors rarely grow larger than 2–3 mm^3. Angiogenesis is tightly controlled by positive and negative regulators of microvascular growth. Tumors may overexpress one or more of the positive regulators of angiogenesis or stimulate normal cells, such as macrophages, to produce angiogenic substances. The most commonly found angiogenic factors are bFGF and vascular endothelial growth factor (VEGF). In addition to the growth-promoting angiogenic factors, there are negative regulators of endothelial cell proliferation that normally balance the effect of the angiogenic factors. For example, the bFGF soluble receptor will act to bind bFGF, thereby inhibiting the effect of the latter. When this balance of positive and negative regulation is tilted towards the positive regulatory factors, uncontrolled angiogenesis may occur. The importance of angiogenesis in colorectal cancer[85–91] has been documented in a variety of studies that have looked at markers of angiogenesis using immunohistochemical techniques and have correlated these findings with patient outcome. Furthermore, in vivo preclinical studies in animals have demonstrated that the use of antiangiogenic compounds in xenografted colon tumors decreased metastasis and increased survival.[92–94] It should be recognized that endothelial cells can themselves produce angiogenic factors. Furthermore, hypoxia, which is commonly found in solid tumors, can stimulate VEGF production.[95] As previously noted, *ras* mutations resulting in constitutive expression of the Ras protein are associated with colorectal cancer in approximately 50% of cases. It has been reported[96,97] that such a *ras* mutation will increase VEGF expression, which would lead to an angiogenic effect.

The central role of angiogenesis in tumor growth and metastasis has led to the development of antiangiogenic compounds. A variety of compounds[98–122] that can interfere with angiogenesis have been identified. These may be categorized as endogenous inhibitors of angiogenesis, which include angiostatin and platelet factor 4; inhibitors of receptor tyrosine kinases involved in angiogenesis, such as VEGF receptors; natural products, such as minocycline and AGM 1470; hormones and vitamins, such as steroids and retinoids; polysulfated and glycosylated compounds such as suramin; and miscellaneous agents, including antibodies to VEGF and the VEGF receptor (see Table 61.2). It should be noted that MMPIs, as discussed previously, might act in part by inhibiting angiogenesis. While studies of many of these agents are still in a preliminary stage, some have undergone phase I testing. The utility of these compounds – either alone or in combination with therapeutic agents – is currently unknown. Preliminary studies[123,124] have explored the feasibility of combining angiogenesis inhibitors with cytotoxic agents. The use of an angiogenesis inhibitor in combination with classical anticancer drugs will have to be carefully evaluated, since adequate

Table 61.2 Angiogenesis inhibitors

Endogenous inhibitors

Platelet factor 4

Thrombospondin-1

Tissue inhibitors of metalloproteinases:
  TIMP-1, TIMP-2, TIMP-3

Prolactin

Angiostatin

Endostatin

bFGF soluble receptor

TGF-β

IFN-γ

Receptor tyrosine kinase inhibitors
  (SU5146, SU6668, ZD4190, PD173073)

Natural products

Minocycline

AGM 1470

Herbimycin A

Tecogalan

Paclitaxel

Hormones and vitamins

Corticosteroids

Medroxyprogesterone

Estrogens

Antiestrogens

Vitamin D analogs

Retinoids

Polysulfated and glycosylated compounds

Suramin

Pentosan polysulfate

Protamine

Cartilage-derived factors

Vitreous extract

Heparin analogs

Sulfated polysaccharide peptidoglycans

Miscellaneous agents

D-Penicillamine

Inhibitors of prostaglandin synthesis

Gold salts

Anti-bFGF monoclonal antibodies

Anti-VEGF monoclonal antibodies

Anti-VEGF receptor monoclonal antibodies

vascular access to tumor cells is critical for drug delivery.

From the variety of new approaches currently being investigated will come many opportunities for clinical trials in patients with colorectal cancer.

MAP KINASE INHIBITORS

Mitogen-activated protein kinases (MAP kinases) are a family of kinases that are involved in signaling through Ras and result in activating transcription factors involved in cell proliferation. They are stimulated by a wide variety of extracellular stimuli.[125-127] There are at least two family members, ERK1 and ERK2, which are activated by Ras through Raf-1 and then MEK. Phosphorylation of MAP kinases results in activation of various transcription factors, including Elf-1, c-Myc, HSF-1, c-Jun, and c-Fos. ERKs are specifically activated by MEK1 through phosphorylation at two sites. The involvement of MAP kinases in colon cancer growth is supported by the results of work by Licato et al[128] and Hoshino et al.[129] Furthermore, MAP kinase activation can play a role in VEGF expression.[130] The central role that MAP kinases play and their selective coupled activation by MEK raises the potential for inhibition of MAP kinase activity through direct inhibition of MEK.[131] Sebold-Leopold recently reported that PD184352 is a potent and selective inhibitor of MEK. This inhibition was associated with growth inhibition in vitro and of colon carcinomas of both mouse and human origin in vivo. Whether the inhibition of signaling at this site in the signaling pathway for cell proliferation will be more selective than at upstream sites such as Ras and Raf will necessitate further evaluation in future trials.

REFERENCES

1. Wysocki AB, Staiano-Coico L, Grinnell F, Wound fluid from chronic leg ulcers contains elevated levels of MMP-2 and MMP-9. *J Invest Derm* 1991; **101**: 64–8.

2. Jeffrey J, Collagen and collagenase: pregnancy and parturition. *Semin Perinatol* 1991; **15**: 118–26.

3. Harris E, Rheumatoid arthritis: pathophysiology and implications for therapy. *N Engl J Med* 1990; **322**: 1277–89.

4. Matrisian L, Metalloproteinases and their inhibitors in matrix remodeling. *Trends Genet* 1990; **6**: 121–5.

5. Ennis BW, Matrisian LM, Matrix degrading metalloproteinases. *J Neuro-Oncol* 1993; **18**: 105–9.

6. Kohn EC, Liotta LA, Molecular insights into cancer invasion: strategies for prevention and intervention. *Cancer Res* 1995; **55**: 1856–62.

7. Pyke C, Ralfkiaer E, Tryggvason K et al, Messenger RNA for two type IV collagenases is located in stromal cells in human colon cancer. *Am J Pathol* 1993; **142**: 359–64.

8. Newell KJ, Witty JP, Rodgers WH et al, Expression and localization of matrix-degrading metalloproteinases during colorectal tumorigenesis. *Mol Carcinog* 1994; **10**: 199–206.

9. Hoyhtya M, Fridman R, Komarek D et al, Immunohistochemical localization of matrix metalloproteinase 2 and its specific inhibitor TIMP-2 in neoplastic sites with monoclonal antibodies. *Int J Cancer* 1994; **56**: 500–5.

10. D'Errico A, Garbisa S, Liotta L et al, Augmentation of type IV collagenase, laminin receptor, and Ki67 proliferation antigen associated with human colon, gastric, and breast carcinoma progression. *Mod Pathol* 1991; **4**: 239–46.

11. Sato H, Motoharu S, Membrane-type matrix metalloproteinases (MT-MMPs) in tumor metastases. *J Biochem* 1996; **119**: 209–15.

12. Sang QX, Birkedal-Hansen H, Van Wart HE, Proteolytic and non proteolytic activation of human neutrophil progelatinase B. *Biochim Biophys Acta* 1995; **1251**: 99–108.

13. Mauviel A, Cytokine regulation of metalloproteinase gene expression. *J Cell Biochem* 1993; **53**: 288–95.

14. Overall CM, Wrana JL, Sodek J, Independent regulation of collagenase, 72-kDA progelatinase, and metalloendoproteinase inhibitor expression in human fibroblasts by transforming growth factor-β. *J Biol Chem* 1989; **264**: 1860–9.

15. Overall CM, Wrana JL, Sodek J, Transforming growth factor-β regulation of collagenase, 72-kDA progelatinase, TIMP and PAI-1 expression in rat bone cell populations and human fibroblasts. *Connect Tissue Res* 1989; **20**: 289–94.

16. Parsons SL, Watson SA, Brown PD et al, Matrix metalloproteinases. *Br J Surg* 1997; **84**: 160–6.

17. Yamagata S, Yoshii Y, Suh JG et al, Occurrence of an active form of gelatinase in human gastric and colorectal carcinoma tissues. *Cancer Lett* 1991; **59**: 51–5.

18. Parsons SL, Watson SA, Collins HM et al, Colorectal cancers overexpress gelatinases (matrix metalloproteinases-2 and -9). *Gastroenterology* 1996; **110**: A574.

19. Murray G, Duncan M, O'Neil P et al, Matrix metalloproteinase-1 is associated with poor prognosis in colorectal cancer. *Nature Med* 1966; **2**: 461–2.

20. Roose JP, Van Noorden CJ, Synthetic protease inhibitors: promising compounds to arrest pathobiologic processes. *J Lab Clin Med* 1995; **125**: 433–41.

21. Brown PD, Giavazzi R, Matrix metalloproteinase inhibition: a review of antitumor activity. *Ann Oncol* 1995; **6**: 967–74.

22. Brown P, Clinical studies with matrix metalloproteinase inhibitors. *APMIS* 1999; **107**: 174–80.

23. Chirivi RG, Garofalo A, Crimmin MJ et al, Inhibition of the metastatic spread and growth of B16-BL6 murine melanoma by a synthetic matrix metalloproteinase inhibitor. *Int J Cancer* 1994; **58**: 460–4.

24. Watson SA, Morris TM, Robinson G et al, Inhibition of organ invasion by the matrix metalloproteinase inhibitor batimastat (BB-94) in two human colon carcinoma metastasis models. *Cancer Res* 1995; **55**: 3629–33.

25. Watson SA, Morris TM, Parson SL et al, Therapeutic effect of the matrix metalloproteinase inhibitor, batimastat, in a human colorectal cancer ascites model. *Br J Cancer* 1996; **74**: 1354–8.

26. Taraboletti G, Garofalo A, Belotti D et al, Inhibition of angiogenesis and murine hemangioma growth by batimastat, a synthetic inhibitor of matrix metalloproteinases. *J Natl Cancer Inst* 1995; **87**: 293–8.

27. Wang X, Fu X, Brown PD et al, Matrix metalloproteinase inhibitor BB-94 (batimastat) inhibits human colon tumor growth and spread in a patient-like orthotopic model in nude mice. *Cancer Res* 1994; **54**: 4726–9.

28. Primrose JN, Bleiberg H, Daniel F et al, Marimastat in recurrent colorectal cancer: exploratory evaluation of biologic activ-

ity by measurement of carcinoembryonic antigen. *Br J Cancer* 1999; **79**: 509–14.

29. Brown PD, Giavazzi R, Clinical trials of a low molecular weight matrix metalloproteinase inhibitor in cancer. *Ann NY Acad Sci* 1994; **732**: 217–21.

30. Drug design at www.agouron.com, 27 July 2001.

31. Shalinsky DR, Brekken J, Zou H et al, Broad antitumor and antiangiogenic activities of AG3340, a potent and selective MMP inhibitor undergoing advanced oncology clinical trials. *Ann NY Acad Sci* 1999; **878**: 236–70.

32. Shalinsky DR, Zou H, McDermott CD, AG3340, a selective MMP inhibitor, has broad antiangiogenic activity across oncology and ophthalmology models in vivo. *Proc Am Assoc Cancer Res* 1999; **38**: 521 (Abst 3547).

33. Collier MA, Yuen GJ, Bansal SK et al, A phase I study of the matrix metalloproteinase (MMP) inhibitor AG3340 given in single doses to healthy volunteers. *Proc Am Assoc Cancer Res* 1997; **38**: 521 (Abst 3547).

34. Bull C, Flynn C, Eberwein D et al, Activity of the biphenyl matrix metalloproteinase inhibitor BAY 12-9566 in murine in vivo models. *Proc Am Assoc Cancer Res* 1998; **39**: 302 (Abst 2062).

35. Erlichman C, Adjei AA, Alberts S et al, Phase I study of BAY 12-9566 – a matrix metalloproteinase inhibitor (MMPI). *Proc Am Soc Clin Oncol* 1998; **17**: 217a.

36. Drummond AH, Beckett P, Bone EA et al, BB-2516: an orally bioavailable matrix metalloproteinase inhibitor with efficacy in animal cancer models. *Proc Am Assoc Cancer Res* 1995; **36**: A595.

37. Santos O, Daniels R, McDermott C et al, Anti-tumor studies with the synthetic matrix metalloproteinase inhibitors AG3319 and AG3340. *Proc Am Assoc Cancer Res* 1996; **37**: 90.

38. Cho KR, Vogelstein B, Genetic alterations in the adenoma-carcinoma sequence. *Cancer* 1992; **70**: 1727–31.

39. Kern SE, Hamilton SR, Vogelstein B, Clinical implications of colorectal tumor mutations. In: *Molecular Foundations of Oncology* (Broder S, ed). Baltimore: Williams & Wilkins, 1991: 381–90.

40. Sidransky D, Tokino T, Hamilton SR et al, Identification of RAS oncogene mutations in the stool of patients with curable colorectal cancer. *Science* 1992; **256**: 102–5.

41. Margolis B, Skolnik EY, Activation of Ras by receptor tyrosine kinases. *J Am Soc Nephrol* 1994; **5**: 1288–99.

42. Gibbs JB, Oliff A, Kohl NE, Farnesyltransferase inhibitors: Ras research yields a potential cancer therapeutic. *Cell* 1994; **77**: 175–8.

43. Cox AD, Garcia AM, Westwick JK et al, The CAAX peptidomimetic compound B581 specifically blocks farnesylated, but not geranylated or myristylated, oncogenic Ras signaling and transformation. *J Biol Chem* 1994; **260**: 19203–6.

44. Garcia AM, Rowell C, Ackermann K et al, Peptidomimetic inhibitors of Ras farnesylation and function in whole cells. *J Biol Chem* 1993; **268**: 18415–18.

45. Graham SL, deSolms SJ, Giuliani EA et al, Pseudopeptide inhibitors of Ras farnesylprotein transferase. *J Med Chem* 1994; **37**: 725–32.

46. Hall CC, Watkins JD, Ferguson SB et al, Inhibitors of farnesyl-transferase and Ras processing peptidase. *Biochem Biophys Res Commun* 1995; **217**: 728–32.

47. Kang MS, Stemerick DM, Zwolshen JH et al, Farnesyl-derived inhibitors of ras farnesyl transferase. *Biochem Biophys Res Commun* 1995; **217**: 245–9.

48. Nigam M, Seong CM, Qian Y et al, Potent inhibition of human tumor p21ras farnesyltransferase by A1A2-lacking p21ras CA1A2Xpeptidomimetics. *J Biol Chem* 1993; **268**: 20695-8.

49. Tamanoi F, Inhibitors of Ras farnesyltransferases. *Trends Biochem Sci* 1993; **18**: 349–53.

50. Gelb MH, Tamanoi F, Yokoyama K et al, The inhibition of protein prenyltransferases by oxygenated metabolites of limonene and perillyl alcohol. *Cancer Lett* 1995; **91**: 169–75.

51. Karlson J, Borgkarlson AK, Unelius R et al, Inhibition of tumor cell growth by monoterpenes in vitro – evidence of a RAS-independent mechanism of action. *Anticancer Drugs* 1996; **7**: 422–9.

52. Bergstrom JD, Kurtz MM, Rew DJ et al, Zaragozic acids: a family of fungal metabolites that are picomolar competitive inhibitors of squalene synthase. *Proc Natl Acad Sci USA* 1993; **90**: 80–4.

53. Jayasuriya H, Ball RG, Zink DL et al, Barceloneic acid A, a new farnesyl-protein transferase inhibitor from a *Phoma* species. *J Nat Prod* 1995; **58**: 986–91.

54. Sepp-Lorenzino L, Ma ZP, Rands E et al, A peptidomimetic inhibitor of farnesyl-protein transferase blocks the anchorage-dependent and -independent growth of human tumor cell lines. *Cancer Res* 1995; **55**: 5302–9.

55. Lerner EC, Qian Y, Blaskovich MA et al, Ras CAAX peptidomimetic FTI-227 selectively blocks oncogenic Ras signaling by inducing cytoplasmic accumulation of inactive Ras–Raf complexes. *J Biol Chem* 1995; **270**: 802–6.

56. Vogt A, Qian Y, Blaskovich MA et al, A non-peptide mimetic of Ras-CAAX: selective inhibition of farnesyltransferase and Ras processing. *J Biol Chem* 1995; **270**: 660–4.

57. Kohl NE, Mosser SD, deSolms SJ et al, Selective inhibition of ras-dependent transformation by a farnesyltransferase inhibitor. *Science* 1993; **260**: 1934–7.

58. Ma Y, Gilbert BA, Rando RR, Inhibitors of the isoprenylated protein endoprotease. *Biochemistry* 1993; **32**: 2386–93.

59. Nagase T, Kawata S, Tamura S et al, Inhibition of cell growth of human hepatoma cell line (Hep G2) by a farnesyl protein transferase inhibitor: a preferential suppression of ras farnesylation. *Int J Cancer* 1996; **65**: 620–6.

60. Nagasu T, Yoshimatsu K, C. R et al, Inhibition of human tumor xenograft growth by treatment with the farnesyl transferase inhibitor B956. *Cancer Res* 1995; **55**: 5310–14.

61. Sebti SM, Tkalcevic GT, Jani JP, Lovostatin, a cholesterol biosynthesis inhibitor, inhibits the growth of human h-RAS oncogene transformed cells in nude mice. *Cancer Commun* 1991; **3**: 141–7.

62. Prendergast GC, Davide JP, DeSolms SJ et al, Farnesyltransferase inhibition causes morphological reversion of ras-transformed cells by a complex mechanism that involves regulation of the actin cytoskeleton. *Mol Cell Biol* 1994; **14**: 4193–202.

63. Kohl NE, Omer CA, Conner MW et al, Inhibition of farnesyl-transferase induces regression of mammary and salivary carcinomas in ras transgenic mice. *Nature Med* 1995; **1**: 792–7.

64. James GL, Brown MS, Cobb MH et al, Benzodiazepine peptidomimetics: potent inhibitors of Ras farnesylation in animal cells. *Science* 1993; **260**: 1937–42.

65. Kothapalli R, Guthrie N, Chambers AF et al, Farnesylamine: an inhibitor of farnesylation and growth of ras-transformed cells. *Lipids* 1993; **28**: 969–73.

66. Kohl NE, Wilson FR, Mosser SD et al, Protein farnesyltrans-ferase inhibitors block the growth of ras-dependent tumors in nude mice. *Proc Natl Acad Sci USA* 1994; **91**: 9141–5.

67. Gibbs JB, Kohl NE, Pompliano DL et al, Selective inhibition of Ras-dependent cell transformation by a farnesyl-protein transferase inhibitor. *FASEB J* 1993; **7**: A1048.

68. Leftheris K, Kline T, Vite GD et al, Development of highly potent inhibitors of Ras farnesylation possessing cellular and in vivo activity. *J Med Chem* 1996; **39**: 224–36.

69. Prendergast GC, Davide JP, Lebowitz PF et al, Resistance of a

variant ras-transformed cell line to phenotypic reversion by farnesyl transferase inhibitors. *Cancer Res* 1996; **56**: 2626–32.

70. Zujewski J, Horak ID, Bol CJ et al, Phase I and pharmaco-kinetic study of farnesyl protein transferase inhibitor R115777 in advanced cancer. *J Clin Oncol* 2000; **18**: 927–41.

71. Hudes GR, Schol J, Baab J et al, Phase I clinical and pharmaco-kinetic trial of the farnesyltransferase inhibitor R115777 on 21-day dosing schedule. *Proc Am Soc Clin Oncol* 1999; **18**: 156a (Abst 601).

72. Soignet S, Yao S-L, Britten C et al, Pharmacokinetics and pharmacodynamics of the farnesyl protein transferase inhibitor (L-778,123) in solid tumors. *Proc Am Assoc Cancer Res* 1999; **40**: 517 (Abst 3413).

73. Britten CD, Rowinsky E, Yao S-L et al, The farnesyl protein transferase (PFTase) inhibitor L-778,123 in patients with solid cancers. *Proc Am Soc Clin Oncol* 1999; **18**: 155a (Abst 597).

74. Adjei AA, Erlichman C, Davis JN et al, A phase I and pharmacologic study of the farnesyl protein transferase (FPT) inhibitor SCH 66336 in patients with locally advanced or metastatic cancer. *Proc Am Soc Clin Oncol* 1999; **18**: 156a (Abst 598).

75. Hurwitz HI, Colvin OM, Petros WP et al, Phase I and pharmacokinetic study of SCH66336, a novel FPTI, using a 2-week on, 2-week off schedule. *Proc Am Soc Clin Oncol* 1999; **18**: 156a (Abst 599).

76. Eskens F, Awada A, Verweij J et al, Phase 1 and pharmacologic study of continuous daily oral SCH 66336, a novel farnesyl transferase inhibitor, in patients with solid tumors. *Proc Am Soc Clin Oncol* 1999; **18**: 156a (Abst 600).

77. Pittler SJ, Fliesler SJ, Fisher PL et al, In vivo requirements of protein prenylation for maintenance of retinal cytoarchitecture and photoreceptor structure. *J Cell Biol* 1995; **130**: 431–9.

78. Dalton MB, Sinensky M, Farnesylation independent processing of p21ras. *FASEB J* 1995; **9**: A1315.

79. Bernhard EJ, Kao G, Cox AD et al, The farnesyltransferase inhibitor FTI-227 radiosensitized H-ras-transformed rat embryo fibroblasts. *Cancer Res* 1996; **56**: 1727–30.

80. Rowinsky EK, Windle JJ, Von Hoff DD, Ras protein farnesyltransferase: A strategic target for anticancer therapeutic development. *J Clin Oncol* 1999; **17**: 3631–52.

81. Cockerill GW, Gamble JR, Vadas MA, Angiogenesis: models and modulators. *Int Rev Cytol* 1995; **159**: 113–60.

82. Folkman J, Ingber D, Inhibition of angiogenesis. *Semin Cancer Biol* 1992; **3**: 89–96.

83. Folkman J, Clinical applications of research on angiogenesis. *N Engl J Med* 1995; **333**: 1757–63.

84. Sipos EP, Tamargo RJ, Weingart JD et al, Inhibition of tumor angiogenesis. *Ann NY Acad Sci* 1994; **732**: 263–72.

85. Bossi P, Viale G, Lee AK et al, Angiogenesis in colorectal tumors: microvessel quantitation in adenomas and carcinomas with clinicopathological correlations. *Cancer Res* 1995; **55**: 5049–53.

86. Frank RE, Saclarides TJ, Leurgans S et al, Tumor angiogenesis as a predictor of recurrence and survival in patients with node-negative colon cancer. *Cancer Res* 1995; **53**: 533–5.

87. Pritchard A, Powe DG, Wilkinson M et al, Tumor vascularity in colorectal carcinoma. *J Pathol* 1992; **168**: 118A.

88. Takebayashi Y, Yamada K, Maruyama I et al, The expression of thymidine phosphorylase and thrombomodulin in human colorectal carcinomas. *Cancer Lett* 1995; **92**: 1–7.

89. Abdalla SA, Behzad F, Bsharah S et al, Prognostic relevance of microvessel density in colorectal tumors. *Oncol Rep* 1999; **6**: 839–42.

90. Vermeulen PB, Van den Eynden GG, Huget P et al, Prospective study of intratumoral microvessel density, p53 expression and survival in colorectal cancer. *Br J Cancer* 1999; **79**: 316–22.

91. Ishigami SI, Arii S, Furutani M et al, Predictive value of vascular endothelial growth factor (VEGF) in metastasis and prognosis of human colorectal cancer. *Br J Cancer* 1998; **78**: 1379–84.

92. Konno H, Tanaka T, Matsuda I et al, Comparison of the inhibitory effect of the angiogenesis inhibitor, TNP-470, and mitomycin C on the growth and liver metastasis of human colon cancer. *Int J Cancer* 1995; **61**: 268–71.

93. Gallegos NC, Smales C, Savage FJ et al, The distribution of matrix metalloproteinases and tissue inhibitor of metalloproteinases in colorectal cancer. *Surg Oncol* 1995; **4**: 111–19.

94. Konno H, Tanaka T, Kanai T et al, Efficacy of an angiogenesis inhibitor, TNP-470, in xenotransplanted human colorectal cancer with high metastatic potential. *Cancer* 1996; **77**: 1736–40.

95. Mukhopadhyay D, Tsiokas L, Zho XM et al, Hypoxic induction of human vascular endothelial growth factor expression through C-SRC activation. *Nature* 1995; **375**: 577–01.

96. Rak J, Mitsuhashi Y, Bayko L et al, Mutant ras oncogenes upregulate VEGF/VPF expression: implications for induction and inhibition of tumor angiogenesis. *Cancer Res* 1995; **55**: 4575–80.

97. Grugel S, Finkenzeller G, Weindel K et al, Both v-Ha-Ras and v-Raf stimulate expression of the vascular endothelial growth factor in NIH 3T3 cells. *J Biol Chem* 1995; **270**: 25915–19.

98. Eckhardt SG, Eckhardt JR, Weiss G et al, Results of a phase I trial of the novel angiogenesis inhibitor, tecogalan sodium. *Proc Am Assoc Cancer Res* 1995; **36**: A628.

99. Kohn E, Reed E, Sarosy G et al, Clinical investigation of a cytostatic calcium influx inhibitor in patients with refractory cancers. *Cancer Res* 1996; **56**: 569–73.

100. O'Reilly M, Holmgren L, Shing Y et al, Angiostatin: a novel angiogenesis inhibitor that mediates the suppression of metastases by a Lewis lung carcinoma. *Cell* 1994; **79**: 315–28.

101. Oktaba AC, Hunter WL, Arsenault AL, Taxol: a potent inhibitor of normal and tumor-induced angiogenesis. *Proc Am Assoc Cancer Res* 1995; **36**: A2707.

102. Belman N, Lipton A, Harvey H et al, rhuPF4: phase I study of an angiogenesis inhibitor in metastatic colon cancer (MCC). *Proc Am Soc Clin Oncol* 1994; **13**: A360.

103. Clapp C, Martial JA, Guzman RC et al, The 16-kilodalton N-terminal fragment of human prolactin is a potent inhibitor of angiogenesis. *Endocrinology* 1993; **133**: 1292–9.

104. Fotsis T, Zhang Y, Pepper MS et al, The endogenous oestrogen metabolite 2-methoxyoestradiol inhibits angiogenesis and suppresses tumour growth. *Nature* 1994; **368**: 237–9.

105. Fotsis T, Pepper M, Adlercreutz H et al, Genistein, a dietary-derived inhibitor of in vitro angiogenesis. *Proc Natl Acad Sci USA* 1993; **90**: 2690–4.

106. Gagliardi A, Collins DC, Inhibition of angiogenesis by antiestrogens. *Cancer Res* 1993; **53**: 533–5.

107. Galardy RE, Grobelny D, Foellmer HG et al, Inhibition of angiogenesis by the matrix metalloprotease inhibitor N-[2R-2-(hydroxamidocarbonylmethyl)-4-methylpentanoyl)]-L-tryptophan methylamide. *Cancer Res* 1994; **54**: 4715–18.

108. Gilbertson-Beadling S, Powers EA, Stamp-Cole M et al, The tetracycline analogs minocycline and doxycycline inhibit angiogenesis in vitro by a non-metalloproteinase-dependent mechanism. *Cancer Chemother Pharmacol* 1995; **36**: 418–24.

109. Hu DE, Fan TP, Suppression of VEGF-induced angiogenesis by the protein tyrosine kinase inhibitor, lavendustin A. *Br J Pharmacol* 1995; **114**: 262–8.

110. Miyadera K, Sumizawa T, Haraguchi M et al, Role of thymidine phosphorylase activity in the angiogenic effect of platelet derived endothelial cell growth factor/thymidine phosphorylase. *Cancer Res* 1995; **55**: 1687–90.

111. Nguyen NM, Lehr JE, Pienta KJ, Pentosan inhibits angiogene-

sis in vitro and suppresses prostate tumor growth in vivo. *Anticancer Res* 1993; **13:** 2143–7.

112. Pluda JM, Wyvill K, Figg WD et al, A phase I study of an angiogenesis inhibitor, TNP-470 (AGM-1470), administered to patients (pts) with HIV-associated Kaposi's sarcoma (KS). *Proc Am Soc Clin Oncol* 1994; **13:** A8.

113. Pluda JM, Shay LE, Foli A et al, Administration of pentosan polysulfate to patients with human immunodeficiency virus-associated Kaposi's sarcoma. *J Natl Cancer Inst* 1993; **85:** 1585–92.

114. Ray JM, Stetler-Stevenson WG, The role of matrix metalloproteases and their inhibitors in tumour invasion, metastasis and angiogenesis. *Eur Respir J* 1994; **7:** 2062–72.

115. Tamargo RJ, Bok RA, Brem H, Angiogenesis inhibition by minocycline. *Cancer Res* 1991; **51:** 672–5.

116. Yamamoto T, Sudo K, Fujita T, Significant inhibition of endothelial cell growth in tumor vasculature by an angiogenesis inhibitor, TNP-470 (AGM-1470). *Anticancer Res* 1994; **14:** 1–3.

117. Yamaoka M, Yamamoto T, Ikeyama S et al, Angiogenesis inhibitor TNP-470 (AGM-1470) potently inhibits the tumor growth of hormone-independent human breast and prostate carcinoma cell lines. *Cancer Res* 1993; **53:** 5233–6.

118. Yamaoka M, Yamamoto T, Masaki T et al, Inhibition of tumor growth and metastasis of rodent tumors by the angiogenesis inhibitor O-(chloroacetyl-carbamoyl)fumagillol (TNP-470; AGM-1470). *Cancer Res* 1993; **53:** 4262–7.

119. Zukiwski A, Gutterman J, Bui C et al, Phase I trial of the angiogenesis inhibitor TNP-470 (AGM-1470) in patients (pts) with androgen-independent prostate cancer (AI PCa). *Proc Am Soc Clin Oncol* 1994; **13:** A795.

120. Danesi R, Del Bianchi S, Soldani P et al, Suramin inhibits bFGF-induced endothelial cell proliferation and angiogenesis in the chick chorioallantoic membrane. *Br J Cancer* 1993; **68:** 932–8.

121. Klohs WD, Hamby JM, Antiangiogenic agents. *Curr Opin Biotechnol* 1999; **10:** 544–9.

122. Drevs J, Droll A, Mross K et al, Angiogenesis inhibition: drugs in clinical trials. *Onkologie* 1999; **22:** 282–90.

123. Devineni D, Klein-Szanto A, Gallo JM, Uptake of temozolomide in a rat glioma model in the presence and absence of the angiogenesis inhibitor TNP-470. *Cancer Res* 1996; **56:** 1983–7.

124. Kato T, Sato K, Kakinuma H et al, Enhanced suppression of tumor growth by combination of angiogenesis inhibitor O-(chloroacetyl-carbamoyl)fumagillol (TNP-470) and cytotoxic agents in mice. *Cancer Res* 1994; **54:** 5143–7.

125. Lewis TS, Shapiro PS, Signal transduction through MAP kinase cascades. *Adv Cancer Res* 1998; **74:** 49–139.

126. Cobb MH, Goldsmith EJ, How MAP kinases are regulated. *J Biol Chem* 1995; **270:** 148431–6.

127. Cobb MH, MAP kinase pathways. *Prog Biophys Mol Biol* 1999; **71:** 479–500.

128. Licato LL, Keku TO, Wurzelmann JI et al, In vivo activation of mitogen-activated protein kinases in rat intestinal neoplasia. *Gastroenterology* 1997; **113:** 1589–98.

129. Hoshino R, Chatani Y, Yarmori T et al, Constitutive activation of the 41-/43-kDa mitogen-activated protein kinase signaling pathway in human tumors. *Oncogene* 1999; **18:** 813–22.

130. Milanini J, Vinals F, Pouyssegur J et al, P42/P44 map kinase module plays a key role in the transcriptional regulation of the vascular endothelial growth factor gene in fibroblasts. *J Biol Chem* 1998; **273:** 18165–72.

131. Sebold-Leopold JS, Dudley DT, Herrera R et al, Blockade of the MAP kinase pathway suppresses growth of colon tumors in vivo. *Nature Med* 1999; **5:** 810–16.

Part 8

New Approaches to Treatment

62

New treatment concepts

Guy A Chung-Faye, Ming-Jen Chen, David J Kerr

INTRODUCTION

Conventional therapy for colorectal cancer has made little impact on 5-year survival figures over the last decade. For most patients with colorectal cancer, the prognosis remains poor, and novel therapeutic concepts are urgently needed. Significant advances in our understanding of the molecular and cellular events that accompany the development of colorectal cancer (see Chapter 1) have identified specific targets for novel therapeutic approaches. Key discoveries have been the adenomatous polyposis coli (APC) and p53 genes and the elucidation of signalling pathways controlling the initiation and progression of tumours, along with a better understanding of the immunological interplay in the development of colorectal cancer. Another critical factor that has facilitated this process has been the concurrent expansion in technological innovations. Although we are just beginning to unravel the complex processes during tumorigenesis, significant progress has been made in the development of novel therapies, such as gene therapy and immunotherapy approaches. The initial results are encouraging, but the work is still at an early stage of development and preclinical studies are only just being translated into clinical trials, which will require evaluation in well-designed randomized controlled trials. This chapter will review the current state of these emerging therapeutic modalities and evaluate their clinical effectiveness.

GENE THERAPY

Several gene therapy approaches have been adopted in colorectal cancer. They are gene correction, virus-directed enzyme–prodrug therapy, and immuno-modulatory approaches. Viral[1] and non-viral[2] vectors have been utilized for gene transfer. The viral vectors commonly used in gene therapy protocols are retroviruses, adenoviruses, herpes simplex viruses, and vaccinia viruses. Non-viral delivery systems, such as liposomes and polymers, have been used, but are generally less efficient in gene transfer than viral vectors. However, even with the most effective viral vector, gene transfer in vivo is low to moderate.

Gene correction

The most logical approach to gene therapy is the correction of a single-gene defect that causes the disease phenotype. This goal is elusive, since malignant transformation is usually accompanied by a series of genetic mutations (see Chapter 1), as well as clonal heterogeneity. However, certain mutations are important for the maintenance or propagation of the malignant phenotype, and the corollary is that correcting these mutations might inhibit tumour growth. Two paradigms are mutations in the p53 tumour suppressor gene and the K-ras oncogene, both of which exert a dominant positive effect on tumour progression. Hence, correcting only one crucial defect in a malignant cell might induce apoptosis or growth arrest. Additionally, while most work has concentrated on the role of genetic mutations in the process of tumorigenesis, it is increasingly being recognized that epigenetic events are also important. An example is the hypermethylation of the promoter regions of tumour suppressor genes, which can inhibit gene transcription, leading to loss of inhibition of tumour growth. This problem is potentially remediable by gene therapy strategies that can restore expression of the tumour suppressor genes.

The p53 gene

Mutation of the *p53* gene is the most common mutation in human cancers, and is present in 20–70% of all colorectal cancers.[3] The *p53* gene is a tumour suppressor gene; it regulates the cell cycle, and can cause G_1 growth arrest or apoptosis in response to DNA damage.[4] Loss of the *p53*-regulated checkpoint in the cell cycle can lead to uncontrolled tumour growth, and, furthermore, restoration of wild-type *p53* in *p53*-mutated colon cancer cell lines causes growth inhibition.[5] In a murine model of *p53*-mutated colon cancer, direct intratumoral injection to subcutaneous tumours with an adenovirus encoding wild-type *p53* showed tumour regression and a doubling of survival times in treated mice compared with controls.[6] There is a correlation between the development of *p53* mutations and chemo/radio-resistance of tumours. Therefore, restoring wild-type *p53* to *p53*-mutated tumours may potentially improve tumour response to chemotherapy/radiotherapy.[7] In immunodeficient mice with subcutaneous *p53*-mutated colon cancer xenografts, there was a synergistic effect with intratumoral injection of an adenovirus encoding wild-type *p53* and intraperitoneal cisplatin.[8]

A phase I trial delivered a single dose of up to 2.5×10^{12} adenovirus particles encoding wild-type *p53*, by hepatic artery infusion, to 16 patients with *p53*-mutated colorectal liver metastases.[9] This procedure was well tolerated, with the main side-effects being fever and transiently deranged liver function. Although transgene expression was detected in subsequently resected tumours by reverse-transcriptase polymerase chain reaction (RT-PCR), no radiological response was seen. A subgroup of patients also received intrahepatic floxuridine-based chemotherapy, in addition to the adenovirus, and 11 out of 12 evaluable patients had partial responses. Possible explanations for the lack of response with *p53* gene therapy as a single agent are the large tumour sizes and the low efficiency of gene transfer.

The K-ras gene

K-*ras* is a dominant proto-oncogene that is often mutated early in colon cancers, as well as many other cancers. The product of the K-*ras* gene mutation is the p21 protein, which is involved in cell signal transduction and the control of proliferation. Thus a potential target for gene correction is inactivation of the K-*ras* oncogene product by antisense mRNA, which eliminates mutant K-*ras* mRNA by binding to it according to Watson–Crick base-pairing. In colon cancer cell lines, antisense oligonucleotides complementary to K-*ras* inhibited cell growth, colony formation, and K-*ras* protein production in a

dose-dependent manner.[10] This effect was only seen in colon cancer cells with activated K-*ras*, but did not affect the normal cells or those colon cancer cells without K-*ras* mutation. This approach is currently in a phase I trial for lung cancer.[11]

Virus-directed enzyme–prodrug therapy (VDEPT) (Figure 62.1)

Systemic chemotherapy regimens can be effective in treating colorectal tumours, but they cause nondiscriminatory cell killing. Their dose-limiting toxicities are due to effects on other rapidly dividing cell populations, such as the bone marrow and the gastrointestinal mucosa. Enzyme–prodrug systems aim to localize this toxicity to the milieu of tumour cells. This involves gene transfer into tumour cells of a bacterial or viral enzyme that converts an inactive prodrug into a toxic metabolite. In vivo, not every tumour cell can be transduced with the therapeutic gene. However, an important feature of enzyme–prodrug systems is the 'bystander effect', where surrounding cells, not expressing the enzyme, are also killed by active metabolites. Enzyme–prodrug combinations include thymidine kinase and ganciclovir, cytosine deaminase and 5-fluorocytosine, and nitroreductase and the prodrug CB1954.

Thymidine kinase–ganciclovir

The herpes simplex viral enzyme thymidine kinase (HSVtk) phosphorylates the antiviral drug ganciclovir into an intermediary metabolite, which is then converted by cellular kinases into a potent inhibitor of DNA polymerase, leading to cell death. Additionally, it has been shown that there is a 'bystander effect', which is mediated principally by transfer of the activated drug via gap junctions.[12] Importantly, the bystander effect has also been shown in vivo in a murine model of colorectal cancer, when complete tumour regression was achieved with only 9% of tumour cells expressing HSVtk.[13]

Cytosine deaminase–5-fluorocytosine[14]

The bacterial enzyme cytosine deaminase (CD) converts the non-toxic antifungal agent 5-fluorocytosine (5-FC) into 5-fluorouracil (5-FU), the most effective chemotherapy agent in colon cancer. 5-FU induces apoptosis during DNA replication by inhibiting the thymidylate synthase enzyme and RNA synthesis. In vitro and in vivo models of CD–5-FC have shown that cells transduced to express CD are very susceptible to 5-FC-mediated cell death. In nude mice with colon cancer xenografts expressing CD, there was a

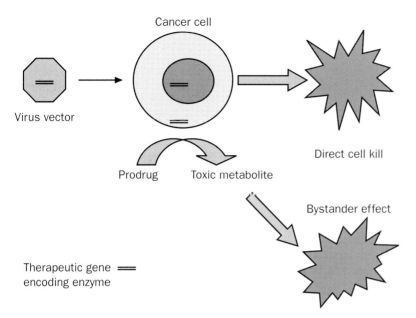

Cancer cell

Virus vector

Prodrug   Toxic metabolite

Direct cell kill

Bystander effect

Therapeutic gene ⹀
encoding enzyme

Figure 62.1 In virus-directed enzyme–prodrug therapy (VDEPT), a viral vector encoding the enzyme (⹀) infects the tumour cell. The cell starts to produce viral proteins, including the enzyme, which converts an inert prodrug into a toxic metabolite. This causes direct tumour cell killing, as well as having a bystander effect, killing non-transfected neighbouring cells.

100% regression and 75% cure rate following systemic administration of 5-FC.[15] Very high intratumoral concentrations of 5-FU (>400 μM) were generated, with few systemic side-effects. In marked contrast, no antitumour response was seen with the maximally tolerated dose of 5-FU. Importantly, there was a profound bystander effect, with significant tumour regression being seen in all mice with colon cancer xenografts treated with 5-FC, when only 2% of cells expressed CD.[16]

There is an ongoing phase I study of the treatment of colorectal liver metastases by direct intratumoral injection of an adenovirus encoding CD, together with oral administration of 5-FC.[17]

Nitroreductase – CB1954

The prodrug CB1954 (5-(aziridin-1-yl)-2,4-dinitrobenzamide) is a weak non-functional alkylating agent. CB1954 is converted by the *Escherichia coli* bacterial enzyme nitroreductase (NTR) to a potent bifunctional DNA-binding agent, which induces cell death by forming interstrand DNA crosslinks. Unlike with many other cytotoxic agents, cell killing by CB1954 metabolites is not cycle-dependent, which is an advantage since only a small proportion of tumour cells are actively replicating at any one time. Additionally, cell killing occurs even in tumours that have acquired resistance to cisplatin. In vitro, NTR-expressing colon cancer cells were markedly sensitized to the prodrug CB1954. A significant bystander effect was seen when only 10% of cells express NTR. In murine models with NTR-expressing pancreatic tumour xenografts, treated with intratumoral injections of virus encoding NTR, long-term remissions were achieved following intraperitoneal administration of CB1954.[18]

At the CRC Institute for Cancer Studies, University of Birmingham, UK, we have commenced a phase I study with an adenoviral vector encoding nitroreductase injected into colorectal hepatic metastases under radiological guidance, followed by intravenous CB1954. Suitable patients will also undergo resection of treated hepatic metastases. The primary objective of this phase I study is to determine the toxicity and efficacy of the VDEPT approach; however, access to resected liver specimens will provide invaluable information on systemic and regional virus distribution, enzyme expression, drug pharmacokinetics, and treatment efficacy. It will also provide a considerable opportunity to demonstrate 'proof of principle'.

IMMUNOTHERAPY

Many cancers can be destroyed by a cell-mediated immune response, usually through cytotoxic T lymphocytes (CTL) (CD8[+]), mediated by T-helper cells (CD4[+]). The activation of this process requires three synergistic signals (see Figure 62.2):

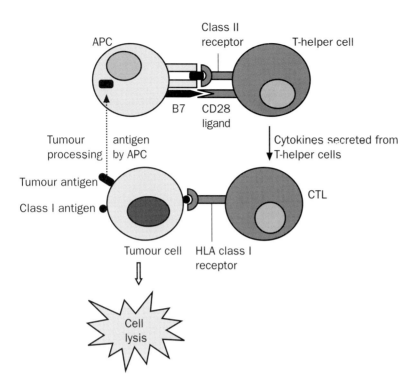

Figure 62.2 Cell-mediated immunity against tumours. Tumour antigens are taken up and processed by antigen-presenting cells (APC), and re-presented to class II receptors on T-helper cells. This requires a co-stimulatory signal, B7, which binds to the CD28 ligand, causing T-helper cell activation. This leads to secretion of cytokines, which in turn activates cytotoxic lymphocytes (CTL) to bind to tumour cells via class I receptors, and causes tumour lysis.

- Presentation of tumour antigen by antigen-presenting cells (APC) to T cells, in conjunction with human leukocyte antigen (HLA) class I (CD8$^+$) and class II (CD4$^+$);
- accessory signals from co-stimulatory molecules such as B7;
- cytokine secretion by stimulated helper T cells.

However, colorectal tumours are poorly immunogenic, and evade immune destruction by a variety of different mechanisms. Many colorectal tumours exhibit a heterogeneous loss of HLA class I antigens, and this failure to present antigen in the context of HLA class I may allow them to evade CD8$^+$-mediated cytolysis.[19] Also, colorectal tumours do not express co-stimulatory signals, such as B7, which may lead to T-cell 'tolerance' to tumour antigens.[20] Colorectal tumours can also downregulate cell-mediated immunity by increasing levels of immune-inhibitory substances such as interleukin (IL)-10 and transforming growth factor β_1 (TGF-β_1).[21] In order to overcome these problems, several immunostimulatory approaches have been advocated to augment the innate immune response against tumours:

- cytokine gene transfer to tumours;
- co-stimulation with B7;
- allostimulation by HLA-B7 gene transfer;
- vaccination utilizing autologous tumour cells;
- vaccination against tumour-associated antigens or epitopes, such as carcinoembryonic antigen (CEA);
- the use of monoclonal antibodies directed against tumour antigens.

Cytokine gene transfer

An antitumour effect can be achieved by activation of CTL and natural killer (NK) cells using cytokines, such as IL-2 and IL-12, or granulocyte–macrophage colony-stimulating factor (GM-CSF), which stimulates the precursors of dendritic cells. However, these cytokines have significant side-effects, which limit their usage systemically. Cytokine transfer directly into tumour cells or into autologous T cells may overcome this problem, by limiting cytokine expression locally. In murine models, antitumour effects have been shown in a colon cancer line transduced with IL-2,[22] in liver metastases of a colon cancer line transduced with an adenovirus encoding IL-12,[23] and with retrovirally mediated GM-CSF transduction of colon cancer cells.[24] A phase I study of autologous tumour cell and IL-2-transduced fibroblast immunization in patients with metastatic colon cancer is ongoing.[25]

Co-stimulation with B7

The co-stimulatory molecules B7.1 (CD80) and B7.2 (CD86) are normally only present on APC, and are required for T-cell activation during antigen presentation. However, expression of B7 on tumour cells may allow direct T-cell stimulation. Colorectal tumours modified to express B7.2 and injected into syngeneic mice were rejected in 50% of cases, whereas all mice in the control group (no B7.2 expression) developed tumours. Both B7.2- and non-B7.2-expressing tumours grew at the same rate in immunodeficient mice, suggesting a T-cell-mediated antitumour effect.[26] However, the effect may be more pronounced when B7 is co-expressed with a cytokine, such as IL-12. In a colon cancer cell line, co-expression of IL-12 and B7.1 prevented tumour formation in mice and, importantly, protected against subsequent tumour re-challenges – which was not seen in tumours with B7.1 or IL-12 alone.[26]

HLA-B7 allostimulation

Animal studies have shown that expression of foreign major histocompatibility complex (MHC) molecules in tumours can elicit a T-cell-mediated immune response, not only against the foreign protein, but also against tumour antigens.[27] A phase I study of direct intratumoral injection of the MHC class I HLA-B7 as a liposome in 15 patients with colorectal liver metastases showed gene expression in over 50% of biopsy specimens. No serious toxicity was observed. Although circulating anti-HLA-B7 specific cytotoxic lymphocytes were generated in 53% of patients, no therapeutic response was seen.[28] This is in contrast to a similar study in melanoma patients, where 4 out of 14 patients had partial responses.[29] Possible explanations for the lack of response are lack of susceptibility of colon cancers to the induced immune response, tumour burden, and the size of the injected lesions. These issues are currently being investigated in a phase II study.

Active specific immunotherapy (ASI)

This approach uses the patient's own tumour (autologous) cells to elicit a cell-mediated immune response against the tumour. In order to increase the efficacy of this response, tumour cells are co-administered with an immunomodulatory adjuvant, such as bacillus Calmette–Guérin (BCG). This approach has been tested in three randomized controlled trials in an adjuvant setting in colorectal cancer (Table 62.1). In all the studies, no serious side-effects were encountered. In the first study, 98 colon and rectal cancer patients were randomized to either surgery alone or surgery and ASI. There was no significant improvement in the recurrence or survival rate in the ASI group, although subgroup analysis of colon cancer patients only showed a statistically significant improvement in survival and disease-free survival in

Table 62.1 Active specific immunotherapy

Study	Design	Results	Statistics
Hoover et al (1993)[30]	98 colon and rectal cancers	No difference in survival overall. Improved survival in colon cancer only subgroup	Not significant $p = 0.02$
Harris J et al (1994)[31]	412 colon cancers, Dukes B/C	No difference between groups	Not significant
Vermorken et al (1999)[32]	254 colon cancers, stage II/III	44% reduction in recurrence rate	7–66% reduction (95% confidence interval)

the ASI-treated group ($p = 0.02$ and $p = 0.039$ respectively).[30] The second study, of 412 colon cancer patients with Dukes stage B and C disease postoperatively randomized to ASI or to no further treatment, showed no significant differences between the two groups.[31] Recently, 254 postoperative patients with stage II and III colon cancer were randomized to ASI or to no further treatment. In contrast to the two previous studies, ASI patients received a fourth booster vaccine after 6 months. In the ASI group, there was a statistically significant reduction in the recurrence rate (44% reduction, 95% confidence interval (CI) 7–66%) and a non-statistically significant increase in overall survival. The main benefit was in stage II disease, with a non-significant reduction in recurrence in stage III disease; the relative lack of efficacy in stage III disease was thought to be due to the increased tumour burden in more advanced stages of disease.[32]

Vaccination against tumour-associated antigens

Another immunostimulatory approach is to vaccinate against a tumour-associated antigen, such as carcinoembryonic antigen (CEA), a cell surface glycoprotein with a putative role in cellular adhesion. CEA is expressed in the fetus, suppressed to low levels in normal adult colon, but overexpressed in 90% of colon cancers, as well as in a variety of other tumours such as lung, ovary, breast, and pancreas. A phase I immunization study of a recombinant vaccinia virus encoding the CEA gene, in patients with advanced colorectal cancer, demonstrated HLA-specific cytolytic T-cell responses to CEA epitopes in vitro.[33] This study did not show any clinical benefit, but several trials are underway using optimized vaccination approaches in patients with minimal residual disease where clinical responses may be observed.

Monoclonal antibodies directed against tumour antigens

Monoclonal antibodies against tumour antigens have been shown to elicit immune responses against the antigens, which may previously have been tolerized. The 17-1A antigen is a surface glycoprotein with a putative role in cell adhesion, and is present in over 90% of colorectal tumours. A study in patients with Dukes stage C colon cancer randomized 189 postsurgical patients to observation only or repeat administrations of a murine monoclonal antibody against the 17-1A antigen.[34] Treatment side-effects were infre-

quent, consisting mainly of mild constitutional and gastrointestinal symptoms. There were four anaphylactic reactions, which necessitated intravenous steroids but no hospital admissions. After 7 years of follow-up, there was a 32% relative reduction in mortality in the treatment group (90 patients) ($p < 0.01$, 95% CI 8–51%), compared with the observation group (99 patients). Following on from these encouraging results, this strategy has progressed to a multicentre phase III study.

FUTURE STRATEGIES IN THERAPY FOR COLORECTAL CANCER

Advances in vector technology

A crucial limiting factor in gene therapy is the low efficiency of gene transfer with the currently available vectors. An additional problem with the commonly used adenoviral vector is the generation of neutralizing antibodies, which reduces the gene transfer efficacy and limits repeat virus administration. However, developments in vector technology, such as the use of helper-dependent adenoviruses, which have most of the viral genes deleted, may address some of these issues. There is also a safety concern regarding viral vectors, especially after the recent death of a young patient with an inherited metabolic disorder, following high-dose hepatic artery adenoviral injection.

Replication-conditional oncolytic adenovirus

An E1B attenuated adenovirus, dl 1520 (ONYX-015), was engineered not to express the E1B 55 kDa viral protein. The virus was initially reported to replicate specifically in cancer cells with *p53* mutation, leading to cell lysis.[35] However, it was subsequently found that this virus could also replicate efficiently in several tumour cell lines with wild-type *p53*. These contradictory results raised doubt about the specificity of the dl 1520-mediated killing effect in *p53*-mutated cells.[36] However, recent data have shown that the loss of p14-mediated Mdm2 inhibition plays an important role in supporting the replication of this virus in tumour cells with wild-type *p53*.[37]

A phase I/II trial combined hepatic artery infusion of ONYX-015 with 5-FU/folinic acid for metastatic gastrointestinal metastasis to the liver.[38] Two courses of a five-day infusion of 5-FU/folinic acid were given concurrently. The virus dose was escalated from 10^7 to 10^{11} plaque-forming units (pfu) per infusion. Most patients developed grade 1/2 fever, and a few developed rigors after viral injection. No dose-limiting toxicities were observed. Preliminary data showed partial responses in two of the four evaluable patients.

Another trial used the same virus administered without chemotherapy via hepatic artery infusion, intravenous infusion, or intratumoral injection in 16 patients with primary or metastatic hepatic tumour (mainly from colorectal primaries).[39] Tumour necrosis after viral injection was seen on computed tomographic scanning and histological analysis in all patients. No severe side-effects were observed at a dose of 3×10^{11} pfu. No alterations of liver or kidney function tests were noted. The use of dl 1520 in combination with chemotherapy (5-FU and cisplatin) has also shown promising results in a trial of head and neck tumours, with a complete response rate of 27% and a partial response rate of 36%.[40]

Recently, a novel E1A attenuated adenovirus was reported to replicate specifically in tumours with pRb checkpoint impairment. Importantly, a more potent antitumour effect was seen compared with dl 1520 in preclinical experiments.[41]

Combination therapy

In order to maximize tumour cell kill, different gene therapy strategies can be combined, such as a VDEPT approach together with cytokine therapy. In a murine model of colon cancer liver metastases, treatment with a combination of adenovirally mediated HSVtk–ganciclovir, IL-2, and GM-CSF led to long-term remission. No long-term survival was seen in mice treated with monotherapy.[42] Another approach is the use of gene therapy to augment conventional treatment, such as *p53* replacement combined with chemotherapy/radiotherapy. Preliminary reports suggest that this dual approach may be clinically effective.[9] It is also possible to envisage the use of vaccination approaches in an adjuvant setting, in combination with chemotherapy, following optimal tumour debulking – a clinical paradigm that would offer the best opportunity of proving the worth of immunomodulation.

Tumour-specific targeting

Other possible areas for development are tumour targeting strategies. One approach exploits the differences in antigen expression between cancer cells and normal cells, such as the expression of CEA, which is overexpressed in 90% of colon cancers. A VDEPT approach with the use of a CEA promoter to control transgene expression provides a considerable degree of tumour specificity, since only cells expressing CEA would activate the promoter, allowing transgene expression.[43] An adenovirus with the CEA promoter driving CD expression has been shown in vitro[44] and in vivo[45] to restrict CD expression and sensitization to 5-FC only to cells expressing CEA, in a dose-dependent manner. However, gene expression with tumour-specific promoters is generally weaker compared with the non-specific cytomegalovirus (CMV) promoter.

NOVEL THERAPEUTIC AGENTS

Anti-VEGF and anti-EGF/EGFR strategies

Angiogenesis is essential for tumour growth. A key component in this process is vascular endothelial growth factor (VEGF). VEGF binds to receptors, such as Flt-1 and Flt-1 KDR, on endothelial cells to induce the formation of capillaries, which are necessary for primary tumour growth, as well as to facilitate metastasis.[46,47] Therefore, anti-VEGF therapies have been used as antiangiogenic strategies in colon cancer. Adenovirally mediated, soluble Flt-1 VEGF receptor gene transfer in mice with CT26.CL25 colonic tumours showed significant reduction in local tumour growth and regional metastases.[48] In another approach, wild-type *p53* gene replacement via an adenoviral vector demonstrated a significant reduction in VEGF expression in colon cancer cells with *p53* mutations and reduced angiogenesis in vivo.[49] The epidermal growth factor receptor (EGFR) is overexpressed in 50–70% of human primary carcinomas of the breast, lung, and colon. Activation of EGFR by epidermal growth factor (EGF) or TGF-α has been proposed to be involved in the regulation of tumour growth[50] and metastasis[51] in colon cancer cells. Antisense oligonucleotides or antisense RNA directed against EGF-like growth factors[50] or EGFR[51] inhibited the growth of colon cancer cells in vitro. These results suggest a potential benefit in disrupting the angiogenic and growth-factor-mediated autocrine loop driving colon cancer growth, and represent an alternative strategy for therapy.

Matrix metalloproteinase inhibitors

The matrix metalloproteinases are a group of enzymes involved in the physiological maintenance of the extracellular matrix. They degrade this matrix and promote the formation of new blood vessels, and are involved in tissue remodelling processes such as wound healing and angiogenesis. However, matrix metalloproteinases are overexpressed in a variety of different tumours, including colorectal cancers, and have been implicated in tumour invasion and metastasis. A matrix metalloproteinase inhibitor, marimastat, has shown reductions in levels of tumour markers in phase I studies,[53] and its clinical efficacy is currently being tested in phase III trials.

Farnesyl transferase inhibitors

Another novel agent is the farnesyl transferase inhibitor, SCH 66336, which inhibits the effects of *ras* oncogenes. Inhibition of farnesylation (addition of a 15-carbon isoprenoid lipid) of Ras proteins disrupts cell membrane localization and ablates its growth-promoting properties.[54] Murine studies have shown regression of colon cancer xenografts after oral administration of SCH 66336.[55] The clinical activity of SCH 66336 is currently being tested in phase I trials.

CONCLUSIONS

The current limitations of conventional therapy for colorectal cancer have prompted a variety of novel therapeutic approaches in attempts to improve disease survival. Certain modalities appear promising, but much work remains to be done. Gene therapy is still at an early stage of development. Preclinical studies have shown promise, and thus have prompted several ongoing clinical studies. Encouragingly, phase I studies of similar gene therapy approaches in tumours of the brain, lung, and head and neck, and in melanoma have reported complete and partial responses in some patients.[56] Although these uncontrolled clinical studies have shown gene therapy to be relatively safe and theoretically feasible, significant problems, such as low gene transfer, need to be addressed. However, future developments in vector technology and gene therapy approaches, in conjunction with conventional treatments, may translate into clinically important benefits. Then, promising gene therapy strategies need to be subjected to large randomized controlled trials. This work is only just beginning.

More promisingly, immunotherapy approaches, such as ASI and the use of monoclonal antibodies, have been shown to be well tolerated and effective in phase III studies as adjuvant treatment for colon can-

cer. Their efficacy in limited-stage disease is comparable to adjuvant 5-FU and folinic acid chemotherapy in Dukes stage C colon cancer, and is now under evaluation in a large randomized, multicentre controlled trial. In more advanced disease, immunotherapy may have a role to play in combination with chemotherapy, and this avenue is being explored in ongoing studies. Novel approaches such as inhibition of Ras or tumour angiogenesis and metastasis are conceptually attractive but their clinical efficacy remains to be proven.

Despite the lack of success in reducing colorectal cancer mortality over the last decade, there is now a concerted effort to explore novel therapeutic avenues, aided by technological advances, which may ultimately provide a major breakthrough to this elusive goal.

REFERENCES

1. Anderson WF, Human gene therapy. *Nature* 1998; **392:** 25–30.
2. Langer R, Drug delivery and targeting. *Nature* 1998; **392:** 5–10.
3. Ozturk M, Ponchel F, Puisieux A, p53 as a potential target in cancer therapy. *Bone Marrow Transplant* 1992; **9:** 164–70.
4. Levine AJ, p53, the cellular gatekeeper for growth and division. *Cell* 1997; **88:** 323–31.
5. Baker SJ, Markowitz S, Fearon ER et al, Suppression of human colorectal carcinoma cell growth by wild-type p53. *Science* 1990; **249:** 912–15.
6. Harris MP, Sutjipto S, Wills KN et al, Adenovirus-mediated p53 gene transfer inhibits growth of human tumor cells expressing mutant p53 protein. *Cancer Gene Ther* 1996; **3:** 121–30.
7. Bunz F, Hwang PM, Torrance C et al, Disruption of p53 in human cancer cells alters the responses to therapeutic agents. *J Clin Invest* 1999; **104:** 263–9.
8. Ogawa N, Fujiwara T, Kagawa S et al, Novel combination therapy for human colon cancer with adenovirus-mediated wild-type p53 gene transfer and DNA-damaging chemotherapeutic agent. *Int J Cancer* 1997; **73:** 367–70.
9. Venook AE, Bergsland EK, Ring E et al, Gene therapy of colorectal liver metastases using a recombinant adenovirus encoding wt p53 (SCH 58500) via hepatic artery infusion: a phase I study. *Proc Am Soc Clin Oncol* 1998; **17:** 431a.
10. Sakakura C, Hagiwara A, Tsujimoto H et al, Inhibition of colon cancer cell proliferation by antisense oligonucleotides targeting the messenger RNA of the Ki-ras gene. *Anti-Cancer Drugs* 1995; **6:** 553–61.
11. Roth JA, Modification of mutant K-ras gene expression in non-small cell lung cancer (NSCLC). *Hum Gene Ther* 1996; **7:** 875–89.
12. Yang L, Chiang Y, Lenz HJ et al, Intercellular communication mediates the bystander effect during herpes simplex thymidine kinase/ganciclovir-based gene therapy of human gastrointestinal tumor cells. *Hum Gene Therapy* 1998; **9:** 719–28.
13. Link CJ Jr, Levy JP, McCann LZ, Moorman DW, Gene therapy for colon cancer with the herpes simplex thymidine kinase gene. *J Surg Oncol* 1997; **64:** 289–94.
14. Mullen CA, Kilstrup M, Blaese RM, Transfer of the bacterial gene for cytosine deaminase to mammalian cells confers lethal sensitivity to 5-fluorocytosine: a negative selection system. *Proc Natl Acad Sci USA* 1992; **89:** 33–7.

15. Austin EA, Huber BE, A first step in the development of gene therapy for colorectal carcinoma: cloning, sequencing, and expression of *Escherichia coli* cytosine deaminase. *Mol Pharmacol* 1993; **43**: 380–7.

16. Huber BE, Austin EA, Richards CA et al, Metabolism of 5-fluorocytosine to 5-fluorouracil in human colorectal tumor cells transduced with the cytosine deaminase gene: significant antitumor effects when only a small percentage of tumor cells express cytosine deaminase. *Proc Natl Acad Sci USA* 1994; **91**: 8302–6.

17. Crystal RG, Hirschowitz E, Lieberman M et al, Phase I study of direct administration of a replication deficient adenovirus vector containing the *E. coli* cytosine deaminase gene to metastatic colon carcinoma of the liver in association with the oral administration of the prodrug 5 fluorocytosine. *Hum Gene Ther* 1997; **8**: 985–1001.

18. McNeish IA, Green NK, Gilligan MG et al, Virus directed enzyme prodrug therapy for ovarian and pancreatic cancer using retrovirally delivered *E. coli* nitroreductase and CB1954. *Gene Therapy* 1998; **5**: 1061–9.

19. Todryk S, Lemoine N, Can immunotherapy by gene transfer tip the balance against colorectal cancer. *Gut* 1998; **43**: 445–9.

20. Harding FA, McArthur JG, Gross JA et al, CD28-mediated signalling co-stimulates murine T cells and prevents induction of anergy in T-cell clones. *Nature* 1992; **356**: 607–9.

21. Kucharzik T, Lugering N, Winde G et al, Colon carcinoma cell lines stimulate monocytes and lamina propria mononuclear cells to produce IL-10. *Clin Exp Immunol* 1997; **110**: 296–302.

22. Fearon ER, Pardoll DM, Itaya T et al, Interleukin-2 production by tumor cells bypasses T helper function in the generation of an antitumor response. *Cell* 1990; **60**: 397–403.

23. Caruso M, Pham-Nguen K, Kwong YL et al, Adenovirus-mediated interleukin-12 gene therapy for metastatic colon carcinoma. *Proc Natl Acad Sci USA* 1996; **93**: 11302–6.

24. Gunji Y, Tagawa M, Matsubara H et al, Antitumor effect induced by the expression of granulocyte macrophage-colony stimulating factor gene in murine colon carcinoma cells. *Cancer Lett* 1996; **101**: 257–61.

25. Sobol RE, Royston I, Fakhrai H et al, Injection of colon carcinoma patients with autologous irradiated tumor cells and fibroblasts genetically modified to secrete interleukin-2 (IL-2): a phase I study. *Hum Gene Ther* 1995; **6**: 195–204.

26. Chong H, Todryk S, Hutchinson G et al, Tumour cell expression of B7 costimulatory molecules and interleukin-12 or granulocyte–macrophage colony-stimulating factor induces a local antitumour response and may generate systemic protective immunity. *Gene Ther* 1998; **5**: 223–32.

27. Plautz GE, Nabel EG, Fox B et al, Direct gene transfer for the understanding and treatment of human disease. *Ann NY Acad Sci* 1994; **716**: 144–53.

28. Rubin J, Galanis E, Pitot HC et al, Phase I study of immunotherapy of hepatic metastases of colorectal carcinoma by direct gene transfer of an allogeneic histocompatibility antigen, HLA-B7. *Gene Ther* 1997; **4**: 419–25.

29. Vogelzang N, Clinical experience in phase I and phase II testing of direct intratumoral administration with Allovectin-7: a gene based immunotherapeutic agent. *Proc Am Soc Clin Oncol* 1996; **17**: 235.

30. Hoover HC Jr, Brandhorst JS, Peters LC et al, Adjuvant active specific immunotherapy for human colorectal cancer: 6.5-year median follow-up of a phase III prospectively randomized trial. *J Clin Oncol* 1993; **11**: 390–9.

31. Harris J, Ryan L, Adams G et al, Survival and relapse in adjuvant autologous tumour vaccine therapy for Dukes B and C colon cancer – EST 5283. *Proc Am Soc Clin Oncol* 1994; **13**: 294.

32. Vermorken JB, Claessen AM, van Tinteren H et al, Active specific immunotherapy for stage II and stage III human colon cancer: a randomised trial. *Lancet* 1999; **353**: 345–50.

33. Tsang KY, Zaremba S, Nieroda CA et al, Generation of human cytotoxic T cells specific for human carcinoembryonic antigen epitopes from patients immunized with recombinant vaccinia-CEA vaccine. *J Natl Cancer Inst* 1995; **87**: 982–90.

34. Riethmuller G, Holz E, Schlimok G et al, Monoclonal antibody therapy for resected Dukes' C colorectal cancer: seven-year outcome of a multicenter randomized trial. *J Clin Oncol* 1998; **16**: 1788–94.

35. Bischoff JR, Kirn DH, Williams A et al, An adenovirus mutant that replicates selectively in p53-deficient human tumor cells. *Science* 1996; **274**: 373–6.

36. Rothmann T, Hengstermann A, Whitaker NJ et al, Replication of ONYX-015, a potential anticancer adenovirus, is independent of p53 status in tumor cells. *J Virol* 1998; **72**: 9470–8.

37. Ries SJ, Brandts CH, Chung AS et al, Loss of p14^{ARF} in tumor cells facilitates replication of the adenovirus mutant dl 1520 (ONYX-015). *Nature Med* 2000; **6**: 1123–33.

38. Reid T, Rubin J, Galanis E et al, Hepatic artery infusion of ONYX-015 in combination with 5-FU/leukovorin for metastatic gastrointestinal cancer metastasis to liver: a phase I/II study (conference abstract of AACR–NCI–EORTC International Conference on Molecular Targets and Cancer Therapeutics, November, 1999). *Clin Cancer Res* 1999; **5**: 3798s.

39. Habib N, Kelly MD, Zhao J et al, E1B-deleted adenovirus gene therapy for liver tumors (conference abstract of First International Meeting on Cancer Gene Therapy, London). *Cancer Gene Ther* 1999; **6**: 389.

40. Khuri FR, Nemunaitis J, Ganly I et al, A controlled trial of intratumoral ONYX-015, a selectively-replicating adenovirus, in combination with cisplatin and 5-fluorouracil in patients with recurrent head and neck cancer. *Nature Med* 2000; **6**: 879–85.

41. Heise C, Hermiston T, Johnson L et al, An adenovirus E1A mutant that demonstrates potent and systemic anti-tumoral efficacy. *Nature Med* 2000; **6**: 1134–9.

42. Chen SH, Kosai K, Xu B et al, Combination suicide and cytokine gene therapy for hepatic metastases of colon carcinoma: sustained antitumor immunity prolongs animal survival. *Cancer Res* 1996; **56**: 3758–62.

43. Richards CA, Austin EA, Huber BE, Transcriptional regulatory sequences of carcinoembryonic antigen: identification and use with cytosine deaminase for tumor-specific gene therapy. *Hum Gene Ther* 1995; **6**: 881–93.

44. Lan KH, Kanai F, Shiratori Y et al, Tumor-specific gene expression in carcinoembryonic antigen-producing gastric cancer cells using adenovirus vectors. *Gastroenterology* 1996; **111**: 1241–51.

45. Lan KH, Kanai F, Shiratori Y et al, In vivo selective gene expression and therapy mediated by adenoviral vectors for human carcinoembryonic antigen-producing gastric carcinoma. *Cancer Res* 1997; **57**: 4279–84.

46. Thomas KA, Vascular endothelial growth factor, a potent and selective angiogenic agent. *J Biol Chem* 1996; **271**: 603–6.

47. Takahashi Y, Kitadai Y, Bucana CD et al, Expression of vascular endothelial growth factor and its receptor, KDR, correlates with vascularity, metastasis, and proliferation of human colon cancer. *Cancer Res* 1995; **55**: 3964–8.

48. Kong HL, Hecht D, Song W et al, Regional suppression of tumor growth by in vivo transfer of a cDNA encoding a secreted form of the extracellular domain of the flt-1 vascular endothelial growth factor receptor. *Hum Gene Ther* 1998; **9**: 823–33.

49. Bouvet M, Ellis LM, Nishizaki M et al, Adenovirus-mediated wild-type p53 gene transfer down-regulates vascular endothelial growth factor expression and inhibits angiogenesis in human colon cancer. *Cancer Res* 1998; **58**: 2288–92.

50. Normanno N, Bianco C, Damiano V et al, Growth inhibition of

human colon carcinoma cells by combinations of anti-epidermal growth factor-related growth factor antisense oligonucleotides. *Clin Cancer Res* 1996; **2:** 601–9.

51. Radinsky R, Risin S, Fan D et al, Level and function of epidermal growth factor receptor predict the metastatic potential of human colon carcinoma cells. *Clin Cancer Res* 1995; **1:** 19–31.

52. Wang HM, Rajagopal S, Chakrabarty S, Inhibition of human colon cancer malignant cell behavior and growth by antisense epidermal growth factor receptor expression vector. *Anticancer Res* 1998; **18:** 2297–300.

53. Primrose JN, Bleiberg H, Daniel F et al, Marimastat in recurrent colorectal cancer: exploratory evaluation of biological activity by measurement of carcinoembryonic antigen. *Br J Cancer* 1999; **79:** 509–14.

54. Beaupre DM, Kurzrock R, RAS and leukemia: from basic mechanisms to gene-directed therapy. *J Clin Oncol* 1999; **17:** 1071–9.

55. Liu M, Bryant MS, Chen J et al, Antitumor activity of SCH 66336, an orally bioavailable tricyclic inhibitor of farnesyl protein transferase, in human tumor xenograft models and wap–ras transgenic mice. *Cancer Res* 1998; **58:** 4947–56.

56. Roth JA, Cristiano RJ, Gene therapy for cancer: What have we done and where are we going? *J Natl Cancer Inst* 1997; **89:** 21–39.

63

Gene therapy

Paul Jacobs, Vincent Richard, Diamon Gangji, Thierry Velu

INTRODUCTION

Gene therapy can be broadly defined as a therapeutic transfer of genetic material in some cells of a patient. Most frequently, this genetic material corresponds to the coding sequences of a gene (cDNA). The objective of the gene transfer is either to correct a mutation-related gene defect or to bring a new function to the cells.

Most gene-transfer clinical protocols submitted so far have involved patients with different types of cancer, including colorectal adenocarcinomas.[1] This reflects in part the inadequacy of conventional treatments for most advanced solid tumours and the fact that novel treatments are considered acceptable in this situation.

To date, 532 gene-therapy protocols have been completed, have started, or are ongoing. They have involved about 3500 patients. Of the protocols, 62%, amounting to 2361 patients, deal with cancers, as can be seen from the online database of the *Journal of Gene Medicine* (http://www.wiley.co.uk/wileychi/genmed/clinical/index.html). Of these trials, 32 are targeting colorectal cancers, following immune or non-immune strategies (Table 63.1), with 78% being performed in the USA and 18% in Europe.

Gene-transfer techniques

A gene-therapy vector (usually called a 'vector') is a system designed to transfer exogenous genetic material, the *transgene*, into a target cell. Gene vectors can either be derived from a virus or have a non-viral backbone. The simplest systems are vectors composed of 'naked DNA', usually in the form of plasmids, designed to contain the gene of interest and regulatory elements that control and enhance its expression. Their use is restricted by their low gene-transfer efficiency and their susceptibility to degradation. To solve these problems, as well as ongoing major efforts to develop non-viral vectors, several viruses have been engineered to carry foreign DNA sequences, and are still presently the most efficient vectors to transduce cells in vivo (Figure 63.1). The critical determinants for choosing a particular vector system for a specific application include the host range and tissue specificity, the ability to transfer genes to dividing versus non-dividing cells, and the capacity to integrate or not into the host genome. The potential immunogenicity of the vector is of fundamental importance if multiple administrations are considered.

Safety and production of vectors

The possible side-effects of transgene expression must be considered, as well as the potential risks of the vector system as a whole. The level of containment required during the production process as well as during clinical trials is determined by the virus from which the vector is derived, the transgene that is to be expressed, the amount of viral sequences retained in the vector, and the relative titre of contaminating replication-competent viruses.

Several guidelines and legal documents in the USA (Food and Drug Administration, FDA) and in Europe (EU Directives) provide a regulatory framework for activities with genetically modified microorganisms under appropriate conditions of containment used to limit their contact with the general population and the environment. Several European countries have incorporated European biotechnology directives, decisions, regulations, and guidelines into national laws. Decisions regarding

Table 63.1 Classification of gene-therapy protocols, depending on tumour type and therapeutic strategy used (immune versus non-immune)

Tumour type	Immune	Non-immune	Total
Melanoma	72	1	73
Breast cancer	20	14	34
Colorectal cancer or other	26	5	31
Brain tumours	6	23	29
Renal carcinoma	21	0	21
Non-Hodgkin's lymphoma	15	6	21
Prostate cancer	10	7	17
Ovarian cancer	5	11	16
Bronchial cancer	10	4	14
Head and neck cancer	6	4	10
Leukaemia	1	8	9
Hepatoma and hepatic metastasis	1	5	6
Neuroblastoma	5	0	5
Multiple myeloma	0	3	3
Mesothelioma	1	2	3
Sarcoma	2	0	2
Cervical cancer	2	0	2
Bladder cancer	0	2	2
Germinoma	0	1	1
Carcinomatous meningitis	0	1	1
Various advanced cancers	11	4	15

authorization by different administrative bodies representing different institutional levels are based on a common science-based biosafety advisory system. In such a system, all regulatory aspects of the uses of genetically modified organisms are assessed in a coordinated way, inside the same procedures, independently of specific regulations. Advice and decisions on biological safety are given on a case-by-case basis.

Clinical trials involving recombinant DNA must be approved by the appropriate authorities and by ethical committees to ensure that they are scientifi-

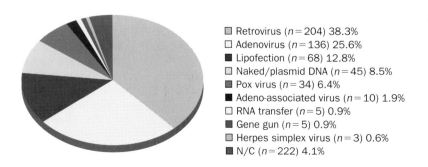

☐ Retrovirus (*n* = 204) 38.3%
☐ Adenovirus (*n* = 136) 25.6%
■ Lipofection (*n* = 68) 12.8%
☐ Naked/plasmid DNA (*n* = 45) 8.5%
■ Pox virus (*n* = 34) 6.4%
■ Adeno-associated virus (*n* = 10) 1.9%
☐ RNA transfer (*n* = 5) 0.9%
■ Gene gun (*n* = 5) 0.9%
☐ Herpes simplex virus (*n* = 3) 0.6%
■ N/C (*n* = 222) 4.1%

Figure 63.1 Gene-therapy protocols according to vector. Reproduced from the *Journal of Gene Medicine*, 2001, with permission from John Wiley & Sons (www.wiley.co.uk/genmed).

cally based, consider the ethical implications of the proposed work, and are not associated with unacceptable health risks to the enrolled patients or the population as a whole. The manufacturing process itself must follow good manufacturing practice (GMP) procedures, it must be carefully analysed with regard to the identity and purity of the vector, and it must ensure that pathogens or toxic materials are not introduced during vector production and that the generated material has sufficient activity to confer the intended therapeutic benefit.

Toxicological studies should address the following points in relevant animal models: (a) toxicity and tumorigenicity of the vector alone; (b) toxicity of transgene expression; (c) occurrence and consequences of transgene expression in non-targeted tissues; (d) occurrence and consequences of immune responses to transgene or vector proteins; and (e) the possibility of germline transduction. Toxicological studies should include doses equivalent to and higher than the intended human dose, and, when appropriate, the toxic dose should be determined in animals. A general schematic diagram for vector production and testing is given in Figure 63.2.

For clinical-grade vector production, manufacturing processes have been defined by regulatory bodies, in GMP guidelines. For most phase I/II clinical trials, a clone is expanded to generate 100–200 vials of cells packaging viral vectors, which are cryopreserved and stored as a master cell bank. Approximately 20 vials are used for certification

assays and 10 are archived. The main tests performed on vector clinical batches include general safety assays, looking for sterility, mycoplasmas, replication-competent viruses, unexpected viruses, producing-cell identity, vector or transgene DNA sequence, and titre.

Gene therapy is a rapidly developing field, and the requirements for toxicological evaluation and certification evolve accordingly. Certification testing in compliance with GMP is the major cost incurred in the production of clinical materials.

Vector systems

As illustrated in Figure 63.1, several vectors have been used in clinical trials of gene therapy. Each has different features that may be advantageous or disadvantageous, depending on the strategy of the trial: for example, transient expression for a cancer vaccine versus stable expression for correction of gene defects (Table 63.2).

Naked DNA, liposomes, and other non-viral vectors

Naked DNA in the form of oligonucleotides can be used to modulate endogenous gene expression. Antisense oligodeoxynucleotides are synthetic nucleotides that are complementary to short sequences of specific mRNAs.[2] They hybridize to their mRNA's counterparts and consequently inhibit their translation. The use of antisense oligonucleotides is limited by their high susceptibility to degradation, inefficient entry into cells, and relatively low mRNA translation-inhibiting efficacy.

Plasmids are circular DNA molecules in which the transgene has been inserted downstream to regulatory sequences promoting and controlling its expression.

Both oligonucleotides and plasmids can be incorporated into cationic liposomes that protect them from nucleases and improve their uptake by targeted cells. Although a priori safer than virus-derived vectors, their in vivo efficiency is nevertheless still too low to supplant the latter.

Retroviral vectors

Retroviral vectors, like their parental murine leukaemia viruses (MLVs), cause little direct toxicity to the infected cell.[3] Since the RNA genome of retroviruses is randomly inserted into the host genome after conversion into DNA by the viral reverse transcriptase, the major safety concern with the clinical use of retroviral vectors is related to the potential

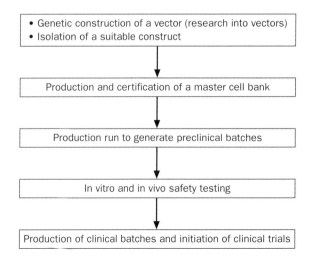

- Genetic construction of a vector (research into vectors)
- Isolation of a suitable construct

↓

Production and certification of a master cell bank

↓

Production run to generate preclinical batches

↓

In vitro and in vivo safety testing

↓

Production of clinical batches and initiation of clinical trials

Figure 63.2 Schematic diagram for vector production and testing.

Table 63.2 Main characteristics of some viral vectors

	Murine retrovirus	Adenovirus	Adeno-associated virus	Herpesvirus	Human lentivirus
Genome[a]	RNA	ds DNA	ss DNA	ds DNA	RNA
Transgene[b]	3–7	7–36	2.0–4.5	10–100	8–9
Proliferation of target	Required	Not required	Improves efficiency	Not required	Improves efficiency
Stable integration	Yes	No	Occasional	No	Yes
Immunogenicity	Low	High	Low	Variable	Not well studied

[a] ds, double-stranded; ss, single-stranded.
[b] Approximate size (in kilobases) of potential transgene.

development of malignancy due to random insertional mutagenesis. This risk becomes significant if replication-competent retroviruses are generated by homologous recombination in vitro during vector preparation. More and more ingeniously engineered packaging cell lines have been generated to reduce the risk of such recombination.

It is nevertheless reassuring that none of the clinical gene-therapy trials performed so far have detected patient exposure to replication-competent retrovirus or any malignancy arising as a consequence of insertional mutagenesis.

Adenoviral vectors

Adenoviruses are non-encapsulated viruses with a double-stranded (ds)-DNA genome.[3,4] The development of adenoviral vectors, as is the case for the other viruses, involved the deletion of genome fragments required for virus replication, opening space for the transgene insertion. The safety of adenoviral vectors for human gene therapy has been less well characterized than that of retroviral vectors. Partly because they still contain several viral genes, adenoviral vectors induce immune responses that may limit the efficiency of their re-administration, and inflammatory responses that can sometimes be life-threatening when injected at high titre. They are characterized by their very high titre, and their capacity to infect non-dividing cells efficiently. Because adenoviral DNA is maintained episomally and rarely integrates into the host genome, the risk of insertional mutagenesis is minimal.[5] Wild-type, replication-competent adenoviruses generally cause only mild upper respiratory infections in immuno-competent humans, and, in fact, the risk of generating replication-competent adenovirus is extremely low because of size constraints.[5]

Thanks to their high titre and high transduction efficiency, adenoviral vectors can be used to transfer clinically relevant genes rapidly in as many as 90% of freshly isolated tumour cells. Adenovirus-mediated gene delivery was reproducibly and significantly more efficient than retroviral transduction, and provides a rationale for genetic immunotherapy for colorectal cancer.[6]

Other vectors

Adeno-associated viruses (AAVs) are small single-stranded (ss)-DNA human parvoviruses. They are not pathogenic, and AAV vectors are generally believed to be among the safest vectors available. In certain circumstances, AAV can integrate into the cellular genome, but at a quite specific site in the presence of the viral Rep gene product. Furthermore, production of AAV vectors generally requires the use of helper adenovirus. AAV are characterized by a titre higher than that of retroviral vectors, by their low immunogenicity thanks to the elimination of most viral sequences, and by their ability to infect non-dividing cells.

Autonomous parvoviruses, such as the minute virus of mice (MVM), constitute another group of potential vectors for cancer therapy, since they are not pathogenic to humans and show a clear tropism and killing activity for cancer cells.[7]

Herpesviruses, such as herpes simplex and varicella zoster viruses, are large enveloped viruses with a ds-DNA genome suitable to transfer large DNA fragments – especially in the nervous system, for which they show a clear tropism.

Vaccinia viruses are also large ds-DNA viruses, which, interestingly, replicate into the cytoplasm, thus avoiding potential mutation during interaction with the cellular genome.

The ability of lentiviruses to infect non-dividing cells and to integrate into the cellular genome prompted much research on their development as vectors, despite the important safety issues related to the serious diseases that they induce. As a consequence, most of the published studies regarding lentiviral vectors are concerned with vector design and careful toxicological studies, especially in non-human primates. To date, these vectors have still not been used in clinical trials.

Ethical issues

The transfer of genetic material to treat serious diseases has not led to major ethical objections from religious, political, or scientific communities. Gene-therapy trials are directed at somatic cells, and most political and religious groups have not objected to gene therapy that does not affect future progeny. In contrast, germline gene therapy has raised major objections, and very few people have argued in its favour. Gene-therapy protocols so far have followed guidelines requiring demonstration of sufficient gene transfer and expression as well as safety in preclinical studies, allowing estimation of the risk-to-benefit ratio. More specifically, the transgene should be transferred to a sufficient number of cells and expressed at a level and for a period of clinical significance, and transgene expression should not exceed levels that could be detrimental.

GENE-TRANSFER APPLICATIONS

The first clinical trial involving human gene transfer started in 1989.[8] The initial rationale for applying gene therapy to cancer derives from the well-established fact that cancers result from genetic lesions in somatic cells. Numerous lesions of several classes of genes, including proto-oncogenes and tumour suppressor genes, have been associated with malignant transformation and progression, and identified in a wide variety of human cancers, during the last 20 years or so. As a consequence, gene therapy has emerged as a new method of therapeutic and possibly preventive intervention against cancer, targeted at the gene level.[9] Indeed, gene-therapy strategies may offer the potential of a much higher

specificity of action than conventional drugs, by virtue of the highly specific control and regulatory mechanisms of gene expression that may be targeted. Research into gene therapy of cancer follows three main directions: mutation compensation, molecular chemotherapy, and genetic immunopotentiation.[10]

- In mutation compensation, gene-therapy techniques are designed to correct the molecular lesions that are aetiologic of malignant transformation; an example is *p53* gene transfer into tumour cells.
- In molecular chemotherapy, methods have been developed to achieve selective delivery or expression of a toxin gene in cancer cells to induce their eradication, or of a gene to increase their sensitivity to concomitant chemotherapy or radiotherapy; an example of the latter approach is the transfer of the suicide gene coding for herpes simplex virus thymidine kinase, followed by administration of ganciclovir.
- Genetic immunopotentiation strategies attempt to achieve active immunization against defined tumour-associated antigens (TAAs) (e.g. MAGE, MUC-1, or CEA) by gene transfer in antigen-presenting cells, or against undefined TAAs by, for example, transfer of a gene coding for a cytokine (e.g. IL-2 or GM-CSF) into tumour cells.

Table 63.3 summarizes the 32 clinical trials that have been undertaken so far to assess the safety of the approach or to treat advanced colorectal cancers or their hepatic metastases.

Genetic immunopotentiation

The major gene-transfer strategy in cancer seeks to induce or increase antitumour immune responses. Indeed, it is obvious that most patients with cancer do not mount an effective immune response to their tumour. This could be due to defects in antigen presentation, co-stimulation, or differentiation of activated T cells into functional effector cells. Gene-therapy strategies are addressing each of these possibilities.

The rationale underlying these strategies is based on preclinical studies that have shown that the immune system can recognize and eliminate malignant tumours cells in vivo.[11–13] Depending on the particular experimental system used, participation of helper effector T cells, cytotoxic T lymphocytes (CTL), natural killer (NK) cells, and other cell types has been implicated.

It is thus assumed that the tolerance or anergy to

Table 63.3 Classification of gene-therapy trials for colorectal cancer[a]

Principal investigator	Phase, number of patients enrolled, type	Type of vector	Transgene	Targeted pathology[b]	Country
Chang AE	Phase II, 22, open	Liposome	HLA-B7, β_2-microglobulin	RCC, MM, BC, CRC, AdC, NHL	USA
Cole D	Phase I, 8, open	Poxvirus	CEA	BC, GI AdC, lung AdC	USA
Crystal RG	Phase I, 6, open	Adenovirus	Cytosine deaminase	CRC, liver metastasis	USA
Curiel DT	Phase I, open	Naked plasmid DNA	CEA + KanaR	Metastatic CRC	USA
Sobol RE	Phase I, open	Naked plasmid DNA	CD80 (B7-1)	CRC	USA
Gilly B	Phase I, 8, open	Adenovirus	IL-2	CRC	France (Transgene)
Marshall JL	Phase I/II, open	Poxvirus	CEA	Unresectable or advanced cancer	USA
Hersh E	Phase II, 102, closed	Liposomes	HLA-B7, β_2-microglobulin	MM, BC, CRC, RCC, NHL	USA
Littler	Phase I, open	N/C		CRC	UK (Wellcome Research Laboratories)
Conry RM			CEA	Metastatic CEA-expressing AdC	USA
Junghans RP	Phase I, open	Retrovirus	Anti-CEA-sFv-Zeta TcR	CEA-expressing AdC	USA
Rosenberg SA	Phase I, 12, open	Retrovirus	IL-2	MM, RCC, CRC	USA
Rosenberg SA	Phase I, 12, open	Retrovirus	TNF + NeoR	MM, RCC, CRC, BC	USA
Rubin J	Phase II, 28, closed	Liposomes	HLA-B7, β_2-microglobulin	MM, RCC, CRC, BC, NHL	USA
Schmidt-Wolf I	Phase I, 20, open	Naked plasmid DNA	IL-7 + IL-2	MM, RCC, CRC, NHL	Germany
Sobol RE	Phase I, 6, open	Retrovirus	IL-2	CRC	USA
Sung MW	Phase I, open	Adenovirus	HSV-TK	Liver metastasis	USA
Venook AP	Phase I, 1, open	Adenovirus	*p53*	Liver metastasis, CRC	USA
Marshall JL	Phase I, 7, open	Poxvirus	CEA	CEA-expressing malignancies	USA
Conry RM	Phase I, open	Poxvirus	CEA	Metastatic CEA-expressing AdC	USA
Venook AP	Phase I/II, open	Retrovirus	CC49-Zeta TcR chimera	CRC expressing TAG-72	USA
Kaufman HL	Phase I, open	Poxvirus	CD80 (B7-1) + CEA	CRC	USA
Bergsland EK	Phase I/II, open	Retrovirus	CC49-Zeta TcR chimera	CRC, liver metastasis	
Suzuki T	Phase I, 5, open		GM-CSF	BC, CRC, H&N cancers, soft tissue sarcoma	USA
Stewart	Phase I, 1, open	Adenovirus	*p53*	GI cancer/malignant cancer ascites	UK
Lotze	Phase I, open	Poxvirus	CEA	CRC	UK
Venook AP	Phase II, open	Adenovirus	*p53*	CRC with hepatic metastasis	USA
Lyerly HK	Phase I, open	RNA transfer	CEA	CEA-expressing malignancies	USA
Eck SL	Phase I, submission	Adenovirus	GA733-2	CRC	USA
Sung MW	Phase I, open	Adenovirus	IL-2 + HSV-TK	Liver metastasis of CRC	USA
Fong Y	Phase I, open	Herpes simplex virus	NV1020	CRC (hepatic metastasis)	USA
Marshall JL	Phase I, submission	Poxvirus	CEA + ICAM-1 + LFA-3	CEA-expressing malignancies	USA

[a] Data from the *Journal of Gene Medicine* database on gene-therapy clinical trials (http://www.wiley.co.uk/wileychi/genmed/clinical/index.html).
[b] AdC, adenoma carcinoma; BC, breast cancer; CRC, colorectal cancer: GI, gastrointestinal; H&N, head and neck; MM, malignant melanoma; NHL, non-Hodgkin's lymphoma; RCC, renal cell carcinoma.

tumour antigens could be reversed by exposing tumour antigens to the immune system in a more favourable context (see Chapter 64).

Genetically modified adoptive cell therapy

The cell-mediated immune reaction plays a central role in the destruction of tumour cells, the regression of established tumours, and the maintenance of anti-tumour immunity. Adoptive transfer therapy aims to promote the cellular immune functions in patients by the administration of cells that have been cultured ex vivo. In adoptive transfer approaches, immune effector cells are collected and cultured, circumventing normal immune-regulatory constraints and potential tumour suppression. Potential agents toxic in vivo can be used ex vivo, in cell culture, to enhance favourable cellular properties. Generally, the activated and expanded effector cells are used to treat the patient in an autologous setting. A phase I clinical trial involving infusion of NK cells genetically modified to express interleukin-2 (IL-2) in patients with metastatic renal cancer, colorectal cancer, and lymphoma[14] showed only mild side-effects and an increase in cytotoxic immune activity, with 1 out of 10 patients developing a complete response.

Active gene immunotherapy using undefined antigens

For many years, irradiated tumour cells, either autologous or allogeneic, have been administered in combination with various adjuvants (e.g. bacillus Calmette–Guérin, BCG). Promising new approaches to antitumour therapeutic vaccines are tumour cells that have been genetically modified to increase their immunogenicity by transfer of a variety of genes, including cytokines or co-stimulatory molecules, and major histocompatibility complex (MHC) molecules. Transfer of the genes coding for IL-2 and granulocyte–macrophage colony-stimulating factor (GM-CSF) into tumour cells appears to be among the most promising strategies. The objective is to induce locally an antitumour immune response directed against undefined TAAs. Nevertheless, it should be stressed that, up to now, no definitive immunological parameter has been correlated with a clear clinical response.

Such vaccines can be based on either autologous tumour cells or allogeneic tumour cell lines. The autologous approach has the advantage that it offers the greatest potential to vaccinate against the spectrum of relevant autologous tumour antigens, but has the disadvantages of being very labour-intensive and being dependent on the variability of gene transfer in cultures derived from primary tumours. The use of allogeneic vaccines is advantageous with regard to these two points, since a single standardized transduced cell line is used for the vaccine preparation, but, to be successful, this technique requires that the transduced cells share the patient's tumour antigens.

Preclinical studies on a mouse model of colon carcinoma have shown a reduction in lung metastasis following administration of IL-2 gene-modified tumour cells.[15] Direct intraperitoneal injection of a retroviral vector expressing IL-2 also prolonged survival significantly in a mouse model of disseminated peritoneal colon carcinoma.[16] On the basis of these and many other preclinical data, several phase I/II clinical trials using human tumour cells expressing cytokines have been initiated. A phase I study involving the infusion of autologous colorectal tumour cells and fibroblasts transfected to express IL-2 has shown that it was well tolerated despite flu-like symptoms and that the frequency of cytotoxic T-cell precursors was increased in two out of six evaluable patients.[17]

Other strategies of active gene immunotherapy with undefined antigens are based on the transfer of genetic material into dendritic cells, which are the most potent antigen-presenting cells. For example, transfer of RNA extracted from tumour cells (and thus containing genetic materials corresponding to TAAs) is able to induce potent and efficient cellular immune response against tumour antigens.

Active gene immunotherapy using defined antigens

The TAA is a key component of active gene-derived immunotherapy (see Chapter 64). Immunotherapies based on defined antigens have an advantage over undefined antigen-based vaccines in that they can be produced with GMP standards, with clear-cut release criteria, and that they may have well-defined immune endpoints for evaluation in clinical trials. Immune responses against these antigens are evaluated using the in vivo delayed-type hypersensitivity (DTH) test, which remains a crude but clinically simple parameter to monitor potential response. Novel in vitro methods for more precise monitoring of immune responses are available, such as assays studying, at the cellular level, the specific production of a cytokine (most frequently interferon-γ, IFN-γ) by T lymphocytes in response to the antigen used in the vaccine (ELISPOT assays, FACS analysis with brefeldin), or searching for lymphocytes with T-cell receptor specific for this antigen (tetramer technology). All of these methods allow early monitoring of an immune response, but their prognostic value and correlation with in vivo clinical responses have not been definitively established.

In addition, this vaccine strategy has used some antigens without knowing whether there are 'the' right tumour-rejection antigens able to induce tumour regression. Another disadvantage of using a small number of defined antigens is the immuno-selection that probably occurs following vaccination. Theoretically, the ability of a given antigen to promote a strong cytotoxic antitumour response is positively correlated with its relevance in vaccine therapy, and immune responses to multiple antigens should result in more significant tumour cell kill.

Several antigens associated with colorectal cancers have been identified (see Chapter 64). They include:

- tumour–testis antigens, expressed only on tumour cells, and not on normal cells (with the exception of testis cells – but these are protected from immune responses since they do not express HLA molecules), such as the MAGE family of antigens, which can be expressed in up to 30% of colorectal cancers;
- antigens generated by mutations in oncogenes or tumour suppressor genes, such as the *ras* proto-oncogene mutated in about 50% of colorectal cancers;
- differentiation antigens, such as carcinoembryonic antigen (CEA) (an oncofetal antigen over-expressed, but not mutated, in most colorectal cancers and other adenocarcinomas) and the mucin antigens (overexpressed in colorectal cancers and other adenocarcinomas, but also expressed on normal tissue);
- overexpressed antigens, such as the *p53* tumour suppressor gene product.

Numerous epitopes binding specifically to different HLA molecules have been identified for several TAAs, and trials are ongoing that evaluate the loading of dendritic cells with antigenic peptides or recombinant proteins. However, the transfer of the *genes* coding for these TAAs should have a number of advantages: the antigens will be expressed and presented for a prolonged period of time; unidentified epitopes can be presented; both HLA class I and II molecules can be targeted, thus stimulating not only CD8[+] T cells but also CD4[+] T cells that could provide essential help for the development of an efficient antitumour immune response.

Recent studies suggest that the genetic modification of dendritic cells to express tumour antigens and/or immunomodulatory proteins improves their capacity to promote an antitumour response. In 1997, Crystal and co-workers[18] showed that in a mouse model, dendritic cells genetically modified by an adenovirus to express a model antigen (*Escherichia coli* β-galactosidase) were able to induce a long-lasting CTL response against the injection of a syngeneic colon carcinoma cell line itself transduced to express β-galactosidase. Later in 2000, they were able to show that mice challenged by subcutaneous administration of tumour cells up to 400 days after immunization and an initial intravenous challenge were still protected.[19]

Cytokine-gene modification of dendritic cells is also under investigation, and has demonstrated improved capacity to prime antigen-specific T-cell responses in vivo.

Virus-directed enzyme prodrug therapy (VDEPT)

'Suicide' genes code for foreign enzymes that convert relatively non-toxic drugs (prodrugs) into active cytotoxic compounds, thus selectively inducing the death of the cell in which they are expressed. The most studied example is the herpes simplex virus thymidine kinase (HSV-TK), which is about 1000-fold more efficient than mammalian thymidine kinases at phosphorylating ganciclovir. Ganciclovir monophosphate can then be converted to ganciclovir triphosphate, which inhibits DNA polymerase and is thus toxic to cells. Systemic administration of ganciclovir after intratumoral injection of fibroblasts transduced with an HSV-TK vector can induce regression of tumours in rats.[20] The efficacy of HSV-TK transduction of tumours followed by ganciclovir therapy has been confirmed in several preclinical models. Tumour regression has been observed despite the fact that only a small fraction of tumour cells are transduced with the HSV-TK gene. The nature of this 'bystander effect' of transduced on non-transduced tumour cells appears to be complex, but includes the participation of immune effector cells. In a rat model of colorectal adenocarcinoma-derived peritoneal carcinomatosis, the efficiency of ganciclovir treatment of cancer cells expressing HSV-TK was demonstrated as early as 1997.[21] Moreover, a synergy has been shown between TK/ganciclovir and a topoisomerase I inhibitor (topotecan)[22] or thymidylate synthase inhibitor (e.g. raltitrexed).[23] Clinical trials are being conducted in which ganciclovir is given after the HSV-TK gene has been introduced into tumour cells in vivo using retroviral or adenoviral vectors.

Another suicide gene under active investigation for cancer therapy is the cytosine deaminase gene from *E. coli*.[24] Cytosine deaminase converts the non-toxic fluoropyrimidine 5-fluorocytosine to 5-fluorouracil (5-FU). 5-FU is converted by endogenous cellular enzymes into fluorodeoxyuridine monophosphate, which inhibits thymidylate synthase activity, and fluorouridine triphosphate, which can be incorporated into RNA and interfere with RNA processing and transcription. Transduction of the cytosine deaminase gene renders tumour cells, such as human colorectal carcinoma cells, exquisitely sensitive to 5-fluorocytosine in vitro and in vivo.[24]

An important aspect of vector design in the context of suicide gene therapy concerns the specificity of its delivery to the cancer cells. One strategy to improve this specificity is to combine a relatively specific vector with a promoter of the transgene expression specific for the tumour cell. To this end, the CEA promoter has been isolated from a CEA-producing human colorectal carcinoma and used in a retroviral vector to drive the expression of the cytosine deaminase gene. It was demonstrated in a nude mouse model that the cytosine deaminase expression was strictly restricted to the colorectal cancer cells after intraperitoneal injection, even though bone marrow cells were equally transfected.[25]

Replacement of defective tumour suppressor genes

Gene transfer techniques can be used to introduce wild-type copies of tumour suppressor genes into malignant cells, thus potentially reversing the neoplastic phenotype. Mutations of the p53 tumour suppressor gene occur commonly in a variety of human cancers, including those of breast, lung, colon, prostate, bladder, and cervix. Transduction of a p53 transgene has been shown to inhibit tumour growth both in vitro and in vivo, and, in some settings, to induce apoptosis.[26–30] In addition, wild-type p53 gene transfer into cancer cells that had a homozygous deletion of p53 markedly increased the cellular sensitivity of these cells to chemotherapeutic drugs, such as cisplatin. Direct injection of the p53–adenovirus construct into H358 tumours implanted into nude mice, followed by intraperitoneal administration of cisplatin, induced massive apoptotic destruction of the tumours, supporting the clinical application of a regimen combining gene replacement using replication-deficient wild-type p53 adenovirus and DNA-damaging drugs for the treatment of human cancer.[31]

However, given the relatively low gene-transfer efficiencies achieved with currently available vectors, and their inability to target tumour cells, it is unlikely that tumour suppressor gene therapy will be very efficacious for bulky or disseminated cancers. Effective replacement of tumour suppressor genes most likely requires technical advances in gene-transfer efficiency.

Several phase I/II clinical trials are currently being performed. In one of them, a p53-expressing recombinant virus is infused into the hepatic artery in order to destroy hepatic metastases from colorectal cancer.[32]

Inhibition of transforming oncogenes

In contrast to tumour suppressor genes, oncogenes promote neoplastic transformation by acquiring dominant or gain-of-function mutations. Thus, disruption of oncogene expression could be therapeutically beneficial. The antisense strategy includes several related approaches for achieving this goal. Antisense oligonucleotides have been shown to efficiently inhibit the activity of several oncogenes, and, consequently, tumorigenesis in murine models.[33,34] Antisense oligonucleotides have also been incorporated into liposomes in an attempt to enhance their delivery to target cells. Point mutations that activate the Ki-ras proto-oncogene are present in approximately 50% of human colorectal tumours. Antisense oligonucleotides complementary to Ki-ras mRNA significantly reduced the growth of colon cancer cells in culture, but not that of normal cells or of cancer cells devoid of Ki-ras mutations.[35] The same type of experiments directed at the epidermal growth factor (EGF)-like growth factors have shown an enhancement of conventional antitumour drug efficacy in human colon cancer cells.[36]

An alternative approach is to transduce cells with vectors encoding antisense RNA. Complementary DNA encoding antisense RNA can be delivered using any of the viral vector systems described above. This approach has been used to successfully inhibit the expression of c-myc and Ki-ras in vitro and to reverse the transformed phenotypes of cell lines in vitro and their tumorigenicity in vivo. Phase I clinical trials of retroviral vectors encoding antisense mRNA specific for Ki-ras are in progress.[37]

Antiangiogenic therapy

Numerous lines of evidence have clearly established that the growth and expansion of tumours and their metastases are dependent on angiogenesis.[38] Endothelial cells also produce a number of paracrine growth factors that stimulate tumour growth.[39]

Several factors that stimulate angiogenesis have been identified and described. These include the acidic and basic fibroblast growth factors (aFGF and bFGF), vascular endothelial cell growth factor/vascular permeability factor (VEGF/VPF), hepatocyte growth factor/scatter factor, transforming growth factor β (TGF-β), proliferin, erythropoieitin, and several others. Numerous inhibitors of angiogenesis have also been described, and the discovery and characterization of these inhibitors has become an area of intense study.

As an alternative to systemic therapy with angiogenesis inhibitors, tumour cells can indeed be transfected with the corresponding genes. To test the feasibility of this approach, Cao and his colleagues[40] transfected an aggressive murine fibrosarcoma (T241) with a cDNA for angiostatin, and observed an 80% inhibition of primary tumour growth. Furthermore, metastases in 70% of mice implanted with the angiostatin-transfected tumours remained in a state of dormancy after primary tumour resection. Thrombospondin-1 expression in human breast and skin carcinomas injected into immunocompromised mice showed similar inhibition of tumour growth.[41]

These studies open the way to new gene-therapy approaches for delivering angiogenesis inhibitors, which often require extended administration.[42]

FUTURE OF GENE THERAPY

As discussed in this chapter, numerous strategies of cancer gene therapy are being developed, taking advantage of the enormous number of basic discoveries in the fields of genetics, immunology, and molecular oncology. Today, we face the challenge of improving the delivery of genetic material into cells. Because of the limited transduction efficiency of presently available vectors, specific active gene immunotherapy of cancer appears to be the most promising strategy in the future, since these antitumour vaccines require transduction of only a small number of cells. Because functional and antigenic heterogeneity is an intrinsic property of all malignancies, polyvalent vaccines are more likely to stimulate a response that can eliminate every cancer cell than are vaccines based on one or a few antigens. Strategies to improve antigen presentation, with dendritic cells, will assume paramount importance in future studies because inability to present an antigen effectively results in an inadequate immune response. Even a small therapeutic benefit would be clinically significant, because cancer vaccines (delivered as proteins or genes) have such minimal toxicity. In the future, better definition of immunogenic tumour antigens, improvements in antigen presentation and in co-stimulatory natural or artificial adjuvants administered with vaccines, development of sophisticated methods to improve antigen presentation, and early identification of non-responders with adjustment of their therapeutic regimens accordingly, will increase the applicability and effectiveness of genetic vaccines.

Although gene therapy is the talk of the town, we should keep in mind that it is still in its infancy. While proof of efficacy has been clearly demonstrated in an inherited disease,[43] major success in cancer gene therapy is still to come. Gene therapy is a remarkably promising and innovative approach for the treatment of cancer – a field where the discovery of efficient treatments remains a permanent challenge. It is now possible to tackle the disease at the genetic level. The simultaneous and interconnected growth of gene therapy and the understanding of cancer pathogenesis provides insights into new approaches.

The general lack of toxicity associated with gene transfer will allow combinations with standard chemotherapy or hormonal therapy, as well as with newer treatments, such as antiangiogenic agents. Gene therapy is intimately linked to various biological therapies, including cell manipulation. The most striking evidence of this interface between cellular and gene therapy is the ex vivo transfer of a therapeutic gene into tumour cells. Those involved in the development of cellular and gene therapy, in academia, clinical practice, and industry, must work together. New ways of thinking, working, and developing clinical trials must be explored in order to create synergy rather than conflicts, in order to make gene therapy a major success of modern medicine. Ultimately, if efficacy can be demonstrated, the lack of toxicity observed in most of these approaches may establish gene therapy as a standard of care.

REFERENCES

1. Zwacka RM, Dunlop MG, Gene therapy for colon cancer. *Hematol Oncol Clin North Am* 1998; **12**: 595–615.
2. Narayanan R, Akhtar S, Antisense therapy. *Curr Opin Oncol* 1996; **8**: 509–15.
3. Leber SM, Yamagata M, Sanes JR, Gene transfer using replication-defective retroviral and adenoviral vectors. *Meth Cell Biol* 1996; **51**: 161–83.
4. Hitt MM, Addison CL, Graham FL, Human adenovirus vectors for gene transfer into mammalian cells. *Adv Pharmacol* 1997; **40**: 137–206.

5. Nanni P, Forni G, Lollini PL, Cytokine gene therapy: hopes and pitfalls. *Ann Oncol* 1999; **10:** 261–6.

6. Diaz RM, Todryk S, Chong H et al, Rapid adenoviral transduction of freshly resected tumour explants with therapeutically useful genes provides a rationale for genetic immunotherapy for colorectal cancer. *Gene Ther* 1998; **5:** 869–79.

7. Clement N, Avalosse B, El Bakkouri K et al, Cloning and sequencing of defective particles derived from the autonomous parvovirus minute virus of mice for the construction of vectors with minimal *cis*-acting sequences. *J Virol* 2001; **75:** 1284–93.

8. Rosenberg SA, Aebersold P, Cornetta K et al, Gene transfer into humans – immunotherapy of patients with advanced melanoma, using tumor-infiltrating lymphocytes modified by retroviral gene transduction. *N Engl J Med* 1990; **323:** 570–8.

9. Anderson WF, Human gene therapy. *Nature* 1998; **392:** 25–30.

10. Gomez-Navarro J, Curiel DT, Douglas JT, Gene therapy for cancer. *Eur J Cancer* 1999; **35:** 2039–57.

11. Boon T, Toward a genetic analysis of tumor rejection antigens. *Adv Cancer Res* 1992; **58:** 177–210.

12. Roth C, Rochlitz C, Kourilsky P, Immune response against tumors. *Adv Immunol* 1994; **57:** 281–351.

13. Cox AL, Skipper J, Chen Y et al, Identification of a peptide recognized by five melanoma-specific human cytotoxic T cell lines. *Science* 1994; **264:** 716–19.

14. Schmidt-Wolf IG, Finke S, Trojaneck B et al, Phase I clinical study applying autologous immunological effector cells transfected with the interleukin-2 gene in patients with metastatic renal cancer, colorectal cancer and lymphoma. *Br J Cancer* 1999; **81:** 1009–16.

15. Tasaki K, Tagawa M, Gunji Y et al, Inhibition of experimental lung metastasis of murine colon carcinoma cells depends on the amount of interleukin-2 secreted from the transduced cells. *Anticancer Res* 1998; **18:** 813–17.

16. Gunji Y, Tasaki K, Tagawa M et al, Inhibition of peritoneal dissemination of murine colon carcinoma cells by administrating retrovirus harboring IL-2 gene. *Cancer Gene Ther* 1998; **5:** 339–43.

17. Sobol RE, Shawler DL, Carson C et al, Interleukin 2 gene therapy of colorectal carcinoma with autologous irradiated tumor cells and genetically engineered fibroblasts: a phase I study. *Clin Cancer Res* 1999; **5:** 2359–65.

18. Song W, Kong HL, Carpenter H et al, Dendritic cells genetically modified with an adenovirus vector encoding the cDNA for a model antigen induce protective and therapeutic antitumor immunity. *J Exp Med* 1997; **186:** 1247–56.

19. Song W, Tong Y, Carpenter H et al, Persistent, antigen-specific, therapeutic antitumor immunity by dendritic cells genetically modified with an adenoviral vector to express a model tumor antigen. *Gene Ther* 2000; **7:** 2080–6.

20. Culver KW, Ram Z, Wallbridge S et al, In vivo gene transfer with retroviral vector-producer cells for treatment of experimental brain tumors. *Science* 1992; **256:** 1550–2.

21. Lechanteur C, Princen F, Lo BS et al, HSV-1 thymidine kinase gene therapy for colorectal adenocarcinoma-derived peritoneal carcinomatosis. *Gene Ther* 1997; **4:** 1189–94.

22. Wildner O, Blaese RM, Morris JC, Synergy between the herpes simplex virus tk/ganciclovir prodrug suicide system and the topoisomerase I inhibitor topotecan. *Hum Gene Ther* 1999; **10:** 2679–87.

23. Wildner O, Blaese RM, Candotti F, Enzyme prodrug gene therapy: synergistic use of the herpes simplex virus–cellular thymidine kinase/ganciclovir system and thymidylate synthase inhibitors for the treatment of colon cancer. *Cancer Res* 1999; **59:** 5233–8.

24. Huber BE, Austin EA, Good SS et al, In vivo antitumor activity of 5-fluorocytosine on human colorectal carcinoma cells genetically modified to express cytosine deaminase. *Cancer Res* 1993; **53:** 4619–26.

25. Cao G, Kuriyama S, Cui L et al, Analysis of the human carcinoembryonic antigen promoter core region in colorectal carcinoma-selective cytosine deaminase gene therapy. *Cancer Gene Ther* 1999; **6:** 572–80.

26. Cai DW, Mukhopadhyay T, Liu Y et al, Stable expression of the wild-type p53 gene in human lung cancer cells after retrovirus-mediated gene transfer. *Hum Gene Ther* 1993; **4:** 617–24.

27. Fujiwara T, Grimm EA, Mukhopadhyay T et al, Induction of chemosensitivity in human lung cancer cells in vivo by adenovirus-mediated transfer of the wild-type p53 gene. *Cancer Res* 1994; **54:** 2287–91.

28. Liu TJ, Zhang WW, Taylor DL et al, Growth suppression of human head and neck cancer cells by the introduction of a wild-type p53 gene via a recombinant adenovirus. *Cancer Res* 1994; **54:** 3662–7.

29. Hsu FJ, Benike C, Fagnoni F et al, Vaccination of patients with B-cell lymphoma using autologous antigen-pulsed dendritic cells. *Nature Med* 1996; **2:** 52–8.

30. Thurner B, Haendle I, Roder C et al, Vaccination with mage-3A1 peptide-pulsed mature, monocyte-derived dendritic cells expands specific cytotoxic T cells and induces regression of some metastases in advanced stage IV melanoma. *J Exp Med* 1999; **190:** 1669–78.

31. Fujiwara T, Grimm EA, Mukhopadhyay T et al, Induction of chemosensitivity in human lung cancer cells in vivo by adenovirus-mediated transfer of the wild-type p53 gene. *Cancer Res* 1994; **54:** 2287–91.

32. Habib NA, Hodgson HJ, Lemoine N, Pignatelli M, A phase I/II study of hepatic artery infusion with wtp53-CMV-Ad in metastatic malignant liver tumours. *Hum Gene Ther* 1999; **10:** 2019–34.

33. Ratajczak MZ, Kant JA, Luger SM et al, In vivo treatment of human leukemia in a scid mouse with c-myb antisense oligodeoxynucleotides. *Proc Natl Acad Sci USA* 1992; **89:** 11823–7.

34. Skorski T, Nieborowska-Skorska M, Campbell K et al, Leukemia treatment in severe combined immunodeficiency mice by antisense oligodeoxynucleotides targeting cooperating oncogenes. *J Exp Med* 1995; **182:** 1645–53.

35. Sakakura C, Hagiwara A, Tsujimoto H et al, Inhibition of colon cancer cell proliferation by antisense oligonucleotides targeting the messenger RNA of the Ki-ras gene. *Anticancer Drugs* 1995; **6:** 553–61.

36. De Luca A, Selvam MP, Sandomenico C et al, Anti-sense oligonucleotides directed against EGF-related growth factors enhance anti-proliferative effect of conventional anti-tumor drugs in human colon-cancer cells. *Int J Cancer* 1997; **73:** 277–82.

37. Stass SA, Mixson J, Oncogenes and tumor suppressor genes: therapeutic implications. *Clin Cancer Res* 1997; **3:** 2687–95.

38. Folkman J, What is the evidence that tumors are angiogenesis dependent? *J Natl Cancer Inst* 1990; **82:** 4–6.

39. Jantscheff P, Herrmann R, Rochlitz C, Cancer gene and immunotherapy: recent developments. *Med Oncol* 1999; **16:** 78–85.

40. Cao Y, O'Reilly MS, Marshall B et al, Expression of angiostatin cDNA in a murine fibrosarcoma suppresses primary tumor growth and produces long-term dormancy of metastases. *J Clin Invest* 1998; **101:** 1055–63.

41. Arienti F, Sule SJ, Belli F et al, Limited antitumor T cell response in melanoma patients vaccinated with interleukin-2 gene-transduced allogeneic melanoma cells. *Hum Gene Ther* 1996; **7:** 1955–63.

42. Folkman J, Antiangiogenic gene therapy. *Proc Natl Acad Sci USA* 1998; **95:** 9064–6.

43. Cavazzana-Calvo M, Hacein-Bey S, de Saint BG et al, Gene therapy of human severe combined immunodeficiency (SCID)-X1 disease. *Science* 2000; **288:** 669–72.

64

Vaccine therapy for colorectal cancer

John L Marshall, Evelyn S Fox

INTRODUCTION

It has been a long-held belief that the immune system has the potential to eradicate cancers in patients. We are all aware of the immune system's power to control most infectious organisms that invade the human body, to recognize and reject foreign tissues, and, most importantly for this chapter, to be stimulated to recognize and remember a particular protein/antigen so that, upon re-exposure, a more potent and rapid response is generated. This last property of the immune system has resulted in the global use of vaccines against infectious organisms and subsequent dramatic reductions in the mortality from them.

Cancer can be generally defined as the clonal expansion of cells that have acquired mutations in key regulatory proteins, resulting in unregulated growth, invasion, and metastasis. During the past decade, significant advances in basic science have given us a much clearer picture of the differences between normal and malignant cells. While retaining the majority of the molecular characteristics of the normal cell, malignant cells nearly always express altered proteins, which not only are important for the malignant behavior of the cell but also could serve as targets for the immune system. These altered proteins should present novel peptide sequences that, if recognized as foreign by the immune system, would stimulate immune-mediated rejection of the mutated cells. While it is hypothesized that the immune system does indeed reject some tumors prior to their becoming clinically evident, and that an impaired immune system leads to an increased rate of cancer development, these theories have been difficult to prove. A large 'alternative therapy' industry has grown out of the hope that certain agents may stimulate the immune system to either prevent or help treat cancer, and the level of interest among patients in immune-based therapies is extremely high.

With all the potential and previous success of harnessing the immune system for medical purposes, why has there been so little success in immunologic therapies of cancer? Of course, the theories are many, but they can be divided into two major categories: suppression of the immune system by the cancer itself (both directly and systemically) and insufficient differences in the mutated proteins to be recognized as foreign. Early attempts at immunotherapy focused mostly on the first category by attempting to enhance the immune response systemically by the addition of agents such as interferon, interleukin-2, levamisole, and BCG. More recent work has focused on enhancing the immune system against a specific tumor-associated antigen(s), and currently many trials are being performed using a combination of both antigen-specific and systemically enhancing immune therapies.

Colon cancer is an ideal setting in which to explore vaccine therapy. First, it is a common disease, which not only improves the rate of accrual to clinical trials but also means that success would translate into benefit for a large portion of the population. Second, there is an urgent need for more effective agents for the disease. Third, there are many clinical situations where immune-based therapy would be logical (adjuvant therapy for Stage II/III, postoperative therapy following resection of metastases, combinations with chemotherapy for advanced disease). Fourth, colon cancer expresses several tumor-specific antigens that have been well characterized and have high potential for immune targeting. In this chapter, we shall review the current experience with immune therapies in colon cancer, dividing the chapter by different approaches: active specific immunotherapy, recombinant gene/virus therapy, monoclonal antibody therapy, anti-idiotype therapy, and peptide-based therapy.

ACTIVE SPECIFIC IMMUNOTHERAPY

Immunotherapy evolution: general to specific

Virtually a century ago, vaccine-activated immune response was first demonstrated to afford effective prophylaxis against infectious pathogens[1] via induction of the B-lymphocyte humoral or antibody response. The current evolutionary stage of this approach for use in the oncology arena includes a more therapeutic aim, via stimulation of the T-lymphocyte cell-mediated cytotoxic immune response. Active non-specific immunotherapy, utilizing agents such as bacillus Calmette–Guérin (BCG), interleukin-2 (IL-2), levamisole, and diphtheria toxoid, has been used to stimulate a systemic or generalized immune response not directed against any specific tumor antigen.[2] This approach has served as the precursor to development of the more recent modalities of active specific immunotherapy (ASI). The endpoint of this newer therapy is to immunize the patient against his/her own cancer, via induction of an immune response able to kill tumor cells.[3]

Cellular-mediated immune response

In order for the immune system to mount a significant T-cell response (Figure 64.1), antigen-presenting cells (APC), such as dendritic cells (DC), monocytes, macrophages, and Langerhans cells,[3] must present the digested antigen on their cell surface as glycoprotein-bound/major histocompatibility complex (MHC)-encoded peptides in conjunction with co-stimulatory molecules. Both CD8+ cytotoxic T lymphocytes (CTL), as well as CD4+ helper T lymphocytes, are stimulated by such APC activity. CTL recognize peptides in the context of MHC class I, proliferate and migrate to tumor, and kill cells expressing the target peptide. The helper T lymphocytes recognize peptides in the context of MHC class II, and encourage CTL proliferation via cytokine production and release.[4]

Tumor antigens

The overall goal of ASI is to surmount the host's inherent immunologic non-responsiveness to cancer. Several mechanisms are likely to be involved in this endogenous acquired resistance, such as immune suppression produced by tumor-derived factors (i.e.

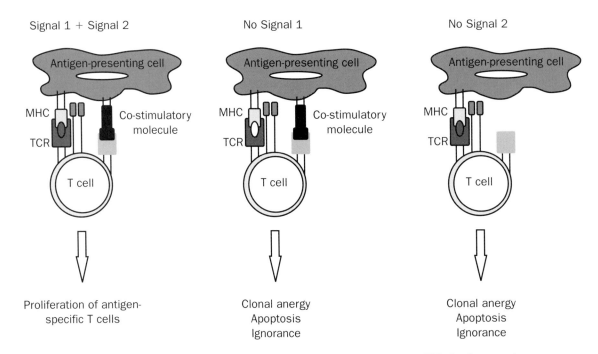

Figure 64.1 T-cell dependence on co-stimulation (MHC, major histocompatibility complex; TCR, T-cell receptor).

inhibitory cytokines), and the inherently weak antigenic properties of tumor-associated antigens (TAA) due to a lack of co-stimulatory molecules (i.e. B7 and IL-12) as well as low expression of MHC molecules, culminating in failure to mount a sufficient cytotoxic immune response.[2] However, such TAA remain therapeutically useful by providing adaptable target antigen for vaccine therapy, as the malignancy remains vulnerable to antitumor immune response via vaccination. An important hypothesis is that tumor cells encode antigens distinct from self-antigen, resulting in generation of a sufficient antitumor immune response. Accordingly, some degree of immunogenicity must be a property of the target utilized in the vaccine, which may be enhanced with the use of systemic immune modulators such as BCG.[1] TAA may occur as an overexpression of a normally occurring antigen, as neo-expression of antigen normally repressed in differentiated tissue, or as neo-expression on tissue where it is not typically present. Additionally, gene products may be considered tumor antigens.[3] ASI focuses on the use of immunogenically enhanced tumor antigens to prompt specific stimulation of the immune system to eradicate tumor cells via generation of both immediate and memory immune response cascades, yet effectively avoid damaging non-tumor tissue.[5]

Whole-cell ASI

A broad definition of ASI includes vaccination with whole-tumor-cell preparations (allogeneic or autologous), which are often combined with systemic immune modulators such as BCG, admixed with virus such as Newcastle disease virus,[6] or even genetically altered to secrete cytokines. Whole-cell preparations possess several distinct qualities compared with other more targeted modalities of ASI. For instance, whole-cell preparations provide all possible tumor antigens together, including all cell-surface as well as intracellular antigens. Additionally, this method affords a high tumor-antigen versus self-antigen ratio. Safety concerns regarding the clinical use of tumor cells include their inherent tumorigenicity; therefore they are irradiated to render them non-tumorigenic. Whole-cell allogeneic vaccines are created utilizing cells from multiple patients and multiple tumor cell lines, with the advantage of enhanced immunogenicity via exposure of the patient to a wider variety of TAA, as well as greater probability for developing standardization, thus making multiple patient therapy a reasonable goal. Whole-cell autologous vaccine preparation requires a fresh sample of the patient's own tumor, either primary or derived from an established tissue culture. Primary tumor is preferred, since cell lines modify the phenotype of the tumor during culture, and such cell lines remain technically difficult to grow.[7] In either case, the inherent heterogeneity of tumors presents the additional problem of possible under-dosing of TAA within the utilized tumor cells.

ASI using whole-cell autologous tumor vaccine was first successfully demonstrated preclinically in a guinea pig hepatocellular tumor model, in which dissociated tumor cells were admixed with BCG and utilized as an intradermal vaccine to stimulate systemic tumor immunity. This led to a prospectively randomized controlled clinical trial of ASI for colorectal carcinoma, in which 74 postsurgical patients received two weekly intradermal injections of autologous irradiated tumor cells admixed with BCG, followed by a third injection of tumor cells alone. Results indicated a significant delay in both death and recurrence (56-month median follow-up time) for colon and rectal cancer patients combined.[8,9] In 1993, Hoover et al demonstrated no statistically significant difference regarding survival or disease-free survival in a 6.5-year median follow-up of patients with Dukes stage B2–C3 colon or rectal cancer treated with resection and autologous tumor-cell–BCG ASI versus resection alone. However, a subsequent cohort analysis did demonstrate statistically significant improvement in both endpoints mentioned above within the colon cancer ASI group.[10] It is unclear why this difference between colon and rectal cancers was seen. This study was soon followed by an Eastern Cooperative Oncology Group (ECOG) trial that examined survival and relapse rates with autologous tumor-cell–BCG ASI versus surgery alone in the setting of Dukes B and C colon cancer. Differences in results between these groups were not statistically significant, yet a subset analysis indicated that further investigation with a heightened vaccination schedule was warranted.[11] Ockert et al compared autologous colon cancer cells infected with Newcastle disease virus versus admixture with BCG, and found statistically significant improved survival at 2 years for the viral ASI group.[7] Most recently, Vemorken et al explored the use of an additional booster immunization to the previous model of adjuvant BCG ASI, in the setting of surgically resected stage II and III colon cancer, with findings at the 5.3-year median follow-up consistent with statistically significant reduction in the rate of tumor recurrences. Further analysis by stage failed to demonstrate any significant benefit of ASI in patients with stage III disease; however, stage II patients had

Table 64.1 Clinical trials with adjuvant whole-cell ASI–BCG for colorectal cancer

Author/Trial	Treatment groups	Number of patients	Response/Results
Hoover et al:[9] prospectively randomized trial of adjuvant ASI immunotherapy for human colorectal cancer	Immunized versus non-immunized	74	Significant benefit in disease-free status and survival
Hoover et al:[10] adjuvant ASI for human colorectal cancer: 6.5-year median follow-up of a phase III prospectively randomized trial	Resection alone versus resection plus ASI	98	Significant benefit in disease-free status and survival in colon cancer subgroup, but none in colon and rectal combined
Harris et al:[11] survival and relapse in adjuvant autologous tumour vaccine therapy for Dukes B and C colon cancer	Post-operative ASI versus no further therapy	412	No significant benefit in disease-free status or survival; however, subset analysis of immunized patients who mounted a substantial immune response showed improved (though not significant) survival
Vemorken et al:[12] ASI for stage II and III human colon cancer, a randomized trial	Post-operative ASI versus no further therapy	254	44% risk reduction for recurrence in the recurrence-free period for all ASI patients. Analysis by stage: • stage III disease: no benefit • stage II disease: significant benefit in recurrence-free period, risk reduction for recurrence, and recurrence-free survival, with trend toward improved overall survival

significantly improved recurrence-free interval, recurrence risk reduction, and recurrence-free survival, as well as a trend toward prolonged overall survival.[12] The results of these clinical trials are summarized in Table 64.1.

TARGETED ASI

Colon cancer in particular is a good model in which to examine targeted ASI, since it has well characterized and most likely a finite number of TAA, such as carcinoembryonic antigen (CEA), 17-1A, and 791Tgp72.[13] However, salient questions remain: are these available agents truly the optimal for utilization, and which is the most optimal? The remainder of this chapter will focus on further exploration of the following approaches to targeted ASI within the setting of colorectal cancer: recombinant viral vector encoding TAA (vaccinia–CEA, ALVAC–CEA); naked DNA encoding TAA; anti-idiotype antibodies that mimic TAA (CEAVac, 17-1A, gp72); monoclonal antibodies (17-1A/Panorex, L6); glycoprotein mucins (Muc-1); peptides encoded by oncogenes (K-*ras*, *p53*); and dendritic cells.

Recombinant viral vaccines

As a means to increase antigen processing and expression in APC and improve the expression of co-stimulatory molecules, recombinant viral-based vaccines have been developed. The pox virus family has been most commonly used (vaccinia, fowlpox), but others such as adenovirus have also been used. Genes encoding TAA are genetically recombined to the virus and then administered. The virus serves as a vector, infecting cells, including APC, and the passenger gene is then transcribed and translated into a full-length protein, then cleaved into smaller peptides (9–10 amino acids in length for MHC class I, 13–15 for MHC class II presentation), and then presented on the cell surface in the context of appropriate co-stimulatory molecules to activate both CD4[+] and CD8[+] T cells.[4]

Phase I clinical trials have been completed for both vaccinia–CEA[14,15] and ALVAC–CEA.[16] These trials both demonstrated significant generation of CEA-specific CTL that were capable of lysing autologous (and allogeneic) tumor. The vaccines were well tolerated, without significant toxicity. Vaccinia is a potent stimulus upon initial vaccination, but subsequent injections add little. Fowlpox, on the other hand, is less potent, but appears to boost the T-cell response with each injection. Therefore, trials combining these two agents are underway.

In comparison with the T-cell responses seen with naked DNA, recombinant therapies appear superior. This is likely due to the increased role of the APC, to the environment created during the 'infection' with the virus, and possibly to avoiding triggering the self-recognition that is often observed with naked DNA therapies.[3] Two strategies are being pursued to further increase the activity of these constructs. First, cytokines (granulocyte–macrophage colony-stimulating factor (GM-CSF), IL-2) are being added to the vaccines in the hopes of increasing co-stimulatory molecule expression (B7) by APC and of increasing the T-cell numbers. Trials have been performed with ALVAC–CEA and GM-CSF, and trials are underway with IL-2 as well. Second, as these viral vectors are easily recombined with multiple genes, the genes for co-stimulatory molecules have been added to the constructs (e.g. fowlpox–CEA–B7).[17] Evidence to date suggests these to be more potent stimulators of T cells, which is likely related to increased expression of the co-stimulatory molecules.

Potential problems with this approach include lower specificity of binding of the virus to the target APC, potential downregulation of class I molecules impairing antigen presentation, induction of antiviral responses that limit subsequent immunizations, and the potential dangers of administering viruses (even though attenuated) to humans.[4]

Other similar approaches include the insertion of an immunostimulatory cytokine (tumor necrosis factor α (TNF-α), IL-2, GM-CSF, interferon-γ (IFN-γ)) instead of the TAA, creating cells that secrete cytokines, and similarly creating cells that overexpress a native or mutated form of the TAA to improve antigen processing.

Naked DNA

The potential of using naked DNA as a vaccine was first established by a trial which demonstrated that naked DNA encoding influenza nucleoprotein could protect animals from influenza challenge.[18] More recently, naked DNA encoding TAA was found to be effective in tumor models.[19] It has been hypothesized that the mechanism for this is that following intramuscular injection, monocytes take up the DNA and express the gene product. The newly formed protein is released and taken up by APC, which then process the protein for presentation and T-cell activation. In intradermal injections, it is hypothesized that Langerhans cells serve as the APC.

Advantages of this approach include easy purification and the fact that DNA may be combined with genes for co-stimulatory molecules. Phase I trials are underway. However, the potency of naked DNA vaccines is likely to be less than that of recombinant viral vaccines. Naked DNA does not have the advantage of the viral promoters, which generate multiple copies of TAA, and nor is it associated with as great an acute inflammatory reaction as that produced with the viral vectors.[20] Despite these theoretical drawbacks, naked DNA remains an exciting vaccine mechanism.

Anti-idiotype antibodies

When a monoclonal antibody is administered, it can serve as an antigen itself, with subsequent generation of an antibody directed against the idiotype. This process, called the idiotype network, was originally hypothesized by Linderman and Jerne[21] (Figure 64.2), and is now the subject of significant basic and clinical research. Several anti-idiotype antibodies are being tested in clinical trials against colon cancer. The lead compounds target CEA, 17-1A, and gp 72.

The generation of anti-idiotype antibodies begins with the immunization of an animal with the TAA of choice (e.g. CEA) and the subsequent production of an antibody against the TAA (named Ab1). Ab1 is then used to generate a series of anti-idiotype antibodies called Ab2. Selected Ab2 antibodies effectively mimic the three-dimensional structure of the

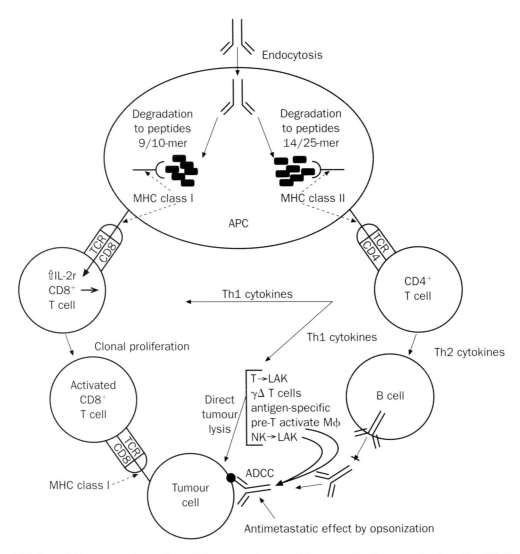

Figure 64.2 Potential immune pathways for anti-idiotype vaccines: anti-idiotype antibodies are endocytosed by APC. They may be degraded to 14/25-mer peptides and presented on MHC class II molecules to CD4+ helper T cells. Activated Th2 CD4+ helper T cells secrete Th2 cytokines, which stimulate B cells that have been directly activated by the anti-idiotype antibody to produce the anti-anti-idiotypic antibody or Ab3 (Abl'), which binds directly to tumor cells. This antibody can mediate complement and ADCC as well as a direct antimetastatic effect by opsonization. In addition, Th1 CD4+ helper T cells secrete Th1 cytokines, which activate T cells, natural killer (NK) cells, and macrophages (Mϕ). The activated macrophages and lymphokine-activated killer (LAK) cells may also serve as effector cells for antibody-dependent cell-mediated cytotoxicity (ADCC). All of these cells may mediate direct tumor lysis. There are also data to suggest that exogenously processed proteins can be degraded to 9/10-mer peptides that can be presented by MHC class I molecules to activate CD8+ cytotoxic T cells. This is enhanced by Th1 cytokines such as IL-2. Activated CD8+ cytotoxic T cells make contact with tumor cells, leading to direct tumor cell lysis. Reproduced from Foon KA et al, *Clin Cancer Res* 1999; **5:** 225–36,[5] with permission.

original TAA, which can then be used as a surrogate for the TAA as an immunogen, with the final result of generating anti-anti-idiotype antibodies.[20] While this may seem like a long way to go to get back to the original antigen, there are significant advantages to this strategy. The primary advantage is that the anti-idiotype represents an exogenous protein that expresses the target antigen, whereas the original antigen itself (e.g. CEA) is a native (self) protein. The native antigen has thus been converted to a foreign protein, which will be endocytosed by APC, processed, and presented to T cells to activate the immunologic activities of CD4[+] and CD8[+] cells. Through this, the production of endogenous cytokines increases, further stimulating the response.[22] This would not be expected from simply vaccinating with the TAA itself.

Foon et al have studied an anti-idiotype antibody directed against CEA called CEAVac. Using this compound in patients with various stages of colon cancer, they have demonstrated that the patients generate high polyclonal anti-CEA responses and idiotypic-specific T-cell responses, 75% of which were CEA-specific. Several patients received 5-fluorouracil (5-FU)-based chemotherapy during the vaccinations, and responses were not adversely affected. Finally, Foon et al have demonstrated the ability to boost the antibody response with monthly injections of CEAVac. While nothing definitive can be said about these patients' clinical response, given the variability in stage and low numbers, seven of eight patients with resected stage IV disease all remain on study without evidence of recurrence (12–33 months).[23]

The anti-idiotypic monoclonal antibody 105AD7 mimics the TAA 791gp72 (CD55), which is expressed on 70–80% of colorectal cancers.[24] CD55 plays a role in signaling between the innate and adaptive immune responses. Absence of the molecule makes the tumor cell susceptible to complement, whereas overexpression results in the antigen being a target for T-cell immunotherapy. A phase I trial in advanced colorectal cancer patients showed the anti-idiotype vaccine to be non-toxic, with a suggestion of improved survival among vaccinated patients compared with historical paired controls.[25] This effect is thought to be mediated by antitumor T-cell responses. To test this theory, 19 patients with colorectal cancer were immunized prior to the resection of the primary tumor. Tumor samples were found to have a significantly higher activated-lymphocyte infiltration compared with non-vaccinated patients. Further analysis of the infiltrating cells showed them to contain a high level of both natural killer (NK) and

CD4[+] cells, and evidence of CD8 activation.[26] This evidence supports further study with this vaccine in colorectal cancer patients, and also demonstrates the value of translational studies in early clinical trials.

Monoclonal antibodies

The ability of the immune system to generate millions of highly specific antibodies that target foreign antigens remains one of the truly awe-inspiring features in the design of living creatures. Hybridoma technology has allowed us to selectively harness this process for broad applicability. Monoclonal antibodies (MoAbs) have been tested extensively for many indications, and a few are now approved for the treatment of cancer and for cancer imaging. MoAbs target and destroy cancer cells through a variety of mechanisms, including complement-dependent cytolysis, antibody-dependent cell-mediated cytotoxicity (ADCC), and apoptosis.[2] Several MoAbs have been conjugated to a variety of agents with the goal of selective delivery of the agent by the antibody.[27]

17-1A
The most extensively studied compound is 17-1A, a murine IgG2a MoAb that targets a 26 kDa polypeptide tumor-associated cell-surface glycoprotein, GA733-2. As a single agent in advanced colon cancer, a 5% response rate was observed, with very little toxicity. It has also been tested in combination with GM-CSF.[28] This agent was tested as adjuvant therapy in patients with stage III colon cancer in a small (189 patients) randomized trial comparing 5 months of 17-1A injections versus observation alone in what may be one day recognized as a landmark study for vaccine therapy.[29]

The primary endpoints of the trial were overall and disease-free survival (Figure 64.3). The results were initially presented after 5 years and re-presented after 7 years, and continue to show a 32% reduced mortality and 23% reduced recurrence rate in the treatment arm. The reduction in metastasis (distant sites) was significant, while local recurrences were not altered between the two arms, but this latter difference could be explained by 11 patients in the control arm receiving radiation with none of the treatment arm receiving it. It also could be explained by some unknown difference in the biology of local and metastatic recurrences. Eighty percent of patients developed human anti-mouse antibodies (HAMA) after the second or third infusion. Regardless, this data was compelling enough for the agent to gain approval in Germany and launch two

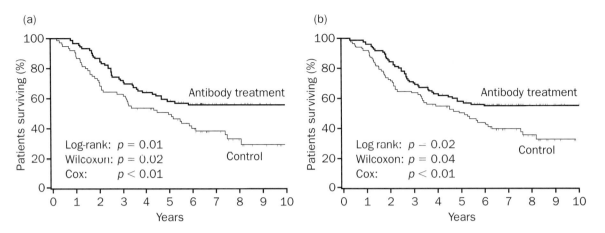

Figure 64.3 Overall survival of (a) 166 eligible patients after 7 years of follow-up, and (b) according to intention-to-treat analysis (185 patients). *p* is adjusted for imbalances in prognostic values with Cox's proportional hazards model; the other *p* values were calculated with the univariate log-rank test and Wilcoxon test.

large randomized trials, 5-FU/leucovorin with or without 17-1A in stage III and 17-1A versus observation in stage II colon cancer. If these trials are positive, this agent is certain to gain US FDA approval, and would represent the first vaccine-type therapy with proven efficacy in solid tumors – and a true breakthrough in cancer medicine.

L6

The murine MoAb L6 is an IgG2a antibody that binds to a poorly characterized antigen on adenocarcinomas and is expressed on the surface of more than 90% of breast, colorectal, ovarian, and non-small cell lung cancers. A phase I study of L6 demonstrated one complete response in a patient with a breast cancer.[30] A second phase I trial was performed in combination with IL-2, again with low toxicity, and with two responses, one in a colon cancer patient.[31] Measures of L6-mediated ADCC activity were increased with the addition of IL-2, which is thought to recruit and expand an effector-cell population essential for ADCC. It was interesting that no dose response was observed for IL-2, suggesting that low doses that result in much less toxicity may be sufficient.

The optimum MoAb should be humanized to avoid HAMA formation. Other approaches to minimize HAMA include the creation of chimeric antibodies and single-change Fv antibodies. These latter constructs consist of light- and heavy-chain variable regions bound by a peptide bridge, and may have the advantage of better tumor penetration because of reduced size.

Mucins

Glycoprotein mucins play an important role in the normal cells of the colon. The observation that mucins from tumor cells are distinct, with a short sugar side chain, suggested a potential immunologic target. Mucin-1 (Muc-1) was found to be ubiquitously expressed in breast cancer and to be highly immunogenic in mice. CTL that were capable of lysing tumors in an unrestricted MHC/Muc-1 system have been isolated from patients' lymph nodes.[32] A phase I study was performed in patients with advanced colon, rectum, breast, and stomach cancers using an Muc-1 fusion protein.[33] The results showed that large amounts of IgG1 anti-Muc-1 antibodies were produced in 13 of 25 patients, T-cell proliferation was found in 4 of 15 patients, and CTL responses were observed in 2 of 10 patients. Thus, this Muc-1-based construct was found to be highly immunogenic in cancer patients, with a dose response observed for antibody production (increased doses lead to higher antibody titers). Previous studies using Muc-1 had demonstrated a relationship between antibody levels and survival in patients, suggesting a need to study these compounds further in larger trials.[34] A phase II study using a Muc-1 peptide admixed with BCG was explored in 30 patients with advanced colon cancer. The observed systemic symptoms and injection-site reactions suggested an activation of the immune system, and 7 of 22 patients tested demonstrated a two- to fourfold increase in CTL.[35]

Peptide vaccines

Tumors express peptides, often encoded by oncogenes, that are unique to the malignant cells. Typically, these proteins are mutated forms of the native protein. While variation in the specific mutations seen would make immunologic targeting difficult across a patient population, several oncogenes share significant homology among patients. For example, K-*ras* is commonly in codon 12 and could serve as a potential target for vaccine development.

Several investigators are testing this hypothesis in patients. The methods include obtaining an individual patient's tumor and determining the presence or absence of a particular oncogene mutation. If one is present, patients are then treated with a vaccine that targets the mutated section of the oncoprotein. The obvious advantage of this approach is that since normal cells do not express the mutated gene, very little systemic toxicity would be expected. However, as with all molecularly targeted therapies, tumor heterogeneity could result in escape for those clones without the specific mutation. Ras and p53 vaccines are currently under clinical investigation.[36] Using a 13-mer mutated Ras peptide reflecting the codon-12 mutations, 3 of 10 evaluable patients generated a mutant Ras CD4[+] and/or CD8[+] T-cell response. No toxicity was observed. The current trial involves a similar strategy, but adds IL-2 and GM-CSF (SN Khleif, personal communication). This approach may provide a unique opportunity for generating a tumor-directed immune therapy.

NEW METHODOLOGY AND TARGETS

Dendritic cells

Dendritic cells (DC) are highly specialized APC that serve as the primary activators of T cells by efficient protein uptake and antigen presentation. The properties of these cells are now well understood, and, given their key role in the immune response, they have become among the most interesting targets for future therapies. One area of interest involves the addition of a cytokine, such as GM-CSF, which will stimulate the number and activity of DC. Alternatively, DC may be harvested by leukaphoresis, expanded ex vivo, activated by specific antigens, and reinfused into patients, ensuring recognition and presentation of the desired antigen.[37] Finally, oncogenes may be transduced into DC to target specific antigens.[38] Much of this work was originally performed in melanoma, but now more is being done in colon and other cancers.

MAGE

MAGE is a tumor-rejection antigen initially identified on melanoma cells, and has proven to be an immunologic target with high potential. Recently, in an attempt to find expression of this antigen on other tumors, MAGE was found on one-third of colon cancers in patients but on none of the normal tissues.[39] In a larger similar study, again MAGE expression was exclusive to the tumor tissue, with at least one of the 10 MAGE antigens tested being present on 70 of the 80 samples. The larger numbers in this study allowed attempts at clinical correlations, with the finding of higher metastatic rates when MAGE 3 was present.[40] Clinical studies are ongoing using MAGE as a vaccine target in colorectal cancers.

SUMMARY

Rigorous testing of new immunologic approaches, built upon the solid foundations of prior knowledge, has brought the field of immune response modification from a primarily non-specific era to a more target-specific realm. Evidence from current prospectively randomized trials clearly indicates the beneficial use of colon cancer vaccine therapy in the adjuvant setting for patients with micrometastatic disease where the goal is prevention of recurrence. Such immunotherapeutic approaches have also shown only minimal adverse reactions. The exciting promise of continued advances in molecular biology encourages our further exploration of vaccine therapy as the latest and one of the most promising weapons in the armamentarium against colorectal cancer. Future utilization of colorectal cancer vaccines will likely include their integration within multimodality regimens for late-stage disease. In fact, prospectively randomized clinical trials for solid tumors utilizing a combination of both active specific and systemically enhancing immune therapies along with standard adjuvant chemotherapy are currently underway.

REFERENCES

1. Rieger P, Immunomodulators, differentiation agents, and vaccines. In: *Clinical Handbook for Biotherapy*. Sudbury: Jones and Bartlett, 1999: 239–62.
2. Maxwell-Armstrong CA, Durrant LG, Scholefield JH,

Immunotherapy for colorectal cancer. *Am J Surg* 1999; **177:** 344–8.

3. Pardoll DM, Cancer vaccines. *Nature Med* 1998; **5:** 525–31.

4. Maxwell-Armstrong CA, Durrant LG, Scholefield JH, Colorectal cancer vaccines. *Br J Surg* 1998; **85:** 149–54.

5. Foon KA, Yannelli J, Bhattacharya-Chatterjee M, Colorectal cancer as a model for immunotherapy. *Clin Cancer Res* 1999; **5:** 225–36.

6. Ockert D, Schirrmacher V, Beck N et al, Newcastle disease virus infected intact autologous tumor cell vaccine for adjuvant active specific immunotherapy of resected colorectal carcinoma. *Clin Cancer Res* 1996; **2:** 21–8.

7. Weber CE, Cytokine modified tumor vaccines: an antitumor strategy revisited in the age of molecular medicine. *Cancer Nurs* 1998; **21:** 167–77.

8. Haspel MV, McCabe RP, Pomato N et al, Coming full circle in immunotherapy of colorectal cancer: vaccination with autologous tumor cells – to human monoclonal antibodies – to development and application of a generic tumor vaccine. In: *Human Tumor Antigens and Specific Tumor Therapy* (Metzgar RS, Mitchell MS, eds). New York: Liss, 1989: 335–44.

9. Hoover HC, Surdyke M, Dangel RB et al, Prospectively randomized trial of adjuvant active-specific immunotherapy for human colorectal cancer. *Cancer* 1985; **55:** 1236.

10. Hoover HC, Brandhurst JS, Peters LC et al, Adjuvant active specific immunotherapy for human colorectal cancer: 6.5 year median follow-up of a phase III prospectively randomized trial. *J Clin Oncol* 1993; **11:** 390–9.

11. Harris J, Ryan L, Adams G et al, Survival and relapse in adjuvant autologous tumour vaccine therapy for Dukes B and C colon cancer-EST 5283. *Proc Am Soc Clin Oncol* 1994; **13:** 294.

12. Vemorken JB, Claessen AM, vanTinteren H et al, Active specific immunotherapy for stage I and stage II human colon cancer: a randomized trial. *Lancet* 1999; **353:** 345–50.

13. Maxwell-Armstrong CA, Durrant LG, Scholefield JH, Colorectal cancer vaccines. *Br J Surg* 1998; **85:** 149–54.

14. Tsang KY, Zaremba S, Nieroda CA et al, Generation of human cytotoxic T cells specific for human carcinoembryonic antigen epitopes from cancer patients immunized with recombinant vaccinia–CEA vaccine. *J Natl Cancer Inst* 1995; **87:** 982–90.

15. McAneny D, Ryan CA, Beazley RN, Kaufman HL, Results of phase I trials of recombinant vaccinia virus that expresses carcinoembryonic antigen in patients with advanced cancer. *Ann Surg Oncol* 1996; **3:** 495–500.

16. Marshall JL, Hawkins MJ, Tsang KY et al, Phase I study in cancer patients of a replication-defective avipox recombinant vaccine that expresses human carcinoembryonic antigen. *J Clin Oncol* 1999; **17:** 332–7.

17. von Mehren M, Davey V, Rivera G et al, Phase I trial of ALVAC–CEAB7.1 immunization in advanced CEA-expressing adenocarcinomas. *Prog Am Soc Clin Oncol* 1999; **18:** 1686.

18. Nomura T, Yasuda K, Yamada T et al, Gene expression and antitumor effects following direct interferon (IFN)-gamma gene transfer with naked plasmid DNA and DC-chol liposome complexes in mice. *Gene Ther* 1999; **6:** 121–9.

19. Irvine KR, Chamberlain RS, Shulman EP et al, Enhancing efficacy of recombinant anticancer vaccines with prime/boost regimens that use two different vectors. *J Natl Cancer Inst* 1997; **89:** 1595–601.

20. Pardoll DM, Beckerley AM, Exposing the immunology of naked DNA vaccines. *Immunity* 1995; **3:** 165–9.

21. Jerne NK, Towards a network theory of the immune system. *Ann Immunol* 1974; **125C:** 373–89.

22. Chatterjee SK, Tripathi PK, Chakraborty M et al, Molecular mimicry of carcinoembryonic antigen by peptides derived from the structure of an anti-idiotype antibody. *Cancer Res* 1998; **58:** 1217–24.

23. Foon KA, Chakraborty M, John WJ et al, Immune response to carcinoembryonic antigen in patients treated with anti-idiotype antibody vaccine. *J Clin Invest* 1995; **96:** 334–42.

24. Spendlove I, Li L, Charmichael J, Durrant LG, Decay accelerating factor (CD55): a target for cancer vaccines? *Cancer Res* 1999; **59:** 2282–6.

25. Buckley DT, Robins AR, Durrant LG, Clinical evidence that human monoclonal anti-idiotypic antibody 105AD7, delays tumor growth by stimulating anti-tumor T-cell responses. *Hum Antibodies Hybridomas* 1995; **6:** 68–72.

26. Maxwell-Armstrong CA, Durrant LG, Robins RA et al, Increased activation of lymphocytes infiltrating primary colorectal cancers following immunisation with the anti-idiotypic monoclonal antibody 105AD7. *Gut* 1999; **45:** 593–8.

27. Goldenberg DM, Monoclonal antibodies in cancer detection and therapy. *Am J Med* 1993; **94:** 297–312.

28. Ragnhammer P, Fagerberg J, Frodin JE et al, Effect of monoclonal antibody 17-1A and GM-CSF in patients with advanced colorectal carcinoma – long lasting complete remissions can be induced. *Int J Cancer* 1993; **53:** 751–8.

29. Riethmuller G, Holz E, Schlimok G et al, Monoclonal antibody therapy for resected Dukes' C colorectal cancer: seven-year outcome of a multicenter randomized trial. *J Clin Oncol* 1998; **16:** 1788–94.

30. Goodman GE, Hellstrom I, Brodzinsky L et al, Phase I trial of murine monoclonal antibody L6 in breast, colon, ovarian and lung cancer. *J Clin Oncol* 1990; **8:** 1083–92.

31. Ziegler LD, Palazzlo P, Cunningham J et al, Phase I trial of murine monoclonal antibody L6 in combination with subcutaneous interleukin-2 in patients with advanced carcinoma of the breast, colorectum and lung. *J Clin Oncol* 1992; **10:** 1470–8.

32. Barnd DL, Lans MS, Metzgar RS, Finn OJ, Specific MHC-unrestricted recognition of tumour-associated mucin by human CTL. *Proc Natl Acad Sci USA* 1989; **86:** 7159–63.

33. Karanikas V, Hwang L, Pearson J et al, Antibody and T cell responses of patients with adenocarcinoma immunized with mannan–MUC1 fusion protein. *J Clin Invest* 1997; **100:** 2783–92.

34. MacLean GD, Reddish MA, Kogantry RR, Longnecker BM, Antibodies against mucin-associated sialyl-Tn epitopes correlate with survival of metastatic adenocarcinoma patients undergoing active specific immunotherapy with synthetic STn vaccine. *J Immunother* 1996; **19:** 59–68.

35. Goydos JS, Elder E, Whiteside TL et al, A phase I trial of a synthetic mucin peptide vaccine. Induction of specific immune reactivity in patients with adenocarcinoma. *J Surg Res* 1996; **63:** 298–304.

36. Khleif SN, Abrams SI, Hamilton JM et al, A phase I vaccine trial with peptides reflecting ras oncogene mutations of solid tumors. *J Immunother* 1999; **22:** 155–65.

37. Chikamatsu K, Nakano K, Storkus WJ et al, Generation of anti-p53 cytotoxic T lymphocytes from human peripheral blood using autologous dendritic cells. *Clin Cancer Res* 1999; **5:** 1281–8.

38. Ishida T, Chada S, Stipanov M et al, Dendritic cells transduced with wild-type p53 gene elicit potent anti-tumerus immune responses. *Clin Exp Immunol* 1999; **117:** 244–51.

39. Mori M, Inove H, Mimori K et al, Expression of MAGE genes in human colorectal carcinoma. *Ann Surg* 1996; **224:** 183–8.

40. Hasegawa H, Mori M, Heraguchi M et al, Expression spectrum of melanoma antigen-encoding gene family members in colorectal carcinoma. *Arch Pathol Lab Med* 1998; **122:** 551–4.

Part 9

Critical Issues in Colorectal Cancer

65

Quality of life and methodology in colorectal cancer studies

Bengt Glimelius

INTRODUCTION

Until the mid-1980s, the influence on tumour size and the patient's quantity of life (QoL) were the paramount measures for determining the value of various therapeutic interventions in cancer. Today, there exists a greater understanding within the health services that an assessment of therapeutic effects may not always be complete unless it also includes the patient's own experience. The qualitative aspects of survival have become particularly important in advanced colorectal cancer, where the effects of any therapy are limited and survival prospects generally poor. The qualitative aspects of life may also be of relevance in the early stages of the disease, since treatments that are more intensive are becoming increasingly available even if the additional curative potential of each of these interventions is limited.

The assessment of the patient's own experience or aspects on QoL has been successively incorporated in clinical trials as an important parameter. The goal of this assessment is to have it serve as an endpoint, complementing the more traditional assessment measures, tumour response, survival, and the physician's opinion concerning patient status. In a bibliographic study covering the period from 1980 to 1997, the proportion of randomized cancer trials incorporating a QoL measure increased from 1.5% to 8.2%.[1]

When the benefits of a new treatment are potentially great (i.e. with possible cure as a result), the side-effects that treatment may involve and the costs of treatment are conceptually easy to accept for both the patient and the health services. When the potential benefits are less pronounced, however, the acceptance level of side-effects declines dramatically. It is assumed that with curative treatments the QoL aspects are of secondary importance. Adjuvant therapy exposes a large group of already-cured patients to unnecessary side-effects that, particularly if persistent, may be of relevance. In the palliative situation, QoL assessments may be very important, and small gains must be weighed against side-effects and other costs to patients to justify the use of the treatment.[2] The European Organization for Research and Treatment of Cancer (EORTC) has given recommendations as to when it may be appropriate to include a QoL assessment in clinical phase III trials (Table 65.1).[3]

Table 65.1 EORTC criteria for inclusion of QoL in clinical trials[3]

QoL aspects can be relevant endpoints in phase III cancer clinical trials if:

- no improvement in overall, recurrence-free, or systemic disease-free survival is expected, but significant changes or differences in (at least) one aspect of QoL are expected
- one treatment results in a better survival but has more toxic effects
- patients have an extremely poor prognosis with or without treatment
- treatment is known to be very burdensome to patients
- a new (invasive) treatment is to be evaluated

The well-being of the patient after curative surgery in colorectal cancer has rarely been systematically studied, but the patient's condition is generally assumed to be satisfactory.[4] Nonetheless, problems after rectal cancer surgery may persist. According to a recent review,[5] only three reports have formally measured QoL after surgery for rectal cancer. These problems[6] and those associated with pre- or postoperative radio(chemo)therapy are discussed in separate chapters. One recent study has explored the QoL after adjuvant 5-fluorouracil (5-FU) levamisole treatment in colon cancer, and found it equivalent to a surgical control group.[7] In advanced colorectal cancer, palliative chemotherapy seemingly increases the patient's well-being and QoL, despite the side-effects of the treatment.[8–13] These studies will be described in greater detail later in the chapter.

DEFINITION OF QoL

Currently, there is no consensus concerning a definition of QoL, and the lack of such a definition is probably related to the complexity of the concept. An overview article on QoL discusses over 10 definitions of QoL in adults.[14] However, the World Health Organization (WHO) definition of health is widely used, and strongly supports the multidimensional aspects of health – health is a state of complete physical, mental, and social well-being, and hence is not merely the absence of disease and infirmity. In health care, most conclude that QoL is a multidimensional concept that includes at least physical, functional, psychological, and social aspects of disease and treatment.[2,14,15] Usually, a global assessment or general dimension of life satisfaction is also included.

METHODS TO DESCRIBE QoL

Attempts to objectively describe the general condition of cancer patients (Karnofsky index) were made as early as 1949.[16] The goal then was to evaluate more accurately new cancer therapies and to define staff workload. The Karnofsky index is not a satisfactory measure of the QoL of cancer patients in trials, since the index, similarly to the ECOG (Eastern Cooperative Oncology Group) scale,[17] only considers the patient's functional status.[18] Furthermore, both scales are completed by the physician, and some studies have shown poor correlation between doctors' and patients' status assessments. There is also wide variation between the assessments of different groups (e.g. doctors, nurses, and relatives).[19] Both

scales yield, however, relevant clinical information on the general condition of the patient, and can be used to exclude groups of patients with low probabilities to respond to and tolerate various treatments. They are also powerful predictors of survival in advanced colorectal cancer, and can be used for stratification in trials. QoL indices, based upon patients' answers to questionnaires (see below), also offer solid prognostic information,[20] but have been much less studied and cannot yet replace performance status for stratification.

It has only been during the past two decades that researchers have addressed patients' experience of their health status/well-being via self-report measures. There are multitudes of different QoL instruments, ranging from short estimates to comprehensive measurements. Although there is no unanimity among researchers concerning a 'gold standard' QoL instrument, such a standard would increase the opportunities for comparisons between studies. An instrument with benchmark quality would require situation-specific modules, which include additional questions concerning the disease or treatment. Several groups of investigators have recommended this approach in cancer trials.[15,21,22]

Patient reporting of QoL issues via various questionnaires is currently the dominant method for QoL assessment in cancer trials. Questionnaires are preferred that are sensitive to changes over time, meet the basic criteria for reliability and validity, are short, easy to understand and complete, and have undergone meticulous translation and back-translation. The latter characteristics are especially important in multicentre studies.

QoL INSTRUMENTS

QoL instruments are both general and cancer-specific. Selected questionnaires constructed specifically for cancer patients and used, or of potential interest to be used, in colorectal cancer trials are described briefly below. The questions in the various questionnaires are answered based on different scale models. The Likert scale, an ordinal scale, is the most common one in oncology trials, and has not been superseded by the VAS (visual analogue scale), despite the great popularity of the latter in different situations.

The *Cancer Rehabilitation Evaluation System (CARES)* focuses on clinical problems, is carefully constructed, and has been repeatedly validated.[23] The longer version (CIPS) comprises 139 questions and the shorter one consists of 59 questions (CARES-SF). Both questionnaires utilize the Likert scale, and include physical, functional, family, emotional, sexual, and social aspects, and satisfaction with treatment and economics. The shorter version, which also contains a global evaluation, has been developed to be used in clinical studies, and has been tested in patients with colorectal cancer.

The *EORTC Quality of Life Questionnaire (EORTC QLQ-C30)* is a general cancer instrument that can be complemented with disease-specific questions for patients with different types of cancer.[21,24] The questionnaire has been translated into several languages. The instrument uses the Likert scale, and includes physical, functional, cognitive, emotional, social, and global domains, as well as various signs and symptoms. Recently, a module for use in colorectal cancer has been developed.[25] The module focuses on aspects of the disease that are more relevant for the primary situation in comparison with the recurrent situation. It is therefore of limited relevance in palliative chemotherapy trials.

The *Functional Assessment of Cancer Therapy (FACT)*[22] has been used in numerous American trials. It has been translated into several languages. FACT comprises a core questionnaire containing 27 questions, to which are added site- or treatment-specific subscales covering all the common solid tumours, including colorectal cancer and treatments. The questionnaire employs Likert-type scoring to measure physical, functional, emotional, and social well-being, and side-effects.

The *Functional Living Index – Cancer (FLIC)* is a well-validated questionnaire.[26] Factor analysis identified two physical and psychological factors that are robust. Although the instrument covers many dimensions, it nevertheless provides a total score. It has been translated into several languages, and includes physical, functional, family, emotional, and social aspects, as well as questions related to treatment satisfaction and economic situation. The patients evaluate 29 questions based on the Likert and analogue scales.

The *Rotterdam Symptom Checklist* is made up of 38 questions, with a Likert-type scoring scale.[27] The instrument comprises two main subscales: a physical and a psychological dimension, together with site-specific questions. The questionnaire has been validated, and is used in many trials of cancer therapy, including colorectal cancer.

OTHER INSTRUMENTS

The *Clinical Benefit Response (CBR)* was developed to be used for the assessment of a cytostatic drug for pancre-

atic cancer.[28] It is not a QoL instrument in the tradiional sense, but is intended to measure physical attributes with a potential influence on QoL. These attributes include pain (assessed by the patient on a VAS scale and by the consumption of pain-relieving drugs), performance status (Karnofsky index), and weight trends. If the patient improves in at least one of these categories without deteriorating in another for at least four weeks, the outcome is scored as a clinical benefit response from the treatment. The instrument has not been validated, and the results have not prospectively been compared with traditional QoL measurements. In a retrospective analysis of data from two randomized trials in metastatic gastrointestinal cancers, CBR criteria and traditional QoL measurements using EORTC QLQ-C30 could discriminate to about the same extent between the two groups. The two evaluation methods, however, did not identify exactly the same patients as having had a benefit from the treatment.[29]

Euroquol is an economic assessment system that permits the computation of *Quality-Adjusted Life Years (QALYs)*, an instrument that may be used to evaluate the financial costs of various procedures and life-maintaining treatments.[30] Although this system is potentially useful when economic parameters are needed, it is less helpful for measuring QoL comprehensively.

Quality-Adjusted Time Without Symptoms or Toxicity (Q-TWiST) is a method to assess the quality of survival, and subtracts from the total survival time the treatment-related time spent in discomfort and the time with side-effects.[31]

PROBLEMS IN THE ASSESSMENT OF QoL

Several QoL questionnaires have come into use over the past 10 years. Consequently, at present, there is little need for the development of additional questionnaires, although new treatment modalities may require new modules. However, a number of methodological issues remain to be resolved.[32] The following are some of the problems that hamper the interpretation of comparative QoL data:

- insufficient sample size;
- the variety of questionnaires used;
- the choice of time points for QoL assessment in relation to various treatment-related events;
- incomplete data, and especially data attrition over time;
- the open design of most trials, which might induce assessment bias;

- the multiplicity of the data obtained from most QoL questionnaires, together with a general lack of predefined endpoints;
- the conceptual difficulties in interpretation of QoL data, not least in the light of prevailing strong psychological defence mechanisms that tend to conserve a general sense of well-being.

The results of QoL measurements address more than the patient's cancer and treatment. Other morbidity, associated treatments, and a number of various events, which deeply affect an individual's sense of well-being, can influence QoL as well. Large randomized studies are preferred as means of minimizing the influence of treatment-unrelated factors on changes in QoL.

In the bibliographic study,[1] it was found that a wide range of instruments were used and that the quality in the reporting of QoL data was often deficient. Typically, many QoL measures have also been added as an afterthought to a clinical trial, and not as an integral component of the protocol from the start of the study. QoL assessments require the same scientific vigour as other clinical outcome measures. Ideally, a predefined hypothesis should determine the instrument to be used. Since the selection of an instrument in a specific study influences both the results and the conclusions, it is essential to select the instrument(s) that has the greatest likelihood of identifying relevant differences between treatment alternatives.

The timing of QoL questionnaires in relation to the administration of cytostatic drugs poses several potential problems. The problem is greatest when two schedules differ in their time intervals. If a fixed time schedule is used, the QoL questionnaires will be completed at different times in relation to chemotherapy administration and the onset of immediate and delayed side-effects. This was illustrated in two trials in advanced colorectal cancer comparing raltitrexed used at 3-week intervals and 5-FU/leucovorin administered every fourth to fifth week.[33] It is not clear how to compare a treatment given on 1 day every 3 weeks with a regimen given for 5 consecutive days every 4–5 weeks. Even if the schedules are comparable when they are administered, differences when the toxicity is expressed may disturb the interpretations. Since QoL measurements in multicentre studies are resource-demanding, the choice of time points during and following treatment should be carefully selected to assure maximal information.

Longitudinal studies have shown that cancer patients adapt to their situation, which might create methodological problems. In comparisons with groups of healthy individuals with temporary disease, cancer patients who previously experienced very severe nausea may indicate, for example, that the nausea was moderate, while moderately ill individuals might assess nausea as more severe.[34] The weight that a patient places on a particular symptom may change in either direction as a result of treatment. Thus, correct interpretations of QoL data would require knowledge of how to weigh various aspects based on patient preferences in various treatment situations.[35]

The weight that patients put on various QoL domains covered by the questionnaires is, with few exceptions, not considered. Some patients place little weight on major problems and others place substantial weight on minor problems. Both the presence of a particular symptom and the weight that patients place on it are of importance for achieving an accurate perception of an individual patient's QoL.[14,22,36] It is rather the investigator who before or, more commonly, after the study, puts the focus on individual functions and symptoms with claims for clinical importance. Methodologically, this is a weak point, and opens the door for mass-significance effects and encourages focusing on QoL domains of less importance. An alternative approach is to ask patients not only to quantify various functions and symptoms but also to express a view on their relative importance. Intuitively, this approach would provide a better basis for the assessment of the clinical relevance of QoL data. However, this increases the length of the questionnaire, and, as will be discussed below, in certain trials it may not be the most relevant task to explore whether an individual patient has improved in his or her QoL. Instead, it would seem more meaningful to study changes in aspects that may be of relevance for the QoL in many patients.

The data attrition experienced in studies concerning the value of palliative chemotherapy for advanced cancer has created major problems when interpreting the data. Dropout is selective and may vary among randomized groups, which precludes conclusions based solely on the mean values of interviewed patients.[21,37–39] Unfortunately, there is no good solution to this problem, although several statistical models have been proposed.[40]

A review of methods to reduce missing data and analyse QoL data in trials can be found in a special edition of *Statistics in Medicine*.[41] Altogether, there is a broad consensus that, besides the selective attrition in trials with a short lifespan, patient-related factors are much less a problem than logistical and administrative problems, particularly staff oversights.[42]

WHAT HAS BEEN LEARNT FROM QoL MEASUREMENTS IN PALLIATIVE COLORECTAL CANCER CHEMOTHERAPY TRIALS?

Until the end of the 1980s, patients with advanced colorectal cancer were often treated with palliative chemotherapy without any scientifically documented knowledge of palliative benefits. It was a clinical impression that, although most patients did not benefit from the treatment, some patients had a striking relief of tumour-related symptoms and a gain in well-being, and their deaths could apparently have been postponed for several months. This knowledge led some doctors to propose active treatment for some patients, whereas others generally refused to treat patients outside clinical trials.

Improvements in tumour-related symptoms paralleling a tumour response or disease stabilization were frequently seen in a phase II trial testing sequential methotrexate, leucovorin rescue, and 5-FU (MFL).[43] In a randomized trial comparing MFL and 5-FU alone, the MFL regimen not only increased response rates and prolonged survival,[44] but also gave a subjective response more often, as evaluated by the physician, and improved QoL.[12] An objective response was associated with a subjective response (improvement in tumour-related symptoms without severe adverse effects from treatment) in virtually all patients. Furthermore, several patients without an objective response, but with disease stabilization for at least four months, also improved subjectively. Patients considered to be improved by their physician generally also improved in the answers to the QoL questionnaire. These correlations between a subjective and an objective response, including disease stabilization (this often means tumour regression, although insufficient to fulfil the criteria of a >50% decrease in tumour surface area), and between physicians' and patients' evaluations, have been repeatedly seen in several Nordic multicentre trials (Tables 65.2 and 65.3).[11,12,45–47] Patients included in the trials all had symptoms from the disease, and they received modulated 5-FU having low toxicity. Thus, the assumption of an improved QoL as a result of symptomatic relief caused by tumour regression is valid – at least when using chemotherapy regimens with low toxicity. If the same low-toxicity regimens are given to asymptomatic patients, their general condition is preserved for a longer time, in contrast to a wait-and-see policy.[48] Whether the same holds for regimens that are more toxic remains to be seen. In a trial in the second-line situation comparing irinotecan with best supportive care,[10] patients randomized to active treatment did not deteriorate during treatment in most QoL dimensions, in spite of the toxicity.

Improvements in various aspects of QoL have also been seen in other trials in advanced colorectal cancer treated with either systemic or regional hepatic chemotherapy.[8,9,13,49–52] Taken together, these trials indicate that the chemotherapy schedules that were available during the 1990s prolonged median survival by about six months and improved well-being for at least a few months (four months in the Nordic trials) in approximately half of the patients. It can be suspected that the combination regimens containing 5-FU/leucovorin and irinotecan or oxaliplatin may

---

Table 65.2 Relations between objective and subjective responses to chemotherapy in advanced colorectal cancer[a]

Subjective response	Objective response[b]			
	CR + PR	SD	PD	All
Improved	40	52	9	101
Unchanged	2	20	6	28
Worse		2	102	104
All	42	74	117	233

[a]Data are pooled from three Nordic trials where symptomatic patients were treated with 5-FU alone or biochemically modulated 5-FU. All responses including disease stabilization (SD) had to last for at least four months.
[b]CR + PR, complete response plus partial response; SD, stable disease; PD, progressive disease.

Table 65.3 Relations between subjective (physician-defined) responses and QoL changes (patient-defined/independently categorized) to chemotherapy in advanced colorectal cancer[a]

Subjective response	Quality of life			
	Improved	Unchanged	Worse	Total
Improved	33	7	2	42
Unchanged	6	5	1	12
Worse	2	6	56	64
Total	41	18	59	118

[a]Pooled Nordic data from three trials (not all centres participated in the associated QoL studies).

improve well-being in a higher proportion of patients. While this is an intriguing hypothesis, it remains to be tested, since the toxicity of these regimens is higher than those used in previous studies exploring QoL.

SOME ASPECTS ON HOW TO PRESENT QoL DATA

The most commonly used way of presenting QoL data from randomized clinical trials is to present mean values in all domains or in selected ones considered more important than others. Mean values or differences in mean values between groups may be difficult for both researchers and clinicians to understand.[53] This is true even if values from reference populations increasingly become available. Recently, for example, data were presented for the EORTC QLQ-C30 questionnaire from the Norwegian and Swedish populations.[54,55] Second, and of particular relevance in palliative trials, mean values may be severely biased because of attrition secondary to patient illness or death resulting from the underlying malignancy.[42] This attrition is selective, and thus it may be different in the two comparative groups. Since compliance with completing a questionnaire decreases with poorer performance, for example because of disease progression, attrition will be higher in groups showing shorter time to progression and survival.[37–39] The QoL in the group showing the poorest survival prospect would naturally be poorer – but this may go undetected in the mean scores, in that only patients in comparatively good shape will answer the questionnaire. There are several ways of handling this problem by imputation of

scores for missing patients, including those who already have died.[56] Although imputation methods may partly overcome the problem of selective attrition, none of these methods is ideal. As a result, it has been suggested that QoL data should be presented in many different ways and that conclusions should only be drawn if they consistently show the same results.[38]

CATEGORIZATION OF QoL DATA

The traditional physician-defined endpoint objective response rate is presented as proportions (e.g. complete response plus partial response rates). Although the objectivity of the response evaluation can be criticized, the rates are easy to understand and are useful in the clinical situation. Alternatively, tumour response data could be presented as mean values of, for example, the surface areas before and during treatment in the trial groups. This particular way of presenting data is feasible, and the results could easily be treated statistically, although again a selective attrition would disturb the longitudinal evaluations. It would be more difficult for the clinician to understand, however. With very few exceptions, QoL data have been presented as mean values before and during treatment. Although some mean values have changed differently between the randomization groups in a few trials, the general pattern in virtually all colorectal cancer trials (and in other cancer trials as well) is that of a stable pattern with, if anything, only small variations.[10,33,50,57] Slightly more pronounced changes have been seen in domains reflecting treatment-specific toxicities, such as nausea/vomiting or diarrhoea. This general pattern of stability is to be expected if about half of the patients have some benefit from the intervention, with improving scores in disease-related domains (although potentially counterbalanced by worsening scores in toxicity domains), and the other half have no benefit and deteriorate from the disease, with generally decreasing scores. This has also been the situation in advanced colorectal cancer treated with chemotherapy during the past decade.

Rather, QoL data should be presented in the same way as objective response rates, namely as proportions reaching certain levels. This requires guidelines on meaningful categorizations that are internationally agreed upon. It is regrettable that the international cooperative groups working with QoL measurements have not devoted more of their research to this issue. In its simplest form, two categories – a favourable and a non-favourable outcome – could be used. A favourable outcome could be present either if QoL scores remain at a certain high level for a fixed minimal period or if they improve at least to or beyond an agreed-upon predetermined level. In all others, including those who do not answer subsequent questionnaires (if no follow-up computed tomography (CT) is available, the patient cannot be referred to the group of responders; no follow-up CT or no QoL questionnaire completed is usually a sign of interrupted treatment because of tumour progression or severe toxicity), a non-favourable outcome is present.

At present, we do not know enough about how to categorize patients into favourable or non-favourable groups in an accurate manner. However, rather than design new questionnaires and test them psychometrically, it is far better to encourage approaches that seek to present QoL data more lucidly. The CBR criteria for use in pancreatic cancer is one very simple example that resulted in yielding meaningful data – at least in the sense that they did result in the general acceptance of gemcitabine as one treatment option in advanced pancreatic cancer.[28] The CBR criteria can be criticized because it is mainly a physician or nurse that defines them and because they are too limited, i.e. they consider only a few physical features. To overcome these limitations, one approach would be to select the most relevant domains of an established QoL questionnaire. The categorization would require predefined cut-off points of relevance for the disease and the specific treatments in the trial. Examples of an arbitrarily defined algorithm using the EORTC QLQ-C30 for a chemotherapy trial in advanced colorectal cancer can be seen in Table 65.4. This algorithm may look somewhat complicated, but it has been tested at the University Hospital in Uppsala on patients participating in two Nordic randomized trials.[58] The algorithm measure was found to yield high correlations with other, more complete, measures. When using such an algorithm, the primary aim is not to evaluate if an individual patient has improved his or her overall well-being (global QoL), but rather to study differences between treatments in QoL aspects that other research has found important for many patients' overall well-being. The focus of QoL research aimed at improving the evaluation of various treatments in clinical trials must be changed from what an individual patient values during the treatment (such as a global score) to what patients generally value. The relevance of what patients generally value must then be explored in separately designed trials. It will probably never be possible to capture in a single questionnaire (and one that can be used in a randomized multicentre trial comparing two chemotherapy regimens) whether an individual's QoL has changed in either direction, because of the complexity of what constitutes QoL. Rather, in clinical trials, the goal must be to arrive at a much more pragmatic approach, including only the most important aspects.

SUMMARY AND CONCLUSIONS

Increasingly, treatments that are more aggressive have led to heightened awareness of the importance of addressing how patients experience and value the impact that treatment has on their overall life situation. Assessment of a patient's QoL is now viewed as an important complement to traditional objective evaluation measures.

QoL assessments have come into wide use, and the number of instruments that have been developed has flourished during the past decade. At present, there is little need for the development of new instruments, although specific treatments may need new modules.

Ideally, a predefined hypothesis should determine the instrument to be used. Since the selection of a QoL instrument in a specific study influences both the results and the conclusions, it is essential to select instruments that have the greatest likelihood of identifying relevant differences between treatment alternatives.

The interpretation of QoL data is more difficult than that of data on endpoints, such as survival time, objective response rates, or toxicity. Despite these difficulties, QoL analyses have provided new insights into the advantages and disadvantages of

---

Table 65.4 Proposal for a limited QoL categorization[a]

QoL outcome	Criteria of the EORTC QLQ-C30 questionnaire (scale 0–100)
Favourable	*Either*
	A. Improvement in at least one of the following four domains:
	1. Physical functioning (PF) increased by at least 20 points
	2. Emotional functioning (EF) increased by at least 17 points
	3. Global health status/QoL (Global) increased by at least 17 points
	4. The sum of the symptom scales fatigue, nausea/vomiting, pain, and the single items appetite and diarrhoea decreased at least 50%, or by at least 50 points if the sum was initially below 100, without any negative change in any of the other domains
	A negative change was present if:
	1. PF decreased by more than 20 points or to 20
	2. EF decreased by more than 17 points or to 34
	3. Global decreased by more than 17 points or to 34
	4. Sum of symptom scales increased by more than 50 points or remained above 200
	Or
	B. The scores of the four domains remain at a high level for at least 4 months:
	1. PF ⩾ 80 points
	2. EF ⩾ 83 points
	3. Global ⩾ 75 points
	4. Sum of symptom scales < 50 points
Non-favourable	All others, including those who did not complete the questionnaires after 2 and 4 months

[a]This algorithm, which follows the principles of the Clinical Benefit Response (CBR) criteria used in pancreatic cancer,[28] has been applied to 120 patients with advanced gastrointestinal cancers answering the EORTC QLQ-C30 questionnaire in randomized trials comparing 5-FU-based therapy with best supportive care.[58] This algorithm is presently being explored in a prospective trial, and should only be looked upon as a proposal as to how to proceed to facilitate the understanding of QoL data in randomized trials involving patients with advanced cancer and a poor prognosis.

various treatments that are not provided by traditional endpoints.

Several palliative treatments in advanced colorectal cancer seem to increase patient well-being and QoL, despite the existence of side-effects and only marginal increases in survival.

To improve the possibilities of understanding QoL data in clinical trials, research must be devoted to categorizing changes into meaningful response groups (in analogy with objective response categories). This is because mean values are more difficult to understand and can be severely biased.

Assessment of QoL is clearly in need of further methodological refinement before this parameter can be regarded as being fully established with respect to its ability to provide useful data unequivocally. Missing data are among a number of serious methodological problems. Thus, QoL data, even from apparently well-performed clinical trials, must be interpreted with caution.

REFERENCES

1. Sanders C, Egger M, Donovan J et al, Reporting on quality of life in randomised controlled trials: bibliographic study. *BMJ* 1998; **317:** 1191–4.

2. American Society of Clinical Oncology, Outcomes of cancer treatment for technology assessment and cancer treatment guidelines. *J Clin Oncol* 1996; **14:** 671–9.

3. Kiebert GM, Kaasa S, Quality of life in clinical cancer trials: experience and perspective of the European Organization for Research and Treatment of Cancer. *J Natl Cancer Inst* 1996; **20:** 91–5.

4. Ramsey SD, Andersen MR, Etzioni R et al, Quality of life in survivors of colorectal carcinoma. *Cancer* 2000; **88:** 1294–303

5. Camilleri-Brennan J, Steele R, Quality of life after treatment for rectal cancer. *Br J Surg* 1998; **85:** 1036–43.

6. Allal AS, Bieri S, Pelloni A et al, Sphincter-sparing surgery after preoperative radiotherapy for low rectal cancers: feasibility, oncologic results and quality of life outcomes. *Br J Cancer* 2000; **82:** 1131–7.

7. Norum J, Adjuvant chemotherapy in Dukes' B and C colorectal cancer has only a minor influence on psychological distress. *Support Care Cancer* 1997; **5:** 318–21.

8. Allen-Mersh TG, Earlam S, Fordy C et al, Quality of life and survival with continuous hepatic-artery floxouridine infusion for colorectal liver metastases. *Lancet* 1994; **344:** 1255–60.

9. Cunningham D, Zalcberg JR, Rath U et al, 'Tomudex' (ZD1694): results of a randomised trial in advanced colorectal cancer demonstrate efficacy and reduced mucositis and leucopenia. The 'Tomudex' Colorectal Cancer Study Group. *Eur J Cancer* 1995; **31A:** 1945–54.

10. Cunningham D, Pyrhönen S, James RD et al, Randomised trial of irinotecan plus supportive care versus supportive care alone after fluorouracil failure for patients with metastatic colorectal cancer. *Lancet* 1998; **352:** 1413–18.

11. Glimelius B, Hoffman K, Graf W et al, Quality of life during chemotherapy in symptomatic patients with advanced colorectal cancer. *Cancer* 1994; **73:** 556–62.

12. Glimelius B, Hoffman K, Olafsdottir M et al, Quality of life during cytostatic therapy for advanced symptomatic colorectal carcinoma. A randomized comparison of two regimens. *Eur J Cancer Clin Oncol* 1989; **25:** 829–35.

13. Scheithauer W, Rosen H, Kornek GV et al, Randomised comparison of combination chemotherapy plus supportive care with supportive care alone in patients with metastatic colorectal cancer. *BMJ* 1993; **306:** 752–5.

14. King C, Haberman M, Berry D et al, Quality of life and the cancer experience. *Oncol Nurses Forum* 1997; **24:** 27–41.

15. Moinpour CM, Measuring quality of life: an emerging science. *Semin Oncol* 1994; **21:** 48–60.

16. Karnofsky D, Burchenal J, The clinical evaluation of chemotherapeutic agents in cancer. In: *Evaluation of Chemotherapeutic Agents in Cancer* (McLeod CM, ed). New York: Columbia University Press, 1949: 191–205.

17. Oken MM, Creech RH, Tormey DC et al, Toxicity and response criteria of the Eastern Cooperative Oncology Group. *Am J Clin Oncol* 1982; **5:** 649–55.

18. Adams SG, Britt DM, Godding PR et al, Relative contribution of the Karnofsky performance status scale in a multi-measure assessment of quality of life in cancer patients. *Psycho-Oncology* 1995; **4:** 239–46.

19. Slevin ML, Plant H, Lynch D et al, Who should measure quality of life, the doctor or the patient? *Br J Cancer* 1988; **57:** 109–12.

20. Earlam S, Glover C, Fordy C et al, Relation between tumor size, quality of life, and survival in patients with colorectal liver metastases. *J Clin Oncol* 1996; **14:** 171–5.

21. Aaronson NK, Ahmedzai S, Bergman B et al, The European Organization for Research and Treatment of Cancer QLQ-C30: a quality-of-life instrument for use in clinical trials in oncology. *J Natl Cancer Inst* 1993; **85:** 365–76.

22. Cella DF, Tulsky DS, Gray G et al, The functional assessment of cancer therapy scale: development and validation of the general measure. *J Clin Oncol* 1993; **11:** 570–9.

23. Schag CA, Ganz PA, Wing DS et al, Quality of life in adult survivors of lung, colon and prostate cancer. *Qual Life Res* 1994; **3:** 127–41.

24. Sprangers MA, Cull A, Bjordal K et al, The European Organization for Research and Treatment of Cancer. Approach to quality of life assessment: guidelines for developing questionnaire modules. EORTC Study Group on Quality of Life. *Qual Life Res* 1993; **2:** 287–95.

25. Sprangers M, te Velde A, Aaronson N, The construction and testing of the EORTC colorectal cancer-specific quality of life questionnaire module (QLQ-CR38). *Eur J Cancer* 1999; **35:** 238–47.

26. Schipper H, Clinch J, McMurray A et al, Measuring the quality of life in cancer patients: the Functional Living Index – Cancer: Development and Validation. *J Clin Oncol* 1984; **2:** 472–83.

27. de Haes JC, van Knippenberg FC, Neijt J, Measuring psychological and physical distress in cancer patients: structure and application of the Rotterdam Symptom Checklist. *Br J Cancer* 1990; **62:** 1034–8.

28. Burris H, Storniolo AM, Assessing clinical benefit in the treatment of pancreas cancer: gemcitabine compared to 5-fluorouracil. *Eur J Cancer* 1997; **33:** 18–22.

29. Hoffman K, Glimelius B, Clinical benefit response compared with quality of life measurements in patients with upper gastrointestinal cancer. *Acta Oncol* 1998; **37:** 651–60.

30. Williams A, Economics of coronary artery bypass grafting. *BMJ* 1985; **291:** 326–9.

31. Gelber RD, Goldhirsch A, A new endpoint for the assessment of adjuvant therapy in postmenopausal women with operable breast cancer. *J Clin Oncol* 1986; **4:** 1772–9.

32. Gunnars B, Nygren P, Glimelius B, Assessment of quality of life during chemotherapy. *Acta Oncol* 2001; **40:** 175–84.

33. Anderson H, Palmer M, Measuring quality of life: impact of chemotherapy for advanced colorectal cancer. Experience from two recent large phase III trials. *Br J Cancer* 1998; **77**(Suppl 2): 9–14.

34. de Haes JC, van Knippenberg FC, The quality of life of cancer patients: a review of the literature. *Soc Sci Med* 1985; **20:** 809–17.

35. Redmond K, Assessing patients' needs and preferences in the management of advanced colorectal cancer. *Br J Cancer* 1998; **77:** 5–7.

36. Gill TM, Feinstein AR, A critical appraisal of the quality of quality-of-life measurements. *JAMA* 1994; **272:** 619–26.

37. Glimelius B, Hoffman K, Sjödén P-O et al, Chemotherapy improves survival and quality of life in advanced pancreatic and biliary cancer. *Ann Oncol* 1996; **7:** 593–600.

38. Hopwood P, Stephens RJ, Machin D, Approaches to the analysis of quality of life data: experiences gained from a Medical Research Council Lung Cancer Working Party palliative chemotherapy trial. *Qual Life Res* 1994; **3:** 339–52.

39. Moinpour CM, Sawyers Triplett J, McKnight B et al, Challenges posed by non-random missing quality of life data in an advanced-stage colorectal cancer clinical trial. *Psychooncology* 2000; **9:** 340–54.

40. Fairclough DL, Summary measures and statistics for comparison of quality of life in a clinical trial of cancer therapy. *Stat Med* 1997; **16:** 1197–209.

41. *Stat Med* 1998; **17:** 517–796.

42. Bernhard J, Cella DF, Coates AS et al, Missing quality of life data in cancer clinical trials: serious problems and challenges. *Stat Med* 1998; **17:** 517–32.

43. Glimelius B, Ginman C, Graffman S et al, Sequential methotrexate–5-FU–leucovorin (MFL) in advanced colorectal cancer. *Eur J Cancer Clin Oncol* 1986; **22:** 295–300.

44. Nordic Gastrointestinal Tumour Adjuvant Therapy Group, Sequential methotrexate/5-fluorouracil/leucovorin (MFL) is superior to 5-fluorouracil alone in advanced symptomatic colorectal carcinoma. A randomized trial. *J Clin Oncol* 1989; **7:** 1437–46.

45. Nordic Gastrointestinal Tumor Adjuvant Therapy Group, Biochemical modulation of 5-fluorouracil: a randomized comparison of sequential methotrexate, 5-fluorouracil and leucovorin versus sequential 5-fluorouracil and leucovorin in patients with advanced symptomatic colorectal cancer. *Ann Oncol* 1993; **4:** 235–41.

46. Glimelius B, Hoffman K, Graf W et al, Cost-effectiveness of palliative chemotherapy in advanced gastrointestinal cancer. *Ann Oncol* 1995; **6:** 267–74.

47. Glimelius B, Jacobsen A, Graf W et al, Bolus injection (2–4 minutes) versus short-term (10–20 minutes) infusion of 5-fluorouracil in patients with advanced colorectal cancer: a prospective randomized trial. *Eur J Cancer* 1998; **34:** 674–8.

48. Glimelius B, Graf W, Hoffman K et al, General condition of asymptomatic patients with advanced colorectal cancer receiving palliative chemotherapy: a longitudinal study. *Acta Oncol* 1992; **31:** 645–51.

49. Poon MA, O'Connell MJ, Moertel CG et al, Biochemical modulation of fluorouracil: evidence of significant improvement of survival and quality of life in patients with advanced colorectal carcinoma. *J Clin Oncol* 1989; **7:** 1407–18.

50. Hill M, Norman A, Cunningham D et al, Impact of protracted venous infusion fluorouracil with or without interferon alfa-2b on tumor response, survival, and quality of life in advanced colorectal cancer. *J Clin Oncol* 1995; **13:** 2317–23.

51. Caudry M, Bonnel C, Floquet A et al, A randomized study of bolus fluorouracil plus folinic acid versus 21-day fluorouracil infusion alone or in association with cyclophosphamide and mitomycin C in advanced colorectal carcinoma. *Am J Clin Oncol* 1995; **18:** 118–25.

52. Earlam S, Glover C, Davies M et al, Effect of regional and systemic fluorinated pyrimidine chemotherapy on quality of life in colorectal liver metastasis patients. *J Clin Oncol* 1997; **15:** 2022–9.

53. Osoba D, Rodrigues G, Myles J et al, Interpreting the significance of changes in health-related quality-of-life scores. *J Clin Oncol* 1998; **16:** 139–44.

54. Hjermstad MJ, Fayers PM, Bjordal K et al, Health-related quality of life in the general Norwegian population assessed by the European Organization for Research and Treatment of Cancer Core Quality-of-Life Questionnaire: the QLQ-C30 (+3). *J Clin Oncol* 1998; **16:** 1188–96.

55. Michelson H, Bolund C, Nilsson B et al, Health-related quality of life measured by the EORTC QLQ-C30 – Reference values from a large sample of the Swedish population. *Acta Oncol* 2000; **39:** 477–84.

56. Fairclough DL, Peterson HF, Cella D et al, Comparison of several model-based methods for analysing incomplete quality of life data in cancer clinical trials. *Stat Med* 1998; **17:** 781–96.

57. Rougier P, Van Cutsem E, Bajetta E et al, Randomised trial of irinotecan versus fluorouracil by continuous infusion after fluorouracil failure in patients with metastatic colorectal cancer. *Lancet* 1998; **352:** 1407–12.

58. Nordin K, Steel J, Hoffman K et al, Alternative methods of interpreting quality of life data in advanced gastrointestinal cancer patients. *Br J Cancer* 2001; in press.

66

Cost assessments in colorectal cancer

Niels Neymark

INTRODUCTION

When the editors of this book asked me to contribute a chapter, they suggested the title 'Cost assessments'. This provides me with the occasion to make an essential and perhaps surprising and somewhat paradoxical statement from the outset: economists are not particularly interested in costs, as such, or in primarily minimizing costs, as is often believed. An economic analysis, in the proper sense of the word, must also include an assessment of which desired outcomes (benefits) are obtained by incurring a certain cost. Economic assessments aim at determining the relation between the costs incurred and the benefits obtained, and a properly conducted economic analysis will give just as much importance to an accurate valuation of the benefits as to the estimation of costs.

In this short chapter, I shall first give a very brief introduction to the fundamental types of economic assessments used to provide information of relevance for medical decision making. Subsequently, I present an up-to-date survey of published economic evaluations of alternative treatment options for patients with colorectal cancer. In trying to summarize the results of the available analyses, I point out their principal shortcomings and suggest possibilities for further research.

ECONOMIC EVALUATION: A BRIEF PRIMER TO THE FUNDAMENTAL IDEAS

At its broadest level, an economic evaluation may be defined as 'a systematic comparison of two or more alternative actions with the same objective taking into account both their benefits and their costs'.[1] The aim of economic evaluation is to provide decision makers with information that enables them to allocate their limited resources efficiently – that is, to achieve the most benefits given the resources available.

An important starting point is an understanding of the economic concept of costs. This derives from a recognition that resources are limited and always will be so relative to the wishes and desires of people. This makes it necessary to choose between alternative ways of using the resources, and economics is often referred to as a science of choice. By using a particular resource for a certain purpose during a given time period, the opportunity of using it for another purpose during the same time period is forgone. The *opportunity cost* of using the resource for the purpose chosen is therefore the benefits that could have been achieved by using it for its next best alternative purpose.

Clearly, this is not a concept that is easily measured, and all economic analyses are forced to use approximations, but it is central for the understanding of economic arguments and methods of analysis. As an example, take the frequently heard proposals of solving the problems due to limited resources available for healthcare by increasing the budget of the healthcare sector. Such ideas will usually be countered by economists pointing to the welfare losses in other sectors or activities that will follow from transferring some of their resources to healthcare. Such losses are the opportunity costs of allocating more resources to healthcare.

Economic evaluation applied to healthcare interventions or treatment options seek to determine the differences between the options in terms of their benefits (outcomes) and costs in order to present this information to the decision makers who have to choose which option to use. A standard situation, to which the following discussion will refer, is that of an established treatment of a particular group of patients, where a new treatment is developed and marketed. How should the decision makers decide whether to adopt the new treatment or to continue using standard care? Most frequently, the new treatment will be claimed to offer certain improvements in clinical outcomes, but this will often be at the expense of increased costs. How may it be decided whether the improvements in outcome are worth the additional costs?

One of the most frequently seen types of economic analysis in healthcare is *cost identification studies* or *cost analyses*. Such analyses typically set out to determine if the increased acquisition costs of a new treatment are balanced or offset by reductions of other derived costs of the treatments compared. An example may be that a new drug leads to fewer and less serious adverse events than the standard care, and therefore also entails less costs due to the management of adverse events. The reduction in derived costs may be estimated to (more than) compensate the higher acquisition costs, leading to a reduction in the overall costs of treatment. However, this assessment is not an economic evaluation properly speaking, because treatment outcomes are not taken into account.

The four common types of actual economic evaluations treat costs in the same way, but differ with regard to the way health outcomes are taken into account. In a *cost-minimization analysis*, the treatments are considered to achieve the outcome of principal interest to the same degree. This is not to say that the outcomes are assumed to be identical in all respects, but differences in other aspects of outcome than the principal (e.g. survival time) are ignored in the analysis. With identical outcomes, the least costly treatment would normally be considered preferable.

In a *cost–effectiveness analysis*, outcomes are measured in natural physical units, such as survival time, number of lives saved, treatment episodes avoided, etc. Again, this selection of one principal outcome for the analysis makes it more tractable at the expense of not attempting a quantitative assessment or valuation of other important dimensions of outcome. Assuming a difference in outcomes, the results of the analysis are usually summarized in an *incremental cost–effectiveness ratio* (ICER), or $\Delta C/\Delta E$, which is a measure of the increase in costs associated with the increase in health effect achieved by changing from the less to the more effective treatment. The results of an analysis of a new treatment that increases survival time at the expense of an increase in costs may thus be expressed in a standardized way as an ICER of XX 000 euro per life-year gained, no matter what the exact estimate of the gain in survival time amounts to. Such standardization of the reporting of results

makes it easier to compare the results of different analyses.

A major attraction of *cost–utility analysis* is that the problems caused by the one-dimensionality of cost–effectiveness analysis are overcome by using a global measure of the patients' health-related quality of life as the outcome. A frequently recommended outcome measure that combines length of survival with health-related quality of life is the *quality-adjusted life-year* (QALY). A QALY may take on values between 1 (perfect health) and 0 (death or worst health state possible), and an ideal outcome measure would be mean quality-adjusted survival time (with continuous quality adjustment). It is not possible here to give an adequate summary of 25 years of heated discussions about the most appropriate way to estimate health-related quality of life, so suffice it to say that there is still no agreement on several vital issues of measurement. Economists generally agree on the relevance and attractiveness of expressing the results of any economic evaluation in terms of the incremental costs per QALY gained. This would enable comparisons across all types of diseases and treatments, and thereby provide information for making resource allocation decisions for the healthcare sector as a whole. It is clear, however, that there is still a lot of work to be accomplished before reliable so-called cost–utility league tables can be established.

In a *cost–benefit analysis*, health outcomes are valued in monetary terms, which makes benefits and costs commensurable and allows determination of the net benefits of a treatment as benefits minus costs per patient. Alternative treatment options can then be compared in terms of their net benefits, just as any comparisons across therapeutic areas can be made directly. Only options with positive net benefits should be considered acceptable, and normally interventions with higher positive net benefits would be preferred to those with smaller. While the theoretical foundation of the other types of economic evaluation is not quite clear, cost–benefit analysis is well founded in the theory of welfare economics, which builds on the premise that societal decisions should be made on the basis of the preferences of the individuals affected by a decision. The value of a good is determined by how much the individuals on the average are willing to pay for it, and cost–benefit analysis was developed as a tool for making decisions about the provision of goods for which no ordinary markets (can) exist.

The principal problem with using cost–benefit analysis for the economic evaluation of healthcare interventions is of course to find ways of valuing the outcomes in monetary terms. The currently favoured method of obtaining such valuations is called *contingent valuation*. This is a survey method, in which the respondents are asked to imagine the contingency of a market existing for the outcome(s) of interest. There are an increasing number of publications using cost–benefit analysis based on contingent valuation to assess healthcare interventions, and a recent review[2] was quite optimistic about the potential for solving remaining problems.

No matter which type of evaluation is used in a particular analysis, the principal task of the analyst is to ensure that the information about each alternative in the comparison is collected, treated and assessed according to *uniform, systematic, and consistent criteria*. The basic steps in any economic evaluation are therefore to systematically identify, quantify, and value all the costs and effects of the alternatives. An account of these, varying in detail, may be found in either of references 1 and 3, since the space allotted here does not allow this. The outline of the fundamental ideas of economic evaluation given above should permit the reader with no prior experience with such analyses to better appreciate the following summary and discussion of published evaluations dealing with treatment options in colorectal cancer.

SURVEY OF RECENT ECONOMIC EVALUATIONS IN COLORECTAL CANCER

In a book published in 1998,[4] I surveyed the literature of economic analyses of cancer therapies published between 1985 and 1996 (inclusive). The survey includes eight studies dealing with colorectal cancer patients, the majority of which are cost analyses. Typically, such studies seek to determine the costs of various diagnostic procedures or to examine whether the treatment costs for a patient from diagnosis to death vary depending on the stage of disease at diagnosis. Such variations might have implications for decisions on initiation of screening programmes, but one of the studies is particularly useful in making it clear that focusing on costs alone may lead to erroneous conclusions. Whynes et al[5] thus compared the treatment costs of two groups of patients, one detected by screening and one detected after presenting with clinical symptoms. Examining patients with low costs of management over a 3-year period, they found that in the control group the main explanation for low costs is the early death of patients, while almost all the screen-detected patients survived the 3-year follow-up period.

Only two of the studies retrieved for the survey are actual economic evaluations, both of the cost–utility type,[6,7] but none of these are very convincing, because the study designs and/or the data used are rather poor. It was clear at the time of writing the survey, however, that many new economic evaluations were to be expected because of the recent or imminent marketing of several new cytotoxics as alternatives to the conventional 5-fluorouracil (5-FU) regimens. This prediction has come true, and I shall focus the following presentation on these studies, while simply noting that screening programmes continue to generate many analyses, just as plain cost–identification studies continue to appear.[8,9] Some recent studies of screening programmes for colorectal (and other) cancer(s) are of great methodological interest, because they break new ground. One study tries to estimate the impact on patients' quality of life of participation in screening programmes,[10] while the other uses contingent valuation methods to determine patients' willingness to pay for participating in a screening programme as a means of assessing the net benefits of the programme.[11] So far, these studies have only been presented as conference abstracts, but both approaches seem very interesting.

Although other new drugs such as oxaliplatin are also under investigation as substitutes for or complements to 5-FU, data for these are not yet mature enough for analysis. Primary interest has accordingly focused on the two drugs raltitrexed and irinotecan, first as second-line therapy in patients with advanced disease and subsequently as first-line therapy as well. Both drugs have been tested against various regimens of 5-FU plus folinic acid (FA, leucovorin), and economic evaluations have been carried out in relation to large phase III randomized controlled trials. In addition, an economic evaluation of infusional versus bolus 5-FU + FA is under preparation in the EORTC Health Economics Unit.[12]

From a clinical point of view, raltitrexed has been extensively studied in several large clinical trials in patients with advanced disease, and its efficacy has been adequately shown. There is no substantial difference in survival when raltitrexed is compared to bolus 5-FU + FA, while raltitrexed may show some advantages in terms of less severe neutropenia and mucositis. But, the acquisition price of raltitrexed is much higher, as shown by Ross et al,[13] who reported a price of £457 versus a price of £74 for 5-FU + FA.

In a cost analysis, Kerr and O'Connor[14] suggested that raltitrexed may reduce costs associated with administration of chemotherapy in advanced colorectal cancer. The total monthly costs may be lower or about the same as other 5-FU-based chemotherapy regimens. It may offer potential savings in terms of physician, nursing and pharmacy time, inpatient, stays and outpatient visits. The patients' and their carers' direct expenses and loss of working time may also be expected to be lower (cf. below).

Ross et al[13] attempted a retrospective audit of the costs of four chemotherapy regimens in advanced colorectal cancer: bolus 5-FU + low-dose FA (Mayo regimen), bolus 5-FU + high-dose FA 24-hour infusion (de Gramont), continuous infusional 5-FU administered through an ambulatory pump, and raltitrexed by 15-minute injection. The retrospective examination of patient charts showed that the use of raltitrexed may entail a lower level of use of some hospital resources, such as outpatient visits, while the median number of inpatient stays per month is higher for raltitrexed. The authors conclude that the total costs of raltitrexed and bolus 5-FU (Mayo regimen) are not significantly different, with results reported as median total costs equal to £959 for raltitrexed and £660 for the Mayo regimen and overlapping 95% confidence intervals.

Groener et al[15] present an economic evaluation of raltitrexed compared with the Mayo regimen of 5-FU. Clinical and resource use data come from an international randomized controlled trial, and they calculate costs by multiplying resource use data from the trial with Dutch unit prices, although the results are reported in US dollars. The main outcome of the trial was survival (measured as survival rates at 6 months and 1 year), while the incidence of severe adverse events was the secondary endpoint. The trial showed equal efficacy of the regimens in terms of survival time, while the incidence of severe adverse events (leucopenia and mucositis) was lower in the raltitrexed group. Given equal efficacy in terms of the principal outcome, a cost-minimization analysis is indicated, but the authors also invent a new outcome measure (patient free of adverse event) to report the results. They report that 80% of the higher acquisition costs of raltitrexed ($3132 per patient) is balanced by savings on other costs due to a more convenient administration scheme. The net incremental cost per patient of raltitrexed compared with the 5-FU regimen is estimated to be $626. When taking the reduced incidence of severe adverse events into account, they report an incremental cost of $396 per additional patient free of any severe events.

Sculpher et al[16] estimate some aspects of treatment costs, which ought to be taken into consideration in an economic evaluation carried out from the societal perspective. Analyses from this viewpoint should comprise all costs incurred by everybody affected by a particular treatment decision, also so-called pro-ductivity costs, which refer to the loss of time for production or other valued activities for the patients and relatives caring for them. It is contentious whether patients' and carers' time costs should simply be added to direct medical costs, but a recommended solution is to report these different types of costs separately.[17] However, such costs are rarely included, even in studies claiming to take a societal viewpoint.

The analysis by Sculpher et al[16] is based on a prospective substudy within a multinational randomized controlled trial of raltitrexed versus infusional 5-FU + FA. The median duration of treatment was 12.7 weeks for raltitrexed and 16.9 weeks for the 5-FU patients. In order to value the costs of the journeys to and from treatment and the time lost from usual activities over the period of therapy, a subset of the patients in the trial were asked to complete a questionnaire necessary to provide the information needed to value travel and time costs in monetary terms. Patients were asked about the distance travelled and the mode of transport, and on this basis average travel cost per patient in each treatment group has been calculated by using price data provided by various transport associations. Patient or carer time that otherwise would have been spent working is valued by the average hourly pay of UK workers, while non-working time is valued at a lower rate, recommended by the Department of Transport for valuation of time spent travelling. Median travel costs for raltitrexed patients are statistically significantly lower than for 5-FU patients, and the same is the case for median time costs. These results are very robust, when assumptions are varied in sensitivity analyses, and it is proposed that the major reason for the differences is the longer treatment periods for the 5-FU + FA patients.

In a multinational randomized controlled trial of irinotecan versus infusional 5-FU (each centre could choose between three different regimens) for patients with metastatic colorectal cancer after 5-FU failure,[18] resource utilization data were collected prospectively. Supplemented with data collected from clinicians' responses to questionnaires, these data have been used for several economic evaluations adapted to the local settings (based on local expert opinions) of specific countries. So far, economic evaluations with British[19] and French[20] data have been published. The clinical trial showed a statistically significant survival gain for irinotecan, with a 1-year survival rate of 44.8% compared with 32.4% in the 5-FU group, and a higher median survival time, 10.8 months versus 8.5 months (but overlapping 95% confidence intervals). For the cost–effectiveness analysis, the gain in survival is estimated as the difference in median survival per year, that is $(10.8 - 8.5)/12 = 0.19$. It is assumed that all three 5-FU regimens are equally effective. The incidence of serious adverse events was significantly higher in the irinotecan group, but a quality-of-life analysis included in the study found no significant differences.

Only the UK data on costs and cost–effectiveness will be presented here, since the French data are similar in tendency, but less clearly presented in the paper. Only direct hospital costs are included, and a separation has been made between costs associated with administration of chemotherapy (including the drugs) and costs associated with complications due to the treatment or the disease. Drug acquisition costs per patient were higher for irinotecan than for any of the 5-FU regimens, £4680 versus a range from £336 to £3358, but these were partly offset by lower costs of administering the drug, that is inpatient stays, day hospital attendance, and catheter and pump costs. Complication costs were also lower for irinotecan patients, mainly because of fewer days being spent in hospital after the treatment period. The total cost per patient of irinotecan (£8253) is midway in the range of cost estimates for the various 5-FU regimens (£5983 – £9981). Compared with the different 5-FU regimens, irinotecan is found either to be a *dominant solution* (more effective and less costly) or to lead to incremental costs per life-year gained of either £7695 or £11 947.

Subsequently, irinotecan + 5-FU/FA has been compared with 5-FU/FA alone as first-line therapy in metastatic colorectal cancer in a randomized controlled trial that showed a statistically significant difference in median survival, with 17.4 months in the combination arm and 14.1 months in the 5-FU/FA arm.[21] As part of the trial that included 387 patients, data on medical resource use were collected prospectively. This was combined with a retrospective data collection to document further chemotherapy and disease complication costs after study treatment failure. Based on these data, Schmitt et al[22] have carried out an economic evaluation from the viewpoint of the French National Health System. Again, costs are broken down in a very informative way, where costs of drug acquisition and administration are distinguished from costs of complications and second-line therapy after study treatment failure. Average total costs per patient are estimated as FFr 182 546 in the irinotecan + 5-FU/FA arm and FFr 123 669 in the 5-FU/FA arm. Using the difference in median survival (3.3 months) as the estimate of the gain in survival from adding irinotecan to 5-FU/FA leads to an estimate of the incremental costs per life-year gained of FFr 214 098.

CONCLUDING REMARKS

It has for some time been thought that mass population screening programmes would prove effective in reducing the mortality of colorectal cancer, for which a close association between stage at detection and survival after diagnosis has been observed. A large variety of screening protocols are feasible, and many of these have been the subjects of cost–effectiveness analyses in many different healthcare settings. Conclusions depend decisively on factors such as the frequency of screening and the age group of the screened population. In general, these analyses have not taken population preferences into account, but this has been done in some of the most recent studies. Thus, Frew et al[11] examined the populations' preferences and willingness to pay for two different protocols, biennial faecal occult blood testing and once-only flexible sigmoidoscopy. For both screening protocols, the average willingness to pay was more than the actual resource cost of the testing.

With regard to the economic evaluations of the treatment options for advanced colorectal cancer, the results for the new cytotoxics compared with various infusional 5-FU regimens turn out somewhat differently in terms of both costs and effectiveness. Raltitrexed has not shown clear advantages in outcomes compared with 5-FU, while it is clearly more costly. By taking into account a reduced incidence of adverse events and a more convenient administration scheme, it is possible to offset substantial parts of the incremental acquisition costs of raltitrexed, but the analyses published will probably not easily convince decision makers to switch to raltitrexed.

For irinotecan, the results of the economic evaluations depend decisively on which infusional 5-FU regimen is used as comparator and on how this is administered. Especially for the de Gramont regimen, there are large differences in administration. In some hospitals, patients are admitted for two full days of hospital stay, while in others the patients receive the infusion in a day clinic without actual hospital admission. The average total cost per irinotecan patient is found to be about midway in the range of average total cost estimated for the various 5-FU regimens, which are all accepted unquestioningly in the healthcare settings where they are practised. As irinotecan results in a significant improvement in survival compared with infusional 5-FU, it may in certain comparisons be a dominant solution, with improved outcomes at lower costs. Compared with other infusional 5-FU regimens, the improvement is achieved at the expense of a certain increase in costs, but the estimated ICER does not seem to be excessive compared with the existing benchmark figures for a critical threshold ($50 000 per QALY is widely cited).

In all of the economic evaluations comparing infusional 5-FU with the new alternatives, the most important cost factors are hospital stays and visits to day hospital clinics, in addition to the acquisition costs of the new drugs and of the modulator folinic acid, while 5-FU is cheap. Several new ways of administering the drug regimens, such as continuous infusion with transportable pumps or by oral intake of tablets, are under development, and the realization of these potentials will require renewed economic evaluations, since this may reduce the costs (particularly of the 5-FU regimens) considerably.

The published economic evaluations show some common deficiencies that should be noted. The first is that many of the studies report only *median* costs. The median may be claimed to be a useful summary descriptive statistic for data with a skewed distribution, but an economic analysis should focus on the mean or average total costs per patient. Decision makers need an estimate of the total incremental costs of changing from one treatment to another, and this is determined by the difference in average costs multiplied by the expected number of patients. The median cost cannot be used for this calculation, and a lot of information is lost, because it ignores most of the cost data available.

Another problem is that the cost–effectiveness analyses[19,20,22] report only survival rates at certain time points and median survival times. Incremental cost–effectiveness ratios are determined by relating differences in average total costs to differences in median survival times. However, the appropriate effect measure in cost–effectiveness analyses of treatments with survival time as the principal outcome is the expected survival. The best estimate of expected survival is the mean survival time, and a given difference in median survival time cannot be interpreted as an equivalent change in expected survival, although this is done in numerous other studies. Because of censoring, mean survival time usually cannot be determined from observed data alone, and other estimation methods are needed. The most appropriate methods for estimating differences in mean survival are the subject of current research,[23] but basically there are two approaches: truncation or extrapolation of the data. The inappropriate use of median instead of mean survival time may be explained but not justified by the difficulties involved in estimating differences in mean survival.

REFERENCES

1. Drummond MF, O'Brien B, Stoddart GL, Torrance GW, *Methods for the Economic Evaluation of Health Care Programmes*, 2nd edn. Oxford: Oxford University Press, 1997.

2. Diener A, O'Brien B, Gafni A, Health care contingent valuation studies: a review and classification of the literature. *Health Econ* 1998; **7**: 313–26.

3. Neymark N, Techniques of health economics analysis in oncology. Parts 1 and 2. *Crit Rev Oncol Hematol* 1999; **30**: 1–11 and 13–24.

4. Neymark N, *Assessing the Economic Value of Anticancer Therapies* (Recent Results in Cancer Research, Vol 148). Heidelberg: Springer-Verlag, 1998.

5. Whynes D, Walker A, Chamberlain J et al, Screening and the costs of colorectal cancer. *Br J Cancer* 1993; **68**: 965–8.

6. Kievit J, van de Velde C, Utility and cost of carcinoembryonic antigen monitoring in colon cancer follow-up evaluation: a Markov analysis. *Cancer* 1990; **65**: 2580–7.

7. Glimelius B, Hoffmann K, Graf W et al, Cost effectiveness of palliative chemotherapy in advanced gastrointestinal cancer. *Ann Oncol* 1995; **6**: 267–74.

8. Brown ML, Riley GF, Potosky AL, Etzioni RD, Obtaining long-term disease specific costs of care. Application to Medicare enrollees diagnosed with colorectal cancer. *Med Care* 1999; **37**: 1249–59.

9. Finkelstein E, Neighbors D, Bradley C, Candrilli S, Medical resource utilization and costs of distinct episodes of colon cancer. *Eur J Cancer* 2000; **36**(Suppl 3): s14.

10. Gyrd Hansen D, Søgaard J, Estimation of utility associated with participation in cancer screening programmes. *Eur J Cancer* 2000; **36**(Suppl 3): s3.

11. Frew E, Wolstenholme JL, Whynes DK, Willingness to pay for colorectal cancer screening: faecal occult blood testing versus flexible sigmoidoscopy. *Eur J Cancer* 2000; **36**(Suppl 3): s9.

12. Roy T, Neymark N, Wils J et al, Chemotherapy as primary treatment in advanced colorectal cancer: economic evaluation of three different 5-FU schedules. *Eur J Cancer* 2000; **36**(Suppl 3): s8.

13. Ross P, Heron J, Cunningham D, Cost of treating advanced colorectal cancer: a retrospective comparison of treatment regimens. *Eur J Cancer* 1996; **32A**(Suppl 5): s13–17.

14. Kerr DJ, O'Connor KM, The costs of managing advanced colorectal cancer: a broad perspective. *Anticancer Drugs* 1996; **8**(Suppl 2): s23–6.

15. Groener MGH, van Inefeld BM, Byttebier G et al, An economic evaluation of Tomudex (raltitrexed) and 5-fluorouracil plus leucovorin in advanced colorectal cancer. *Anticancer Drugs* 1999; **10**: 283–8.

16. Sculpher M, Palmer MK, Heyes A, Costs incurred by patients undergoing advanced colorectal cancer therapy. A comparison of raltitrexed and fluorouracil plus folinic acid. *Pharmaco-Economics* 2000; **17**: 361–70.

17. Neymark N, Kiebert W, Torfs K et al, Methodological and statistical issues of QoL and economic evaluation in cancer clinical trials: report of a workshop. *Eur J Cancer* 1998; **34**: 1317–33.

18. Rougier P, Van Cutsem E, Bajetta E et al, Phase III trial of irinotecan versus infusional fluorouracil in patients with metastatic colorectal canceer after fluorouracil failure. *Lancet* 1998; **352**: 1407–12.

19. Iveson TJ, Hikisch T, Schmitt C, van Cutsem E, Irinotecan in second-line treatment of metastatic colorectal cancer: improved survival and cost-effect compared with infusional 5-FU. *Eur J Cancer* 1999; **35**: 1796–804.

20. Levy-Piedbois C, Durand-Zaleski I, Juhel H et al, Cost–effectiveness of second-line treatment with irinotecan or infusional 5-flurorouracil in metastatic colorectal cancer. *Ann Oncol* 2000; **11:** 157–61.

21. Douillard JY, Cunningham D, Roth AD et al, Irinotecan combined with fluorouracil compared with flourouracil alone as first-line treatment for metastatic colorectal cancer: a multicentre randomised trial. *Lancet* 2000; **355:** 1041–7.

22. Schmitt C, Levy-Piedbois C, Frappé M, Durand-Zaleski I, Cost–effectiveness analysis of irinotecan (Campto®) as first-line therapy in advanced colorectal cancer. *Eur J Cancer* 2000; **36**(Suppl 3): s24.

23. Neymark N, Gorlia T, Estimating differences in mean survival in studies where survival time is the principal outcome: a systematic assessment of the relative performance of extrapolation and restricted means methods. *Med Decision Making* 2000; **20:** 500.

67

Critical issues in colorectal cancer randomized trials and meta-analysis

Jean-Pierre Pignon, Marc Buyse, Pascal Piedbois

'More usually, advances in therapeutics will come to consist of a succession of small improvements ... When such small differences are to be established, only carefully conducted trials will be able to provide definite information'

Schwartz, Flamant, and Lellouch (1980)

INTRODUCTION

The purpose of this chapter is to present critical issues in randomized clinical trials and meta-analyses of therapies for colorectal cancer. Early-phase clinical trials are therefore outside the scope of the present chapter. Randomized trials of preventive interventions raise specific methodological questions that also fall beyond the scope of this chapter, which focuses on treatment evaluation.

RANDOMIZED TRIALS IN PATIENTS WITH RESECTABLE COLORECTAL CANCER

Sample size

Table 67.1 gives some examples of observed relative risks of death of patients receiving chemotherapy compared with those receiving no adjuvant therapy in colon cancer, and the sample size needed to detect such relative risks.

Table 67.1 Relative risks of death observed in a large trial or a meta-analysis of adjuvant chemotherapy versus none, and sample sizes needed to detect such relative risks

Trial reference	Population	Treatment	Relative risk (95% CI[a])	Sample size:[b] No. of patients	(No. of events)
				C stages	B stages
Moertel et al[1]	Colon, stage III	5-FU + levamisole	0.67 (0.53–0.84)	500 (200)	750 (200)
IMPACT[2]	Colon, stages II and III	5-FU + leucovorin	0.78 (0.62–0.97)	1200 (475)	1700 (475)

[a]95% confidence interval.
[b]Based on a 55% survival rate in stage III without adjuvant treatment and a 70% survival rate in stage II; two-sided logrank test with 80% power and 5% significance level.

When a trial is contemplated for all patients after tumour resection, the number of patients needed to detect a given difference is higher if both stage II (UICC) and stage III tumours are included than if only stage III tumours are included, because the survival rate of patients with stage II tumours is higher (Table 67.1). The sample size increases even further if a comparison between different active treatments is contemplated (rather than between an experimental group and an untreated control group) because the expected difference is a priori smaller. Sample size calculations have been reviewed elsewhere.[3–5] For all analyses of time-dependent events such as survival, it is the number of events and not the number of patients that is critical.

An erroneous interpretation of the results of inconclusive trials is quite frequent.[6] When a trial concludes that there is no statistically significant benefit in favour of a new treatment, it does not follow that there is in truth no benefit, but merely that the trial failed to show it. In the past, trial sizes tended to be too small to detect a moderate and yet clinically relevant treatment effect.[7–10] For example, among the nine randomized trials included in the meta-analysis of adjuvant portal vein 5-fluorouracil (5-FU) chemotherapy, six had included less than 300 patients.[11]

Design issues

The design of a clinical trial is crucial, since a faulty design may makes meaningful analyses of the trial results difficult and a proper interpretation of its results impossible. For a general review of trial designs, see Simon,[12] Pocock,[3] and Buyse.[13]

In oncology, a common design is to include between 100 and 300 patients in two equally sized treatment groups. Such moderately sized developmental trials are needed to evaluate new treatments and new routes of treatment administration. Usually they include selected patients with poor prognosis. These trials are time-consuming and potentially costly. Their cost is due to one or several of the following factors: (a) patient selection based on new or expensive tests; (b) systematic collection of prognostic covariates, toxicity data, compliance, and secondary endpoints; (c) careful monitoring of treatment quality and data collection. According to the type of treatment evaluated and its stage of development, some or all of these factors are essen-

tial to the trial design. It is, however, often possible and desirable to simplify the trial procedures either to reduce the overall cost of the trial or to increase its sample size.[14] Really large-scale trials (or megatrials) can be considered for the reliable detection of small but worthwhile benefits obtained with widely available treatments such as adjuvant portal vein chemotherapy.[15]

A design that is worth special mention in the context of oncology is the *factorial design*. Peto[16] and Byar and Piantadosi[17] advocated a wider use of factorial designs, in particular the *2 × 2 design*, which answers two questions instead of one with little or no extra difficulties or cost. To compare two treatments, A and B, versus no treatment, patients can be randomized into four groups: neither treatment, A or B alone, or both together. To study the effect of A, for example, the results of the comparison A + B versus B and A versus no treatment will be combined. This design is useful when the effect of A is essentially the same in the presence or in the absence of B. If such were not the case, an 'interaction' between treatments A and B would be observed. The statistical tests required to detect interactions have very low power, and therefore the absence of an interaction must be assumed at the time of trial planning.[12,17] One difficulty in oncology is that it is not always possible to give no treatment or both.[18] For example, when chemotherapy and radiotherapy are combined, it may be necessary to lower the treatment doses because of overlapping toxicity. When a significant interaction is present, the trial must be analysed as a four-arm trial, and as a result there is a substantial loss in statistical power.[19] Examples of factorially designed trials include the AXIS trial, which tests the value of portal vein 5-FU and of radiotherapy in patients with rectal cancer.[15] The EORTC trial 40911 compares 'early' regional chemotherapy (portal vein or peritoneal 5-FU) with none and two 'late' systemic chemotherapy regimens (5-FU plus leucovorin versus 5-FU plus levamisole). An NCCTG trial compares two chemotherapy regimens (5-FU plus levamisole versus 5-FU plus levamisole plus leucovorin) as well as two chemotherapy durations (6 months versus 12 months).[20]

Stratification

Stratification consists of using prognostic information at the time of randomization in order to guarantee that the treatment groups are well balanced. Pure randomization achieves such a balance only in the long run, while 'stratified' randomization ensures it even in small samples.[21] This balance is not strictly necessary, as any imbalance can be adjusted for in the analysis, but trials that show a reasonable balance among treatment groups are far more convincing and easier to analyse and interpret. The advantages of using stratified randomization are that: (a) trial results are more credible when prognostic factors are balanced among the treatment arms; (b) there is no need for adjusted analyses that would be called for if an imbalance occurred; (c) the power of the analysis is optimum. With the advent of centralized and computerized randomization, it has become easy to take multiple prognostic factors into account by using techniques such as minimization.[22]

Stratification factors should have an established independent prognostic value, and should be easily and reliably obtainable before randomization. Dukes stage or TNM stage are the most important prognostic factors for potentially resectable colorectal cancer. When adjuvant trials include all stages, it is advisable to stratify them for stage. In fact, the stratification may include a change in treatment policy, because systemic chemotherapy is now standard therapy for UICC stage III colon cancer, while its use is still controversial for stage II and even more so for stage I. Active research is ongoing to refine the prognostic information within each stage, but at present stage is the only prognostic factor for which stratification is absolutely called for. Another factor that should be taken into account in rectal cancer is the administration of preoperative or postoperative radiotherapy. The investigational centre is often taken as a stratification factor for administrative convenience.

Endpoints for adjuvant treatments

The endpoint of interest in trials of adjuvant treatments is usually the period of time from the date of randomization to the occurrence of some well-defined event indicating treatment failure, such as death or disease relapse. Patients who have not yet failed at the time of the analysis constitute so-called *censored observations*, because their time to failure will eventually be longer than that observed at the time of the analysis. *Overall survival* is the time period between randomization and patient death, whatever

its cause. Randomized trials have often failed to show survival differences between treatment groups because the sample size has been insufficient to show the small benefits in mortality that are achievable with adjuvant therapy. Small survival differences are swamped by random errors due to patient heterogeneity.

Cancer survival is the time period between randomization and patient death if its cause is malignant disease. Patients who die from other causes, such as intercurrent diseases, are regarded as censored observations. Cancer survival is a more sensitive indicator of treatment effect than overall survival, particularly if the competing risks of dying from other causes are high, as is the case among the old age groups that typically present with colorectal cancer. The analysis of cancer survival may provide valuable insight into the effects of treatment, but any evidence thus obtained may be biased. Indeed, causes of death are notoriously difficult to ascertain, and misclassification between cancer and non-cancer causes may occur. Moreover, if treatment affected the non-malignant causes of death (perhaps because of some toxicity), an analysis of cancer survival could be misleading: for instance, an aggressive treatment might cure more patients of their cancer but kill them because of toxicity, resulting in no net benefit. In such cases, the overall survival analysis would correctly conclude no benefit, while the cancer survival analysis would show a treatment benefit. Both analyses would have to be considered simultaneously for a reliable and informative conclusion to be drawn.

Disease-free interval is the time between randomization and a clear-cut relapse of the disease. Patients who die without evidence of disease are regarded as censored observations. *Disease-free survival* is defined as disease-free interval, but with all deaths considered failures. Disease-free interval is in most cases a worthwhile endpoint in addition to survival. Just as for cancer survival, it is a more sensitive biological marker of treatment effect, but a less reliable indicator of net benefit to the patient. The type of relapse can yield useful information on the disease process. Therefore disease-free interval is usually subdivided into *time to local progression* (with distant progressions regarded as censored observations) and *time to distant progression* (with local relapses regarded as censored observations). These times can be equally relevant as survival if disease recurrence has a major impact on the patient condition and if no treatment is available on recurrence: for instance, time to local recurrence is an important endpoint after radical surgery of rectal cancer, because recurrences in the pelvis may be very painful and difficult to remove surgically.

To demonstrate the efficacy of chemotherapy in stage II is difficult because of the low rate of events observed in patients treated by surgery only. The most straightforward approach to demonstrate a benefit is to perform a large randomized trial such as the CALGB 69581 trial.[23] Two other approaches used patients randomized in previous trials. The IMPACT B2 investigators[24] pooled five similar randomized trials comparing 5-FU plus folinic acid with nil. This study included only 1016 patients, and 218 deaths were observed. It failed to demonstrate any effect of chemotherapy. Including the 1057 stage III patients randomized in these trials and comparing the efficacy of chemotherapy in stage II and stage III patients would have increased the power of the study. This approach was adopted by Mamounas et al,[25] who showed that the relative benefit of therapy was at least as large in stage II as in stage III patients. Unfortunately, their analyses included trials with no chemotherapy arm and trials comparing two chemotherapy regimens. Moreover, the chemotherapy regimens were quite different, and so it is difficult to draw a definitive conclusion from these results. More patients will be needed to confirm the small benefits observed in these studies.[26]

Large-scale trials and prospective pooled analysis

To detect a 5-year survival benefit of less than 10% in the adjuvant setting implies performing trials in which more than 1000 patients are included, because the survival rates are higher than 40% for most cases of resectable colorectal tumours.[9] An improvement of less than 10% is small, but could have major consequences on public health for such a common disease as colorectal cancer. For treatments with mild toxicity (e.g. portal vein 5-FU), even a 5% improvement in survival would be definitely worthwhile.[11,15] Toxicity, quality of life, and costs should be carefully considered when the expected benefit on survival is small. Table 67.2 shows several examples of trials with more than 1000 patients in colorectal cancer. The National Surgical Adjuvant Breast and Bowel Project (NSABP), for example, has for years performed medium- to large-scale trials in colorectal cancer.

The cost of performing large trials can be prohibitive, and the experience gained in cutting costs in cardiovascular disease could be usefully translated to trials in oncology.[36] Large-scale trials in cardiovascular disease have been possible through a drastic simplification of the inclusion criteria and through the small amount of data collected (few covariates, main endpoints). Only trials addressing important questions are likely to succeed in including a large number of patients. In this type of trial, broad inclusion criteria can be used, with some variation from one centre to another and a broad definition of treatments (e.g. range of doses of chemotherapy or radiotherapy), to facilitate intergroup collaboration.[7,37] Eligibility criteria are loose and mainly based on the 'uncertainty principle', i.e. the clinicians' own uncertainty.[38,39] The uncertainty as to exactly which patients need to be randomized will change from one physician to another; for example, in the AXIS trial comparing portal vein 5-FU versus no adjuvant treatment,[15] some surgeons will randomize only UICC stages II and III, while others might randomize even stage I patients. Because of the large sample size, the entire spectrum of patients will be included and the trial will answer both general and specific questions. Trials with loose inclusion criteria can include a large number of unselected patients in a short period of time. Their results are easy to extrapolate to a large population.

An alternative to large-scale trials and intergroup trials is the prospective pooling of several similar average-sized trials performed in parallel.[2,40] With this design, close collaboration between the data processing centres must be organized. Collaboration between different organizations, each running its own trial, can result in lower trial costs. It is also useful when detailed information on toxicity, compliance, and secondary endpoints is needed.

RANDOMIZED TRIALS IN PATIENTS WITH ADVANCED COLORECTAL CANCER

Place of randomized trials

Therapeutic progress in oncology depends primarily on the identification of new compounds with better clinical efficacy. Screening for new promising drugs is done through phase II trials, the purpose of which is to reject from further research compounds that do not reach a minimum level of activity. While such

Table 67.2 Examples of randomized trials of adjuvant treatment in colorectal cancer including more than 500 patients by arm or more than 1000 patients in a 2 × 2 factorial design

Trial	Population	Treatments randomized[a]	Number of patients included or planned
Swedish Rectal Cancer Trial[27]	Rectum	Preoperative radiotherapy vs surgery alone	1168
AXIS[15]	Colon and rectum, stages I, II, and III	5-FU PVI vs surgery alone	4000
EORTC-GIVIO[28]	Colon and rectum, stages I, II, and III	5-FU PVI vs surgery alone	1235
INTACC[29]	Colon, stages II and III	5-FU + levamisole vs 5-FU/LV + levamisole	1680
INT-0089[30]	Colon, stages II and III	Surgery alone vs 5-FU/LV low dose vs 5-FU/LV high dose, initially; then 5-FU + levamisole vs 5-FU/LV low dose vs 5-FU/LV high dose vs 5-FU/LV low dose + levamisole	3759
EORTC 40911[31]	Colon and rectum stages I, II, and III	Systemic chemotherapy (5-FU/LV vs 5-FU + levamisole) vs systemic chemotherapy + regional chemotherapy	2000
NSABP C-04[32]	Colon, stages II and III	5-FU/LV vs 5-FU + levamisole vs 5-FU/LV + levamisole	2151
QUASAR[33]	Colon and rectum stages I, II, and III	(1) Chemotherapy vs no chemotherapy, or (2) 5-FU/LV high dose vs 5-FU/LV high dose + levamisole vs 5-FU/LV low dose vs 5-FU/LV low dose + levamisole	8000
NSABP C-05[34]	Colon, stages II and III	5-FU/LV vs 5-FU/LV + IFN-α2a	2176
NSABP C-06[35]	Colon, stages II and III	5-FU + calcium folinate vs UFT + calcium folinate	1500
CALGB 69581[23]	Colon, stage II	MoAb 17-1A vs none	2100

[a]PVI, portal vein infusion; LV, leucovorin; IFN-α2a, interferon-α2a; MoAb, monoclonal antibody.

phase II trials are needed, they can be highly misleading because the selection of patients is often a far more important predictor of the therapeutic results than the activity of the compound tested. In colorectal cancer in particular, it has been shown that the therapeutic response observed with cytotoxic agents goes down in successive trials – a phenomenon that can probably be explained by changes in patient selection over time. Clinical trials of interferon-α (IFN-α) in advanced colorectal cancer offer a typical example of the phenomenon, as shown in Table 67.3.

Early phase II trials exhibited extremely high response rates, which led to a large number of confirmatory phase II trials, and later to randomized comparisons of 5-FU plus IFN-α with either 5-FU alone or 5-FU modulated by leucovorin. The response rate went down from 81% (13 responses in 16 patients!) in the first reported phase II trial[41] to 20% in the large-scale confirmatory trials.[44] This example illustrates the need for randomized trials in the search for new regimens in advanced colorectal cancer. Phase II trials undoubtedly have a role to play in drug development, since it would be inappropriate to commit large series of patients to phase III trials of drugs that have insufficient activity. The number of patients entered in non-randomized phase II trials should, however, be limited to the bare minimum needed to screen for efficacy, so that a promising drug is pushed as early as possible to the phase III setting. Alternatively, it is often possible to carry out randomized phase II trials, the purpose of which is *not* to carry out a statistical comparison of a new drug to a standard one but rather to make sure that the new drug has been fairly tested through an *informal* comparison with a group of patients receiving a well-known treatment.[45] In a randomized phase II trial, some of the patients receive a standard regimen and some receive a new regimen. The response rate on the standard regimen is a rough but useful indicator of the patient population entered in the trial; if this response rate is close to what was expected from previous experience, it is likely that the new regimen was given a fair chance of showing its activity. Randomization may also be used when several dose regimens or routes of administration are studied in a single phase II trial.[46]

Endpoints in advanced disease

Clinical endpoints in advanced disease are contrasted in Table 67.4.

Response to treatment is a relevant endpoint in assessing treatment effectiveness against measurable advanced disease. Objective criteria for the assessment of response were proposed in the early 1980s; even though these criteria have been refined and adapted for some tumours since then, they still serve as the basis for evaluating the efficacy of new drugs in advanced cancer.[47] Several cooperative groups have recently proposed to simplify the assessment of response by measuring tumour masses unidimensionally instead of bidimensionally.[48] While this proposal has yet to permeate clinical practice, it does have the potential of making the assessment of tumour response easier and more reliable – a real advantage in multicentric studies. The achievement of a response is an important marker of biological therapeutic effect, and is often associated with both objective and subjective improvements in the patient condition. However, the achievement of a higher response rate is not sufficient per se to establish treatment superiority. The net therapeutic benefit to the patient must also take account of treatment toxicities and of the duration of survival or other time-related endpoints.

Overall survival is regarded as the most important endpoint to establish treatment benefit. Experience shows, however, that it is extremely hard to prolong survival in advanced colorectal cancer. Even treatment regimens that achieve a substantial increase in tumour response may fail to affect survival to any significant extent.[49] Therefore overall survival may not be the best primary endpoint in randomized clinical trials, although obviously it should always be included as a secondary endpoint.

Time to progression is often considered an endpoint in advanced disease. It is a more sensitive marker of treatment efficacy than overall survival, but it is difficult to ascertain. In addition, it is not obvious how to define time to progression for patients whose disease progression is not at least stabilized by treatment. The difficulty of an objective assessment of tumour progression is compounded by the fact that patients are often switched to other therapies (including experimental therapies) upon progression. Finally, it is as yet unclear that tumour response or time to progression can be used as surrogate endpoints for survival. There is some evidence to the contrary, but more quantitative evidence is required before this question is satisfactorily settled.[50,51]

Quality of life is an important endpoint in trials of

Table 67.3 Response rates to 5-FU plus IFN-α in successive trials in advanced colorectal cancer

Trials	Overall response rate (95% CI[a])	Range of response rates	Ref
Initial small phase II trial	13/16 = 81% (57–93%)	81%	41
Confirmatory phase II trials (15 trials)	118/387 = 30% (26–35%)	3–63%	42 (Table 1)
Medium-sized phase III trials (5 trials)	54/244 = 22% (17–28%)	6–41%	42 (Table 3) 43
Large phase III trial	50/245 = 20% (16–26%)	20%	44

[a]95% confidence interval.

Table 67.4 Pros and cons of different clinical endpoints in advanced disease

Endpoint	Pros	Cons
Tumour response	• Measured early • Measured easily • Biologically relevant	• Assessment prone to error • Assessment prone to bias • Complete response very infrequent • Response rate lumps together stable and progressive disease • Disease not always measurable • Limited impact on survival
Time to progression	• Sensitive to differences in treatment efficacy • Unaffected by competing risks • Closely related to quality of life • Strong impact on survival, but validity as a surrogate unclear	• Measured late • Assessment subjective • Assessment prone to bias • Assessment influenced by therapeutic implications
Overall survival	• Most meaningful • Most objective	• Measured very late • Hard to affect • Affected by second-line treatments • Affected by competing risks • Insensitive to short-term benefits

aggressive therapy with minimal chances of cure (only 3% of all patients treated for advanced colorectal cancer enjoy a complete response, and their response may be short-lived[49]). Several quality-of-life scales have been validated and are routinely used.[52]

Stratification

Just as for trials of adjuvant treatments, it may be desirable to stratify the randomization of trials in advanced disease. Stratification factors that can usefully be considered include the investigational centre, the patient's performance status, and the measurability of the tumour (non-measurable disease contributing to analyses of survival but not of response). Other factors such as baseline liver function abnormalities or the percentage of liver parenchyma involved are of prognostic value (for patients with metastases confined to the liver), but may not be known with certainty at the time of randomization and are therefore less good candidates for stratification. In the near future, it is likely that tumour markers and genetic patterns associated with high-risk cases will be added to the well-known clinical factors that are routinely used as stratification factors today.

Design issues

Randomized clinical trials should be designed to provide a reliable answer to one question (or perhaps to several questions, when factorial designs are feasible). Trials with two arms – one receiving standard therapy and the other the experimental therapy – are generally preferable to trials with multiple arms (except in a factorial design, as discussed above). Consider a three-arm design, in which a control group (C) is compared with two experimental therapies (A and B). What is the comparison of interest in this design? Is it A versus C, B versus C, A versus B, or all of these? Is it C versus A + B? A proper three-arm design should clearly state the hypothesis of interest, and stick to this hypothesis in the analysis, even if the observed results suggest that some other hypothesis might have been more appropriate! Statistically, the major drawback of multiple-arm designs is the multiplicity of possible comparisons, which increases the number of patients required. The number of patients required per arm in three-arm designs is larger than in their simpler two-arm counterparts; for instance, if 100 patients were needed *per arm* in a two-arm study, then 123 patients would be needed *per arm* in a three-arm study having the same statistical power.[4] An extreme case of multiplicity was the so-called 'Octopus' trial, in which patients were randomized to no less than seven (not eight!) treatment options.[53] This trial yielded very confusing results in spite of 620 patients having been randomized. Fortunately, this trial could contribute useful information to meta-analyses of some of the questions it had addressed.

META-ANALYSES OF RANDOMIZED TRIALS

Principles of meta-analysis

Randomized clinical trials are undoubtedly the best tool to evaluate experimental treatments,[54] but their results are seldom fully convincing on their own. Large trials can easily identify major treatment effects, such as major increases in response rates, but are usually too small to reliably establish small benefits, such as small prolongations in survival times. However, as stated above, small benefits may have major impacts on public health. These small benefits, which are difficult to identify reliably in individual clinical trials of limited power, can be better assessed in meta-analyses.

A *meta-analysis* is a method for combining in one analysis the results of several randomized clinical trials.[55] The goal of such an analysis is to bring a quantitative and global answer to the question at hand. The advantages of properly conducted meta-analyses over 'reviews of the literature' are obvious. Meta-analyses avoid publication bias and provide a quantitative evaluation of treatment effect. However, the term 'meta-analysis' refers to a wide range of approaches in the medical literature. Approaches based on summary data extracted from published papers may sometimes be useful to provide a first impression or to address non-therapeutic questions, but they are rarely adequate to provide reliable answers on the effects of experimental therapies.[56] In our opinion, the term 'meta-analysis' applied to randomized trials should therefore be restricted to analyses based on individual patient data from all published and unpublished trials.[57–59] Such meta-analyses should be conducted by an independent secretariat in collaboration with all investigators involved in the individual trials.

Role of meta-analyses in colorectal cancer

In colorectal cancer, advances in therapeutics have so far been made step by step, producing only small benefits. On the other hand, colorectal cancer is also a major healthcare problem in developed countries on account of its frequency and mortality. Meta-analyses are worthwhile to evaluate the value of therapeutic approaches in both adjuvant treatment and treatment of metastatic colorectal cancer. They can also generate hypotheses to be tested in future clinical trials.

In 1988, a first meta-analysis pointed out the need for large-scale adjuvant clinical trials in patients with resected colorectal cancer.[60] That meta-analysis showed that the reason why uncertainty still prevailed as to the value of adjuvant therapy was mainly the relatively small number of patients included in previously performed clinical trials. Interestingly, the meta-analysis suggested that long-term administration of 5-FU could improve survival compared with no adjuvant treatment after curative surgery. Most of the new-generation clinical trials reported in the 1990s used 5-FU-based chemotherapy regimens administered over 6–12 months. Meanwhile, clinical trials became much larger, including hundreds or even thousands of patients (see Table 67.2 above).

It is now largely admitted that adjuvant radiotherapy significantly reduces the risk of local recurrences after surgery in patients with Dukes B and C rectal cancer, and that systemic chemotherapy based on 5-FU is a useful adjuvant treatment for patients with stage C colon cancer. However, some pending questions are still difficult to answer in individual trials, and are currently under investigation in ongoing meta-analyses. These questions, which require very large numbers of patients, include the influence of radiotherapy on survival in patients with resectable rectal cancer, and the role of chemotherapy in Dukes B colon cancer.

The role of locoregional adjuvant treatment also remains debatable, despite hundreds of patients being included in clinical trials comparing 5-FU portal vein infusion versus no postoperative treatment. In a meta-analysis performed recently, the value of liver infusion chemotherapy has been confirmed and quantified.[11] It has been shown that the benefit of portal vein infusion over no postoperative treatment was small (13% reduction in the relative risk of mortality, or 4% improvement in the overall 5-year survival), despite a very promising individual trial initially reported. Considering the much more impressive results achieved by adjuvant systemic chemotherapy, this meta-analysis does not indicate that portal vein infusion 5-FU should be given routinely to patients with resected colorectal cancer, and will not change clinical practice. However, the meta-analysis established the rationale for clinical trials testing the interest of adding a locoregional treatment to a systemic chemotherapy in patients with resected colorectal cancer.

The usefulness of meta-analyses in metastatic can-cer is less evident, since the power of individual trials to demonstrate differences in response rates can be considered sufficient. However, the numbers of patients included in individual trials are rarely large enough to address reliably the impact of experimental treatments on survival. Meta-analyses of trials performed in metastatic cancer can therefore be useful not only to address time-dependent endpoints, but also to study the relationship between response and survival, to quantify tumour response differences, to compare toxicity profiles, to study prognostic factors for efficacy and toxicity, and to generate hypotheses that can help in the design of future trials. Such meta-analyses can also serve as a basis for cost–effectiveness analyses. These possibilities have been explored by the *Meta-Analysis Group in Cancer* in the fields of advanced colorectal cancer in the last 10 years, and are illustrated in the following.

The meta-analysis of trials comparing 5-FU alone versus 5-FU plus leucovorin (5-FU/LV) illustrates the use of meta-analyses to provide a quantitative estimation of the value of an experimental treatment.[49] This meta-analysis was based on 1381 patients. A 'review of the literature' would probably have come to the conclusion that the tumour response rate with 5-FU alone was between 3% and 18%, and that the response rate with the 5-FU/LV combination was higher, between 13% and 40%. As far as survival was concerned, the conclusion would have been that there was a trend in favour of patients receiving 5-FU/LV. In contrast, the main conclusions of the meta-analysis were that the modulation of 5-FU by leucovorin led to a doubling of tumour response rates without demonstrable influence on survival. The tumour response rate was 11% in patients allocated to 5-FU alone, compared with 23% in patients allocated to 5-FU/LV. This difference was highly significant (odds ratio 0.45; 95% confidence interval (CI) 0.34–0.60). The advantage of the meta-analysis over a simple review of the literature was to provide quantitative results based on all the randomized evidence. The fact that the achievement of a partial response in colorectal cancer cannot be claimed to be associated with an improved survival seemed clear from the meta-analysis, whereas it was far from evident in the previously published results of individual trials.

The meta-analysis of all trials comparing 5-FU alone versus 5-FU plus methotrexate (5-FU/MTX) confirmed that biomodulation of 5-FU was possible and efficient.[61] This meta-analysis was based on individual data of 1178 patients included in eight randomized clinical trials. The tumour response rate was 10% for patients allocated to 5-FU alone, compared with 19% for patients allocated to 5-FU/MTX. These numbers were very close to those reported in the leucovorin meta-analysis, and here again the difference between 5-FU alone and modulated 5-FU was highly significant. The median overall survival times were 9.1 months in the 5-FU-alone group, and 10.7 months in the 5-FU/MTX groups. This difference was also statistically significant, with an overall survival odds ratio of 0.87 (95% CI 0.77–0.98) ($p = 0.024$). Interestingly, an advantage in terms of survival was observed in only one trial. This illustrates the power of meta-analysis to identify differences that are too small to be picked up in individual clinical trials.

Meta-analyses also permit the reliable study of prognostic factors, since such analyses usually require large numbers of patients. This concerns prognostic factors not only for efficacy (tumour response and survival) but also for toxicity. For example, the Meta-analysis Group in Cancer published a meta-analysis of all trials comparing 5-FU bolus versus 5-FU continuous infusion, in which randomized treatment and performance status were significant predictors of tumour response, whereas the same plus primary tumour site were independent significant predictors of survival.[62] In the same data set, we also reported that independent prognostic factors were age, sex, and performance status for non-haematologic toxicities, performance status and treatment for haematologic toxicities, and age, sex, and treatment for hand–foot syndrome.[63] Meta-analyses can therefore confirm and quantify toxicity profiles, and allow the identification of clinical predictors of toxicity. Because meta-analyses reliably quantify differences between treatments, it is logical to use them in cost–effectiveness studies. The Meta-analysis Group in Cancer has conducted a meta-analysis of all trials comparing bolus intravenous 5-FU versus hepatic arterial infusion floxuridine (FUDR),[64] and then a cost–effectiveness study based on the same data,[65] in which we showed that the cost–effectiveness of localized chemotherapy for colorectal liver metastases is within the range of accepted treatments for serious medical conditions.

A final role for meta-analysis is to suggest hypotheses that are worth testing in future trials.[66] As such, meta-analysis will soon become an indispensable instrument not only to review past data, but also to help in the planning of future trials.

CONCLUSIONS

Clinical research has been very fruitful in the past 20 years in the field of colorectal cancer. This research, based on a deeper understanding of tumour biology and on a faster identification of new drugs, has matured through classical phase I to phase III clinical trials, and more recently through meta-analyses. The potential worth of phase III trials and meta-analyses applied to colorectal cancer have been presented briefly in this chapter. These tools will continue to be essential for a reliable evaluation of therapeutic progress.

REFERENCES

1. Moertel CG, Fleming TR, Macdonald JS et al, Fluorouracil plus levamisole as effective adjuvant therapy after resection of stage III colon carcinoma: a final report. *Ann Intern Med* 1995; **122:** 321–6.
2. International Multicentre Pooled Analysis of Colon Cancer Trials, Efficacy of adjuvant fluorouracil and folinic acid in colon cancer. *Lancet* 1995; **345:** 939–44.
3. Pocock SJ, *Clinical Trials. A Practical Approach.* Chichester: Wiley, 1983.
4. George SL, The required size and length of a phase III clinical trial. In: *Cancer Clinical Trials. Methods and Practice* (Buyse ME, Staquet MJ, Sylvester RJ, eds). Oxford: Oxford University Press, 1988: 287–310.
5. Simon RM, Design and analysis of clinical trials. In: *Cancer: Principles and Practice of Oncology*, 5th edn (DeVita VT, Hellman S, Rosenberg SA, eds). Philadelphia: JB Lippincott, 1997: 513–27.
6. Freiman JA, Chalmers TC, Smith H Jr, Kuebler RR, The importance of beta, the type II error and sample size in the design and interpretation of the randomized controlled trial. Survey of 71 'negative' trials. *N Engl J Med* 1978; **299:** 690–4.
7. Yusuf S, Collins R, Peto R, Why do we need some large, simple randomized trials? *Stat Med* 1984; **3:** 409–20.
8. Buyse M, Potential and pitfalls of randomized clinical trials in cancer research. *Cancer Surv* 1989; **8:** 91–105.
9. Freedman LS, The size of clinical trials in cancer research – What are the current needs? *Br J Cancer* 1989; **59:** 396–400.
10. Deacon J, Peto J, Clinical trial design and evaluation of combined chemotherapy and radiotherapy. In: *Combined Radiotherapy and Chemotherapy in Clinical Oncology* (Horwich A, ed). London: Edward Arnold, 1992: 1–13.
11. Liver Infusion Meta-Analysis Group, Portal vein infusion of cytotoxic drugs after colorectal cancer surgery: a meta-analysis of 10 randomized studies involving 4000 patients. *J Natl Cancer Inst* 1997; **89:** 497–505.
12. Simon R, A critical assessment of approaches to improving the efficiency of cancer clinical trials. In: *Recent Results in Cancer Research*, Vol III (Scheurlen H, Kay R, Baum M, eds). Heidelberg: Springer-Verlag, 1988: 18–26.
13. Buyse M, Clinical trial methodology. In: *Oxford Textbook of Oncology* (Peckham M, Pinedo H, Veronesi U, eds). Oxford: Oxford University Press, 1995: 2377–95.

14. Buyse M, Regulatory versus public health requirements in clinical trials. *Drug Inf J* 1993; **27**: 977–84.

15. Gray R, James R, Mossman J, Stenning S, AXIS – A suitable case for treatment. *Br J Cancer* 1991; **63**: 841–5.

16. Peto R, Clinical trial methodology. *Biomedicine* 1978; **28**: 24–36.

17. Byar DP, Piantadosi S, Factorial designs for randomized clinical trials. *Cancer Treat Rep* 1985; **69**: 1055–63.

18. Crowley J, Discussion. *Cancer Treat Rep* 1985; **10**: 1079–80.

19. Simon R, Statistical tools for subset analysis in clinical trials. In: *Recent Results in Cancer Research*, Vol III (Scheurlen H, Kay R, Baum M, eds). Heidelberg: Springer-Verlag, 1988: 55–66.

20. O'Connell MJ, Laurie JA, Shepherd L et al, A prospective evaluation of chemotherapy duration and regimen as adjuvant treatment for high risk colon cancer. A collaborative trial of the North Central Cancer Treatment Group and the National Cancer Institute of Canada Clinical Trials Group. *Proc Am Soc Clin Oncol* 1996; **15**: 478.

21. Pocock SJ, Simon R, Sequential treatment assignment with balancing for prognostic factors in the controlled clinical trial. *Biometrics* 1975; **31**: 103–15.

22. Simon R, Importance of prognostic factors in cancer clinical trials. *Cancer Treat Rep* 1984; **68**: 185–92.

23. Conley BA, Smiley JK, Cheson BD, Clinical trials referral resource. NCI clinical trials in colon cancer. *Oncology* 1999; **13**: 814–20.

24. International Multicentre Pooled Analysis of B2 Colon Cancer Trials (IMPACT B2) Investigators, Efficacy of adjuvant fluorouracil and folinic acid in B2 colon cancer. *J Clin Oncol* 1999; **17**: 1356–63.

25. Mamounas E, Wieand S, Wolmark N et al, Comparative efficacy of adjuvant chemotherapy in patients with Dukes' B versus Dukes' C colon cancer: results from four National Surgical Adjuvant Breast and Bowel Project Adjuvant studies (C-01, C-02, C-03, and C-04). *J Clin Oncol* 1999; **17**: 1349–55.

26. Pignon JP, Ducreux M, Rougier Ph, More patients needed in stage II colon cancer trials. *J Clin Oncol* 2000; **18**: 235.

27. Swedish Rectal Cancer Trial, Improved survival with preoperative radiotherapy in resectable rectal cancer. *N Engl J Med* 1997; **336**: 980–7.

28. Rougier P, Sahmoud T, Nitti D et al, Adjuvant portal-vein infusion of fluorouracil and heparin in colorectal cancer: a randomised trial. *Lancet* 1998; **351**: 1677–81.

29. Intergruppo Nazionale Terapia Adjuvante Carcinoma Colon (INTACC), 5-Fluorouracil (5FU) + levamisole (Leva) vs 5FU + 6-S-leucovorin (6-S-LV) + Leva: an Italian intergroup study of adjuvant therapy for resected colon cancer. *Proc Am Soc Clin Oncol* 1995; **14**: 205.

30. Haller DG, Catalano PJ, Macdonald JS, Mayer RJ, Fluorouracil (FU), leucovorin (LV) and levamisole (Lev) adjuvant therapy for colon cancer: preliminary results of INT-0089. *Proc Am Soc Clin Oncol* 1996; **15**: 486.

31. Wils J, Bleiberg H, Rougier P, Adjuvant treatment of colon cancer. A plea for a large-scale European trial. *Eur J Cancer* 1994; **30A**: 578–9.

32. Wolmark N, Rockette H, Mamounas E et al, Clinical trial to assess the relative efficacy of fluorouracil and leucovorin, fluorouracil and levamisole, and fluorouracil, leucovorin, and levamisole in patients with Dukes' B and C carcinoma of the colon: results from National Surgical Adjuvant Breast and Bowel Project C-04. *J Clin Oncol* 1999; **17**: 3553–9.

33. QUASAR Collaborative Group, Comparison of fluorouracil with additional levamisole, higher-dose folinic acid, or both, as adjuvant chemotherapy for colorectal cancer: a randomised trial. *Lancet* 2000; **355**: 1588–96.

34. Wolmark N, Bryant J, Smith R et al, Adjuvant 5-fluorouracil and leucovorin with or without interferon alpha-2a in colon carcinoma: National Surgical Adjuvant Breast and Bowel Project C-05. *J Natl Cancer Inst* 1998; **90**: 1810–16.

35. Smith R, Wickerham LD, Wieand HS et al, UFT plus calcium folinate vs 5-FU plus calcium folinate in colon cancer. *Oncology* 1999; **13**(Suppl 3): 44–7.

36. Wittes J, Duggan J, Held P, Yusuf S, Proceedings of cost and efficiency in clinical trials. *Stat Med* 1990; **9**: 1–199.

37. Souhami R, Large-scale studies. In: *Introducing New Treatments for Cancer. Practical, Ethical and Legal Problems* (Williams CJ, ed). Chichester: Wiley, 1992: 173–87.

38. Stenning S, 'The uncertainty principle': selection of patients for cancer clinical trials. In: *Introducing New Treatments for Cancer. Practical, Ethical and Legal Problems* (Williams CJ, ed). Chichester: Wiley, 1992: 161–72.

39. Collins R, Doll R, Peto R, Ethics of clinical trials. In: *Introducing New Treatments for Cancer. Practical, Ethical and Legal Problems* (Williams CJ, ed). Chichester: Wiley, 1992: 49–65.

40. Pater J, Zee B, Myles J et al, A proposal for a new approach to intergroup cancer trials. *Eur J Cancer* 1995; **31A**: 1921–3.

41. Wadler S, Schwartz EL, Goldman M et al, Fluorouracil and recombinant alfa-2a-interferon: an active regimen against advanced colorectal carcinoma. *J Clin Oncol* 1995; **7**: 1769–75.

42. Raderer M, Scheithauer W, Treatment of advanced colorectal cancer with 5-fluorouracil and interferon-α: an overview of clinical trials. *Eur J Cancer* 1995; **31A**: 1002–8.

43. Greco FA, Figlin R, York M et al, Phase III randomized study to compare interferon alfa-2a in combination with fluorouracil versus fluorouracil alone in patients with advanced colorectal cancer. *J Clin Oncol* 1996; **10**: 2674–81.

44. Corfu-A Study Group, Phase III randomized study of two fluorouracil combinations with either interferon alfa-2a or leucovorin for advanced colorectal cancer. *J Clin Oncol* 1995; **13**: 921–8.

45. Simon R, A decade of progress in statistical methodology for clinical trials. *Stat Med* 1991; **10**: 1798–817.

46. Buyse M, Randomized designs for early trials of new cancer treatments – an overview. *Drug Inf J* 2000; **34**: 387–96.

47. *WHO Handbook for Reporting results of Cancer Treatment.* Geneva: WHO Offset Publication No. 48, 1979.

48. James K, Eisenhauer E, Christian M et al, Measuring response in solid tumors: unidimensional versus bidimensional measurement. *J Natl Cancer Inst* 1999; **91**: 523–8.

49. Advanced Colorectal Cancer Meta-analysis Project, Modulation of 5-fluorouracil by leucovorin in patients with advanced colorectal cancer: evidence in terms of response rate. *J Clin Oncol* 1992; **10**: 896–903.

50. Buyse M, Piedbois P, On the relationship between response to treatment and survival. *Stat Med* 1996; **15**: 2797–812.

51. Ellenberg SS, Hamilton JM, Surrogate endpoints in clinical trials: cancer. *Stat Med* 1989; **8**: 405–13.

52. Aaronson NK, Beckmann JH (eds), *The Quality of Life of Cancer Patients*. New York: Raven Press, 1987.

53. Leichman CG, Fleming TR, Muggia FM et al, Phase II study of fluorouracil and its modulation in advanced colorectal cancer: a Southwest Oncology Group study. *J Clin Oncol* 1995; **13**: 1303–11.

54. Pignon JP, Arriagada R, Treatment evaluation. In: *Comprehensive Textbook of Thoracic Oncology* (Aisner J, Arriagada R, Green MR et al, eds). Baltimore: Williams & Wilkins, 1996: 188–214.

55. Buyse M, Piedbois P, Carlson RW, Piedbois Y, Meta-analysis: methods, strengths and weaknesses. *Oncology* 2000; **14:** 437–43.

56. Piedbois P, Buyse M, Recent meta-analyses in colorectal cancer. *Curr Opin Oncol* 2000; **12:** 362–7.

57. Stewart LA, Clarke MJ, on behalf of the Cochrane Working Group on meta-analysis using individual patient data, Practical methodology of meta-analyses using updated individual patient data. *Stat Med* 1995; **14:** 2057–79.

58. Pignon JP, Hill C, Meta-analysis of randomised clinical trials in oncology. *Lancet Oncology* 2001; **2:** 475–82.

59. Clarke M, Stewart L, Pignon JP, Bijnens L, Individual patient data meta-analyses in cancer. *Br J Cancer* 1998; **77:** 2036–44.

60. Buyse M, Zeleniuch-Jacquotte A, Chalmers TC, Adjuvant therapy of colorectal cancer: why we still don't know. *JAMA* 1988; **259:** 3571–8.

61. Advanced Colorectal Cancer Meta-analysis Project, Meta-analysis of randomized trials testing the biochemical modulation of 5-fluorouracil by methotrexate in metastatic colorectal cancer. *J Clin Oncol* 1994; **12:** 960–9.

62. Meta-analysis Group in Cancer, Efficacy of intravenous continuous infusion of 5-fluorouracil compared with bolus administration in advanced colorectal cancer. *J Clin Oncol* 1998; **16:** 301–8.

63. Meta-analysis Group in Cancer, Toxicity of 5-fluorouracil in patients with advanced colorectal cancer: effect of administration schedule and prognostic factors. *J Clin Oncol* 1998; **16:** 3537–41.

64. Meta-analysis Group in Cancer, Reappraisal of hepatic arterial infusion in the treatment of nonresectable liver metastases from colorectal cancer. *J Natl Cancer Inst* 1996; **88:** 252–8.

65. Durand-Zaleski I, Roche B, Buyse M et al, Economic implications of hepatic arterial infusion chemotherapy in treatment of nonresectable colorectal liver metastases. *J Natl Cancer Inst* 1997; **89:** 790–5.

66. Le Péchoux C, Cojean I, Arriagada R et al, From the results of the meta-analysis evaluating the role of chemotherapy in non-small cell lung cancer (NSCLC) to the IALT project. *Eur J Cancer* 1995; **31A**(Suppl 5): S221.

Index